WOUND HEALING

Biochemical &
Clinical Aspects

WOUND HEALING

Biochemical & Clinical Aspects

W. B. SAUNDERS COMPANY
Harcourt Brace Jovanovich, Inc.

Philadelphia   London   Toronto   Montreal   Sydney   Tokyo

I. Kelman Cohen, M.D.

Professor and Chairman
Division of Plastic and Reconstructive Surgery
Department of Surgery
Medical College of Virginia
Virginia Commonwealth University
Richmond, Virginia

Robert F. Diegelmann, Ph.D.

Associate Professor
Division of Plastic and Reconstructive Surgery
Department of Surgery
Medical College of Virginia
Virginia Commonwealth University
Richmond, Virginia

William J. Lindblad, Ph.D.

Associate Professor
Department of Pharmaceutical Sciences
Wayne State University
Detroit, Michigan

W. B. SAUNDERS COMPANY
Harcourt Brace Jovanovich, Inc.

The Curtis Center
Independence Square West
Philadelphia, PA 19106

Library of Congress Cataloging-in-Publication Data

Wound healing : biochemical and clinical aspects / [edited by]
I. Kelman Cohen, Robert F. Diegelmann, William J. Lindblad.—1st ed.

p.   cm.

ISBN 0–7216–2564–9

1. Wound healing.   I. Cohen, I. Kelman.   II. Diegelmann,
   Robert F.   III. Lindblad, William J.   [DNLM: 1. Wound
   Healing.   WO 185 W93825]

RD94.W69 1992   617.1—dc20

DNLM/DLC   91–18290

Editor: Jennifer Mitchell
Designer: Maureen Sweeney
Production Manager: Linda R. Garber
Manuscript Editors: Tina K. Rebane and Ellen Murray
Illustration Coordinator: Peg Shaw
Indexer: Ruth Low
Cover Designer: Michelle Maloney

Wound Healing: Biochemical & Clinical Aspects   ISBN 0–7216–2564–9

Last digit is the print number: 9   8   7   6   5   4   3   2

This book is dedicated to our families.

I.K.C.
R.F.D.
W.J.L.

CONTRIBUTORS

Oscar M. Alvarez, Ph.D.
Director, University Wound Healing Clinic, New Brunswick, New Jersey
  Wound Dressings: Design and Use

Peter C. Amadio, M.D.
Associate Professor of Orthopedic Surgery and Consultant in Hand Surgery and
Orthopedic Surgery, Mayo Clinic, Rochester, Minnesota
  Tendon and Ligament

Simon J. Archibald, Ph.D.
Research Associate, Division of Neurosurgery, Duke University Medical Center,
Durham, North Carolina
  Peripheral Nerve Injury

Adrian Barbul, M.D.
Associate Professor, Department of Surgery, Johns Hopkins School of Medicine;
Assistant Surgeon-in-Chief, Sinai Hospital of Baltimore, Baltimore, Maryland
  Role of the Immune System

Merton R. Bernfield, M.D.
Clement A. Smith Professor of Pediatrics, Professor of Anatomy and Cellular
Biology, and Director, Joint Program in Neonatology, Harvard Medical School;
Chief, Division of Newborn Medicine, Children's Hospital; Chairman, Department
of Newborn Medicine, Brigham and Women's Hospital; Chairman, Department of
Newborn Medicine, Beth Israel Hospital, Boston, Massachusetts
  Proteoglycan Glycoconjugates

Peter B. Bitterman, M.D.

Associate Professor and Chief, Division of Pulmonary and Critical Care Medicine, Department of Medicine and Minnesota Heart and Lung Institute, University of Minnesota, Minneapolis, Minnesota
Acute Lung Injury

Peter Blomquist, M.D., Ph.D.

Department of Surgery, University of Lund; Attending Surgeon, Malmö Hospital, Malmö, Sweden
The Alimentary Canal

Joseph V. Boykin, Jr., M.D.

Clinical Assistant Professor, Department of Surgery, Medical College of Virginia; Medical Director, St. Mary's Hospital Burn Program, Richmond, Virginia
Burn Scar and Skin Equivalents

Scott Brenman, M.D.

Assistant Clinical Professor, University of Pennsylvania, School of Medicine; Attending, Hospital of the University of Pennsylvania, Philadelphia, Pennsylvania
Factitious Problems in Wound Healing

Henry Brown, M.D.

Associate Clinical Professor, Department of Surgery, The Harvard Medical School; Attending Surgeon, New England Deaconess Hospital, Boston, Massachusetts; Chief, Hand Clinic and Rehabilitation Medicine, Veterans Administration Medical Center, Manchester, New Hampshire; Formerly Assistant Director and Chief, Hand Surgery, Harvard Surgical Unit, Boston City Hospital, Boston, Massachusetts
Wound Healing Research Through the Ages

Steven R. Buchman, M.D.

Assistant Clinical Instructor in Surgery, Division of Plastic Surgery, University of Pennsylvania, Philadelphia, Pennsylvania
Bone and Cartilaginous Tissue

Kenneth R. Cutroneo, Ph.D.

Professor of Biochemistry, College of Medicine, University of Vermont, Burlington, Vermont
Pharmacological Interventions

Jeffrey M. Davidson, Ph.D.

Professor, Department of Pathology, Vanderbilt University School of Medicine; Associate Research Career Scientist, Nashville Veterans Administration Medical Center, Nashville, Tennessee
Elastin Repair

Achilles A. Demetriou, M.D., Ph.D.

Professor of Surgery and Assistant Professor of Molecular Physiology and Biophysics, Vanderbilt University School of Medicine; Chief of Surgery, Nashville Veterans Administration Medical Center; Attending Surgeon, Vanderbilt University Medical Center, Nashville, Tennessee
> *Metabolic Factors*

Richard F. Edlich, M.D.

Distinguished Professor of Plastic Surgery and Biomedical Engineering, University of Virginia School of Medicine, Charlottesville, Virginia
> *Surgical Devices in Wound Healing Management*

H. Paul Ehrlich, Ph.D.

Associate Professor of Pathology, Harvard Medical School; Associate Biochemist in Pathology and Surgery, Massachusetts General Hospital, Boston, Massachusetts
> *Wound Contraction and Scar Contracture*

George C. Fuller, Ph.D.

Dean and Professor of Pharmacology, College of Pharmacy and Allied Health Professions, Wayne State University, Detroit, Michigan
> *Pharmacological Interventions*

Steffen Gay, M.D.

Professor of Medicine, School of Medicine, University of Alabama at Birmingham Medical Center, Birmingham, Alabama
> *Collagen Structure and Function*

M. Gabriella Giro, Ph.D.

Associate Professor in Histology and Embryology, University of Padoua Medical School, Italy; Visiting Associate Professor, Department of Pathology, Vanderbilt University School of Medicine, Nashville, Tennessee
> *Elastin Repair*

William H. Goodson III, M.D.

Associate Professor of Surgery, Department of Surgery, School of Medicine, University of California at San Francisco, San Francisco, California
> *Traumatic Injury*

Richard J. Goss, Ph.D.

Professor of Biology, Division of Biology and Medicine, Brown University, Providence, Rhode Island
> *Regeneration Versus Repair*

Martin F. Graham, M.D.

Associate Professor of Pediatrics, Medical College of Virginia, Virginia Commonwealth University; Attending Pediatrician, Division of Pediatric Gastroenterology

and Nutrition, Department of Pediatrics, Children's Medical Center of the Medical College of Virginia Hospitals, Richmond, Virginia
The Alimentary Canal

Frederick Grinnell, Ph.D.

Professor, Department of Cell Biology and Neuroscience, University of Texas Southwestern Medical School, Dallas, Texas
Cell Adhesion

Gary R. Grotendorst, Ph.D.

Associate Professor, Department of Ophthalmology, University of South Florida Eye Institute, Tampa, Florida
Chemoattractants and Growth Factors

Keith R. Harmon, M.D.

Assistant Professor, Division of Pulmonary and Critical Care Medicine, Department of Medicine and Minnesota Heart and Lung Institute, University of Minnesota, Minneapolis, Minnesota
Acute Lung Injury

John P. Heggers, Ph.D.

Professor of Microbiology and Surgery, University of Texas Medical Branch; Chief, Microbiology, Shriners Burns Institute, Galveston, Texas
Eicosanoids, Cytokines, and Free Radicals

Marshall I. Hertz, M.D.

Assistant Professor, Division of Pulmonary and Critical Care Medicine, Department of Medicine and Minnesota Heart and Lung Institute, University of Minnesota, Minneapolis, Minnesota
Acute Lung Injury

Thomas K. Hunt, M.D.

Professor and Vice Chairman of Surgery, University of California at San Francisco; Attending, University of California at San Francisco Medical Center, San Francisco, California
Wound Microenvironment

Zamir Hussain, Ph.D.

Associate Research Biochemist, Department of Stomatology, School of Dentistry, University of California at San Francisco, San Francisco, California
Wound Microenvironment

John J. Jeffrey, Ph.D.

Professor, Division of Hematology, Albany Medical College, Albany, New York
Collagen Degradation

Christian Krarup, M.D., Ph.D.

Co-Director of Clinical Neurophysiology, University Hospital, Copenhagen, Denmark

Peripheral Nerve Injury

Thomas M. Krummel, M.D.

Professor of Surgery and Pediatrics, Pennsylvania State University College of Medicine; Chief, Division of Pediatric Surgery, Milton S. Hershey Medical Center, Hershey, Pennsylvania

Tissue Repair in the Mammalian Fetus

W. Thomas Lawrence, M.D.

Assistant Professor, Division of Plastic and Reconstructive Surgery, University of North Carolina; Attending Surgeon, University of North Carolina Hospital, Chapel Hill, North Carolina

Clinical Management of Nonhealing Wounds

E. Carwile LeRoy, M.D.

Professor of Medicine, Medical University of South Carolina; Attending Physician, Medical University Hospital, Charleston, South Carolina

Scleroderma (Systemic Sclerosis): Comparison with Wound Healing

Stanley M. Levenson, M.D.

Professor Emeritus, Albert Einstein College of Medicine, Yeshiva University; Attending Surgeon, Bronx Municipal Hospital Center; Director, Surgical Intensive Care–Burn Unit, Jacobi Hospital, Bronx Municipal Hospital Center, Bronx, New York

Metabolic Factors

Roger Madison, Ph.D.

Assistant Professor of Experimental Neurosurgery and Neurobiology, Duke University; Attending, Duke University Medical Center, Durham, North Carolina

Peripheral Nerve Injury

Raji Malhotra, M.D.

Associate Professor, University of Massachusetts Medical School; Attending, University of Massachusetts Medical Center, Worcester, Massachusetts

Epithelialization

George R. Martin, Ph.D.

Scientific Director, National Institute on Aging; Director, Gerontology Research Center, Baltimore, Maryland

Current Perspectives in Wound Healing

Bruce A. Mast, M.D.

Research Fellow, Department of Surgery, Medical College of Virginia, Virginia Commonwealth University, Richmond, Virginia

Tissue Repair in the Mammalian Fetus; The Skin

Edward J. Miller, Ph.D.

Professor of Biochemistry, University of Alabama at Birmingham, Birmingham, Alabama
Collagen Structure and Function

Joseph A. Molnar, M.D., Ph.D.

Fellow, Division of Plastic and Reconstructive Surgery, Medical College of Virginia, Richmond, Virginia
Burn Scar and Skin Equivalents

Claudia J. Morgan, Ph.D.

Assistant Professor, Department of Surgery, Ohio State University, School of Medicine, Columbus, Ohio
Fibroblast Proliferation

John C. Murray, M.D.

Assistant Professor of Medicine, Division of Dermatology, Duke University; Attending, Duke University Medical Center, Durham, North Carolina
Keloids and Excessive Dermal Scarring

Jeffrey M. Nelson, M.D.

Fellow, Division of Plastic Surgery, University of California at San Diego, San Diego, California
Tissue Repair in the Mammalian Fetus

Erle E. Peacock, Jr., M.D.

Formerly Professor and Head, Department of Surgery, University of Arizona College of Medicine; Courtesy Staff, University of North Carolina Hospitals, Chapel Hill, North Carolina
Current Perspectives in Wound Healing

Charlotte Phillips, Ph.D.

Research Associate, Department of Medicine, Duke University Medical Center, Durham, North Carolina
Biosynthetic and Genetic Disorders of Collagen

Sheldon R. Pinnell, M.D.

J. Lamar Callaway Professor of Dermatology, Division of Dermatology, Department of Medicine, Duke University, Durham, North Carolina
Keloids and Excessive Dermal Scarring

W. Jack Pledger, Ph.D.

Professor of Cell Biology, Vanderbilt University School of Medicine, Nashville, Tennessee
Fibroblast Proliferation

Daniela Quaglino, Jr., Ph.D.

Ricercatrice, Institute of General Pathology, University of Modena, Modena, Italy
   Elastin Repair

Rajendra Raghow, Ph.D.

Professor of Pharmacology, University of Tennessee at Memphis, The Health
Sciences Center; Research Service, Veterans Administration Medical Center, Memphis, Tennessee
   Hepatic Fibrosis

Martin C. Robson, M.D.

Truman G. Blocker Jr. Distinguished Professor of Surgery and Professor of Microbiology, University of Texas Medical Branch; Chief, Division of Plastic Surgery,
University of Texas Medical Branch Hospitals; Director, Surgical Services, Shriners
Burns Institute, Galveston, Texas
   Eicosanoids, Cytokines, and Free Radicals

George T. Rodeheaver, Ph.D.

Research Professor of Plastic Surgery, University of Virginia School of Medicine,
Charlottesville, Virginia
   Surgical Devices in Wound Healing Management

David T. Rovee, Ph.D.

The Rovee Group, Princeton, New Jersey
   Wound Dressings: Design and Use

Ross Rudolph, M.D.

Head, Division of Plastic Surgery, Scripps Clinic and Research Foundation, La
Jolla; Associate Clinical Professor of Plastic Surgery, University of California at San
Diego, San Diego, California
   Wound Contraction and Scar Contracture

Donald Serafin, M.D.

Professor of Surgery, Division of Plastic, Reconstructive, Maxillofacial and Oral
Surgery, Duke University; Chief of Plastic Surgery, Duke University Medical
Center, Durham, North Carolina
   Factitious Problems in Wound Healing

Jerome M. Seyer, Ph.D.

Professor of Biochemistry, University of Tennessee at Memphis, the Health Sciences
Center; Veterans Administration Medical Center, Memphis, Tennessee
   Hepatic Fibrosis

Linda S. Snyder, M.D.

Assistant Professor, Division of Pulmonary and Critical Care Medicine, Department
of Medicine and Minnesota Heart and Lung Institute, University of Minnesota,
Minneapolis, Minnesota
   Acute Lung Injury

Kurt S. Stenn, M.D.

Professor, Yale School of Medicine; Attending, Yale New Haven Hospital, New Haven, Connecticut
Epithelialization

John G. Thacker, Ph.D.

Professor of Mechanical and Aerospace Engineering, University of Virginia, Charlottesville, Virginia
Surgical Devices in Wound Healing Management

Jerry Vande Berg, Ph.D., M.Sc., B.Sc.

Assistant Professor, University of California at San Diego; Director, Core Clinical and Research Electron Microscope Facility, Veterans Administration Medical Center, San Diego, California
Wound Contraction and Scar Contracture

Larry M. Wahl, Ph.D.

Senior Investigator, National Institute of Dental Research, National Institutes of Health, Bethesda, Maryland
Inflammation

Sharon M. Wahl, Ph.D.

Chief, Cellular Immunology Section, National Institute of Dental Research, National Institutes of Health, Bethesda, Maryland
Inflammation

Michael Weitzhandler, Ph.D.

Senior Research Biochemist, Dionex Corporation, Sunnyvale, California
Proteoglycan Glycoconjugates

Richard J. Wenstrup, M.D.

Assistant Professor of Pediatrics and Medicine, Duke University; Assistant Professor of Pediatrics and Medicine, Duke University Medical Center, Durham, North Carolina
Biosynthetic and Genetic Disorders of Collagen

Giles F. Whalen, M.D.

Assistant Professor, Department of Surgery, New York Hospital, Cornell Medical Center, New York, New York
Angiogenesis

David M. Wiseman, Ph.D., M.R. Pharm. S.

Research Scientist, Johnson & Johnson Medical Inc., North Brunswick, New Jersey
Wound Dressings: Design and Use

Isaac L. Wornom III, M.D.

Assistant Professor of Surgery, Division of Plastic Surgery, Medical College of Virginia, Richmond, Virginia
Bone and Cartilaginous Tissue

Bengt Zederfeldt, M.D., Ph.D.

Department of Surgery, University of Lund; Attending and Chief of Surgery, Malmö Hospital, Malmö, Sweden
The Alimentary Canal

Bruce R. Zetter, Ph.D.

Associate Professor, Departments of Physiology and Surgery, Harvard Medical School; Attending, Children's Hospital Medical Center, Boston, Massachusetts
Angiogenesis

PREFACE

Our understanding of the mechanisms involved in tissue repair underwent unprecedented expansion in the decade of the 1980s. From studies at the molecular level to the use of newly developed wound care products at the bedside, there is a new air of excitement about the progress being made in this field. Yet much remains ahead, as the basic mysteries of this complex and dynamic phenomenon of wound healing are just beginning to yield to a myriad of new investigative techniques.

This surge in wound healing knowledge results in no small part from studies conducted jointly by basic health scientists and clinical investigators. It is our hope that this book will foster communication between these groups and lead to more intellectual fermentation and hence understanding.

This book was planned to attract a diverse audience, which in part reflects the broad range of scientific and clinical disciplines concerned with how mammals repair damaged tissue. Consequently, we have brought together biochemists, immunologists, pharmacologists, internists, and surgeons to share their unique perspectives on tissue repair. From this amalgam, we hope the reader may obtain new insights into the processes of reepithelialization, wound contraction, and extracellular matrix deposition, all of which are critical to healing damaged tissue. In addition, several authors address the process of regeneration and how this form of repair could ultimately be stimulated to prevent many of the problems associated with healing by scar formation.

Although Hippocrates practiced medicine using many of the basic principles of good wound care, one should remember that much of our knowledge of the basic biological processes of wound healing has been determined only within the last 50 to 100 years. It was in 1858 that Rudolf Virchow (1821–1902) published *Cellular-Pathologie*, establishing the significance of the cellular nature of disease. Eli Metchnikoff (1845–1916) was working at the Pasteur Institute about 100 years ago, elucidating the importance of phagocytic leukocytes in bodily defense, an extremely important process in controlling wound healing as we know it today. And it was just 80 years ago that Alexis Carrel (1873–1944), one of this century's greatest investigators of wound healing, was studying the ability of crushed animal tissue to enhance wound healing. He subsequently applied these findings to tissue culture systems, enabling him to propagate cells for years, and today we are applying these tissue factors, now in more purified form, onto patients. Carrel went on to conduct applied clinical research at Temporary Hospital No. 21 near Compiegne, France, during World War I, where, in collaboration with chemist Henry Dakin, he developed the well-known treatment for contaminated wounds by a continuous flushing of the wound with Carrel-Dakin solution. Also at that hospital, Carrel worked with Lecomte de Nouy, a biologist interested in the mathematical study of the rate of healing. De Nouy developed the method of tracing the outline of a wound on transparent cellophane and then calculating the area of the wound. This approach could be used to precisely define the time course needed for the wound to close. The number of basic findings and methodologies developed by Carrel and associates in the early decades of this century is remarkable.

Since Carrel, many individuals have provided crucial insights into the processes of tissue repair. Although it is beyond the scope of this preface to list all of these researchers, we feel that several individuals stand out among the investigators of the latter half of the twentieth century. One such individual is Jerome Gross, who has been a driving force in developmental biology and wound healing for the last 40 years. During this time he identified the first vertebrate collagenase, and he continues to examine various aspects of its regulation. He was also one of the first persons to develop a clear model for the process of wound contraction. And in some ways of greater importance, from his Developmental Biology Laboratory at the Massachusetts General Hospital has come a steady flow of investigators who have become leaders in their respective fields. Another individual who has greatly influenced the field of wound healing is Erle E. Peacock, Jr., a keen observer of the surgical wound and one of the first people to examine the dynamics of collagen metabolism in the healing wound. He conducted the first clinical studies of β-aminopropionitrile, an agent that had been known for many years to alter collagen crosslinking in experimental animals. His precepts have been transferred to numerous clinicians in training who have subsequently gone on to investigate the means to control the scarring process in humans. These are but two of many investigators who have helped to push the field of wound healing forward.

Wound Healing is divided into five major blocks that are meant to facilitate organization of the material, not to impart artificial boundaries between areas. A historical perspective of wound healing research and clinical practice serves as an introduction. The chapters in the first block (Section I) deal with the basic biological processes that are encompassed by the term *wound healing*. In addition, a discussion of the regenerative process is presented that contrasts this phenomenon with the general mechanism of healing employed by mammals, i.e., repair by scar.

The chapters in the next section on the structural and regulatory components of wound healing (Section II) exemplify areas that have undergone a tremendous increase in knowledge base during the 1980s. Today, collagen is no longer considered an inert extracellular structural element, but rather a dynamic multigene family of proteins that provide everything from structure to specific signals to determine cellular phenotype. The growth factors produced from an impressive array of cells during tissue repair impinge on almost every discussion in the book. Yet a decade ago these agents were still for the most part crude extracts.

In Section III, a number of factors that mediate the rapidity and magnitude of the wound repair response are discussed. Of considerable interest are the advances in the area of fetal wound healing. In this context, the mammal does not repair by scar deposition, but rather by a modified regenerative response. How this information can be utilized to facilitate wound healing in the adult is but one of many questions to arise from these chapters.

Next, Section IV provides a discussion of tissue repair in different organs. Here one finds that the basic processes of repair are present in all tissues; however, the manifestation of each varies significantly. It is intriguing to contrast the problems of gut repair, where a hollow organ containing bacteria must be prevented from losing structural integrity, and repair in the lung, which requires an exquisitely thin basement membrane to facilitate oxygen exchange. Whereas the different organs utilize many of the same processes and mediators to accomplish repair, each is forced to modify the process to maintain unique organ-specific functions.

Section V, Clinical Management of Healing Tissues, the final block of chapters, will hold the attention of the basic health scientist as well as that of the clinician. Since one of our goals for this book is to facilitate communication between the research and clinical communities, we have attempted to use illustrative clinical problems that require further basic studies to arrive at an optimal treatment solution.

We are very excited about the future of wound healing research and the translation of these basic studies into clinical reality. The decade of the 1990s holds great promise for opening up new horizons in this field, which we hope this book will help to facilitate.

I. KELMAN COHEN, M.D.
ROBERT F. DIEGELMANN, PH.D.
WILLIAM J. LINDBLAD, PH.D.

CONTENTS

II
STRUCTURAL AND REGULATORY COMPONENTS OF WOUND HEALING

V
CLINICAL MANAGEMENT OF HEALING TISSUES

34
Wound Dressings: Design and Use 562
David M. Wiseman, Ph.D., M.R. Pharm. S., David T. Rovee, Ph.D.,
and Oscar M. Alvarez, Ph.D.

35
Surgical Devices in Wound
Healing Management 581
Richard F. Edlich, M.D., George T. Rodeheaver, Ph.D.,
and John G. Thacker, Ph.D.

Index 601

CURRENT PERSPECTIVES IN WOUND HEALING

George R. Martin, Ph.D., and Erle E. Peacock, Jr., M.D.

Trauma elicits diverse and potent processes that lead to the removal of damaged tissue and the recruitment of cells that deposit a collagen-rich matrix that forms a scar in all tissues except bone.[1] A fully developed skin scar is a rather acellular, poorly organized replica of normal dermis covered by a basement membrane and a relatively normal epidermis. However, scars vary depending on the tissue, type of injury, genetic factors, and the presence of systemic disease in the host. A scar that exceeds the height of the surrounding tissue is termed a *hypertrophic* scar; one that exceeds both the height and the boundaries of the surrounding tissue and that recurs after excision is known as a *keloid*.

Despite its importance in wound healing, scarring is associated with severe sequelae. Injury to internal organs results in the deposition of an excess of collagen with a loss of tissue architecture and function. For example, an alkali burn of the esophagus elicits an enormous scarring reaction that occludes the lumen and prevents peristaltic movements. Similarly, the damage caused by alcohol or other liver toxins may be followed by fibrosis and the permanent loss of normal hepatic structure and function. Scarring is one of the major factors responsible for the low rate of nerve regeneration following injury. On the other hand, wound healing is impaired in many patients, such as diabetics, the physically disabled, those with impaired circulation, and those receiving steroids or cytotoxic drugs. Thus, the events elicited in wound healing, while not completely defined, are central to many significant diseases and disorders. Research in this area focuses on understanding and controlling the scarring process.

CURRENT CONCEPTS IN WOUND HEALING

The processes that terminate bleeding generate byproducts that initiate the repair process.

Repair is carried out by a variety of cells that are drawn to the wound in a regular and highly coordinated procession. Initially there is a rapid entrance of platelets, neutrophils, and macrophages into the damaged area to debride the wound, destroy contaminating microorganisms, and in the case of platelets and macrophages, serve as a source of growth mediators[2-4] for fibroblasts and endothelial cells. The latter cells replace the lost and damaged matrix and blood supply, while epidermal cells migrate out from the margins of the wound and cover the lesion. It is likely that the rate at which these cells enter a wound and proliferate determines the rate at which the wound will heal.[5] Such cellular migrations and rapid proliferation are dependent on the presence of chemoattractants and growth factors.

Chemoattractants are substances, often peptides, proteins, or fragments of proteins, that can induce cells to move in the direction of their source, i.e., along a concentration gradient. The response of a cell to a chemoattractant is dependent on the cell's possessing high-affinity receptors for the factor. Often different cells respond to different factors and this allows their independent recruitment.

Growth factors are proteins or peptides that acting alone, or more often in combination, induce cells to initiate DNA synthesis and to divide. A number of growth factors have been well characterized including platelet-derived growth factor (PDGF), fibroblast growth factors acidic and basic (FGFs), epidermal growth factor (EGF), the transforming growth factors (TGF-α and TGF-β), and the insulin-like growth factors (IGF_1 and IGF_2). This is not an exclusive list and many other growth factors with important physiological roles probably exist. As mentioned, the ability of a cell to respond to a growth factor at relatively low concentrations (1–10 ng/ml) is dependent on the cell's possessing high-affinity receptors for the factor. Thus, PDGF acts on fibroblastic but not endothelial cells, while the FGFs act on both cell types. It should also be noted that certain growth factors also exhibit chemotactic activity,

1

and such dual activity would be particularly valuable in wound healing. Factors with these two activities are sometime referred to as mitoattractants. Chemotaxis and mitogenesis must share some early intracellular events elicited by growth factors, but the later responses associated with DNA synthesis are not needed for chemotaxis.

Chemoattractants are released in the wound as a byproduct of the clotting process, with aggregated platelets a particularly rich source of these factors.[5] Therefore, it is not unexpected that cytotoxic drugs that reduce the number of circulating platelets virtually abolish wound healing,[6] as does antibody prepared against macrophages.[2] In addition, it is thought that other cells entering the wound, including macrophages,[2, 3] fibroblasts,[7] and endothelial cells,[3, 8] also produce mitogens and chemoattractants that sustain cellular activities.

There is a considerable history of attempts to stimulate healing by supplementing wounds with extracts of various tissues. More recently, a realization of the essential role and the potency of growth factors has led to many studies using them as wound supplements. Due to problems involved in sustaining active levels of growth factors after injection into the wound, very large doses have been employed. There is as yet no reason to believe that these large doses are systemically active or produce adverse effects. Nor have there been reports of hypertrophic scars forming in wounds treated with such supplements, although such an excess might be expected to be causative. Of course, the growth factors that have been utilized are those that are available in quantity. The growth factors and attractants that actually regulate wound healing have not been identified, and these might be even more effective than a foreign factor.

The regaining of tensile strength in a wound is critically dependent on the synthesis and deposition of collagen, which in turn are related to the numbers of fibroblasts in the wound. Collagen synthesis is also determined by the oxygen tension in the wound and by the availability of ascorbic acid and other nutritional factors.[9] Growth factors increase cell numbers in the wound and thereby indirectly increase collagen synthesis. However, most growth factors stimulate the production of collagenase and thereby favor the degradation of collagen.[10, 11] In contrast, TGF-β, a potent and ubiquitous factor stored in platelets and produced by many cells, strongly stimulates collagen formation.[12, 13] In addition, TGF-β has other related activities such as attracting macrophages and suppressing degradative reactions that would be expected for a key regulator of wound healing, particularly of the steps associated with fibroses.

SOME AREAS FOR FUTURE RESEARCH

Two factors that have limited progress in wound healing research are the lack of relevant animal models for abnormal scar formation and the lack of sensitive methods to quantitate events in the wound. For example, skin wounds heal at a rapid, near maximal rate in rodents. Thus, factors added to the wound often show only marginal effects, while in an impaired wound they could be critical. It is clear that better models, even those that do not exactly mimic human disorders, would allow significant events to be identified and could be used to evaluate the potency of important mediators.

Repair has classically been evaluated by histologic evaluation, by quantitation of contracture and collagen deposition, and by tensile properties. None of these parameters is particularly sensitive to cellular activities and except in scurvy, where collagen synthesis is reduced, do not allow identification of the defective step. In contrast, the techniques used in molecular biology with recombinant DNA probes are ideally suited for quantitating cellular events in the healing wounds. These methods, which can be used to measure mRNA levels in the wound, are simpler and more sensitive than the conventional methods. Since each of the major populations of cells entering the wound (i.e., macrophages, fibroblasts, endothelial and epidermal cells) produce one or more cell-specific proteins, it should be possible to monitor these cells based on the mRNAs coding for these proteins. This technology has been developed to the point where the levels of various growth factor mRNAs have been measured in single macrophages isolated from wounds using the polymerase chain reaction.[4] One could envision using such technology on small biopsies isolated from human wounds as well as in animal studies.

It is well known that the degradation of collagen requires a specific enzyme, collagenase, that is produced in significant amounts in wounds.[14] Collagenase is produced by neutrophils, macrophages, epidermal cells, fibroblasts, and endothelial cells and is involved in the removal of damaged tissue and the remodeling of the scar. While there are several natural inhibitors of collagenase, the enzyme also binds to collagen fibers and causes a slow but continual degradation. The tearing open of wounds in scorbutic sailors was probably the result of continued collagen breakdown in the absence of synthesis. Thus a failure to control collagenase could be a factor in chronic ulcers and other problem wounds. Since inhibitors of collagenase are available, they might produce positive effects on chronic skin ulcers in which an excess of collagenase may be involved in the maintenance of the lesion.

Remarkable progress has been made in culturing and characterizing epidermal cells and even in using such cultured cells for skin grafts.[15] However, the factors activating the migration and proliferation of epidermal cells and the interaction between epidermal cells and other cells in the wound are not well defined. In addition, since some models of granulation tissue formation utilize subcutaneous implants, research on the role of epidermal cells has been neglected. Since epithelial and mesenchymal cells communicate during development and epithelial-mesenchymal interactions are critical during organogenesis, they may be similarly important, particularly in skin wounds.

Regeneration is common in phylogeny and occurs in fractured bone and probably in wounds in fetal animals. It should be considered whether scarring represents an evolutionary adaption to the regeneration process; that is, trauma in the lower species may trigger regeneration which is sidetracked in higher species by scarring, a more rapid process. Thus the addition of a single factor such as TGF-β could circumvent regeneration and cause a scar. Areas of study in which to explore this possibility include healing in lower organisms, wound healing in fetal versus adult animals, and repair of tissues such as liver and bone that have a high capacity for regeneration. Indeed one might predict that antagonists of the fibrotic growth factors would enhance regeneration. The regeneration of nervous tissue seems a prime candidate for clinical applications.

We believe that a variety of clinical disorders call for research with the possibility of significant clinical impact. Defective wound healing is common in diabetics, in the aged, and in individuals treated with steroids or chemotherapy. As noted, methods are available for following the activities transpiring in a wound to determine if a growth factor supplement induces a positive response. Unfortunately methods to deliver such supplements to wounds in physiological amounts over extended periods are not well established. If high levels of colla-

genase or other proteases contribute to the failure to heal skin ulcers, inhibitors of these proteases are available and might encourage the healing of chronic wounds.[16]

Excessive scarring is common and occurs in cirrhosis, arteriosclerosis, scleroderma, and a number of other diseases characterized by an abnormal deposition of collagen. A variety of approaches are available for intercession. For example, colchicine prevents the deposition of collagen and may also activate collagenase, and improved survival has been noted in cirrhotic patients treated with this alkaloid.[17] Other inhibitors of collagen synthesis show promise in preventing the scarring reaction in the liver, thus allowing the retention of normal histology and function.[18] Inhibitors of collagen crosslinking, such as β-aminopropionitrile and penicillamine, have been found to suppress fibrosis in the alkali-burned esophagus.[19] In this case, it is likely that such compounds prevent the physical changes in the tissue caused by accumulation of crosslinked fibers. It should also be noted that the actions of these inhibitors have been well known for some time, but this information has not been incorporated into common medical practice.

In summary, we view with enthusiasm the recent expansion of research on wound healing. Time will tell if growth factor therapy will reach general usage in surgery and medicine; however, one would hope that recalcitrant injuries would show a response to such factors. An important development is the introduction of recombinant DNA technology in this area with its potential for evaluating the cellular and molecular basis for defective repair in the patient with the application of appropriate and specific therapy. At this time, the emphasis is on research rather than application, with the biology of the wound healing process the first area to be mastered.

References

1. Peacock EE, Van Winkle WV: Surgery and Biology of Wound Repair, 2nd ed. Philadelphia, WB Saunders, 1976, pp 145–203.
2. Leibovich SJ, Ross R: The role of the macrophage in wound repair: A study with hydrocortisone and antimacrophage serum. Am J Pathol 78:71–91, 1975.
3. Martinet Y, Bitterman PB, Mornex JF, et al: Activated human monocytes express the c-sis protooncogene and release a mediator showing PDGF-like activity. Nature 319:158–160, 1986.
4. Rappolee DA, Mark D, Banda MJ, et al: Wound macrophages express TGF (alpha) and other growth factors in vivo: Analysis by an RNA phenotyping. Science 241:708–712, 1988.

5. Grotendorst GR, Pencev D, Martin GR, et al: Molecular mediators of tissue repair. In Hunt TK, Heppenstall RB, Pines E, et al (eds): Soft and Hard Tissue Repair: Biological and Clinical Aspects. New York, Praeger, 1984, pp 20–40.
6. Lawrence WT, Norton JA, Sporn MB, et al: The reversal of an adriamycin induced healing impairment with chemoattractants and growth factors. Ann Surg 203:142–147, 1986.
7. Mensing H, Pontz BF, Muller PK, et al: A study on fibroblast chemotaxis using fibronectin conditioned medium as chemoattractants. Eur J Cell Biol 29:268–273, 1983.
8. Ross R, Raines EW, Bowen-Pope DF: The biology of platelet derived growth factor. Cell 46:155–169, 1986.
9. Hunt TK, Knighton DR, Thakral KK, et al: Cellular control of repair. In Hunt TK, Heppenstall RB, Pines E, et al (eds): Soft and Hard Tissue Repair: Biological and Clinical Aspects. New York, Praeger, 1984, pp 3–19.
10. Chua CC, Geiman DE, Keller GH, et al: Induction of collagenase secretion in human fibroblast cultures by growth promoting factors. J Biol Chem 260:5213–5216, 1985.
11. Bauer EA, Cooper TW, Huang JS, et al: Stimulation of in vitro human skin collagenase expression by platelet derived growth factor. Proc Natl Acad Sci USA 82:4132–4136, 1985.
12. Roberts AB, Sporn MB, Assoian RK, et al: Transforming growth factor-β: Rapid induction of fibrosis and angiogenesis in vivo and stimulation of collagen formation in vitro. Proc Natl Acad Sci USA 83:4167–4171, 1986.
13. Sporn MB, Roberts AB, Wakefield LM, et al: Transforming growth factor-β: Biological functions and chemical structure. Science 233:532–534, 1986.
14. Mignatti P, Welgus HG, Rifkin DB: Role of degradative enzymes in wound healing. In Clark RAF, Henson PM (eds): The Molecular and Cell Biology of Wound Repair. New York, Plenum Press, 1988, pp 497–523.
15. Green H, Kehinde G, Thomas J: Growth of cultured human epidermal cells into multiple epithelia suitable for grafting. Proc Natl Acad Sci USA 76:5665–5668, 1979.
16. Reich R, Thompson E, Iwamoto Y, et al: Effects of inhibitors of plasminogen activator, serine proteinases, and collagenase IV on the invasion of basement membranes by metastatic cells. Can Res 48:3307–3312, 1988.
17. Kershenobich D, Vargas F, Garcia-Tsao G, et al: Colchicine in the treatment of cirrhosis of the liver. N Engl J Med 318:1709–1713, 1988.
18. Gunzler V, Hanauska-Abel HM, Myllyla K, et al: Time dependent inactivation of chick embryo prolyl 4-hydroxylase by coumalic acid. Biochem J 242:163–169, 1987.
19. Davis WM, Madden JM, Peacock EE Jr: Prevention of esophageal stenosis with induced lathyrism. Surg Forum 22:193–198, 1971.

1

WOUND HEALING RESEARCH THROUGH THE AGES

Henry Brown, M.D.

"Tertiam esse medicinae partem, quae manu curet, et vulgo notum et a me propositum est."
[The third part of medicine is that which cures by hand and indeed it is common knowledge.]

CELSUS
De Medicina, Proemium 9, Book VII (circa 25 A.D.)[1]

The theme common to all wound healing research has been an open mind, humility, and honesty. Celsus was a scholar who possessed these attributes. Those who strayed from these precepts in later life, as did Galen, often clouded their good works with insufferable dogma.

The treatment and healing of wounds is an art old as humanity. Vivid evidence of trauma and its consequences comes to us from archeological finds, under the heading of paleopathology. Use of plants in healing, often described as folklore, was universal among all early peoples. The similarity of the armamentaria from this source among the different cultures is striking even for different groups in diverse geographic areas. Examples of ancient plant remedies are boundless. The Chinese currently use a bread mold in folk medicine to treat small burns, which is undoubtedly timeless but dates back in written record at least 2000 years.[2] Penicillin, associated with Alexander Fleming's brilliant discovery in modern times,[3] indeed

may have been very long known before its modern "discovery."

The equally ancient treatment of "cupping" (Figs. 1–1 and 1–2) and "moxibustion" originated from the same Chinese culture that teaches us the virtues of bread mold and continues to be used to treat neurologic and muscular lesions.[2, 4] "Moxibustion" sounds to be very uncomfortable, but its popularity among the Chinese speaks for its acceptance. In brief, smoldering burning soft wormwood leaves or moss and incense are applied at acupuncture sites (Fig. 1–3) in treating such lesions. According to their writings, by using meticulous cleanliness combined with an excellent knowledge of anatomy, the Chinese folk practitioners report almost no untoward results or complications and some rather extravagant therapeutic results.[2, 4] This lack of complications is surprising in light of numerous complications, including pneumothorax and spinal cord injury, when acupuncture methodology has been adapted in Western clinics.[5, 6] The disparity in outcome from many folk remedies may hinge on unwritten but important technical points unknown and hence omitted in application of methods, for example, in this country.

The classic 1975 work of Professor Guido Majno while at Harvard, *The Healing Hand*,[7] and Dr. R. Ted Steinbock's 1976 *Paleopathological Diagnosis and Interpretation*,[8] largely written while he was a medical student at the same university, are both rich sources of information about wound healing in antiquity. The two works are in a sense complementary. Dr.

The author acknowledges with particular thanks Mr. Richard Wolf and Mrs. Ellen Wolf, curators of rare books at the Countway, Harvard–Boston Medical Library for many helpful suggestions and for making available centuries-old texts.

5

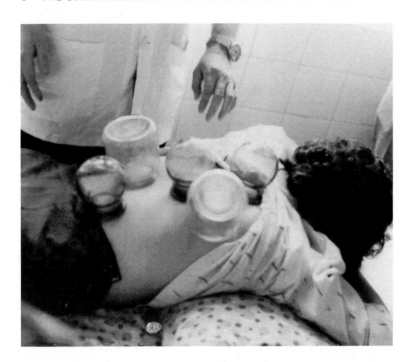

Figure 1–1. Cupping to relieve back pain. A flame within the cup consumes oxygen, forming a partial vacuum that draws up blood with the flesh in a mound at the cup orifice. (From the Zuong Cho School of Chinese Traditional Medicine, Gangzhou (Canton), China.)

Steinbock's work is a fine, painstakingly described and systematized compendium of lesions, many having been wounds, from archaeologic finds from all over the world. Dr. Majno's writings give an account of the methodology in different ancient cultures for managing such wounds. Much of the following is drawn from original sources as well as from these two superb references.

WOUND HEALING IN ANTIQUITY

Animals treat each other's wounds. Their methods undoubtedly antedate the coming of humans. Often they lick wounds, but treatment may extend, for example, to tooth extractions or removal of a foreign body from the eye by chimpanzees.[7] Steinbock's description of fractures among American Indian remains as old as 4000 years suggests a great deal about treatment among these people. Often fracture reduction was minimal, yet healing often occurred with obviously satisfactory function, as evidenced by survival in that very difficult competitive early environment.[8]

The Edwin Smith[9] and Ebers[10] Papyri, discovered among Egyptian antiquities by men of those names in the nineteenth century, have given us our best view of ancient Egyptian medicine. The Smith scroll is almost 16 feet long. Numberless hours of patient, scholarly study spent in translation of these papyri have yielded the historic treasures hidden in their lines.

SWNW was the ancient Egyptian word for physician. It was perhaps pronounced "soonoo," but we may never know since written ancient Egyptian words have come down to us with consonants but without vowels.[7] Estes, after extensive study, pessimistically concluded that Egyptian physicians optimally permitted wounds to heal by themselves, even though they had both medicinal and magical remedies, a substantial number of which continue to be used in various cultures today.[11] Further, the patients usually lived too short a life span to develop the degenerative diseases we know today. The *swnw* had no help for the more serious diseases at any age and probably could do little to alter public health problems. The reader must decide from reading the original texts, however, whether Estes' view of Egyptian medicine as having so many limitations is justified. Even Estes' writings on the papyri and other documents indicate that at least some Egyptian physicians systematically categorized facts about patients to make rational decisions concerning diagnosis, prognosis, and therapy. They wrote the first known Western medicine texts and compiled observations of human anatomy, rudimentary as they were. They also gave

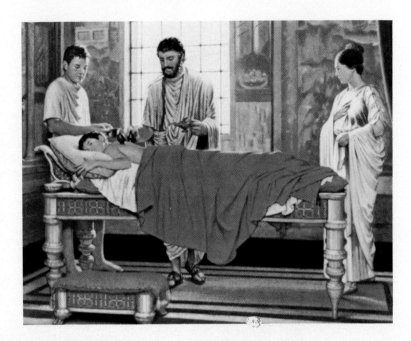

Figure 1–2. Galen. He, like the ancient Chinese, practiced cupping. (From Bender GA, Thom RA: Great Moments in Medicine. Detroit, Northwood Institute Press, 1965, p 57.)

us some of the first surgical methods, drug therapies, and splints and bandages. Importantly, they gave us the first medical vocabulary. Whether the Egyptians or the inhabitants of Mesopotamia, two contemporary cultures, were first to contribute these gifts to medicine is arguable.[11]

A few general remarks are in order as regards the Smith or, more formally, the Edwin Smith Surgical Papyrus as an indication of the medical prowess of ancient Egyptians, particularly in regard to wound care. We have a seventeenth century B.C. copy of the original document written in the Pyramid Age, about 3000 to 2500 B.C. The beginning and end have been lost, and the original author is unknown. Twenty-seven original column-texts were written in pictorials called hieroglyphs. The writing itself, slow and difficult to perform, was known as hieroglyphics.[9] Hieratic was the more rapid, cursive form of signs used for day-to-day writing in business and government. This hieratic script is the form in which the Smith Papyrus has come to us. Since its discovery, it has been translated once again into hieroglyphics.[9]

Well-written case summaries of surgical wounds in the Smith Papyrus have a detail worthy of modern clinics, even though the methodology described may fall short. As an example, consider the patient with a lacerated ear (Case 23, Text VIII, lines 18–27):

Examination—If thou examinest a man having a wound in the ear, cutting though its flesh, the injury being in the lower part of the ear [and] confined to the flesh, thou should draw [it] together for him with stitching behind the hollow of his ear. *Treatment*— A slit in the outer ear. If thou findest the stitching of that wound loose [and] sticking in the two lips of his wound, thou should make for him stiff rolls of linen [and] pad the back of his ear therewith. Thou shouldst treat it afterwards [with] grease, honey [and] lint every day until he recovers.

Their method of splinting the wound and its dressing suggest that the ancient Egyptians understood wound healing and care very well even though their pharmacopeia may not suggest such advanced knowledge. Note the use of honey. Majno[7] points out that *byt*, or honey, was by far the most popular Eygptian "drug," being mentioned about 500 times in 900 remedies. It is an ingredient that is practically harmless to the tissue and probably aseptic, antiseptic, and antibiotic. It prevents adherence to the tissues and draws fluid from wounds, being hypertonic.

Ebbell translated the Ebers Papyrus calling it "the greatest Egyptian medical document."[10] All manner of prescriptions for healing wounds are described but only one will be discussed here. It suggests again that the ancient Egyptian medical formulary had not kept pace with the development of surgical techniques. As an example, the surgical disease cystoid enlargement was to be treated by a dressing that breaks the suppurating membrane: "Acacia seyal, *thwi*, fruit of *szms*, blood of the *hwr* bird, fly's blood, *szsz*, honey, *'mzw*, and sory northern salt are ground, mixed together and [it] is bandaged therewith." Many other such prescriptions are

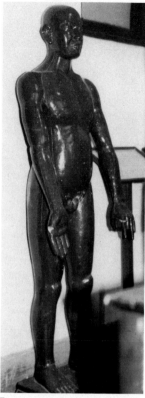

Figure 1–3. Brown ceramic mannequin, a model of one used to teach the art of acupuncture 800 years ago. Mercury was placed in the holes in the mannequin made for acupuncture. If the mercury was retained, the site was proper for acupuncture to relieve pain, but if the mercury came out, the site was improper. (From the Zuong Cho School of Chinese Traditional Medicine, Gangzhou (Canton), China.)

given. Also, a section at the paragraphs of a prescription gives incantations or recitals to be said before medical treatment begins.

Intermixed with the mystique of incantations, the early Egyptians in the Smith and Ebers Papyri nevertheless speak of draining suppuration from wounds and of diseased and not diseased wounds, yet they antedate Halsted's aseptic techniques for wound management by several millennia. For all of their care in handling wounds, the sages of the papyri tell us that it is good for a wound to "rot" a bit, planting the seeds in the Middle Ages and Renaissance of the dictum of "laudable pus." They believed pus to be helpful so long as it was not excessive.[7] The doctrine stated in Latin, "Pus bonum et laudible," remained until it was finally condemned 3000 years later in the works of the French surgeon Ambroise Paré.

Trephination, also called trepanation, an operation to relieve intracranial pressure, by drilling and removing bone from the skull, was widely reported in antiquity for treating head wounds. This procedure was accepted in many cultures, including the ancient Egyptian and American Indian, and often had a successful outcome.[7, 8] It has been reported to have been done as long ago as 10,000 years.[8]

The ancient Indian culture has left us a rich legacy in surgical technique and wound care. Much of it comes to us in the script of the learned Sanskrit text known as *Sushrata Samhita* or simply *Sushrata*.[12] Most of the learning, however, was transmitted by oral tradition in an unbroken line from antiquity. Unfortunately, much of this oral lore has been irretrievably lost through the ages. Two surviving examples of ancient Indian surgical teaching and wound management are cited as illustrative. On rhinoplastic operations:

Now I shall deal with the process of affixing an artificial nose. First the leaf of a creeper, long and broad enough to cover the whole of the severed [nose] is clipped off. Part should be gathered, and a patch of living flesh equal in dimension to the preceding leaf should be sliced off (from down upward) from the region of the cheek and after scarifying it with a knife, swiftly adhered to the severed nose. Then the cool headed physician should steadily tie it up with a bandage decent to look at and perfectly sealed to the end for which it has been employed (Sadher Vandha). . . . The adhesioned part should be dusted with powders of Pattenya, Yashtimadhiekam and Rasannjana pulverized together and the nose should be enveloped in Karpase cotton and several times sprinkled with the refined oil of pure sesamum.

Regarding an ear that has been lost:

A surgeon well-versed in the knowledge of surgery (Shastras) should slice off a patch of living flesh from the cheek. Then the part where the artificial ear lobe is to be made should be slightly scarified (with a knife) and the living flesh full of blood and sliced off as previously directed should be adhesioned to it (so as to resemble a natural ear lobe in shape).

The volumes provide detailed directions on dieting and postoperative management in addition to extensive discussions of all manner of disease treatments

Of the many distinguished thinkers and philosophers of the classical period of Greek medical practice (460 to 136 B.C.),[13] only two, Hippocrates and Herophilus, will be discussed.

Hippocrates (circa 460 to 370 B.C.) is known as the Father of Medicine, who gave us much of our ethical heritage and the scientific spirit. He is a role model physician for all times (Fig. 1–4).[13–15] A contemporary of Socrates and Plato at the zenith of Athenian democracy, Hippocrates is believed to have been born on the

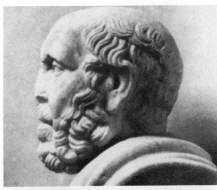

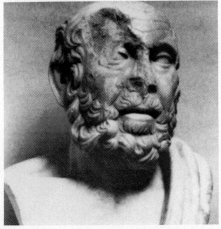

Figure 1–4. Hippocrates. (From Richards DW: Hippocrates of Ostia. JAMA 204:1055, 1968. Courtesy of Johannes Felbermeyer.)

Greek island of Cos, where he later headed a great school of medicine.

The teachings of Hippocrates give us fundamental tenets in treatment of wounds. He emphasized that the physician should use good light and be comfortable when examining the patient, and, very importantly, that the injured part or site should be compared to the corresponding uninjured part. He recognized the importance of cleanliness and asepsis and recommended irrigation of wounds only with clean or river water, preferably boiled water for the latter. He believed rest and immobilization to be better for the wound than bandages and splints. He avoided greasy ointments, preferring a dry wound, and believed that medicaments were better placed around rather than in wounds. The modern theme of adequate documentation is stressed in his case histories, forty-two of which fortunately are extant in his book on epidemics. They are the only clinical cases that have come to us from ancient Greece. The cases are reported with sincerity and without embellishment, and regardless of whether the result was successful or fatal. They are very objective. About 70 works are ascribed to Hippocrates from his great school at Cos. He himself probably wrote only a half dozen or so of these case reports. The absence of self-aggrandizement and his honesty and humility truly fit the oath he gave to medicine. With his passing went the open-minded investigative clinical spirit of his school, and centuries of lesser medical thought and dogma were ushered in.

Herophilus of Chalcedin-Bythnia (circa 335 to 280 B.C.) (Fig. 1–5), grandson of Aristotle, was educated by Praxagorus.[16] The latter succeeded Diocles as the leader of the Dogmatic School of philosphy and represented the antithesis of Hippocratic teaching. Praxagorus was equally well known for his knowledge of anatomy. He had dissected a human body, a most unusual privilege at that time, and he made a fine and lasting impression on his pupil.

Herophilus founded the great school of anatomy at Alexandria, where he became known as the "Father of Anatomy." His contribution to wound healing was in helping to give us an anatomical basis on which to systematically establish that discipline. Of his many contributions, most remembered are his important dealings with head wounds and their healing and his description of the confluence of venous sinuses at the occiput in the floor of the skull. That structure is still known as the "torcular herophili." Also in regard to the cranial vault, he recognized the key role of the central nervous system not only in our mechanical functioning but in our mental functioning as well. He located the seat of the soul or psyche in the fourth ventricle, with the ventricular fluid being an essential element, an idea not discredited for centuries. Even though he was among the

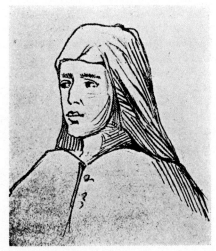

Figure 1–5. Herophilus,"Father of Anatomy." (From Gordon BL: Medicine Throughout Antiquity. Philadelphia, FA Davis, 1949, p 594).

first to be recorded as having this view, undoubtedly this teaching long preceded him and was part of the reasoning of a long line of distinguished philosophers and physicians. The latter included Galen of Pergamon and the celebrated late eighteenth century neuroanatomist, Samuel Thomas von Soemmering,[17] who also established the number of cranial nerves as twelve.[18] As if this were not enough to occupy several lifetimes of study, Herophilus also became the first medical obstetrician recorded in Western history.

In accepting the code of mores of his time, it is not surprising that he practiced human vivisection.[16] That route of study was believed necessary, i.e., that anatomy could only be learned from the living. It is difficult even at this distance in time to understand such cruelty or how it could be accepted and condoned as punishment for heretics and criminals. Even Celsus, who generally vehemently disapproved of vivisection, believed it to be acceptable in some circumstances. Fortunately strong personalities did condemn the practice, as, for example, the philosopher Tertullian, who wrote: "Herophilus, that physician or butcher who dissected six hundred men [HB: without anesthesia] in order to learn the structure of their frame could not . . . since they did not die a natural death, but expired amidst all the agonies of death to which the curiosity of the anatomists had subjected them."

Aurelius Cornelius Celsus (25 B.C. to A.D. 50), known as the "Latin Hippocrates," was one of the great patrician Roman scholars. He wrote on many subjects and very prominently on medicine. Among his extant writings are the books of his encyclopedic work, *De Medicina*. In a sense, his work is a bridge between Hippocrates and the Roman civilization. He continued many of the Hippocratic precepts and teachings in his own writing.[1, 19]

Meinecke observed that Celsus ". . . wrote *De Medicina* with independent judgement and that thereby he originated a new medical nomenclature."[19] He made the timeless statement repeated by Cicero that ". . . the physician cannot apply the proper therapeutics without a correct diagnosis."[20] Many students of history and of Latin classics nevertheless believe that Celsus was a lay person, not a member of the medical profession.[19] I find it difficult to accept that he was not a physician because his learning in medicine and particularly wound healing goes far beyond the laity. He wrote of management of head and neck cancer and carcinoma of the nose and of the dangers of incomplete

treatment and uselessness of others,[*,21] hypertrophic scar, and proper dressing for many lesions, all of which have a modern ring![1] His books are recommended to the reader for many thoughts far ahead of their time.

We know much of Galen's life (see Fig. 1–2), since he left extensive autobiographical notes. He is referred to here because of his absolute dominance of Western medicine for 1500 years. No other recorded dogma has been so permanent. As Majno states, Galen literally left a monument to himself in his 35 extant volumes, which probably represent only two thirds of all his writings.[7]

Galen, born in 130 A.D. in Pergamon on the Mediterranean Sea in Asia Minor, now part of Turkey, had the advantage of a great library second only to that of Alexandria. Nikon, his father, was a rich influential architect who died when Galen was 20. Nikon began his son's education in philosophy at age 14 and after a dream made him study medicine, which was then largely taught by Hebrew slaves who had been expelled from Jerusalem by the Romans after the failure of the Barkochba uprising (132 to 135 A.D.).[22] Galen studied anatomy for 10 years (147 to 157 A.D.) in various cities, including Smyrna, said to be the most beautiful city in Asia Minor, and for five years in Alexandria, where human autopsy was tolerated and where it was occasionally possible to obtain bodies of executed criminals from the river for dissection. With his background, it is difficult to rationalize the lore that he was well grounded in animal, i.e., pig, but not human anatomy. His observations on living and partly dissected animals, however, did include apes, goats, pigs, sheep, lions, cows, wolves, dogs, mice, serpents, fish, and birds, as well as an elephant heart. After he once again returned to his native Pergamon, Galen cared for wounded gladiators for 3 years and thus gained much opportunity to learn human anatomy, undoubtedly by observing many wounds of the skull, thorax, abdomen, and extremities. He had ample opportunity to study the heart in motion as well as to repair blood vessels.

With this opportunity Galen came to understand the venous and arterial circulations, evident in his later advice for treating iatrogenic

*Celsus on carcinoma of the nose and its treatment: "Again at the angle next to the nostrils [HB: here Celsus is speaking of eye lesions], there opens a sort of small fistula, due to some lesion through which rheum persistently drips; the Greeks call it aiglops." "Of these affections it is dangerous to treat those which resemble carcinoma, for that even hastens death. Again it is useless to treat those which penetrate the nostril, for they never heal."

arterial injury to the arm to prevent an aneurysm. His understanding of wound care, the dressings required, and follow-up care needed is clearly indicated by his advice, even though grandiose, to the physician responsible for the difficulty.[23] An uprising in Pergamon at the end of those three years convinced him to leave and to go to Rome.

Galen's services to Emperor Marcus Aurelius are well known and were well regarded until he was unhappily banished in a changing political climate. After studying the Methodists, the Empiricists, and the Dogmatists, he wrote: "The best physician has also to be a philosopher." Like Einstein, Galen had a love of the perfection and simplicity of nature that was like religion, though he was an atheist.

The recording of so many of Galen's astute obervations makes it difficult to rationalize his teaching of unfounded dogmas, such as his theory of pores in the ventricular septum permitting passage of blood from right to left heart. Since modesty was not one of his virtues, and since his clinical success was enormous, he came to look on his theories as truths even when unsupported by objective evidence.

THE MIDDLE AGES

According to Walsh, the Middle Ages began in 476 A.D. with the deposition of Romulus Augustus and ended in 1453 with the fall of Constantinople.[24] During that period Arabic was the language of medicine in the Empire of Islam as Latin was in Western Europe. Persians and Nestorians taught in the East, and Spaniards and Jews in the West. Campbell is of the opinion that Yacub Ebn Ishak el-Kindi (813 to 873 A.D.), known in Europe as Alkindus, was the only prominent Arab writer of pure Arabian lineage whose writings have survived.[25]

Much of the writings of Hippocrates and Galen came to us first from Arabic translations and later from Latin translations from the Arabic. The Scholars were in Asia Minor initially and later in Europe. Syracuse in Sicily and Cordova and particularly Toledo in the "Caliphate" in Spain were seats of Arabic learning.[25]

Abulcasis (circa 936 to 1013 A.D.) wrote of many surgical procedures, and his comprehensive work was translated from Arabic into Latin in 1541.[26] He describes cauterization of the lacrimal duct of the eye for fistula, head fractures, fractures of the feet and hands, and the management of a phlegmon and a carbuncle. The original Arabic text has been lost.

The medical school of Salerno, the first in "modern" Europe, actually was founded in the eighth century A.D. but not formally organized until the tenth century A.D.[24] The school reached its intellectual zenith two hundred years later. Although the school was associated with the Benedictine order, myth or fact has it that the four founders were a Jewish rabbi, Elinus (Elias); a Greek, Pontus (Ganopontus); a Saracen, Adale (Abdullah); and an unnamed native of Salerno. Each lectured in his own tongue. The new school had the advantage of already having a fine academic atmosphere, being influenced by the nearby school of the great Mother House at Monte Cassino. Regimens mostly for diet and health were written in verse for the laity rather than for physicians. The teachings of respect, humility, and primary concern for the patient undoubtedly came directly from Hippocrates. Even though credited with great advances in surgery, a science said to be founded by Roland and Roger of the Four Masters,[24] little detail has been uncovered by this writer.

The next great school was founded probably in the tenth century at Montpelier in southern France near the Mediterranean. The school was steeped in Christian tradition. Guy, or Guido, of the Brothers of the Holy Ghost founded the Holy Ghost Hospital in Montpelier.[24] It became a model for Pope Innocent III's hospital in Rome and those hospitals he wished to build throughout the Christian lands.

The distinguished thirteenth century physician Arnold de Villanova (1235 to 1311) was from Catalonia, Spain.[24] He is also known as Rainaldus or Reginaldus. His writings and aphorisms, widely published during the Renaissance, have appropriate surgical wisdom and wound healing skills for this present volume:[24] "The lips of a wound will glue together of themselves if there is no foreign substance between them, and in this way the natural appearance of the part will be preserved." "In large wounds sutures should be used and silk thread tied at short distances make the best sutures." "A collection of pus is best dissolved by incision and cleaning out the purulent material." "To put off the opening of an abscess brings many dangers with it." The aphorism "where veins and arteries are notably large, incision and deep cautery should be avoided" suggests that Arnold de Villanova may have had experience with esophageal varices, since alcohol consumption was as common then as now.

Many medical historians consider Guy de Chauliac (1300 to 1370) of France as the great surgical authority of the Renaissance prior to Ambroise Paré. He wrote *Wounds and Frac-*

tures, published in 1363.[27] This book concerns all manner of wounds, particularly those caused by foreign bodies such as arrows. He writes authoritatively on bandaging, suturing, compresses, and drains. Regarding repair of cicatrices, "... all of the superfluity may be trimmed away with a razor, or it may be removed with a cautery and the place then treated with fowl fat or with mastic. . . ." He further quotes Galen's *Third Therapeutics (Medicus Medendi)*: "the removal of the superabundance is by medicaments alone and not by nature." He probably well understood the difficulties of treating keloids.[27]

The other great surgeon of that era, also French, was Henri de Mondeville (1260 to 1368), who again speaks of wounds and particularly of abscess.[28]

EARLY PHYSIOLOGY AND BIOMECHANICS

Two late Renaissance nonphysician scholars who had a profound influence on the art of wound healing were René Descartes[29] (1596 to 1650) (Fig. 1–6) and Giovanni Alfonso Borelli[30] (1608 to 1679) (Fig. 1–7). Oddly both were also wards of the nonconventional Queen Christina of Sweden. Descartes, with his superb classical Jesuit education, rebelled against his comfortable merchant class family in Maine, France, and left his native land to become a soldier of fortune-philosopher, never to return. Along

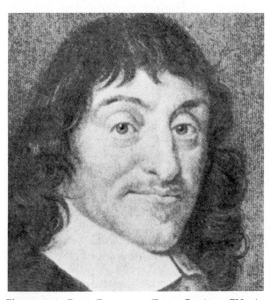

Figure 1–6. René Descartes. (From Garrison FH: An Introduction to the History of Medicine. Philadelphia, WB Saunders, 1929, p 258.)

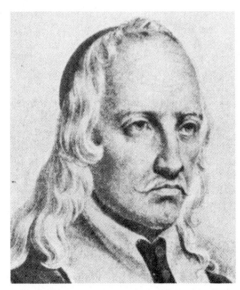

Figure 1–7. Giovanni Alfonso Borelli. (From Garrison FH: An Introduction to the History of Medicine. Philadelphia, WB Saunders, 1929, p 259.)

with his classic *Discourse on Reason*, and his new analytical geometry, Descartes also wrote probably the first physiology text in the Western world, *De Homine* (Fig. 1–8). Even though the book is very different from recent texts, its principles for many of the organ systems include much of medical art and science, of which wound healing is an important part. Descartes spent his last days in Stockholm as philosopher-teacher to Queen Christina. There, unhappily, her strict 5 A.M. daily teaching schedule and the rigors of a severe Swedish winter were more than Descartes' leisurely French constitution could tolerate, and he succumbed to pneumonia at age 54, less than six months after his arrival in Sweden.

The other scholar, Borelli, originally from Naples, was a student of Galileo. He was a mathematician turned philosopher-physiologist and had a keen mind but both a difficult personality and life. He spoke out with unpopular arguments and bitter invective against his colleagues, particularly Malpighi, even while his mentor, Galileo, was having his books burned.[30] Like the writings of Descartes, Borelli's writings on the circulation, respiration, secretion of fluids, nervous activity, and the mechanistic theory of muscle action, even with their many imperfections, underlie much of our modern thinking on treatment. His patron, Queen Christina, was erratic with him, probably with good reason. Borelli died in December 1679 in poverty and in political exile, teaching elementary mathematics in Rome. Late that year, however, Christina agreed to bear publication

RENATUS DES CARTES

DE

HOMINE

FIGURIS,

ET

LATINITATE DONATUS

A

FLORENTIO SCHUYL,

Inclytæ Urbis Sylvæ-Ducis Senatore, & ibidem.
Philosophiæ Professore.

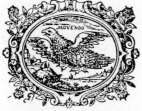

LVGDVNI BATAVORVM,

Ex Officinâ HACKIANA,

cIɔ Iɔc LxIv.

Figure 1–8. Frontispiece from René Descartes' physiology text *De Homine*, which was published posthumously because Descartes wished to avoid conflict with the church, particularly over his views of separation of body and soul. (Courtesy of the Countway, Harvard—Boston Medical Library.)

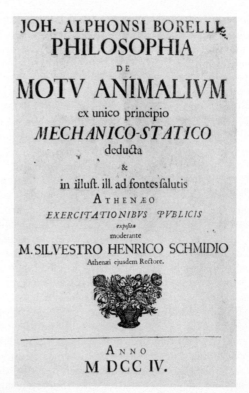

Figure 1–9. Frontispiece from Borelli's *De Motu Animalium*. (Courtesy of the Countway, Harvard—Boston Medical Library.)

costs for his famous *De Motu Animalium* (Fig. 1–9). It details in difficult Latin and mathematics but with simple strikingly effective line drawings the physiologic principles enumerated above.[31]

The French surgeon Ambroise Paré (1510 to 1590) insisted on gentleness in handling tissues[32, 33] several hundred years before William Stuart Halsted insisted on his surgical dictum early in the twentieth century at Johns Hopkins Medical School. Paré was appalled at the barbarous practice of pouring boiling oil into battle wounds to cauterize them while causing suppuration or "laudable pus," methodology from the time of the Smith Papyrus of Pyramid Egypt. Rather, Paré practiced gentleness, meticulous cleanliness, and conservation of tissues, much as Celsus had directed in his writings 1500 years earlier. On his statue are the immortal words "Je le pansey. Dieu le guarit." [I make the wound, God heals it.] Paré recognized the need for specialization. He wrote that at first healers knew surgery, diet, and pharmacy, but since life is not long enough to "learn and exercise all of them, the workmen divided themselves." His favor for the surgeon may be noted in his writing "that none ought to be accounted a surgeon [chirurgeon], . . .

[who] can perform his duty without the knowledge of diet and pharmacy. But both the others can perform their parts without surgery [chirurgery] if we may believe Galen." He speaks of nearly every surgical condition and its management, including toothache, finger dislocations, cataract, bladder stone, and leprosy.

SURGICAL ANATOMISTS

Of the great surgical anatomists of the fifteenth to the twentieth centuries, only a few of whom will be mentioned, all contributed to the surgical principles of wound healing. Andreas Vesalius[34] (1514 to 1564) and Bernhard Siefried Albinus[35] (1697 to 1770) come to mind for the concept of dynamic anatomy and Josais Weitbrecht[36] (1702 to 1747) for importance of ligaments. Richard Quain[37] (1800 to 1887) stressed the importance of the vasculature, an area so critical to the wound healing theme of this text. Sir Charles Bell[38] (1774 to 1887) and, a century later, Ramon Y. Cajal[39] (1852 to 1934) contributed knowledge of neural function, which eventually led to knowledge of the importance of axonal transport and neurotrophic factors in tissue development and homeostasis. Julius Casserius[40] (1545 to 1616) wrote about comparative anatomy in his great early seventeenth century text on the neck and provided plates of the cat and leopard to help us understand differences among species in survival from physical insult. The prolific writings of John Hunter[41] (1728 to 1793), expanding on the same subjects, included the term *healing by primary and secondary intention* and discussed the role of granulation tissue in healing. Another of Hunter's imaginative thoughts raised the possibility of tissue acceptance of transplants because of acceptance of foreign tissue by a "free-martin." The last term refers to a female calf, born as the nonidentical twin of a male, which matures into a sterile cow lacking immunogenicity against its twin; this gave an early clue to Joseph Murray that identical twins would accept each other's kidneys without rejection.[42]

Rudolf Virchow's[43] (1821 to 1902) contributions to microscopic and especially cellular pathology have been of immeasurable value. His observations and methods, following centuries of macroscopic examination of this process, directly led to the examination and understanding of wound healing at the cellular level.

Skin grafting by such nineteenth century surgeons as Karl Thiersch[44] (1822 to 1895) revived an ancient art found in the *Sushrata* and undoubtedly in many other ancient writings. Again perfection of technical detail in the nineteenth century, as of suturing by Lembert[45] or irrigation by sterile solutions early in the twentieth century by Carrel and Dakin,[46] are direct adaptations of the methods of Celsus and probably of many other earlier practitioners.

Philip Ignaz Semmelweis[47] (1818 to 1865) observed the high incidence of often lethal puerperal sepsis ("child-bed fever") that occurred when physicians did not wash their hands when coming from an autopsy to deliver a child and concluded that this might constitute the cause of the fever. His idea met with derision and rejection. In contrast, Oliver Wendell Holmes[48] (1809 to 1894) had the same notion and his ideas met with support in the United States.

MODERN SURGERY, ANESTHESIA, PHYSIOLOGY, AND BIOCHEMISTRY

The events discussed above immediately preceded the description of antiseptic techniques by Joseph Lister (1827 to 1912),[49, 50] who early on had accepted Louis Pasteur's controversial germ theory of infection. Lister made the fascinating observation that the river water of Glasgow receiving effluent from a chemical plant was clear whereas the remaining river water remained cloudy and visibly polluted. On consulting his friend Mr. Anderson in the chemistry department at the same university in Glasgow; Lister learned that phenol wastes were clearing the water and that gypsies had used a phenol-containing tar for centuries to treat small open wounds. The wards in the infirmary at the University of Glasgow where Lister was professor of surgery were literally overrun with infection. This led Lister to adopt his famous antiseptic technique of spraying carbolic acid to kill germs in the operating room and on the wards, thus changing the science and art of surgery (Fig. 1–10). This idea, like that of Semmelweis, met with derision and rejection, forcing Lister to leave Glasgow, but eventually he triumphantly prevailed as Professor at Edinburgh.

Physicians who have changed painful dressings, as of burns, know how merciful anesthesia can be. Dr. William T. G. Morton[51] (1819 to 1868), a Boston dentist, was challenged by the agonizing, sometimes fatal, pain associated with dental treatment and began experimenting with anesthesia on himself and the family dog. Dr. Morton first used ether anesthesia for a human patient for removal of a tumor at the Massachusetts General Hospital on October 16, 1846.

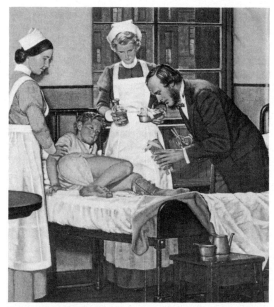

Figure 1–10. Joseph Lister (1827 to 1912). (From Bender GA, Thom RA: Great Moments in Medicine. Detroit, Parke Davis Company, 1965, p 269.)

The patient, Gilbert Abbott, after opening his eyes following the ether vapor anesthesia, said "I have experienced no pain." After this success, Dr. Morton decided to patent ether anesthesia, he said to prevent its abuse. A long legal wrangle ensued with Dr. Charles Jackson, who claimed to have given Morton the idea, and with Morton's former colleague and office partner, Dr. Horace Wells. The latter claimed he had anesthetized 14 or 15 dental patients long before Morton had demonstrated ether anesthesia. As a result of the embroglio, Dr. Morton died in poverty on August 15, 1868, while in New York, having unsuccessfully appealed his case in person years before to President Pierce at the White House.

The development of safe and effective antimicrobial agents in this century represents another advance in our ability to reduce morbidity due to wound infections. The first of these agents, sulfanilamide, was released for clinical use in the United States in about 1936 and was followed by penicillin five years later. Alexander Fleming (1881 to 1955) devoted his professional career mostly to investigating human defenses to control bacterial infection. His eventual recognition came later in life. In 1945, he received the Nobel Prize in medicine, as did Chain and Florey, for his 1928 discovery of penicillin from the mold *Penicillium notatum* on a culture plate surrounded by lysed colonies of staphylococci.[52] The quick acceptance and great benefit derived from the discovery of penicillin and other immunologic work, when combined with proper surgical technique, has led to far better wound healing with much lower morbidity, especially in trauma. Fleming's nimble and versatile mind is further exemplified by his extensive writing on lysozyme. He named it lysozyme after discovering nasal mucus dissolving a yellowish colony on a culture plate of *Micrococcus lysodeikticus*. Collaborating with J. D. Allison, he also found lysozyme in human blood, serum, tears, saliva, and milk.[52]

The work of Fleming and the army of researchers that followed in the study and development of antibiotics was complemented by equally elegant research by an earlier Nobel laureate (1908), the eminent Russian biologist Elie Metchnikoff (1845 to 1916).[53] Metchnikoff, having observed leukocytes engulfing foreign particles, named the process *phagocytosis* and the cells *phagocytes*. He noted the location of phagocytes in the reticuloendothelial system and discovered humoral factors in immunity. These findings have been crucial in combating infection, one of the major obstacles to satisfactory wound healing.

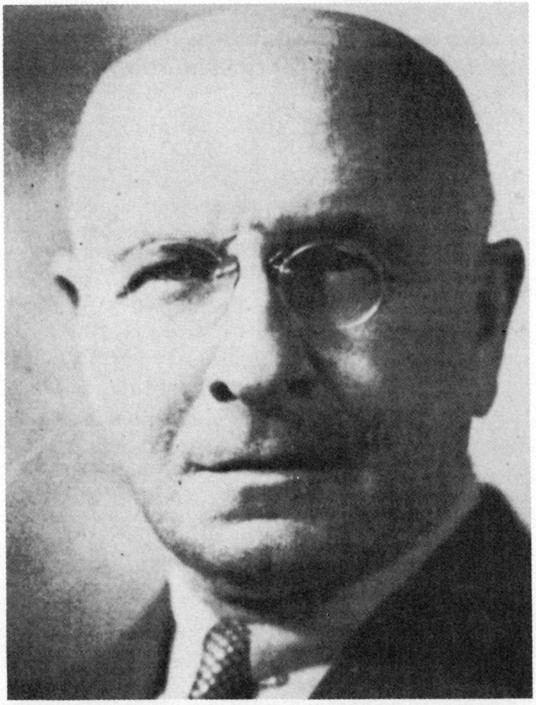

Figure 1–11. Alexis Carrel. (From Brieger GH: The development of surgery. In Sabiston DC (ed): Textbook of Surgery, 14th ed. Philadephia, WB Saunders, 1991, p 15.)

Alexis Carrel (1873 to 1944) (Fig. 1–11) was born in France and worked as a researcher early in this century at the Rockefeller Institute in New York. He added another crucial facet, transplantation surgical techniques, to the unknown mosaic of wound healing. Along with Guthrie, he not only maintained isolated perfused organs but also successfully transplanted a kidney from one cat to another for a short period. His tricornered vascular stitch, developed for the transplantation of blood vessels alone as well as for transplantation of small organs, has remained one of the best methods for anastomosing small vessels. The Nobel Academy cited Alexis Carrel for the Nobel Prize for Medicine or Physiology in 1912, "for his work in vascular suturing and on the grafting of blood vessels and organs."[54]

Alexis Carrel, as a major in the French Army Medical Corps in World War I, assisted in formulating the widely used Carrel-Dakin solution for irrigation of deep wounds.[46, 55] In 1935, with Col. Charles A. Lindbergh, Carrel told of developing a mechanical "heart." Organs such as the heart or the kidney could remain viable for study by perfusing them with "artificial blood" in glass chambers.

Biochemistry plays such a crucial role in wound healing research that it would be remiss not to credit some of the fine minds that have brought about progress in this area. Basic studies on proteins and nucleic acids will be the focus. The little remembered work of the Russian Michael Tswett (published circa 1907) introduced the chromatographic method, now one of the mainstays in analysis of proteins and nucleic acids.[56] Paul Ehrlich's theories of immunology that led to immunoassays are an equally important complement to Michael Tswett's work for analytical methods.[57] Martin and Synge, working in a unheated garage in Leeds, England, during the German air raids of World War II, developed partition chromatography first on silica gel and then on filter paper to separate amino acids.[58, 59] This methodology had an almost explosive effect on protein chemistry and on molecular biology, of which protein chemistry is an important part. Prior to their work, amino acid separation and quantitative estimates for each amino acid in a hydrolysate of a protein required on the order of three years to perform by the Dakin fractional butanol distillation method.[60, 61] Martin and Synge made it possible to semiquantitatively estimate the amino acid content in 48 hours by two-dimensional filter paper chromatography using the solvents phenol and collidine. Within eight years (1951), Frederick Sanger (Fig. 1–12), having only the elegant 1905 Fisher-Hofmeister[62] theory of peptide linkage but little else to guide him, employed the fluorodinitrobenzene terminal amino acid labelling technique suggested by Chibnall[63] to discern the complete amino acid sequence of the protein

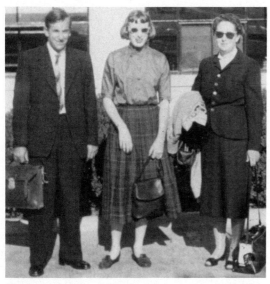

Figure 1–12. Frederick Sanger, along with Julie Brown and Joan Sanger, University of California at Berkeley, October, 1955.

insulin.[64, 65] Parenthetically, the terminal amino group labelling idea was not a new one. Abderhalden and Styx in 1923 had used dinitrochlorobenzene to label free amino groups of individual amino acids with a yellow color, but they had little success identifying free amino groups of proteins.[63] The fluoro-derivative of the same compound, being far more reactive than its chloro-analogue, enjoyed considerable success in Sanger's hands.[63] Myles Partridge employed displacement column chromatography to separate pure amino acids in quantity from protein hydrolysates, using the mechanism from a mechanical alarm clock to operate his fraction collector.[66] Moore and Stein used ion exchange chromatography to isolate and identify amino acids while refining the earlier methods.[67] Rodney Porter and many others gave us much of the structure and function of immunoglobulins.[68] This work demonstrated the wisdom and utility of Paul Ehrlich's earlier lock-and-key theory of antigen–antibody recognition, imperfect as it was.[57] The sum of their work has led to a far better understanding of the immunochemical principles of wound healing.

With all of these tools, it is commonplace to sequence proteins, following identification by immunologic methods, and to synthesize their active peptides or centers. Many growth and other nutritional factors important in wound healing have been so synthesized.

The complement of protein chemistry has been the chemistry of nucleic acid constituents of DNA and RNA. Jesse P. Greenstein, one of the great minds in protein and cancer biochemistry of the World War II era, cautioned me at that time on the enormous difficulties and hence hazards for any young investigator to embark on a career of either protein or nucleic acid chemistry. Kossel,[69] Nobel laureate in 1910, found that nucleic acids consisted of two parts: protein and nucleotide polymers. The latter in turn consisted of hexose, phosphoric acid, and nitrogen-containing compounds. Some readers interpreted his writings as foretelling nucleic acids as repositories and transmitters of genetic information. Concurrently and later, Levene at the Rockefeller Institute persisted in classic studies of nucleotides and nucleosides,[70] with others following doggedly. Watson and Crick,[71] across the street from Sanger's laboratory at the University of Cambridge in the early 1950s, wrote their very accurate and useful double helix theory for the configuration of DNA. Equally remarkable was that later Sanger once again solved the methodologic enigma of sequencing nucleic acids, a solution as difficult and believed to be as nearly impossible as sequencing a protein.[65] Gilbert[72] at Harvard simultaneously devised another method, and others subsequently have greatly improved these techniques. The procedures are so standardized and available as to be widely applied not only to wound healing problems but also to most areas of study currently in biology.

Eriksson, for example, is currently sorting out some of the variables in wound healing with an in vivo "chamber" technique.[73] This methodology and the many new biochemical, histochemical, and immunologic methods are very promising for the future.[73] They will enable us to better understand mechanisms of wound healing, which ultimately and most importantly will lead to better patient care.

References

1. Celsus: De Medicina, vols I and II. Trans WG Spencer. Cambridge, MA, Harvard University Press, 1939.
2. Lecture in Chinese traditional medicine. Gangzhou (Canton), China, Zuong Cho School of Chinese Traditional Medicine, May, 1984.
3. Flemming A: Streptococcal meningitis treated with penicillin. Lancet 2:434–438, 1943.
4. Yihuang K, Jai W: An introduction to the study of moxibustion in China. J Traditional Chin Med 5:67–76, 1985.
5. Mazal DA, King T, Harvey J, et al: Bilateral pneumothorax after acupuncture. N Engl J Med 302:1365–1366, 1980.
6. Shiraishi S, Goto I, Kuroiwa Y, et al: Spinal cord injury as a complication of an acupuncture. Neurology 8:1188–1190, 1979.
7. Majno G: The Healing Hand: Man and Wound in the Ancient World. Cambridge, MA, Harvard University Press, 1975.
8. Steinbock RT: Paleopathological Diagnosis and Interpretation (Bone Diseases in Ancient Human Populations). Springfield, IL, Charles C Thomas, 1976.
9. Breasted JH: The Edwin Smith Surgical Papyrus. Chicago, University of Chicago Press, 1930.
10. Ebbell B: The Papyrus Ebers. The Greatest Egyptian Medical Document. London, Oxford University Press, 1937.
11. Estes JW: The Medical Skills of Ancient Egypt. Canton, Science History Publications USA, 1989, pp 119–121.
12. Sushrata Samhita, vols 1 to 3. Trans KK Bhishagratna. Varanasi, India, Chowkhambra Sanskrit Office, 1963.
13. Garrison FH: An Introduction to the History of Medicine. Philadelphia, WB Saunders, 1929, pp 92–101.
14. Richards DW: Hippocrates of Ostia. JAMA 204:1049–1056, 1968.
15. The Genuine Works of Hippocrates. Trans F Adams. London, 1849.
16. Gordon BL: Medicine Throughout Antiquity. Philadelphia, FA Davis, 1949, pp 548, 594–598.
17. von Soemmering ST: Über das Organ der Seele. Konigsberg, 1776. In Riese W: The Hundred Fiftieth Anniversary of ST von Soemmering's Organ of the Soul. Bull Hist Med 20:310–321, 1946.
18. von Soemmering ST: Dissertatia Inaugeralis Anatomia de Basi Encephali et Originibus Nervorum Cranio

Egredientium. Goettingae, Prostat Apud abr. Vandenhoeck Vidiam, 1778.
19. Meinecke B: Aulus Cornelius Celsus. Plagiarist or artifix medicinae. Bull Hist Med 10:288–298, 1941.
20. Meinecke B: Cicero's principles of hygiene for mental and physical health. The medical connection of a Roman layman. Class J 41:113–118, 1945.
21. Celsus, op cit, vol III, pp 334–335.
22. Siegel RE: Galen's System of Physiology and Medicine. Basil, Karger, 1960.
23. Halsted WS: Ligations of the left subclavian artery in its first portion. Johns Hopkins Rep 21:1–96, 1921.
24. Walsh JL: Medieval Medicine. London, R&C Black, 1920.
25. Campbell D: Arabian Medicine. London, Kegan, Paul, Trench, Trubner and Co, 1926.
26. Abulcasis: Methodus medendi. 1541.
27. Guy de Chauliac: On Wounds and Fractures. Trans WA Brennan, Chicago, 1923.
28. Cumston CG: Henri de Mondeville and his writings. Buffalo Med J 11:1–50, 1903.
29. Garrison, op cit, p 258.
30. Garrison, op cit, p 259.
31. Borelli GA: De Motu Animalium. Leg. Batorum, 1685.
32. Johnson T: The Works of That Famous Chirurgion Ambrose Parey. London, R Cotes and W Du-gaard, 1649.
33. Garrison, op cit, pp 224–26.
34. Vesalius A: De corporis humani structura libri sept. Basileae ex officina Joan. Opporini, 1555.
35. Albinus BS: Historia Musculorum Hominis. Leidal Batavorum, Apud T Hoak and M Mulhovium, 1734.
36. Weitbrecht J: Syndesmologia sive Historia Ligamentum Corporis Humani. Petropoli, 1742.
37. Quain R: Anatomy of the Arteries of the Human Body. London, Taylor and Walton, 1844.
38. Bell C: The Nervous System of the Human Body. London, Longman, 1830.
39. Cajal RY: Degeneration and Regeneration of the Nervous System. Trans and ed RM May. New York, Shafner, 1959.
40. Casserius J: Tabulae Anatomica LXXIIX. Venetiis, Apud Euangelistam Deuchinum, 1627.
41. Hunter J: The Blood, Inflammation and Gunshot Wounds. Philadelphia, James Webster, 1823.
42. Murray JE: Transplantation: Reflections on the past and a view of the future. Lecture, Surgical Grand Rounds, Brigham and Women's Hospital, Boston, June 1, 1991.
43. Virchow RLK: Cellular Pathology as Based upon Physiological and Pathological Histology. Trans F Chance. London, John Churchill, 1860.
44. Orr TG: Operations of General Surgery. Philadelphia, WB Saunders, 1944, p 55.
45. Ibid, p 17.
46. Carrel A: Carrel-Dakin solution. JAMA 67:1777–1778, 1916.
47. Semmelweis IF: The Etiology, the Concept and the Prophylaxis of Childhood Fever. Trans FF Murphy. Medical Classics, vol 5, no 5, Huntington, N.Y., RH Krieger Publishing Co., 1941.
48. Holmes OW: The contagiousness of puerperal fever. N Engl J Med Surg, April, pp 25–60, 1843.
49. Lister J: Illustrations of the antiseptic treatment in surgery. Lancet 2:668–669, 1867.
50. Lister J: On the antiseptic principle of the practice of surgery. Read in the surgical section before the annual meeting of the British Medical Association in Dublin on August 9th, 1867. Classics in Medicine and Surgery. New York, Dover Publications, 1959, pp 9–21.
51. Woodward GS: The Man Who Conquered Pain. A

biography of William Thomas Green Morton. Boston, Beacon Press, 1962.

52. Dolmain CE: Alexander Fleming. In Gillespie CC (ed): Dictionary of Scientific Biography, vol V. New York, Charles Scribner & Sons, 1972, pp 28–31.

53. Garrison, op cit, pp 584–585.

54. Sourkes TL: Nobel Prize Winners in Medicine and Physiology, 1901–1965. New York, Abeland-Shuman, 1966, p 74.

55. Schlessinger BS: The Who's Who of Nobel Prize Winners. Phoenix, Oryx Press, 1986, p 83.

56. Tswett M: Zur Chemie des Chlorphylis, über Phylloxanthin, Phyllocyanin und die Chlorophyllane. Biochem Z 5:6–32, 1907.

57. Himmelweit F: The Collected Papers of Paul Ehrlich, vols 1–4. New York, Pergamon Press, 1956–1958.

58. Martin AJP, Synge RLM: A new form of chromatogram employing two liquid phases. 1. A theory of chromatography. 2. Application of the microdetermination of the higher monoamino acids in proteins. Biochem J 35:1358–1368, 1941.

59. Gordon AH, Martin AJP, Synge RLM: Chromatography in the study of protein constituents. Biochem J 27:79–86, 1944.

60. Dakin HD: XXVI On amino acids. Biochem J 12:290–317, 1918.

61. Schmidt CLA: The Chemistry of the Amino Acids and Proteins, 2nd ed. Springfield, IL, Charles C Thomas, 1944, pp 142–146.

62. Ibid, pp 301–303.

63. Sanger F: The free amino groups of insulin. Biochem J 39:507–515, 1945.

64. Brown H, Sanger F, Kitai R: The structure of pig and sheep insulins. Biochem J 60:556–565, 1955.

65. Sanger F: Sequences, sequences, and sequences. Ann Rev Biochem 57:1–28, 1988.

66. Partridge SM, Brimley RC, Pepper KW: Displacement chromatography on synthetic ion exchange resins. 5. Separation of the basic amino acids. Biochem J 46:334–340, 1950.

67. Moore S, Stein WM: Chromatography of amino acids on sulfonated polystyrene resins. J Biol Chem 192:663–681, 1951.

68. Porter RR: Biochemistry and genetics of complement. A discussion. London, Royal Society, 1984.

69. Sclessinger, op cit, p 82.

70. Sweet JE, Levene FA: Nuclein metabolism in a dog with Eck's fistula. J Exp Med 9:229–239, 1907.

71. Watson JD, Crick FHC: Molecular structure of nucleic acids. A structure for deoxyribose nucleic acid. Nature 171:737–738, 1953.

72. Kolata GB: The Nobel prize in chemistry. Science 210:887–889, 1980.

73. Eriksson E, Lui PY, Zeckel Y, et al: In vivo cell culture accelerates reepithelialization. J Surg Res (In press).

I
BIOLOGICAL PROCESSES INVOLVED IN WOUND HEALING

2

REGENERATION VERSUS REPAIR

Richard J. Goss, Ph.D.

"The organism changes geometrically so as to remain the same physiologically."

BRODY (1945)

Perhaps the most important attribute of living organisms is their capacity for self-repair. This implies the ability to monitor one's normal self in order to recognize any deviations from that norm. In its most ubiquitous form, self-repair is accomplished through the physiological adaptations of the body in an effort to maintain a steady state. These adaptations, which occur at virtually all levels of organization, are achieved by classic negative feedback loops. Imbalance at the molecular level is corrected by appropriate equilibrium shifts in chemical reactions. At the cell and tissue level, proliferation or atrophy serves to maintain the status quo. At higher levels of organization, some creatures are capable of regenerating entire fractions of themselves or appendages thereof.

As they are commonly considered, repair and regeneration are usually thought of in morphological terms, but they are also functional. They must carry on the same physiological activities performed by the original structures. Otherwise, regrowth would be a useless and expensive drain on the system. Clearly, there is an essential functional dimension to repair and regeneration, a dimension inseparable from the morphological one.

It might be asked, which comes first, structure or function? In embryogenesis, structural development precedes physiological competence. In regeneration, which is an example of postembryonic development, the distinction between morphology and physiology is not so well defined. To be sure, nothing can function until its material substrate is in place, yet nature has contrived that no structure shall regenerate unless it will become functional. Not only is regeneration a morphological outgrowth from the adult, it is also a functional restoration. Thus, in the very initiation of regeneration there has evolved a dependence on physiological influences that integrate the activities of the future regenerate with those of the rest of the body. This utilitarian imperative ensures that useless structures shall not grow at the expense of more important processes.

These principles, however, are not perfectly implemented. For example, an organism may be starving to death but will still repair injuries or regenerate lost appendages. There seems never to have evolved a "safety valve" designed to turn off, or at least postpone, regeneration when more essential processes should have priority. Similarly, certain kinds of vertebrate appendages depend on adequate innervation if they are to form a blastema, or bud, from which the missing parts regrow. This would appear to be nature's strategy to avoid regenerating paralyzed appendages. Yet if the motor/sensory nerves remain intact but the spinal cord is severed anteriorly, the appendage will be paralyzed but will grow back anyway. Even if the animal is chronically anesthetized, it will nonetheless replace missing appendages.[2] It would seem that natural selection has avoided the outgrowth of useless structures but has failed to anticipate the schemes of experimental zoologists.

20

SPECTRUM OF GROWTH MECHANISMS

There are many ways by which organisms repair themselves, depending on the level of organization and the nature of the defect (Fig. 2–1), but in every case it is achieved in much the same way in which normal developmental processes take place. Each such mode of repair has evolved so as best to promote physiological recovery.

Turnover

Fundamental to all such mechanisms is turnover, or physiological regeneration. This is a ubiquitous phenomenon at the molecular level whereby virtually all compounds are constantly replaced in accordance with their individual half-lives. At the cellular level, renewing tissues such as epidermis and blood cells maintain homeostasis as their proliferation in the germinative compartments makes up for the equal and opposite loss of cells in the differentiated compartment.[3] Turnover may occur even at the histological level as new ovarian follicles, for example, are produced to replace those lost at ovulation. Expanding organs that do not normally express mitotic activity are nevertheless capable of doing so following reduction in mass or increased functional demand; many of the visceral organs and the various glands of the body fall into this category. There are other tissues (e.g., nerves and muscle) that tend to be mitotically static and must therefore maintain themselves by turnover limited to the subcellular levels of organization.

In all types of turnover, whether occurring at the molecular, cellular, or histological level of organization, it is important for synthesis and degradation to be held in equilibrium. The fundamental problem of growth, then, is to identify such mechanisms as may operate to sustain this balance, for when it is not accurately controlled, pathological conditions supervene. Indeed, it is by no means clear whether rates of destruction are reactions to prevailing synthetic mechanisms or if production is regulated by rates of destruction.

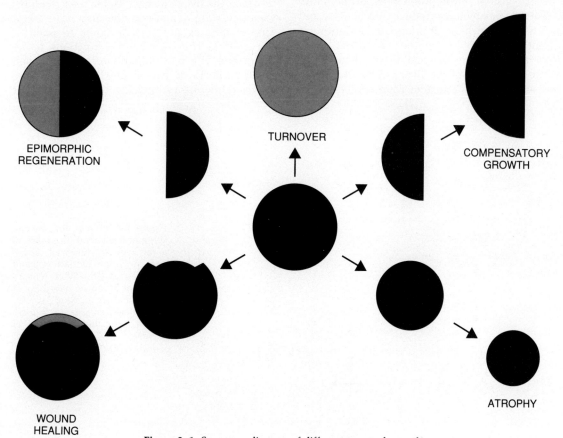

EPIMORPHIC REGENERATION

TURNOVER

COMPENSATORY GROWTH

WOUND HEALING

ATROPHY

Figure 2–1. Summary diagram of different types of growth.

Compensatory Growth

Closely related to physiological turnover is the phenomenon of compensatory growth. Practically every organ and tissue in the body is capable of such compensation, although each may express it differently. Basically, organs and tissues adjust their dimensions to the physiological needs impinging on them: overuse promotes hypertrophy; disuse leads to atrophy.[4]

The question of mass versus function has been a perennial one in studies of compensatory growth. Part of an organ may be removed, as in partial hepatectomy, or one member of a paired organ may be resected, as in unilateral nephrectomy. Is the subsequent enlargement of the remaining parts triggered by the reduction in mass per se or by the concomitant increase in functional demand? In other words, is compensatory growth an attempt to make up for morphological loss or physiological deficiency? As in the riddle of the chicken and the egg, perhaps the correct answer is "both," because there can be no function without structure—and presumably no structure without function. The task, then, is to separate these two dimensions of the problem experimentally.

Partial hepatectomy reduces both mass and function in the liver. It stimulates an outburst of mitotic activity in the otherwise intact lobes, thus restoring the original mass (though not shape) (Fig. 2–2) of the liver.[5] Repeated hepatectomies lead to repeated rounds of liver regeneration by compensatory hyperplasia.[6] Indeed, this remarkable organ appears to be capable of infinite regeneration, given the opportunity. The question is what turns on liver growth after partial resection, and more importantly, what turns it off once the original hepatic mass has been restored? It could very well be the increased demand for hepatic function when the organ's mass has been reduced. The liver is so physiologically versatile that it is almost impossible to eliminate its functions. Therefore, one of the most rewarding approaches to the problem of liver regeneration has been to heighten its functional activity without resorting to surgical deletion experiments. One important function of the liver is that of processing various compounds enzymatically as they enter the liver via the hepatic portal vein; this includes detoxifying poisons. For example, administration of phenobarbital to immature animals induces the liver to produce demethylase and other enzymes designed to break down the drug.[7] Under such conditions, the liver enlarges as its cells increase their synthesis of proteins, replicate their DNA, and undergo mitotic activity. These reactions parallel on a modest scale what happens after partial hepatectomy. The extent to which the liver enlarges under these circumstances is dose dependent and may represent a kind of miniregeneration designed to readjust the mass of the liver to the functions to be performed. It is tempting to interpret the much greater effects of partial hepatectomy as the sum of numerous physiological stimuli, each set

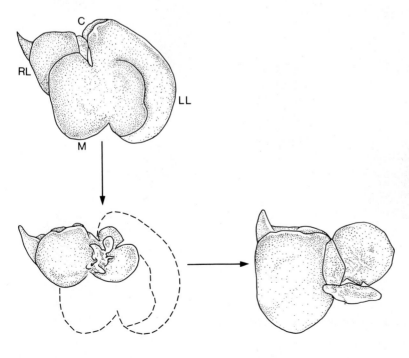

Figure 2–2. When the median (M) and left lateral (LL) lobes of a rat liver are removed *(broken line)*, only the caudate (C) and right lateral (RL) lobes remain, representing about one third of the original organ. After 3 weeks, these lobes enlarge to a mass equivalent to the original size of the liver.

in motion by the functional deficiencies following operation.

Compensatory renal growth following removal of one kidney is achieved by a combination of cellular hyperplasia and hypertrophy, accompanied by the usual increases in RNA, DNA, and protein synthesis.[8] Although the remaining kidney does not completely double its mass, it nevertheless increases its excretory and resorptive activities to meet the normal needs of the body. Is this compensatory growth attributable to the 50 percent reduction in total kidney mass or to the twofold increase in functional demands placed upon the remaining organ? This question can be answered by incapacitating one kidney without removing it, thereby doubling the functional load on the opposite partner without altering the total mass of renal tissue. Ligation of one ureter compromises the physiological activity of the affected kidney, but before it becomes hydronephrotic and in due course degenerates, the contralateral kidney exhibits compensatory growth and function. Thus, it is possible to elicit compensatory growth without reducing the total mass of renal tissue simply by increasing physiological activity.

Even in organs that do not lend themselves to surgical deletion, the phenomenon of compensatory growth can be produced by the appropriate increase in functional overload. The heart is a case in point. The normal asymmetry of this double organ reflects the inequity in the physiological tasks performed by the two ventricles. As pointed out in 1628 by William Harvey,[10] the fetal heart is like "the double kernels of a nut," reflecting the equal work load of the two ventricles before birth. At parturition, when the right ventricle is suddenly relieved of part of its task at the expense of the left, the latter compensates by accelerated growth until it is twice the size of its counterpart.[11] Experimentally it is possible to increase the size of the left ventricle by aortic stenosis, or of the right ventricle by pulmonary arterial constriction or hypoxia, or of both of them by increased exercise (Fig. 2–3). Thus, the "half-hearted hypertrophy" exhibited by the cardiac ventricles closely parallels their respective physiological responses to altered workloads.

Atrophy

Organs capable of hypertrophy are also subject to atrophy. In the case of the exocrine pancreas, for example, the administration of appropriate doses of ethionine, an analogue of

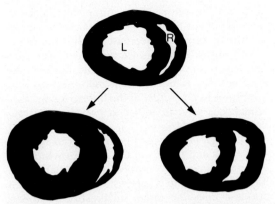

Figure 2–3. Selective hypertrophy of cardiac ventricles as viewed in cross section. In a normal rat heart *(top)* the left ventricle (L) is about twice as large as the right one (R). Hypertension or aortic constriction causes the left ventricle to enlarge *(lower left)*. Hypoxia or pulmonary arterial constriction promotes right ventricular hypertrophy *(lower right)*.

the essential amino acid methionine, results in the wholesale destruction of pancreatic acinar cells[12] and consequent tissue degeneration. Only when treatment is discontinued do cells redifferentiate into secretory units containing zymogen granules. This example illustrates degeneration more clearly than the atrophy that occurs when normal functional activities of a tissue are interfered with. Atrophy is defined more accurately as the absence of tissue growth rather than tissue degeneration.

Erythropoiesis illustrates the relationship between atrophy and functional demand.[13] Red blood cells represent a renewing population dependent upon the proliferation and differentiation of precursor cells in the bone marrow. Normally, the rate of production equals the rate of destruction, resulting in a stable blood count. However, under conditions of low oxygen tension, the rate of erythropoiesis increases until the number of circulating red cells is sufficient to supply the oxygen needs of the body. This reaction is mediated by the production of the hormone erythropoietin, produced in the kidneys. When exposed to high levels of oxygen or increased atmospheric pressure, the body finds itself with a superabundance of red cells and therefore decelerates the rate of erythropoiesis until the natural demise of circulating cells restores the balance. In this sense, anemia represents atrophy of the erythropoietic system, but in reality it is the body's way of maintaining homeostasis between supply and demand.

Atrophy of a different sort may be observed in skeletal muscle, the morphological maintenance of which depends on adequate exercise. If the nerves are cut, the muscle atrophies from disuse.[14] The entire organ diminishes in size as its component fibers become attenuated, which in turn is due to a decrease in the number of myofibrils and filaments in the sarcoplasm. Subsequent reinnervation may restore muscle mass in much the same way that increased exercise promotes hypertrophy of the fibers. Again, morphology is seen to adjust to prevailing physiological demands.

Although atrophy can be induced in virtually all organs and tissues of the body in which one can experimentally reduce or eliminate functional demand, it is interesting to note that in no case does the organ in question disappear altogether. Such organs may waste away to a shadow of their former selves but a remnant remains. It is as if nature, ever optimistic, always allows for the possibility of renewed growth should physiological competence return.

The failure of total atrophy to occur under conditions of complete disuse (provided this extreme condition can in fact actually be achieved) argues against the theory of growth regulation by functional demand. Similarly, it is difficult to explain how organs can develop in the embryo before there is any need for them. Presumably the anlagen of organs are programmed to differentiate on their own, beyond which their subsequent hypertrophy cannot occur except under the influence of physiological demands. In the case of adult animals, there is a severalfold redundancy in most organs that is not consistent with the functional demand theory. It is convenient that we have more of each tissue in the body than may be needed for bare survival, but how can this be reconciled with the notion that organs grow to sizes needed to fulfill their function when only a fraction of each organ is working at any one time? One can only surmise that this represents an adaptation to the need for a margin of safety such that physiology can adapt readily to the vicissitudes of environmental demands. In this sense, there are some adaptations that are of a genetic nature and are the results of natural selection. Others are physiological adaptations whereby the organism can adjust its function (and its organ sizes) to changing conditions. Thus, the red cell count in the blood may be no more absolute than the boiling point of water, because it is not the number of cells that is inherited but the capacity of the marrow to adjust its output according to environmental needs.

WOUND HEALING

All tissues and organs of the body, with the possible exception of teeth, are capable of re-

pairing injuries.[15, 16] An injury may be defined as an interruption in the continuity of tissues, and it is repaired by reestablishing that continuity. This is achieved primarily by proliferation, migration, and differentiation of involved cells. Each cell type is believed to give rise to its own kind in the process of repair. Such dedifferentiation as may occur is limited to the modulation of cells to less specialized conditions; these cells cannot redifferentiate into other histological types.

Epithelial tissue heals primarily by cellular migration, presumably because its structure is basically two-dimensional. In the case of many mesodermal tissues, however, the three-dimensional configuration is correlated with a somewhat different mode of repair that takes the form of an aggregate of cells that migrate into the lesion where they eventually redifferentiate into the tissue in question. These repair aggregates may take the form of granulation tissue in the case of dermis, fracture callus in the case of broken bones, or comparable accumulations of cells between the cut ends of a severed tendon. They are derived from local sources adjacent to the lesion and are programmed to redifferentiate into the same tissues from which they originated. As differentiation proceeds, the morphogenesis of the tissue mass conforms to that of the components being reunited. Tendons and bones, for example, are reconstituted along their longitudinal axes. Dermis, on the other hand, is repaired as a sheet of scar tissue without significant polarity. Tissue repair, therefore, is a stopgap reaction designed to reestablish continuity of interrupted tissues. The gap traversed by this mechanism is very limited. Tissue forms only between the severed parts, without differentiating totally new elements. This, basically, is what distinguishes tissue repair from epimorphic regeneration.

EPIMORPHIC REGENERATION

Epimorphic regeneration is the replacement of an amputated appendage by a direct outgrowth from the severed cross section.[16–23] In a newt limb, regeneration may give rise to a functional replacement within a few months (Fig. 2–4). However, regeneration can take place only when a remnant of the amputated appendage is left behind from which regrowth can occur. If the entire territory of the appendage is extirpated, regeneration fails to take place because no cells remain that are endowed with

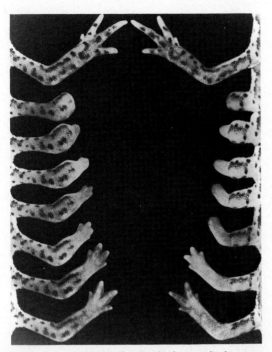

Figure 2–4. Montage of individual newt limbs amputated across lower or upper arms, as photographed after 7, 21, 25, 28, 32, 42, and 70 days of regeneration (From Goss RJ: Principles of Regeneration. New York, Academic Press, 1969.)

the capacity to produce that particular appendage. Such regeneration territories are therefore defined by the distribution of cells capable of participating in their regeneration. The territories of different types of appendages do not overlap, a condition that presumably evolved to obviate the regeneration of chimeric appendages.

Another prerequisite for epimorphic regeneration is the infliction of a wound. An appendage may be defined as a mesodermal structure enveloped in skin. This is important, because

without epidermis and the healing thereof, epimorphic regeneration cannot take place. The wound must include a sufficient cross section of the appendage itself and, of course, must interrupt the continuity of the epidermis. These conditions are essential for regeneration because they lead to epidermal wound healing across the severed ends of the injured internal tissues, and unless this occurs, no blastema can be formed. It is believed that the overlying wound epidermis interacts in an inductive way with the subjacent mesodermal tissues.[24] The cells of the latter lose their specialized characteristics and migrate distally to contribute to the formation of the blastema. This develops between the wound epidermis and the amputated mesodermal tissue—the same location where a scar forms in a nonregenerating appendage (Fig. 2–5).

These events at the cell and tissue levels are accompanied by metabolic changes at the molecular level.[20] Not only does the rate of DNA synthesis increase as a prelude to the proliferative activity of blastema cells, but protein synthesis also accelerates. The latter occurs even during dedifferentiation, presumably as proteolytic enzymes, including cathepsins, peptidases, collagenase, and acid phosphatase, are produced to mediate the process of histolysis. In the postamputation stump, vascular interruption and the attendant depletion of oxygen are correlated with prevailing anaerobic metabolism. The pH declines with increased autolytic activity. Skeletal muscle fibers become depleted of their glycogen as its anaerobic catabolism gives rise to lactic acid.

Once the blastema forms, metabolic pathways become aerobic again. Lactate dehydrogenase declines and the Krebs cycle is restored. Many structural proteins are synthesized as blastema cells differentiate and morphogenesis proceeds,

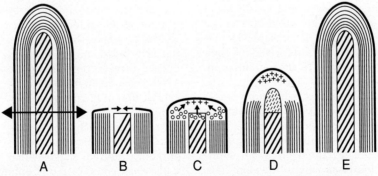

Figure 2–5. Schematic representation of how a vertebrate appendage regenerates. Following amputation (A), the epidermis migrates across the severed mesodermal tissues (B). The cells of the latter dedifferentiate distally (circles), and migrate into the blastema where they proliferate (+) (C). As the blastema elongates, its more proximal cells redifferentiate while a zone of proliferation persists distally (D). Regeneration ceases when all of the blastema cells have differentiated (E).

including actin and myosin in muscles and collagen in connective tissue. Morphological recovery is accompanied by comparable molecular and metabolic changes in each component tissue.

The blastema is made up of many nondescript cells of diverse origins representing practically all anatomical structures in the stump. When their population reaches a certain size, differentiation commences proximally in continuity with the histological counterparts in the stump. Cartilage forms off the ends of the bones, and myogenesis takes place adjacent to the severed muscles. Meanwhile, proliferation continues in the apical growth zone to provide the cells destined to become progressively more distal structures in the regenerate. Morphogenesis thus occurs in a proximodistal direction and comes to a halt when the tip of the missing appendage has differentiated.

Regeneration is a complicated developmental process, the details of which cannot be left to chance. The regenerate corresponds in number, size, and orientation to the parts that are replaced. It forms only those structures lying distal to the level of amputation (except under experimental conditions, when retinoic acid may promote the formation of reduplications).[25] It is usually a flawless replica of the original, but heteromorphic and hypomorphic regeneration are not uncommon. Sometimes that which is replaced is structurally different from the original, as in the case of lizard tails that regenerate an unsegmented cartilaginous tube in place of the original segmented bony vertebrae. Above all, the resulting regenerate must be functional.

The Utilitarian Imperative

In the case of many regenerating appendages, such as the limbs, tails, fins, and taste barbles of lower vertebrates, no regrowth occurs unless an adequate nerve supply is present. Denervated limbs as well as tails deprived of their spinal cords fail to regenerate after amputation. This neurotrophic influence depends upon the presence of intact neurons whose processes innervate the appendage. Even when surgically isolated from the central nervous system, they can still promote regeneration. It is only when the axons or dendrites themselves are interrupted that the blastema fails to develop. This phenomenon is nonspecific, being promoted by either motor or sensory nerves or even by nerves experimentally deviated from other parts of the body. It is not abolished by pharmacologically interfering with the conduction of nerve impulses, nor is it attributable to such common neurotransmitters as epinephrine and acetylcholine. Nerves may be the key in understanding how the regenerative process is turned on, at least in amphibian limbs.[26] Experiments have shown that nerves are necessary for DNA synthesis to occur in amputated limbs. Nerves act primarily at the G_1 phase of the cell cycle, and thereby promote the formation of the blastema. Evidence suggests that the neurotrophic factors responsible for these effects may belong to the family of mitogenic peptides isolated from the nervous systems of higher vertebrates.

The role of nerves in regeneration is an example of the utilitarian imperative. In addition to the aforementioned prerequisites, such as wound epidermis and a source of regenerative mesodermal cells, most appendages also depend upon physiological influences often emanating from elsewhere in the body, influences correlated with the specific function of the appendage to be regenerated. In limbs, fins, and taste barbles, it is the presence of adequate innervation, while in the case of tails, it is the spinal cord that is necessary. Crustacean claws do not regenerate in the absence of molting hormone.[27] Presumably this is because without this a new hardened shell cannot be produced on the flaccid regenerate. Deer antlers do not develop in fawns that have been castrated because secondary sex characteristics are useless in infertile animals.[28] Thus, in most, if not all, regenerating structures there has evolved a means to ensure that the new outgrowths will be useful, a provision that clearly illustrates the economy of nature.

Blastema Formation

It is interesting that very much the same mechanism is utilized in the epimorphic regeneration of all appendages. In each case, be it the fin of a fish, the limb of an amphibian, the tail of a lizard, or the antler of a deer, regeneration is made possible by the development of a blastema. Even in nonhomologous organs, the establishment of regenerative abilities has been achieved by the same developmental mechanism, which must have evolved independently in each case. This remarkable example of convergent evolution suggests that the existence of a blastema is indicative of epimorphic regeneration.

In this regard, it is interesting that epimorphic regeneration is not achieved by the coordinated repair of individual tissues in the stump. This hypothetically alternate mode of regeneration seems never to have evolved. Instead, all mesodermal tissues in the stump pool their cells in a blastema, the developmental potential of which far exceeds the cellular aggregates seen in the repair mechanisms of individual mesodermal tissues.

Epimorphic Regeneration Versus Tissue Repair

These considerations raise the question of whether epimorphic regeneration is simply an exaggerated version of tissue repair or is a qualitatively distinct developmental process.[29] The best way to answer this question is to compare epimorphic regeneration with tissue repair to determine if the differences outweigh the similarities.

Similarities abound. Both processes are initiated by trauma. Whether due to amputation or an internal lesion, anatomical continuity is interrupted in both cases, and as a result, restorative reactions are directed toward the reestablishment of normal structure and function. Epimorphic regeneration and tissue repair are also alike in that they cannot take place unless appropriate tissues remain from which renewal can proceed. Both processes are achieved by a combination of cell migration, proliferation, and redifferentiation. They both produce aggregates of developmentally potent cells from which the new parts will differentiate. Thus, these two kinds of growth have both put to good use certain basic cellular processes upon which all development depends.

Nevertheless, these similarities are outnumbered by the differences that distinguish epimorphic regeneration from tissue repair. Not the least of these is the involvement of the epidermis. Internal tissues of the body repair injuries in the absence of epidermal participation, but amputated appendages cannot undergo epimorphic regeneration unless epidermal wound healing occurs.

The loss of cellular specialization in tissue repair is not so great as to enable the cells to redifferentiate into something entirely different. In regenerating appendages, however, the degree of dedifferentiation is remarkable. Although cells may usually redifferentiate in the blastema into more or less the same type of tissues from which they came, there is always the possibility of metaplasia, the phenomenon by which a cell may under unusual circumstances change into another histological type.

The regeneration blastema superficially resembles the "repair aggregate" characteristic of healing wounds in mesodermal tissues. The blastema, however, must be enveloped in epidermis if it is to fulfill its developmental potential. The repair aggregate is neither associated with nor dependent upon epidermis.

Epimorphic regeneration always occurs in a proximodistal direction. Even if a stump's polarity is reversed such that it is induced to regenerate from a proximally facing cross section, it will give rise only to structures lying distal to that level of amputation. In tissue repair, differentiation in such morphogenesis as may occur reflects no such proximodistal polarity: it proceeds as well distally as it does proximally, and more commonly differentiates simultaneously in all locations.

In epimorphic regeneration the development of new parts is not limited to the extensions of those existing in the stump. Entirely new structures are formed, each in its own appropriate location, as regeneration proceeds. New bones and muscles, for example, develop as the limb itself is replaced. This is not the case in tissue repair, which completes the continuity of interrupted parts and nothing more. The extent to which it can do even this is not unlimited. Gaps that are too wide may be imperfectly repaired, as in the nonunion of fractured bones.

Nerves (or other physiologically significant influences) are required for epimorphic regeneration as a means to ensure the functional competence of the new structures. In tissue repair, on the other hand, no such utilitarian imperative prevails. Denervated limbs can still heal their fractures, reunite their severed tendons, and heal integumental lesions. Even skeletal muscles can repair themselves while undergoing denervation atrophy. Tissue repair is designed to reconstruct morphological integrity; epimorphic regeneration is designed to restore function.

Finally, these two processes can be distinguished on the basis of their distribution. Tissue repair is universal. There is hardly an organ or tissue in the human body, or in any other organism, that lacks this very basic biological process. Its ubiquity reflects the essential nature of wound healing in virtually all organs and organisms. Epimorphic regeneration, in contrast, is a luxury. Its spotty distribution in the animal kingdom reflects the adaptive nature of this phenomenon, which has been selected for or against during the course of evolution. Animals can live without epimorphic regeneration but not without tissue repair.

Judging from the foregoing enumeration of

similarities and differences, the conclusion is inescapable that these two kinds of regeneration differ in kind, not just degree. While they share much in common, epimorphic regeneration cannot properly be regarded as an exaggerated example of tissue repair. Although it is capable of achieving far more spectacular feats of development than tissue repair, it is the latter that is the more essential of the two.

MAMMALIAN REGENERATION

It has been said that even if we were to discover how to promote limb regeneration in human beings, we would still not have solved the basic problem of regeneration, which is to understand the morphogenetic mechanisms responsible for the development of the blastema into a flawless replica of the limb that has been replaced. Nevertheless, there is little doubt that discovering the secret of mammalian regeneration would be a tour de force worthy of a Nobel prize. Indeed, one regenerationist claimed that he would give his right arm to solve the problem!

The lack of regenerative ability in mammals is not unique. Many other vertebrates have appendages that do not regenerate, and among the invertebrates hardly a phylum exists without its nonregenerative members. This nonuniform distribution of regenerative abilities has prompted many phylogenetic explanations. For example, the presence or absence of regenerative ability has been variously attributed to phylogenetic position, complexity of the organism, liability to injury, and adaptation. All of these notions may contain some truth but the trouble is that they rely on subjective factors. "At the present time," wrote Vorontsova and Liosner, "not a single investigator would be willing to predict the nature of regeneration in a species of unknown regenerative powers from its known position in the taxonomic scale."[18]

Seeking animal models in which to investigate the absence of regeneration in mammals, investigators have sought out organisms that exhibit both the presence and the absence of regeneration. Only in such situations would it be possible to compare regenerating and nonregenerating appendages with a view to discovering how they differ. One such model is the metamorphosing frog: the tadpole replaces amputated limbs but the postmetamorphic froglet does not. In this model, the tacit assumption is that the ontogenetic decline in regeneration

recapitulates its phylogenetic loss in higher vertebrates, an assumption that may or may not be true. Still another model depends upon the inhibition of regeneration by experimental means. For example, denervation of a salamander's leg prevents it from regenerating after amputation, the implication being that the evolutionary extinction of regenerative ability might be due to insufficient innervation. Such models as these depend upon extrapolation from amphibian to mammal, which may not necessarily lead to valid conclusions.

The ideal would be to discover a species of mammal (or bird) capable of regenerating its limbs. Such a creature could then be compared in detail with the most closely related available species that is not capable of regeneration to pinpoint the differences between regenerative and nonregenerative appendages, in the hope that one or more of them might be causally related.

It is necessary to assume that the inability of mammals to regenerate appendages is not inherent in "mammal-ness." The existence of certain exceptions to the rule that mammals cannot regenerate (to be described later) testifies to the fact that the cells and tissues of mammals cannot be categorically ruled out of the game of regeneration. It follows, therefore, that mammals apparently possess a latent potential for regeneration that has been secondarily inhibited in some way. This encouraging conclusion suggests that if we can identify the inhibitor we might then be able to interfere with it in such a way as to allow regeneration to proceed unchecked.

Why Mammals Do Not Regenerate

In the course of vertebrate evolution there have been two great advances. The first was the successful transition from aquatic to terrestrial habitats, and the second was the elevation of metabolic rates to establish the homeothermic condition. These two advances could only have arisen in sequence.

It sometimes seems that adaptation to the land environment has been correlated with a decline in regenerative abilities. Fishes and aquatic amphibians regenerate rather nicely, but terrestrial forms do not. Indeed, anurans lose their regenerative prowess when they metamorphose from aquatic tadpole to terrestrial frog—just when one might think they would need it most! Yet lizards, which are terrestrial, are adept at replacing lost tails (but not lost legs). And mammals do not regenerate limbs at all.

Despite the superficial impression that aquatic life is more conducive to regeneration than is terrestrial existence, there is no direct evidence that water per se promotes regeneration nor that desiccation prevents it. It could be related to the fact that regeneration is more prevalent among cold-blooded vertebrates, which tend to be aquatic, or it might be correlated with the derivative condition that terrestrial vertebrates must walk on land where their limbs are vulnerable to more mechanical abuse than were those of their aquatic ancestors. A regenerating leg subject to repeated trauma would not grow back normally, if at all. Perhaps this is why tadpoles can replace lost legs while frogs cannot (except for *Xenopus*, in which the adults remain aquatic), or why lizards cannot grow back legs but can regenerate their tails, which are not used in ambulation. Indeed, the only mammalian appendages capable of regeneration, as will be reviewed below, are ones that are not weight bearing. It would seem that regenerative appendages can be replaced only when they are protected from injuries during the delicate stages of regrowth. Thus, there would has been little selective pressure to regenerate legs that must be walked on.

Regenerative ability may also have evolved, or disappeared, for deeper, more metabolic reasons. When vertebrates invented the warm-blooded condition, they could have done so only after leaving the aquatic environment where the unfavorably high specific heat of water would have militated against it. In no other phylum, including terrestrial arthropods, has this ability to maintain an independent body temperature evolved; yet it did so at least twice in the vertebrates. Is this sufficient reason to explain the extinction of regeneration in birds and mammals?

There are two important consequences of being a warm-blooded animal. One is that body fluids make optimal culture media for bacteria, particularly in open lesions. It is to the animal's advantage, therefore, to heal wounds with alacrity in order to reduce the chances of infection. Integumental lesions are sealed not only by epidermal migrations, but also by wound contraction. The prompt development of granulation tissue forecasts the repair of the interrupted dermal tissues to produce a scar. In addition to providing tensile strength, scars are believed to be a barrier to regeneration, probably by interfering with inductive interactions between the wound epidermis and the underlying mesoder-

mal tissue. However advantageous it may have been to evolve the capacity to heal wounds with such efficiency, our ancestors may have had to sacrifice their regenerative abilities in order to do so.

The other disadvantage of being warm-blooded is that the elevated metabolic rate requires frequent feeding. Depending upon their sizes, mammals are in jeopardy of starving to death within days or weeks, particularly if water is not available. A mammal that has lost a leg is at high risk. If it is a herbivore, it becomes easy game for the predators it cannot outrun; if it is a carnivore, it cannot catch its prey. Either way, crippled mammals live on borrowed time, victims of their own metabolic clock.

If warm-blooded animals had inherited the capacity to regenerate their limbs, what good would it do? It would probably take months for them to replace a lost leg, and they would starve or be killed long before the missing leg would have been restored (Fig. 2–6). From this perspective, it is difficult to see how there could have been much selective advantage to perpetuating the regeneration of legs in warm-blooded vertebrates: there is no sense trying to grow back a structure if one cannot survive long enough to use it.[31]

The Hypothetical Regenerative Mammal

If the capacity to regenerate legs were to have evolved in a mammal, under what ecological conditions would it be expected to have occurred? First of all, it would have to be a mammal whose legs were not vitally essential. This would rule out practically all terrestrial forms whose legs are important for locomotion

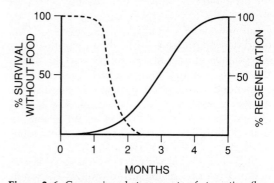

Figure 2–6. Comparison between rate of starvation (*broken line*) in a mammal and degree of regeneration (*solid line*). In approximate units, demise as a result of starvation would occur well before a limb might be expected to regrow.

either for capture or escape. Of course, if there were no predators, as might be the case in certain island fauna, it is not inconceivable that a herbivorous terrestrial mammal might have benefited from a mutation enabling it to replace lost or injured limbs.

Legs are less important to aquatic mammals than to terrestrial ones. Animals that swim do so in large measure by bodily undulations. Such a creature would still be able to escape predators and to find its own food even after it had lost one of its legs. In special circumstances, one can imagine this hypothetical mammal surviving long enough to grow back its missing limb. Such a limb, however, could not be entirely useless or there would be no selective advantage for retaining the ability to replace it. Let us assume, therefore, that such a limb might be important for courtship rituals or for some other functional role that is convenient, but not essential.

There is yet another way a mammal might have escaped the metabolic imperative. If it could reduce its metabolic requirements for a prolonged period of time, might it not buy the time needed to replace a lost limb? Hibernation comes to mind, but when the body temperature is drastically lowered all physiological functions slow down, including growth. On the other hand, what if our hypothetical mammal were to sustain itself on body fat, in a sequestered environment, without substantially lowering its body temperature. This is what bears do in temperate latitudes when they den up. Such creatures survive the winter without eating, defecating, or urinating for a number of months. Bears are not known to regenerate their limbs, but if they could, winter would be the time to do it.

Alternatively, it would be convenient if an injured mammal were able to become lethargic for prolonged periods of time in any season of the year. A torpid state akin to estivation, or "summer sleep," could be the answer. This condition might have evolved in a mammal that was highly vulnerable to injury and in which the stress of amputation might trigger a sort of suspended animation, perhaps by neural or hormonal mechanisms. Such a physiologically altered state of consciousness might resemble that exhibited by opossums when they feign death in response to sudden fright.

This adaptation would be enhanced if the mammal were capable of autotomy. Common among crustaceans and lizards, autotomy is the mechanism by which a limb or tail is spontaneously amputated in response to being grasped by a predator. It is a marvelous mechanism for self-preservation because the wiggling of the discarded segments distracts the predator just long enough for its prey to escape. Wherever autotomy has evolved, it is almost always accompanied by the ability to regenerate. It is not known to occur in mammals, at least when triggered by a nervous reflex. But there are two mammalian phenomena that resemble autotomy. One is the spontaneous shedding of deer antlers each year before the new ones begin to regenerate. This occurs by the action of osteoclasts at the interface between the living bone of the skull and the dead bone of the antler. The other case is in the rat. When held firmly by the end of its tail, a rat will tend to twist violently in circles. As a result, a sleeve of skin sometimes slips off the tail enabling the rat to get away. Of course, the denuded part of the tail dries up and is eventually lost, but it is not replaced. Nevertheless, if a mammal possessed preformed breakage planes in its legs designed to separate only upon violent exertion when the distal part had been caught, one can imagine a heightened ability to regenerate from the proximal stump at the level of autotomy just as occurs in lobster claws and lizard tails. This adaptation would not only allow the animal to escape by means of its partial self-immolation, but could be accompanied by other adaptations enabling it to regenerate the missing part and to survive long enough to do so.

It might make sense for a regenerative mammal to be small rather than large. On an absolute scale, small appendages would be expected to grow back faster than those of a large mammal. Further, a large animal would be in greater danger of bleeding to death following amputation. Blood clotting cannot be relied upon to stem the flow from a large artery, but it could suffice in the homologous artery of a small animal. Yet another adaptation that might evolve would be the reflex contraction of smooth muscles in the tunica media of arteries. This mechanism, known to occur in the blood vessels of umbilical cords and deer antlers (both of which are deciduous), is used to good advantage when excessive blood loss is to be avoided.

One might further expect a regenerative mammal to inhabit tropical latitudes, preferably without wide climatalogical variations. This would liberate it from the need to survive winters, droughts, and rainy seasons. Such an optimal habitat would be important to an animal required, on occasion, to regenerate.

The existence of this mammal would seem improbable but not impossible. One would look for a small, tropical, aquatic herbivore capable of storing fat in its body or food in its nest and endowed with the capacity to survive torpor for a number of months. Such a mammal might be expected to be unusually vulnerable to loss of limb, yet to have evolved behavioral and physiological adaptations enabling it to escape its predators (if any), to avoid exsanguination (possibly coupled with an autotomy reflex), and to possess the instinct to sequester itself during the period of recovery. It is unfortunate that no such mammal exists, because if it did we might be able to find out how its amputated appendages differ from those of its nonregenerative cousins. Whatever this might be, it would probably be something that happens (or doesn't happen) in the early stages of regeneration when the tendency toward scar formation must be diverted to the pathway of blastema production.

The Case of the Rabbit Ear

In inquiring why mammals do or do not regenerate, an ideal model system is the external ear of the rabbit. These appendages fill in full thickness holes that have been punched through them. They do so by producing a circular blastema around the margins that grows centripetally to obliterate the aperture (Fig. 2–7). In doing so, it usually regenerates the sheet of cartilage that is sandwiched between the inner and outer integuments.

This remarkable process was first discovered in the rabbit ear by Markelova in 1953, and was subsequently described by Vorontsova and Liosner in 1960.[18] It was rediscovered in the mid-1960s by Joseph and Dyson, at Guy's Hospital in London.[32] They were studying wound healing by epidermal migration, and in order to exclude the possibility of wound contraction they sought a system in which the skin was firmly adherent to an underlying skeletal substrate. The rabbit ear fulfilled these prerequisites because its skin is difficult to detach from the sheet of auricular cartilage. To obtain biopsies of healing wounds it was convenient simply to cut out full-thickness pieces of the ear for histological preparation. It was later noted that the perforated ears of "used rabbits" had filled in the holes with new ear tissue.

The discovery of rabbit ear regeneration stimulated further research into this remarkable phenomenon.[33, 34] Its mechanism resembles that in the appendages of lower vertebrates. Epidermal wound healing proceeds from both inner and outer integuments to seal the lesion. Then a blastema forms, albeit a circular one rather than a conical bud as is produced on the end of an amphibian limb stump. Proliferation of cells on the leading edge of this blastema is responsible for its elongation in a radial direction. Concomitantly, the cells left behind at the margins undergo chondrogenesis in continuity with the cartilaginous sheet in the surrounding ear tissue. As regeneration nears completion, the new cartilage formed just inside the original margins of the hole may sometimes undergo endochondral ossification. Although the regenerated tissues may be a replica of the original,

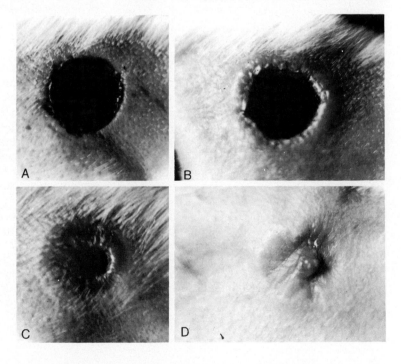

Figure 2–7. Regeneration of ear tissue in a rabbit as viewed 1 day (A), 1 week (B), 4 weeks (C), and 16 weeks (D) after cutting a full-thickness hole 1 cm in diameter. A circular blastema converges from the margins, obliterating the opening in about 8 weeks. (From Goss RJ, Grimes LN: Tissue interactions in the regeneration of rabbit ear holes. Am Zool 12:151, 1972.)

they are not an exact copy. Hair follicles are not usually replaced, despite the fact that those in healing skin wounds elsewhere on the body may be differentiated de novo when wound contraction is prevented.[35]

How is it that the rabbit ear can regenerate tissue in this way while the ears of most other mammals cannot? To seek an explanation one would do well to compare, stage by stage, the sequence of events that occur following injury. Only in this way is it possible to identify in time and space such differences as may occur. Logically, one might suspect any dissimilarities as may be identified to be responsible for the promotion or inhibition of regeneration.

To carry out this comparison, the ears of sheep and dogs, which do not regenerate, have been selected because they are approximately the same thickness as those of rabbits.[34] Histological preparations were made of ear tissue at successive intervals after punching full-thickness holes through the ears. These sections, made at right angles to both the surface of the ears and the margins of the holes cut through them, show in detail how the various components of the ear respond to wounding and how they interact in the process of regeneration. Immediately after a hole is cut through the ear, bleeding results in the formation of a scab. Some of the tissues subjacent to the scab die as a result of desiccation, forming a further protective layer over the underlying viable tissues. Next, epidermal wound healing commences. Cells from both the inner and the outer epidermis begin to migrate toward each other, always creeping along the interface between the living and the dead cells at the margins of the wound. It may take more than a week for these migrating sheets of epidermis to meet in the middle. During this time they must make their way through the intervening barriers, not the least of which is the sheet of cartilage sandwiched between the inner and outer ear skins (Fig. 2–8). Here the cells insinuate themselves through the tissue in close association with the surviving chondrocytes, thus separating the distal segment of dead cartilage from the surviving proximal tissues. These events take place in both regenerative and nonregenerative ears. Subsequently, in the ears of sheep and dogs scar tissue develops beneath the wound epidermis. This scar is established in continuity with the cut edges of the dermis and in fact represents regenerated dermal tissue. Once scar formation occurs, no further developmental events take place.

By contrast, scar formation is omitted in the rabbit ear. Instead, cells of unknown origin

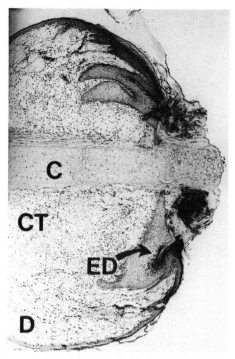

Figure 2–8. Radial section through the edge of a rabbit ear hole 8 days after injury. Epidermis is migrating from both sides, separating the dried out tissue *(right)* from the surviving cartilage (C) and connective tissue (CT). Conspicuous epidermal downgrowths (ED) have formed adjacent to the interrupted dermis (D). (From Goss RJ, Grimes LN: Epidermal downgrowths in regenerating rabbit ear holes. J Morphol 146: 533, 1975.)

migrate to positions between the wound epidermis and the severed edge of the cartilaginous sheet. Here they multiply until a rounded blastema is produced. This pushes out the overlying wound epidermis, maintaining intimate contact between the proliferating blastema cells and their epidermal envelope. Sometime prior to the completion of epidermal wound healing something presumably occurs that deflects the natural tendency to scar formation into the direction of blastema production.

In searching for the earliest visible difference between regenerating and nonregenerating ear wounds, it became clear that epidermal wound healing was not the same in both cases. In the ears of sheep and dogs, epidermis migrated straight in from both sides to complete its continuity, after which scar formation took place. In rabbit ears, the sheets of epidermis, while migrating toward each other, also grew downward into the underlying tissues more or less at right angles to the surface.[34] These tongues of epidermis, visible in histological sections made about 5 to 12 days after injury, are at first solid downgrowths of epidermal cells. Later on, after the wound is sealed and a

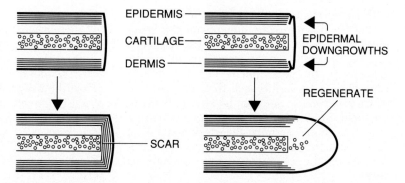

Figure 2–9. Diagrams showing how regenerative ear *(right)* differs from nonregenerative one *(left)*. In the latter, the dermis regenerates a scar that effectively precludes blastema formation. In the former, epidermal downgrowths block scar formation and allow a blastema to develop. (Modified from Goss RJ: Why mammals don't regenerate—or do they? News Physiol Sci 2:112, 1987.)

blastema begins to form, the innermost cells of these downgrowths become keratinized (Fig. 2–8), leading to the formation of clefts lined with fully differentiated epidermal cells. Shortly afterward, the expanding blastema, presumably exerting pressure on its overlying epidermis, stretches the downgrowth into flattened configurations in much the same way that pleats in a fabric will disappear when pulled on both sides.

There is no conclusive evidence that these epidermal downgrowths have anything to do with the regeneration of rabbit ear tissue. We have only a correlation between the existence of these curious structures and the presence of subsequent regeneration (Fig. 2–9). Nevertheless, the circumstantial evidence is compelling.

Their location puts them in a position to interfere with the regeneration of the dermis itself. The time of their appearance corresponds to when the "decision" is being made whether to form a scar or a blastema. They are conspicuous by their absence in the ears of dogs and sheep, neither of which is capable of regenerating missing tissue. This does not necessarily mean that such downgrowths are specifically responsible for promoting regeneration, but the possibility is worth further exploration. They are in the right place at the right time in the right species to be a factor in promoting regeneration. Nevertheless, it is important to determine whether or not they develop in rabbit ears themselves under experimental conditions designed to inhibit regrowth.

One way to inhibit ear regeneration is to remove the sheet of cartilage from the area of the ear through which a hole is to be cut.[33] A three-sided flap of skin is resected, the exposed cartilage is excised, and the skin flap is replaced. This results in an area of the ear with inner and outer layers of skin back to back with no cartilage in between. After allowing the operated area to heal, one can then cut a hole through the operated part of the ear such that there is no cartilage in the vicinity of the margins of the hole. When cartilage has been previously re-

moved from an otherwise intact area of the ear it is not regenerated. Consequently, the hole punched through the double layers of skin remains permanently without adjacent cartilage, and under these circumstances, no regeneration occurs (Fig. 2–10). The layers of skin heal to each other by epidermal migration, but blastema formation fails to occur in the absence of cartilage. Histological examination of the edges of such holes reveals that no epidermal downgrowths develop. Thus, it is possible that regeneration from the margins of such holes depends upon the formation of epidermal downgrowths, which in turn depends upon the proximity of the severed cartilaginous sheet.

It is instructive that when part of the cartilaginous sheet in the ear is removed internally, it does not reconstitute itself, yet when part of the cartilage is removed along with the overlying integument, it is capable of regeneration. Clearly, the reaction of the cartilaginous sheet to injury depends upon its close association

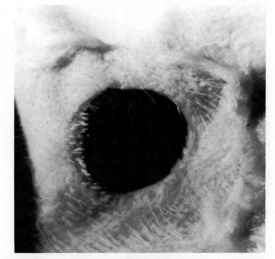

Figure 2–10. Nonregenerating rabbit ear. Following prior resection of the cartilaginous sheet, a 1 cm hole cut through the remaining layers of skin fails to fill in after injury, by which time an ear retaining its cartilage would have completed its regeneration.

with an overlying epidermal wound. Whether epidermal downgrowths depend on the presence of cartilage or chondrogenesis depends on the proximity of epidermal downgrowths remains to be determined. Perhaps it is a synergistic relationship such that the presence of cartilage might induce the downgrowth of the epidermis, which in turn, by preventing scar formation, permits the development of blastema cells capable of undergoing chondrogenesis off the cut edge of the cartilaginous sheet.

Deer Antlers

The only mammalian appendage capable of being completely replaced is the deer antler.[36, 37] These remarkable appendages that adorn the heads of male deer (and both male and female reindeer and caribou) are replaced spontaneously each year. In most species they grow during the spring and summer months after the previous year's antlers have been cast

off (Fig. 2–11). Once they have attained their full dimensions, internal ossification eventually curtails venous return, bringing about ischemic necrosis. As a result, the outer skin, or velvet, becomes desiccated and is actively shed to reveal the mature dead bony antlers at the end of the summer. This process anticipates the autumn mating season when the fully developed antlers are used to good advantage by competing males. They are destined to drop off the following year to be replaced by another set.[39]

As secondary sex characteristics, deer antlers are profoundly affected by levels of testosterone. If a fawn is castrated early in life, he will not grow antlers as an adult.[28] It is the rising levels of testosterone in juvenile males that cause the frontal bones on the skull to develop pedicles, the stumps from which the antlers themselves regenerate. The yearling's first antlers are not, strictly speaking, a case of regeneration because there is nothing to be replaced. Nevertheless, they represent a remarkable example of generation in that they sprout from

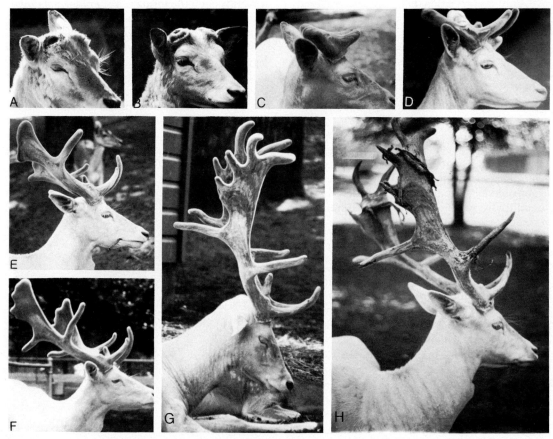

Figure 2–11. Successive stages in the regeneration of fallow deer antlers as photographed on April 23 *(A)*, May 5 *(B)*, May 23 *(C)*, June 5 *(D)*, July 2 *(E)*, July 19 *(F)*, Aug. 7 *(G)*, and Aug. 26 *(H)*. The rate of elongation at the steepest inflection of the growth curve exceeds 0.6 cm per day. (From Goss RJ: Chondrogenesis in regenerating systems. In Hall BK (ed): Cartilage. Biomedical Aspects. New York, Academic Press, 1983.)

the pedicles by the same mechanism involved in subsequent annual rounds of regeneration. The onset of antler growth is correlated with reduced levels of testosterone. Indeed, it is the decline in testosterone that is responsible for the detachment of the old antlers from the frontal pedicles. The regeneration of antlers occurs at a time of year when testosterone levels are normally minimal and when the testes are aspermatogenic. The onset of antler growth occurs 6 months out of phase from the mating season, and coincides with the infertile phase of the reproductive cycle. Maturation of the antlers, involving solidification of the bone and shedding of the velvet, is triggered by rising levels of testosterone and forecasts the fertile phase of the reproductive cycle.

If male hormone is administered to a deer that has not yet shed his antlers, he will retain these antlers as long as exogenous testosterone is available.[40] If the hormone is injected into a male that has recently dropped his old antlers and has begun to grow new ones, the elongation of the regenerates ceases, ossification occurs, and within a few weeks the velvet is shed. These aborted antlers may later be lost and replaced if no further hormones are administered. Thus, by artificially altering the hormone levels of different seasons, it is possible to induce two sets of antlers in 1 year.

Castration yields opposite effects, depending on when it is carried out. If an adult deer is castrated while in velvet, the antlers will fail to mature and will remain permanently viable and in velvet. If he is castrated in the fall when his antlers are bony, they will be shed in several weeks, to be followed by regeneration even at the wrong time of year. These antlers may grow to normal length but they are unable to complete their development in the absence of testosterone. They too remain permanently viable and in velvet. When the next growing season arrives, castrated deer will still have their last year's antlers yet will be stimulated to grow new ones. As a result, the antlers may grow laterally or may even sprout supernumerary outgrowths around the base. After several years, depending upon the species, some of these antlers may develop bizarre protuberances that resemble tumors (Fig. 2–12). These "antleromas" are not known to be cancerous or malignant but may be capable of growing into massive swellings that hang in festoons from the sides of the antler. Histologically, they are made up of nondescript tissue with no evidence of bone or cartilage.

In some respects antleromas are reminiscent of hypertrophic scars or keloids, a condition for

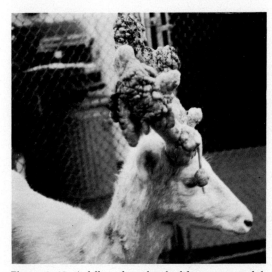

Figure 2–12. A fallow deer that had been castrated for several years and held indoors to prevent freezing of the antlers. Grotesque amorphous outgrowths have developed from the sides of the permanently viable antlers. Note the pendulous "antleroma" dangling in front of the right eye.

which they may in fact be a convenient animal model for experimental investigation. They also resemble the neurofibromas of von Recklinghausen's disease. If a castrated deer with such antlers is treated with testosterone, the antleromas will die and drop off as the velvet is shed.

The normal regeneration of antlers may begin even before the old ones have been cast off. This is first evident as a swelling in the pedicle skin around the base of the old antler. When the latter is detached, a process mediated by osteoclastic erosion, the raw wound on the end of the pedicle forms a scab beneath which the pedicle epidermis migrates in the process of wound healing. Epidermal migration is accompanied by the invasion of masses of mesodermal cells of uncertain origin. Such cells appear to originate in the skin or associated connective tissues around the pedicle bone, but deletion and transplantation experiments have thus far failed to identify their precise histogenesis. Whatever their derivation, they rapidly invade the pedicle wound where their increasing numbers push up into a rounded bud. This antler bud has all the characteristics of regeneration blastemas found in other systems. It is made up of undifferentiated cells capable of proliferation. Its subsequent elongation is achieved by the activities of an apical growth zone, and as elongation and branching proceed, the cells left behind undergo differentiation. They first develop into cartilage, which subsequently becomes calcified and replaced by bony trabeculae

(Fig. 2–13). This sequence of temporal events can be visualized spatially in a longitudinal section cut through the end of a growing antler. The bone that is first formed is cancellous, being made up of intricate trabeculae interspersed with blood vessels. The rapidly elongating antler is well vascularized. The arteries in the velvet skin convey a copious supply of blood to the growing tips, and a cascade of capillaries travels downward through the central core of the antler. Even the cartilage is honeycombed with blood vessels.

The velvet is particularly interesting. It is adorned with numerous hairs that protrude at right angles from the skin, the follicles of which are equipped with sebaceous glands. New hair follicles are constantly being produced at the tip of the rapidly growing antler where they differentiate and are left behind on the sides of the shaft as the growth zone advances. The velvet is easily distinguished from the fur elsewhere on the pedicle and scalp and is destined to die and peel off once the antler is fully formed. Experiments have shown that if velvet skin is transplanted elsewhere, it is not shed when the antler matures.[42] Therefore, the demise of the antler velvet would appear to be a case of murder, rather than suicide.

It is a curious thing that these cephalic appendages are so readily regenerated while other amputated structures in the deer are not. Why does the pedicle form an antler blastema instead of a scar? There appear to be no epidermal downgrowths such as have been documented in the regenerating rabbit ear. The dermis of the pedicle skin gives every indication of contributing cells to the antler bud, yet these cells do not develop into a scar. Indeed, the tissues that elsewhere in the body would produce a fibrous barrier to regeneration appear to be the very ones that give rise to the antler on the end of the pedicle. One wonders if the deer has evolved a mechanism of antler regeneration that deflects its cells from scar formation to blastema production. If so, the antler itself might be regarded as nothing more than an exaggerated morphological version of scar formation.

Although the histogenesis of regenerating antlers remains unknown, that of the original pedicle in the fawn has been convincingly demonstrated by two experimental approaches. Deletion experiments have shown that if the periosteum is removed from the frontal bones in the region of the presumptive pedicle, neither pedicle nor antler subsequently develops.[43] Transplantation experiments, in which disks of periosteum from the pedicle region of a fawn's frontal bones have been transplanted beneath the skin elsewhere on the body, have yielded ectopic antlers.[44–46] Such antlers have been induced to sprout from the forehead, hip, front and hind legs, ear, and cornea. In all such locations, the transplanted piece of periosteum undergoes ossification, after which it induces the overlying skin to transform into antler velvet. Such antlers may grow less than a centimeter during the first year but sometimes achieve lengths of up to 7 cm in subsequent

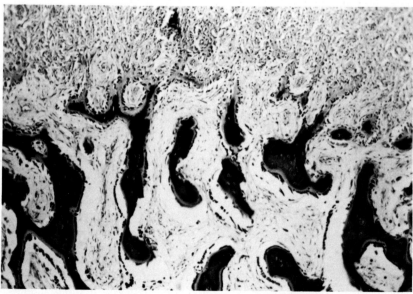

Figure 2–13. Cancellous bone in an antler while still in velvet. The trabeculae are surrounded by osteoblasts that will subsequently lay down appositional bone under the influence of testosterone. (From Goss RJ: Problems of antlerogenesis. Clin Orthop 69:227, 1970.)

years (Fig. 2–14). They are replaced in synchrony with the deer's normal antlers.

The results of these transplantation experiments prove that the skin, while indispensable for antler development, is not specifically predetermined to form velvet. Skin from many areas of the body can be induced to undergo velvet transformation, even though it may have been fully differentiated previously. Whatever the inductive mechanism may be, it operates through several layers of connective tissue, from periosteum to epidermis, traversing over a millimeter of tissue thickness. How this is achieved is not known, but it is probably by the same mechanism that operates in the yearling as its pedicle bone induces antlerogenesis in the overlying scalp.

The importance of epidermis in antler development cannot be overemphasized. As in all other examples of epimorphic regeneration, the epidermis plays an indispensable role in blastema formation. If an amphibian limb stump is stripped of its skin and inserted internally into the body, it will not regenerate, and if full-thickness skin is ligated over the end of an amputation stump, no regeneration ensues. Similarly, when an antler pedicle is sealed by flaps of full-thickness skin, no antler can be produced from it.[42] Hence, an integumental wound is essential for regeneration because only in this way can wound epidermis be produced. This is consistent with the definition of an

appendage as an outgrowth covered with skin. A blastema is not a blastema unless it is enveloped in epidermis.

If deer had never evolved antlers, there would be little reason to expect mammals to regenerate anything epimorphically. The fact that these remarkable appendages actually do exist and are capable of epimorphic regeneration challenges us to explain how they could have evolved in the first place. While other ungulates evolved horns with cornified sheaths or fur-covered appendages such as those carried by giraffes, early members of the deer tribe grew headpieces that died spontaneously and were shed and regrown each year. One wonders what might have been the selective pressures responsible for antler evolution.

About 30 million years ago in the Miocene some of the early deer in tropical habitats in what is now Mongolia evolved cephalic outgrowths that, because they were secondary sex characteristics carried by aggressive males, were probably subject to repeated injuries. They may well have evolved mechanisms of repair that went beyond the usual stopgap measures of wound healing, and any mutation that favored the replacement of missing branches might have had a strong selective advantage.

When some of these early cervids migrated to temperate zones (or when the previously tropical climate of their habitat changed), their

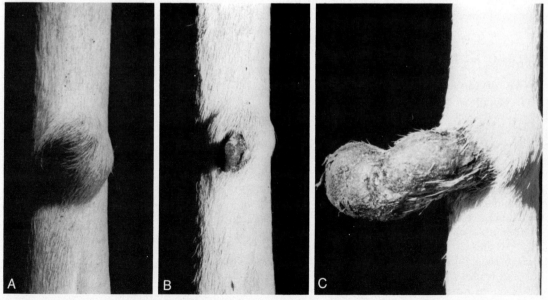

Figure 2–14. When a disc of antlerogenic periosteum is grafted subcutaneously to the foreleg, it differentiates into a bony nodule that pushes out the overlying leg skin (A). The latter subsequently transforms into antler velvet and is shed in the early autumn, revealing a small antler composed of dead bone (B). This is detached in the following spring and replaced by a larger antler (C).

viable "horns" would have frozen in the winter. This is exactly what happens to the castrate antlers of temperate zone deer living outdoors in the winter. There are two ways to solve this problem. One is to grow the antlers during the winter months when the rich flow of blood would prevent freezing. This is what the roe deer does today, except that such a schedule is in conflict with the gestation period. While most deer must mate in the fall in order to ensure spring births, roe deer mate in the summer, undergo delayed implantation until December, whereupon the resumption of gestation in the female and the onset of antler growth in the male coincide. All other species solve the problem in a different way by linking the antler production cycle to the cycle of testosterone secretion, such that the hormone causes the antler to die before it can be killed by frostbite. This adaptation, anticipating seasonal freezing, served the purpose of providing the males with hard formidable weapons for use in display and combat.[47] These structures were a considerable improvement over living fur-covered appendages, particularly if they were to be used in fighting. In no other known animal is the existence of dead tissue tolerated as it is in deer antlers. Their ability to be shed and regrown makes it possible for them to repair injury not by piecemeal outgrowths of missing branches, but by the wholesale renewal of the entire structure. Annual replacement also enables deer to enlarge their antlers to keep pace with overall body growth, similar to the way diminutive teeth of young animals are replaced by adult-sized ones during maturation.

Human Limb Regeneration

What are the prospects for the regeneration of human appendages?[48] Inasmuch as arms and legs were essential parts of the body for our primitive ancestors, it is not difficult to understand why they are unable to replace themselves. Nevertheless, there seems to be two possible exceptions to the rule that such appendages cannot regenerate. In both cases the phenomena have strained the definition of epimorphic regeneration.

The phenomenon of bone overgrowth is perhaps not unrelated to regeneration.[49] It tends to occur in children following amputation of a limb and is characterized by the gradual extension of bones from their original levels of transection. The result is a protuberance from the amputation stump due mainly to the internal elongation of the bone. Such overgrowths may require surgical removal in order to maintain a stump morphology conducive to being fitted to a prosthesis. Bone overgrowth is reminiscent of the epiphyseal regeneration that has been studied in rodents.[50] When the head of a long bone in a young rat is resected, including the epiphysis and cartilaginous plate, a new growth plate may sometimes be formed. This kind of regeneration resembles the epimorphic type in that it is polarized in a proximodistal direction. Unlike appendage regeneration, however, it does not involve the skin nor is a blastema responsible for the development of the new bone. On the other hand, bone overgrowth goes beyond simple tissue repair. It does not just complete the continuity of interrupted components but actually gives rise to new histological structures. Its significance is an enigma.

The other possible example of mammalian regeneration is the famous case of fingertip replacement in young children. If the finger is lost distal to the last articulation in a sufficiently young child there is a possibility that regrowth may occur. This typically includes the reconstitution of the fingernail and the bony extension of the amputated phalanx. According to Illingworth, this kind of development takes place when the finger stump is not sealed with full-thickness skin.[51] When the lesion is not surgically treated in this way healing can occur by epidermal migration, which presumably permits the establishment of conditions necessary for regeneration. Because the histology of this phenomenon has not been investigated, it is impossible to say whether or not a true blastema is produced from which the missing fingertip may develop. Nor is it certain that the replacement of the fingernail occurs de novo because the original nailbed actually extends proximally very close to the joint. Because of this it is unlikely that a fingertip would be lost without leaving behind at least part of the nail bed in the stump. Why it is that the fingertips of children (and mice too)[52] can be regenerated in this way while those of adults are not is not understood. Nor do we know why it is limited to the distal tip of the finger. Nevertheless, such exceptions to the rule that regeneration does not occur in mammals encourage continued investigations in this area.

References

1. Brody S: Bioenergetics and Growth. Princeton, Van Nostrand-Reinhold, 1945.
2. Hui F, Smith A: Regeneration of the amputated amphibian limb: Retardation by hemicholinium-3. Science 170:1313–1314, 1970.

3. Bizzozero G: An address on the growth and regeneration of the organism. Br Med J 1:728–732, 1894.

4. Goss RJ: The Physiology of Growth. New York, Academic Press, 1978.

5. Bucher NLR, Malt RA: Regeneration of Liver and Kidney. Boston, Little, Brown, 1971.

6. Ingle DJ, Baker BL: Histology and regenerative capacity of liver following multiple partial hepatectomies. Proc Soc Exp Biol Med 95:813–815, 1957.

7. Argyris TS, Miller A: Liver hepatocyte mitotic activity after a single injection of phenobarbital in immature male rats. Anat Rec 185:447–451, 1976.

8. Nowinski WW, Goss RJ: Compensatory Renal Hypertrophy. New York, Academic Press, 1969.

9. Dicker SE, Shirley DG: Compensatory renal growth after unilateral nephrectomy in the new-born rat. J Physiol 228:193–202, 1973.

10. Harvey W: Movement of the Heart and Blood in Animals. Oxford, Blackwell, 1957.

11. Alpert, NR: Cardiac Hypertrophy. New York, Academic Press, 1971.

12. Fitzgerald PJ, Herman L: Degeneration and regeneration of the pancreas. Bull NY Acad Med 41:804–810, 1965.

13. Jacobson LO, Doyle M: Erythropoiesis. New York, Grune & Stratton, 1962.

14. Gutmann E, Hnik P: The Effect of Use and Disuse on Neuromuscular Functions. Amsterdam, Elsevier, 1963.

15. McMinn RMH: Tissue Repair. New York, Academic Press, 1969.

16. Needham AE: Regeneration and Wound-healing. London, Methuen, 1952.

17. Morgan TH. Regeneration. New York, Macmillan, 1901.

18. Vorontsova MA, Liosner LD: Asexual Propagation and Regeneration. London, Pergamon Press, 1960.

19. Hay ED: Regeneration. New York, Holt, Rinehart & Winston, 1966.

20. Schmidt AJ: Cellular Biology of Vertebrate Regeneration and Repair. Chicago, University of Chicago Press, 1968.

21. Goss RJ: Principles of Regeneration. New York, Academic Press, 1969.

22. Wallace H: Vertebrate Limb Regeneration. New York, John Wiley & Sons, 1981.

23. Sicard RE: Regulation of Vertebrate Limb Regeneration. New York, Oxford University Press, 1985.

24. Thornton CS: The effect of apical cap removal on limb regeneration in Amblystoma larvae. J Exp Zool 134:357–382, 1957.

25. Thoms SD, Stocum DL: Retinoic acid–induced pattern duplication in the regenerating forelimbs of urodeles. Dev Biol 103:319–328, 1984.

26. Singer M. Nervous mechanisms in the regeneration of body parts in vertebrates. In Rudnick D (ed): Developing Cell Systems and Their Control. New York, Ronald Press, 1960, pp 115–133.

27. Passano LM, Jyssum S: The role of the Y-organ in crab proecdysis and limb regeneration. Comp Biochem Physiol 9:195–213, 1963.

28. Zawadowsky MM: Bilateral and unilateral castration in *Cervus dama* and *Cervus elaphus*. Trans Lab Exp Biol Zoopark, Moscow 1:18–43, 1926.

29. Goss RJ: Epimorphic regeneration in mammals. In Hunt TK, Heppenstall RB, Pines E, et al: Soft and Hard Tissue Repair. New York, Praeger, 1984, pp 554–573.

30. Butler EG: Regeneration of the urodele forelimb after reversal of its proximodistal axis. J Morphol 96:265–281, 1955.

31. Goss RJ: Why mammals don't regenerate—or do they? News Physiol Sci 2:112–115, 1987.

32. Joseph J, Dyson M: Tissue replacement in the rabbit's ear. Brit J Surg 53:372–380, 1966.

33. Goss RJ, Grimes LN: Tissue interactions in the regeneration of rabbit ear holes. Am Zool 12:151–157, 1972.

34. Goss RJ, Grimes LN: Epidermal downgrowths in regenerating rabbit ear holes. J Morphol 146:533–542, 1975.

35. Breedis C: Regeneration of hair follicles and sebaceous glands from the epithelium of scars in the rabbit. Cancer Res 14:575–579, 1954.

36. Brown RD: Antler Development in Cervidae. Kingsville, TX, Caesar Kleberg Wildlife Research Institute, 1983.

37. Goss RJ: Deer Antlers: Regeneration, Function, and Evolution. New York, Academic Press, 1983.

38. Goss RJ: Chondrogenesis in regenerating systems. In Hall BK (ed): Cartilage: Biomedical Aspects, vol 3. New York, Academic Press, 1983, pp 267–307.

39. Goss RJ: The deciduous nature of deer antlers. In Sognnaes R (ed): Mechanisms of Hard Tissue Destruction. Washington, DC, AAAS Publ No. 75, 1963, pp 339–369.

40. Goss RJ: Inhibition of growth and shedding of antlers by sex hormones. Nature 220:83–85, 1968.

41. Goss RJ: Problems of antlerogenesis. Clin Orthop 69:227–238, 1970.

42. Goss RJ: Wound healing and antler regeneration. In Maibach HI, Rovee DT (eds): Epidermal Wound Healing. Chicago, Year Book, 1972, pp 219–228.

43. Hartwig H: Verhinderung der Rosenstock- und Stangenbildung beim Reh, *Capreolus capreolus*, durch Periostausschaltung. Zool Garten 35:252–255, 1968.

44. Hartwig H, Schrudde J: Experimentelle Untersuchungen zur Bildung der primaren Stirnauswuchse beim Reh *(Capreolus capreolus* L). Z Jagdwiss 20:1–13, 1974.

45. Goss RJ, Powel RS: Induction of deer antlers by transplanted periosteum. I. Graft size and shape. J Exp Zool 235:359–373, 1985.

46. Goss RJ: Induction of deer antlers by transplanted periosteum. II. Regional competence for velvet transformation in ectopic skin. J Exp Zool 244:101–111, 1987.

47. Coope GR: The evolutionary origins of antlers. Deer 1:215–217, 1968.

48. Goss RJ: Prospects for regeneration in man. Clin Orthop 151:270–282, 1980.

49. Speer DP: Pathogenesis of amputation stump overgrowth. Clin Orthop 159:294–307, 1981.

50. Nunnemacher RF: Experimental studies on the cartilage plates in the long bones of the rat. Am J Anat 65:253–290, 1939.

51. Illingworth CM: Trapped fingers and amputated finger tips in children. J Pediatr Surg 9:853–858, 1974.

52. Borgens RB: Mice regrow the tips of their foretoes. Science 217:747–750, 1982.

3

INFLAMMATION

Larry M. Wahl, Ph.D., and Sharon M. Wahl, Ph.D.

Inflammation is a progression of complex, interrelated events that occur in response to tissue injury induced by trauma or an immune response to a foreign object. The initial changes that occur following injury include altered vascular permeability, the exudation of plasma components, the aggregation of platelets, and the activation of the coagulation and fibrinolytic cascades.[1] Subsequently, peripheral blood leukocytes are recruited to the site in response to a variety of chemotactic agents. These cells, through the release of soluble mediators, interact to regulate their own biological responses as well as those of other cells, such as fibroblasts and endothelial cells. The interactions of cells and their products lead to the degradation of damaged tissue as well as the restoration of the tissue architecture.

The inflammatory response is essential for the repair and restoration of structural and functional integrity of damaged tissue. Moreover, depending on the specific circumstances of the wound, certain cellular elements can be shown to be critical in the ultimate healing of the tissue. In the absence of infection or a specific antigen, the process leading to normal wound healing can occur in an animal treated to deplete red blood cells,[2, 3] lymphocytes,[4] neutrophils,[5] or complement.[6] However, if the monocyte/macrophage population is depleted, there is a retardation of the normal tissue repair process.[7] Thus the involvement of the various cellular and molecular components in inflammation is in part dependent on the causative and complicating agents involved in the wound site.

Irrespective of the nature of the inciting events, the wound healing response follows a predictable pattern. These events can be divided into early or acute inflammation, a proliferative phase characterized by fibroblast and endothelial cell proliferation, and finally, matrix synthesis and scar formation. In the event of a persistent inflammatory stimulus the response may be chronic, resulting in pathological disruption of the tissue architecture.

ACUTE INFLAMMATION

Hemostasis

The tissue injury incurred in a wound results in damage to blood vessels leading to the extravasation of blood components into the tissue space (Fig. 3–1). This tissue insult, which causes a disruption in the endothelial integrity of the vessels, results in the exposure of the subendothelial structure and its various connective tissue components. Exposure of types IV and V collagen found in the subendothelium promotes binding and aggregation of platelets to these structural proteins.[8–11] The adhesion of platelets to collagen in the subendothelium involves a platelet membrane glycoprotein (GIb) receptor that binds von Willebrand factor (vWF), a 220 to 225 kDa protein, and multimers of the vWF bind to collagen, thus serving as a mediator of adhesion between platelets and collagen.[12] Endothelial cells and platelets secrete vWF when exposed to collagen and other activating agents.[13, 14] In addition to vWF, activated platelets also release a variety of other products from their α and dense granules including fibronectin, serotonin, platelet-derived growth factor (PDGF), adenosine diphosphate (ADP), platelet-activating factor (PAF), factor V, 12-hydroxyeicosatetranoic acid (12-HETE), and thromboxane A_2 (TxA$_2$), which promote inflammation.[15]

Following activation, the platelet undergoes

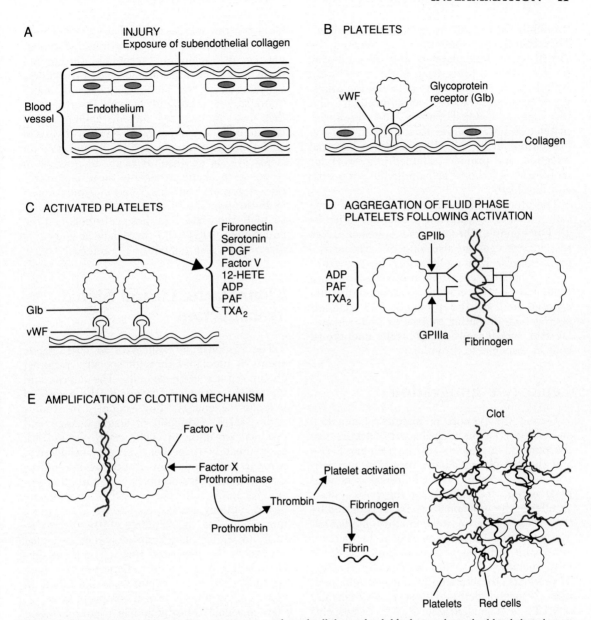

Figure 3–1. The process of hemostasis requires a number of cellular and soluble factors from the blood that change this complex suspension into a solid. These factors interact in several stages to produce a mature clot. vFW = von Willebrand factor; PDGF = platelet-derived growth factor; 12-HETE = 12-hydroxyeicosatetranoic acid; ADP = adenosine diphosphate; PAF = platelet-activating factor; TXA_2 = thromboxane A_2; GPIIb = glycoprotein IIb; GPIIIa = glycoprotein IIIa.

a series of structural and functional changes that are involved in coagulation (see review in reference 15). The activated platelet changes shape from a smooth disk to a sphere from which spiny pseudopods project. This change in shape results in increased stickiness and promotes binding of other platelets. Aggregation is further enhanced by the secretion of ADP, PAF, and TXA_2, which activates and causes coaggregation of fluid phase platelets. Also promoting aggregation is the induction on the surface of activated platelets of a heterodimer complex composed of glycoprotein IIb (GPIIb) and glycoprotein IIIa (GPIIIa), which serve as a receptor for fibronectin.[16–18]

In addition to aggregation, activation stimulates rearrangement of the phospholipids in the platelet membrane, enabling clotting factor V to bind to the platelets and to subsequently interact with clotting factor X. This interaction results in the generation of membrane-bound prothrombinase activity, which increases thrombin production by several thousandfold. Thrombin further potentiates aggregation by directly activating platelets and by catalyzing the formation of fibrin from fibrinogen. Fibrin strands, which form a mesh between the aggregated platelets, trap red cells, forming a clot that is impermeable to plasma. Thus, this fibrin-platelet structure serves to seal off the injury, preventing further bleeding as well as bacterial infection, and provides a lattice framework for mobilized endothelial cells, inflammatory cells, and fibroblasts.

The process of hemostasis is a series of intricate and well-coordinated events (see Fig. 3–1). For example, thromboxane A_2 which causes platelet aggregation, also induces vasoconstriction, thereby limiting bleeding by two pathways. Platelet aggregation and coagulation are regulated by the amount of subendothelium exposed and by the production of platelet-aggregation–inhibiting molecules such as prostacyclin, which is produced by the endothelial cells in response to thrombin.

Leukocyte Emigration

During the process of platelet aggregation and clotting, factors are released that influence the permeability of the surrounding capillaries and the subsequent chemoattraction and activation of leukocytes. The adherence of neutrophils to the endothelium of the postcapillary venules in the inflammatory site is increased by the local release of inflammatory mediators. Mediators that have been shown to increase neutrophil adherence to endothelial cells in vitro include C5a and C5a des arg, bacterial products characterized by the synthetic peptide N-formyl-methionyl-leucyl-phenylalanine (FMLP), and leukotriene B_4.[19–22] These also function as chemoattractants. Additionally, endothelial cells, in response to thrombin and leukotrienes C_4 and D_4, release PAF, which can enhance neutrophil adhesion to endothelial cells.[23–25] Other factors that promote endothelial cell–neutrophil adherence are interleukin-1 (IL-1) and tumor necrosis factor (TNF), products of monocytes and endothelial cells themselves.[26–29]

The release of chemotactic factors in the local inflammatory site serves as a migration signal for the adhering cells. In response to a concentration gradient of the chemoattractants, the adherent or marginated neutrophils begin the process of diapedesis, or migration, between the endothelial cells into the inflammatory site. Diapedesis of the neutrophils is further facilitated by the increased capillary permeability following the release of a spectrum of vasodilating agents, including serotonin, histamine, bradykinin, and arachidonic acid metabolites. In addition to the chemotactic ligands mentioned above, other leukocyte chemoattractants that may be involved include kallikrein and plasminogen activator, factors involved in coagulation and fibrinolysis; PDGF; and platelet factor IV. As neutrophils begin to migrate in response to chemoattractants there is a secretion of granule contents,[30] and enzymes stored in these granules such as elastase, which may facilitate the passage of these cells between the endothelial cells.[31] (For a review of leukocyte margination and diapedesis see reference 32.)

Chemotactic Ligand Signal Transduction

The response of leukocytes to chemotactic agents is mediated through specific receptors on the surface of these cells. The degree and type of the response depends on the degree of receptor occupancy. For example, in studies with FMLP, induction of shape change and maximal elevation in cyclic AMP occurs with approximately 10 percent receptor occupancy, whereas peak production of superoxide requires maximum receptor occupancy.[33] While the specific receptors differ for individual chemotactic ligand,[34] the events involved in signal transduction, following the binding of the ligand to receptor, are similar. Transmission of the signal appears to be mediated through guanine nucleotide–binding proteins (G-proteins), which are linked to the receptor,[35] as described in many cell systems.[36] (For a comprehensive review of signal transduction in neutrophils see reference 35.)

In addition to the chemotactic ligand receptors, neutrophils also express Fc, CR1 and CR3 receptors that recognize immunoglobulin G (IgG), and the complement proteins C3b and C3bi, respectively. During the course of the host immune response to microorganisms, the microorganisms may become opsonized with IgG, C3b, or C3bi. Thus the receptors for these molecules on the neutrophil provide the basic mechanism by which these cells recognize and phagocytize microorganisms. Moreover, during neutrophil stimulation there is an increase in the expression of CR1 and CR3 receptors on the cell surface.[37–42] Increased expression of these receptors not only permits more efficient binding of the appropriately coated microorganisms but is also essential for the CR3-ligand complex to be internalized.[42]

Oxygen-Dependent Microbicidal Activity

A primary function of neutrophils is to serve as the first line of defense against microorganisms that may be introduced into the host. Neutrophils can kill bacteria intra- or extracellularly by both oxygen-dependent and oxygen-independent mechanisms. Intracellular killing occurs in the phagosome subsequent to the binding and internalization of the microorganisms.

When stimulated, neutrophils exhibit a significant increase in oxygen consumption with the generation of oxygen radicals (Fig. 3–2). This respiratory burst involves the action of NADPH (nicotinamide adenine dinucleotide) oxidase on NADPH, which serves as the primary electron donor for the reduction of oxygen.[43–46] The NADPH oxidase system is found in the membrane with the NADPH binding site extending into the cytoplasm.[47, 48] This system consists of a number of components, particularly flavoproteins (see review in reference 49), which are involved in transmembrane electron transport to the extracellular fluids or into phagosomes where superoxide anion (O_2^- is formed when oxygen accepts a single electron. Interaction of two O_2^- molecules results in the oxidation of one and the reduction of the other to form oxygen and hydrogen peroxide (H_2O_2). This reaction can occur spontaneously, but more likely it is catalyzed by superoxide dismutase (SOD).[50] Moreover, the inhibition of microbicidal activity by the addition of SOD provides evidence for the role of O_2^- in this process.[51]

The generation of H_2O_2 by dismutation of O_2^- is also important in the microbicidal activity of neutrophils. H_2O_2 may be degraded by catalase, glutathione peroxidase, or myeloperoxidase (MPO). The microbicidal or cytotoxic effect of H_2O_2 can be enhanced by interaction of this oxygen metabolite with MPO released from the azurophilic granules of the neutrophil during phagocytosis or in response to antibody-coated organisms or soluble stimuli. In an interaction between MPO and H_2O_2, the halides iodide, bromide, and chloride become oxidized. The oxidation of chloride to hypochlorous acid (HOCl) by MPO and H_2O_2 has been demonstrated to occur in neutrophils and appears to be the major halide oxidation product.[52, 53] HOCl is a potent oxidant that can rapidly attack a variety of chemical sites on the microorganism, resulting in the loss of membrane transport function, which is associated with loss of viability.[54–56] The bactericidal effect of the MPO/H_2O_2/chloride system can be blocked by taurine (2-aminoethanesulfonic acid),[57, 58] which appears to be a competitive inhibitor as a result of the formation of taurine chloramine.

In addition to O_2^-, H_2O_2, and HOCl, another toxic product derived from oxygen metabolism is the hydroxyl radical ($\cdot$OH). Formation of $\cdot$OH occurs as a result of a metal-catalyzed (most likely iron) reaction between H_2O_2 and O_2^-, termed the Haber-Weiss reaction.[59] Lactoferrin, a source of iron, enhances $\cdot$OH production by neutrophils.[60] Moreover, lactoferrin is found in the specific granules released into the phago-

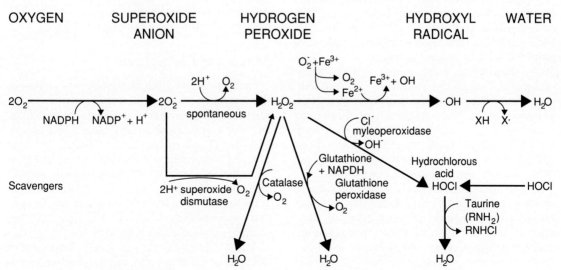

Figure 3–2. Pathway for the production of various activated oxygen species.

somes or extracellularly in response to soluble stimuli. The potent oxidant capability of ·OH suggests that, in addition to its bactericidal effect, it may also be toxic to the neutrophil and surrounding cells and tissues.[49]

Oxygen-Independent Microbicidal Mechanisms

Neutrophils have also been shown to kill microorganisms through oxygen-independent mechanisms. This was first demonstrated by the ability of a protein fraction from acid-extracted neutrophils, termed phagocytin, to kill both gram-negative and gram-positive bacteria.[61, 62] Subsequent purification of these neutrophil extracts led to the identification of several proteins with antimicrobial properties. An antimicrobial protein isolated from human and rabbit neutrophils was given the descriptive name of bactericidal/permeability increasing protein (BPI). This protein, with a molecular weight of approximately 50,000 to 60,000 daltons[63] is found in the primary granules of the neutrophil.[64] BPI is a potent bactericidal protein that selectively kills gram-negative bacteria but has no effect on gram-positive bacteria. Binding of BPI to gram-negative bacteria occurs through an electrostatic interaction with surface sites that have a negative charge and as a result displaces Ca^{2+} and Mg^{2+}, resulting in the destabilization of the outer lipopolysaccharide layer and the membrane phospholipid structure.[65, 66] Subsequent to binding, BPI induces an irreversible, but undefined, sequence of events leading to loss of bacterial viability.

Another acid-extracted neutrophil fraction contains arginine- and cystine-rich proteins with antimicrobial properties.[67, 68] Purification of these cationic proteins reveals them to be small peptides with a molecular weight of less than 4000 daltons that share a high degree of homology and can be isolated from different species. For example, three peptides with close homology have been purified and sequenced from human neutrophils.[69, 70] Due to their antimicrobial effect these peptides have been named defensins. The mechanism by which defensins kill microorganisms is unknown.

The primary granules of the neutrophil also contain several enzymes that may kill microorganisms by a mechanism unrelated to their enzyme activity. One of these, cathepsin G, which is a chymotrypsin-like protease, has been shown to destroy both gram-negative and gram-positive bacteria.[71] Although its enzymatic activity can be abolished by heating, the protein maintains its microbicidal capabilities.

Extracellular Release of Degradative Enzymes

As a result of stimulation, phagocytosis, or lysis, neutrophils may release the contents of their granules into the extracellular space. Among these granule contents are enzymes that can degrade the connective tissue found at the site of the wound. Elastase,[72] collagenase,[73] and other hydrolytic enzymes likely contribute to removal of damaged tissue, but also may cause further injury. As is the case with other granule contents, these enzymes are synthesized in the early or myeloid stages of neutrophil development, and therefore, stimulation of the neutrophils triggers the release of preformed enzymes without additional enzyme synthesis.

Monocytes/Macrophages

Subsequent to the early events that occur following the initial trauma and neutrophil accumulation, mononuclear cells become evident in the inflammatory site. These cells remain at the wound site for days to weeks, during which time they participate in debridement, microbicidal events, and orchestration of the events involved in tissue repair. Monocytes/macrophages carry out many of these processes through release of soluble molecules that act on other inflammatory cells and on mesenchymal cells to regulate their phenotype and function. Some of these biological mediators and their relevance in inflammation and wound healing are described in the following sections.

Monocyte Chemotaxis

Like the neutrophil, the monocyte arrives at the site of the wound in response to chemoattractants, such as bacterial products and C5a, for which specific receptors have been identified on the cell surface.[34, 74, 75] One of the most potent chemotactic agents that can be found in an inflammatory site is transforming growth factor-beta (TGF-β), a product of platelets, neutrophils,[76] monocytes, and lymphocytes. Monocytes express high-affinity TGF-β receptors and migrate to femtomolar concentrations of this peptide.[77] Lymphocytes produce one or more other factors that are also chemotactic for monocytes. These chemoattractants, at higher concentrations than required for chemotaxis, can also activate the monocytes. For example, TGF-β in the femtomolar range is chemotactic, whereas when added to monocytes in the nanomolar range, TGF-β stimulates monocytes to produce monokines, including interleukin-1, which contribute to the inflammatory network.[78] Monocytes are also activated during phagocytosis at the wound site and/or by exposure to products, such as lipopolysaccharide, from microorganisms that might infect the tissues. As a result of these various stimuli, monocytes are induced to release a number of biologically relevant molecules that have regulatory effects on inflammation and tissue repair.

Reactive Oxygen Intermediates

Similar to neutrophils, activated monocytes/macrophages release the reactive oxygen intermediates O_2^-, H_2O_2, and ·OH, which function in a microbicidal capacity. The formation of oxygen radicals by monocytes does not differ substantially from that described previously for neutrophils. However, monocyte-reactive oxygen intermediate generation can also be regulated by the T-cell product interleukin-2 (IL-2). When monocytes are activated by bacterial products or interferon-γ, they express receptors for IL-2.[79–81] The addition of exogenous IL-2 to these IL-2 receptor–bearing monocytes then results in an increase in O_2^- release and killing of certain microorganisms.[81] This IL-2 regulation of monocyte microbicidal activity exemplifies the network of interactions involved in augmentation and perpetuation of the inflammatory response.

Arachidonic Acid Metabolites

Activation of monocyte/macrophages also results in the induction of a membrane-associated enzyme, phospholipase, that releases arachidonic acid from the phospholipids in the cell membrane. The arachidonic acid is metabolized through two separate pathways, the cyclooxygenase pathway leading to the formation of the prostaglandins and the lipoxygenase pathway from which the leukotrienes and monohydroxyeicosatetranoic acids (HETEs) are formed. The prostaglandins released by the monocyte/macrophage include 6-keto-prostaglandin $F_{1\alpha}$ (6-keto-$PGF_{1\alpha}$) and thromboxane B_2 (TxB_2), the stable products of prostacyclin (PGI_2) and thromboxane A_2 (TxA_2), respectively; prostaglandin E_2 (PGE_2) and $F2_\alpha$ ($PGF_{2\alpha}$).[82] Included in the lipoxygenase products released by mono-

cytes/macrophages are leukotriene B_4 (LTB_4) and C_4 (LTC_4) and 15- and 5-HETE.[82] These lipid metabolites have multiple effects on the various cellular functions involved in inflammation.

Of the prostaglandins, PGE_2 is possibly the most relevant mediator since it is a stable compound that, like PGI_2, causes an elevation in the intracellular levels of cyclic adenosine monophosphate (cAMP). The effects of PGE_2 result in feedback regulation of the monocyte/macrophage. For example, PGE_2 is an inhibitor of macrophage adherence, spreading, and migration,[83] production of macrophage-derived colony-stimulating factor activity,[84] clonal proliferation of macrophage stem cells,[85] Ia expression on macrophages that is also inhibited by PGI_2,[86] and macrophage IL-1 production.[87] Conversely, PGE_2 also enhances certain monocyte/macrophage functions, including collagenase production[88] and phagocytosis.[89] The effect of PGE_2 on lymphocytes is predominantly immunosuppressive with inhibitory effects on migration, lymphokine synthesis, and proliferation.[90–92]

Products from the lipoxygenase pathway, primarily LTB_4, also modulate inflammatory responses. LTB_4 has been shown to be a potent chemoattractant for neutrophils in vitro and in vivo where a rapid accumulation of leukocytes occurs following intradermal or intraperitoneal injection of LTB_4.[93] Moreover, LTB_4 has been shown to increase neutrophil adherence to endothelial cells[93] and to enhance neutrophil microbicidal activity through a complement-dependent mechanism.[94]

Lipoxygenase products can modulate lymphocyte function to either enhance or suppress the immune response.[95] LTB_4 inhibition of human peripheral blood lymphocyte proliferation[96–98] is apparently due to the induction of $CD8^+$ lymphocyte proliferation (suppressor/cytotoxic subset) with concomitant inhibition of $CD4^+$ lymphocyte proliferation (helper/inducer subset).[98, 99] Subsequent studies demonstrated that LTB_4 directly stimulated $CD8^+$ lymphocytes, whereas the inhibition of $CD4^+$ cells was dependent on monocytes and their prostaglandin products.[100] Moreover, LTB_4 was reported to induce suppressor cells from either the $T4^+$ or $T8^+$ lymphocyte subsets.[100] Other products of the lipoxygenase pathway including 15-HPETE, 15-HETE, LTD_4, and LTE_4 also inhibit lymphocyte proliferation.[101–103] LTB_4 has also been shown to inhibit lymphocyte inhibitory factor (LIF) production[96, 104] and the mixed lymphocyte response (MLR).[105]

Lipoxygenase products are also capable of

enhancing the immune response as evidenced by the ability of LTB_4, LTC_4, and LTD_4 to replace T-helper cells or IL-2 in the induction of interferon-γ in the murine system.[106] LTB_4 has also been shown to enhance natural killer (NK) or natural cytotoxic (NC) function.[107, 108] Thus, arachidonic acid metabolites from the cyclooxygenase and lipoxygenase pathways appear to be intricately involved in all phases of the regulation of the inflammatory response.

Collagenase Production and Regulation

Damaged tissue and debris at a site of tissue injury must be degraded and cleared before healing can proceed. Collagen is one of the major connective tissue components found in damaged tissue, and degradation of this protein is dependent upon the enzyme collagenase, since the triple helical structure of collagen can be cleaved only by this enzyme. Macrophages[109–112] and monocytes[113–116] are a source of collagenase, and the large numbers of macrophages in an inflammatory site most likely, along with neutrophils and fibroblasts, contribute to the degradation and removal of collagen from the damaged tissue.

The ability of macrophages to synthesize and secrete collagenase is dependent upon activation of the cells by stimuli such as lipopolysaccharide (LPS)[109] or products from activated lymphocytes.[117] Following exposure to a primary signal, macrophages generate PGE_2, which induces an elevation in the intracellular levels of cAMP.[88, 116, 118] Subsequent to this increase in PGE_2 and cAMP, the ornithine decarboxylase pathway is triggered and its polyamine product putrescine further regulates the activation sequence leading to collagenase production.[119]

Monocyte/macrophage collagenase synthesis can be pharmacologically interrupted at several points in the activation sequence. Due to its dependence on the PGE_2-cAMP pathway, collagenase synthesis is susceptible to inhibition by indomethacin and other cyclooxygenase inhibitors.[88, 116] Dexamethasone, an anti-inflammatory corticosteroid, inhibits monocyte/macrophage collagenase production,[116, 120, 121] likely by blocking the turnover of phospholipids required for PGE_2 synthesis. Although initial studies suggested that dexamethasone induced the synthesis of a protein, lipocortin, that directly inhibited phospholipase A_2,[122, 123] recent evidence indicates that lipocortin binds to the phospholipids in the cell membrane, thereby blocking phospholipase activity by a substrate depletion mechanism.[124] Other anti-inflammatory agents that appear to diminish monocyte/macrophage collagenase production include colchicine and retinoic acid.[116, 121] Regulation of monocyte/macrophage collagenase may provide an important mechanism for controlling excessive enzymatic degradation of connective tissue in destructive inflammatory lesions.

Interleukin-1

Monocytes are a major secretory cell with the capability of secreting more than 100 different molecules.[125] Among these secretory products are numerous polypeptide molecules that are central to the initiation, amplification, and resolution of an inflammatory response. Of these monokines, interleukin-1 (IL-1) is possibly the most well studied. The production of IL-1 by activated monocytes/macrophages plays an important role in the early events in inflammation, which are collectively called "acute phase responses," as well as the later events (Fig. 3–3). cDNA cloning of IL-1 demonstrated that this molecule is produced in two protein forms that have been identified as IL-1α and IL-1β.[126–130] These molecules differ in their separation on isoelectric focusing with a pI of 5.2 for IL-1α and 7.0 for IL-1β.[131, 132] While the amino acid sequence homology of these two forms of IL-1 is only 27 to 33 percent,[133, 134] they exhibit similar biological activities,[135] which can be accounted for by their binding to the same receptor.[136] Both IL-1α and IL-1β are synthesized as 31,000 dalton precursor molecules that are proteolytically modified to the 17,000 dalton biologically active forms.[137, 138]

Originally the term "interleukin-1" was used to rename "lymphocyte-activating factor," a molecule that augmented T-cell responses to mitogens or antigens[139]; however, this protein has since been linked to a vast array of biological responses. One of these responses is the induction of fever. In the 1940s and 1950s investigators described an endogenous pyrogen found in acute exudate fluid that caused fever.[140–142] This endogenous pyrogen was subsequently linked to IL-1 by its ability to cause lymphocyte activation.[143, 144] Confirmation of the pyrogenic role of IL-1 was obtained in studies demonstrating the ability of human recombinant IL-1 to cause a febrile response in rabbits and mice.[145] IL-1 induces fever by stimulating prostaglandin synthesis in the hypothalamus, which in turn increases the temperature set point.[146]

IL-1 has been shown to have direct effects on endothelial cell functions involved in hemostasis, including induction of the vasodilators PGI_2 and PGE_2,[147, 148] increased adhesiveness

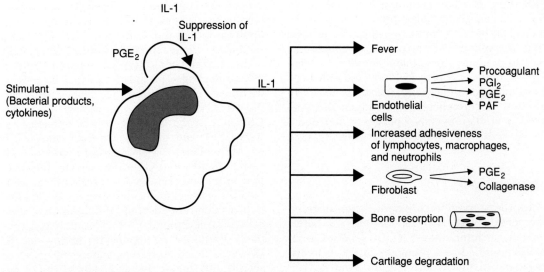

Figure 3–3. Functional effects of monocyte/macrophage-derived interleukin-1. Following an appropriate stimulus, this cell can modulate the phenotypic expression of multiple cell types due to the secretion of this interleukin. PGE_2 = prostaglandin E_2; IL-1 = interleukin-1; PGI_2 = prostacyclin; PAF = platelet-activating factor.

for lymphocytes, monocytes, and neutrophils,[26] and stimulation of procoagulant activity and platelet-activating factor.[148] In addition to monocyte-derived IL-1 at the wound site, endothelial cells also produce IL-1 in response to endotoxin and tumor necrosis factor[149] with the potential for self-regulation of hemostasis functions.

Particularly relevant to the dynamics of the structural changes in the damaged tissue is the effect of IL-1 on connective tissue metabolism. Studies with stimulated human peripheral blood mononuclear cells initially demonstrated that supernatants from these cultures contained a factor, mononuclear cell factor (MCF), that enhanced PGE_2 and collagenase production by synovial adherent cells.[150] Subsequent work demonstrated that MCF could be isolated from purified monocytes,[151] and furthermore that the same effect could be induced with partially purified IL-1[152] and with human recombinant IL-1.[153] Additionally, a monocyte/macrophage factor, likely IL-1, stimulates chondrocytes to degrade their cartilage matrix[154–156] by increasing the production of metalloproteinase.[157] IL-1, which shares amino acid sequence identity with osteoclast-activating factor (OAF),[158] mediates bone resorption when added to bone cultures.[159] While these biological effects of IL-1 may promote degradation of damaged tissues at a site of tissue injury, IL-1 is also instrumental in regulating repair of the damaged tissue. IL-1 enhances fibroblast proliferation[160, 161] by stimulating fibroblasts to produce PDGF, which acts in an autocrine fashion to induce fibroblast

DNA synthesis.[162] IL-1 is also important in modulating matrix synthesis.[161] However, overproduction of IL-1 as a result of continued stimulation of the monocyte/macrophage may result in the exaggerated destruction of normal tissue and/or excessive fibrosis responsible for the histopathology associated with certain chronic inflammatory lesions.

IL-1, as the name implies, is involved in the interaction of immunocompetent cells to bring about normal immune functions. Normal activation of T cells requires the presentation of antigen by monocytes/macrophages in the context of the major histocompatibility complex (MHC) and IL-1. B-cell functions may also require IL-1 acting as a cofactor with IL-4 or B-cell–stimulating factor to regulate B-cell antibody production and proliferation.[163, 164]

Tumor Necrosis Factor/Cachectin

Supernatants from monocytes/macrophages exposed to microbial products, such as endotoxin, were shown to contain a factor that caused the necrosis of tumor cells[165, 166] and a factor that suppressed lipoprotein lipase, thereby preventing normal uptake of triglycerides by fat cells, resulting in wasting of the body, or cachexia.[167–169] Purification and subsequent DNA sequencing of both factors revealed that they were homologous and that this single 17,000 dalton protein accounted for the bioactivities previously ascribed to both tumor necrosis factor (TNF) and cachectin.[170–172] Many of the bioactivities induced by TNF/cachectin overlap with those of IL-1, including induction of fever,[173] enhanced fibroblast production of PGE_2 and collagenase,[174] stimulation of cartilage[175] and bone resorption,[176, 177] activation of endothelial cells to produce procoagulant activity[178, 179] and platelet-derived growth factor,[180] and enhanced neutrophil adherence and degranulation.[27] In addition, TNF/cachectin can induce the production of IL-1 by macrophages[181] and endothelial cells[149, 182] and act synergistically with IL-1.[183]

Interleukin-6

Another monocyte/macrophage–derived polypeptide with IL-1–like activities is interferon-β_2, or interleukin-6 (IL-6). IL-6 was originally described as a promoter of B-cell hybridoma and plasmacytoma cell line growth,[184, 185] but, like IL-1, it also induces T-cell proliferation,[186] acute phase proteins,[187] and fever[188] and increases class I human leukocyte antigen (HLA) expression on fibroblasts.[189] Furthermore, IL-1 and IL-6 synergize to induce T-cell proliferation and the release of acute phase proteins.[188] IL-1 induces IL-6 production in fibroblasts,[190] thymocytes, and endothelial cells,[188] further contributing to the complex network of cell-cell interactions in an inflammatory lesion.

Platelet-Derived Growth Factor

Platelet-derived growth factor (PDGF), originally described as a 27 to 31 kDa glycoprotein from activated platelets, is also produced by activated macrophages[191] as a dimer of two polypeptide chains, A and B. PDGF purified from platelets consists predominantly of the A-B isoform, but A-A and B-B dimers have been isolated from other sources.[192, 193] Originally the PDGF glycoprotein receptor[194, 195] was thought to exist as two classes,[196] but the receptor is now known to be a dimer of either α or β subunits.[196] The α subunit binds only the A chain of the PDGF dimer, and the β subunit binds the B chain.

Functionally, PDGF displays chemotactic properties for neutrophils, fibroblasts, and macrophages at low concentrations,[197, 198] whereas at higher concentrations it is a potent mitogen.

Colony-Stimulating Factors

The differentiation of hematopoietic cells from stem cells to progenitor cells and ultimately to mature granulocytes, monocytes/macrophages, and lymphocytes is dependent on specific glycoproteins referred to as colony-stimulating factors (CSFs). In addition to their ability to induce differentiation, these CSFs also modulate various functions of inflammatory cells and as a result may have an important role in wound healing. The four CSFs that have been identified, characterized, and cloned are granulocyte CSF (G-CSF), macrophage CSF (M-CSF or CSF-1), granulocyte-macrophage CSF (GM-CSF), and multilineage CSF (multi-CSF or interleukin-3).[133, 199] Monocytes produce G-CSF, M-CSF, and GM-CSF, which may function in an autocrine and/or paracrine manner. G-CSF, with a molecular weight of 19 kDa, induces differentiation and proliferation of stem cells into neutrophils[133, 199, 200] and is constitutively produced by monocytes at low levels. However, upon activation, monocytes produce significantly higher levels of G-CSF.[201] In addition to growth regulation, G-CSF also increases antibody-dependent cell-mediated cytotoxicity and oxidative metabolism by neutrophils exposed to FMLP.[201]

The monocyte/macrophage also produces the macrophage-specific growth factor M-CSF, a glycosylated 70 to 90 kDa homodimer. In addition to its proliferative and differentiative functions, M-CSF modulates monocyte functions as evidenced by increased RNA synthesis and protein synthesis and the induction of antibody-dependent cell-mediated cytotoxicity.[202, 203] M-CSF also increases macrophage production of PGE, proteinases, IL-1, and TNF.[202, 203]

GM-CSF promotes colony formation by neutrophil, monocyte, eosinophil, and erythroid progenitors.[204] In addition to monocytes/macrophages,[205] this 20 kDa glycoprotein is also produced by activated B cells,[206] virally infected fibroblasts,[207] vascular endothelium,[208, 209] and epidermal cells.[210] Studies with recombinant human GM-CSF have identified many cellular functions that are enhanced when this cytokine is added prior to or with a primary stimulus.[211] For example, while GM-CSF has no direct effect on neutrophil oxidative metabolism, it causes a significant increase in O_2^- production by neutrophils in response to stimulants such as FMLP, C5a, or LTB_4.[212, 213] Neutrophil antibody-dependent cell-mediated cytotoxicity and phagocytosis of opsonized staphylococci are also enhanced by GM-CSF.[214] In addition to promoting neutrophil activity, GM-CSF augments certain monocyte/macrophage functions represented by increased tumoricidal[215] and microbicidal activity,[211] PGE_2 synthesis,[216] and accessory cell function.[211]

Transforming Growth Factors

Transforming growth factors α and β (TGF-α and TGF-β), originally identified as products of other cell types, are also released by activated monocytes.[217, 218] TGF-β is a 25 kDa disulfide-linked homodimeric molecule that was originally defined by its ability to induce anchorage-independent growth of cells that were normally anchorage-dependent[219] but was subsequently shown to have a plethora of biological activities, many of which are important to the sequence of events in inflammation and repair. TGF-$β_1$ and its homologue (70%) TGF-$β_2$ appear in numerous mammalian tissues and are constituents of a family of related peptides, of which TGF-$β_1$ through TGF-$β_6$ have so far been characterized.[335] Three different surface receptors have been identified for TGF-β, including type I (65 kDa), type II (85 to 95 kDa), and type III (250 to 350 kD), which may reflect different functional signaling mechanisms.[220, 221] Monocytes constitutively express mRNA for TGF-β, and when activated these cells synthesize and release TGF-β,[217] which can upregulate its own gene expression in an autocrine fashion.[77, 222] Additionally, picomolar concentrations of TGF-β can initiate monocyte mRNA expression for other growth-promoting peptides, such as TNF-α, IL-1, and PDGF.[222] Since TGF-β is released by macrophages and other cells in latent form, it is likely that a cell-derived enzyme may cleave the latent form to generate biologically active TGF-β. TGF-β appears to inhibit certain macrophage functions such as release of reactive oxygen intermediates[223] while not influencing others such as phagocytosis.

At femtomolar concentrations, TGF-β is a potent chemoattractant for monocytes.[222, 224] Thus TGF-β produced by platelets and monocytes can attract additional monocytes to the site of inflammation. As the monocytes enter the wound they are exposed to increasing concentrations of TGF-β and other cytokines and become activated to produce growth factor and other mediators. These monocyte products, among their other activities, stimulate fibroblasts and smooth muscle cells to proliferate and generate matrix-facilitating connective tissue repair and angiogenesis. Moreover, TGF-β has been shown to directly stimulate fibroblasts to produce collagen and fibronectin in vitro[225–227] and in vivo.[225, 228, 229] Administration of TGF-β to animals promotes formation of granulation tissue[225, 336] and the healing of incisional wounds in rats.[230]

Although TGF-α shares a common nomenclature with TGF-β, these two macrophage-derived peptides are functionally and structurally distinct. TGF-α does, however, have substantial amino acid sequence homology and shares its biological activities with epidermal growth factor (EGF)[231] likely due to their commonality of receptors.[219] EGF stimulates epidermal growth and keratinization, angiogenesis in rabbit cornea models,[232] and proliferation and differentiation of various mesenchymal cell types (for a review see reference 233). Whether TGF-α and EGF mediate the same biological effects in vivo is not clear, although they both increase the rate of angiogenesis and wound repair[234, 235] with TGF-α being more potent.

The macrophage-derived factors discussed thus far have been, for the most part, both mitogenic and chemotactic for a variety of cell types including the cells responsible for angiogenesis and tissue repair. Macrophage-derived interferon-α (IFN-α), on the other hand, appears to inhibit the chemotaxis of fibroblasts exposed to known chemoattractants such as PDGF.[236] Interestingly, IFN-α does not inhibit chemotaxis of actively growing fibroblast populations (i.e., low-density conditions), which may allow for the preferential selection of fibroblast populations with unique phenotypic characteristics that are compatible with the wound healing process.

Monocytes/macrophages produce a host of additional inflammatory mediators, enzymes, adhesion molecules, and cytokines, all of which contribute to the network of cellular and molecular interactions responsible for the orderly sequence of inflammation and tissue repair. Disruption of this complex series of interlinking molecules can presumably lead to impaired healing and potential pathological sequelae.

Lymphocytes

In the absence of an overt infection or other antigenic stimulus, the role of the lymphocyte in nonspecific tissue injury and inflammation is likely not crucial to its resolution. (A detailed discussion of the role of lymphocytes in wound healing is given in Chapter 17.) If, however, the injury is precipitated by a foreign antigen or subject to secondary infection, the lymphocyte becomes an important constituent of the initiation, amplification, and resolution of the inflammatory response. The arrival of lymphocytes at the wound site coincides with that of monocytes, and their activation is dependent on an interaction with these monocytes/macrophages. This interaction involves the processing of foreign antigens or modified host proteins by macrophages and the presentation of these antigens to the lymphocytes initiating lymphocyte proliferation and the secretion of lymphocyte-derived cytokines, which play an important regulatory role in the immune process. These cytokines have been reviewed in detail elsewhere[237] and will be discussed only briefly in this chapter.

Interferon-γ

Gamma interferon (IFN-γ) was the first T-cell cytokine to be described[238] and subsequently sequenced and cloned.[239] Both T-helper/inducer and cytotoxic/suppressor lymphocytes produce IFN-γ, also called immune IFN, following stimulation with mitogens or antigens.[240, 241] When natural IFN-γ was purified from human peripheral blood lymphocytes and run on SDS gels under reducing conditions, two forms, a 25 kDa and a 20 kDa species, were detected.[242] However, when IFN-γ was cloned and expressed in bacterial vectors, the recombinant molecule had an apparent molecular weight of 17 kDa.[239, 243] The differences in molecular weight are related to the carbohydrate levels due to lack of glycosylation on the recombinant IFN-γ. Lymphocytes also produce IFN-α, but IFN-γ accounts for a greater percentage of the cellular protein and has many defined biological activities, in addition to its ability to inhibit viral replication, that are relevant to inflammation (Fig. 3–4).

One of the main targets for IFN-γ is the monocyte/macrophage.[244] Modulation of human monocyte functions by this cytokine occurs through its interaction with specific monocyte receptors.[245] Subsequent to this receptor-ligand interaction, IFN-γ enhances monocyte antimicrobial activity and the release of reactive oxygen intermediates.[246] Additionally, IFN-γ stimulates the secretion of a cascade of monocyte/macrophage products, most notably TNF-α,[247, 248] IL-1,[248, 249] plasminogen activator,[248] and 1,25-dihydroxyvitamin D_3.[250, 251] Interferon-γ also enhances Fc,[252–254] Ia,[255] and IL-2 receptors[79, 81] on monocytes. Moreover, IFN-γ also induces monocytes to form giant cells.[256]

Although IFN-γ is a potent promoter of monocyte activation, it appears to selectively inhibit certain monocyte functions. The ability of IFN-γ to decrease prostaglandin synthesis[257–260] may account for the enhancement of some of the functions mentioned previously, since prostaglandins, particularly PGE_2, suppress many monocyte activities. It should be noted that under certain experimental conditions, IFN-γ can also increase prostaglandin

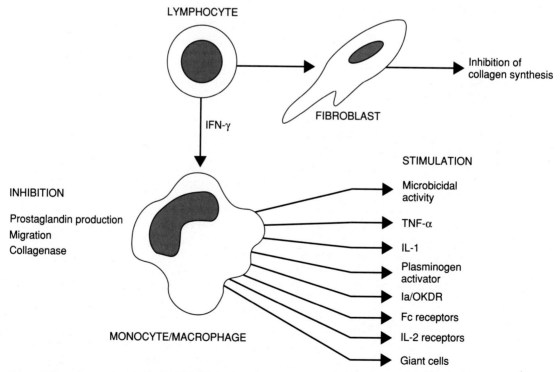

Figure 3–4. Effect of lymphocyte-derived interferon-γ on monocyte/macrophage and fibroblast function. IFNγ = interferon-γ; TNFα = tumor necrosis factor-α; IL-1 = interleukin-1; IL-2 = interleukin-2.

synthesis.[261] An additional effect of IFN-γ is the inhibition of monocyte migration,[262] which may promote the retention of these cells at the inflammatory site.

In addition to monocytes, IFN-γ also modulates the functions of other target cells. Increased Fc receptor expression on neutrophils following IFN-γ treatment[254] facilitates antibody-dependent cytotoxicity.[263] Endothelial Ia expression[264] and glycosaminoglycan synthesis[265] are increased by IFN-γ. The ability of IFN-γ to suppress fibroblast collagen synthesis[266-268] suggests that this cytokine may regulate the amount of collagen synthesized in the wound repair process.

Interleukin-2

In 1976, a T-cell growth factor (TCGF) that stimulated the proliferation of antigen- or lectin-induced T-lymphocyte blasts and sustained normal T cells in long-term culture was first identified.[269] Purification revealed that what had previously been considered as several different mitogenic lymphokines had the same molecular weight and were actually the same factor, then termed interleukin-2 (IL-2).[270] Subsequently, IL-2 was cloned and cDNA expressed for this molecule.[271, 272] Synthesized initially as a 17,632 dalton molecule, IL-2 is then converted to a 15,420 dalton protein as a result of the loss of a 20 amino acid signal peptide. Both helper/inducer (CD4) and cytotoxic/suppressor (CD8) T cells produce IL-2,[273] which is required to promote the transition from G_1 to the S phase of the cell cycle of activated T cells.[274] In addition to its primary growth-promoting effect on T cells, IL-2 stimulates T cell–derived B-cell growth factor[275] and IFN-γ synthesis,[276] augmenting the cascade effect of this cytokine. IL-2 also enhances tumoricidal activity of lymphocytes and natural killer cells.[277]

Structure-function analysis of the T-cell receptor (Tac) for IL-2 was facilitated through the use of a monoclonal antibody directed against this antigen (anti-Tac).[278, 279] The receptor identified by anti-Tac has a molecular weight of 55 kDa[280, 281] and activated T cells, but not resting T cells, contain both high-affinity (2 to 50 pM) and low-affinity (10 to 30 nM) receptors.[282] Although the high-affinity receptors constitute only 2 to 10 percent of the total IL-2 receptors, ligand binding to these receptors transduces the growth-promoting IL-2 signal[282, 283] and regulates the internalization of IL-2.[284, 285] In addition to the Tac protein, another IL-2 binding protein with a molecular weight of 70 to 75 kDa (p70 protein) has recently been identified.[286-288]

Cells that express only low-affinity binding may have either Tac or the p70 protein, whereas cells with the high-affinity binding express both proteins.[288, 289] These observations suggest a multichain model for the high-affinity interaction of Tac and p70 with IL-2.[288]

Not only T cells can be induced to express IL-2 receptors: upon activation, B cells become IL-2 receptor–positive[290, 291] with IL-2 dependent regulation of maturation and immunoglobulin secretion. As previously discussed, monocytes that are stimulated by bacterial products or IFN-γ transcribe and translate IL-2 receptors and become susceptible to IL-2–dependent regulation of microbicidal activity[81] and IL-1 synthesis.[292]

Interleukins-3 Through 8

Activated lymphocytes generate a host of additional lymphokines that are involved in the amplification and regulation of the host immune response. According to current nomenclature, these have been designated interleukins-3 through 8. Interleukin-3 (IL-3), or multilineage-CSF (multi-CSF), stimulates the replication of pluripotent stem cells as well as precursor cells of all hematopoietic lineages.[133] This 20 kDa molecule is expressed in low levels by activated T cells.[133]

Interleukin-4 (IL-4) was originally identified as a T-cell–derived B-cell growth factor and termed B-cell stimulatory factor 1 (BSF-1).[293] This 20 kDa cytokine causes resting B cells to enter S phase in response to certain stimuli,[294] express Ia antigen,[295-297] and increase their secretion of IgG₁ and IgE in the presence of lipopolysaccharide.[298, 299] IL-4 can co-stimulate growth of resting T cells[300] and stimulate T-cell and mast cell line growth.[301] Another important function of IL-4 is its ability to increase monocyte/macrophage expression of major histocompatibility class II antigen[302, 303] as well as receptors for C3bi and p150.95 antigen, which are two members of the lymphocyte function–associated antigen (LFA). Evidence suggests that IL-4 decreases monocyte IL-1 production.[303] Receptors for BSF-1/IL-4 have been demonstrated on B and T cells, macrophages, mast cells, and undifferentiated hematopoietic cell lines,[304] favoring its potential widespread functional impact.

The term interleukin-5 (IL-5) encompasses activities originally defined under T-cell–replacing factor (TRF)[305, 306] and B-cell growth factor-II (BCGF-II).[307] Activities ascribed to this lymphokine include B-cell differentiation and regulation of proliferation. Although IL-5 induces the secretion of IgA by B cells, unlike IL-4, IL-5 has no effect on IgG subclasses or IgM synthesis.[308–310] Less well characterized biological effects of IL-5 include acting on T cells to induce cytotoxic T-cell generation.[305]

Interleukin-6 (IL-6), produced by both lymphocytes[311] and monocytes,[311, 312] has multiple biological effects in immune regulation. IL-6, identical to interferon-β_2[190] and B-cell stimulatory factor-2 (BSF-2),[313, 314] induces the final maturation of activated B-cells into antibody-producing cells.[315, 316] Interleukin-6 also functions in the regulation of differentiation of hematopoietic stem cells similar to multi-CSF,[317] stimulation of hepatocytes,[318] enhancement of myeloma growth,[319] as a second signal for IL-2 production by T cells,[320] and as a helper factor in the induction of cytotoxic T cells.[321, 322] Furthermore, IL-6 may contribute to the fibroblastic response associated with inflammatory lesions.[323]

Interleukin-8 (IL-8) was originally isolated from LPS-activated peripheral blood monocytes and shown to be a potent chemoattractant for neutrophils.[324] It is a 72 amino acid residue protein (8000 daltons) and is synonymous with monocyte-derived neutrophil chemotactic factor (MDNCF) and neutrophil-activating peptide (NAP-1). IL-8 is induced by IL-1 and TNF-α, as well as LPS.[325] In addition, other cells have been shown to produce IL-8,[326] and it is capable of mediating additional functions of neutrophils, including the stimulation of lysozyme release and the oxidative burst.[327] This protein has been shown to be active in vivo, where it can produce plasma leakage from the vasculature and promote neutrophil accumulation.[328] The receptor for this interleukin has recently been cloned.[329]

CHRONIC INFLAMMATION

The acute inflammatory response includes altered vascular permeability, the release of inflammatory mediators, and the infiltration of leukocytes to sequester and eliminate injured tissue and/or foreign antigens. As the leukocytes engulf and degrade the damaged tissue, they also release inflammatory mediators necessary for the infiltration and activation of mononuclear cells. If these cellular elements succeed in eliminating the inflammatory stimulus, tissue repair begins with resolution of the inflammation. If the inflammatory stimulus persists, continued recruitment and activation of mononuclear cells occurs with the development of a chronic inflammatory lesion.

Continued activation of the mononuclear cells causes the chronic secretion of inflammatory cytokines, which amplify and perpetuate the inflammatory response. Secretion is a major function of the mononuclear phagocytes and the release of neutral proteases, hydrolases, complement components, coagulation factors, and polypeptide hormones contributes not only to the protective, but also the detrimental, aspects of inflammation. In a chronic lesion, macrophages continue to generate many of the products that were secreted in the acute phase of the response, but the accumulation of these molecules may alter the outcome of the host response, often leading to pathological tissue destruction.[78] Monocyte products contribute to lymphocyte accumulation and activation with lymphokine secretion. Lymphokines, in turn, augment monocyte cytokine synthesis, characteristic of the cyclic, self-perpetuating nature of these responses. Exposure of peripheral blood monocytes to lymphokines (IFN-γ, GM-CSF) or bacterial products (endotoxin) triggers an increase in steady state levels of mRNA for IL-1, TNF, and certain other monokines.[330] Thus, many of these monocyte-derived mediators are inducible, not being expressed and secreted until the cells are exposed to inflammatory stimuli in vitro or in vivo. In a cell-mediated immune response, lymphokines are particularly important to the regulation of macrophage function and the evolution of the lesion.

In addition to the enzymes, inhibitors, and lipid molecules generated by macrophages within a chronic inflammatory locus, these persistently activated cells release an array of polypeptide hormones that interact with various target tissues and cells in an endocrine, paracrine, and/or autocrine fashion. These cytokines contribute to the activation of the other cell populations and the chronicity of these lesions.

CONNECTIVE TISSUE RECONSTITUTION

Tissue repair begins as the host sequesters and degrades the inflammatory stimulus (a process reviewed elsewhere in this book). Although fibroblast accumulation becomes obvious only late in the response, the stage was set for these events from the onset of the inflammation. Inflammatory products released by the complement system, activated platelets, and endothelial cells contribute to fibroblast recruitment and proliferation. Platelets release platelet factor 4, PDGF, and TGF-β, which contribute to fibroblast recruitment. Infiltrating monocytes and lymphocytes generate additional chemotactic factors including LDCF-F, LTB$_4$, PDGF, and TGF-β to recruit fibroblasts.[330]

Accumulation of fibroblasts is the result of recruitment and of proliferation regulated by fibroblast growth factors. Platelets, lymphocytes, and monocytes/macrophages produce a series of polypeptide growth factors that are mitogenic for fibroblasts and for endothelial cells. These growth factors are produced following activation of the cells by various stimuli in the inflammatory environment. IL-1 plays a role in neovascularization and tissue repair in collaboration with TNF-α.[331] Monocytes also produce PDGF,[191, 332] which has chemotactic activity for leukocytes and fibroblasts and also promotes fibroblast growth following binding to its high-affinity protein kinase receptor.[198] Monocyte-derived basic FGF,[333] PDGF,[332] and TGF-β promote angiogenic activity necessary for the formation of granulation tissue,[334] fibroblast proliferation, and matrix synthesis.

Transforming growth factor-β and many of the other growth factors in addition to regulating growth stimulate formation of collagen, fibronectin, and other matrix components by fibroblasts and have potent angiogenic activity.[225] Further stimulation of fibroblast matrix synthesis by IL-1, TNF, and PDGF leads to scar formation and repair of the tissue injury. Remodeling of scar tissue depends on collagenase produced by fibroblasts and macrophages, and normally this is accomplished with minimal or no scarring. In a chronic inflammatory response this healing process can become excessive due to continued secretion of fibroblast-active cytokines with the potential for tissue pathology. Exaggerated matrix deposition is characteristic of certain chronic inflammatory lesions and granulomatous responses, exemplified by schistosomiasis, pulmonary fibrosis, and hepatic cirrhosis. Chronic secretion of inflammatory cell–derived enzymes and mediators in certain other sites can result in destruction of the tissue, such as in arthritis.

CONCLUSION

Inflammation is a complex tissue response to injury or antigen, which comprises (1) increased vasodilation and vascular permeability with extravasation of fluids and (2) emigration of leukocytes from the circulation to the tissues where they proliferate and are activated to regulate healing and repair. Regardless of the inciting agent, the mechanisms of host defense are amazingly consistent and are manifested clinically as pain, heat, redness, and swelling. The inflammatory response functions to degrade, eliminate, or sequester pathogens or injured tissue as the leukocytes mobilize to protect the host from injury. A network of cell-cell interactions propelled by peptide and lipid molecular signals initiates and maintains inflammation by acting on endothelial cells, triggering leukocyte recruitment, and augmenting the biochemical, endocytic, and synthetic activities of the phagocytic leukocytes. Furthermore, when the inflammatory stimulus is antigenic in nature, T cells and their secreted products add another level of amplification and complexity to the host response. Continued definition of these cascading mediator-cell and cell-cell interactions will contribute important insight into the physiological and pathological events associated with inflammation and repair.

References

1. Ross R: Wound healing. Sci Am 220:40–55, 1969.
2. Hugo NE, Thompson LW, Zook EG, et al: Effect of chronic anemia on the tensile strength of healing wounds. Surgery 66:741–745, 1969.
3. Macon WL, Pories WJ: Effect of iron deficiency anemia on wound healing. Surgery 69:792–796, 1967.
4. Stein JM, Levenson SM: Effect of the inflammatory reaction on subsequent wound healing. Surg Forum 17:484–485, 1966.
5. Simpson DM, Ross R: The neutrophilic leukocyte in wound repair. A study with antineutrophil serum. J Clin Invest 51:2009–2023, 1972.
6. Wahl SM, Arend WP, Ross R: The effect of complement depletion on wound healing. Am J Pathol 74:73–83, 1974.
7. Leibovich SJ, Ross R: The role of the macrophage in wound repair: A study with hydrocortisone and anti-macrophage serum. Am J Pathol 78:71–91, 1975.
8. Barnes MJ, Bailey AJ, Gordon JL, et al: Platelet aggregation by basement membrane–associated collagens. Thromb Res 18:375–388, 1980.
9. Chiang TM, Mainardi CL, Seyer JM, et al: Collagen platelet interaction. Type V (A-B) collagen induces platelet aggregation. J Lab Clin Med 95:99–107, 1980.
10. Tryggvason K, Oikarinen J, Viinikka L, et al: Effects of laminin, proteoglycan and type IV collagen, components of basement membranes, on platelet aggregation. Biochem Biophys Res Commun 100:233–239, 1981.
11. Legrand YJ, Fauvel F, Arbeille B, et al: Activation of platelets by microfibrils and collagen. A comparative study. Lab Invest 54:566–573, 1986.
12. Meyer D, Baumgartner HR: Role of von Willebrand factor in platelet adhesion to the subendothelium. Br J Haematol 54:1–9, 1983.
13. Jaffe EA, Hoyer LW, Nachman RL: Synthesis of von Willebrand factor by cultured human endothelial cells. Proc Natl Acad Sci USA 71:1906–1909, 1974.
14. Jaffe EA: Endothelial cells. In Gallin JI, Goldstein IM, Snyderman R (eds): Inflammation: Basic Principles and Clinical Correlates. New York, Raven Press, 1988, pp 559–576.

15. Weksler BB: Platelets. In Gallin JI, Goldstein IM, Snyderman R (eds): Inflammation: Basic Principles and Clinical Correlates. New York, Raven Press, 1988, pp 543–557.

16. Bennett JS, Vilaire G: Exposure of platelet fibrinogen receptors by ADP and epinephrine. J Clin Invest 64:1393–1401, 1979.

17. Pidard D, Montgomery RR, Bennett JS, et al: Interaction of AP-2, a monoclonal antibody specific for the human platelet glycoprotein IIb-IIIa complex, with intact platelets. J Biol Chem 258:12582–12586, 1983.

18. Baldassare JJ, Kahn RA, Knipp MA, et al: Reconstitution of platelet proteins into phospholipid vesicles: Functional proteoliposomes. J Clin Invest 75:35–39, 1985.

19. Hoover RL, Briggs RT, Karnovsky MJ: The adhesive interaction between polymorphonuclear leukocytes and endothelial cells in vitro. Cell 14:423–428, 1978.

20. Smith RPC, Lackie JM, Wilkinson PC: The effects of chemotactic factors on the adhesiveness of rabbit neutrophil granulocytes. Exp Cell Res 122:169–177, 1979.

21. Gimbrone MA Jr, Brock AF, Schafer AI: Leukotriene B₄ stimulates polymorphonuclear leukocyte adhesion to cultured vascular endothelial cells. J Clin Invest 74:1552–1555, 1984.

22. Tonnesen MG, Smedly LA, Henson PM: Neutrophil-endothelial cell interactions: Modulation of neutrophil adhesiveness induced by complement fragments C5a and C5a des Arg and formyl-methionyl-leucyl-phenylalanine. J Clin Invest 74:1581–1592, 1984.

23. Bussolino F, Breviaro F, Tetta C, et al: Interleukin 1 stimulates platelet-activating factor production in cultured human endothelial cells. J Clin Invest 77:2027–2033, 1986.

24. McIntyre TM, Zimmerman GA, Prescott SM: Leukotrienes C4 and D4 stimulate human endothelial cells to synthesize platelet-activating factor and bind neutrophils. Proc Natl Acad Sci USA 83:2204–2208, 1986.

25. Prescott SM, Zimmerman GA, McIntyre TM: Human endothelial cells in culture produce platelet-activating factor (1-alkyl-2-acetyl-sn-glycero-3-phosphocholine) when stimulated with thrombin. Proc Natl Acad Sci USA 81:3534–3538, 1984.

26. Bevilacqua MP, Pober JS, Wheeler ME, et al: Interleukin 1 acts on cultured human vascular endothelium to increase the adhesion of polymorphonuclear leukocytes, monocytes, and related leukocyte cell lines. J Clin Invest 76:2003–2011, 1985.

27. Gamble JR, Harlan JM, Klebanoff SJ, et al: Stimulation of the adherence of neutrophils to umbilical vein endothelium by human recombinant tumor necrosis factor. Proc Natl Acad Sci USA 82:8667–8671, 1985.

28. Pohlman TH, Stanness KA, Beatty PG, et al: An endothelial cell surface factor(s) induced in vitro by lipopolysaccharide, interleukin 1, and tumor necrosis factor-α increases neutrophil adherence by a CDα18-dependent mechanism. J Immunol 136:4548–4553, 1986.

29. Schleimer RP, Rutledge BK: Cultured human vascular endothelial cells acquire adhesiveness for neutrophils after stimulation with interleukin 1, endotoxin, and tumor-promoting phorbol diesters. J Immunol 136:649–654, 1986.

30. Wright DG, Gallin JI: Secretory responses of human neutrophils: exocytosis of specific (secondary) granules by human neutrophils during adherence in vitro and during exudation in vivo. J Immunol 123:285–294, 1979.

31. Janoff A: Elastase in tissue injury. Ann Rev Med 36:207–216, 1985.

32. Malech HL: Phagocytic cells: Egress from marrow and diapedesis. In Gallin JI, Goldstein IM, Snyderman R (eds): Inflammation: Basic Principles and Clinical Correlates. New York, Raven Press, 1988, pp 297–308.

33. Sklar A, Jesaitis AJ, Painter RG: The neutrophil N-formyl peptide receptor: Dynamics of ligand-receptor interaction and their relationship to cellular responses. Contemp Top Immunobiol 14:29–82, 1984.

34. Ohura K, Katona IM, Wahl LM, et al: Co-expression of chemotactic ligand receptors on human peripheral blood monocytes. J Immunol 138:2633–2639, 1987.

35. Snyderman R, Uhing RJ: Phagocytic cells: Stimulus-response coupling mechanisms. In Gallin JI, Goldstein IM, Snyderman R (eds): Inflammation: Basic Principles and Clinical Correlates. New York, Raven Press, 1988, pp 309–323.

36. Gilman AG: G proteins and dual control of adenylate cyclase. Cell 36:577–579, 1984.

37. Kay AB, Glass J, Salter DM: Leucoattractants enhance complement receptors on human phagocytic cells. Clin Exp Immunol 38:294–299, 1979.

38. Fearon DT, Collins LA: Increased expression of C3b receptors on polymorphonuclear leukocytes induced by chemotactic factors and by purification procedures. J Immunol 130:370–375, 1983.

39. Berger M, O'Shea J, Cross AS, et al: Human neutrophils increase expression of C3bi as well as C3b receptors upon activation. J Clin Invest 74:1566–1571, 1984.

40. Todd RF III, Arnaout MA, Rosin RE, et al: Subcellular localization of the large subunit of Mol (Mol; formerly gp 110), a surface glycoprotein associated with neutrophil adhesion. J Clin Invest 74:1280–1290, 1984.

41. O'Shea JJ, Brown EJ, Seligmann BE, et al: Evidence for distinct intracellular pools of receptors for C3b and C3bi in human neutrophils. J Immunol 134:2580–2587, 1985.

42. Wright SD, Meyer BC: Phorbol esters cause sequential activation and deactivation of complement receptors on polymorphonuclear leukocytes. J Immunology 136:1759–1764, 1986.

43. Rossi F, Zatti M: Biochemical aspects of phagocytosis in polymorphonuclear leukocytes: NADH and NADPH oxidation by the granules of resting and phagocytizing cells. Experientia 20:21–23, 1964.

44. Babior BM, Curnutte JT, Kipnes RS: Pyridine nucleotide-dependent superoxide production by a cell-free system from human granulocytes. J Clin Invest 56:1035–1042, 1975.

45. Gabig TG, Babior BM: The O_2^- forming oxidase responsible for the respiratory burst in human neutrophils: Properties of the solubilized enzyme. J Biol Chem 254:9070–9074, 1979.

46. Nakamura M, Baxter CR, Masters BSS: Simultaneous demonstration of phagocytosis-connected oxygen consumption and corresponding NAD(P)H oxidase activity: Direct evidence for NADPH as the predominant electron donor to oxygen in phagocytizing human neutrophils. Biochem Biophys Res Commun 98:743–751, 1981.

47. Green TR, Shaefer RE, Makler MT: Orientation of the NADPH dependent superoxide generating oxidoreductase of the outer membrane of human PMNs. Biochem Biophys Res Commun 94:262–269, 1980.

48. Babior GL, Rosin RE, McMurrich BJ, et al: Arrangement of the respiratory burst oxidase in the plasma membrane of the neutrophil. J Clin Invest 67:1724–1728, 1981.

49. Klebanoff SJ: Phagocytic cells: products of oxygen

metabolism. In Gallin JI, Goldstein IM, Snyderman R (eds): Inflammation: Basic Principles and Clinical Correlates. New York, Raven Press, 1988, pp 391–444.

50. Rabani J, Klug D, Fridovich I: Decay of the HO_2^- and O_2^- radicals catalyzed by superoxide dismutase: A pulse radiolytic investigation. Isr J Chem 10:1095–1106, 1972.

51. Halliwell B, Gutteridge JMC: The role of transition metals in superoxide-mediated toxicity. In Oberley LW (ed): Superoxide Dismutase, vol III. Boca Raton, FL, CRC Press, 1985, pp 45–82.

52. Weiss SJ, Klein R, Slivka A: Chlorination of taurine by human neutrophils: Evidence for hypochlorous acid generation. J Clin Invest 70:598–607, 1982.

53. Thomas EL, Grisham MB, Jefferson MM: Myeloperoxidase-dependent effect of amines on functions of isolated neutrophils. J Clin Invest 72:411–454, 1983.

54. Klebanoff SJ, Clark RA: The Neutrophil: Function and Clinical Disorders. Amsterdam, North Holland, 1978.

55. Sips HJ, Hamers MN: Mechanism of the bactericidal action of myeloperoxidase: Increased permeability of the *Escherichia coli* cell envelope. Infect Immun 31:11–16, 1981.

56. Albrich JM, Gilbaugh JH III, Callahan KB, et al: Effects of the putative neutrophil-generating toxin, hypochlorous acid, on membrane permeability and transport systems of *Escherichia coli*. J Clin Invest 78:176–184, 1986.

57. Strauss RR, Paul BB, Jacobs AA, et al: Role of the phagocyte in host parasite interactions. XXVII. Myeloperoxidase-H_2O_2-Cl^--mediated aldehyde formation and its relationship to antimicrobial activity. Infect Immun 3:595–602, 1971.

58. Thomas EL: Myeloperoxidase–hydrogen peroxide–chloride antimicrobial system: Effect of exogenous amines on antibacterial action against *Escherichia coli*. Infect Immun 25:110–116, 1979.

59. Haber F, Weiss J: The catalytic decomposition of hydrogen peroxide by iron salts. Proc R Soc Lond 147:332–357, 1934.

60. Ambruso DR, Johnston RB: Lactoferrin enhances hydroxyl radical production by human neutrophils, neutrophil particulate fractions, and an enzymatic generating system. J Clin Invest 67:352–360, 1981.

61. Hirsch JC: Phagocytin: A bactericidal substance from polymorphonuclear leukocytes. J Exp Med 103:589–611, 1956.

62. Hirsch JG: Antimicrobial factors in tissues and phagocytic cells. Bacteriol Rev 21:133–147, 1960.

63. Weiss J, Ooi CE, Elsbach P: Structural and immunological dissection of highly conserved neutrophil bactericidal/permeability-increasing proteins. Clin Res 34:537A, 1986.

64. Weiss J, Olsson I: Cellular and subcellular localization of the bactericidal/permeability-increasing protein of neutrophils. Blood 69:652–659, 1987.

65. Elsbach P, Weiss J: A reevaluation of the roles of the O_2-dependent and O_2-independent microbicidal systems of phagocytes. Rev Infect Dis 5:843–853, 1983.

66. Elsbach P, Weiss J: Oxygen-dependent and oxygen-independent mechanisms of microbicidal activity of neutrophils. Immunol Lett 11:159–163, 1985.

67. Zeya HI, Spitznagel JK: Cationic proteins of polymorphonuclear leukocytes. II. Composition, properties and mechanisms of antibacterial action. Acta Chem Scand 91:755–762, 1966.

68. Zeya HI, Spitznagel JK: Arginine-rich proteins of polymorphonuclear leukocyte lysosomes. Antimicrobial specificity and biochemical heterogeneity. J Exp Med 127:927–941, 1968.

69. Ganz T, Selsted ME, Szklarek D, et al: Natural peptide antibiotics of human neutrophils. J Clin Invest 76:1427–1435, 1985.

70. Selsted ME, Harwig SSL, Ganz T, et al: Primary structures of three human neutrophil defensins. J Clin Invest 76:1436–1439, 1985.

71. Odeberg H, Olsson I, Venge P: Antibacterial cationic proteins of human granulocytes. J Clin Invest 56:1118–1124, 1975.

72. Janoff A, Scherer J: Mediators of inflammation in leukocyte lysosomes. IX. Elastinolytic activity in granules of human polymorphonuclear leukocytes. J Exp Med 128:1137–1155, 1968.

73. Lazarus GS, Brown RS, Daniels JR, et al: Human granulocyte collagenase. Science 159:1483–1485, 1968.

74. Chenoweth DE, Hugli TE: Demonstration of a specific receptor for human C5a anaphylatoxin on murine macrophages. J Exp Med 156:68–78, 1982.

75. Van Epps DE, Chenoweth DE: Analysis of the binding of fluorescent C5a and C3a to human peripheral blood leukocytes. J Immunol 132:2862–2867, 1984.

76. Grotendorst GR, Smale G, Pencer D: Production of transforming growth factor-β by human peripheral blood monocytes and neutrophils. J Cell Physiol 140:396–402, 1989.

77. Wahl SM, Hunt DA, Wakefield LM, et al: Transforming growth factor type β induces monocyte chemotaxis and growth factor production. Proc Natl Acad Sci USA 84:5788–5792, 1987.

78. Wahl SM: Acute and chronic inflammation. In Asherson GL, Zembala M (eds): Human Monocytes. New York, Academic Press, 1989, pp 361–371.

79. Herrmann F, Cannistra SA, Levine H, et al: Expression of interleukin 2 receptors and binding of interleukin 2 by gamma interferon–induced human leukemic and normal monocytic cells. J Exp Med 162:1111–1116, 1985.

80. Holter W, Grunow R, Stockinger H, et al: Recombinant interferon-γ induces interleukin 2 receptors on human peripheral blood monocytes. J Immunol 136:2171–2175, 1986.

81. Wahl SM, McCartney-Francis N, Hunt DA, et al: Monocyte interleukin 2 receptor gene expression and interleukin 2 augmentation of microbicidal activity. J Immunol 139:1342–1347, 1987.

82. Parker CW: Mediators: Release and function. In Paul WE (ed): Fundamental Immunology. New York, Raven Press, 1984, pp 697–747.

83. Cantarow WD, Cheung HT, Sundharadas G: Effects of prostaglandins on the spreading, adhesion and migration of mouse peritoneal macrophages. Prostaglandins 16:39–46, 1978.

84. Moore RN, Urbaschek R, Wahl LM, et al: Prostaglandin regulation of colony-stimulating factor production by lipopolysaccharide-stimulated murine leukocytes. Infect Immun 26:408–414, 1979.

85. Kurland JI, Broxmeyer HE, Pelus LM, et al: Role for monocyte-macrophage–derived colony-stimulating factor and prostaglandin E in the positive and negative feedback control of myeloid stem cell proliferation. Blood 52:388–407, 1978.

86. Snyder DS, Beller DI, Unanue ER: Prostaglandins modulate macrophage Ia expression. Nature 299:163–165, 1982.

87. Kunkel SL, Chensue SW: Arachidonic acid metabolites regulate interleukin-1 production. Biochem Biophys Res Commun 128:892–897, 1985.

88. Wahl LM, Olsen CE, Sandberg AL, et al: Prostaglandin regulation of macrophage collagenase production. Proc Natl Acad Sci USA 74:4955–4958, 1977.

89. Razin E, Bauminger S, Globerson A: Effect of prostaglandins on phagocytosis of sheep erythrocytes by mouse peritoneal macrophages. J Reticuloendothel Soc 23:237–242, 1978.

90. Gordon D, Bray M, Morley J: Control of lymphokine secretion by prostaglandins. Nature 262:401–407, 1976.

91. Goodwin JS, Messner RP, Peake GT: Prostaglandin suppression of mitogen-stimulated lymphocytes in vitro. J Clin Invest 62:753–760, 1978.

92. Van Epps D: Suppression of human lymphocyte migration by PGE_2. Inflammation 5:81–87, 1981.

93. Ford-Hutchinson AW: Leukotriene B_4 and neutrophil function: A review. J R Soc Med 74:831–833, 1981.

94. Moqbel R, Sass-Kuhn SP, Goetzl EJ, et al: Enhancement of neutrophil- and eosinophil-mediated complement-dependent killing of schistosomula of Schistosoma mansoni in vitro by leukotriene B4. Clin Exp Immunol 52:519–527, 1983.

95. Rola-Pleszczynski M: Immunoregulation by leukotrienes and other lipoxygenase metabolites. Immunol Today 6:302–307, 1985.

96. Rola-Pleszczynski M, Borgeat P, Sirois P: Leukotriene B_4 induces human suppressor lymphocytes. Biochem Biophys Res Commun 108:1531–1537, 1982.

97. Payan DG, Goetzl EJ: Specific suppression of human lymphocyte function by leukotriene B_4. J Immunol 131:551–553, 1983.

98. Gualde N, Atluru D, Goodwin JS: Effect of lipoxygenase metabolites of arachidonic acid on proliferation of human T cells and T cell subsets. J Immunol 134:1125–1129, 1985.

99. Payan DG, Missirian-Bastian A, Goetzl EJ: Human T-lymphocyte subset specificity of the regulatory effects of leukotriene B_4. Proc Natl Acad Sci USA 81:3501–3505, 1984.

100. Rola-Pleszczynski M: Differential effects of leukotriene B_4 on $T4^+$ and $T8^+$ lymphocyte phenotype and immunoregulatory functions. J Immunol 135:1357–1360, 1985.

101. Goodman MG, Weigle WO: Modulation of lymphocyte activation. Inhibition by an oxidation product of arachidonic acid. J Immunol 125:593–600, 1980.

102. Bailey JM, Bryant RW, Low CE, et al: Regulation of T lymphocyte mitogenesis by the leukocyte product 15-hydroxyeicosatetranoic acid (15-HETE). Cell Immunol 67:112–120, 1982.

103. Webb DR, Nowowiejski I, Healy C, et al: Immunosuppressive properties of leukotriene D_4 and E_4 in vitro. Biochem Biophys Res Commun 104:1617–1622, 1982.

104. Svenson M, Bisgaard H, Bendtzen K: Effects of leukotrienes on neutrophil migration, and on production and action of lymphokines. Allergy 39:481–484, 1984.

105. Myers MJ, Ades EW, Jackson WT, et al: Possible in vivo modulation of the immune system by the leukotriene, LTB_4. J Clin Lab Immunol 15:205–209, 1984.

106. Johnson HM, Torres BA: Leukotrienes: Positive signals for regulation of gamma-interferon production. J Immunol 132:413–416, 1984.

107. Rola-Pleszczynski M, Gagnon L, Sirois P: Leukotriene B_4 augments human natural cytotoxic cell activity. Biochem Biophys Res Commun 113:531–533, 1983.

108. Rola-Pleszczynski M, Gagnon L, Sirois P: Natural cytotoxic cell activity enhanced by leukotrienes (LT) A_4 and B_4, but not by stereoisomers of LTB_4 or HETEs. Prostaglandins Leukotrienes Med 13:113–117, 1984.

109. Wahl LM, Wahl SM, Mergenhagen SE, et al: Collagenase production by endotoxin activated macrophages. Proc Natl Acad Sci USA 71:3598–3601, 1974.

110. Werb Z, Gordon S: Secretion of a specific collagenase by stimulated macrophages. J Exp Med 142:346–360, 1975.

111. Horowitz AL, Crystal RG: Collagenase from rabbit pulmonary alveolar macrophages. Biochem Biophys Res Commun 69:296–303, 1976.

112. Birkedal-Hansen H, Cobb CM, Taylor RE, et al: In vivo and in vitro stimulation of collagenase production by rabbit alveolar macrophages. Arch Oral Biol 21:21–25, 1976.

113. Evans CH, Mears DC, Cosgrove JL: Release of neutral proteinases from mononuclear phagocytes and synovial cells in response to cartilaginous wear particles in vitro. Biochem Biophys Acta 677:287–294, 1981.

114. Wahl LM: Collagenase production by human monocytes. J Dent Res 63:338a, 1984.

115. Louie JS, Weiss J, Ryhänen KM, et al: The production of collagenase by adherent mononuclear cells cultured from human peripheral blood. Arthritis Rheum 27:1397–1404, 1984.

116. Wahl LM, Lampel LL: Regulation of human peripheral blood monocyte collagenase by prostaglandins and anti-inflammatory drugs. Cell Immunol 105:411–422, 1987.

117. Wahl LM, Wahl SM, Mergenhagen SE, et al: Collagenase production by lymphokine-activated macrophages. Science 187:261–263, 1975.

118. McCarthy JB, Wahl SM, Rees J, et al: Mediation of macrophage collagenase production by 3′-5′ cyclic adenosine monophosphate. J Immunol 124:2405–2409, 1980.

119. Prosser FH, Wahl LM: Involvement of the ornithine decarboxylase pathway in macrophage collagenase production. Arch Biochem Biophys 260:218–225, 1988.

120. Werb Z: Biochemical actions of glucocorticoids on macrophages in culture. Specific inhibition of elastase, collagenase, and plasminogen activator secretion and effects on other metabolic functions. J Exp Med 147:1695–1712, 1978.

121. Wahl LM, Winter CC: Regulation of guinea pig macrophage collagenase production by dexamethasone and colchicine. Arch Biochem Biophys 230:661–667, 1984.

122. Hirata F, Schiffmann E, Venkatasubramanian K, et al: A phospholipase A_2 inhibitory protein in rabbit neutrophils induced by glucocorticoids. Proc Natl Acad Sci USA 77:2533–2538, 1980.

123. Blackwell GJ, Carnuccio R, DiRosa M, et al: Macrocortin: A polypeptide causing the anti-phospholipase effect of glucocorticoids. Nature 287:147–149, 1980.

124. Davidson FF, Dennis EA, Powell M, et al: Inhibition of phospholipase A_2 by "lipocortins" and calpactins: An effect of binding to substrate phospholipids. J Biol Chem 262:1698–1705, 1987.

125. Nathan CF: Secretory products of macrophages. J Clin Invest 79:319–326, 1987.

126. Auron PE, Webb AC, Rosenwasser LJ, et al: Nucleotide sequence of human monocyte interleukin-1 precursor cDNA. Proc Natl Acad Sci USA 81:7907–7911, 1984.

127. Lomedico PT, Gubler U, Hellmann CP, et al: Cloning and expression of murine interleukin-1 in Escherichia coli. Nature 312:458–462, 1984.

128. March CJ, Mosley B, Larsen A, et al: Cloning, sequence and expression of two distinct interleukin-1 complementary DNAs. Nature 315:641–647, 1985.

129. Furutani Y, Notake M, Yamayoshi M, et al: Cloning and characterization of the cDNAs for human and rabbit interleukin-1 precursor. Nucleic Acids Res 13:5869–5882, 1985.

130. Gray PW, Glaister D, Chen E, et al: Two interleukin-1 genes in the mouse: Cloning and expression of the cDNA for murine interleukin-1-beta. J Immunol 137:3644–3648, 1986.

131. Schmidt JA: Purification and partial biochemical characterization of normal human interleukin 1. J Exp Med 160:772–787, 1984.

132. Bayne EK, Rupp EA, Limjuco G, et al: Immunocytochemical detection of interleukin 1 within stimulated human monocytes. J Exp Med 163:1267–1280, 1986.

133. Clark SC, Kamen R: The human hematopoietic colony-stimulating factors. Science 236:1229–1237, 1987.

134. Furutani Y, Notake M, Fukui T, et al: Complete nucleotide sequence of the gene for human interleukin-1-alpha. Nucleic Acids Res 14:3167–3179, 1986.

135. Oppenheim JJ, Kovacs E, Matsushima K, et al: There is more than one interleukin 1. Immunol Today 7:45–56, 1986.

136. Dower SK, Urdal DL: The interleukin-1 receptor. Immunol Today 8:46–51, 1987.

137. Giri JG, Lomedico PT, Mizel SB: Studies on the synthesis and secretion of interleukin 1. I. A 33,000 molecular weight precursor for interleukin 1. J Immunol 134:343–349, 1985.

138. Limjuco G, Galuska S, Chin J, et al: Antibodies of predetermined specificity to the major charged species of human interleukin 1. Proc Natl Acad Sci USA 83:3972–3976, 1986.

139. Gery I, Waksman BH: Potentiation of the T-lymphocyte response to mitogens. II. The cellular source of potentiating mediator(s). J Exp Med 136:143–155, 1972.

140. Menkin V: Chemical basis of injury in inflammation. Arch Pathol 36:269–288, 1943.

141. Beeson PB: Temperature-elevating effect of a substance obtained from polymorphonuclear leucocytes. J Clin Invest 27:524A, 1948.

142. Atkins E, Wood WB Jr: Studies on the pathogenesis of fever. J Exp Med 102:499–576, 1955.

143. Rosenwasser LJ, Dinarello CA, Rosenthal A: Adherent cell function in murine T-lymphocyte antigen recognition. IV. Enhancement of murine T-cell antigen recognition by human leukocytic pyrogen. J Exp Med 150:709–714, 1979.

144. Murphy PA, Simon PL, Willoughby WF: Endogenous pyrogens made by rabbit peritoneal exudate cells are identical with lymphocyte activating factors made by rabbit alveolar macrophages. J Immunol 124:2498–2501, 1980.

145. Dinarello CA, Cannon JG, Mier JW, et al: Multiple biological activities of human recombinant interleukin-1. J Clin Invest 77:1734–1739, 1986.

146. Dinarello CA, Wolff SM: Molecular basis of fever in humans. Am J Med 72:799–819, 1982.

147. Rossi V, Breviario F, Ghezzi P, Dejana E, et al: Interleukin-1 induces prostacyclin in vascular cells. Science 229:1174–1176, 1985.

148. Dejana E, Brevario F, Erroi A, et al: Modulation of endothelial cell function by different molecular species of interleukin-1. Blood 69:695–699, 1987.

149. Libby P, Ordovas JM, Auger KR, et al: Endotoxin and tumor necrosis factor induce interleukin-1 gene expression in adult human vascular endothelial cells. Am J Pathol 124:179–186, 1986.

150. Dayer J-M, Breard J, Chess L, et al: Participation of monocytes-macrophages and lymphocytes in the production of a factor that stimulates collagenase and prostaglandin release by rheumatoid synovial cells. J Clin Invest 64:1386–1392, 1979.

151. Dayer J-M, Stephenson ML, Schmidt E, et al: Purification of a factor from human blood monocyte-macrophages which stimulates the production of collagenase and prostaglandin E_2 by cells cultured from rheumatoid synovial tissues. FEBS Lett 124:253–256, 1981.

152. Mizel SB, Dayer J-M, Krane SM, et al: Stimulation of rheumatoid synovial cell collagenase and prostaglandin by partially purified lymphocyte-activating factor (interleukin-1). Proc Natl Acad Sci USA 78:2474–2477, 1981.

153. Dayer J-M, de Rochemonteix B, Burrus B, et al: Human recombinant interleukin 1 stimulates collagenase and prostaglandin E_2 production by human synovial cells. J Clin Invest 77:645–648, 1986.

154. Deshmukh-Phadke K, Lawrence M, Nanda S: Synthesis of collagenase and neutral proteases by articular chondrocytes: Stimulation by a macrophage-derived factor. Biochem Biophys Res Commun 85:490–496, 1978.

155. Ridge SC, Oronsky AL, Kerwar SS: Induction of the synthesis of latent collagenase and latent neutral protease in chondrocytes by a factor synthesized by activated macrophages. Arthritis Rheum 23:448–454, 1980.

156. Trechsel U, Dew G, Murphy G, et al: Effects of products from macrophages, blood mononuclear cells or retinol on collagenase secretion and collagen synthesis in chondrocyte culture. Biochem Biophys Acta 720:364–370, 1982.

157. Schnyder J, Payne T, Dinarello CA: Human monocyte or recombinant interleukin-1s are specific for the secretion of a metalloproteinase from chondrocytes. J Immunol 138:496–503, 1987.

158. Dewhirst FE, Stashenko PP, Mole JE, et al: Purification and partial sequence of human osteoclast-activating factor: Identify with interleukin 1β. J Immunol 135:2562–2568, 1985.

159. Thomson BM, Saklatvala J, Chambers TJ: Osteoblasts mediate interleukin 1 responsiveness of bone resorption by rat osteoclasts. J Exp Med 164:104–112, 1986.

160. Schmidt JA, Mizel SB, Cohen D, et al: Interleukin 1, a potential regulator of fibroblast proliferation. J Immunol 128:2177–2182, 1982.

161. Canalis E: Interleukin-1 has independent effects on DNA and collagen synthesis in cultures of rat calvariae. Endocrinology 118:74–81, 1986.

162. Raines EW, Dower SK, Ross R: Interleukin-1 mitogenic activity for fibroblasts and smooth muscle cells is due to PDGF-AA. Science 243:393–396, 1989.

163. Lipsky PE: Role of interleukin-1 in human B-cell activation. Contemp Top Mol Immunol 10:195–217, 1985.

164. Muraguchi A, Kehrl JH, Butler JL, et al: Regulation of human B-cell activation, proliferation, and differentiation by soluble factors. J Clin Immunol 4:337–347, 1984.

165. Männel DN, Moore RN, Mergenhagen SE: Macrophages as a source of tumoricidal activity (tumor-necrotizing factor). Infect Immun 30:523–530, 1980.

166. Matthews N: Tumor-necrosis factor from the rabbit. V. Synthesis in vitro by mononuclear phagocytes from various tissues of normal and BCG-injected rabbits. Br J Cancer 44:418–424, 1981.

167. Kawakami M, Cerami A: Studies of endotoxin-induced decrease in lipoprotein lipase activity. J Exp Med 154:631–639, 1981.

168. Kawakami M, Pekala PH, Lane MD, et al: Lipoprotein lipase suppression in 3T3-L1 cells by an endotoxin-induced mediator from exudate cells. Proc Natl Acad Sci USA 79:912–916, 1982.

169. Beutler B, Greenwald D, Hulmes JD, et al: Identity of tumor necrosis factor and the macrophage-secreted factor cachectin. Nature 316:552–554, 1985.

170. Pennica D, Hayflick JS, Bringman TS, et al: Cloning and expression in *Escherichia coli* of the cDNA for murine tumor necrosis factor. Proc Natl Acad Sci USA 82:6060–6064, 1985.

171. Caput D, Beutler B, Hartog K, et al: Identification of a common nucleotide sequence in the 3′-untranslated region of mRNA molecules specifying inflammatory mediators. Proc Natl Acad Sci USA 83:1670–1674, 1986.

172. Beutler B, Cerami A: Cachectin and tumor necrosis factor: Two sides of the same biological coin. Nature 320:584–588, 1986.

173. Dinarello CA, Cannon JG, Wolff SM, et al: Tumor necrosis factor (cachectin) is an endogenous pyrogen and induces interleukin-1. J Exp Med 163:1433–1450, 1986.

174. Dayer J-M, Beutler B, Cerami A: Cachetin/tumor necrosis factor stimulates collagenase and prostaglandin E_2 production by human synovial cells and dermal fibroblasts. J Exp Med 162:2163–2167, 1985.

175. Saklatvala J: Tumor necrosis factor α stimulates resorption and inhibits synthesis of proteoglycan in cartilage. Nature 322:547–549, 1986.

176. Bertolini DR, Nedwin GE, Bringman TS, et al: Stimulation of bone resorption and inhibition of bone formation *in vitro* by human tumor necrosis factors. Nature 319:516–518, 1986.

177. Thomson BM, Mundy GR, Chambers TJ: Tumor necrosis factors α and β induce osteoblastic cells to stimulate osteoclastic bone resorption. J Immunol 138:775–779, 1987.

178. Nawroth PP, Stern DM: Modulation of endothelial cell hemostatic properties by tumor necrosis factor. J Exp Med 163:740–745, 1986.

179. Bevilacqua MP, Pober JS, Majeau GR, et al: Recombinant tumor necrosis factor induces procoagulant activity in cultured human vascular endothelium: Characterization and comparison with the actions of interleukin 1. Proc Natl Acad Sci USA 83:4533–4537, 1986.

180. Hajjar KA, Hajjar DP, Silverstein RL, et al: Tumor necrosis factor–mediated release of platelet-derived growth factor from cultured endothelial cells. J Exp Med 166:235–245, 1987.

181. Bachwich PR, Chensue SW, Larrick JW, et al: Tumor necrosis factor stimulates interleukin 1 and prostaglandin E_2 production in resting macrophages. Biochem Biophys Res Commun 136:94–101, 1986.

182. Nawroth PP, Bank I, Handley D, et al: Tumor necrosis factor/cachectin interacts with endothelial cell receptors to induce release of interleukin 1. J Exp Med 163:1363–1375, 1986.

183. Elias JA, Gustilo K, Baeder W, et al: Synergistic stimulation of fibroblast prostaglandin production by recombinant interleukin 1 and tumor necrosis factor. J Immunol 138:3812–3816, 1987.

184. Aarden LA, Lansdorp PM, DeGroot ER: A growth factor for B cell hybridomas produced by human monocytes. Lymphokines 10:175–186, 1985.

185. Lansdorp PM, Aarden LA, Calafat J, et al: A growth factor–dependent B cell hybridoma. Curr Top Microbiol Immunol 132:105–113, 1986.

186. Houssiau FA, Coulie PG, Olive D, et al: Synergistic activation of human T cells by interleukin 1 and interleukin 6. Eur J Immunol 18:653–656, 1988.

187. Marinkovic S, Jahreis GP, Wong GG, et al: IL-6 modulates the synthesis of a specific set of acute phase plasma proteins in vivo. J Immunol 142:808–812, 1989.

188. Helle M, Brakenhoff JPJ, DeGroot ER, et al: Interleukin 6 is involved in interleukin 1–induced activities. Eur J Immunol 18:957–959, 1988.

189. May LT, Helfgott DC, Seghal PB: Anti-β-interferon antibodies inhibit the increased expression of HLA-B7 mRNA in tumor necrosis factor–treated human fibroblasts: Structural studies of the β2 interferon involved. Proc Natl Acad Sci USA 83:8957–8961, 1986.

190. Zilberstein A, Ruggieri R, Korn JH, et al: Structure and expression of cDNA and genes for human interferon beta 2, a distinct species inducible by growth-stimulating cytokines. EMBO J 5:2529–2537, 1986.

191. Shimokado K, Raines EW, Madtes DK, et al: A significant part of macrophage-derived growth factor consists of at least two forms of PDGF. Cell 43:277–286, 1985.

192. Johnsson A, Heldin CH, Wasteson A, et al: The c-sis gene encodes a precursor of the B chain of platelet-derived growth factor. EMBO J 3:921–928, 1984.

193. Heldin C-H, Johnsson A, Wennergren S, et al: A human osteosarcoma cell line secretes a growth factor structurally related to a homodimer of PDGF A-chains. Nature 319:511–514, 1986.

194. Glenn K, Bowen-Pope DF, Ross R: Platelet-derived growth factor. III. Identification of a platelet-derived growth factor receptor by affinity labelling. J Biol Chem 257:5172–5176, 1982.

195. Heldin C-H, Backstrom G, Ostman A, et al: Binding of different dimeric forms of PDGF to human fibroblasts: Evidence for two separate receptor types. EMBO J 7:1387–1393, 1988.

196. Gronwald RGK, Grant FJ, Haldeman BA, et al: Cloning and expression of a cDNA coding for the human platelet-derived growth factor receptor: Evidence for more than one receptor class. Proc Natl Acad Sci USA 85:3435–3439, 1988.

197. Deuel TF, Senior RM, Huang JS, Griffin GL: Chemotaxis of monocytes and neutrophils to platelet-derived growth factor. J Clin Invest 69:1046–1049, 1982.

198. Deuel TF, Huang JS: Platelet-derived growth factor. Structure, function and roles in normal and transformed cells. J Clin Invest 74:669–676, 1984.

199. Metcalf D: The granulocyte-macrophage colony–stimulating factors. Science 229:16–22, 1985.

200. Metcalf D, Nicola NA: Proliferative effects of purified granulocyte colony-stimulating factor (G-CSF) on normal mouse hemopoietic cells. J Cell Physiol 116:198–206, 1983.

201. Souza LM, Boone TC, Gabrilove J, et al: Recombinant human granulocyte colony-stimulating factor: Effects on normal and leukemic myeloid cells. Science 232:61–65, 1986.

202. Moore RN, Hoffeld JT, Farrar JJ, et al: Role of colony-stimulating factors as primary regulators of macrophage functions. In Pick E (ed): Lymphokines, vol 3. New York, Academic Press, 1981, pp 119–148.

203. Stanley ER: The macrophage colony-stimulating factor, CSF-1. Methods Enzymol 116:564–587, 1985.

204. Metcalf D: The Hematopoietic Colony Stimulated Factors. Amsterdam, Elsevier, 1984.

205. Thorens B, Mermod JJ, Vassali P: Phagocytosis and inflammatory stimuli induce GM-CSF mRNA in macrophages through posttranscriptional regulation. Cell 48:671–679, 1987.

206. Bickel M, Amstad P, Tsuda H, et al: Induction of granulocyte-macrophage colony-stimulating factor by lipopolysaccharide and anti-immunoglobulin M-stimulated murine B cell lines. J Immunol 39:2984–2988, 1987.

207. Koury MJ, Pragnell IB: Retroviruses induce granulocyte-macrophage colony-stimulating activity in fibroblasts. Nature 299:638–640, 1982.

208. Ascensao JL, Vercellotti HS, Jacob H, et al: Role of endothelial cells in human hematopoiesis: Modulation of mixed colony growth in vitro. Blood 63:553–558, 1984.

209. Bagby GC, Dinarello CA, Wallace P, et al: Interleukin 1 stimulates granulocyte-macrophage colony-stimulating activity release by vascular endothelial cells. J Clin Invest 78:1316–1323, 1986.

210. Koury MJ, Balmain A, Pragnell IB: Induction of granulocyte-macrophage colony-stimulating activity in mouse skin by inflammatory agents and tumor promoters. EMBO J 2:1877–1882, 1983.

211. Smith PD, Lamerson CL, Wahl SM: Granulocyte-macrophage colony-stimulating factor augmentation of leukocyte effector cell function. J Cell Biochem 105:137–141, 1989.

212. Weisbart RH, Golde DW, Clark SC, et al: Human granulocyte-macrophage colony-stimulating factor is a neutrophil activator. Nature 314:361–363, 1985.

213. Weisbart RH, Kwan L, Golde DW, et al: Human GM-CSF primes neutrophils for enhanced oxidative metabolism in response to the major physiologic chemoattractants. Blood 69:18–21, 1987.

214. Fleischmann J, Golde DW, Weisbart RH, et al: Granulocyte-macrophage colony-stimulating factor enhances phagocytosis of bacteria by human neutrophils. Blood 68:708–711, 1986.

215. Grabstein KH, Urdal DL, Tushinski RJ, et al: Induction of macrophage tumoricidal activity by granulocyte-macrophage colony-stimulating factor. Science 232:506–508, 1986.

216. Hancock WW, Pleau ME, Kobzik L: Recombinant granulocyte-macrophage colony-stimulating factor down-regulates expression of IL-2 receptor on human mononuclear phagocytes by induction of prostaglandine. J Immunol 140:3021–3025, 1988.

217. Assoian RK, Fleurdelys BE, Stevenson HC, et al: Expression and secretion of type β transforming growth factor by activated human macrophages. Proc Natl Acad Sci USA 84:6020–6024, 1987.

218. Rappolee DA, Mark D, Banda MJ, et al: Wound macrophages express TGF-α and other growth factors in vivo: Analysis by mRNA phenotyping. Science 241:708–712, 1988.

219. Todaro GJ, Fryling C, DeLarco JE: Transforming growth factors produced by certain human tumor cells: Polypeptides that interact with epidermal growth factor receptors. Proc Natl Acad Sci USA 77:5258–5262, 1980.

220. Massague J, Cheifetz S, Ignotz R, et al: Multiple type-beta transforming growth factors and their receptors. J Cell Physiol (Suppl) 5:43–48, 1987.

221. Cheifetz S, Bassols A, Stanley K, et al: Heterodimeric transforming growth factor β: Biological properties and interaction with three types of cell surface receptors. J Biol Chem 263:10783–10789, 1988.

222. Wahl SM, Hunt DA, Wong HL, et al: Transforming growth factor-β is a potent immunosuppressive agent that inhibits IL-1–dependent lymphocyte proliferation. J Immunol 140:3026–3032, 1988.

223. Tsunawaki S, Sporn M, Ding A, et al: Deactivation of macrophages by transforming growth factor-β. Nature 334:260–262, 1988.

224. Wiseman DM, Polverini PJ, Kamp DW, et al: Transforming growth factor-beta (TGF-β) is chemotactic for human monocytes and induces their expression of angiogenic activity. Biochem Biophys Res Commun 157:793–800, 1988.

225. Roberts AB, Sporn MB, Assoian RK, et al: Transforming growth factor type-β: Rapid induction of fibrosis and angiogenesis and stimulation of collagen formation in vitro. Proc Natl Acad Sci USA 83:4167–4171, 1986.

226. Ignotz RA, Massagué, J: Transforming growth factor-β stimulates the expression of fibronectin and collagen and their incorporation into the extracellular matrix. J Biol Chem 261:4337–4345, 1987.

227. Raghow R, Postlethwaite AE, Keski-Oja J, et al: Transforming growth factor-β increases steady state levels of type 1 procollagen and fibronectin messenger RNAs posttranscriptionally in cultured human dermal fibroblasts. J Clin Invest 79:1285–1288, 1987.

228. Sporn MB, Roberts AB, Shull JH, et al: Polypeptide transforming growth factors isolated from bovine sources and used for wound healing in vivo. Science 219:1329–1331, 1983.

229. Lawrence WT, Norton JA, Sporn MB, et al: The reversal of an Adriamycin induced healing impairment with chemoattractants and growth factors. Ann Surg 203:142–147, 1986.

230. Mustoe TA, Pierce GF, Thomason A, et al: Accelerated wound healing of incisional wounds in rats by transforming growth factor-β. Science 237:1333–1338, 1987.

231. Marquardt H, Hunkapillar MW, Hood LE, et al: Rat transforming growth factor type I: Structure and relation to epidermal growth factor. Science 223:1079–1082, 1984.

232. Gospodarowicz D, Bialecki H, Thakral TK: The angiogenic activity of the fibroblast and epidermal growth factor. Exp Eye Res 28:501–514, 1979.

233. Carpenter G, Cohen S: Epidermal growth factor. Ann Rev Biochem 48:193–216, 1979.

234. Schreiber AB, Winkler ME, Derynck R: Transforming growth factor-α: A more potent angiogenic mediator than epidermal growth factor. Science 232:1250–1253, 1987.

235. Schultz GS, White M, Mitchell R, et al: Epithelial wound healing by transforming growth factor-α and vaccinia growth factor. Science 235:350–352, 1987.

236. Adelmann-Grill BC, Heinz R, Wach F, et al: Inhibition of fibroblast chemotaxis by recombinant human interferon-γ and interferon-α. J Cell Physiol 130:270–275, 1987.

237. Smith PD, Wahl SM: The role of cytokines in the immune response. In Nelson DS (ed): Natural Immunity. New York, Academic Press, 1989, pp 241–283.

238. Wheelock EF: Interferon-like virus inhibitor induced in human leukocytes by phytohemagglutinin. Science 149:310–311, 1965.

239. Gray P, Goeddel DV: Structure of the human immune interferon gene. Nature 298:859–863, 1982.

240. Kirchner H, Marucci F: Interferon production by leukocytes. In Vilcek J, DeMaeyer E (eds): Interferons and the Immune System, vol 2. Amsterdam, Elsevier, 1984, pp 7–34.

241. Epstein LB: The special significance of interferon-gamma. In Vilcek J, DeMaeyer E (eds): Interferons and the Immune System, vol 2. Amsterdam, Elsevier, 1984, pp 185–220.

242. Rinderknecht E, O'Connor BH, Rodriguez H: Natural human interferon-γ: Complete amino acid sequence and determination of sites of glycosylation. J Biol Chem 259:6790–6797, 1984.

243. Gray PW, Leung DW, Derynck R, et al: Expression of human immune interferon cDNA in E. coli and monkey cells. Nature 295:503–508, 1982.

244. Nathan C, Yoshida R: Cytokines: Interferon-γ. In Gallin JI, Goldstein IN, Snyderman R: Inflammation: Basic Principles and Clinical Correlates. New York, Raven Press, 1989, pp 229–251.

245. Finbloom DS, Hoover DL, Wahl LM: The characteristics of binding of human recombinant interferon-γ

to its receptor on human monocytes and human monocyte-like cell lines. J Immunol 135:300–305, 1985.

246. Nathan CF, Murray HW, Wiebe ME, et al: Identification of interferon-γ as the lymphokine that activates human macrophage oxidative metabolism and antimicrobial activity. J Exp Med 158:670–689, 1983.

247. Nedwin GE, Svedersky LP, Bringman TS, et al: Effect of interleukin 2, interferon-gamma, and mitogens on the production of tumor necrosis factors alpha and beta. J Immunol 135:2492–2497, 1985.

248. Collart MA, Belin D, Vassali J-D, et al: Interferon enhances macrophage transcription of the tumor necrosis factor/cachectin, interleukin 1, and urokinase genes, which are controlled by short lived repressors. J Exp Med 164:2113–2118, 1986.

249. Arenzana-Seisdedos F, Virelizier JL, Fiers W: Interferons as macrophage activating factors. III. Preferential effect of interferon-γ on the interleukin 1 secretory potential of fresh or aged human monocytes. J Immunol 134:2444–2448, 1985.

250. Adams JS, Gacod MA: Characterization of 1-α-hydroxylation of vitamin D3 sterols by cultured alveolar macrophages from patients with sarcoidosis. J Exp Med 161:755–765, 1985.

251. Koeffler HP, Reichel H, Bishop JE, et al: Gamma-interferon stimulates production of 1,25-dihydroxyvitamin D3 by normal human macrophages. Biochem Biophys Res Commun 127:596–603, 1985.

252. Guyre PM, Morganelli PM, Miller R: Recombinant immune interferon increases immunoglobulin G Fc receptors on cultured human mononuclear phagocytes. J Clin Invest 72:393–397, 1983.

253. Ezekowitz RAB, Bampton M, Gordon S: Macrophage activation selectively enhances expression of Fc receptors for IgG2a. J Exp Med 157:807–812, 1983.

254. Perussia B, Dayton ET, Lazarus R, et al: Immune interferon induces the receptor for monomeric IgG1 on human monocytic and myeloid cells. J Exp Med 158:1092–1113, 1983.

255. Steeg PS, Moore RN, Johnson M, et al: Regulation of murine macrophage Ia antigen expression by a lymphokine with immune interferon activity. J Exp Med 156:1780–1793, 1982.

256. Weinberg JB, Hobbs MM, Misukonis MA: Phenotypic characterization of gamma interferon–induced human monocyte polykaryons. Blood 66:1241–1246, 1985.

257. Dore-Duffy P, Perry W, Kuo H-H: Interferon-mediated inhibition of prostaglandin synthesis in human mononuclear leukocytes. Cell Immunol 79:232–239, 1983.

258. Boraschi D, Censini S, Bartalini M, et al: Interferon inhibits prostaglandin biosynthesis in macrophages. Effects on arachidonic acid metabolism. J Immunol 132:1987–1992, 1984.

259. Boraschi D, Censini S, Bartalini M, et al: Regulation of arachidonic acid metabolism in macrophages by immune and nonimmune interferons. J Immunol 135:502–505, 1985.

260. Rachmilewitz D, Karmeli F, Panet A: Interferon inhibits prostaglandin E₂ synthesis and stimulates (2′-5′) oligoadenylate synthetase activity in peripheral blood mononuclear cells of inflammatory bowel disease patients. J Interferon Res 5:629–635, 1985.

261. Hamilton TA, Ribsbee JE, Scott WA, et al: Gamma-interferon enhances the secretion of arachidonic acid metabolites from murine peritoneal macrophages stimulated with phorbol diesters. J Immunol 134:2631–2636, 1985.

262. Thurman GB, Braude IA, Gray PW, et al: MIF-like activity of natural and recombinant human interferon-

263. Shalaby MR, Aggarwal BB, Rinderknecht E, et al: Activation of human polymorphonuclear neutrophil functions by interferon-gamma and tumor necrosis factors. J Immunol 135:2069–2073, 1985.

264. Pober JS, Gimbrone MA Jr, Cotran RS, et al: Ia expression by vascular endothelium is inducible by activated T cells and human γ interferon. J Exp Med 157:1339–1353, 1983.

265. Montesano R, Mossez A, Ryser J-E, et al: Leukocyte interleukins induce cultured endothelial cells to produce a highly organized glycosaminoglycan-rich pericellular matrix. J Cell Biol 99:1706–1715, 1984.

266. Duncan MR, Berman B: Gamma interferon is the lymphokine and beta interferon the monokine responsible for inhibition of fibroblast collagen production and late but not early fibroblast proliferation. J Exp Med 162:516–527, 1985.

267. Jimenez SA, Freundlich B, Rosenbloom J: Selective inhibition of human diploid fibroblast collagen synthesis by interferons. J Clin Invest 74:1112–1116, 1984.

268. Stephenson ML, Krane SM, Amento EP, et al: Immune interferon inhibits collagen synthesis by rheumatoid synovial cells associated with decreased levels of the procollagen mRNAs. FEBS Lett 180:43–50, 1985.

269. Morgan DA, Ruscetti FW, Gallo RC: Selective in vitro growth of T lymphocytes from normal human bone marrows. Science 193:1007–1008, 1976.

270. Aarden LA, Brunner TK, Cerottini J-C, et al: Revised nomenclature for antigen-nonspecific T cell proliferation and helper factors. J Immunol 123:2928–2929, 1979.

271. Taniguchi T, Matsui H, Fujita T, et al: Structure and expression of a cloned cDNA for human interleukin 2. Nature 302:305–310, 1983.

272. Devos R, Plaetinck G, Cheroutre H, et al: Molecular cloning of human interleukin 2 cDNA and its expression in E. coli. Nucleic Acids Res 11:4307–4323, 1983.

273. Luger TA, Smolen JS, Chused TM, et al: Human lymphocytes with either the OKT4 or OKT8 phenotype produce interleukin 2 in culture. J Clin Invest 70:470–473, 1982.

274. Smith KA: T-cell growth factor. Immunol Rev 51:337–357, 1980.

275. Howard M, Matis L, Malek TR, et al: Interleukin 2 induces antigen reactive T cell lines to secrete BCGF-1. J Exp Med 158:2024–2039, 1983.

276. Farrar JJ, Benjamin WR, Hilfiker ML, et al: The biochemistry, biology, and role of interleukin 2 in the induction of cytotoxic T cell and antibody forming B cell responses. Immunol Rev 63:129–166, 1982.

277. Brooks CG, Henney CS: Interleukin-2 and regulation of natural killer activity in cultured cell populations. Contemp Top Mol Immunol 10:63–92, 1985.

278. Leonard WJ, Depper JM, Uchiyama T, et al: A monoclonal antibody that appears to recognize the receptor for human T cell growth factor: partial characterization of the receptor. Nature 300:267–269, 1982.

279. Leonard WJ, Depper JM, Robb RJ, et al: Characterization of the human receptor for T cell growth factor. Proc Natl Acad Sci USA 80:6957–6961, 1983.

280. Leonard WJ, Depper JM, Crabtree GR, et al: Molecular cloning and expression of cDNAs for the human interleukin-2 receptor. Nature 311:631–635, 1984.

281. Nikaido T, Shimizu A, Ishida N, et al: Molecular cloning of cDNA encoding human interleukin-2 receptor. Nature 311:631–635, 1984.

282. Robb RJ, Greene WC, Rusk CM: Low and high

affinity cellular receptors for interleukin 2. Implications for the level of Tac antigen. J Exp Med 160:1126–1146, 1984.

283. Robb RJ, Munck A, Smith KA: T-cell growth factor receptors: Quantification, specificity, and biological relevance. J Exp Med 154:1455–1474, 1981.

284. Weissman AM, Harford JB, Svetlik PB, et al: Only high affinity receptors for interleukin-2 mediate internalization of ligand. Proc Natl Acad Sci USA 83:1463–1466, 1986.

285. Fujii M, Sugamura K, Sano K, et al: High-affinity receptor-mediated internalization and degradation of interleukin 2 in human T cells. J Exp Med 163:550–562, 1986.

286. Kuo LM, Rusk CM, Robb RJ: Structure-function relationships for the IL 2 receptor system. II. Localization of an IL 2 binding site on high and low affinity receptors. J Immunol 137:1544–1551, 1986.

287. Sharon M, Klausner RD, Cullen BR, et al: Novel interleukin-2 receptor subunit detected by cross-linking under high affinity conditions. Science 234:859–863, 1986.

288. Tsudo M, Kozak RW, Goldman CK, et al: Demonstration of a non-Tac peptide that binds interleukin-2: A potential participant in a multichain interleukin-2 receptor complex. Proc Natl Acad Sci USA 83:9694–9698, 1986.

289. Teshigawara K, Wang H-M, Kato K, et al: Interleukin-2 high affinity receptor expression requires two distinct binding proteins. J Exp Med 165:223–238, 1987.

290. Tsudo M, Uchiyama T, Uchino H: Expression of Tac antigen on activated normal human B-cells. J Exp Med 160:612–617, 1984.

291. Waldmann TA, Goldman CK, Robb RJ, et al: Expression of interleukin-2 receptors on activated human B-cells. J Exp Med 160:1450–1466, 1984.

292. Herrmann F, Lindemann A, Cannistra SA, et al: Monocyte interleukin-1 secretion is regulated by the sequential action of gamma interferon and interleukin-2 involving monocyte surface expression of interleukin-2 receptors. Hematol Bulttransfus 32:299–315, 1989.

293. Howard M, Farrar J, Hilfiker M, et al: Identification of a T cell derived B cell growth factor distinct from IL-2. J Exp Med 155:914–923, 1982.

294. Rabin EM, Ohara J, Paul WE: B-cell stimulatory factor 1 activates resting B cells. Proc Natl Acad Sci USA 82:2935–2939, 1985.

295. Noelle RJ, Krammer PH, Ohara J, et al: Increased expression of Ia antigens on resting B cells: An additional role for B-cell growth factor. Proc Natl Acad Sci USA 81:6149–6153, 1984.

296. Noelle R, Kramer PH, Ohara J, et al: Increased expression of Ia antigens on resting B cells: An additional role for B-cell growth factor. Proc Natl Acad Sci USA 81:6149–6153, 1984.

297. Roehm NW, Liebson HJ, Zlotnik A, et al: Interleukin-induced increase in Ia expression by normal mouse B cells. J Exp Med 160:679–694, 1984.

298. Vitetta ES, Ohara J, Myers C, et al: Serological, biochemical, and functional identity of B cell–stimulatory factor 1 and B cell differentiation factor for IgG1. J Exp Med 162:1726–1731, 1985.

299. Coffman RL, Ohara J, Bond MW, et al: B cell stimulatory factor-1 enhances the IgE response of lipopolysaccharide-activated B cells. J Immunol 136:4538–4541, 1986.

300. Hu-Li J, Shevach EM, Mizuguchi J, et al: B cell stimulatory factor 1 (interleukin 4) is a potent costimulant for normal resting T lymphocytes. J Exp Med 165:157–172, 1987.

301. Lee F, Yokota T, Otsuka T, et al: Isolation and characterization of a mouse interleukin cDNA clone that expresses B-cell stimulatory factor 1 activities and T-cell and mast-cell stimulating activities. Proc Natl Acad Sci USA 83:2061–2065, 1986.

302. Crawford RM, Finbloom DS, Ohara J, et al: B cell stimulatory factor-1 (interleukin 4) activates macrophages for increased tumoricidal activity and expression of Ia antigens. J Immunol 139:135–141, 1987.

303. Te Velde AA, Klomp JPG, Yard BA, et al: Modulation of phenotypic and functional properties of human peripheral blood monocytes by IL-4. J Immunol 140:1548–1554, 1988.

304. Ohara J, Paul WE: Receptors for B-cell stimulatory factor-1 expressed on cells of haematopoietic lineage. Nature 325:537–538, 1987.

305. Takatsu K, Kikuchi Y, Takahashi T, et al: Interleukin 5, a T-cell-derived B-cell differentiation factor also induces cytotoxic T lymphocytes. Proc Natl Acad Sci USA 84:4234–4238, 1987.

306. Takatsu K, Tominaga A, Hamaoka T: Antigen-induced T cell-replacing factor (TRF). I. Functional characterization of a TRF-producing helper T cell subset and genetic studies on TRF production. J Immunol 124:2414–2422, 1980.

307. Swain SL, Howard M, Kappler J, et al: Evidence for two distinct classes of murine B cell growth factors with activities in different functional assays. J Exp Med 158:822–835, 1983.

308. Bond MW, Shrader B, Mosmann TR, et al: A mouse T cell product that preferentially enhances IgA production. II. Physiochemical characterization. J Immunol 139:3691–3696, 1987.

309. Coffman RL, Shrader B, Carty J, et al: A mouse T cell product that preferentially enhances IgA production. I. Biologic characterization. J Immunol 139:3685–3690, 1987.

310. Murray PD, McKenzie DT, Swain SL, et al: Interleukin 5 and interleukin 4 produced by Peyer's patch T cells selectively enhanced immunoglobulin A expression. J Immunol 139:2669–2674, 1987.

311. Hori Y, Muraguchi A, Suematsu S, et al: Regulation of BSF-2/IL-6 production by human mononuclear cells macrophage-dependent synthesis of BSF-2/IL-6 by T cells. J Immunol 141:1529–1535, 1988.

312. Tosato G, Seamon KB, Goldman ND, et al: A monocyte-derived human B cell growth factor identified as interferon-β_2 (BSF-2, IL-6). Science 239:502–504, 1988.

313. Hirano T, Ysukawa K, Harada H, et al: Complementary DNA for a novel human interleukin (BSF-2) that induces B lymphocytes to produce immunoglobulin. Nature 324:73–76, 1986.

314. Sehgal PB, May LT, Tamm I, et al: Human β_2 interferon and B-cell differentiation factor BSF-2 are identical. Science 235:731–732, 1987.

315. Hirano T, Taga T, Nakano N, et al: Purification to homogeneity and characterization of human B-cell differentiation factor (BCDF or BSFp-2). Proc Natl Acad Sci USA 82:5490–5494, 1985.

316. Kishimoto T, Hirano T: Molecular regulation of B lymphocyte response. Ann Rev Immunol 6:485–512, 1988.

317. Ikebuchi K, Wong GG, Clark SC, et al: Interleukin-6 enhancement of interleukin-3-dependent proliferation of multipotential hemopoietic progenitors. Proc Natl Acad Sci USA 84:9035–9039, 1987.

318. Gauldie J, Richards C, Harnich D, et al: Interferon $\beta2$/BSF-2 shares identity with monocyte derived hepatocyte stimulating factor (HSF) and regulates the major acute phase protein response in liver cells. Proc Natl Acad Sci USA 84:7251–7255, 1987.

319. Kawano M, Hirano T, Matsuda T, et al: Autocrine generation and essential requirement of BSF-2/IL-6 for human multiple myelomas. Nature 332:83–85, 1988.

320. Garman RD, Jacobs KA, Clark SC, et al: B-cell-stimulatory factor 2 (β_2 interferon) functions as a second signal for interleukin 2 production by mature murine T cells. Proc Natl Acad Sci USA 84:7629–7633, 1987.

321. Takai Y, Wong GG, Clark SC, et al: B cell stimulatory factor-2 is involved in the differentiation of cytotoxic T lymphocytes. J Immunol 140:508–512, 1988.

322. Okada M, Kitahara M, Kishimoto S, et al: IL-6/BSF-2 functions as a killer helper factor in the in vitro induction of cytotoxic T cells. J Immunol 141:1543–1549, 1988.

323. Kohase M, Henriksen-DeStefano D, May LT, et al: Induction of β2-interferon by tumor necrosis factor: A homeostatic mechanism in the control of cell proliferation. Cell 45:659–666, 1986.

324. Yoshimura T, Matsushima K, Oppenheim JJ, et al: Neutrophil chemotactic factor produced by lipopolysaccharide (LPS)-stimulated human blood mononuclear leukocytes: Partial characterization and separation from interleukin-1 (IL-1). J Immunol 139:788–793, 1987.

325. Matsushima K, Morishita K, Yoshimura T, et al: Molecular cloning of a human monocyte-derived neutrophil chemotactic factor (MDNCF) and the induction of MDNCF mRNA by interleukin 1 and tumor necrosis factor. J Exp Med 167:1883–1893, 1988.

326. Larsen CG, Anderson AO, Oppenheim JJ, et al: Production of interleukin-8 by human dermal fibroblasts and keratinocytes in response to interleukin-1 or tumor necrosis factor. Immunology 68:31–36, 1989.

327. Thelen M, Peveri P, Kernen P, et al: Mechanism of neutrophil activation by NAF, a novel monocyte-derived peptide agonist. FASEB J 2:2702–2706, 1988.

328. Rampart M, Van Damme J, Zonnekeyn L, et al: Granulocyte chemotactic protein/interleukin-8 induces plasma leakage and neutrophil accumulation in rabbit skin. Am J Pathol 135:21–25, 1989.

329. Grob PM, David E, Warren TC, et al: Characterization of a receptor for human monocyte-derived neutrophil chemotactic factor/interleukin-8. J Biol Chem 265:8311–8316, 1990.

330. Wong HL, Wahl SM: Tissue repair and fibrosis. In Asherson GL, Zembala M (eds): Human Monocytes. New York, Academic Press, 1989, pp 383–394.

331. Vilcek J, Palombella VJ, Henriksen-DeStefano D, et al: Fibroblast growth enhancing activity of tumor necrosis factor and its relationship to other polypeptide growth factors. J Exp Med 163:632–643, 1986.

332. Martinet Y, Bitterman PB, Mornex JF, et al: Activated human monocytes express the c-sis proto-oncogene and release a mediator showing PDGF-like activity. Nature 319:158–160, 1986.

333. Baird A, Mormede P, Bohlen P: Immunoreactive fibroblast growth factor in cells of peritoneal exudate suggests its identity with macrophage-derived growth factor. Biochem Biophys Res Commun 126:358–364, 1985.

334. Folkman J, Klagsburn M: Angiogenic factors. Science 235:442–447, 1987.

335. Roberts AB, Sporn MB: The transforming growth factor-betas. In Sporn MB, Roberts AB (eds): Peptide Growth Factors and Their Receptors, vol 1. Heidelberg, Springer-Verlag, 1990, pp 425–472.

336. Allen JB, Manthey CL, Hand AR, et al: Rapid onset synovial inflammation and hyperplasia induced by TGF-β. J Exp Med 171:231–247, 1990.

4

FIBROBLAST PROLIFERATION

Claudia J. Morgan, Ph.D., and W. Jack Pledger, Ph.D.

In normal, uninjured tissue, fibroblasts are sparsely distributed and generally quiescent throughout the connective tissue matrix. After injury, fibroblasts are activated to migrate from adjacent tissue into the wound site, where they proliferate and produce collagen, elastin, and proteoglycans, which will reconstruct the connective tissue. Fibroblast function in wound healing is controlled by the interaction of a number of factors released locally by several different cell types that make up the wound healing module. These regulatory factors include both stimulatory and inhibitory activities and in some cases modulate more than one fibroblast function, for example, proliferation and chemotactic migration. The fibroblast response to a given factor may depend on the proliferative state of the fibroblast, the concentration of the mediator, or the presence of other regulatory substances. Understanding and controlling these events in the appropriate context will be of great clinical importance.

Tissue injury is rapidly followed by the adherence and activation of platelets in the area of injury and the release of growth factors and chemotactic agents contained in the platelet α granules. Within a few hours, granulocytes and mononuclear phagocytes migrate into the site, apparently in response to platelet factors. Shortly thereafter, the site is infiltrated by fibroblasts, whose migration and proliferation are stimulated by both platelet and mononuclear phagocyte products. Growth modulating factors present in normal plasma act synergistically with one or more of the factors released by platelets and mononuclear phagocytes to promote proliferation. The activated fibroblasts produce and secrete β-interferon, which acts as an autocrine growth inhibitor. Other cells involved in immune regulation, such as T lymphocytes, produce factors that stimulate fibroblast proliferation, as well as activators and inhibitors of fibroblast chemotaxis.

This chapter describes the biochemistry and biological action of factors affecting fibroblast proliferation in the context of a model for the regulation of fibroblast growth by the combined action of two classes of growth factors, competence factors and progression factors. A brief outline of growth inhibition is presented and implications for the control of fibrogenesis are discussed.

THE CELL CYCLE

In vitro, an exponentially growing population of fibroblasts goes through cell division every 18 to 20 hours, on the average. The interval between consecutive mitoses has been termed the cell cycle; during the cell cycle, an ordered sequence of events appears to be necessary for a newly derived daughter cell to proceed to the next mitosis. As an experimental construct designed to categorize the events involved in cell replication, the cell cycle has been subdivided into phases bounded by the two most easily observable events, DNA synthesis (S phase) and mitosis (M) (Fig. 4–1). The remainder of the cycle consists of two relatively undefined times gaps: G_1, between mitosis and the onset of DNA synthesis, and G_2, between S phase and mitosis. Historical and current perspectives of the cell cycle and its regulation are presented in excellent reviews by Baserga and Pres-

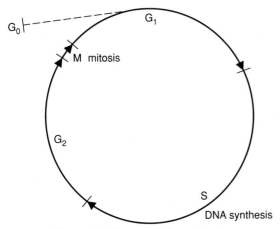

Figure 4–1. The mammalian cell cycle.

cott,[1-3] and much of this section is based on these reviews.

The cellular DNA content is replicated during a discrete interval of the cell cycle, the S phase. The amount of time required to replicate the entire DNA complement of a mammalian cell, based on measured rates of bacterial DNA replication, should be only 20 to 30 minutes. The duration of the S phase, however, is consistently close to 8 hours in cultured cells, indicating that at any given time at most only 5 to 15 per cent of the DNA undergoes replication. In fact, different segments of DNA appear to be replicated in a temporal order that is retained from cycle to cycle. Protein synthesis occurs throughout S phase and is required for DNA synthesis. At the onset of S phase, a substantial increase occurs in most of the enzymes involved in DNA synthesis and metabolism, including polymerases, ligases, and thymidine kinase, as well as the histones and ribonucleotide reductase. However, there is no consistent correlation between the time of expression of these proteins and the onset or duration of S phase.

During the mitotic phase, which lasts 30 minutes to an hour, protein synthesis is substantially decreased and RNA synthesis ceases entirely. The morphology of the cell surface membrane changes markedly, temporarily resembling that of a transformed cell, and the cell becomes rounded and less tightly attached to the culture surface.

During the course of each cell cycle, the cell doubles its mass in preparation for division. The G_1 and G_2 phases are characterized by active RNA and protein synthesis, both of which are required throughout most of each period for transit through to the G_1/S or G_2/M boundaries. The products of this synthetic activity contribute to the doubling of cell mass as well as to components that may be required for cell cycle regulation. Baserga has proposed that although an increase in cell size appears to be coordinated with DNA synthesis, the two processes are experimentally dissociable and are, therefore, under different controls.[4]

Although the average cell cycle time varies widely among different cell types, the composite length of the S, G_2, and M phases is a surprisingly consistent 10 to 12 hours, with differences among cell types confined primarily to differences in the duration of the G_1 phase. Historically, this observation led to the suggestion that transit through the cell cycle was regulated by events occurring in the G_1 phase. This suggestion was supported by the fact that when cells that have been arrested in culture by high culture density or nutrient or serum deprivation are stimulated to resume proliferation, they enter the cell cycle in the G_1 phase. Studies of the nature of cell cycle control have focused primarily on the entry of arrested cells into G_1 and the biochemical events occurring in G_1 and for the most part have adopted the bias that regulatory events may be differentiated from processes that are required for the bulk duplication of cellular components in preparation for cell division.

CELL CYCLE REGULATION

Normal cells become growth arrested in vitro when they reach confluent density on the culture surface. Cells may also be arrested at subconfluent density by depriving them of serum growth factors. Cells that have become growth arrested by high density or serum deprivation enter a quiescent phase, designated G_0, that lies outside the G_1 phase of the cell cycle (see Figure 4–1). The G_0 state is a reversible, nontoxic state, and cells can remain viable in G_0 arrest for extended periods. In vivo, cells may be classified into three populations: continuously dividing cells, nondividing postmitotic cells, and cells reversibly growth arrested in G_0, which can be induced to reenter the proliferative cycle. There are ample cases of the stimulation of cell cycle transit and DNA synthesis in arrested cells in vivo, such as the regeneration of liver after partial hepatectomy and the immune activation of lymphocytes, as well as the activation of several cell types during wound repair.

The nature of the distinction between G_0 and

G_1 has been investigated by studying the factors and events involved in the transit of cells through the prereplicative stage of the cell cycle to the onset of DNA synthesis and commitment to cell division. When G_0-arrested fibroblasts are stimulated to reenter the cell cycle in vitro, there is a characteristic delay of 12 to 15 hours before the onset of DNA synthesis. This delay is longer than the G_1 period of continuously cycling cells; exponentially growing murine Balb/c-3T3 fibroblasts proliferate with a 6 hour G_1 phase, compared with the 12 hours required for density-arrested Balb/c-3T3 cells to enter S phase after serum stimulation.[5] Serum can be fractionated into two classes of components that regulate two different aspects of cell function, the initiation of cell proliferation and the stimulation of G_0/G_1 traverse.[5] The factors required for maintenance of cell viability are contained in defibrinogenated platelet-poor plasma, a fraction prepared from unclotted blood, which does not stimulate cell replication. Platelet-derived growth factor (PDGF), released from platelets into serum during the clotting process, is the serum factor that stimulates proliferation.[6] The identification of these two classes of serum factors provided the experimental basis for a model of cell cycle regulation in which the process of commitment to cell division can be separated into two discrete stages governed by the two classes of factors.

Transient exposure of density-arrested Balb/c-3T3 fibroblasts to PDGF renders them "competent" to transit the cell cycle in response to factors present in plasma.[5] In the absence of plasma factors, PDGF-treated cells do not progress through G_1 but remain competent to do so for at least 13 hours after PDGF removal. Exposure of competent cells to plasma results in the initiation of DNA synthesis 12 hours after plasma addition. The presence of plasma is required throughout the 12 hour G_1 phase, and the sequential order of exposure to PDGF and plasma must be preserved: transient exposure to plasma followed by PDGF does not stimulate DNA synthesis.

These observations are consistent with a model of cell cycle control presented in Figure 4–2. Quiescent cells are made competent to proliferate by transient exposure to PDGF. The acquisition of competence is associated with the entry of G_0 cells into early G_1, but no further progression into G_1 occurs. Progression factors present in plasma are able to stimulate competent cells to undergo replication. The designation of a mitogen as a competence factor is based on the satisfaction of three criteria: (1) the factor acts synergistically with plasma to

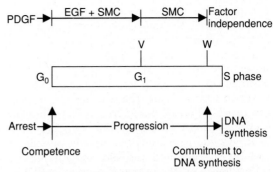

Figure 4–2. The G_0/G_1 phase of the cell cycle.

stimulate DNA synthesis; (2) transient exposure to the factor is sufficient to induce competence; and (3) cells made competent by the factor remain temporally 12 hours from the onset of S phase. Fibroblast growth factor (FGF) and precipitates of calcium phosphate are also classified as competence factors by these criteria. Competence factors do not cause progression, and progression factors, which include the insulin-like growth factors (see below), do not induce competence (Table 4–1).[7, 8]

This model for the dual control of fibroblast proliferation offers a paradigm for the regulation of fibroblast function in vivo, in which fibroblasts remain in a reversible quiescent state in the presence of a constant supply of the progression factors present in plasma in concentrations sufficient to support cell growth. The transition to cell replication may be initiated by a single stimulus, the release of competence factors, conferring the ability to proliferate in the presence of plasma. This mode of regulation would allow for the specific stimulation of cell proliferation in areas of tissue injury by the localized release of competence factors by activated cells, such as platelets, mononuclear phagocytes, and lymphocytes, at the affected site.

PLATELET-DERIVED GROWTH FACTOR

The serum dependence of fibroblast and smooth muscle cell proliferation in vitro reflects

Table 4–1. COMPETENCE AND PROGRESSION FACTORS IN THE FIBROBLAST SYSTEM

Competence Factors
    Platelet-derived growth factor (PDGF)
    Fibroblast growth factor (FGF)
    Calcium phosphate precipitates

Progression Factors
    Insulin-like growth factor-1 (IGF-1)
    Epidermal growth factor (EGF)
    Other plasma factors

the requirement for platelet-derived growth factor (PDGF), the major mitogenic component of serum for fibroblastic cells.[9, 10] (PDGF is also discussed in detail in Chapter 14.) Human serum contains approximately 770 pg of PDGF per mg of protein, while normal plasma contains levels of PDGF below that needed to support the proliferation of Balb/c-3T3 cells or human fibroblasts in vitro.[6] PDGF has been shown to be produced by several different cells, including endothelial cells and vascular smooth muscle cells;[11] however, the principal sources of PDGF in vivo are probably platelets and activated mononuclear phagocytes. In the platelet, PDGF is stored in the α granules, the storage site of other growth modulators such as epidermal growth factor (EGF) or an EGF-like growth factor[12] and transforming growth factor-β (TGF-β).[13, 14]

Immediately after tissue injury, localized platelet activation occurs in response to thrombogenic stimuli. The contents of the platelet α granules are released, and local concentrations of these growth modulators, including PDGF, increase. Within hours after injury, mononuclear phagocytes migrate into the site of the wound in response to the chemotactic activity of factors such as PDGF and TGF-β released by platelets. Cultured alveolar and peritoneal macrophages,[15] macrophagelike cell lines,[16] and activated blood monocytes, but not resting monocytes,[17] have been shown to synthesize and secrete PDGF or a PDGF-like substance. The secretion of PDGF by activated mononuclear phagocytes in the wound may function to maintain a continued localized supply of PDGF that can induce migration into the wound and proliferation of fibroblasts over an extended period.

PDGF is a heat stable, cationic glycoprotein of approximately 30,000 daltons. The protein core of PDGF is a disulfide-linked dimer composed of two distinct but homologous polypeptides, A and B, which are encoded by different genes. PDGF exists in vivo in homodimeric and heterodimeric form, and homodimers of both A chains[18] and B chains[19] as well as heterodimers[20] have been shown to be biologically active. The human genes that encode the A and B chains are located on different chromosomes—the A chain gene on chromosome 7 and the B chain gene on chromosome 22. Complementary DNA (cDNA) clones of both the A[21] and B[22] chains of human PDGF have been isolated. The A chain cDNA encodes a 211 amino acid precursor protein containing a 20 amino acid propeptide followed by the 125 amino acid mature A chain. Human PDGF exhibits size microheterogeneity due to small changes in the electrophoretic mobility of the A chain, which may be indicative of additional proteolytic processing at the C terminus of the mature A peptide. A single site for N-linked glycosylation is present in the A chain sequence; the mature B chain protein contains no glycosylation sites.

The B chain of PDGF is the gene product of the proto-oncogene c-sis, the cellular homologue of the v-sis transforming gene of the simian sarcoma retrovirus (SSV).[23, 24] Acute transforming retroviruses appear to have arisen by the substitution of cellular gene sequences involved in the control of cell proliferation for viral genes required for normal viral replication. As a result, cellular genes become activated, due to inappropriate expression or structural mutation, to induce cellular transformation.[25] NIH 3T3 fibroblasts and NRK fibroblasts transformed by SSV secrete the viral form of PDGF, p28[sis], which stimulates proliferation of these cells by an autocrine mechanism. Injection of SSV-transformed cells into nude mice results in tumor growth at a rate directly proportional to the levels of p28[sis] secreted by the transformed cells.[26] Unregulated expression of the normal sis protein in cells expressing functional PDGF receptors also causes transformation. Introduction of the normal genomic[27] or cDNA[22] sequences encoding the human proto-oncogene c-sis into NIH 3T3 cells induces transformation when transcription of the introduced sequences is activated.

The c-sis/PDGF B chain gene codes for a precursor protein that is approximately 40 percent homologous to the human A chain precursor. The mature A and B proteins show somewhat higher homology, with tightly conserved cysteine residues, indicating that the disulfide bonding structure of the A and B chains is similar. The resulting homology in tertiary structure would be consistent with the ability of both AA dimers and BB dimers to bind to the PDGF receptor.

PDGF Receptor

The initial interaction of PDGF with its target cells is by noncovalent binding to a cell surface receptor with high affinity and selectivity for PDGF. PDGF receptors have been identified in fibroblasts, smooth muscle cells, glial cells, and chondrocytes, and responsiveness to PDGF is strictly correlated with the presence of PDGF receptor.[28] The three isoforms of PDGF bind with different affinities to two highly homologous forms of PDGF receptor, α and β. The sequences of cDNAs encoding the PDGF-α and PDGF-β receptor forms indicate that the proteins are synthesized with signal peptides that are cleaved to produce mature proteins of approximately 1070 amino acids.[29, 30, 31] The amino acid sequences deduced from cDNA account for 120,000 daltons of the 180,000 dalton mature receptors. The remaining mass of the receptors may be contributed by N- and O-linked carbohydrate and covalently associated ubiquitin. Enzymatic removal of sialic acid and N-linked oligosaccharide moieties from purified PDGF receptor has shown that these components represent 30,000 to 40,000 daltons of the mature receptor form. An additional 8000 daltons are contributed by covalently bound ubiquitin, a 76 amino acid protein whose primary structure is invariant in higher eukaryotes. Ubiquitin is found in all eukaryotic cells, either free or conjugated to selected cellular proteins at α or ε amino groups. Ubiquitination has been implicated in the targeting of cellular proteins for ATP-dependent, nonlysosomal degradation.[32] However, the presence of ubiquitin bound to the PDGF receptor and other plasma membrane proteins suggests that it may play a role in other cellular events. Recent evidence of intrinsic proteolytic activity in purified ubiquitin may relate to this role.[33]

The PDGF receptors are bisected by a single transmembrane domain. The extracellular domains are 30 percent homologous and are composed of five immunoglobulin-like domains defined by cysteine residues. The intracellular domains contain tyrosine kinase activity in two 80 percent homologous domains separated by 100 amino acid inserts that may determine the substrate specificity of the receptor kinases.[34] A family of structurally related proteins includes the two PDGF receptor forms, the receptor for the colony-stimulating factor CSF-1 and c-kit, a putative receptor for an unidentified ligand.[29]

The PDGF-α receptor binds all isoforms of PDGF; the PDGF-β receptor binds only the BB and AB forms. It is not known whether the two receptor forms mediate different activities of PDGF. It has been proposed that the PDGF receptor dimerizes at the cell surface to become active.[35]

PDGF Action

The induction of competence by PDGF requires only transient exposure of cells to the factor.[4] It is still unclear what biochemical events lead to the establishment of competence and whether competence is correlated with an identifiable molecular state of the cell. The question has been studied by defining changes in gene expression and the more rapid biochemical changes that occur in fibroblasts in response to PDGF (Fig. 4–3).[36-38]

Binding of PDGF to its cell surface receptor is followed within minutes by rapid receptor autophosphorylation and the phosphorylation on tyrosine of a number of endogenous proteins, possibly by the PDGF receptor/tyrosine kinase.[39, 40] Protein domains with tyrosine kinase activity are common to many oncogene-encoded proteins in addition to growth factor receptors, and there are strong structural homologies among these domains,[41] which suggests that tyrosine phosphorylation may be an important biochemical step in the transmission of the mitogenic signal.

PDGF activates a phosphatidylinositol-specific phospholipase C, which hydrolyzes plasma membrane phosphatidylinositol diphosphate (PIP_2) to form inositol trisphosphate (IP_3) and diacylglycerol.[42, 43] Recent evidence suggests that the activation of phospholipase C may occur by direct association of an isoform of phospholipase C with a complex of the PDGF receptor, the Raf-1 serine-threonine kinase and the phosphatidylinositol-3 kinase.[44] Inositol trisphosphate can cause the release of calcium ion from an intracellular pool. The resulting increase in the cytoplasmic calcium ion concentration would be expected to modulate the activity of calcium/calmodulin-dependent and other calcium-dependent enzymes including protein kinases and proteases.[45] High intracellular calcium concentrations may also activate an amiloride-sensitive plasma membrane Na^+/H^+ antiporter, leading to cellular alkalinization as a result of the exchange of intracellular hydrogen ion for extracellular sodium ion, an event that has been correlated with the stimulation of DNA synthesis.[46]

Diacylglycerol (DAG) generated by the hydrolysis of PIP_2 is an activator of the serine/threonine-specific protein kinase C, which in turn is capable of phosphorylating a number of intracellular proteins including growth factor receptors,[47, 48] cytoskeletal components[49, 50] and ribosomal subunit S6.[51] Protein kinase C activation has been shown to stimulate amiloride-sensitive Na^+/H^+ exchange and cellular alkalinization in several cell lines.[52, 53] Protein kinase C is directly activated by the tumor promoter 12-0-tetradecanoyl phorbol-13-acetate (TPA), an analogue of DAG that has been used experimentally to define the role of protein kinase C in cell cycle regulation. Recent evidence, how-

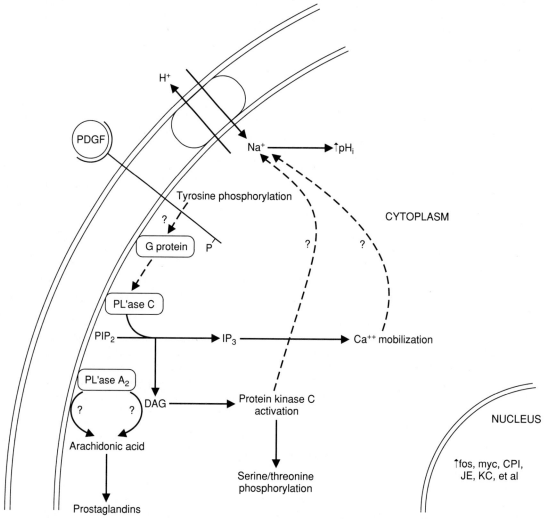

Figure 4–3. Early responses to platelet-derived growth factor (PDGF) resulting in the transcription of multiple genes including fos, myc, CPI, JE, and KC. PIP_2 = phosphatidylinositol bisphosphate; IP_3 = inositol triphosphate; DAG =diacylglycerol; PL'ase C = phospholipase C; PL'ase A_2 = phospholipase A_2; CPI = the competence-related protein pI identified by Pledger et al[63]; JE and KC = early response genes identified by Cochran et al.[65]

ever, suggests that TPA may have primary effects on other cellular events,[54] and the role of protein kinase C in the control of cell proliferation based on studies using TPA may have been somewhat overstated.

In addition to activation of protein kinase C, diacylglycerol may serve as a substrate for diacylglycerol lipase to generate monoacylglycerol and arachidonic acid in response to PDGF. Addition of PDGF to quiescent Swiss 3T3 fibroblasts causes rapid PIP_2 hydrolysis and a transient increase in cellular diacylglycerol levels. After 10 minutes, cellular diacylglycerol decreases, with a concomitant increase in the levels of monoacylglycerol and arachidonic acid in the cell and medium.[42] The released arachidonic acid may be reincorporated into newly synthesized phospholipid or converted to prostaglandins, the synthesis and release of which are stimulated in Swiss 3T3 cells by PDGF.[55, 56] The importance of stimulated prostaglandin synthesis in PDGF action is unclear, however; inhibitors of both the cyclo-oxygenase and lipoxygenase pathways of arachidonic acid metabolism do not interfere with PDGF-induced DNA synthesis.[55]

An early event in the response of most cell types to a variety of growth-promoting substances is the induction of expression of the cellular proto-oncogenes c-fos and c-myc. These genes encode proteins of approximately 53,000 to 69,000 daltons[57] and 62,000 daltons[58], respectively, based on electrophoretic mobility. The expression of c-fos and c-myc, as well as a number of other early genes (see further on) in response to growth factors is not prevented by inhibitors of protein synthesis. This indicates that the induction of transcription of these genes is a primary response to growth factor addition; that is, stimulation of their expression does not require synthesis of a protein mediator after growth factor binding. The c-fos and c-myc proteins localize to the cell nucleus and have been shown to bind to DNA.[59, 60] Expression of c-fos in response to PDGF occurs within minutes, and the amount of c-fos mRNA is maximal at 30 to 60 minutes after stimulation. The mRNA turns over with a relatively short half-life (20 to 30 minutes), and the half-life of the protein is also short (30 to 60 minutes). The c-fos protein rapidly becomes hyperphosphorylated on serine in response to serum and the phosphoryl groups are turned over rapidly (half-life less than 15 minutes).[57]

The induction of c-myc transcription by growth factors occurs within 1 hour and is maximal at around 2 hours after stimulation. Unlike c-fos, stimulated cells maintain elevated transcription of c-myc for more than 10 hours. The c-myc protein, however, is rapidly degraded (half-life of 30 to 60 minutes).

Although the induction of c-fos and c-myc expression is an early event common to stimulation by several growth-promoting substances, the role of these proteins in the regulation of transit through all the cell cycle is unknown. Microinjection of c-myc protein into nuclei of Swiss 3T3 cells has been shown to render these cells competent to respond to progression factors with stimulated DNA synthesis,[61] suggesting that c-myc functions in the G_0 to G_1 transition associated with competence. Alternatively, addition of a c-myc antisense oligonucleotide (complementary to the "sense," or coding strand, of c-myc mRNA) to T lymphocytes has been suggested to cause inhibition of c-myc protein synthesis and DNA synthesis in response to lectin, but not to prevent the G_0 to G_1 transition or progression into late G_1.[58] Moreover, the rapid turnover of the c-fos and c-myc proteins seems inconsistent with stability of the competent state, which decays with a half-life of approximately 16 hours.[62]

The bulk of data currently suggests that the expression of early transcribed genes is required for the induction of competence in stimulated cells but is insufficient to induce progression through DNA synthesis and cell division.

In an effort to identify other gene products that are required for the induction of competence in fibroblasts, several investigators have studied changes in gene expression induced in arrested cells by PDGF. Pledger and associates[63] compared specific protein synthesis in PDGF- versus platelet-poor plasma-treated Balb/c-3T3 fibroblasts and identified five proteins that were preferentially synthesized in cells stimulated with PDGF. Four proteins were detected within 1.5 hours after PDGF stimulation, while one, pI, was observed within 40 minutes. Two of these proteins, pI and pII, were found to be synthesized constitutively by a spontaneously transformed variant of Balb/c-3T3 that had lost the requirement for PDGF for stimulation of growth, supporting the association of these proteins with the PDGF-induced competent state. The pI protein was found to be preferentially associated with the nucleus, where it persisted for 12 to 15 hours after a brief (2.5 hours) treatment with PDGF.[64] Synthesis of pI was stimulated by the competence factors FGF and calcium phosphate in addition to PDGF but was not affected by progression factors (plasma, EGF, insulin).

Stiles and co-workers[65] identified five gene sequences whose transcriptional products were increased in abundance in the presence of PDGF by differential screening of a cDNA library prepared from PDGF-treated Balb/c-3T3 cells. Two of the cDNAs, JE and KC, were induced ten to twenty fold within 1 hour after PDGF treatment and could be translated in vitro to produce polypeptides of approximately 19,000 and 10,000 daltons, respectively. Neither sequence appeared to correspond to any of the five PDGF-induced proteins identified by Pledger and co-workers.[63]

Lau and Nathans[66] identified ten genes whose expression is induced rapidly in Balb/c-3T3 by serum, PDGF, or FGF. The oncogenes c-fos and c-myc were not represented in this set of genes, nor did the sequences of these genes correspond to those of other early genes whose sequences have been determined. Like c-fos and c-myc and the early genes identified by Stiles and co-workers, inhibitors of protein synthesis such as cycloheximide do not prevent transcription of the early genes studied by Lau and Nathans in response to growth stimulation. Rather, inhibition of protein synthesis has consistently been observed to cause superinduction of early response genes. The mechanism of superinduction appears to be twofold: the decay of transcribed mRNA is retarded by inhibitors of protein synthesis, and the shut-off of transcriptional activation of these genes at later times after stimulation seems to be inhibited.[66] The rapid transcriptional response to growth stimulation and the lack of effect of protein synthesis inhibitors on transcriptional activation implies that cells arrested in G_0 are poised for immediate activation of gene expression in response to growth stimulation. These results also suggest that synthesis of a protein or proteins is required to shut off the early response to stimulation by competence factors. Early gene transcription is a transient response to competence factors and is followed by the expression of other late gene products, a process that may be regulated by one or more of the transiently activated early response genes.

PROGRESSION FACTORS

In the presence of PDGF, quiescent Balb/c-3T3 fibroblasts become competent to respond to progression factors normally present in platelet-deficient plasma. Subsequent culture in plasma allows competent cells to initiate DNA synthesis after 12 hours; this lag time represents the minimum time required for density arrested cells to transit the G_1 phase of the cell cycle. Although a transient exposure to PDGF is sufficient to render cells competent to proliferate, continuous exposure to plasma is necessary for cells to complete transit of the entire G_1 phase. The requirement for platelet-deficient plasma in the culture medium can be met by substitution of two growth factors: epidermal growth factor (EGF) and somatomedin C/insulin like growth factor-1 (IGF-1). IGF-1 is indeed one of the progression factors present in plasma.[8] However, the identity of the second activity has not been established; EGF may be replacing an EGF-like activity present in platelet-deficient plasma. Pharmacological concentrations of insulin can replace IGF-1 in stimulating progression; at these concentrations, insulin has been shown to cross-react with the IGF-1 receptor.[67]

In order to identify events involved in the regulation of progression, the G_1 phase has been subdivided by the introduction of several experimentally induced arrest points. By manipulating the time of exposure to plasma, two arrest points within G_1 have been defined: the V point, which occurs 6 hours before the onset of DNA synthesis, and the W point, immediately prior to DNA synthesis (Fig. 4–2).[68] The W point appears to be the point of commitment to DNA synthesis and cell division: the cell requires plasma components to become committed to DNA synthesis; however, beyond this point no growth factors are required to stimulate transit through DNA synthesis, G_2, and mitosis.[69] Competent cells cultured in defined media (lacking serum or plasma) require both EGF and IGF-1 to reach the V point, which bisects the G_1 phase, but IGF-1 (or pharmacological levels of insulin) alone is sufficient for transit from the V point to the G_1/S boundary.

Epidermal Growth Factor

EGF is a 6000 dalton polypeptide growth factor that was first isolated by Cohen from the murine submaxillary gland as an inducer of precocious eyelid opening and tooth eruption in newborn mice.[70] The receptor for EGF is expressed in a wide variety of cell types and mediates the binding and biological activity of EGF and two related polypeptides, type α transforming growth factor (TGF-α) and a vaccinia virus growth factor (VGF).[71] The EGF receptor is a 170,000 dalton glycoprotein that, like the PDGF receptor, has a cytoplasmic tyrosine kinase domain that is capable of autophosphorylation as well as phosphorylation of several cellular substrates, such as the lipocortins, in response to EGF. Although EGF is mitogenic in many cell types, density arrested Balb/c-3T3 fibroblasts are EGF-unresponsive. Moreover, many fibroblast lines that do respond mitogenically to EGF require EGF concentrations at least an order of magnitude greater than that found in 10 per cent plasma- or serum-supplemented medium. Treatment with PDGF causes the EGF-insensitive Balb/c-3T3 cells to acquire responsiveness to EGF, and in C3H 10T$_{1/2}$ cells, which respond to relatively high concentrations of EGF, treatment with PDGF has been found to increase by more than tenfold the sensitivity to EGF-stimulated DNA synthesis.[72]

The induction of competence by PDGF, therefore, is associated with an increase in cellular responsiveness to EGF. The mechanism of PDGF induction of increased EGF responsiveness is unclear. It has been observed that differential sensitivity of fibroblast cell lines to EGF is correlated with differences in intracellular cyclic AMP levels and that induction of intracellular cyclic AMP accumulation enhances EGF responsiveness.[73] PDGF, however, does not appear to influence intracellular cyclic AMP concentrations. Paradoxically, treatment of cells with PDGF causes a decrease in the number of high-affinity receptors for EGF. Decreased EGF binding and receptor tyrosine kinase activity also follows activation of protein kinase C by phorbol esters, apparently as a result of phosphorylation of threonine 654 of the EGF receptor.[71] Although PDGF also induces phosphorylation of threonine 654, the effects of PDGF on EGF binding and mitogenic activity have been shown to be independent of the activation of protein kinase C.[74]

Somatomedin C/IGF-1

Somatomedin C is a 7000 dalton polypeptide that is identical to insulinlike growth factor-1 (IGF-1), or NSILA, one of two peptides originally identified as nonsuppressible insulinlike activity.[75] The major source of circulating IGF-1 appears to be the liver, and circulating IGF-1 levels are regulated by growth hormone. A wide range of cell types including chondrocytes, granulosa, smooth muscle cells, and lymphocytes appear to respond to IGF-1, and in many cases IGF-1 affects differentiated functions as well as proliferation in these tissues.[76]

In tissue culture, human fibroblasts release a large (20,000 daltons) IGF-1–like peptide that is immunologically cross-reactive with plasma IGF-1. These cells are able to proliferate in culture in the presence of PDGF in IGF-1–deficient plasma, suggesting that in vitro, the IGF-1–like peptide produced by human fibroblasts may support growth by an autocrine mechanism. Addition of monoclonal antibody directed against IGF-1 inhibits the proliferation of these cells and of Balb/c-3T3 fibroblasts in medium to which IGF-1 has been added.[8, 77]

The receptor for IGF-1 is expressed in a wide variety of tissues and is modulated developmentally in some tissues.[75] The IGF-1 receptor is structurally similar to the insulin receptor, shares some antigenic determinants with the insulin receptor, and binds insulin, albeit with a relatively low affinity.

The expression of the IGF-1 receptor in fibroblasts is influenced by PDGF.[78] Transient exposure of arrested cells to PDGF followed by platelet-poor plasma causes a twofold increase in IGF-1 binding, reflected in an increase in the number of IGF-1 binding sites per cell, with no change in binding affinity. This effect is dependent upon sequential exposure to PDGF and plasma: incubation with plasma followed by PDGF is ineffective. The factor in plasma necessary for the enhancement of IGF-1 binding is a nondialyzable component that is distinct from IGF-1 itself, since hypopituitary plasma is as effective as normal plasma. These observations suggest that the induction of competence by PDGF may sensitize the cell to respond to IGF-1.

The availability of techniques for arresting cells at the V point in mid-G_1 has facilitated studies of IGF-1 action. Campisi and Pardee[79] demonstrated that exponentially growing cells, in contrast to cells stimulated from G_0 arrest, require only IGF-1 for cell cycle traverse, suggesting that the 6 hour G_1 phase observed in cycling Balb/c-3T3 fibroblasts is equivalent to the 6 hours between the V point and the G_1/S boundary in arrested cells, during which IGF-1 alone is sufficient for progression. Treatment of cells in early or late G_1 with inhibitors of protein and RNA synthesis has shown that although protein synthesis is required throughout most of the G_1 period, the traverse of cells through late G_1 is relatively refractory to inhibition of RNA synthesis.[79–81] Moreover, progression from the V point to S phase does not appear to require increased overall protein synthesis, nor does IGF-1 appear to stimulate synthesis of specific proteins detectable by two-dimensional electrophoresis of ^{35}S-methionine-labeled cellular extracts. A possible posttranslational role for IGF-1 is indicated by changes observed in the isoelectric point of several preexisting proteins in the presence of the factor.[81] These observations are consistent with the idea that once cells stimulated from G_0 have reached mid G_1 phase, transcription of additional mRNA is not needed for traverse through late G_1 and initiation of DNA synthesis. The requirement for IGF-1 in late G_1 may be posttranscriptional and may reflect a role in the stabilization of preexisting mRNA,[82] or in posttranslational modification of preexisting proteins that may be required for commitment to DNA synthesis.

TRANSFORMING GROWTH FACTOR-β

The platelet α granules are a major storage site for transforming growth factor-β (TGF-β), which is released with PDGF upon platelet activation. Mammalian TGF-β occurs in multiple forms that are 70 to 80 percent homologous, although they represent different gene products with tissue-specific expression. Mature TGF-β is a 25,000 dalton polypeptide composed of two identical disulfide-linked subunits formed by cleavage of a larger precursor.[83–85] In human platelets, this form is bound in a noncovalent complex with the disulfide-linked dimer of the amino-terminal portion of the inactive precursor, which is in turn covalently associated with a dimeric protein of approximately 150,000 daltons. Activation of precursor TGF-β can be induced by a number of denaturing treatments and may correspond to the dissociation of already cleaved precursor peptide from the active TGF-β dimer.

Three forms of receptor for TGF-β have been identified.[85] Type I, a 65,000 dalton affinity-labeled peptide, has been identified in all cells examined. Types II and III, approximately 100,000 and 300,000 daltons, respectively, bind TGF-β but have not been shown to mediate TGF-β activity. The ubiquitous nature of both TGF-β and its receptor suggests that the activation of the TGF-β precursor in vivo, by a mechanism that is still speculative, may be an important step in the regulation of TGF-β action.

The biological activity of TGF-β is highly cell type– and context-dependent. TGF-β is a growth inhibitor for most cell types, including lymphocytes and epithelial cells as well as several types of malignant cells, and is similar or identical to the growth inhibitor (GI) isolated by Holley and co-workers.[86, 87] However, TGF-β is a growth stimulator for mesenchymal cells[88] and accelerates experimental wound healing in Schilling-Hunt chambers in rats.[89] Single application of TGF-β has been found to accelerate healing in gastric wounds in rabbits[90] and to reverse glucocorticoid-induced wound healing deficiency in rats.[91] The mechanism of stimulation by TGF-β of fibroblast proliferation is unclear. TGF-β induces expression of c-sis/PDGF B chain mRNA in mouse embryo-derived AKR-2B fibroblasts;[92] however, this response may not strictly be correlated with proliferation in response to TGF-β. It has been suggested that TGF-β enhances wound healing by direct stimulation of the synthesis of connective tissue by fibroblasts and indirect stimulation of fibroblast proliferation mediated by PDGF.[91]

TUMOR NECROSIS FACTOR

Tumor necrosis factor (TNF-α) was originally defined by its antitumor activity in vivo and in vitro; it is now recognized as a modulator of growth and differentiated function in many cell types involved in inflammation.[96] The major source of TNF-α is mononuclear phagocytic cells, which synthesize it as a 233 amino acid precursor from which the amino terminal portion is cleaved prior to secretion to produce a 157 amino acid mature peptide of 17,000 daltons.[93] Lymphotoxin, a T-lymphocyte product now called TNF-β, is also tumoricidal and acts through the same cell surface receptor as TNF-α. The TNFs are 50 per cent homologous but are not immunologically crossreactive. The genes for TNF-α and TNF-β are closely linked in mouse and human in the regions of chromosomes 17 and 6, respectively, which also contain the genes of the major histocompatibility complex.[93]

Like TGF-β, the biological activity of TNF is highly cell-type–specific. In vitro, TNF induces growth, cytotoxicity, or no effect depending on the target cell type.[93, 94] In several fibroblast cell lines, Vilcek and associates demonstrated an increase in cell number and DNA synthesis in response to recombinant TNF-α.[94] When tested against a battery of cultured cell lines derived from various human tumors, TNF was cytotoxic or cytostatic to two thirds of the cell lines and without effect on the remainder.[95] The pattern of inhibition of TNF-α action by different monoclonal antibodies directed against TNF-α indicates that the same epitope is responsible for both growth stimulation in FS-4 cells and cytotoxicity in L929 fibroblasts, and a single high-affinity receptor for TNF apparently mediates both activities.[94] The effect of TNF on a given cell type may be dependent upon the capacity of the cell to respond at the subcellular level and/or the presence of other factors in the local environment of the cell.

INHIBITION OF CELL PROLIFERATION

Although the existence of substances that inhibit cell proliferation has been recognized for some time, the consideration of growth inhibitors as an integral part of the mechanism for control of cell proliferation is a relatively recent development. Two growth factors, TGF-β and tumor necrosis factor (TNF),[96] have been found to be growth inhibitory for selected cell types. The best characterized inhibitor, however, is interferon, which appears to act as an autocrine growth modulator in fibroblasts and in a large variety of other cell types.[97]

Six to eight hours after exposure to PDGF, Balb/c-3T3 fibroblasts produce mRNA encoding β-fibroblast interferon (IFN-β), and mRNA levels remain high for as long as 12 hours after stimulation.[98] Exposure of Balb/c-3T3 cells to IFN-β results in inhibition of DNA synthesis and cell division.[99] Addition of IFN-β to arrested cells stimulated with PDGF and plasma results in inhibition only if IFN-β is added within the first 6 hours after PDGF stimulation, suggesting that IFN-β inhibits events involved in the G_0/G_1 transition associated with the induction of competence.[99] Consistent with this idea is the observation that IFN-β inhibits the overall stimulation of protein synthesis by PDGF and suppresses the production of the competence-related proteins pI and pII identified by Pledger and co-workers.[63] Addition of IFN-β to PDGF-stimulated cells also suppresses the induction of other early response genes including c-myc, c-fos, and ornithine decarboxylase. However, unlike the induction of these genes by PDGF, suppression of c-myc induction by IFN-β appears to be partially dependent on protein synthesis.[100] Recent work has focused on mechanisms of active growth inhibition that may be mediated by specific genes expressed under conditions leading to growth arrest.[101, 102]

CLINICAL CONTROL OF FIBROBLAST PROLIFERATION

Currently, clinical modulation of wound repair generally involves the use of relatively nonspecific activators or inhibitors of cell proliferation and collagen production. Advances in the understanding of cell cycle regulation provide a theoretical basis for the development of more target-directed manipulation of the wound healing process.

The apparent complexity of the regulatory machinery of wound repair reflects the multifunctional involvement of several cell types, including platelets, mononuclear phagocytes, endothelial cells, and fibroblasts, which are activated to perform replication, directed migration, phagocytosis, proteolysis, and synthesis and deposition of specific proteins. Not unexpectedly, disturbances of wound repair appear in a broad range of clinical contexts and reflect both repair deficiencies and uncontrolled fibrogenic processes. Pathological fibrogenic processes (e.g., keloids, encapsulation of breast implants, and entrapment of tendons after tendon repair) as well as postoperative obstruction due to peritoneal adhesion, may be controllable by treatments aimed at inhibiting fibroblast proliferation. Alternatively, conditions in which wound repair is suppressed, such as in patients with inborn errors of metabolism or diabetes, patients on immunosuppressive regimens, such as transplant recipients, and patients on steroid or chemotherapy, may be treatable by localized stimulation of fibroblast proliferation.

Current understanding of the regulation of fibroblast proliferation suggests that the one means to specifically stimulate fibroblast prolif-eration is by application of factors such as PDGF and TGF-β that cause entry of fibroblasts into the cell cycle. Clinically, this could be accomplished by treatment with exogenous growth factors or by induction of the release and/or activation of PDGF and TGF-β. The widespread tissue distribution of fibroblasts capable of proliferation militates against the management of wound repair disorders by systemic application of growth regulatory factors. Ideally, treatment to modulate repair should be localized to the wound site. The application of TGF-β immobilized in bovine collagen to linear skin incisions in rats has been found to enhance wound tensile strength.[103] The effect was noted in the first few days after injury and was limited to the local area of TGF-β application. Treatment of incisions with TGF-β in saline solution had no effect on tensile strength. Histologically, incisions treated with immobilized TGF-β showed local increases in the numbers of mononuclear phagocytes and fibroblasts and in the synthesis of new collagen. Similarly, in a porcine mid-dermal thermal wound model, TGF-α and vaccinia growth factor (VGF) applied in a water-miscible antibiotic cream were found to increase the area of regenerated epithelium in second degree burns.[104] Interestingly, both TGF-α and VGF appeared to be more potent than EGF in this system, although these factors all appear to act through the EGF receptor.

The mononuclear phagocyte is probably the major source of both PDGF and TGF-β after platelet activation has occurred and may also be responsible for the activation of TGF-β secreted by platelets and other cells. Thus, targeted activation of the mononuclear phagocyte might be an approach to the generation of an endogenous stimulus to fibroblast proliferation. Alternatively, negative modulation of fibroblast proliferation might be accomplished by inhibition of the release and/or activation of PDGF and TGF-β or by stimulation of the endogenous release of inhibitory substances, such as IFN-β. IFN-β–induced growth inhibition appears to be an autocrine effect mediated by IFN-β produced and released by the mitogen-stimulated fibroblast; hemopoietic cells also produce β-related IFNs that apparently function as autocrine inhibitors.[105] IFN-β shares a single receptor with IFN-α that is distinct from the IFN-γ receptor; however, both IFN-α and IFN-β may synergize with IFN-γ to inhibit growth.[97] The three IFN families are biologically active in a wide range of cell types, potentially complicating their use for modulation of wound repair.

The clinical management of wound disorders should exploit the fact that the healing process itself is the net result of the balance of both stimulatory and inhibitory signals, the localized release and/or activation of which causes locally restricted and temporally regulated activation of cells within the wound site.

References

1. Baserga R: Multiplication and Division in Mammalian Cells. New York, Marcel Dekker, 1976.
2. Baserga R: The Biology of Cell Reproduction. Cambridge, Harvard University Press, 1985.
3. Prescott CM: Reproduction of Eukaryotic Cells. New York, Academic Press, 1976.
4. Baserga R: Growth in size and cell DNA replication. Exp Cell Res 151:1–5, 1984.
5. Pledger WJ, Stiles CD, Antoniades HN, et al: Induction of DNA synthesis in Balb/c-3T3 cells by serum components. Reevaluation of the commitment process. Proc Natl Acad Sci USA 74:4481–4485, 1977.
6. Antoniades HN, Scher CD: Radioimmunoassay of a human serum growth factor for Balb/c-3T3 cells: Derivation from platelets. Proc Natl Acad Sci USA 74:1973–1977, 1977.
7. Stiles CD, Capone GT, Scher CD, et al: Dual control of cell growth by somatomedins and platelet-derived growth factor. Proc Natl Acad Sci USA 76:1279–1283, 1979.
8. Russell WE, Van Wyk JJ, Pledger WJ: Inhibition of the mitogenic effects of plasma by a monoclonal antibody to somatomedin C. Proc Natl Acad Sci USA 81:2389–2392, 1984.
9. Ross R, Glomset JA, Kariya B, et al: A platelet dependent serum factor that stimulates the proliferation of arterial smooth muscle cells in vitro. Proc Natl Acad Sci USA 71:1207–1210, 1974.
10. Kohler N, Lipton A: Platelets as a source of fibroblast growth-promoting activity. Exp Cell Res 87:297–301, 1974.
11. Ross R, Raines EW, Bowen-Pope DF: The biology of platelet-derived growth factor. Cell 46:155–169, 1986.
12. Oka Y, Orth DN: Human plasma epidermal growth factor/β-urogastrone is associated with blood platelets. J Clin Invest 72:249–259, 1983.
13. Childs CB, Proper JA, Tucker RF, et al: Serum contains a platelet-derived transforming growth factor. Proc Natl Acad Sci USA 79:5312–5316, 1982.
14. Assoian RK, Komoriya A, Meyers CA, et al: Transforming growth factor-β in human platelets: Identification of a major storage site, purification, and characterization. J Biol Chem 258:7155–7160, 1983.
15. Shimokado K, Raines EW, Madtes DK, et al: A significant part of macrophage-derived growth factor consists of at least two forms of PDGF. Cell 43:277–286, 1985.
16. Wharton W, Gillespie GY, Russell SW, et al: Mitogenic activity elaborated by macrophage-like cell lines acts as competence factor(s) for Balb/c-3T3 cells. J Cell Physiol 110:93–100, 1982.
17. Martinet Y, Bitterman PB, Mornex J-F, et al: Activated human monocytes express the c-sis protooncogene and release a mediator showing PDGF-like activity. Nature 319:158–160, 1986.
18. Sejersen T, Betsholtz C, Sjolund M, et al: Rat skeletal myoblasts and arterial smooth muscle cells express the gene for the A chain, but not the gene for the B chain (c-sis) of platelet-derived growth factor (PDGF) and produce a PDGF-like protein. Proc Natl Acad Sci USA 83:6844–6848, 1986.
19. Kelley JD, Raines EW, Ross R, et al: The B chain of PDGF alone is sufficient for mitogenesis. EMBO J 4:3399–3405, 1985.
20. Nister M, Hammacher A, Mellström K, et al: A glioma-derived PDGF A chain homodimer has different functional activities from a PDGF AB heterodimer purified from human platelets. Cell 52:791–799, 1988.
21. Betsholtz C, Johnsson A, Heldin C-H, et al: cDNA sequence and chromosomal localization of human platelet-derived growth factor A chain and its expression in tumor cell lines. Nature 320:695–699, 1986.
22. Clarke MF, Westin E, Schmidt D, et al: Transformation of NIH 3T3 cells by a human c-sis cDNA clone. Nature 308:464–467, 1984.
23. Waterfield MD, Scrace GT, Whittle N, et al: Platelet-derived growth factor is structurally related to the putative transforming protein p28sis of simian sarcoma virus. Nature 304:35–39, 1983.
24. Doolittle RF, Hunkapiller MW, Hood LE, et al: Simian sarcoma virus onc gene, v-sis, is derived from the gene (or genes) encoding a platelet-derived growth factor. Science 221:275–277, 1983.
25. Bishop M: Cellular oncogenes and retroviruses. Ann Rev Biochem 52:301–354, 1983.
26. Huang JS, Huang SS, Deuel TF: Transforming protein of simian sarcoma virus stimulates autocrine growth of SSV-transformed cells through PDGF cell-surface receptors. Cell 39:79–87, 1984.
27. Gazit A, Igarashi H, Chiu I-M, Srinivasan A, et al: Expression of the normal human sis/PDGF-2 coding sequence induces cellular transformation. Cell 39:89–97, 1984.
28. Bowen-Pope DF, Rosenfeld ME, Seifert RA, et al: The platelet-derived growth factor receptor. Int J Neurosci 26:141–153, 1985.
29. Yarden Y, Escobedo JA, Kuang W-J, et al: Structure of the receptor for platelet-derived growth factor helps define a family of closely related growth factor receptors. Nature 323:226–232, 1986.
30. Matsui T, Heidaran M, Miki T, et al: Isolation of a novel receptor cDNA establishes the existence of two PDGF receptor genes. Science 24:800–804, 1989.
31. Claesson-Welsh L, Eriksson A, Westermark B, et al: cDNA cloning and expression of the human A-type platelet-derived growth factor (PDGF) receptor establishes structural similarity to the B-type receptor. Proc Natl Acad Sci USA 86:4917–4921, 1989.
32. Hershko A, Ciechanover A: The ubiquitin pathway for the degradation of intracellular proteins. Prog Nucl Acid Res Mol Biol 33:19–56, 1986.
33. Fried VA, Smith HT, Hildebrandt E, et al: Ubiquitin has intrinsic proteolytic activity: Implications for cellular regulation. Proc Natl Acad Sci USA 84:3685–3689, 1987.
34. Escobedo JA, Williams LT: A PDGF receptor domain essential for mitogenesis but not for many other responses to PDGF. Nature 335:85–87, 1988.
35. Seifert RA, Hart CE, Phillips PE, et al: Two different subunits associate to create isoform-specific platelet-derived growth factor receptors. J Biol Chem 264:8771–8778, 1989.
36. Olashaw NE, Pledger WJ: Mechanisms initiating cellular proliferation. In Ford RJ, Maizel AL (eds): Mediators in Cell Growth and Differentiation. New York, Raven Press, 1985, pp 31–44.
37. Rosengurt E: Early signals in the mitogenic response. Science 234:161–166, 1986.
38. Stiles CD: The molecular biology of platelet-derived growth factor. Cell 33:653–655, 1983.
39. Cooper JA, Bowen-Pope DF, Raines E, et al: Similar effects of platelet-derived growth factor and epidermal

growth factor on the phosphorylation of tyrosine in cellular proteins. Cell 31:263–273, 1982.

40. Cooper JA, Sefton BM, Hunter T: Diverse mitogenic agents induce the phosphorylation of two related 42,000 dalton proteins on tyrosine in quiescent chick cells. Mol Cell Biol 4:30–37, 1984.

41. Hunter T, Cooper JA: Protein-tyrosine kinases. Ann Rev Biochem 54:897–930, 1985.

42. Habenicht AJR, Glomset JA, King WC, et al: Early changes in phosphatidylinositol and arachidonic acid metabolism in quiescent Swiss 3T3 cells stimulated to divide by platelet-derived growth factor. J Biol Chem 256:12329–12335, 1981.

43. Berridge M: Inositol phosphate and diacylglycerol: Two interacting second messengers. Ann Rev Biochem 56:159–194, 1987.

44. Morrison DK, Kaplan DR, Rhee SG, et al: Platelet-derived growth factor–dependent association of phospholipase C-8 with the PDGF receptor signalling complex. Mol Cell Biol 10:2359–2366, 1990.

45. Rassmussen H, Kojima I, Kojima K, et al: Calcium as intracellular messenger: Sensitivity modulation, C-kinase pathway, and sustained cellular response. Adv Cyclic Nucleotide Res Prot Phosphor 18:159–193, 1984.

46. L'Allemain G, Paris S, Pouyssegur J: Growth factor activation and intracellular pH regulation in fibroblasts: Evidence for a major role of the Na$^+$/H$^+$ antiport. J Biol Chem 259:5809–5815, 1984.

47. Downward J, Waterfield MD, Parker PJ: Autophosphorylation and protein kinase C phosphorylation of the epidermal growth factor receptor: Effect on tyrosine kinase activity and ligand binding affinity. J Biol Chem 260:14538–14546, 1985.

48. Bollag GE, Roth RA, Beaudoin J, et al: Protein kinase C directly phosphorylates the insulin receptor in vitro and reduces its protein tyrosine kinase activity. Proc Natl Acad Sci USA 83:5822–5824, 1986.

49. Litchfield DW, Ball EH: Phosphorylation of the cytoskeletal protein talin by protein kinase C. Biochem Biophys Res Comm 134:1276–1283, 1986.

50. Werth DK, Niedal JE, Pastan I: Vinculin, a cytoskeletal substrate of protein kinase C. J Biol Chem 258:11423–11426, 1983.

51. Blenis J, Spivak JG, Erikson RL: Phorbol ester, serum, and Rous sarcoma virus transforming gene product induce similar phosphorylations of ribosomal subunit S6. Proc Natl Acad Sci USA 81:6408–6412, 1984.

52. Besterman JM, Cuatrecasas P: Phorbol esters rapidly stimulate amiloride-sensitive Na$^+$/H$^+$ exchange in a human leukemic cell line. J Cell Biol 99:340–343, 1984.

53. Moolenaar WH, Tertoolen LGJ, de Laat SW: Phorbol ester and diacylglycerol mimic growth factors in raising cytoplasmic pH. Nature 312:371–374, 1984.

54. Ways DK, Dodd RC, Earp HS: Dissimilar effects of phorbol ester and diacylglycerol derivative on protein kinase C activity in the monoblastoid U937 cell. Cancer Res 47:3344–3350, 1987.

55. Shier WT, Durkin JP: Role of stimulation of arachidonic acid release in the proliferative response of 3T3 mouse fibroblasts to platelet-derived growth factor. J Cell Physiol 112:171–181, 1982.

56. Habenicht AJR, Dresel HA, Goerig M, et al: Low density lipoprotein receptor–dependent prostaglandin synthesis in Swiss 3T3 cells stimulated by platelet-derived growth factor. Proc Natl Acad Sci USA 83:1344–1348, 1986.

57. Barber JR, Verma IM: Modification of fos proteins: Phosphorylation of c-fos, but not v-fos, is stimulated by 12-tetradecanoyl-phorbol-13-acetate and serum. Mol Cell Biol 7:2201–2211, 1987.

58. Heikkila R, Schwab G, Wickstrom E, et al: A c-myc antisense oligonucleotide inhibits entry into S phase but not progress from G$_0$ to G$_1$. Nature 328:445–449, 1987.

59. Sambucetti LC, Curran T: The fos protein complex is associated with DNA in isolated nuclei and binds to DNA cellulose. Science 234:1417–1419, 1986.

60. Hann SR, Abrams HD, Rohrschneider LR, et al: Proteins encoded by v-myc and c-myc oncogenes: Identification and localization in acute leukemia virus transformants and bursal lymphoma lines. Cell 34:789–798, 1983.

61. Kaczmarek L, Hyland JK, Watt R, et al: Microinjected c-myc as a competence factor. Science 228:1313–1315, 1985.

62. Bravo R, Burckhardt J, Muller R: Persistence of the competent state in mouse fibroblasts is independent of c-fos and c-myc expression. Exp Cell Res 160:540–543, 1985.

63. Pledger WJ, Hart CA, Locatell KL, et al: Platelet-derived growth factor-modulated proteins: Constitutive synthesis by a transformed cell line. Proc Natl Acad Sci USA 78:4358–4362, 1981.

64. Olashaw NE, Pledger WJ: Association of platelet derived growth factor–induced proteins with nuclear material. Nature 306:272–274, 1983.

65. Cochran BH, Reffel AC, Stiles CD: Molecular cloning of gene sequences regulated by platelet derived growth factor. Cell 33:939–947, 1983.

66. Lau LF, Nathans D: Expression of a set of growth-regulated immediate early genes in Balb/c-3T3 cells: Coordinate regulation with c-fos or c-myc. Proc Natl Acad Sci USA 84:1182–1186, 1986.

67. Van Wyk JJ, Underwood LE, Baseman JB, et al: Exploration of the insulin-like and growth-promoting properties of somatomedin by membrane receptor assays. Adv Metab Disord 8:127–150, 1975.

68. Pledger WJ, Stiles CD, Antoniades HN, et al: An ordered sequence of events is required before Balb/c-3T3 cells become committed to DNA synthesis. Proc Natl Acad Sci USA 75:2839–2843, 1978.

69. Wharton W: Hormonal regulation of discrete portions of the cell cycle: Commitment to DNA synthesis is commitment to cellular division. J Cell Physiol 117:423–429, 1983.

70. Carpenter G, Cohen S: Epidermal growth factor. Ann Rev Biochem 48:193–216, 1979.

71. Carpenter G: Receptors for epidermal growth factor and other polypeptide mitogens. Ann Rev Biochem 56:881–914, 1987.

72. Wharton W, Leof EB, Olashaw NE, et al: Mitogenic response to epidermal growth factor is modulated by platelet derived growth factor. Exp Cell Res 147:443–448, 1983.

73. Olashaw NE, Leof EB, Okeefe EJ, et al: Differential sensitivity of fibroblasts to epidermal growth factor is related to cyclic AMP concentration. J Cell Physiol 118:291–297, 1984.

74. Olashaw NE, Okeefe EJ, Pledger WJ: Platelet derived growth factor modulates epidermal growth factor receptors by a mechanism distinct from that of phorbol esters. Proc Natl Acad Sci USA 83:3834–3838, 1986.

75. Baxter RC: The somatomedins: Insulin-like growth factors. Adv Clin Chem 25:49–115, 1986.

76. Van Wyk JJ, Russell WE, Underwood LE, et al: Action of somatomedins on cell growth: Effect of selective neutralization of somatomedin C (IGF-1) with a monoclonal antibody. In Raiti S, Tolman RA (eds): Human Growth Hormone. New York, Plenum, 1986, pp 585–599.

77. Clemmons DR, Van Wyk JJ: Evidence for a functional role of endogenously produced somatomedin-like peptides in the regulation of DNA synthesis in cultured human fibroblasts and porcine smooth muscle cells. J Clin Invest 75:1914–1918, 1985.

78. Clemmons DR, Van Wyk JJ, Pledger WJ: Sequential addition of platelet factor and plasma to Balb/c-3T3 fibroblast cultures stimulates somatomedin C binding early in cell cycle. Proc Natl Acad Sci USA 77:6644–6648, 1980.

79. Campisi J, Pardee AB: Post-transcriptional control of the onset of DNA synthesis by an insulin-like growth factor. Mol Cell Biol 4:1807–1814, 1984.

80. Yang HC, Pardee AB: Insulin-like growth factor-1 regulation of transcription and replicating enzyme induction necessary for DNA synthesis. J Cell Physiol 127:410–416, 1986.

81. Olashaw NE, Van Wyk JJ, Pledger WJ: Control of late G_0/G_1 progression and protein modification by somatomedin C/insulin-like growth factor-1. Am J Physiol Cell Physiol 22:C575–C579, 1987.

82. Coppock DL, Pardee AB: Control of thymidine kinase mRNA during the cell cycle. Mol Cell Biol 7:2925–2932, 1987.

83. Keski-Oja J, Leof EB, Lyons RM, et al: Transforming growth factors and control of neoplastic cell growth. J Cell Biochem 33:95–107, 1987.

84. Sporn MB, Roberts A: Peptide growth factors and inflammation, tissue repair and cancer. J Clin Invest 78:329–332, 1986.

85. Nilsen-Hamilton M: Transforming growth factor-β and its actions on cellular growth and differentiation. Curr Top Dev Biol 24:95–136, 1990.

86. Holley RW, Armour R, Baldwin JH: Density-dependent regulation of growth of BCS-1 cells in cell culture: Growth inhibitors formed by the cells. Proc Natl Acad Sci USA 75:1864–1866, 1978.

87. Tucker RF, Shipley GD, Moses HL, et al: Growth inhibitor from BSC-1 cells closely related to platelet type-β transforming growth factor. Science 226:705–707, 1984.

88. Shipley GD, Tucker RF, Moses HL: Type β transforming growth factor/growth inhibitor stimulates entry of monolayer cultures of AKR-2B cells into S phase after a prolonged prereplicative interval. Proc Natl Acad Sci USA 82:4147–4151, 1985.

89. Sporn MB, Roberts AB, Shull JH, et al: Enhancement of wound healing in rats by a bovine transforming growth factor. Science 291:1329–1331, 1983.

90. Mustoe TA, Landes A, Cromack DT, et al: Differential acceleration of healing of surgical incisions in the rabbit gastrointestinal tract by platelet-derived growth factor and transforming growth factor, type beta. Surgery 108:324–330, 1990.

91. Pierce GF, Mustoe TA, Lingelbach J, et al: Transforming growth factor β reverses the glucocorticoid-induced wound-healing deficit in rats: Possible regulation in macrophages by platelet-derived growth factor. Proc Natl Acad Sci USA 86:2229–2233, 1989.

92. Leof EB, Proper JA, Goustin AS, et al: Induction of c-sis mRNA and activity similar to platelet-derived growth factor by transforming growth factor β. A proposed model for indirect mitogenesis involving autocrine activity. Proc Natl Acad Sci USA 83:2453–2457, 1986.

93. Wanebo HJ: Tumor necrosis factors. Semin Surg Oncol 5:402–413, 1989.

94. Vilcek J, Palombella VJ, Henriksen-DeStefano D, et al: Fibroblast growth-enhancing activity of tumor necrosis factor and its relationship to other polypeptide growth factors. J Exp Med 163:632–643, 1986.

95. Yamamoto A, Williamson BD, Carswell EA, et al: In Homma JY, Kanegasaki S, Lueaderitz O (eds): Bacterial Endotoxin: Chemical, Biological and Clinical Aspects. Basel, Verlag Chemie, 1984, pp 223–234.

96. Old LJ: Tumor necrosis factor (TNF). Science 230:630–632, 1985.

97. Taylor-Papadimitriou J, Rosengurt E: Interferons as regulators of cell growth and differentiation. In Taylor-Papadimitriou J (ed): Interferons. Their impact in biology and medicine. Oxford, Oxford University Press, 1985, pp 81–98.

98. Zullo JN, Cochran BH, Huang AS, et al: Platelet-derived growth factor and double-stranded ribonucleic acids stimulate expression of the same genes in 3T3 cells. Cell 43:793–800, 1985.

99. Lin SL, Kikuchi T, Pledger WJ, et al: Interferon inhibits the establishment of competence in G_0/S phase transition. Science 233:356–359, 1986.

100. Einat M, Resnitsky D, Kimchi A: Inhibitory effects of interferon on the expression of genes regulated by platelet derived growth factor. Proc Natl Acad Sci USA 82:7608–7612, 1985.

101. Schneider C, King RM, Philipson L: Genes specifically expressed at growth arrest of mammalian cells. Cell 54:787–793, 1988.

102. Whyte P, Buchkovich KJ, Horowitz JM, et al: Association between an oncogene and an anti-oncogene: The adenovirus E1A proteins bind to the retinoblastoma gene product. Nature 334:124–129, 1988.

103. Mustoe TA, Pierce GF, Thomason A, et al: Accelerated healing of incisional wounds in rats induced by transforming growth factor β. Science 237:1333–1336, 1987.

104. Schultz G, White M, Mitchell R, et al: Epithelial wound healing enhanced by transforming growth factor α and vaccinia growth factor. Science 235:350–352, 1987.

105. Kimchi A, Zipori D, Resnitsky D: Autocrine IFN controls the reduction of c-myc mRNA and growth arrest during hematopoietic cell differentiation. In Stewart WE, Schellekens H (eds): The Biology of the Interferon System. Amsterdam, Elsevier, 1986.

5

ANGIOGENESIS

Giles F. Whalen, M.D., and Bruce R. Zetter, Ph.D.

The normal progression of neovascularity in a healing wound is evident to any careful observer. Shortly after wounding, the skin edges become erythematous. Within several days the wound bed develops a crimson base that bleeds readily when touched. The scar of a newly healed wound is thick, pink, and blanches with pressure. As the scar strengthens, it becomes thin and pale. Such gross observations have drawn attention to the importance of new vessel formation, termed angiogenesis, in healing.[1, 2]

The process of wound healing is often described as comprising a series of discrete events or phases.[3–5] Factors involved in blood clotting lead directly to the phase of acute inflammation. Macrophages are attracted to the wound during this acute phase but do not begin to predominate until the third day. The granulation tissue phase begins shortly thereafter. This phase is characterized by the migration of myofibroblasts and capillary sprouts into the wound behind the macrophages. Just behind this advancing edge, near newly functioning capillary loops, fibroblasts divide and deposit quantities of fibrillar collagen (Fig. 5–1). When the wound space is filled with new tissue, some capillaries involute, while others differentiate into arterioles and venules. The wound matrix becomes progressively less cellular, and the freshly deposited collagen is remodeled, providing greater tensile strength.

The vascular growth that occurs in wound healing requires endothelial cell migration and proliferation, events that occur rarely in the normal adult. Unlike the hematopoietic elements or intestinal epithelium, endothelial cells in mature blood vessels do not divide or migrate actively. Their doubling time is measured in years or decades,[6] as opposed to days for the intestinal epithelium.[7] Capillaries normally proliferate only during embryonic development, ovulation, menstruation, inflammation, and tissue repair. New vessels generally do not grow

in adults except in those situations, and in some pathological ones, but the vascular system is almost instantly responsive to proper angiogenic signals. Activation of this quiescent system is reminiscent of the physiological processes involved in blood clotting; a local stimulus starts a cascade of cellular events that results in the formation of new vessels where they are needed. As with clotting, the angiogenic process normally remains localized to the wound area and stops when the healing is complete.

NEOVASCULARIZATION IN WOUNDS

Over 50 years ago, Sandison along with Clark and Clark published a remarkable series of elegant drawings based on their observations of vessel ingrowth, primarily in rabbit ear chambers.[8–10] Their description of the angiogenic response in healing wounds is the foundation on which our current understanding of vascular development rests. Under a light microscope they observed that new capillaries developed as buds or sprouts from pre-existing vessels. Endothelial cells were seen to migrate and proliferate within the wound site. They further described a process in which vascular "threads" could make contact with other sprouts or with established blood vessels, leading to the formation of vascular loops through which blood could flow (Fig. 5–2). Capillaries without blood flow regressed within 24 hours, whereas those vessels with the greatest apparent blood flow later differentiated into arteries and veins.

With the advent of electron microscopy, Cliff[11] and Schoefl[12] were able to confirm many of the earlier morphological findings and to begin to describe the cellular and subcellular aspects of vascular growth. In these now classic studies, they demonstrated that newly formed

77

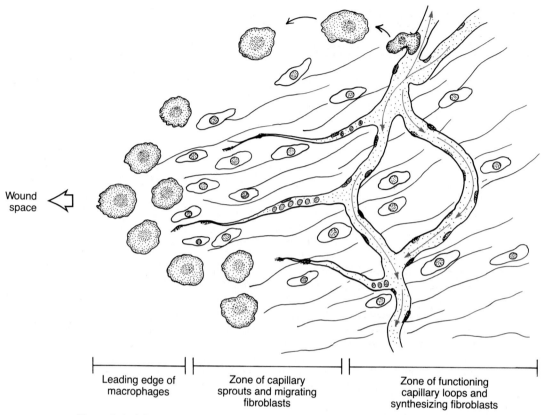

Wound
space

Leading edge of	Zone of capillary	Zone of functioning
macrophages	sprouts and migrating	capillary loops and
	fibroblasts	synthesizing fibroblasts

Figure 5–1. Advancing module of reparative tissue during granulation tissue phase.

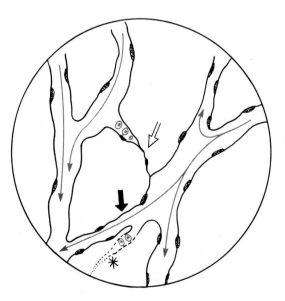

Figure 5–2. Light microscopic view of growing capillaries in a wound chamber. One sprout has contacted a functioning vessel but has not yet established flow *(open arrow)*. Another sprout has recently established flow between two functioning channels *(closed arrow)*. Its neighbor, thereby robbed of flow, is regressing *(asterisk)*.

capillaries lacked the well-formed basement membranes characteristic of mature vessels. The investigators speculated that this deficiency in basement membrane components might account for the increased permeability characteristic of growing blood vessels. As the new vessels matured, the endothelial cells became surrounded by a layer of perivascular cells (pericytes), and both cell types eventually were embedded in new basement membrane.[13] More recently, sophisticated studies using modern image analysis systems have quantified this wound angiogenesis in the rabbit ear chamber.[14, 15]

MODELS FOR THE STUDY OF ANGIOGENESIS

In addition to the rabbit ear chamber, a variety of other experimental models have been used to study angiogenesis. Angiogenesis assays have been employed by investigators interested in neovascularization associated with development and tumors as well as wound healing, since these processes all have a known angiogenic component. In general, the commonly used angiogenic assays fall into two classes: in vivo bioassays and in vitro assays using cultured vascular cells.

In vivo assays that have been used to study angiogenesis include the rabbit ear chamber,[8-10] the Algire chamber in which a transparent plastic window is placed in the dorsal subcutaneous tissue of a mouse,[16] the hamster cheek pouch,[17, 18] the corneal pocket,[19, 20] and the chick chorioallantoic membrane assay.[21] The Algire chamber and the rabbit ear chambers are particularly useful for determining the number and length of new vessels and how they develop over a period of days because it is possible to examine precisely the same microscopic area by positioning the chamber in the same orientation on a microscope stage. The somewhat less cumbersome rabbit corneal pocket assay is usually used to determine whether a putative angiogenic factor placed in an incision in the middle of the cornea has the ability to attract vessel outgrowth from the limbus into the avascular corneal stroma (Fig. 5–3). The relative acellularity and transparency of the cornea make it easy to see the new vessels. While daily observation of vessel growth is possible in the corneal pocket assay, it is difficult to maintain a constant point of reference from day to day so that quantitative

measurements of vessel ingrowth tend to be gross ones (estimations of vessel length and density). The assay is also potentially costly since one rabbit is required for every two experimental points. Nevertheless, the sensitivity and reliability of this method make it the assay of choice for simple determination of angiogenic activity in vivo.

Substances placed onto the chick chorioallantoic membrane (CAM) can also elicit new blood vessel growth. The chick embryo CAM assay is the least costly and cumbersome and is therefore useful for studies requiring a large number of experimental determinations. The CAM is, however, very sensitive to inflammatory agents and has a relatively high background of normal vessels that grow on the membrane as the embryo develops. This latter problem is not all bad, however, as it has allowed the development of the chick CAM as an assay for angiogenesis *inhibition*. Application of inhibitory agents to the normal CAM at day 6 of development results in an avascular zone that is visible by day 9. Although quantitation of angiogenesis on the CAM is possible,[22] it is difficult due to the high background. Consequently the assay is most frequently used for rapid, inexpensive analysis of angiogenic or angiostatic activity of a factor on a large number of CAMs (Fig. 5–4).

Although the in vivo angiogenesis assays are relatively easy to perform, some caution is required in their interpretation due to the fact that inflammatory agents cause an angiogenic response, probably due to angiogenic factors being produced by inflammatory cells such as macrophages. Consequently, a molecule can be considered to cause angiogenesis directly only if the angiogenic response occurs in the absence of inflammatory cells, which can be checked by careful histological examination of the test tissue. Alternatively, angiogenesis assays can be conducted in the presence of anti-inflammatory agents such as steroids or antilymphocyte serum,[23] although these agents can themselves modulate the angiogenic response[24] and thus complicate the interpretation of the results. A second caveat regarding these assays is that the vascular growth that occurs in specialized test sites such as the CAM or cornea may not be identical to the angiogenesis that occurs normally during wound healing in other tissues. The cornea, for example, is naturally avascular, a property normally shared by only a few other tissues such as the lens and mature cartilage. The CAM is a tissue undergoing rapid vascular and cellular growth. Thus assays for angiogenic inhibition are best conducted on the rapidly

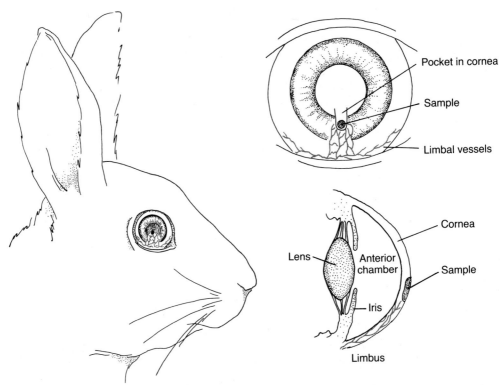

Figure 5–3. Corneal pocket assay. The test material is placed into a pocket raised via an incision into the corneal stroma. To monitor the progression of vessels from the limbus to the sample, the eye is proptosed and examined through a slit lamp.

vascularizing day 6 CAM, whereas studies on angiogenic stimulation are better carried out on later embryos (day 10) when vascularization in the CAM is slowing down. If these considerations are heeded, the in vivo bioassays can provide solid, interpretable data on the relative angiogenic activity of a variety of factors.

Although angiogenic factors are usually defined as such by their ability to induce neovascularity in one of these in vivo models, our current knowledge of the biochemical nature of the signals that cause angiogenesis has been largely derived from in vitro studies employing cultured vascular endothelial cells. Earlier studies employed endothelial cells derived from a variety of large and small blood vessels, but since angiogenesis is a process of *capillary* growth, capillary endothelial cells are now considered the optimal test cell for angiogenesis studies.[25, 26]

In vitro endothelial cell assays have now been developed for several of the cellular components of the angiogenic process. These include assays for endothelial production of hydrolytic enzymes such as collagenase and plasminogen activator,[27–29] assays for endothelial cell migration[30] and proliferation,[31] and novel assays for the formation of capillary tubes in vitro.[32]

These assays have been directly responsible for the purification of a variety of angiogenic factors that have been identified, purified, sequenced, and cloned.[33] One important concept that has emerged from the use of these assays is that not all of the angiogenic factors affect endothelial cells in the same way; some stimulate activity in all of the assays mentioned above, some stimulate only cell migration or proliferation, and some potent angiogenic factors have *no* apparent effects on endothelial cells in vitro. These latter factors may act by causing accumulation of accessory cells that in turn secrete active angiogenic factors.

CELLULAR COMPONENTS OF THE ANGIOGENIC PROCESS

Histological examination and autoradiography of the early events of angiogenesis in the rabbit cornea have demonstrated the biological importance of several distinct cellular events that occur temporally in the angiogenic process. New capillaries usually begin as outgrowths from pre-existing *venules*. Within several hours

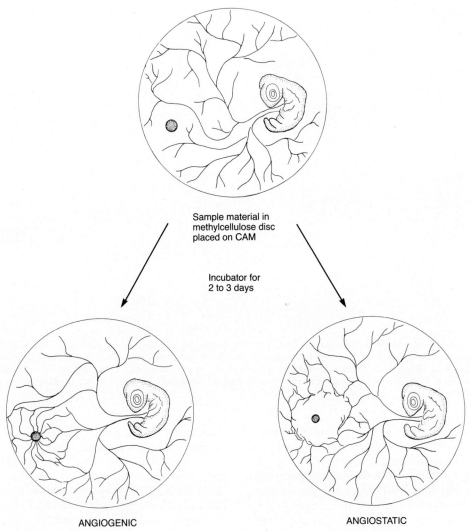

Sample material in
methylcellulose disc
placed on CAM

Incubator for
2 to 3 days

ANGIOGENIC

ANGIOSTATIC

Figure 5–4. The chick chorioallantoic membrane (CAM) assay for angiogenic and angiostatic activity. The sample material in a methylcellulose disc is placed on the CAM surface and incubated for 2 to 3 days.

of exposure to an angiogenic stimulus, the endothelial cells in the pre-existing vessels begin to produce enzymes that degrade the vascular basement membrane *only on the side facing the stimulus.* After 24 hours, the endothelial cells begin to migrate across the degraded basement membrane in the direction of the angiogenic stimulus. Behind the leading tip of migrating cells, trailing endothelial cells divide and differentiate to form a tubular lumen. Eventually the sprouts connect to form branching vascular networks, and as the vessels mature, extracellular matrix components are deposited to form a new basement membrane (Fig. 5–5).[34, 35]

Skin flaps, like any soft tissue wound, reproduce this angiogenic format all along the cut margins. Here, capillary sprouts advance across the wound space from each edge, eventually connecting with each other and with established vessels on the opposing side. Blood flow is established across the wound and the vascular network undergoes extensive remodeling. This is a rapid process: in rats, new vascular channels across the wound margins can be demonstrated by India ink perfusion within 3 days of raising a flap.[36, 37] If the flap has a functioning vascular pedicle, the distal end is more ischemic and induces a relatively greater angiogenic response across the wound than does the better perfused proximal end. The result is that the distal end of the flap can survive pedicle division several days sooner than the proximal end.[38, 39] The entire flap will survive pedicle division by day 7.

Angiogenesis is a critical component of normal bone formation,[40] and a similar angiogenic

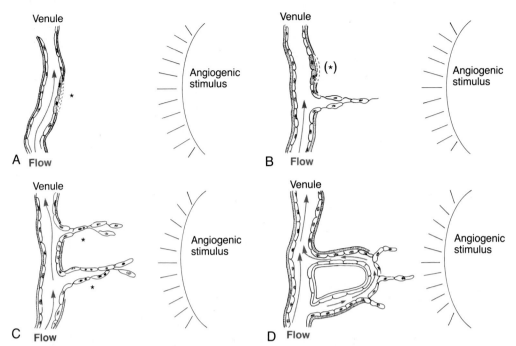

Figure 5–5. Sequential steps in angiogenesis. *A,* Basement membrane is degraded by activated endothelial cells (*). *B,* Endothelial cells migrate through gap in basement membrane toward angiogenic stimulus. The basement membrane at another site is being degraded (*). *C,* Behind the migrating tip, trailing endothelial cells divide (*) and form a lumen. *D,* Flow is established through the new lumen and the basement membrane is deposited as the capillary loop matures.

process can be observed in healing fractures.[41] Capillary sprouts originate from the disrupted ends of the periosteal and medullary circuits and grow into the fracture hematoma along with osteochondrogenic cells from the periosteum. Those cells deposit collagen and, depending on the local environment, differentiate into cartilage or bone. Unless the fracture ends are firmly apposed and immobilized, new bone is generated by the process of endochondral osteogenesis. Invasion of newly formed cartilage by capillary sprouts from the periosteal circuit is temporally related to the further differentiation into bone in this process. Re-establishment of the medullary circulation follows thereafter.

Vascularization in vivo can be divided in two general classes based on the eventual morphology of the new vascular network. In development and in wound healing, there is active remodeling of the new vascular network in which some vessels form and then regress. Many of these capillaries eventually differentiate into arteries and veins. The mechanism whereby some vessels regress whereas others remain and expand is completely unknown. Speculation has centered on the role of blood flow in enhancing vessel development since capillaries with poor blood flow typically involute while those with active flow are usually maintained or expand into larger vessels.[8–12] In recent studies, increased blood flow, subsequent to prolonged exercise[42] and vasodilators,[43] has been associated with the development of new capillaries. This may be due to mechanical factors such as the direct effect of shear force or stretch caused by increased flow in the pre-existing vessels.[44, 45] Alternatively, changes in blood flow may modulate the exposure of vessels to circulating angiogenic factors or inhibitors. In any event, the vasculature formed in wound healing and development is usually permanent and has a characteristic arborizing morphology that is considered "normal": a new capillary network served by its own arterioles and drained back into the existing circuit by its own venules.

In some pathological situations such as tumors, arteriovenous malformations, and hemangiomas, the vasculature may have a morphology distinctly different from the "normal" pattern seen in development and wound healing. Undifferentiated tumors, in particular, can induce a vasculature with a strange morphology, including tortuous thin-walled vessels, dilated endothelial-lined lacunae, and copious arteriovenous connections.[46] Clinically, this is often appreciated as a "tumor blush" on angiography. The reasons why tumor angiogenesis may lead to such an abnormal morphology are not known, and the following explanations are purely speculative. A tumor may secrete large amounts of one type of angiogenic factor resulting in the relative overgrowth of one component of the vascular wall (e.g., endothelium). A second possibility is that a rapidly growing tumor surrounds and engulfs the existing host vasculature[47] and thus confuses migrating endothelial cells about the direction of the angiogenic stimulus. A third possibility is that an effective remodeling step based on blood flow is thwarted because blood flow through a tumor is completely inhomogeneous.[48, 49] Remodeling of the newly formed capillaries in a tumor might also fail to occur because tumor matrix sometimes does not evolve much beyond the initial fibrin/fibronectin clot as it does in a healing wound.[50] The abnormal tumor vasculature remains intact only so long as the tumor itself continues to produce angiogenic factors; removal of the tumor causes rapid and complete regression of the new capillaries.[51]

In summary, the angiogenic cascade in wound healing parallels that seen in development and, to a lesser extent, in tumors. With the exception of the most primitive embryonic vessels, new vessels arise as capillaries from pre-existing venules in response to a combination of humoral and mechanical factors. These components of the angiogenic process are identical: basement membrane degradation followed by endothelial cell migration, proliferation, and lumen formation. When functional vessels are formed, they undergo a process of remodeling and pattern formation that results in a typical vascular network. Although some vessels regress and disappear, others become permanent components of the vasculature.

ANGIOGENIC FACTORS

Evidence for the presence of soluble angiogenic factors has been accumulating for the past 40 years,[52–54] yet until recently, progress in identifying and isolating any of these factors has been extremely slow. Only in the past decade has the development of long-term cultures of capillary endothelial cells[32] and the advent of the sensitive cell culture assays described previously allowed more rapid progress in angiogenic factor purification. Our problem now is completely different from that of 10 years ago. Where there were once no well-characterized angiogenic factors, there now appear to be almost too many.[33] The challenge now is to determine the physiological role of

any or all of these factors in the normal and pathological conditions associated with angiogenesis in situ.

The angiogenic factors that have been identified fall into two general classes: those that have a direct effect on endothelial cell migration and/or proliferation and those that have no apparent in vitro effect on endothelial cells. The first class (direct-acting angiogenic factors) have been isolated by techniques utilizing assays for endothelial cell stimulation. The second class (indirect angiogenic factors) are generally molecules that have been isolated on the basis of other biological activities and are later shown to be angiogenic in the rabbit cornea or chick CAM assays. Direct-acting angiogenic factors include the basic and acidic forms of fibroblast growth factor, transforming growth factor-α, tumor necrosis factor-α (cachectin), and another macrophage-derived growth factor, wound angiogenesis factor (WAF). Indirect angiogenic factors include angiogenin and transforming growth factor-β. There are a number of small molecular weight angiogenic substances such as nicotinamide, copper-carrying peptides, hyaluronic acid, and E-series prostaglandins that probably also work indirectly.[55] The mechanism of action for the indirect angiogenic factors is not yet known, but it is possible that they act by causing the accumulation of other cell types such as platelets and/or macrophages that then release direct-acting factors (Fig. 5–6).

Heparin-Binding Angiogenic Factors

The role of heparin in the angiogenic process was first suggested by studies demonstrating that heparin could stimulate the migration of capillary endothelial cells in vitro.[56] Shortly thereafter, Taylor and Folkman demonstrated that heparin could potentiate the activity of angiogenic factors both in vivo[57] and, as further demonstrated by Thornton and colleagues, in vitro.[58] These studies suggested a potential interaction between heparin and angiogenic growth factors. Consequently, Shing and colleagues attempted to use heparin affinity as a means to purify angiogenic factors.[59] The enormous success of this approach has led to rapid advances in the isolation and characterization of an important class of angiogenic factor. Several previously undefined factors that had been named for their source of origin were soon discovered to be members of this class. These included tumor angiogenesis factor (TAF),[54] en-

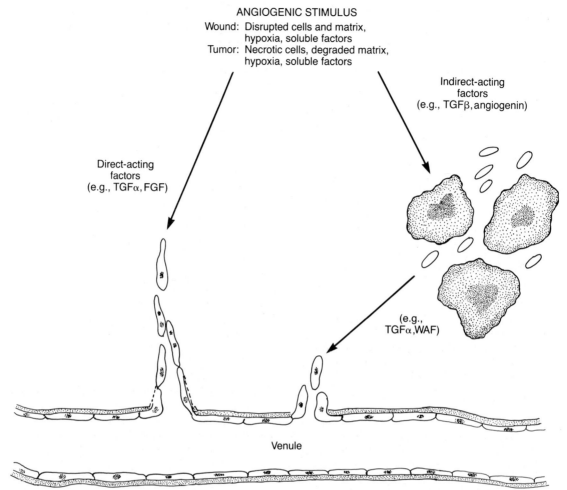

ANGIOGENIC STIMULUS
Wound: Disrupted cells and matrix,
            hypoxia, soluble factors
Tumor: Necrotic cells, degraded matrix,
            hypoxia, soluble factors

Indirect-acting
factors
(e.g., TGFβ, angiogenin)

Direct-acting
factors
(e.g., TGFα, FGF)

(e.g.,
TGFα, WAF)

Venule

Figure 5–6. Direct versus indirect angiogenic activity. Some factors exert their angiogenic effects through other cells, like macrophages, while others are able to act directly on capillary endothelial cells. TGFα = transforming growth factor-α; FGF = fibroblast growth factor; TGFβ = transforming growth factor-β; WAF = wound angiogenesis factor.

dothelial cell growth factor (ECGF),[60] retinal and eye-derived growth factors (RDGF; EDGF),[61, 62] and cartilage-derived growth factor (CDGF).[63] It is now apparent that all of these factors are related and share the property of high-affinity binding to heparin.

The heparin-binding angiogenic factors can be further divided into two classes on the basis of their isoelectric points. The acidic form has a pI of approximately 5.0, whereas the basic form has a pI of approximately 9.5. Virtually all of the factors appear to have molecular weights between 15,000 and 18,000 daltons. These factors have been purified[59, 61–68] and sequenced[69, 70] and their genes cloned.[71, 72] The acidic and basic forms of the heparin-binding growth factors appear to be equivalent to acidic and basic fibroblast growth factors (FGFs), mitogens previously isolated from neural tissue.[66–72] Acidic FGF is found primarily in neural tissue,

whereas basic FGF is nearly ubiquitous in normal and neoplastic tissue. Basic FGF made by cultured endothelial cells is not secreted into the culture media but is deposited into the extracellular matrix secreted by the cells.[73] Regulation of angiogenesis in vivo may consequently involve the selective release of growth factors from extracellular matrix deposits. Because FGF may be bound to heparin or heparan sulfate residues in the basement membrane, heparin-degrading enzymes released by platelets and tumor cells[74–77] may act to release FGF and consequently start the angiogenic cascade. In support of a role for FGF in wound healing is the recent finding by Davidson and colleagues that antibodies to basic FGF retard the early stages of the wound response in rats implanted with subcutaneous polyvinyl alcohol sponges. Histological and biochemical evaluation of the granulation tissue that infiltrated the sponges showed a reduction in DNA, protein, and collagen content relative to controls.[77]

Transforming Growth Factor-α

Transforming growth factor-α (TGF-α) is a polypeptide originally discovered and defined by its ability to confer anchorage-independent growth to normal cells suspended in semisolid medium.[78] It has been completely purified, and its amino acid and nucleotide sequences determined.[79] TGF-α does have a 35 percent homology with epidermal growth factor (EGF) and it binds to the cellular EGF receptor.[80] EGF and TGF-α are equipotent at inducing in vitro endothelial cell proliferation and bind equally well to endothelial cell EGF receptors. TGF-α, however, is approximately ten times more potent than EGF at inducing angiogenesis in vivo.[81] Because tumor cells secrete ample amounts of TGF-α, and because TGF-α is a potent direct-acting angiogenic factor, this molecule is a prime candidate for a "tumor angiogenesis factor" that can attract new capillaries to a site of solid tumor growth.

Tumor Necrosis Factor-α

Tumor necrosis factor-α (TNF-α) was originally isolated as an agent that could cause necrosis and subsequent regression of certain solid tumors.[82] More recently, TNF-α has been shown to stimulate angiogenesis in two types of in vivo bioassays.[83, 84] In addition, TNF-α has been shown to promote endothelial cell chemotaxis and capillary tube formation in vitro.[84] Because activated macrophages have been shown to produce substantial quantities of TNF-α, this molecule is considered likely to play a central role in the macrophage-induced angiogenesis that accompanies inflammation and wound healing. One paradox of the multiple actions of TNF-α is that this agent causes tumor regression whereas angiogenic factors are considered to *promote* tumor growth. Perhaps, as Folkman and Klagsbrun have suggested,[85] the differential activity of this factor is dictated by its localization relative to the blood vessels. When delivered to the intravascular compartment, TNF-α promotes coagulation, hemorrhage, and eventual necrosis. When presented to the exterior of the blood vessel, its effect is to cause endothelial migration and new capillary formation. Thus, the in vivo activity of TNF-α

may depend on its source and route of delivery to a given tissue.

Transforming Growth Factor-β

Transforming growth factor-β (TGF-β) is a 25,000 molecular weight homodimeric polypeptide, first isolated on the basis of its ability to induce anchorage-independent growth of normal rat fibroblasts.[86] TGF-β has a variety of effects on cultured cells including stimulation of cell motility and cell proliferation in some cell types and inhibition of these same processes in other cells.[87] TGF-β has a somewhat paradoxical effect on angiogenesis: in vivo, it stimulates angiogenesis,[88] yet in vitro, it blocks both endothelial proliferation and motility.[89] Of the two best characterized forms of TGF-β the inhibitory activity for endothelial cells is expressed by TGF-β_1 and not by TGF-β_2.[90] These effects of TGF-β appear to be dependent on the composition of the extracellular matrix that supports the cultured cells. TGF-β induces formation of three-dimensional capillary-like networks of endothelial cells grown in collagen gels but not of endothelial cells grown on tissue culture plastic.[91] Because cell motility and proliferation are both important components of the angiogenic process, it is clear that the environment in vivo in some way reduces the inhibitory activity of TGF-β and is permissive for its stimulatory activities. Among these activities is the ability to attract monocytes,[92] which suggests that the angiogenic activity of TGF-β may be due in part to the elaboration of direct-acting angiogenic factors from monocytes attracted to the tumor site by the activity of the growth factor.

TGF-β is also chemotactic for fibroblasts[93] and may be expected to promote fibroblast accumulation and fibrosis in the healing process. TGF-β has potent effects on matrix synthesis, giving rise to increased production of collagen and fibronectin[87, 94] and reduced production of matrix-degrading enzymes.[95, 96] For this reason, it is not completely clear whether administration of exogenous TGF-β to a healing wound would result in accelerated normal healing or simply increased fibrosis and scar formation.

It is likely that a balance exists between the inhibitory effects of TGF-β and the stimulatory effects of other factors in vivo. TGF-β is released in an inactive form in most tissues and can be activated in vitro by acidification or by proteolytic cleavage.[97] Thus the net effect of TGF-β will be modulated by both the level of activated TGF-β present and by the levels of other growth factors present in the same location. Recently, D'Amore and colleagues have shown that vascular pericytes and smooth muscle cells release large quantities of activated TGF-β.[98] This result implies that in mature blood vessels, the presence of activated TGF-β and the absence of many other growth factors[99–103] may lead to a net inhibition of endothelial cell proliferation. In a wound, however, the presence of many other cell growth factors and angiogenic factors may lead to a balance that favors new capillary growth over inhibition.

Angiogenin

Angiogenin, a 14,400 molecular weight angiogenic peptide isolated from a human adenocarcinoma,[104] has been purified, sequenced, and cloned.[104–106] While not directly related to any of the other known angiogenic molecules, angiogenin shares a 35 percent sequence homology with a family of pancreatic ribonucleases and is able to cleave 28S and 18S ribosomal RNA.[107] In mice, angiogenin gene expression is greatest in the adult liver and lower in fetal tissue and in regenerating liver, suggesting that it is primarily a product of mature liver tissue.[108] Angiogenin has no known direct effect on the growth or migration of vascular endothelial cells, suggesting that it, too, may act indirectly on vessel growth by causing the accumulation of other cell types that can then release other angiogenic factors.

Lipids and Prostaglandins

Although most of the known angiogenic agents are polypeptides, certain lipids also possess angiogenic activity. The first reports were of angiogenic effects associated with prostaglandins E_1 and E_2, which stimulate angiogenesis in the chick CAM and rabbit cornea bioassays.[109–111] Lipids are natural candidates for the potent angiogenic activity secreted by adipocytes.[112] After prolonged investigation, the active agent in adipocyte-induced angiogenesis has been found to be 1-butyryl-glycerol.[113] This agent may possibly have a role in other lipid-mediated angiogenic events such as the cardiac-associated angiogenesis attributed to fatty deposits around the heart.[114]

CELL TYPES THAT INDUCE ANGIOGENESIS DURING WOUND HEALING

The process of inflammation and wound healing involves the recruitment of a variety of accessory cells that may produce angiogenic modulators. Now that the identities and sources of several angiogenic factors are known, it is possible to describe a potential sequence for the production of angiogenic factors during wound healing (Fig. 5–7). One of the earliest consequences of tissue damage is, of course, the release of granule constituents from activated *platelets* at the site of vascular rupture. Besides provoking the coagulation cascade, these granules also contain large quantities of TGF-β that can subsequently act to attract monocytes and macrophages to the wound site.[88, 115] Platelets also release a platelet-derived growth factor (PDGF) that although not angiogenic does stimulate growth of vascular smooth muscle cells.[116] In addition, PDGF is also a potent chemoattractant for macrophages and monocytes[117] and may help to recruit these important accessory cells. Finally, platelets release enzymes that can liberate angiogenic factors stored in the basement membrane.[73–75] Recent work by Knighton and colleagues has described a major role for platelet products in facilitating the wound healing process,[118, 119] but the molecules that mediate this response are not yet known.

Macrophages play a central role in wound repair[120, 121] and are known to promote both wound and tumor-associated angiogenesis.[122–124] Although neither neutrophils nor lymphocytes produce significant amounts of angiogenic factor, macrophages produce several potent, direct-acting angiogenic factors including TNF-α,[84] basic fibroblast growth factor (FGF)[101] and additional, as yet unsequenced molecules that stimulate capillary endothelial cell migration and are potent angiogenic factors.[99, 103, 125]

Mast cells are also found in increased quantities around sites of neovascularization including wounds, tumors, and hemangiomas.[126–128] While mast cells are not *essential* for angiogenesis since there are no mast cells in the retina even when rapid pathological vascularization of the retina is taking place,[129] they do, however, release a number of biological response modifiers such as histamine and heparin that may be expected to potentiate the angiogenic process when other angiogenic factors are present[5, 130]

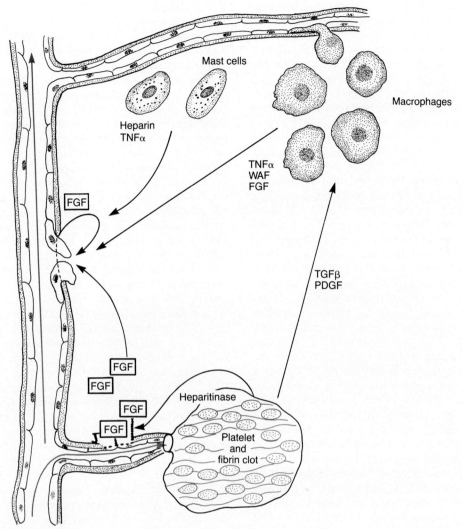

Figure 5–7. Some of the cells that can affect wound healing angiogenesis. TNFα = tumor necrosis factor-α; WAF = wound angiogenesis factor; FGF = fibroblast growth factor; TGFβ = transforming growth factor-β; PDGF = platelet-derived growth factor.

as well as a TNF-α-like factor.[131] Finally, angiogenesis may be modulated by cells directly damaged in an injury. Lysed or ischemic cells release a variety of intracellular products that could also include intracellular growth factors such as FGF.

Some cells found in a wound may influence angiogenesis in an inhibitory manner by helping to slow capillary sprouting and inducing vessel differentiation. This event is most important as the healing process nears completion and the vessels cease proliferation and begin to mature. The work of Orlidge and D'Amore suggests that the vascular pericyte may act to block vascular cell proliferation and induce differentiation.[135] In healing wounds, pericytes appear shortly after the new sprouts are formed and are enveloped by the capillary basement membrane.[11–13, 132] They are often absent where there is pathological neovascularization as in diabetic retinopathy[133] or angiomatous tumors.[134] Orlidge and D'Amore have now shown convincingly that pericytes and vascular smooth muscle cells inhibit capillary endothelial cell proliferation in vitro.[135]

EXTRACELLULAR MATRIX MOLECULES THAT MODULATE ANGIOGENESIS

It is being increasingly appreciated that cellular behavior is directly influenced by the composition of the extracellular matrix on which the cells rest.[136] In development, differentiation, and a variety of pathological conditions, changes in extracellular matrix composition bring about profound changes in cellular organization. These alterations are mediated by the effects of distinct matrix components on cell growth, cell migration, and cell differentiation. These new findings are particularly important for our understanding of angiogenesis in wound healing because the matrix composition changes so dramatically during the course of the healing process.

The first matrix material found at a wound site, by virtue of its role in blood clotting, is *fibrin*. Kadish and associates[137] originally demonstrated that exposure of cultured endothelial cells to fibrin will cause the cells to retract and migrate, resulting in a disorganization of the normal endothelial monolayer. A role for fibrin in promoting angiogenesis has been convincingly made by Dvorak and co-workers. In recent studies, this group has shown that when plastic chambers with one porous surface were filled with fibrin and implanted into the subcutaneous space in guinea pigs, growth of new vessels into the chambers occurred within 4 days.[138] The intensity of the angiogenic response was enhanced when zymosan-activated serum, an N-formylmethionine tripeptide, or PDGF was included in the fibrin matrix. No similar angiogenic activity was seen when agarose or type I collagen was placed in the chambers in place of fibrin. Because tumors constitutively produce procoagulants and vascular permeability factors[139, 140] that result in constant extravascular fibrin deposition, fibrin deposits in solid tumors may be important in promoting tumor angiogenesis as well as accounting for some of the differences between the eventual morphology of tumor neovascularity and that seen in healed wounds.[50, 141]

In a healing wound, the distribution of extracellular matrix molecules undergoes progressive change. Among the other molecules that accumulate in early wound matrix are hyaluronic acid and fibronectin. Hyaluronic acid predominates in early granulation tissue but is steadily replaced between the fifth and tenth days by more highly sulfated proteoglycans such as chondroitin sulfate and dermatan sulfate.[142] Fibronectin is a high molecular weight glycoprotein that contains binding sites for cells, collagen, and heparin.[143] In wounds, fibronectin is deposited from plasma[144] with fibrin and is produced in increased quantities by injured endothelial cells[145] and by macrophages.[146] Fibronectin is a major component of early wound extracellular matrix,[147–150] and it appears to be the initial structural fibril secreted by wound fibroblasts acting as the template for deposition of collagen fibrils and organization of the fibronexus.[151, 152] Thus the stage is set for further maturation into a collagenous stroma.

Surgeons have long known that collagen deposition and cross linking coincide with the restoration of tensile strength in a wound[153] and have appreciated the dynamic nature of that process.[154] However, the important role played by collagen deposition in cell migration and differentiation is much less appreciated. It may be that modulation of collagen synthesis and degradation controls angiogenesis by altering endothelial basement membrane composition or extracellular matrix attachments. Tube formation, which has been considered a marker of differentiation in cultured capillary endothelial cells,[32] can be rapidly induced by placing endothelial cells into a three-dimensional collagen matrix,[155] or by culturing them on a substratum of basement membrane (types IV and V) collagen.[156] Both degradation of collagen by endothelial cell collagenases and synthesis of endothelial cell collagen have been shown to facilitate normal endothelial cell migration.[157, 158] Several direct-acting angiogenic factors induce both collagenase production and cell migration by vascular endothelial cells.[27–29, 84] Suppression of basement membrane synthesis with inhibitors of collagen deposition has been shown to prevent the normal morphogenetic growth of branching structures in the lung, salivary glands, breast, and thyroid gland.[159–161] Use of those inhibitors has also caused the involution of *growing* capillaries in vivo, and this has been correlated with dissolution of the capillary basement membrane.[162, 163] These results clearly show that angiogenesis is dependent on the deposition of the vascular extracellular matrix and that modulation of this matrix can be used to regulate the angiogenic process.

Perhaps the greatest body of information on the role of a matrix molecule in regulating angiogenesis derives from studies on the proteoglycan *heparin*. While heparin is capable of dramatically affecting angiogenesis, it is not at present clear what role it plays in regulating angiogenesis in vivo or the mechanism by which it acts. The evidence for heparin's involvement in angiogenesis is as follows: (1) Heparin promotes migration of capillary endothelial cells in vitro.[56] (2) Heparin potentiates the activity of low doses of angiogenic factor when tested on the chick chorioallantoic membrane assay.[57] (3) Heparin binds tightly to potent angiogenic factors.[59–68] (4) Heparin binding growth factors can be released from biological matrices by enzymes that degrade heparin or heparan sulfate, suggesting that these factors are bound to heparin in biological matrices in vivo.[164] (5) Heparin potentiates the in vitro activity of the acidic form of heparin-binding growth factor.[58] (6) Heparin prolongs the half-life of acidic and basic FGF.[165] (7) Heparin increases the affinity of a heparin-binding growth factor for its receptor on human endothelial cells.[166] (8) Heparin antagonists, such as protamine or platelet factor IV, block angiogenesis in vivo.[57]

Although heparin can act to potentiate the activity of angiogenesis factors both in vivo and in vitro, there are other circumstances in which heparin can act to *inhibit* angiogenesis. The combination of heparin with hydrocortisone, for example, blocks tumor-induced angiogenesis as well as normal developmental angiogenesis.[24] Other steroid analogues that possess no known biological activity also act in concert with heparin to block angiogenesis.[167] Among these is tetrahydrocortisol, a known metabolite of cortisone that circulates in the bloodstream and may act physiologically to suppress unwanted angiogenesis in vivo.

MODULATION OF WOUND ANGIOGENESIS BY OXYGEN

Normal wound healing requires an adequate supply of oxygen; the poor healing seen in ischemic limbs is a common clinical example of the effects of oxygen deprivation. Experimentally, increasing the supply of oxygen permits more rapid accumulation of collagen, enhances the angiogenic response, and accelerates healing.[168–170] Nevertheless, the wound environment is normally hypoxic,[171] and ischemic tissue seems to promote angiogenesis relatively more than nonischemic tissue.[38, 39] Both Hunt and Knighton postulated that the low oxygen tension in the wound space is a signal for angiogenesis and that such a signal would be self regulating since wound hypoxia should diminish as neovascularization proceeded.[172, 173] They have demonstrated that fluid taken from the dead space is angiogenic and that this property is due to a factor secreted by wound macrophages.[99, 124] Furthermore, they have demonstrated that oxygen tension regulates the secretion of this factor by the macrophages.[174]

Although the role of oxygen in regulating wound angiogenesis might appear paradoxical (both hypoxia and hyperoxia promote neovascularization), there is a plausible explanation. Wound oxygen tension depends primarily on blood flow and only secondarily on the concentration of inspired oxygen.[175] Although the inspired oxygen concentration can be made very high in a hyperbaric chamber, the nonvascularized center of a closed wound will remain hypoxic, and therefore able to stimulate angiogenesis, until new vessels grow into this area. In the same hyperbaric environment, wounded areas with blood flow, however marginal, might be expected to have higher oxygen tensions than usual; this may allow a more rapid local accumulation of matrix and consequently more new vessel growth.

CLINICAL APPLICATIONS OF ANGIOGENESIS RESEARCH

In the past decade, enormous strides have been made in our understanding of the biochemical and molecular nature of several angiogenic factors and of the cells that produce these factors. For all of our increased understanding, however, the fruits of angiogenesis research have been only partially available in the clinic. Nevertheless, clinically useful applications of the principles discussed in this chapter are possible now. For example, healing may be improved in a thrombocytopenic patient simply by replenishing platelets.[118] Sufficient oxygenation is critical to neovascularization in wound healing, and Hunt has consequently emphasized the importance of blood flow in maintaining wound PO_2 at a sufficiently high level to permit healing.[176] He has further stressed the sensitivity of wound PO_2 to changes in a patient's volume status. Often tissue PO_2 is surprisingly low in patients who have reasonable arterial PO_2 and appear adequately hydrated by other parameters such as urine output.[175, 176] While healing proceeds quite well in most situations without sophisticated monitoring, bedside measurement of tissue PO_2 can help guide drug therapy, volume replacement, and respiratory care in critically ill patients in whom healing must be optimized.[177] Furthermore, oxygen can act as an effective antibiotic when prophylaxis against wound infection is advisable.[178]

Direct use of currently available growth factors on wounds in order to accelerate healing is a clinical application that is just emerging from the experimental stages. It is logical to assume that angiogenic factors in particular would accelerate healing, and a number of experimental studies have shown this to be the case. Not every study, however, has confirmed this finding,[179] and there are several issues to consider when observations of the effects of such factors on wound healing confound expectation. First, normal healing proceeds rapidly without any additional intervention, and when extra help is warranted, simple measures (preventing desiccation of the wound, for example) may have as large an impact on the rate of healing as the addition of an exogenous growth factor. Secondly, the effectiveness of a particular growth factor as a wound healing agent can be influenced by the type of wound model used. Epithelial growth factor (EGF), for example, is a potent epithelial mitogen that has been shown to be especially effective in accelerating re-epithelialization of split-thickness skin wounds,[180] but alone it is less effective at promoting collagen deposition in subcutaneously implanted wound chambers than some other growth factors.[181] Conversely, the effect of an experimental factor may be obscured if the animals are able to lick their wounds, since growth factors are present in rodent saliva.[182] Finally, while the amount of collagen deposited in a wound chamber normally correlates with structural healing,[183] this correlation may be skewed when specific factors are being tested. Some factors may, for example, be merely contributing to the intensity of an experimental foreign-body reaction. Increased angiogenesis might not then necessarily lead to faster healing or a structurally superior union. The assumption that it does is currently being investigated.

There are, however, many recent publications that attest to the ability of angiogenic factors such as EGF,[184] FGF,[185-187] and TGF-β[88, 188] to promote both angiogenesis and collagen deposition at the wound site. Furthermore, some of these factors clearly accelerate structural repair either by increasing the rate of epithelial closure[180] or by increasing the gain in tensile strength of an incised wound.[189] From a clinical standpoint, the demonstration that healing can be promoted in compromised hosts with these factors is very important. TGF-β is able to partially reverse the retarded healing seen in rats pretreated with Adriamycin,[181] and PDGF (although it is not an angiogenic factor) has been shown to be capable of reversing the retarded healing seen in diabetic rats.[190] Interestingly, the most effective treatments currently in use are those that involve using either combinations of different growth factors or crude preparations that contain a variety of factors.[181, 191] One such preparation of a crude platelet extract has been successfully used by Knighton to heal chronic skin ulcers.[119] Another such preparation in clinical use is demineralized bone powder, which induces bone formation where it is implanted and is used to close skeletal defects.[192, 193] The efficacy of crude growth factor preparations or combinations of factors reflects the fact that there is a complex mixture of signals in a healing wound and that our understanding of the function of these factors and how they act is still nascent. It will be important to investigate whether certain combinations of these factors will preferentially lead to the production of functional differentiated tissue as opposed to a scar. TGF-β, for example, changes the character of wound matrix in fetal tissue to a more adult inflammatory pattern,[194] whereas basic FGF can induce mesodermal differentiation in the embryo.[195] Modulating the end result of the healing process may be possible and more worthwhile than simply accelerating it. Understanding the "cross-talk" between the various cellular elements in a vessel wall should provide insight into the control of growth and differentiation of complex tissue in adults.

Revolutionary clinical applications, therefore, await a clearer appreciation of the molecular signals directing angiogenesis in situ. However, it is apparent now that the use of angiogenic factors in clinical situations, especially in chronic, nonhealing wounds, will expand and prove even more valuable in the years to come.

References

1. Hunt TK: Wound Healing and Wound Infection: Theory and Surgical Practice. New York, Appleton-Century-Crofts, 1980.
2. Madden JW, Arem AJ: Wound Healing: Biological and Clinical Features. In Sabiston, DC (ed): Textbook of Surgery, 12th ed. Philadelphia, WB Saunders, 1981, pp 265–286.
3. Ross R, Benditt EP: Wound healing and collagen formation. Sequential changes in components of guinea pig skin wounds observed in the electron microscope. J Biophys Biochem Cytol 11:677–750, 1961.
4. Hunt TK, Van Winkle W Jr: Fundamentals of Wound Management in Surgery: Wound Healing: Normal Repair. South Plainfield, NJ, Chirugecom, 1976.
5. Clark RAF: Cutaneous tissue repair: Basic biologic considerations. I. J Am Acad Dermatol 13:701–725, 1985.
6. Hobson B, Denekamp J: Endothelial proliferation in tumours and normal tissues: Continuous labelling studies. Br J Cancer 49:405–413, 1984.
7. Bloom W, Fawcett D: A Textbook of Histology, 10th ed. Philadelphia, WB Saunders, 1975, pp 83–107.
8. Sandison JC: Observations on the growth of blood

vessels as seen in the transparent chamber introduced in the rabbit's ear. Am J Anat 41:475–496, 1928.

9. Clark ER, Clark EL: Observations on changes in blood vascular endothelium in the living animal. Am J Anat 57:385–438, 1935.

10. Clark ER, Clark EL: Microscopic observations on the growth of blood capillaries in the living mammal. Am J Anat 64:251–301, 1939.

11. Cliff WJ: Observations on healing tissue: A combined light and electron microscopic investigation. Philos Trans R Soc Lond Ser B (Biol Sci) 246:305–325, 1963.

12. Schoefl GI: Electron microscopic observations on the regeneration of blood vessels after injury. Ann NY Acad Sci 116:789–802, 1964.

13. Rhodin JA: Ultrastructure of mammalian venous capillaries, venules and small collecting veins. J Ultrastruct Res 25:452–500, 1968.

14. Dudar TE, Jain RK: Microcirculatory flow changes during tissue growth. Microvasc Res 25:1–21, 1983.

15. Hashimoto H, Prewitt RL: Microvascular density changes during wound healing. Int J Microcirc Clin Exp 5:303–310, 1987.

16. Algire GH: An adaptation of the transparent chamber technique to the mouse. J Natl Cancer Inst 4:1–11, 1943.

17. Sanders AG, Shubik P: A transparent window for use in the Syrian hamster. Israel J Exp Med 11:118a, 1964.

18. Goodall CM, Sanders AG, Shubik P: Studies of vascular patterns in living tumors with a transparent chamber inserted in a hamster cheek pouch. J Natl Cancer Inst 35:497–521, 1965.

19. Langham ME: Observations on the growth of blood vessels into the cornea. Application of a new experimental technique. Br J Ophthalmol 37:210–222, 1953.

20. Gimbrone MA, Cotran RS, Leapman SB, et al: Tumor growth and neovascularization: An experimental model using the rabbit cornea. J Natl Cancer Inst 52:413–427, 1974.

21. Auerbach R, Kubai L, Knighton D, et al: A simple procedure for the long term cultivation of chicken embryos. Dev Biol 41:391–394, 1974.

22. Jakob W, Voss K: Utilization of image analysis for the quantification of vascular responses in the chick chorioallantoic membrane. Exp Pathol 26:93–99, 1984.

23. Chodak GW, Haudenschild C, Gittes RF, et al: Angiogenic activity as a marker of neoplastic and preneoplastic lesions of the human bladder. Ann Surg 192:762–771, 1980.

24. Folkman J, Langer R, Linhardt RJ, et al: Angiogenesis inhibition and tumor regression caused by heparin or a heparin fragment in the presence of cortisone. Science 221:719–725, 1983.

25. Zetter BR: The endothelial cells of large and small blood vessels. Diabetes (Suppl 2) 30:24–28, 1981.

26. Zetter BR: Endothelial heterogeneity: Influence of vessel size, organ localization, and species specificity on the properties of cultured endothelial cells. In Ryan U (ed): Endothelial Cells. Orlando, FL, CRC Press, 1988, pp 63–80.

27. Gross JL, Moscatelli D, Rifkin DB: Increased capillary endothelial cell protease activity in response to angiogenic stimuli in vitro. Proc Natl Acad Sci USA 80:2623–2627, 1983.

28. Glaser BM, Kalebic T, Garbisa S, et al: Degradation of basement membrane components by vascular endothelial cells: Role in neovascularization. In Development of the Vascular System. Ciba Foundation Symposium 100. London, Pitman, 1983, pp 150–162.

29. Moscatelli D, Presta M, Rifkin DB: Purification of a factor from human placenta that stimulates capillary endothelial cell protease production, DNA synthesis and migration. Proc Natl Acad Sci USA 83:2091–2095, 1986.

30. Zetter BR: Migration of capillary endothelial cells is stimulated by tumour-derived factors. Nature 285:41–43, 1980.

31. Folkman J, Haudenschild CC, Zetter BR: Long term culture of capillary endothelial cells. Proc Natl Acad Sci USA 76:5217–5221, 1979.

32. Folkman J, Haudenschild CC: Angiogenesis in vitro. Nature 288:551–556, 1982.

33. Folkman J, Klagsbrun M: Angiogenic factors. Science 235:442–447, 1987.

34. Ausprunk DH, Folkman J: Migration and proliferation of endothelial cells in preformed and newly formed blood vessels during tumor angiogenesis. Microvasc Res 14:53–65, 1977.

35. Ausprunk DH, Boudreau CL, Nelson DA: Proteoglycans in the microvasculature. II. Histochemical localization in proliferating capillaries of the rabbit cornea. Am J Pathol 103:367–375, 1981.

36. Nakajima T: How soon do venous drainage channels develop at the periphery of a free flap? A study on rats. Br J Plast Surg 31:300–308, 1978.

37. Tsur H, Danniler A, Strauch B: Neovascularization of skin flaps: Route and timing. Plast Reconstr Surg 66:85–93, 1980.

38. Gatti JE, LaRossa D, Brousseau DA, et al: Assessment of neovascularization and timing of flap division. Plast Reconstr Surg 73:396–402, 1984.

39. Semashko D, Song Y, Silverman DG, et al: Ischemic induction of neovascularization: A study by fluorometric analysis. Microsurg 6:244–248, 1985.

40. Caplan AL, Pechak DG: The cellular and molecular embryology of bone formation. In Peck WA (ed): Bone and Mineral Research, vol 5. Elsevier, Amsterdam, 1987, pp 117–183.

41. Heppenstall RB: Fracture healing. In Hunt, TK, Heppenstall RB, Pines E, et al (eds): Soft and Hard Tissue Repair. Biological and Clinical Aspects. Surgical Science Series, vol 2. New York, Praeger, 1984, pp 101–142.

42. Myrhage R, Hudlicka O: Capillary growth in chronically stimulated adult skeletal muscle as studied by intravital microscopy and histological methods in rabbits and rats. Microvasc Res 16:73–90, 1978.

43. Ziada AM, Hudlicka O, Tyler K, et al: The effect of long-term vasodilation on capillary growth and performance in rabbit heart and skeletal muscle. Cardiovasc Res 18:724–732, 1984.

44. Huklicka O, Tyler KR: Angiogenesis. The growth of the vascular system. New York, Academic Press, 1986, pp 165–169.

45. Waxman AM: Blood vessel growth as a problem in morphogenesis: A physical theory. Microvasc Res 22:32–42, 1981.

46. Warren BA: The vascular morphology of tumors. In Peterson HI (ed): Tumor Blood Circulation. Angiogenesis, Vascular Morphology and Blood Flow of Experimental and Human Tumors. Boca Raton, FL, CRC Press, 1979, pp 34–47.

47. Thompson WD, Shiach KJ, Fraser RA, et al: Tumors acquire their vasculature by vessel incorporation, not vessel ingrowth. J Pathol 151:323–332, 1987.

48. Endrich B, Reinhold HS, Gross JF, et al: Tissue perfusion inhomogeneity during early tumor growth in rats. J Natl Cancer Inst 62:387–395, 1979.

49. Jain RK: Transport of macromolecules in tumor microcirculation. Biotechnol Prog 1:81–84, 1985.

50. Dvorak HF: Tumors: Wounds that do not heal. Similarities between tumor stroma generation and wound healing. N Engl J Med 315:1650–1659, 1986.

51. Ausprunk DH, Falterman K, Folkman J: The sequence of events in the regression of corneal capillaries. Lab Invest 38:284–294, 1978.

52. Algire GH, Chalkey HW: Vascular reactions of normal and malignant tissues in vivo. I. Vascular reactions of mice to wounds and to normal and neoplastic transplants. J Natl Cancer Inst 6:73–85, 1945.

53. Greenblatt M, Shubik P: Tumor angiogenesis; Transfilter diffusion studies in the hamster by the transparent chamber technique. J Natl Cancer Inst 41:111–124, 1968.

54. Gimbrone M, Leapman S, Cotran R, et al: Tumor dormancy in vivo by prevention of neovascularization. J Exp Med 136:261–276, 1972.

55. D'Amore P, Braunhut SJ: Stimulatory and inhibitory factors in vascular growth control. In Ryan U (ed): The Endothelial Cell. Boca Raton, FL, CRC Press, 1988, pp 13–36.

56. Azizkhan RG, Azizkhan JC, Zetter BR, et al: Mast cell heparin stimulates migration of capillary endothelial cells *in vitro*. J Exp Med 152:931–944, 1980.

57. Taylor S, Folkman J: Protamine is an inhibitor of angiogenesis. Nature 297:307–312, 1982.

58. Thornton SC, Mueller SN, Levine EM: Human endothelial cells: Use of heparin in cloning and long term serial cultivation. Science 222:623–625, 1983.

59. Shing Y, Folkman J, Sullivan R, et al: Heparin affinity: Purification of a tumor derived capillary endothelial cell growth factor. Science 223:1296–1298, 1984.

60. Maciag T, Mehlman T, Friesel R, et al: Heparin binds endothelial cell growth factor, the principal mitogen in the bovine brain. Science 225:932–935, 1984.

61. D'Amore PA, Klagsbrun M: Endothelial cell mitogens derived from retina and hypothalamus: Biochemical and biological similarities. J Cell Biol 99:1545–1549, 1984.

62. Courty J, Loret C, Moenner M, et al: Bovine retina contains three growth factor activities with different affinity to heparin: Eye derived growth factor I, II, III. Biochemistry 67:265–269, 1985.

63. Sullivan R, Klagsbrun M: Purification of cartilage-derived growth factor by heparin-affinity chromatography. J Biol Chem 260:2399–2403, 1985.

64. Lobb RR, Fett JW: Purification of two distinct growth factors from bovine neural tissue by heparin affinity chromatography. Biochemistry 23:6295–6299, 1984.

65. Conn G, Hatcher VB: The isolation and purification of two anionic endothelial cell growth factors from human brain. Biochem Biophys Res Commun 124:262–268, 1984.

66. Gospodarowicz D, Cheng J, Liu GM, et al: Isolation of brain fibroblast growth factor by heparin-sepharose affinity chromatography: Identity with pituitary fibroblast growth factor. Proc Natl Acad Sci USA 81:6963–6967, 1984.

67. Klagsbrun M, Shing Y: Heparin affinity of anionic and cationic endothelial cell growth factors: Analysis of hypothalamus-derived growth factors and fibroblast-growth factors. Proc Natl Acad Sci USA 82:805–809, 1985.

68. Lobb R, Sasse J, Sullivan R, et al: Purification and characterization of heparin-binding endothelial cell growth factors. J Biol Chem 261:1924–1928, 1986.

69. Esch R, Baird A, Ling N, et al: Primary structure of bovine pituitary basic fibroblast growth factor (FGF) and comparison with the amino-terminal sequence of bovine brain acidic FGF. Proc Natl Acad Sci USA 82:6507–6511, 1985.

70. Gimenez-Gallego G, Rodkey J, Bennett C, et al: Brain-derived acidic fibroblast growth factor: Complete amino acid sequence and homologies. Science 230:1385–1388, 1985.

71. Abraham JA, Mergia A, Whang JL, et al: Nucleotide sequence of a bovine clone encoding the angiogenic protein, basic fibroblast growth factor. Science 233:545–548, 1986.

72. Jaye M, Howk R, Burgess W, et al: Human endothelial cell growth factor: Cloning, nucleotide sequence, and chromosome localization. Science 233:541–548, 1986.

73. Vlodovsky I, Folkman J, Sullivan R, et al: Endothelial cell–derived basic fibroblast growth factor: Synthesis and deposition into subendothelial extracellular matrix. Proc Natl Acad Sci USA 84:2292–2296, 1987.

74. Oosta GM, Favreau LV, Beeler DL, et al: Purification and properties of human platlet heparitinase. J Biol Chem 257:11248–11255, 1982.

75. Yahalom J, Eldor A, Biran S, et al: Platelet tumor cell interaction with the extracellular matrix: Relationship to cancer metastasis. Radiother Oncol 3:211–225, 1985.

76. Maniglia CA, Loulakis PP, Sartorelli AC: Interference with tumor cell–induced degradation of endothelial matrix on the antimetastatic action of Nafazatrom. J Natl Cancer Inst 76:739–744, 1986.

77. Broadley KN, Aquino AM, Woodward SC, et al: Monospecific antibodies implicate basic fibroblast growth factor in normal wound repair. Lab Invest 61:571–575, 1989.

78. Marquadt H, Hunkapiller MW, Hood LE, et al: Rat transforming growth factor type I: Structure and relationship to epidermal growth factor. Science 223:1079–1082, 1984.

79. Derynck R, Roberts AB, Eaton DH, et al: Human transforming growth factor-alpha: Precursor sequence, gene structure and heterologous expression. In Feramisco J, Ozanne B, Stiles C (eds): Cancer Cells, vol 3. Growth Factors and Transformation. Cold Spring Harbor, NY, Cold Spring Harbor Press, 1985, pp 79–86.

80. Delarco JE, Todaro GJ: Sarcoma growth factor (SGF): Specific binding to epidermal growth factor (EGF) membrane receptors. J Cell Physiol 102:267–277, 1980.

81. Schreiber AB, Winkler ME, Derynck R: Transforming growth factor-α: A more potent angiogenic mediator than epidermal growth factor. Science 232:1250–1253, 1980.

82. Carswell EA, Old LJ, Kassel RL, et al: An endotoxin-induced serum factor that causes necrosis of tumors. Proc Natl Acad Sci USA 72:3666–3670, 1975.

83. Frater-Schroder MF, Risau W, Hallmann R, et al: Tumor necrosis factor type-α, a potent inhibitor of endothelial cell growth *in vitro*, is angiogenic in vivo. Proc Natl Acad Sci USA 84:5277–5281, 1987.

84. Leibovich SJ, Polverini PJ, Shepard HM, et al: Macrophage-induced angiogenesis is mediated by tumour necrosis factor-alpha. Nature 329:630–632, 1987.

85. Folkman J, Klagsbrun M: A family of angiogenic peptides. Nature 329:671–672, 1987.

86. Roberts AB, Anzano MA, Lamb LC, et al: New class of transforming growth factors potentiated by epidermal growth factor: Isolation from non-neoplastic tissues. Proc Natl Acad Sci USA 78:5339–5343, 1981.

87. Sporn MB, Roberts AB: Peptide growth factors are multifunctional. Nature 332:217–219, 1988.

88. Roberts AB, Sporn MB, Assoian RK, et al: Transforming growth factor type beta: Rapid induction of fibrosis and angiogenesis in vivo and stimulation of collagen formation in vitro. Proc Natl Acad Sci USA 83:4167–4171, 1983.

89. Muller G, Behrens J, Nussbaumer U, et al: Inhibitory action of transforming growth factor beta on endothelial cells. Proc Natl Acad Sci USA 84:5600–5604, 1987.

90. Jennings JC, Mohan S, Linkhart TA, et al: Comparison of the biological actions of TGF beta-1 and TGF beta-2: Differential activity in endothelial cells. J Cell Physiol 137:167–172, 1985.

91. Madri JA, Pratt BM, Tucker AM: Phenotypic modulation of endothelial cells by transforming growth factor-beta depends upon the composition and organization of the extracellular matrix. J Cell Biol 106:1375–1384, 1988.

92. Wahl SM, Hunt DA, Wakefield IM, et al: Transforming growth factor-beta (TGF-β) induces monocyte chemotaxis and growth factor production. Proc Natl Acad Sci USA 84:5788–5792, 1987.

93. Postelthwaite AE, Keski-Oja J, Moses HL, et al: Stimulation of the chemotactic migration of human fibroblasts by transforming growth factor-beta. J Exp Med 165:251–256, 1987.

94. Ignotz R, Endo T, Massague J: Regulation of fibronectin and type I collagen mRNA levels by transforming growth factor-beta. J Biol Chem 262:6443–6446, 1987.

95. Edwards DR, Murphy G, Reynolds JJ, et al: Transforming growth factor-beta modulates the expression of collagenase and metalloproteinase inhibitor. EMBO J 6:1899–1904, 1987.

96. Matrisian LM, Leroy R, Ruhlmann C, D'Amore P: Isolation of the oncogene and epidermal growth factor induced transin gene: Complex control in rat fibroblasts. Mol Cell Biol 6:1679–1686, 1986.

97. Lawrence DA, Pircher R, Julien P: Conversion of a high molecular weight latent beta-TGF from chicken embryo fibroblasts into a low molecular weight active beta-TGF under acidic conditions. Biochem Biophys Res Commun 133:1026–1034, 1985.

98. Antonelli-Orlidge A, Saunders KB, Smith SR, et al: An activated form of TGF-β is produced by co-cultures of endothelial cells and pericytes. Proc Natl Acad Sci USA 86:4544–4548, 1989.

99. Banda MJ, Knighton DR, Hunt TK, et al: Isolation of a nonmitogenic angiogenesis factor from wound fluid. Proc Natl Acad Sci USA 79:7773–7777, 1982.

100. Banda MJ, Dwyer KS, Beckmann A: Wound fluid angiogenesis factor stimulates the directed migration of capillary endothelial cells. J Cell Biochem 29:183–193, 1985.

101. Baird A, Mormede P, Bohlen P: Immunoreactive fibroblast growth factor in cells of peritoneal exudate suggests its identity with macrophage-derived growth factor. Biochem Biophys Res Commun 126:358–364, 1985.

102. Shimokado K, Raines EW, Madtes DK, et al: A significant part of macrophage-derived growth factor consists of at least two forms of PDGF. Cell 43:277–286, 1985.

103. Hockel M, Beck T, Wissler JH: Neomorphogenesis of blood vessels in rabbit skin induced by a highly purified monocyte-derived polypeptide (monocyte-angiotropin) and associated tissue reactions. Int J Tiss Reac 6:323–331, 1984.

104. Fett JW, Strydom DS, Lobb RR, et al: Isolation and characterization of angiogenin, an angiogenic protein, from human carcinoma cells. Biochemistry (Wash) 24:5480–5486, 1985.

105. Strydom DJ, Fett JW, Lobb RR, et al: Amino acid sequence of human tumor derived angiogenin. Biochemistry (Wash) 24:5486–5499, 1985.

106. Kurachi K, Davie EW, Strydam DJ, et al: Sequence of the cDNA and gene for angiogenin, a human angiogenesis factor. Biochemistry (Wash) 24:5494–5499, 1985.

107. Shapiro R, Riordan JF, Vallee BL: Characteristic ribonucleolytic activity of human angiogenin. Biochemistry (Wash) 25:3527–3532, 1986.

108. Weiner HL, Weiner LH, Swain JL: Tissue distribution and developmental expression of the messenger RNA encoding angiogenin. Science 237:280–282, 1987.

109. Ben Ezra D: Neovasculogenic ability of prostaglandins, growth factors and synthetic chemoattractants. Am J Ophthalmol 86:455–461, 1978.

110. Ziche M, Jones J, Gullino P: Role of prostaglandin E1 and copper in angiogenesis. J Natl Cancer Inst 69:475–482, 1982.

111. Form DM, Auerbach R: PGE_2 and angiogenesis. Proc Soc Exp Biol Med 172:214–218, 1983.

112. Castellot JJ Jr, Karnovsky MJ, Spiegelman BM: Potent stimulation of vascular endothelial cell growth by differentiated 3T3 adipocytes. Proc Natl Acad Sci USA 77:6007–6011, 1980.

113. Dobson EE, Kambe A, Block E, et al: 1-Butyrlglycerol: A novel angiogenesis factor secreted by differentiating adipocytes. Cell 61:223–230, 1990.

114. Silverman KJ, Lund DP, Zetter BR, et al: Angiogenic activity of adipose tissue. Biochem Biophys Res Commun 153:347–352, 1988.

115. Childs CB, Proper JA, Tucker RF, et al: Serum contains a platelet-derived transforming growth factor. Proc Natl Acad Sci USA 79:5312–5316, 1982.

116. Ross R, Raines EW, Bowen-Pope DF: The biology of platelet-derived growth factor. Cell 46:155–169, 1986.

117. Deuel TF, Senior RM, Huang JS, et al: Chemotaxis of monocytes and neutrophils to platelet-derived growth factor. J Clin Invest 69:1046–1049, 1982.

118. Knighton DR, Hunt TK, Thakral KK, et al: Role of platelets and fibrin and the healing sequence: An in vivo study of angiogenesis and collagen synthesis. Ann Surg 196:379–388, 1982.

119. Knighton DR, Ciresi KF, Fiegel VD, et al: Classification and treatment of chronic nonhealing wounds. Successful treatment with autologous platelet derived wound healing factors. Ann Surg 104:322–330, 1986.

120. Leibovich SJ, Ross R: The role of the macrophage in wound repair: A study with hydrocortisone and anti-macrophage serum. Am J Pathol 78:71–100, 1975.

121. Diegelman RF, Cohen K, Kaplan AM: The role of macrophages in wound repair: A review. Plast Reconstr Surg 68:107–113, 1981.

122. Polverini PJ, Cotran RS, Gimbrone MA, et al: Activated macrophages induce vascular proliferation. Nature 269:804–806, 1977.

123. Polverini PJ, Leibovich SJ: Induction of neovascularization in vivo and endothelial proliferation in vitro by tumor associated macrophages. Lab Invest 51:635–642, 1984.

124. Hunt TK, Knighton DR, Thakral KK, et al: Studies on inflammation and wound healing: Angiogenesis and collagen synthesis stimulated in vivo by resident and activated wound macrophages. Surgery 96:48–54, 1984.

125. Hockel M, Sasse J, Wissler JH: Purified monocyte-derived angiogenic substance (angiotropin) stimulates migration, phenotypic changes, and tube formation but not proliferation of capillary endothelial cells in vitro. J Cell Physiol 133:1–13, 1987.

126. Yurt RW: Role of mast cells in trauma. In Dineen P, Hildick-Smith G (eds): The Surgical Wound. Philadelphia, Lea and Febiger, 1981, pp 37–62.

127. Kessler DA, Langer RS, Pless NA, et al: Mast cells and tumor angiogenesis. Int J Cancer 18:703–709, 1976.

128. Dethlefsen SM, Mulliken JB, Glowacki J: An ultrastructural study of mast cell interactions in hemangiomas. Ultrastruct Pathol 10:175–183, 1986.

129. Lopez R, Rand LI, Zetter BR: Absence of mast cells in diabetic retinopathy. Microvasc Res 24:87–93, 1982.
130. Roche WR: The nature and significance of tumour-associated mast cells. J Pathol 148:175–182, 1986.
131. Young JD, Liu CC, Butler G, et al: Identification, purification, and characterization of a mast cell–associated cytotoxic factor related to tumor necrosis factor. Proc Natl Acad Sci USA 84:9175–9179, 1987.
132. Crocker DJ, Murad TM, Greer JC: Role of the pericyte in wound healing. An ultrastructural study. Exp Mol Pathol 13:51–65, 1970.
133. Kuwabara T, Cogan DG: Retinal vascular patterns. VI. Mural cells of the retinal capillaries. Arch Ophthal NS 69:492–502, 1963.
134. Feldman PS, Shneidmann D, Kaplan C: Ultrastructure of hemangioendothelioma of the liver. Cancer 42:521–527, 1978.
135. Orlidge A, D'Amore P: Inhibition of capillary endothelial cell growth by pericytes and smooth muscle cells. J Cell Biol 105:1455–1461, 1987.
136. Hay ED: Cell Biology of the Extracellular Matrix. New York, Plenum Press, 1981.
137. Kadish JL, Butterfield CE, Folkman J: The effects of fibrin on cultured vascular endothelial cells. Tissue Cell 11:99–108, 1979.
138. Dvorak HF, Harvey VS, Estrella P, et al: Fibrin containing gels induce angiogenesis. Implications for tumor stroma generation and wound healing. Lab Invest 57:673–686, 1987.
139. Dvorak HF, Van DeWater L, Bitzer AM, et al: Procoagulant activity associated with plasma membrane vesicles shed by cultured tumor cells. Cancer Res 43:4434–4442, 1983.
140. Dvorak HF, Senger DR, Dvorak AM: Fibrin as a component of the tumor stroma: Origins and biological significance. Cancer Metast Rev 2:41–73, 1983.
141. Dvorak HF: Thrombosis and cancer. Human Pathol 18:275–284, 1987.
142. Bently JP: Rate of chondroitin sulfate formation in wound healing. Ann Surg 165:186–190, 1967.
143. Akiyama SK, Yamada KM: Fibronectin. Adv Enzymol 59:1–57, 1987.
144. Yamada KM: Fibronectin and other structural proteins. In Hay ED (ed): Cell Biology of the Extra Cellular Matrix. New York, Plenum Press, 1981, pp 95–114.
145. Clark RAF, Quinn JH, Winn HJ, et al: Fibronectin is produced by blood vessels in response to injury. J Exp Med 156:646–651, 1982.
146. Alitatlo K, Hovi T, Vaheri A: Fibronectin is produced by human macrophages. J Exp Med 151:602–613, 1980.
147. Viljanto J, Penttinen R, Raekallio J: Fibronectin in early phases of wound healing in children. Acta Chir Scand 147:7–13, 1981.
148. Grinnell F, Billingham RE, Burgess L: Distribution of fibronectin during wound healing in vivo. J Invest Dermatol 76:181–189, 1981.
149. Holund B, Clemmensen I, Junker P, et al: Fibronectin in experimental granulation tissue. Acta Pathol Microbiol Immunol Scand 90:159–165, 1982.
150. Kurkinen M, Vaheri A, Roberts PJ, et al: Sequential appearance of fibronectin and collagen in experimental granulation tissue. Lab Invest 43:47–51, 1980.
151. McDonald JA, Kelley DG, Brockelmann TJ: Role of fibronectin in collagen deposition: F'ab to the gelatin-binding domain of fibronectin inhibits both fibronectin and collagen organization in fibroblast extracellular matrix. J Cell Biol 92:485–492, 1982.
152. Singer II, Kawka DW, Kazazis DM, et al: In vivo co-distribution of fibronectin and actin fibers in granulation tissue: Immunofluorescence and electron microscope studies of the fibronexus at the myofibroblast surface. J Cell Biol 98:2091–2106, 1984.
153. Levenson SM, Geever EG, Crowley LV, et al: The healing of rat skin wounds. Ann Surg 161:293–308, 1965.
154. Madden JW, Peacock EE: Studies on the biology of collagen synthesis and deposition in cutaneous wounds of the rat. Surgery 64:288–294, 1968.
155. Montesano R, Orci L, Vassalli P: In vitro rapid organization of endothelial cells into capillary-like networks is promoted by collagen matrices. J Cell Biol 97:1648–1652, 1983.
156. Madri JA, Williams SK: Capillary endothelial cell cultures: Phenotypic modulation by matrix components. J Cell Biol 96:153–165, 1983.
157. Kalebic T, Garbisa S, Glaser B, et al: Basement membrane collagen: Degradation by migrating endothelial cells. Science 221:281–282, 1983.
158. Madri JA, Stenn KS: Aortic endothelial cell migration. I. Matrix requirements and composition. Am J Pathol 106:180–186, 1982.
159. Spooner BS, Faubion JM: Collagen involvement in branching morphogenesis of embryonic lung and salivary gland. Dev Biol 77:84–102, 1980.
160. Wicha MS, Liotta LA, Vonderhaar BK, et al: Effects of inhibition of basement membrane collagen deposition on rat mammary gland development. Dev Biol 80:253–266, 1980.
161. Hilfer SR, Pakstis GL: Interference with thyroid histogenesis by inhibitors of collagen synthesis. J Cell Biol 75:446–463, 1977.
162. Ingber DE, Folkman J: Inhibition of angiogenesis through modulation of collagen metabolism. Lab Invest 59:44–51, 1988.
163. Ingber DE, Madri JA, Folkman J: A possible mechanism for inhibition of angiogenesis by angiostatic steroids: Induction of capillary basement membrane dissolution. Endocrinology 119:1768–1775, 1986.
164. Folkman J, Klagsbrun M, Sasse J, et al: A heparin-binding angiogenic protein—basic fibroblast growth factor—is stored within basement membrane. Am J Pathol 130:393–400, 1988.
165. Gospodarowicz D, Cheng J: Heparin protects basic and acidic FGF from inactivation. J Cell Physiol 128:475–484, 1986.
166. Schreiber AB, Kenney J, Kowalski WJ, et al: Interaction of endothelial cell growth factor with heparin: Characterization by receptor and antibody recognition. Proc Natl Acad Sci USA 82:6138–6142, 1985.
167. Crum R, Szabo S, Folkman J: A new class of steroids inhibits angiogenesis in the presence of heparin or a heparin fragment. Science 230:1375–1378, 1985.
168. Hunt TK, Pai MP: Effect of varying ambient oxygen tension on wound metabolism and collagen synthesis. Surg Gynecol Obstet 135:561–567, 1972.
169. Ninikoski J: Effect of oxygen supply on wound healing and formation of experimental granulation tissue. Acta Physiol Scand (Suppl 78) 334:1–72, 1980.
170. Meltzer T, Meyers B: The effect of hyperbaric oxygen on the bursting strength and rate of vascularization of skin wounds in the rat. Am Surg 52:659–662, 1986.
171. Silver IA: The measurement of oxygen tension in healing tissue. Prog Resp Res 3:124–135, 1969.
172. Hunt TK, Conolly WB, Aronson SB, et al: Anaerobic metabolism and wound healing: An hypothesis for the initiation and cessation of collagen synthesis in wounds. Am J Surg 135:328–332, 1978.
173. Knighton DR, Silver IA, Hunt TK: Regulation of wound healing angiogenesis: Effect of oxygen gra-

dients and inspired oxygen concentration. Surgery 90:262–270, 1981.

174. Knighton DR, Hunt TK, Scheunstuhl H, et al: Oxygen tension regulates expression of angiogenesis factor by macrophages. Science 221:1283–1285, 1983.

175. Jensen JA, Jonsson K, Hunt TK: Epinephrine lowers subcutaneous wound oxygen tension. Curr Surg 42:472–474, 1985.

176. Hunt TK: Can repair processes be stimulated by modulators (cell growth factors, angiogenic factors, etc.) without adversely affecting normal processes. J Trauma (Suppl) 24:39–47, 1984.

177. Chang N, Goodson WH, Gottrup F, et al: Direct measurement of wound and tissue oxygen tension in postoperative patients. Ann Surg 197:470–478, 1983.

178. Hunt TK, Halliday B, Knighton DR, et al: Impairment of microbicidal function in wounds: Correction with oxygen. In Hunt TK, Heppenstall RB, Pines E, et al (eds): Soft and Hard Tissue Repair. Biological and Clinical Aspects. Surgical Science Series, vol 2. New York, Praeger, 1984, pp 455–468.

179. Leitzel K, Cano C, Marks JG, et al: Growth factors and wound healing in the hamster. J Dermatol Surg Oncol 11:617–622, 1985.

180. Brown GL, Schultz G, Brightwell JR, et al: Epidermal growth factor enhances epithelialization. Surg Forum 25:565–567, 1984.

181. Lawrence WT, Norton JA, Sporn MB, et al: The reversal of an Adriamycin induced healing impairment with chemoattractants and growth factors. Ann Surg 203:142–147, 1986.

182. Li AKC, Koroly MJ, Schattenerk M, et al: Nerve growth factor: Acceleration of the rate of wound healing in mice. Proc Natl Acad Sci USA 77:4379–4381, 1980.

183. Viljanto J: Biochemical basis of tensile strength in wound healing. Acta Chir Scand (Suppl) 333:1–91, 1964.

184. Laoto M, Niinikiski J, Lebel L, et al: Stimulation of wound healing by epidermal growth factor. A dose dependent effect. Ann Surg 203:379–381, 1986.

185. Davidson JM, Klagsbrun M, Hill KE, et al: Accelerated wound repair, cell proliferation, and collagen accumulation are produced by a cartilage-derived growth factor. J Cell Biol 100:1219–1227, 1985.

186. Buntrock P, Jentzch KD, Heder G: Stimulation of wound healing, using brain extract with fibroblast growth factor (FGF) activity. Exp Pathol 21:62–67, 1982.

187. Fourtanier AY, Courty J, Muller E, et al: Eye-derived growth factor isolated from bovine retina and used for epidermal wound healing in vivo. J Invest Dermatol 87:76–80, 1986.

188. Sporn MB, Roberts AB, Shull JH, et al: Polypeptide transforming growth factors isolated from bovine sources and used for wound healing in vivo. Science 219:1329–1331, 1983.

189. Mustoe TA, Pierce GF, Thomason A, et al: Accelerated healing of incisional wounds in rats induced by transforming growth factor-beta. Science 237:1333–1336, 1987.

190. Grotendurst GR, Martin GR, Pencev D, et al: Stimulation of granulation tissue formation by platelet-derived growth factor in normal and diabetic rats. J Clin Invest 76:2323–2329, 1985.

191. Lynch SE, Nixon JC, Colvin RB, et al: Role of platelet derived growth factor in wound healing: Synergistic effects with other growth factors. Proc Natl Acad Sci USA 84:7696–7700, 1987.

192. Glowacki J, Kaban LB, Murray JE, et al: Application of the biological principle of induced osteogenesis for craniofacial defects. Lancet 1:959–963, 1981.

193. Kaban LB, Mulliken JB, Glowacki J: Treatment of jaw defects with demineralized bone implants. J Oral Maxillo Surg 40:623–626, 1982.

194. Krummel TM, Nelson JM, Diegelmann RF, et al: Fetal response to injury and its modulation with transforming growth factor-beta. Surg Forum 28:622–623, 1987.

195. Slack JMW, Darlington BG, Heath JK, et al: Mesoderm induction in early xenopus embryos by heparin binding growth factors. Nature 326:197–200, 1987.

6

WOUND CONTRACTION AND SCAR CONTRACTURE

Ross Rudolph, M.D., and Jerry Vande Berg, Ph.D.;
and H. Paul Ehrlich, Ph.D.

Wound contraction has been defined as the mechanisms by which the edges of a wound are drawn toward the center, due to forces generated within that wound.[1] Wound contraction is a basic biological process necessary for survival. An open wound that results from trauma, such as burn or attack by a carnivore, must be capable of being closed, else the animal will succumb to infection. When occurring in a location where there is sufficient tissue mobility, wound contraction can be a most effective mechanism for wound closure (Fig. 6–1A–D). Specifically, in areas where tissue loss is relatively small, where deformity will not occur as a consequence of skin edges being drawn together, or where tissue loss is not across a joint, wound contraction is a surgically acceptable means of wound closure.

On the other hand, scar contracture can produce scar deformities, some of which can be horrendous.[2] The inexorable shrinkage of a scar can pull a healed chin down to the chest or cause dislocating traction on joints (Fig. 6–2). The unfortunate consequences of scar contracture are naturally most obvious on the body surface, yet the same deleterious effects of connective tissue contracture can occur underneath the skin surface or involve the deep vital organs. Well-known examples are the contraction of the palmar fascia in Dupuytren's contracture and the contraction of a capsule around

a silicone breast implant. An occasional patient with a cardiac pacemaker will experience constant unremitting pain and extrusion of the implant. This problem appears to be due to a process of scar contracture that is similar to that around breast implants.[3]

Contraction of collagenous connective tissue with consequent scar contracture can occur even in more internal tissues. For example, contracted fibrotic scar bundles within the cirrhotic liver may compress intrahepatic vessels and contribute to portal hypertension (Fig. 6–3). The constriction of hepatic scar may explain the nodularity of cirrhosis and may impair the ability of liver cells to regenerate due to the formation of rigid confined spaces.[4] Other viscera can undergo contractures, such as in duodenal ulcer stricture, the contracture of cardiac valves in rheumatic heart disease, and urethral strictures in trauma.

The contractile process can also be seen in certain malignant conditions. In scirrhous carcinoma of the breast a stromal tissue contracture can pull on the surrounding tissues, causing skin dimpling that may be an early sign of carcinoma. Adenocarcinoma of the colon produces a constriction that may produce bowel obstruction, also an early sign of malignancy.

An important distinction is made between wound contraction and scar contracture. *Wound contraction* is a normal healing process that

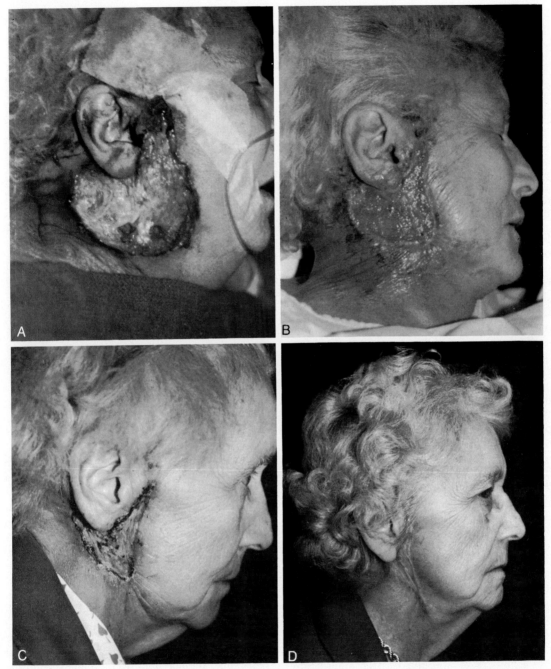

Figure 6–1. *A,* Large cheek wound due to tissue slough caused by extravasated calcium solution. *B,* Wound contraction. *C,* Wound covered with split-thickness skin graft and still shrinking. *D,* Fully contracted wound.

closes a wound and protects the organisms from its hostile environment. *Scar contracture* is the result of the contractile process occurring in a healed scar and often resulting in an undesirable fixed, rigid scar that can cause functional and/or cosmetic deformity. In general, wound contraction occurs in an incompletely epithelialized defect, while scar contracture occurs in an epithelialized covered defect.

THEORIES OF WOUND CONTRACTION

Multiple theories have been proposed to explain the process of wound contraction. In this chapter, two theories are presented, one of which highlights the contribution of a specialized population of contractile cells termed myo-

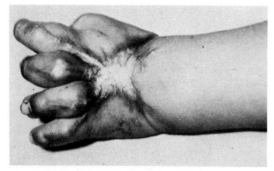

Figure 6–2. Stellate scar on a child's hand due to circular untreated skin slough. (From Rudolph R, Fisher JC, Ninneman JL: Skin Grafting. Boston, Little, Brown, 1979.)

fibroblasts, while the other examines the fibroblast, whose locomotion within the extracellular matrix produces tissue contraction. While these two concepts are considered separately, one should not infer that they are mutually exclusive; rather each may represent a component in the overall process of wound contraction.*

Wound contraction was formerly believed to be dependent on the connective tissue matrix at the healing site.[5] Collagen fibers developing in the granulation tissue of healing wounds were thought to generate some of the forces responsible for wound contraction. However, this hypothesis was questioned by Abercrombie and co-workers who demonstrated that wounds still contracted in scorbutic guinea pigs, suggesting that the cells in this granulation tissue produced the forces responsible for wound contraction.[6] These findings were supported by studies using lathyritic rats.[7] Another theory, termed the push theory, suggested that the mechanism of wound contraction is operant when the skin at the wound edge pushes itself into and over the defect. That force was said to be generated in the skin surrounding the defect. Edwards proposed that the pulsation of blood vessels at the wound edge pushed the skin over the defect.[8] However, if the wound edge is excised during the process of contraction, the skin retracts from the wound edge and the central granulation tissue contracts inward to the center of the wound.[9] This shows that the skin surrounding the healing wound does not push inward; instead, it pulls away.

The idea that a structure similar to a sphincter

*The authors of this chapter reflect the diversity of opinion on the mechanism of wound contraction. Drs. Rudolph and Vande Berg have extensively examined the myofibroblast and its contribution to the contraction process, whereas Dr. Ehrlich has studied the role that individual fibroblasts may play, thereby questioning the direct involvement of myofibroblasts in this process.

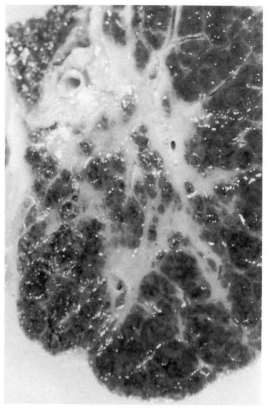

Figure 6–3. Contracted scar tissue in the cirrhotic liver. (Courtesy of G. Bordin, M.D.)

muscle develops at the wound edge that can close the wound by a "purse-string" mechanism was labeled the sphincter wound edge theory.[1] This idea was short-lived when it became clear that circular wounds close more slowly than rectangular ones, since the purse-string theory had postulated that circular wounds would close faster than square or rectangular ones.[10] Another theory, centered on dehydration, was predicated on the fact that covered wounds showed less contraction than open ones,[9] leading to the hypothesis that wounds that permitted dehydration of the scab contracted faster than those that did not.[9] However, most of these theories failed to account for the observation that viable cells within the wound or the wound edges are required for the process of contraction to occur.[6, 11–13]

Grillo, Watts, and Gross offered the picture frame theory, which stated that cells located at the wound edge generate forces that pull the normal skin over the defect.[9, 12, 14] This hypothesis was based on experiments showing that removing the central area of the contracting wound did not halt contraction, whereas disrupting the wound edge did. In contrast, Abercrombie and co-workers reported a pull theory whereby cells throughout the granulation tissue generate the forces responsible for contraction.[6] According to this theory, fibroblasts in the granulation tissue produce the forces to close wounds. Billingham and Medawar provided another example of granulation tissue as the producer of contractile forces when they showed that a central intact island of skin in a large open wound in a rabbit expanded instead of contracted.[15] The picture frame theory holds that the inward movement of granulation tissue toward the center of the wound should prevent outward growth from the central area of skin. These theories differ in their premises as to the location in the contracting wound of the cell responsible for generating those forces. Arguments in support of and in opposition to these theories are well presented in Van Winkle's review.[1]

MYOFIBROBLASTS AND FIBROBLASTS IN WOUND CONTRACTION

Myofibroblast Characterization

In the early 1970s, Gabbiani, Majno, and others characterized a fibroblast-like cell by electron microscopy and functional experiments that appeared to be the long-sought cell of wound contraction.[16] Because the ultrastructure of the cell combined characteristics of both fibroblasts and smooth muscle cells, the term "myofibroblast" was coined.

The most compelling electron microscopic evidence for the myofibroblast is the presence within the cell of long bundles of 60 to 80 angstrom microfilaments that are joined by electron-dense bodies (Fig. 6–4). These structures are similar in appearance to actin-myosin filaments (actomyosin) that occur in mammalian smooth muscle cells. In early granulating wounds, the microfilament bundles in myofibroblasts tpically appear as thin bundles lying parallel to the long axis of the cell. In later granulating wounds, the bundles increase in size and extend to the cell membrane.[17]

Adding to these identifiable features, Gabbiani and colleagues[16] observed the presence of convoluted nuclear membranes and associated this finding with cells in contraction. Other hallmarks of myofibroblasts were the presence of a basal lamina and intracellular connections such as hemidesmosomes and gap junctions. The latter structures can interconnect neighboring cells, allowing them to exert tension on each other and possibly to communicate through ionic exchange (perhaps to the point of creating a synchronized tensional force).[18]

Other electron microscopic studies have delineated further characteristics of the myofibroblasts. Rudolph and Woodward noted the presence of many microtubules in myofibroblasts.[19] These microtubules frequently occur parallel to the long axis of the cell, interdigitating with the meshwork of microfilament bundles at the end of the cell. Occasionally, the microtubules cross at angles, suggesting a bracing function. Rudolph[20] and others noted that the microfilament bundles, particularly at the ends of the myofibroblasts, appeared to extend out into the surrounding tissue stroma, suggesting a mechanism by which myofibroblasts could connect to collagen in the extracellular space.[3, 20]

Ryan and co-workers first observed cell-stroma linkages as microfilaments between myofibroblasts and basal lamina surrounding the cell membrane.[21] They suggested that these "microtendons" possibly functioned in transmitting cellular contraction to newly synthesized collagen. Singer described the "fibronexus" as a connection between intracytoplasmic 5 mm microfilaments and the extracellular matrix.[22] Subsequent immunochemical studies demonstrated that actin[22] and vinculin[23] were the principal cytoplasmic components while fibronectin and collagen types I and III were the primary constituents in the bordering extracellular matrix.[24] Extracellular fibrillar material on the surface of myofibroblasts was named myofibroblast anchoring substance (MAS) by Baur and associates.[25]

Are Myofibroblasts Really Necessary?

Evidence from Ehrlich's laboratory suggests that the cellularly generated contractile forces that close wounds do not require a specialized cell.[26] It is proposed instead that fibroblast locomotion provides the force for wound closure. Rather than cellular contraction providing the force necessary for wound contraction, it is the movement of the fibroblast as a single unit through the matrix that results in the reorganization of the connective tissue fibers.

The major difference between myofibroblast and fibroblast-generated contractile forces is based on the following premise: Myofibroblasts are said to act as multicellular units that undergo cell contraction resulting in a re-

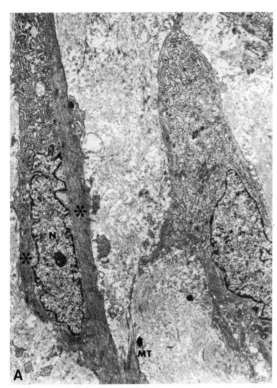
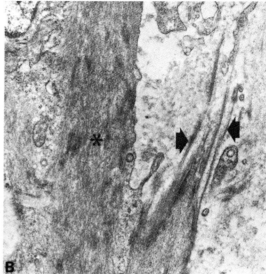

Figure 6–4. *A,* Electron micrographs of a classic myofibroblast from a contracted pacemaker pocket. Note convoluted nucleus, suggesting contraction (N). Large bundles of microfilaments with electron-dense bodies are typical (*). Filamentous "microtendons" (MT), also called "fibronexus" and "myofibroblast anchoring substance," connect cell to surrounding stroma (×3,800). (From Rudolph R: Contraction and the control of contraction. World J Surg 4:279–287, 1980.) *B,* Higher power view of "microtendon" *(arrows)* shown in *A* (×15,250).

arrangement of the surrounding connective tissue matrix.[27] The fibroblast theory suggests that the movement of individual fibroblast units in the matrix causes the rearrangement of the surrounding connective tissue matrix.

Arguments in support of both premises are based upon animal wound healing studies and upon in vitro tissue culture models whose local environments are well controlled. The cytoplasm of nonmuscle cells such as the fibroblast have a cytoskeletal contractile muscle structure rich in actin and myosin filaments. In the myofibroblast, these filaments form thick fibers, called stress fibers.[28] Those fibers are thought to contract and cause cell contraction. Because the cytoskeletal structure of fibroblasts is fine and filamentous, cell contraction is thought not to occur. However, fibroblasts in monolayer cultures become highly dense, show contact inhibition, and have cytoplasmic stress fibers. These cells, which maintain a fibroblast phenotype, should at that point be able to produce cell contraction.

In vivo studies have noted that stress fibers, as determined morphologically by electron microscopy, can be used to identify myofibroblasts in contracting rat wounds at 7 days.[27] Their appearance in contracting wounds is difficult to discern any earlier than 7 days, at which time full-excision wounds in rats have contracted by as much as 50 percent.[29] With wound contraction in rats having progressed that far, one would expect to find an abundance of myofibroblasts before 7 days. Fibroblasts have been observed to migrate into healing wounds as early as 2 to 3 days, when wound contraction is first evident.[10]

A model that has been used to support the role of fibroblasts in wound contraction is full-excision wounds in the tight skin mouse, a specialized genetic strain that exhibits a delay in wound closure, usually of about 3 weeks.[30] After that period, wounds close at a rate equal to that seen in normal mice where closure commences soon after trauma. One, two, and three weeks after injury, before wound contraction commences in tight skin mice, actin-stained cytoplasmic stress fibers are evident, indicating myofibroblasts in high density throughout the granulation tissue.[31] At 4 and 5 weeks, when tight skin mouse wounds are contracting, fewer cytoplasmic stress fibers are present and the resident cell populations are primarily fibroblasts and the density of myofibroblasts is greatly diminished. Myofibroblasts disappeared when wound contraction commenced. When contraction is complete in 6-week-old tight skin mice wounds, cells with abundant cytoplasmic stress fibers are present in great density, signaling the return of myofibroblasts.[31] While the appearance of fibroblasts is indicative of wound contraction, the reappearance of myofibroblasts is, in this model, the hallmark of the termination of active wound contraction. However, the use of this genetically altered animal to provide information on normal human wound contraction must be viewed with caution.

An in vitro model, the fibroblast populated collagen lattice (FPCL),[32] can be used to compare the generation of contractile forces by the myofibroblast, a multicellular contractile unit, or by the fibroblast, a single unit. An FPCL is made from fibroblasts freshly isolated from monolayer tissue culture by trypsinization and mixed rapidly with culture medium containing serum and cold native collagen solution. Following incubation at 37° C, the collagen polymerizes in less than 90 seconds and entraps the fibroblasts in the newly generated matrix.[32] This FPCL eventually undergoes a reduction in size, referred to here as lattice contraction (Fig. 6–5). The rate and degree of that contraction is directly proportional to cell number and is inversely proportional to the concentration of collagen. Two cell populations emerge during active lattice contraction. One, found in the center of the lattice, has cells with a random orientation, is surrounded by collagen, and has few actin-rich stress fibers (Fig. 6–6). These are fibroblasts. Cells in the other group, located in the periphery of the FPCL, have parallel orientation to each other, little collagen surrounding them, many cell-cell contacts, and an abundance of cytoplasmic actin-rich stress fibers (Fig. 6–6). These are myofibroblasts.

If myofibroblasts are responsible for lattice contraction, the outer edge of the FPCL should show greater contractile ability. If a wedge cut from a contracting lattice includes one edge rich in myofibroblasts, one would expect greater contraction in that edge than in the other two edges of the FPCL wedge (Fig. 6–7). If a wedge were cut in such a way that all three edges contained fibroblasts and myofibroblasts were found only at one apex, less contraction would be expected. Figure 6–7 shows that after 48 hours, the edge rich in myofibroblasts contracts less than the edges with plentiful fibroblasts. In this model, the area populated by myofibroblasts demonstrates the least degree of lattice contraction, while the edges with a larger proportion of fibroblasts contract more.

Additional experiments in vitro have compared fibroblast contraction with fibroblast locomotion. A model of cell contraction was used to demonstrate the contractility of stress fibers and microfilaments. After 24 hours in monolayer at low densities, fibroblasts showed fewer stress fibers than confluent, highly dense cultures of fibroblasts after 48 hours in culture (Fig. 6–8). Both preparations were treated with descending concentrations of glycerol (50% to 5%) to permeabilize the cell membrane.[33] Adding ATP and cofactors Ca^{+2}, Mg^{+2}, and KCl to these permeabilized preparations induced cell contraction resulting from the sliding of actinmyosin filaments. In this case, fibroblasts (microfilaments) and myofibroblasts (stress fi

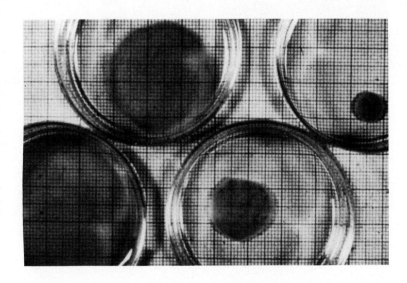

Figure 6–5. Lattice contraction. The dynamic reorganization of a rapidly polymerized collagen matrix by resident human fibroblasts at 24 hours. *Left to right,* Four fibroblast populated collagen lattices (FPCLs) made with varying cell numbers. The FPCL at far right has 100,000 fibroblasts, the one at near right has 70,000, near left has 50,000, and the FPCL at far left has 10,000 cells. The FPCL made with the highest number of cells contracted the most.

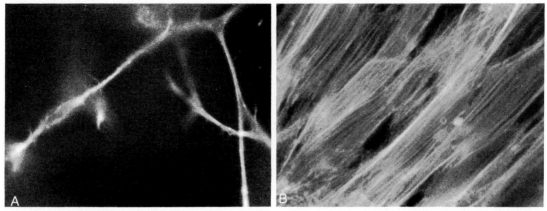

Figure 6–6. Human fibroblast morphology in an FPCL at 48 hours. An FPCL was fixed in 4% paraformaldehyde and stained with NBD-phallicidin, which binds specifically to F-actin. *A*, Fibroblasts in the center of the FPCL are elongated and have a cytoplasmic structure of uniformly stained F-actin filaments. *B*, Fibroblasts at the periphery of the FPCL show clearly definable stress fibers, rich in F-actin, in parallel arrangements with many cell-cell contacts. They are myofibroblasts.

bers) contracted equally, and there appeared to be no difference between the contractile abilities or the degree of contraction between these cells (Fig. 6–8). During cell contraction, the actin-rich cytoskeletons of these treated cells contracted to form aggregates. These contracted filaments pulled the cells inward to compact the cell. Compacted cells containing aggregates of actin were not found in the granulation tissue

of contracting healing wounds or in fibroblasts at the edge or in the center of the FPCL. The rate and degree of cell contraction in wound and lattice contraction suggest that compacted actin clumps in the cytoplasm should be common. This was not the case, however. It could be argued that cell contraction by the aggregation of the entire cytoskeletal muscle is not the mechanism by which the connective tissue ma-

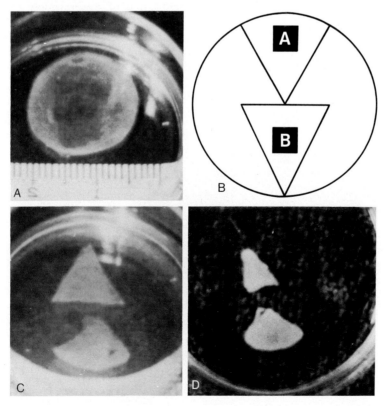

Figure 6–7. The wedge experiment. *A*, A 24-hour-old FPCL. *B*, A schematic of how two wedges would be cut from an FPCL. Wedge A has a side with myofibroblasts, while wedge B has only an apex with myofibroblasts. *C*, Two wedges have been cut from an FPCL. Wedge A is at the bottom, wedge B at the top. *D*, At 48 hours, wedge B *(top)* shows greater contraction, and wedge A *(bottom)* less contraction, particularly in the edge rich in myofibroblasts.

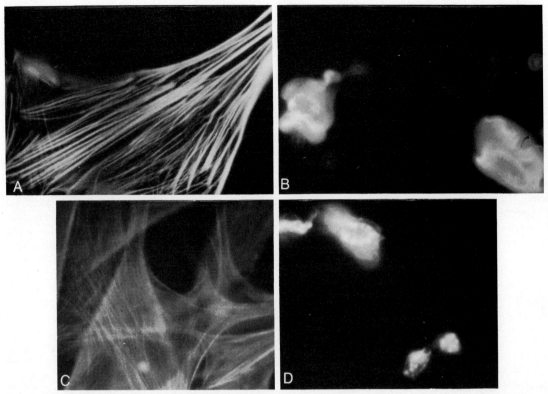

Figure 6–8. ATP-induced cell contraction. Fibroblasts in monolayer culture are permeabilized by treatment with glycerol. Adding ATP and the required cofactors promotes myosin ATPase activity and the sliding action of actin and myosin filaments. The sliding filaments provide the mechanical force that results in cell contraction. These cellular preparations were fixed and stained with rhodamine phalloidin. *A,* Fibroblasts grown at low density for 18 hours were treated with glycerol, fixed, and stained. They show fine, diffuse actin-rich microfilaments. *B,* The same cells as described in *A,* 10 minutes after the addition of ATP. Cells contract and microfilaments aggregate. *C,* Cells in culture at 48 hours initially plated in high density show a myofibroblast-like morphology. Note the large actin-rich stress fibers in these monolayer culture cells, which have been permeabilized with glycerol. *D,* Cells from the same cultures as in *C,* 10 minutes after the addition of ATP and cofactors. Note the cell contraction associated with the aggregation of actin-rich stress fibers. The ability of microfilaments and stress fibers to show cell contraction and actin filament aggregation appears to be equivalent. There is no evidence of a unique cell, such as the myofibroblast, being responsible for producing contractile forces.

trix of granulation tissue and FPCL is rearranged.

Fibroblast locomotion has been demonstrated by Harris and co-workers.[34] Fibroblasts plated onto a thin film of heat-polymerized silicone oil will cause that surface to wrinkle when they attempt to move across it. The fibroblast does not move; the surface moves. When wrinkles appear under this cell, this cell does not lose its flattened, elongated appearance (Fig. 6–9).

In dynamic models of cell-generated contractile forces, the fibroblast is prominent, whereas the myofibroblast is prominent under conditions of static motion or at the termination of the contractile process. Ehrlich has proposed that the fibroblast, acting as a single cellular unit, reorganizes the surrounding connective tissue matrix, consolidating the tissue into a smaller unit and pulling surrounding skin with it. When the connective tissue matrix becomes

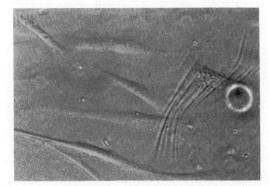

Figure 6–9. Fibroblast-generated thin film surface wrinkling. Silicone oil was placed on a glass coverslip and its surface was flamed briefly to produce a thin polymerized surface that floats the oil. Fibroblasts readily attach to this surface, spread out, and try to move. This attempted cell movement results in the wrinkling of that thin surface. Harris[34] proposes that this wrinkling is due to cell tractional forces and not cell contraction.

highly organized and fibroblasts become increasingly dense making cell-cell contact, contact inhibition occurs. Fibroblast proliferation and cell locomotion cease, and cytoplasmic stress fibers form. This occurrence can be demonstrated in monolayer fibroblast culture as well as in the outer edge of the FPCL. Cell-cell contacts, which inhibit cell locomotion, lead to the formation of thick actin-myosin filaments, or stress fibers. These cells are no longer capable of organizing a connective tissue matrix. Morphologically, they are myofibroblasts; they are static and can no longer participate in wound contraction, lattice contraction, or surface wrinkling.

Speculation as to the role of myofibroblasts in wound closure might lead one to conclude that these cells are fibroblasts in a transitional state. Fibroblasts move into the defect early in wound healing, proliferate, lay down a new connective tissue matrix, and rearrange that matrix. At the conclusion of wound closure, fibroblast density in that area is greatly reduced, which is characteristic of the remodeling period, the last phase of the wound healing process. Remodeling is characterized by a great reduction in cell density and a consolidation of connective tissue into scar. It is also notable that there is far less vascularization in that area than is seen in granulation tissue. Since fibroblast necrosis is not evident, it appears that these cells migrate from the healed space. The myofibroblast may represent the terminus of cell migration to and the initiation of fibroblast migration from the healed wound space; therefore, myofibroblasts may be a transitional state of fibroblasts in granulation tissue. The low cell density characteristic of normal scar may be predicated on cell migration from the healed wound.

The connective tissue matrix is another important component of the contractile process. Experimental evidence from both in vivo and in vitro models demonstrates a governing role for connective tissue in wound contraction. Full-excision wounds in rats contract faster than full-thickness burns, and the reason may be the need for complete debridement of the burn wound prior to contraction. Denatured connective tissue matrix and necrotic cellular components, both of which result from thermal trauma, are pushed up into the scab covering the defect by the increasing volume of granulation tissue, and this debris must be removed before contraction can proceed. The defect in full-excision wounds removes all cellular and connective tissue components and is initially replaced by a fibrin clot that is more readily and rapidly replaced by granulation tissue than is the necrotic tissue left by burn injury.

Freeze injuries, in contrast to burn and full-excision wounds, show little or no contraction. Cells are killed by freeze injury but little damage occurs in the connective tissue matrix. Healing proceeds, therefore, by islands of granulation tissue repopulating the residual connective tissue matrix.[11] A stable matrix will resist the cellular contractile forces responsible for local distortion and reorganization.

The FPCL has also been used to demonstrate control by the connective tissue matrix of fibroblast-generated contractile forces. FPCLs containing fibroblasts grown out from contracting scar excised during reconstructive surgery are equal to FPCLs containing identical numbers of fibroblasts from normal static dermis in the rate of lattice contraction and ultimate size.[26] This again suggests that a specialized cell is not required to produce contraction in scar tissue. In contrast, lattice contraction is different in an FPCL made from collagen from contracting scar compared with one made with normal dermal collagen. FPCLs made with pepsin-extracted collagen from contracting scar contract faster and to a greater degree than ones made with pepsin-extracted collagen from normal dermis.[26] Hence, the collagen composition of an FPCL can control the rate and extent of lattice contraction (Fig. 6–10). FPCL made with collagens in equal concentrations but differing types are vastly different.[35] FPCLs made with type III collagen contract faster and to a greater degree than those made with type I, and those made from type II collagen contract the slowest and to the least degree (Fig. 6–10).

These findings support the idea that fibroblasts organize a type III collagen matrix more rapidly and to a greater degree than matrices made from other collagen types. The reason for this is not known, but it may be that fibroblasts can move more type III collagen fibers than any other type on their cell surface at any one time. Another possibility is that the fibroblast can compress type III collagen fibers more densely than other types. It should be noted that granulation tissue is rich in type III collagen, and this enrichment is present during wound contraction, while mature scar tissue has reduced amounts of type III collagen.

Wound contraction is a dynamic process requiring the interaction of cells and matrix. Normal skin surrounding a defect must have enough elasticity and mobility to be pulled over that defect. The fibroblast-generated contractile forces developing in the healing defect appear to be directly related to the organization of the connective tissue matrix. That matrix becomes condensed during this remodeling process, re-

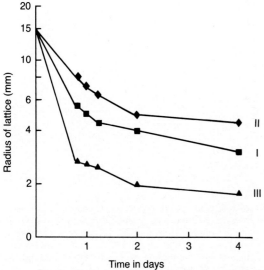

Figure 6–10. Diagram showing differences in lattice contraction. Fibroblast populated collagen lattices were made under identical conditions except for alterations in human collagen composition. Types I, II, and III collagen were used at 1.25 mg per ml per lattice. Lattices made with type II collagen contracted the least and at the slowest rate. Lattices made from type I contracted faster and to a greater degree. Lattices made from type III collagen contracted the fastest and to the greatest degree. (From Ehrlich HP: Wound closure: Evidence of cooperation between fibroblasts and collagen matrix. Eye 2:149–157, 1988.)

sulting in a reduction in volume and the drawing in of surrounding normal skin.

It is proposed from these studies that fibroblast locomotion is the mechanism that generates the contractile forces of wound contraction. The connective tissue matrix is important in controlling these forces. It is suggested that the histological existence of myofibroblasts is related to a transitional state of fibroblasts in granulation tissue wherein they prepare to migrate from the healed wound.

Observations to Support the Role of Myofibroblasts

Evidence to support the hypothesis that myofibroblasts are related to wound contraction comes from their reported occurrence in large numbers during the time that wound contraction takes place in certain animal species. In studies utilizing 5×5 cm full-thickness wounds on the backs of minipigs, contraction occurred over a 6 to 8 week period, very similar to what would occur in a human wound of similar size (Fig. 6–11A). Frequent biopsies were processed for electron microscopy and showed that from 2 to 8 weeks, when the rate of contraction was most vigorous, 80 to 90 percent of the fibroblasts within the granulating wounds had typical myofibroblast characteristics (Fig. 6–11B).[16] A similar finding of myofibroblast prominence at the same time as the active phase of wound contraction was found by McGrath and Hundahl.[46] In contrast, studies using the tight skin mouse have determined that myofibroblast prominence did not correlate with the period of maximal wound contraction.[31]

Additional life cycle studies on the inhibition of myofibroblasts by skin grafts showed a direct correlation between myofibroblast activity with the wound contraction phenomenon.[36] In rats, 2 $\times$ 4 cm skin wounds were produced and allowed to form granulation tissue or were immediately covered with split-thickness or full-thickness skin grafts. As is typical of rat wounds, full-thickness grafts inhibited contraction completely, whereas split-thickness grafts inhibited contraction only partially (Fig. 6–12A). Electron microscopic observations of wound biopsies at frequent intervals showed that regardless of the types of wound cover, large numbers of fibroblasts had myofibroblast characteristics by ap-

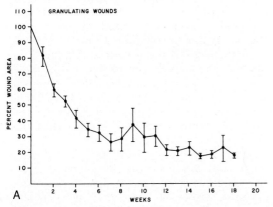
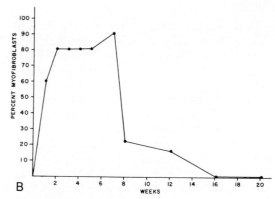

Figure 6–11. A, Contraction of pig wounds with time. B, Population of myofibrolasts in contracting pig wounds shown in A. (From Rudolph R, Guber S, Suzuki M, et al: The life cycle of the myofibroblast. Surg Gynecol Obstet 145:389–394, 1977. By permission of Surgery, Gynecology, and Obstetrics.)

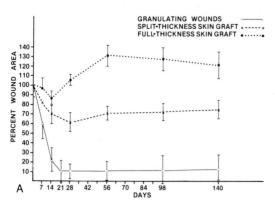

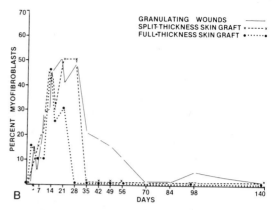

Figure 6–12. *A,* Contraction of rat skin wounds with time. Granulating wounds contracted most, while full-thickness grafted wounds did not contract. Split-thickness grafted wounds contracted less than granulating wounds but more than full-thickness grafted wounds. *B,* Myofibroblast populations in wounds shown in *A.* In each type of wound, the myofibroblast population rises equally. However, the myofibroblast population drop-off is fastest in full-thickness grafted wounds, intermediate in split grafted wounds, and slowest in granulating wounds. (From Rudolph R: Inhibition of myofibroblasts by skin grafts. Plast Reconstr Surg 63:473–480, 1979.)

proximately 2 weeks after wounding. However (Fig. 6–12*B*), the myofibroblast population dropped off fastest under the full-thickness skin grafts, disappeared less rapidly under split-thickness grafts, and lasted longest in the granulating wounds.

Using biochemical methods, Bertolami and Donoff found that there was a minimal amount of actomyosin present in wounds grafted with full-thickness skin as opposed to considerable actomyosin in granulating wounds.[37] However, even in the granulating wounds the actomyosin content was less than that found in uterine smooth muscle. They theorized that perhaps moving fibroblasts (which would have less actomyosin) rather than stationary but contracting myofibroblasts provided the motive force for wound contraction.[37]

Location of Myofibroblasts in Humans and Experimental Animals

Myofibroblasts have been visualized with electron microscopy in many tissues that form contracting and/or nodular scars. Myofibroblasts also occur in many human and animal pathological conditions in which contracted fibrotic tissue is present. For example, in examining scar capsules around silicone breast implants, Rudolph and colleagues obtained 49 specimens from 29 patients having a variety of implant types.[38] Of the 49 specimens, 25 implant capsules were contracted and 24 were noncontracted. Myofibroblasts were found in 36 of the 49 specimens, 28 from around gel implants and 8 from saline. Interestingly, the myofibroblasts were found in 20 hard and 16 soft capsules. The

presence of myofibroblasts thus appeared not to correlate directly with hardness but instead with whether there had been recent surgery or manual capsulotomy of contracted capsules. Myofibroblasts were not necessarily found in every hard capsule, since as noted previously they have a well-defined life cycle. Myofibroblasts could have led to the initial capsular contraction which was fixed by collagen synthesis after which the myofibroblasts would disappear, leaving behind a rigid contracted capsule.

Bhathal has reported myofibroblasts in samples from four patients with hepatic cirrhosis.[39] Owing to an ongoing study of acute operative intervention in bleeding esophageal varices, Rudolph and associates were able to obtain biopsies of cirrhotic liver.[4] At surgery, 12 specimens were obtained from patients who had been alcoholics for many years and subsequently developed acute bleeding from esophageal varices. Tissue specimens from these patients were compared to biopsies from three noncirrhotic livers and to three liver specimens obtained at autopsy. Electron microscopy showed typical myofibroblasts in 9 of the 12 cirrhotic livers. It was theorized that myofibroblasts in the actively contracting scar tissue of the liver could compress hepatic vessels and contribute to portal hypertension. In addition, contracting scar could prevent the liver tissue from regenerating normally and produce the nodularity so common in cirrhosis.

Many microtubules were seen via electron microscopy within the myofibroblasts in cirrhosis. Of interest is that Rojkind has treated cirrhosis, with some success, using colchicine, based on the premise that interference with fibroblast microtubules might interfere with collagen synthesis and deposition in the cirrhotic scar tissue.[40] An alternate explanation for the reported success of cirrhosis treatment with colchicine is that microtubules within myofibroblasts became disrupted.

Dupuytren's contracture is a disease process that can cause severe disabling contractures of the palm and digits. Several investigators have found active appearing myofibroblasts in the nodules, but not the cords, of Dupuytren's contracture.[41–43] Fibroblasts, myofibroblasts, and adjacent extracellular matrix formed a whorled appearance, suggesting a capstanlike effect of the contracting nodule in the active Dupuytren's contracture.[44]

Vande Berg and co-workers also studied the relationship of nodule and cord to palmar skin when it is drawn into the Dupuytren's contracture.[44] Using light and electron microscopy, myofibroblasts were identified in a layer directly underneath the dermis of the contracted skin, but no myofibroblasts were seen within the dermis itself. Previous studies had indicated that recurrence of Dupuytren's contracture was most likely in those patients having active myofibroblasts in the disease nodules.[41] The presence of myofibroblasts at the junction with dermis suggested that recurrence was also likely when skin was adherent to a nodule and that skin excision should be accomplished regionally. Since full-thickness skin grafts taken from other areas of the body will inhibit recurrent Dupuytren's contracture, there may be a defect in the quality of the regional palm skin in patients with Dupuytren's contracture that prevents palmar skin from inhibiting the contraction process.

Location of Wound Contraction Force

Location of myofibroblasts has also been studied by electron microscopy to determine the location of the wound contraction force. Past theories have centered on "picture frame" versus "pull" mechanisms, in which wound contraction was due either to force at the granulation tissue periphery or to force exerted throughout the wound substance. Using both pig and rat models, Rudolf showed that myofibroblasts were present throughout the granulating wound substance at the same time active contraction was occurring.[71] Myofibroblasts could also be seen at the wound edges but appeared approximately 1 week later in both animal species. Using myofibroblasts as a marker of contraction, this study showed that the force of contraction is generated uniformly throughout the contracting wound, rather than being localized at the wound margins.[71]

McGrath and Hundahl came to a similar conclusion, finding myofibroblasts throughout the substance of granulating pig wounds at four weeks.[46] They suggested that myofibroblasts appeared to be derived from inflammatory foci. After 1 week, pig wounds showed localized aggregations of myofibroblasts (identified by immunoperoxidase staining for actin) around areas of inflammation. By 4 weeks, the myofibroblasts were more uniformly distributed through the granulation tissue but were concentrated at the surface. The authors speculated that inflammatory cells are most likely the biological mediators of myofibroblast induction.

Myofibroblast-Derived Cell Lines

A logical development of electron microscopic studies on the identification of myofibroblasts in contracted tissues was to evaluate myofibroblast cell lines and their growth kinetics in tissue culture. Standard tissue culture techniques have been used by Vande Berg and co-workers to obtain growth curves of myofibroblasts from granulating tissue in animals, from contracted tissues from eleven patients with Dupuytren's contracture, from three scirrhous breast cancers, and from four human granulating wounds.[42, 45, 48] In initial studies of cultured cells from the human granulating wounds, two salient points emerged. First, there was preservation of microanatomy of myofibroblasts in tissue culture, and second, there was slower growth of myofibroblast-derived cell lines from granulating and contracting tissues as opposed to cell lines from normal dermis fibroblasts.

A tissue culture of fibroblasts has some similarities to an open wound. A space exists supplied with nutrients within which fibroblasts move, multiply, and manufacture collagen. Because of these similarities, cell culture of fibroblasts may be well suited to the study of wound contraction.

Fibroblasts in culture have the ability to move, divide, and in plastic culture dishes develop intracellular "stress" filaments composed of actin and myosin. In both human and animal culture studies performed by Vande Berg and associates,[42, 45, 48] myofibroblast-derived cell lines had extensively developed bundles of 60 to 80 angstrom microfilaments with electron-dense bodies. In contrast, cultured cells derived from normal dermal fibroblasts had looser, smaller microfilament bundles. The myofibroblasts from granulating wounds were also larger in tissue culture, measuring 20 to 24 μ versus fibroblasts from intact dermis (20 to 22μ) and from skin grafts (16 to 20μ).

Tissue culture showed a significant decrease in the growth rate of myofibroblast-derived cell lines as opposed to fibroblast-derived cell lines (Fig. 6–13). This was most apparent in early passages. In late passages, the growth rate difference and the distinction between sizes of microfilament bundles began to disappear. In humans, it was difficult to grow the myofibroblast-derived cell lines beyond 15 passages, by which time the growth rates were becoming similar to those of fibroblast-derived cell lines. In rats, in which cells remained viable at least until passage 30, the difference between early and late passage was more striking. At three passages, myofibroblasts from granulating wounds grew significantly more slowly than did fibroblasts from rat dermis. However, by 30

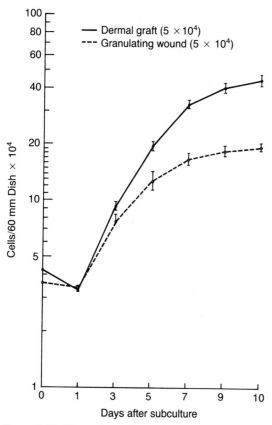

Growth curves of human cultured fibroblasts from dermal graft and granulating wound

— Dermal graft (5×10^4)
--- Granulating wound (5×10^4)

Cells/60 mm Dish × 10^4

Days after subculture

Figure 6–13. Comparison of growth rates between fibroblasts from uninjured human dermis *(solid line)* and myofibroblasts from a granulating wound *(dashed line)*. (From Rudolph R, Vande Berg JS, Woodward M: Growth dynamics of tissue-cultured myofibroblasts from granulating wounds. Surg Forum 33:579–581, 1982. Copyright 1982 American College of Surgeons.)

passages, selection had probably occurred in favor of faster growing cells and the growth rates were similar.[72]

Differences between fibroblast and myofibroblast actin concentration were recently reported.[45] Paired populations of fibroblasts from normal dermis and granulating wound myofibroblasts were obtained from three patients. The average actin content was significantly greater in the myofibroblasts (24 to 62 pg/cell) than in the paired normal fibroblasts (3 to 47 pg/cell). These data suggest that myofibroblasts have an increased availability of monomeric actin for synthesis of contractile microfilament bundles.

Cell culture studies have shown that both fibroblasts and myofibroblasts synthesize type I and III procollagen.[47] More recently, these same researchers noted that early-passage myofibroblasts produce three times more type I and III procollagen compared with the same passage fibroblasts. However, these differences became less pronounced at later passages.[48] Only myofibroblasts demonstrated prominent type V procollagen staining, as well as staining with anti-muscle actin antibodies. It was concluded that the myofibroblast is an active secretory form of fibroblast, which, although possessing properties of both smooth muscle cells and fibroblasts, is most likely a modified fibroblast that has undergone a phenotypic change in response to specific signals from the extracellular matrix.

From these data, it would appear that the myofibroblast is not a separate cell line but rather a differentiated fibroblast that can modulate back to fibroblast characteristics or possibly degenerate when the stimulus for wound contraction has ceased. Although it is difficult to make functional comparisons between in vivo and in vitro, the modulation of fibroblast growth rates from slow growing to normal parallels the observed electron microscopic disappearance of myofibroblasts in a stable wound that has ceased contracting.

Tissue Culture Studies of Tension Exerted in Fibroblasts

The ability of cultured fibroblasts to move, to form intracellular actomyosin-containing stress filaments thought similar to those of in vivo myofibroblasts, and to functionally exert contraction has been studied.[49, 50] Krebs and Birchmeier injected cultured fibroblasts with rhodamine-labeled smooth muscle actin, which became incorporated into the stress fibers, and showed that these labeled fibers contracted in response to Mg-ATP.[51] They concluded that stress fiber sarcomeres of cultured fibroblasts are contractile, and theorized that this occurs via an actin-myosin system.

In an ingenious series of experiments, Harris and colleagues demonstrated that tissue-cultured fibroblasts are capable of exerting tensional forces on the underlying stroma.[34] By seeding cultured fibroblasts onto extremely thin sheets of polymerized silicone rubber, Harris was able to demonstrate wrinkling of the underlying silicone sheet, which he theorized was due to traction forces exerted by the cells. Harris further theorized that in attempting to move across the substrate, the cell instead caused the substrate to wrinkle underneath the cell margin.

In reviewing Harris' studies, Burridge noted that this wrinkling was most likely to occur under stationary cells.[52] He noted that stress fibers, most likely identical to the actomyosin-containing microfilament bundles first identified by Gabbiani in myofibroblasts, do not occur in migrating cells, but rather in stationary cells. He stated that the more strongly a cell adheres to the substrate, the greater is the tension and the larger the development of the resulting stress fibers. In interpreting Harris' data, Burridge concluded that stress fibers are contractile but are adapted to develop isometric rather than isotonic contraction. Probably tension generated at a tight attachment to the underlying substrate causes the formation of actomyosin microfilament bundles within the fibroblasts.

Extensive studies have further interpreted Harris' data and have led Ehrlich to the conclusion that wound contraction is more likely due to cell locomotion than to cell contraction.[26] This theory is based on the observed contraction of a collagen gel lattice seeded with actively growing tissue cultured fibroblasts. It was noted that contraction of the gel lattice occurred during a phase of cell movement when the cells did not contain stress filaments. Once contraction had ceased and the cells were not moving, then stress filaments developed. It was concluded that the stress filaments in the gel-cultured fibroblast mark an end-stage cell that has nothing to do with wound contraction.

A theory that can potentially accommodate both the fibroblast locomotion studies and the myofibroblast hypothesis relates to differential development of "muscle" bundles in response to demands. An analogy can be drawn between different types of athletic muscle toning: isotonic activity results from using weights with multiple repetitions over distances, while isometric contraction involves muscle contraction against a nonmoving surface.

It is possible that early wound contraction is due to the process described by Ehrlich, in which not cell contraction but abortive cell locomotion piles up collagen fibers under the cell membrane due to tractional forces.[53] Thus, a fibroblast not containing stress filaments, enmeshed in a collagen grid, attempts to move by mobilizing its plasma membrane. This results in the collagen being piled together much as a loose rug would pile up under a walker's foot.

While this process is occurring in vivo, there is continued outward tension on wound edges. In response to this, the fibroblasts may develop the larger muscle-type bundles that are visible by electron microscopy, and that correspond to the actin-myosin stress filaments of fibroblasts that are adherent to plastic in tissue culture. These larger muscle-type bundles would preserve the fibroblasts and the collagen matrix against the constant outward pull of the surrounding tissue.

An ingenious experiment by Bellows and co-workers, who were studying tooth eruption, has suggested that this scenario may in fact be true.[54, 55] They placed a gel matrix with cultured fibroblasts between two portions of demineralized bone and tooth. The collagen gel reorganized in a linear fashion between the solid structures. Once reorganization had been accomplished and the cells were no longer moving, the fibroblasts developed linear alignment. When the attachment was removed at one end, the collagen gel retracted further and the cells rounded up suggesting that in fact these cells were exerting isometric tension. Gels to which colcemid or cytochalasin D had been added had minimal contraction. Since colcemid is an inhibitor of microtubules and cytochalasin D is an inhibitor of microfilaments, Bellows concluded that both microtubules and microfilaments were necessary for cell alignment and for development of tension in the collagen gels.

Fleischer and Wohlfarth-Bottermann had shown in 1975 that isometric contraction does cause development of longitudinally oriented microfilament bundles in protoplasmic strands.[56] Additional studies have further substantiated the effect of cultured fibroblast microfilament bundles in isometric tension.[57] Fibroblasts were cultured in collagen gel attached to glass coverslips. The cultured fibroblasts developed prominent microfilaments while they were exerting enough tension to tear the gel from the glass and to contract the released gel. Farsi and Aubin noted that their data "support a role for contractile microfilament bundles during collagen fiber alignment and isometric contraction of the attached collagen gels, and the loss of these large bundles during an isotonic phase when the gel is no longer attached to the substratum."[57]

Thus, the myofibroblast with its microfilament bundles may be a marker of isometric contraction. Initial wound contraction may occur via the mechanism proposed by Ehrlich in which cell membrane movement piles up collagen matrix. The wound centrifugal tensions that must be resisted by the collagen matrix and the fibroblasts cause the fibroblasts to develop muscle-type bundles that develop isometric tension and keep the wound contracted.

Direct support for this theory has been offered by Squier, whose study examined the role of mechanical tension (stretching) and wound healing as an event capable of stimulating the formation of myofibroblasts in mouse skin.[58] He observed that stretching produced essentially no inflammation at any time, but myofibroblasts were observed at 4 days and were abundant at 6 days. Skin that had been stretched and wounded was inflamed and contained some myofibroblasts but fewer than in skin subjected to stretching alone. Squier concluded that the effect of mechanical tension alone may be the stimulus for myofibroblast formation.

CLINICAL CONTROL OF SCAR CONTRACTURE AND WOUND CONTRACTION

In spite of these extensive electron microscopy and tissue culture studies, manipulation of wound contraction remains at this stage mechanical and surgical. The surgeon may wish to *facilitate* wound contraction in some situations and to *inhibit* it in others.

Wound contraction is a satisfactory mechanism when tissue loss is small, not in a critical area, and surrounded by mobile tissue. Thus a small third degree burn on a thigh may heal satisfactorily by contraction and epithelization. Similarly, a dorsally angled tissue loss on a fingertip will contract and pull normal pulp tissue into a desired location.

Currently, no commonly accepted therapeutic approach exists to speed the normal process of wound contraction. However, infection and necrotic tissue can slow the contraction process. Surgical and chemical debridement along with judicious antibiotic usage can facilitate contraction by reducing inhibition due to infection. A thick leathery eschar can splint a wound open and should be removed to allow normal wound

contraction. Alternatively, in a setting where wound contraction will produce a poor result, *inhibition* of wound contraction may be sought.

The physician has available for prevention of pathological scar contraction five therapeutic approaches: (1) prolonged splinting, (2) range of motion exercises, (3) pressure, (4) full-thickness skin grafting, and (5) judicious planning of surgical procedures.

Splinting. Wounds that have been covered with split-thickness grafts, particularly of the thin variety, will contract dramatically over the course of months, and grotesque deformities can result, particularly in patients whose large burns had to be covered with thin or meshed skin grafts. Where contraction cannot be prevented by the use of full-thickness skin grafting or flaps, and split skin grafting is essential, splinting has been used to reduce contracture.

In an experimental setting, splints fixed to wound margins will prevent wound contraction. If the splints are removed while granulation tissue is still present, the wound rapidly contracts, suggesting that the effect of splinting is mechanical rather than due to modification of the contraction process.[59]

Molded splints, such as clinically used by Cronin, can reduce the total amount of contraction if used faithfully and continuously for a prolonged period of time until a stable wound occurs. Cronin found that constant use of a molded neck splint prevented a grafted wound from contracting.[60] Owing to the constant pull of the contracting wound, pressure ulcers can develop at bony pressure points and must be guarded against by judicious padding. The splint helps to keep the tissue stretched mechanically during the active phase of wound contraction.

Range of Motion Exercises. During the phase of wound contraction, the active cellular process is locked into position by increasing amounts of rigid collagenous scar. In its initial deposition, this scar contains large amounts of type III collagen and more soluble collagen and is therefore malleable. Frequent, gentle exercises can be used to put an extremity joint through a full range of motion and keep the newly developing scar tissue stretched and remodeled. Presumably the malleable scar tissue stretches in response to the effect of the range of motion. Frequent use of the range of motion exercises is important to keep the developing and contracting scar tissue from becoming a rigid, fixed scar contracture. Range of motion exercises ignore the contraction of the wound bed and instead concentrate on remodeling the newly laid collagen before it develops into a rigid scar contracture.

Pressure. The plasticity of new scar tissue is also affected by pressure garments applied to hypertrophic and thickened scars. These will remodel over the course of 6 months with the continuous use of pressure garments. The mechanism by which this occurs is unknown; however, hypertrophic scars have been found to be hypoxic possibly because of constriction of scar tissue around microvessels, and the oxygen tension in the tissues returns to normal as the hypertrophic scar flattens.[61]

Skin Grafting to Prevent Wound Contraction. One of the most effective ways to control the contraction of a surface wound is through the application of a full-thickness skin graft. Contraction is inhibited both when grafts are applied to fresh wounds and when they are placed into a release of a contracted scar. Clinically, full-thickness skin grafts inhibit contraction almost completely and will grow with a growing child. Full-thickness skin grafts also have the advantage of a more normal appearance than that of split-thickness skin grafts. Thus, full-thickness skin grafting is done in a wound of the face or in a pediatric wound, particularly in a web space contracture.

Unfortunately, contaminated wounds should be grafted with split skin grafts to encourage graft take and to minimize tissue loss if infection occurs. Large wounds must be covered with split-thickness skin grafts so that donor sites can be allowed to heal and sometimes be reharvested. When skin is in exceedingly short supply, it has to be expanded by meshing, a process by which multiple slits are cut in the graft and then expanded. While this provides protection, the wound is largely covered with epithelium in the interstices of the mesh graft.

Clinically it has been thought that the thicker the graft, the more it will inhibit contraction. However, the total percentage of the dermal thickness grafted determines how much contraction will be inhibited. Clinically full-thickness skin grafts are taken from the thinnest possible areas of the body, i.e., the upper eyelid, postauricular area, thin skin of the upper inner arm, and the thin hairless skin of the lateral groin.[62] Split skin grafts that include the majority of the dermis, such as Padgett's three-fourths thickness skin graft, will inhibit contraction far better than thinner split-thickness grafts. Wound coverage achieved by seeding with epithelium alone produces wounds that contract as though no skin grafting had been applied and are clinically unsatisfactory.

Greater understanding of the importance of the deep dermis in skin grafting has been achieved by studying animal grafts in which precise percentages of graft skin can be determined. In studies by Klein and Rudolph, full-thickness skin grafts of .25 ± standard deviation (SD) .10 mm (.010 ± .004 inches) inhibited contraction completely, even though they were thinner than standard split-thickness skin grafts of .38 ± .07 mm (.015 ± .003 inches).[63]

Studies by Corps clearly documented that the percentage of the dermis that was grafted is most important in determining how much the wound will contract.[64] Corps found that 0.2 mm split-thickness grafts taken from thicker dermis contracted more than 0.2 mm grafts taken from thinner dermis. He also found that 0.2 mm full-thickness grafts did not contract at all. Thus, what makes a full-thickness graft effective in inhibiting wound contraction is the inclusion of the total deep dermis, not merely the absolute thickness of the skin that is grafted.

Experimentally, the life cycle of the myofibroblast parallels the behavior of skin grafts in wound contraction. In rat skin grafts, the myofibroblast population increases whether the wounds are granulating or covered with split-thickness of full-thickness skin. In wounds covered with full-thickness skin, the myofibroblast population drops off rapidly, whereas in granulating wounds it persists for a long time. In wounds covered with split-thickness skin, contraction is intermediate and the myofibroblast population drops off at an intermediate rate. These studies suggest that skin grafts inhibit contraction by speeding up the life cycle of the myofibroblast rather than by preventing its development. It would appear that the wound in some way recognizes the quality of the overlying skin and this reduces the stimulus to wound contraction.

This effect does not appear to depend on living cells or even on biological tissue. Li and associates have pointed out that in freeze injuries in which the collagen matrix is not coagulated but cells are killed, the wound does not contract.[65] Myofibroblasts do develop underneath the freeze wound, but possibly their life cycle is speeded up in the same fashion as underneath a full-thickness graft.

Even artificial tissue can inhibit contraction. Frank and associates have pointed out that Biobrane, a plastic membrane covering a nylon fiber mesh coated with collagen, will inhibit contraction in both animals and humans.[66] Artificial skins for burn treatment, composed of shark glycosaminoglycans and bovine collagen and seeded with epidermal cells can be engineered to prevent contraction as well. The collagen gels used by Ehrlich also prevent wound contraction in vivo.[67] While the ideal clinical goal would be to find a way to make split-thickness grafts behave like full-thickness grafts, this may not be possible. Ultimately, engineered artificial skin may provide a more suitable method for controlling wound contraction in large burn scars.

Delayed application of skin grafts does not inhibit contraction as effectively as immediate grafting. Stone and Madden noted that in open wounds, immediate application of split-thickness skin grafting will moderately reduce wound contraction.[68] If in contrast, the split grafts are not applied until the wound has begun actively granulating and contracting, the inhibitory effect of the split-thickness graft is lost. Donoff and Grillo did show that delayed full-thickness skin grafting of open wounds in rabbits inhibited contraction.[69] However, it is clinically uncommon for full-thickness grafts to be applied to contracting wounds, primarily because of the bacterial surface contamination that makes the full-thickness graft's survival more precarious.

Operative Design. The final method by which the surgeon can prevent scar contracture is by judicious preplanning of incisions. An incision placed longitudinally across a joint such as a wrist or elbow is likely to produce a thick hypertrophic scar that will contract and restrict joint range of motion. Placing that same scar in the joint crease will reduce the likelihood of scar contracture. The reason for this is not clear but it probably results from the nature of the compressive forces applied to the longitudinally oriented wound as opposed to the different forces applied when that same wound is placed in the flexion crease.[70]

CONCLUSION

As is apparent from this chapter, much is still unknown concerning the mechanisms by which wound contraction occurs. Are myofibroblasts the important cell type in this process? Ehrlich, Rudolph, and Vande Berg give supporting evidence for and against their direct involvement. Of particular interest is the attempt to combine the two sets of data to arrive at another hypothesis. This theory states that non–stress fiber containing fibroblasts produces early wound contraction events, whereas the development of stress fiber–rich myofibroblasts is due to an attempt by the fibroblasts in the wound edge to resist the outward tension on the wound edges. Further studies to reconcile the data already obtained are essential to understand the basic biology of the process that results in multiple pathologic wound healing conditions.

References

1. Van Winkle W Jr: Wound contraction. Surg Gynecol Obstet 125:131–142, 1967.
2. Peacock EE Jr, Van Winkle W Jr: Wound Repair, 2nd ed. Philadelphia, WB Saunders, 1976, pp 54–80.
3. Rudolph R, Utley J, Woodward M: Contractile fibroblasts (myofibroblasts) in a painful pacemaker pocket. Ann Thorac Surg 31:373–376, 1981.
4. Rudolph R, McClure W, Woodward M: Contractile fibroblasts in cirrhosis. Gastroenterology 76:704–709, 1979.
5. Chu J: Studies on wound healing and tissue regeneration. I. Contraction in the healing skin wounds in rats. Acta Exp Biol Sinica 4:293–339, 1955.
6. Abercrombie M, Flint MH, James DW: Wound contraction in relation to collagen formation in scorbutic guinea pigs. J Embryol Exp Morphol 4:167–175, 1956.
7. Craven JL: Wound contraction in lathyritic rats. Arch Pathol 89:526–530, 1970.
8. Edwards LC: Inflammation and wound healing. In Tiecke RW (ed): Oral Pathology. New York, McGraw-Hill, 1965, p 12.
9. Cuthbertson AM: Contraction of full-thickness skin wounds in the rat. Surg Gynecol Obstet 108:421–432, 1959.
10. Billingham RE, Russell PS: Studies on wound healing with special reference to the phenomenon of contracture in experimental wounds in rabbits' skin. Ann Surg 144:961–981, 1956.
11. Ehrlich HP, Hembry RM: A comparative study of fibroblasts in healing freeze and burn injuries in rats. Am J Pathol 117:218–224, 1984.
12. Grillo HC, Watts GT, Gross J: Studies in wound healing. I. Contraction and the wound contents. Ann Surg 148:145–152, 1958.
13. Higton DIR, James DW: The effect of potassium cyanide on wound contraction, studied in vitro. Br J Surg 51:698–701, 1964.
14. Watts GT, Grillo HC, Gross J: Studies in wound healing. II. The role of granulation tissue in contraction. Ann Surg 148:153–160, 1958.
15. Billingham RE, Medawar PB: Contracture and intussusceptive growth in the healing of extensive wounds in mammalian skin. J Anat (Lond) 89:114–123, 1955.
16. Gabbiani G, Ryan GB, Majno G: Presence of modified fibroblasts in granulation tissue and possible role of wound contraction. Experientia 27:549, 1971.
17. Rudolph R, Guber S, Suzuki M, et al: The life cycle of the myofibroblast. Surg Gynecol Obstet 145:389–394, 1977.
18. Gabbiani G, Chaponnier C, Huttner I: Cytoplasmic filaments and gap junctions in epithelial cells and myofibroblasts during wound healing. J Cell Biol 76:561, 1978.
19. Rudolph R, Woodward M: Spatial orientation of microtubules in contractile fibroblasts in vivo. Anat Rec 191:169–182, 1978.
20. Rudolph R: Contraction and the control of contraction. World J Surg 4:279–287, 1980.
21. Ryan GB, Cliff WJ, Gabbiani G, et al: Myofibroblasts in human granulation tissue. Hum Pathol 5:55–67, 1974.
22. Singer II: The fibronexus: A transmembrane association of fibronectin-containing fibers and bundles of 5 nm microfilaments in hamster and human fibroblasts. Cell 16:675, 1979.
23. Singer II, Pardiso PR: A transmembrane relationship between fibronectin and vinculin (130 kd protein):

Serum modulation in normal and transformed hamster fibroblasts. Cell 24:481–492, 1981.

24. Furcht LT, Wendelschafer-Crabb G, Mosher DF, et al: An axial periodic fibrillar arrangement of antigenic determinants for fibronectin and procollagen on ascorbate treated human fibroblasts. J Supramol Struct 13:15–33, 1980.

25. Baur PS, Barratt G, Linares HA, et al: Wound contractions, scar contractures, and myofibroblasts: A classical case study. J Trauma 18:8–22, 1978.

26. Ehrlich HP: Wound closure: Evidence of cooperation between fibroblasts and collagen matrix. Eye 2:149–157, 1988.

27. Majno G, Gabbiani G, Hirschel BJ, et al: Contraction of granulation tissue in vitro: Similarity to smooth muscle. Science 173:548–550, 1971.

28. Hirschel BJ, Gabbiani G, Ryan GB, et al: Fibroblasts of granulation tissue: Immunofluorescent staining with anti-smooth muscle serum. Proc Soc Exp Biol Med 138:466–469, 1971.

29. Ehrlich HP, Grislis G, Hunt TK: Evidence of the involvement of microtubules in wound contraction. Am J Surg 135:706–711, 1977.

30. Ehrlich HP, Needle AL: Wound healing in tight skin mice: Delayed enclosure of excised wounds. Plast Reconstr Surg 72:190–196, 1983.

31. Hembry RM, Bernanke DH, Hayakashi K, et al: Morphologic examination of mesenchymal cells in healing wounds of normal and tight skin mice. Am J Pathol 125:81–89, 1986.

32. Bell E, Ivarson B, Merrill C: Production of a tissue-like structure by contraction of collagen lattice by human fibroblast of different proliferative potential in vitro. Proc Natl Acad Sci USA 76:1274–1278, 1979.

33. Ehrlich HP, Rajartnam JBM: ATP-induced cell contraction in dermal fibroblasts: Effects of cAMP and myosin light chain kinase. J Cell Physiol 128:223–230, 1986.

34. Harris AK, Wild P, Stopak D: Silicone rubber substrate: A new wrinkle in the study of cell locomotion. Science 280:177–179, 1980.

35. Ehrlich HP: The modulation of contraction of fibroblast populated collagen lattices by types I, II, and III collagen. Tiss Cell 20:47–50, 1988.

36. Rudolph R: Inhibition of myofibroblasts by skin grafts. Plast Reconstr Surg 63:473–480, 1979.

37. Bertolami C, Donoff RB: The effect of full thickness skin grafts on the actomyosin content of contracting wounds. J Oral Surg 37:471–476, 1979.

38. Rudolph R, Abraham J, Vecchione T, et al: Myofibroblasts and free silicon around breast implants. Plast Reconstr Surg 62:185–196, 1978.

39. Bhathal PS: Presence of modified fibroblasts in cirrhotic livers in man. Pathology 4:139–144, 1972.

40. Kershenobich D, Uribe M, Suarez CI, et al: Treatment of cirrhosis with colchicine: A double-blind randomized trial. Gastroenterology 77:532–536, 1979.

41. Gelberman RH, Amiel D, Rudolph R, et al: Dupuytren's contracture. An electron microscope, biochemical and clinical correlative study. J Bone Joint Surg 62A:425–432, 1980.

42. Vande Berg JS, Gelberman, R, Rudolph R, et al: Dupuytren's contracture: Comparative growth dynamics and morphology between cultured myofibroblasts (nodule) and fibroblasts (cord). J Orthop Res 2:247–256, 1984.

43. Hueston JT, Hurley JV, Whittingham S: The contracting fibroblast as a clue to Dupuytren's contracture. Hand 8:10–12, 1976.

44. Vande Berg JS, Rudolph R, Gelberman R, et al: Ultrastructural relationship of skin to nodule and cord in Dupuytren's contracture. Plast Reconstr Surg 69:835–844, 1982.

45. Vande Berg JS, Rudolph R, Poolman WL, et al: Comparative growth dynamics and actin concentrations between cultured human myofibroblasts from granulating wounds and dermal fibroblasts from normal skin. Lab Invest 61:532–538, 1989.

46. McGrath MH, Hundahl SA: The spatial and temporal quantification of myofibroblasts. Plast Reconstr Surg 69:975–985, 1982.

47. Oda D, Gown AM, Vande Berg JS, et al: The fibroblast-like nature of myofibroblasts. Exp Mol Pathol 49:316–329, 1988.

48. Oda D, Gown AM, Vande Berg JS, et al: Instability of the myofibroblast phenotype in culture. Exp Mol Pathol 52:221–234, 1990.

49. Skalli O, Vandekorckhove J, Gabbiani G: Actin-isoform pattern as marker of normal or pathological smooth muscle and fibroblastic tissues. Differentiation 33:232–238, 1987.

50. Skalli O, Gabbiani G: The biology of the myofibroblast in relation to wound contraction and fibrocontractive diseases. In Clark RAF, Henson PM (eds): The Molecular and Cellular Biology of Wound Repair. New York, Plenum, 1988, pp 373–402.

51. Krebs TE, Birchmeier W: Stress fiber sarcomeres of fibroblasts are contractile. Cell 22:555–561, 1980.

52. Burridge K: Are stress fibers contractile? Nature 294:691–692, 1981.

53. Stopak D, Harris AK: Connective tissue morphogenesis by fibroblast traction. I. Tissue culture observations. Dev Biol 90:383–398, 1982.

54. Bellows CG, Melcher AH, Aubin JE: Association between tension and orientation of periodontal ligament fibroblasts and exogenous collagen fibers in collagen gels in vitro. J Cell Sci 58:125–138, 1982.

55. Bellows CG, Melcher AH, Bhargava U, et al: Fibroblasts contracting three dimensional collagen gels exhibit ultrastructure consistent with either contraction or protein secretion. J Ultrastruct Res 78:178–192, 1982.

56. Fleischer M, Wohlfarth-Bottermann KE: Correlation between tension force generation, fibrillogenesis and ultrastructure of cytoplasmic actomyosin during isometric and isotonic contractions of protoplasmic strands. Cytobiologie 10:339–365, 1975.

57. Farsi JMP, Aubin JE: Microfilament rearrangements during fibroblast-induced contraction of three-dimensional hydrated collagen gels. Cell Motility 4:29–40, 1984.

58. Squier CA: The effect of stretching on formation of myofibroblasts in mouse skin. Cell Tiss Res 220:325–335, 1981.

59. McGrath M: Healing of the open wound. In Rudolph R (ed): Problems in Aesthetic Surgery. Biological Causes and Clinical Solutions. St. Louis, CV Mosby, 1986, pp 13–48.

60. Cronin TD: The use of a molded splint to prevent contracture after split skin grafting on the neck. Plast Reconstr Surg 27:7–18, 1961.

61. Berry RB, Tan OT, Cooke ED, et al: Transcutaneous oxygen tensions as an index of maturity in hypertrophic scars treated by compression. Br J Plast Surg 38:163–173, 1985.

62. Rudolph R, Fisher JC, Ninneman JL: Skin Grafting. Boston, Little, Brown, 1979.

63. Klein L, Rudolph R: ^{3}H-collagen turnover in skin grafts. Surg Gynecol Obstet 135:49–57, 1972.

64. Corps BVM: The effect of graft thickness, donor site, and graft bed on graft thickness in the hooded rat. Br J Plast Surg 22:125–133, 1969.

65. Li AKC, Ehrlich HP, Trelstad RL, et al: Differences in healing of skin wounds caused by burn and freeze injuries. Ann Surg 191:244–248, 1980.

66. Frank DH, Brahme J, Vande Berg JS: Decrease in rate of wound contraction with the temporary skin substitute Biobrane. Ann Plast Surg 12:519–524, 1984.

67. Bell E, Ehrlich HP, Buttle DJ, et al: Living tissue formed in vitro and accepted as skin-equivalent tissue of full thickness. Science 211:1052–1054, 1981.

68. Stone PA, Madden JW: Effect of primary and delayed split skin grafting on wound contraction. Surg Forum 25:41–44, 1974.

69. Donoff RB, Grillo HC: The effects of skin grafting on healing open wounds in rabbits. J Surg Res 19:163–167, 1975.

70. Brody GS: The biomechanical properties of tissue. In Rudolph R (ed): Problems in Aesthetic Surgery. Biological Causes and Clinical Solutions. St. Louis, CV Mosby, 1986, pp 49–64.

71. Rudolph R: Location of the force of wound contraction. Surg Gynecol Obstet 148:547–551, 1979.

72. Vande Berg JS, Rudolph R, Woodward M: Comparative growth dynamics between cultured myofibroblasts from granulating wounds and dermal fibroblasts. Am J Pathol 114:187–200, 1984.

7

EPITHELIALIZATION

Kurt S. Stenn, M.D., and Raji Malhotra, M.D.

All organisms and organs are separated from their environment, and thus defined, by a simple or complex layer of cells that forms a protective and impermeable wrapping. When this layer, referred to as epithelium, is compromised after external injury, it must regenerate rapidly in order to reestablish the integrity of the underlying tissues. Characteristic of all epithelia are two features: (1) tight cell junctions and (2) a specialized bed, referred to as the basement membrane zone, upon which the layer of cells sits.

This chapter reviews the properties of this very special tissue with particular regard to how it repairs and regenerates itself after injury. Because of its importance to mammals and, therefore, to clinical medicine, the emphasis will be on skin, the structure of the epidermis, and the mechanisms of epidermal wound closure. It is recognized, however, that the principles illustrated here are similar for other repairing epithelial systems, including gastrointestinal mucosa, respiratory lining, and mesentery. Other recent reviews of this field are available.[1-3]

EPIDERMIS

Covering the mammalian body over all areas and separating it from the outer environment is the skin. The outer region of the skin is a multilayered, stratified squamous epithelium, the epidermis. As its outer cover, the epidermis bestows on the body protection from physical trauma, electromagnetic radiation, fluid loss or gain, and bacterial invasion. Moreover, it contains elements that support the early phases of the immune response.

Although there is a conservation of epidermal function throughout the animal kingdom, not all animals are covered by a stratified squamous

epidermis. In fact, the multilayered epidermis does not appear before the vertebrates on the evolutionary tree. The invertebrates are covered by an epidermis that is single-layered but usually amplified by glandular secretions such as mucus (snails), chitin (insects), calcareous material (bivalve molluscs), and collagen and proteoglycans (nematodes).[4, 5]

The adult vertebrate epidermis is multilayered and shows a complex stratification that reflects its regenerative and differentiative properties (Fig. 7–1). For mammals, the epidermis interfaces with the musculoskeletal framework by means of the dermis, a connective tissue layer, and the subcutis, a fibrofatty layer. The epidermis interdigitates and attaches to the dermis by means of broad downfoldings, the epidermal rete ridges. Epidermal cell growth occurs among the cells of the lowest epidermis, namely, those cells that rest on the basement membrane zone or just above it. Moreover, the dividing cells appear to be concentrated in the region of the lower rete.[6] To maintain a constant thickness, cell growth in the lower epidermis balances the loss of cells from the outer epidermis. One daughter cell from every mitotic division leaves the basal layer and begins the trip outward; concomitantly, it begins to differentiate. The process of selecting which cell will move up is as yet unknown, but two hypothetical mechanisms have been suggested: The first requires growth pressure provided by the dividing basal cells to push the differentiating cell outward passively, and the second, based on the facts that these cells contain actin and migrate quite well in tissue culture, requires that the cells become motile and actively migrate upward.[7] Once a cell leaves the basal layer it takes about 14 days to reach the granular layer and another 14 days to desquamate.

The basal cell (Fig. 7–2) is cuboidal, but as it moves upward it becomes progressively flattened, forming a 14-sided, hexagonal-faceted

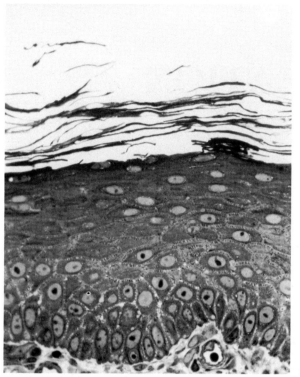

Horny layer

Granular layer

Spinous layer

Basal layer
Basal lamina

Figure 7–1. Photomicrograph of epidermis showing progressive maturation of keratinocytes from the basal layer to the keratin layer (1 μ thick toluidine blue staining, ×600).

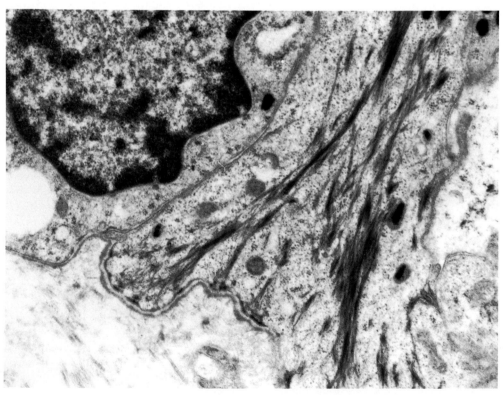

Figure 7–2. Electron micrograph of normal epidermal basal cell, basement membrane zone, and upper dermis (×7100).

structure. Above the basal layer, the epidermal cells begin to accumulate keratin filaments and concomitantly desmosomes (by light microscopy the desmosomes extending from cell to cell appear as "prickles" and thus the name "prickle cell layer," or "stratum spinosum"). The keratin filaments belong to the family of intermediate filaments found in all cells (vimentin, desmin, glial fibrillary acidic protein, neurofilament protein, lamin, and keratin). Keratin filaments basket the epidermal cell nucleus (interacting with nuclear lamins) and extend outward to the desmosomes in the cell periphery. Each keratin filament is made of two different keratin proteins. There are about 20 distinct keratin proteins in human cells, each derived from a different gene, which range in molecular weight from 40 to 70 kDa. The keratin types found vary with the type of epithelial tissue and its state of differentiation. It is therefore not surprising that the keratin types present in the lower generating epidermal cells (keratin types K5 and K14) differ from those in the upper differentiated cells (keratin types K1 and K10).[8] Because epidermal cells accumulate more keratin as they move upward, they are often referred to as keratinocytes. In the upper stratum spinosum the epidermal cells acquire granules, or keratohyalin, which are composed in large part of a protein termed filaggrin that appears to play a role in the aggregation of keratin filaments and/or in the hydration properties of the epidermis.[9] Above the granular layer, keratinocytes lose their cytoplasmic organelles and become filled with keratin filaments and surrounded by an inner wall, the cornified envelope, which is made of a protein, involucrin, that is highly crosslinked by the action of a unique transglutaminase. In the upper epidermis the intercellular space becomes filled with organized lipids. Finally, the intercellular cohesions are broken and the outer epidermis breaks apart into individual desquamating cells.

The development of the human epidermis parallels, to some extent, epidermal phylogeny. In the earliest embryo the epidermis consists of a single layer of flat epithelial cells; subsequently a second short-lived but secretory outer distinct epithelial layer, the periderm, forms. With time a third layer develops between these two layers (stratum intermedium) and, finally, by about 6 months the epidermis becomes fully stratified and keratinized.

The fully mature epidermis is referred to as keratinized or cornified. In this review, as in the literature, these two words are used interchangeably, but there is potential for confusion in the use of the words "keratin" and "keratin-ized." The former refers to the proteins that make up keratin filaments; the latter refers to a complex mixture of molecules (including keratin but also other proteins, lipids, and proteoglycans) that characterize the fully differentiated epidermal cell.[10]

BASEMENT MEMBRANE ZONE

The epidermis imparts fluid impermeability and traumatic and radiative resistance to the skin. Although the strength of the dermis is crucial to the structural properties of the skin, the epidermis protects against the invasion of pathogenic organisms and the loss of body fluids. The basement membrane zone (BMZ) (Fig. 7–3) serves as a structural support and means of attachment of the epidermis to the dermis. Because the BMZ plays a central role in cutaneous function, after injury it must be reestablished and maintained in short order by the repairing epidermis.

By light microscopy the BMZ appears as a well-defined, thin, glycoprotein-rich layer (periodic acid Schiff stain positive) immediately below the epithelium. However, using electron microscopy and antibody techniques, this zone can be seen to be quite elaborate: below the basal layer successively are (1) an electron-clear layer, the lamina lucida; (2) an electron-dense layer, the lamina densa; and (3) a series of fibrillar structures interfacing with the upper dermis. The molecular structure of this zone is currently being elucidated (see Figures 7–2 and 7–3).[11]

The basal cell attaches to the BMZ by means of hemidesmosomes, which have the morphology of a half desmosome and are found only on the basal side of the basal epidermal cell. This complex structure within the cytoplasm and the basal cell membrane of that cell comprises an attachment plate to which keratin filaments (also referred to as tonofilaments) insert. Within the area of the attachment plate is the bullous pemphigoid antigen, a glycoprotein of 220 to 240 kDa[12, 13] to which patients with a generalized bullous disorder have circulating antibodies. Extending from the hemidesmosome to the lamina densa and coursing perpendicularly through the lamina lucida are anchoring filaments that presumably serve as mooring strands that join the intermediate filament cytoskeleton to the extracellular dermis. The chemical nature of the anchoring filaments is not yet known. An important constituent of the lamina lucida is

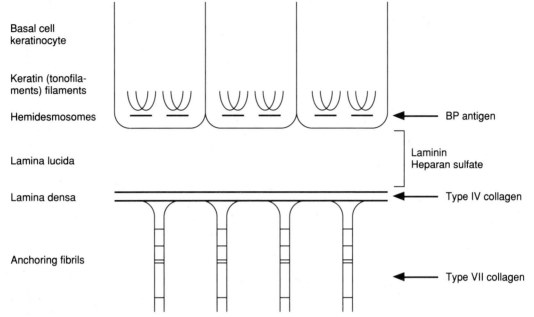

Figure 7–3. The epidermal basement zone. This illustration shows structures identified by electron microscopy (*left*) and antigens identified by immunological methods (*right*).

laminin, a large cruciate glycoprotein of about one million molecular weight.

The lamina densa contains at least one type of collagen, type IV, that forms a netlike quarternary structure and provides a broad two-dimensionality to this layer. As other noncollagenous proteins (e.g., KF-1 antigen, nidogen) and proteoglycans (heparan sulfate) are found in this layer, it is recognized that the lamina densa is not entirely collagenous. Extending from the lamina densa into the dermis are anchoring fibrils that form under the regions of the hemidesmosomes. These fibrils show a very characteristic periodicity and are made up of type VII collagen.[14] From the lamina densa the anchoring fibrils splay out into the underlying dermis and apparently form stable attachments to the dermal collagen bundles.

The BMZ serves to moor the epidermis to the dermis, binding the cytoskeleton of the keratinocyte to the collagen bundles of the dermis by means of vertically arranged fibrillar structures and horizontally arranged broad layers. Although the actual BMZ molecules with which the resting basal cells interact have not been identified, they play an important structural role in maintaining the integrity of the epidermis and a supportive role in its repair, as will be discussed later.

Having considered the nature of the stationary epidermis and its interface with the dermis, one might next ask what happens to this structure when it is wounded and stimulated to regenerate itself?

MORPHOLOGY OF EPITHELIAL CELL MOVEMENT

After a rent occurs in the epidermis it becomes critical to survival that access of the environment to the dermis is blocked without delay. In this event the body effects wound closure in two temporally related steps: within minutes by the formation of a blood clot, which reestablishes a temporary barrier, and then within hours to days by the movement of residual epithelium below the clot and over the underlying dermis—the process of reepithelialization. The first step, involving blood clot formation and its dependence on vessel wall, platelets, and coagulation proteins, is the subject of a recent review[15] and will not be further considered.

Characteristic of all epithelial cells is the propensity to cover a free surface. Clearly, in order to cover a denuded surface, epithelial cells must either (1) move or (2) grow over that wounded area. Although both processes are stimulated by wounding, the more important process in early wound closure is cell migration, which is independent of cell division.[16–20] Indeed, under experimental conditions, blocking of cell division has no effect on the rate of epithelial cell movement or wound closure.[21–23] The migrating cells arise from the residual epithelium at the periphery of the rent or, more often, from the residual hair or sweat structures at the wound base. In large, deep cutaneous lesions, the epithelium that covers the rent arises from the wound periphery; in small, superficial cutaneous wounds, however, most of the epithelium arises from the residual pilosebaceous or eccrine structure.[19, 24, 25] Recent observations suggest, however, that under some circumstances mesenchymal cells may transform and become part of the regenerating epithelium;[26] however, that phenomenon probably plays a minor role in the closure of most wounds.

Reepithelialization occurs most rapidly over a superficial wound that leaves the BMZ intact. In the repair of a suction blister, for example, in which the floor of the wound consists of an intact lamina densa (suction causes the separation of the epidermis from the dermis within the lamina lucida), short tongues of epithelial cells rapidly (within 12 to 24 hours) grow out from the residual epithelial structures.[27] By 24 to 72 hours, most of the wound base is covered by a thin layer of epithelium and by 4 days it is covered by layered keratinocytes.[27, 28]

In all systems it is the basal cell, i.e., the cell attached to the substratum, that responds to wounding and initiates migration. These marginal cells flatten out in the direction of the wound and send out cytoplasmic projections over the substratum.[29, 30] In preparation for their movement, the epithelial cells loosen their intercellular and substratum attachments. They lose hemidesmosomal junctions, their tonofilaments withdraw from the cell periphery, and the BMZ becomes less well defined.[27, 31–33] In addition, the cells at the leading edge become actively phagocytic, picking up tissue debris and erythrocytes. This phagocytic property of epidermal cells can be illustrated in the laboratory using fluoroscein-coated beads or Thorotrast particles, which are taken up by epidermal cells.[30, 31, 34] This property is enhanced by the fibronectin in wound fluid.[35]

Within 1 or 2 days the epithelial cells behind the migrating front begin to proliferate, generating new populations of cells to cover the wound.[20, 27] Once epithelialization is complete and the rent is covered, the epithelial cells revert to their normal phenotype and reassume their intercellular and basement membrane contacts.

MODELS OF EPIDERMAL SHEET MIGRATION

Reepithelialization over any wound will occur, like an unrolling carpet or a military phalanx, by the movement of epithelial cells as a sheet. Considering the tight intercellular cohesions that epithelial cells share, it is not surprising that these cells do not migrate over a wound as single cells but, instead, as small clusters or sheets. When sheets of epithelial cells have been observed directly, the cells at the margin of the moving sheet appeared to be actively motile while the cells behind (or above, in a stratified layer) the marginal cells were passively dragged along.[36, 37] If attachment of the marginal cells to the substrate is disturbed, the migrating sheet, under tension, will withdraw. This mode of sheet movement, referred to as the sliding model of wound closure, has been demonstrated directly for epithelial cells in tissue culture,[36] for embryonic epithelial movement,[38] for amphibian wound closure,[37] and for corneal wound closure.[39]

It is much more difficult to study mammalian cutaneous wound closure directly because of the thickness and opacity of the dermis. Moreover, the migrating epithelial sheet of mammalian epidermis is multilayered and thus more complex than those systems illustrating the sliding model. For the repairing mammalian epidermis, Winter[40] proposed the leap frog model of epidermal sheet movement (Fig. 7–4). This model was deduced indirectly from ultrastructural morphological data that suggested that cells at the migrating front adhere to the substrate only to be replaced at the front, in turn, by the cells above and behind it: successively, then, submarginal cells are conceived to crawl over the newly adherent basal cells in a "leap frog" fashion. Cell marker studies have been presented in support of this model wherein keratin antigens found in suprabasal cells of the intact epidermis (K10, K1) are found in the basal cells of the migrating tip. Although one may ascribe these results to cell movement, these changes may also be explained by the ability of keratinocytes to switch their differentiation pattern after injury to express a keratin that normally is not found among the cells in the basal layer.[28] Although the data are indirect, the leap frog model of mammalian epidermal wound closure has many proponents.[20, 27, 41–44] As the issue is not yet resolved, it is currently reasonable to contend that simple epithelium moves by the sliding model while multilayered epithelium may manifest a more complex pattern. In mammals, either or both mechanisms (sliding and leap-frogging) may function in wound closure depending on the state and character of the epithelium affected.[3]

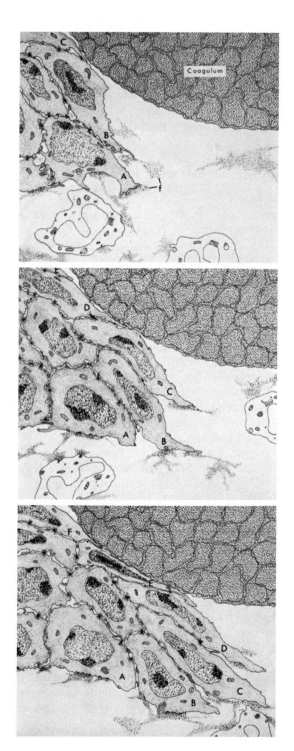

Figure 7–4. Leap frog model of wound closure. The progressive movement of keratinocytes covering a wound is shown. The cells are believed to move below a clot by translocating over one another. (From Krawczyk WS: A pattern of epidermal cell migration during wound healing. Reproduced from the Journal of Cell Biology, 1971, 49:247–263 by copyright permission of the Rockefeller University Press.)

BIOCHEMICAL PARAMETERS OF MIGRATING EPITHELIUM

For epithelium, like other wounded differentiated tissues, the reacting cells show features of a less mature state, usually manifesting the growth properties, metabolism, and cell markers of a growing or developing cell population. The responding cells are less differentiated, have fewer cell junctions, have a higher metabolic rate, and are more motile. Moreover, they manifest receptors that enhance interactions with the wound environment. With time they secrete constituents that enhance wound closure and repair, reconstruct their tissue structure, and finally become quiescent once again.

As the epidermal sheet begins to move in response to a wound, the cells acquire an increased number of gap junctions, structures implicated in cell-cell communication. At the same time, the distal portion of the cytoplasmic projections and the peripheral areas of the marginal cells stain for actin and myosin;[45] in addition, the migrating cells show increased amounts of cytoplasmic actin.[28, 33, 46] That there is a direct correlation between gap junction density and contractile protein content in the motile cells suggests a coordinated response of the regional epidermis to injury.[46]

Moving as a complete, one to two cell thick sheet, the marginal epidermal cells migrate until the rent is covered and neighboring contacts are reestablished. As mentioned, if the BMZ remains intact, wound closure is rapid, but if the BMZ is destroyed, closure is much slower, apparently because the migrating reparative epithelium must then reconstruct its own BMZ as it covers the wound. That pattern of BMZ regeneration by the repairing epidermis is similar in various mammalian systems (rodent, swine, guinea pig, primate, human).[28, 47–53] Initially, the substratum is coated with host fibronectin, apparently arising from wound fluids. Of the basement membrane components, the migrating, or marginal, tip demonstrates only bullous pemphigoid antigen and type V collagen. Later, and further back from the tip, laminin and type IV collagen reappear and fibronectin produced by the migrating cells is secreted. (Primates other than adult humans may show a variation of this pattern in that bullous pemphigoid antigen returns later than laminin, type IV collagen, and fibronectin.[52]) Antigens associated with mature epidermis (e.g., filaggrin, involucrin, *Ulex europeus* ligand, transglutaminase) are usually not found in the motile cells and reappear only in the repaired, nonmigratory epithelium. With time the repaired epidermis loses its expression of basal fibronectin and a morphologically mature BMZ reforms.

While the migrating cells are forming new BMZ by secreting basement membrane components (e.g., fibronectin, collagen, laminin), they are also expressing fibronectin receptors, losing some surface markers,[54] and releasing such proteases as collagenase[55–57] and plasminogen activator.[58] As indicated, the motile cells apparently use secreted fibronectin as a temporary BMZ and use collagenase and plasminogen activators to facilitate their dissection through reparative connective tissue.[59]

Within 12 to 16 hours after injury the wounded cells show a qualitative increase in protein synthesis and a quantitative difference in proteins synthesized compared to the resting cell. For example, in the early phase of repair, the synthesis of some keratins (K-1, K-2, and K-10) decreases while that of others (K-6 and K-16) increases over control values.[28] By 48 hours after wound closure, the keratin pattern begins to return to normal.

Although the molecular mechanisms of cell migration in general, and epithelial cells in particular, are currently being actively studied, they remain poorly understood.[60, 61] However, it is known that in order for a cell to move it must (1) establish some bond or adhesion to a surface (substrate), (2) sense a signal to initiate movement in a given direction for a given extent, and (3) manifest cytoskeletal machinery that will produce movement. Having identified these ordered phases it is important to note that it is not always possible to cleanly separate such phases experimentally; e.g., cell adhesion requires cytoskeletal machinery and the signal to move may require no more than cell adhesion.

BIOCHEMICAL AND BIOPHYSICAL FACTORS AFFECTING EPITHELIAL CELL ADHESION AND SPREADING

The wounded epidermal cell is exposed to blood and its products (cells, plasma, serum), components of the BMZ, and dermis. Within the blood are two substrate-active proteins, fibronectin and vitronectin (serum spreading

Table 7–1. BASEMENT MEMBRANE ZONE- OR SUBSTRATUM-ASSOCIATED MOLECULES
INFLUENCING EPIDERMAL WOUND CLOSURE

Molecule	Molecular Weight	Source	Location and Action	References

Collagen Type I	300 kDa
	Triple helical
	3 subunits
		Fibroblast	Dermis
			Supports epidermal
			  cell attachment and
			  spreading
				69

Collagen Type IV	540 kDa	Epidermal cell,
		  fibroblast
			Lamina densa
			Supports epidermal
			  cell attachment and
			  spreading
				69

Collagen Type V	300 kDa Triple helical	Epidermal cell	Basement membrane zone ? Function	47

Fibronectin	250 kDa dimer
	RGDS sequence
		Diploid fibroblasts,
		  macrophage,
		  serum
			Basement membrane
			  zone in wounds
			Supports epidermal
			  cell adhesion and
			  spreading
				74, 75

Laminin	100 kDa
	RGDS sequence
		Epidermal cell	Lamina lucida
			Epidermal cells adhere
			  but migration is
			  inhibited
				76, 77

Vitronectin	75 kDa
	RGDS sequence
		Serum	? Location
			Promotes cell
			  adhesion and
			  spreading
				64, 78

factor, epibolin), each of which has been shown to support epidermal cell spreading. Fibronectin and vitronectin are related but distinct surface active glycoproteins of 440 kDa and 75 kDa molecular weight, respectively. Both molecules contain the same "RGDS" cell binding domain (ArgGlyGluSer).[62, 63] This sequence, and its specific cell receptors, are important to the cell adhesive functions of these molecules.[64] The action of vitronectin on epidermal cells differs from that of fibronectin in that it is enhanced by a second serum protein that copurifies with albumin,[65] but that alone does not support cell spreading; moreover, this cofactor appears to act through a protein kinase C mechanism.[66] Epidermal cells in tissue culture have been found to spread as well on fibronectin as on collagen types I, III, IV, laminin, and vitronectin.[67–72] Epidermal cells appear to use any one of these molecules efficiently in order to effect adhesion and spreading. Since blocking protein synthesis does not affect the character of epidermal cell spreading on these proteins, it is generally accepted that no one of these molecules alone is necessary for epidermal cell spreading and that epidermal cells can spread as well on various other substrates. Such "promiscuity" favors the movement of these cells, and thus wound closure, over many different substrata after sundry injuries. Quantitatively, however, there may be a difference in the response of these cells to purified substrate molecules. It appears that fibronectin, probably not a constituent of the intact BMZ, supports better cell movement than constituents of the BMZ, such as laminin. Experimentally, epithelial sheet spread is greater on interstitial collagens (types I and II) and fibronectin than on basement membrane constituents (laminin, type IV collagen).[73] It should be noted, however, that these studies and their conclusions refer to early wound closure, since after a time the responding cells acquire the ability to synthesize fibronectin and thus form their own optimal surface. Some of the BMZ molecules influencing wound closure are listed in Table 7–1.

Recently scientists have become aware that cells within the wound environment (including blood cells such as platelets and macrophages and tissue cells such as endothelial cells, smooth muscle cells, and epithelial cells) release molecules that are not necessarily associated with the BMZ but can influence the repair process itself. Such molecules, referred to as cytokines, are liberated by cells to stimulate certain processes in other cells distant, vicinal, or even parental.

Some cytokines imputed to influence wound closure are listed in Table 7–2. Certain of these cytokines, such as interleukin-1 and basic fibroblast growth factor, may arise within the epidermis itself while others originate within cells of the inflammatory cell infiltrate, such as the

Table 7–2. MOLECULES OF THE WOUND ENVIRONMENT THAT MAY INFLUENCE EPIDERMAL WOUND CLOSURE

Molecule	Molecular Weight	Source	Action	References
Basic fibroblast growth factor	18 kDa	Keratinocyte, fibroblasts	Stimulates epidermal cell growth	79, 80
Calcium	111 daltons (CaCl$_2$)	Milieux	Stimulates differentiation in high concentration, stimulates proliferation in low concentration	81
Epidermal growth factor (EGF)	6 kDa Single chain	Salivary gland	Stimulates epidermal cell proliferation	82–85
Hypothalamic keratinocyte growth factor	~ 1.7 kDa	Hypothalamus	Stimulates epidermal cell growth	86
Interleukin-1	31 kDa	Macrophages, epidermal cells	Stimulates epidermal growth and motility	87, 88
Platelet-derived growth factor	Dimer of 30–32 kDa and 14–18 kDa	Platelets, endothelium	Stimulates epidermal hyperplasia in combination with EGF	89
Placental growth factor	Nondialyzable, heat sensitive	Placenta	Enhances keratinocyte growth	90
Scatter factor	50 kDa	Fibroblasts	Stimulates epidermal cell motility	91
Transforming growth factor-α	5.6 kDa	Transformed cells, placenta, embryonic tissue	Stimulates epidermal growth	92, 93
Transforming growth factor-β	23–25 kDa (two subunits that may combine as TGF-β$_1$, TGF-β$_2$, or TGF-β$_{1.2}$)	Fibroblasts, platelets	All forms inhibit epidermal cell proliferation but stimulate motility	77, 94–97

platelet or macrophage, and still others arise in distant sites, such as the liver or placenta. These factors influence both epithelial cell motility and growth. It is notable that at least one factor, transforming growth factor-β, blocks epithelial cell growth. Calcium is included in this list to emphasize its potential in vivo role in controlling these phenomena: calcium has been demonstrated to have a profound influence on the growth and differentiation of these cells in vitro. A complete discussion of the influences of cytokines on wound healing is presented in Chapters 3 and 14.

In addition to skin, many growing and developing mammalian and amphibian tissues demonstrate a steady transtissue current. Injury alters the normal voltage found across the skin.[98] Within epidermal wounds, voltage gradients can be measured and thus have been implicated in epidermal cell motility and wound closure.[99] Laboratory studies have suggested that applied electrical currents across healing nerve or bone can accelerate that process and that electrical

fields may be a necessary component of the repair process.

Although most of these studies have been indirect, it has been reported that a current of 50 to 300 µA delivered to the superficial skin wound of pigs speeds reepithelialization by 50 percent.[100] Further work on this aspect of epithelial wound closure is merited.

INITIATION OF EPITHELIAL CELL MOVEMENT

While the specific signals or stimuli for re-epithelialization are unknown, evidence for physical and chemical stimuli has been gathered experimentally. It is generally held that a free edge is all epithelium needs to initiate movement. The concept of "contact inhibition of cell movement" asserts that physical contact alone prevents cell movement. However, that concept may be too simple,[69, 101, 102] since primary epidermal cells not adapted to culture will not spread in tissue culture unless the substratum is optimal even though the cells have a free edge (are not confluent). In contrast, adapted, nonconfluent epidermal cells actively growing in tissue culture will spread in the absence of added protein even on tissue culture plastic. This effect is a function of cell sociology since cells arising from confluent cultures are once again dependent on substrate proteins in order to spread. Because this effect is inducible by growing cells under confluent and subconfluent conditions (analogous to a nonwounded and a wounded situation), it appears likely that a free edge may provide the external stimulus to spread, but with time the wounded cell acquires the ability to spread independently of environmental proteins, a function that is dependent upon acquiring the ability to synthesize substrate proteins[101] and their receptors.[103] While primary epidermal cells do not synthesize substrate-active molecules, such as fibronectin, as these same cells grow in culture they acquire the ability to secrete fibronectin and exhibit fibronectin receptors.[50, 104–107] Once the epidermal lesion is repaired (or the cells become confluent), the cells no longer express the fibronectin receptor.[106] That the wounded cell may manifest either a nonspreading (and nonsecretory) or a spreading mode begs the question of how the epidermal cell rests in situ under normal and nonpathological states. Although the experiment has not been done, one would assume that the normal epidermal basal cell would be present in a nonspreading mode and would thus need a free edge as well as an appropriate substratum in order to begin moving. With time this cell would acquire the ability to produce its own substratum and thus become independent of the wound environment until it could form a confluent sheet once again. Following complete reepithelialization (i.e., wound closure), epidermal cells proliferate, stratify, deposit new basement membrane, and finally restore the original epidermal structure.

CYTOSKELETAL MACHINERY IN REEPITHELIALIZATION

Once a cell is wounded it subsequently migrates. As indicated previously, what actually "turns on" the cellular machinery of movement, be it physical or chemical, is still not known. Little work has been done on the cytoskeletal

mechanisms of epidermal cell motility, but it is recognized that epidermal cells in all strata of the epidermis contain actin and that the motile machinery probably involves the actin-myosin contractile system. A cytoskeletal model of epidermal cell motility has been proposed by Bereiter-Hahn and associates[45] in which the motive force is generated by directed contractions of the actomyosin system, forcing cytoplasm into a peripheral focus that produces a cytoplasmic protrusion in the direction of movement. Soluble actin and myosin enter the protrusion to form a lamellipodium that adheres to the substratum. In this model, directed regional cytoplasmic contractions induce the formation of processes that propel the marginal cell.

CONCLUSION

An epithelial wound is primarily repaired by the movement of a tightly coherent cell sheet. That this repair occurs by cells in a sheet allows the maximal preservation of the environmental barrier during the recovery period. To effect this cover the wounded cells must be stimulated to move, to activate the appropriate cell machinery to effect that move, and to adhere to an appropriate surface at the proper time. The molecules of the substratum change with the stage of wound closure: in the early stage fibronectin, and probably vitronectin, play an important role, and with time the responding cells acquire the ability to synthesize their own BMZ constituents. Later, when the epidermal cells rest upon reconstituted BMZ molecules they cease moving and resynthesize and restructure a mature BMZ. The reepithelialization process is influenced, and perhaps orchestrated, by a bath of cytokines arising from cells in the wound environment and in distant tissues. Currently, we have a good phenomenological idea of wound closure. In the future we must learn more about the molecules influencing this process and the mechanisms controlling their expression.

REFERENCES

1. Bereiter-Hahn J: Epidermal Cell Migration and Wound Repair. In Biology of the Integument. II. Vertebrates. Bereiter-Hahn J, Matoltsy AG, Richards KS (eds): Berlin, Springer-Verlag, 1986, pp 443–471.
2. Donaldson DJ, Mahan JT: Keratinocyte migration and the extracellular matrix. J Invest Dermatol 90:623–628, 1988.
3. Stenn KS, DePalma L: Re-epithelialization. In Clark RAF, Henson PM (eds): The Molecular and Cellular

Biology of Wound Repair. New York, Plenum Press, 1988, pp 321–335.

4. Spearman RIC: The Integument: A Textbook of Skin Biology. Cambridge, Cambridge University Press, 1973.

5. Bereiter-Hahn J, Matoltsy AG, Richards KS: Biology of the Integument. I. Invertebrates. Berlin, Springer-Verlag, 1984.

6. Wright N, Alison M: The Biology of Epithelial Cell Populations, vol I. Oxford, Clarendon Press, 1984, pp 283–345.

7. Etoh H, Taguchi YH, Tabachnick J: Movement of beta irradiated epidermal basal cells to the spinous-granular layers in the absence of cell division. J Invest Dermatol 64:431–435, 1975.

8. Cooper D, Schermer A, Sun T-T: Classification of human epithelia and their neoplasms using monoclonal antibodies to keratins: Strategies, applications and limitations. Lab Invest 52:243–256, 1985.

9. Scott IR, Harding CR, Barrett JG: Histidine-rich protein of the keratohyalin granules: Source of the free amino acids, urocanic acid and pyrrolidone carboxylic acid in the stratum corneum. Biochem Biophys Acta 719:110–117, 1982.

10. Stenn KS, Bhawan J: The normal histology of skin. In Farmer ER, Hood AF (eds): Dermatopathology. East Norwalk, CT, Appleton-Century-Crofts, 1990, pp 3–29.

11. Fine J-D: The skin basement membrane zone. East Norwalk, CT, Adv Dermatol 2:283–304, 1987.

12. Westgate GE, Weaver AC, Couchman JR: Bullous pemphigoid antigen localization suggests an intracellular association with hemidesmosomes. J Invest Dermatol 84:218–224, 1985.

13. Stanley JR, Hawley-Nelson P, Yuspa S, et al: Characterization of bullous pemphigoid antigen: A unique basement membrane protein of stratified squamous epithelia. Cell 24:897–903, 1981.

14. Sakai LY, Keene DR, Morris NP, et al: Type VII collagen is a major structural component of anchoring fibrils. J Cell Biol 103:2499–2509, 1986.

15. Clark RAF, Henson PM: The Molecular and Cellular Biology of Wound Repair. New York, Plenum Press, 1988.

16. Arey LB: Wound healing. Physiol Rev 16:327–406, 1936.

17. Marks R, Nishikawa T: Active epidermal movement in human skin in vitro. Brit J Dermatol 86:481–490, 1973.

18. Kuwabara T, Perkins DG, Cogan DG: Sliding of the epithelium in experimental corneal wounds. Invest Ophthalmol 15:4–14, 1976.

19. Pang SC, Daniels WH, Buck RC: Epidermal migration during the healing of suction blisters in rat skin: A scanning and transmission electron microscopic study. Am J Anat 153:177–191, 1978.

20. Winter GD: Epidermal regeneration studied in the domestic pig. In Maibach HI, Rovee DT: Epidermal Wound Healing. Chicago, Year Book, 1972, pp 71–112.

21. DiPasquale A: Locomotion of epithelial cells. Exp Cell Res 95:425–439, 1975.

22. Dunlap MK, Donaldson DJ: Inability of colchicine to inhibit newt epidermal cell migration or prevent concanavalin A–mediated inhibition of migration studies. Exp Cell Res 116:15–19, 1978.

23. Gipson IK, Westcott MJ, Brooksby NG: Effects of cytochalasins B and D and colchicine on migration of corneal epithelium. Invest Ophthalmol Vis Sci 22:633–642, 1982.

24. Gillman T, Penn J, Brooks D, et al: Reactions of healing wounds and granulation tissue in man to auto-thiersch, autodermal and homodermal grafts. Brit J Plast Surg 6:153–223, 1963.

25. Hinshaw, JR, Miller ER: Histology of healing split-thickness, full thickness autogenous skin grafts and donor sites. Arch Surg 91:658–670, 1965.

26. Chong ASF, Hendrix MJC, Misiorowski RL: Expression of cytokeratins in fibroblasts is induced by reconstituted basement membrane. J Cell Biol 105:49a, 1987.

27. Krawczyk WS: A pattern of epidermal cell migration during wound healing. J Cell Biol 49:247–263, 1971.

28. Mansbridge JN, Knapp AM: Changes in keratinocyte maturation during wound healing. J Invest Dermatol 89:253–263, 1987.

29. Odland G, Ross R: Human wound repair. I. Epidermal regeneration. J Cell Biol 39:139–151, 1968.

30. Fejerskov O: Excision wounds in palatal epithelium in guinea pigs. Scan J Dent Res 80:139–154, 1972.

31. Gibbins JR: Migration of stratified squamous epithelium in vivo. Am J Pathol 53:929–941, 1968.

32. Andersen L, Fejerskov O: Ultrastructure of initial epithelial cell migration in palatal wounds of guinea pigs. J Ultrastructure Res 48:313–324, 1974.

33. Gabbiani G, Ryan GB: Development of a contractile apparatus in epithelial cells during epidermal and liver regeneration. J Submicr Cytol 6:143–157, 1974.

34. Betchaku T, Trinkaus JP: Contact relations, surface activity and cortical microfilaments of marginal cells of the enveloping layer and of the yolk synctial and yolk cytoplasmic layers of Fundulus before and during epiboly. J Exp Zool 206:381–426, 1978.

35. Takashima A, Grinnell F: Human keratinocyte adhesion and phagocytosis promoted by fibronectin. J Invest Dermatol 83:352–358, 1984.

36. Vaughan RB, Trinkaus JP: Movements of epithelial cell sheets in vitro. J Cell Sci 1:407–413, 1966.

37. Radice G: The spreading of epithelial cells during wound closure in Xenopus larvae. Develop Biol 76:26–46, 1980.

38. Bellairs R: Differentiation of the yolk sac of the chick studied by electron microscopy. J Embryol Exp Morphol 11:201–225, 1963.

39. Buck RC: Cell migration in repair of mouse corneal epithelium. Invest Ophthalmol Vis Sci 18:767–784, 1979.

40. Winter GD: Movement of epidermal cells over the wound surface. Dev Biol Skin 5:113–127, 1964.

41. Ortonne JP, Loning T, Schmitt D, et al: Immuno-morphological and ultrastructural aspects of keratinocyte migration in epidermal wound healing. Virchow Arch A 392:217–230, 1981.

42. Beerens EGT, Slot TW, Van de Leun JC: Rapid regeneration of the dermal-epidermal junction after partial separation by vacuum. An electron microscopic study. J Invest Dermatol 65:513–521, 1975.

43. Sciubba JJ: Regeneration of the basal lamina complex during epithelial wound healing. J Periodont Res 12:204–217, 1977.

44. Gibbins JR: Epithelial migration in organ culture. A morphological and time lapse cinematographic analysis of migrating stratified squamous epithelium. Pathology 10:207–218, 1978.

45. Bereiter-Hahn J, Strohmeier R, Kunzenbacher I, et al: Locomotion of Xenopus epidermis cells in primary culture. J Cell Sci 52:289–311, 1981.

46. Gabbiani G, Chaponnier C, Huttner I: Cytoplasmic filament and gap junctions in epithelial cells and myofibroblasts during wound healing. J Cell Biol 76:561–568, 1978.

47. Stenn KS, Madri JA, Roll FJ: Migrating epidermis produces AB2 collagen and requires continual collagen synthesis for movement. Nature 277:229–232, 1979.

48. Stanley JR, Alvarez OM, Aere EW, et al: Detection of basement membrane zone antigens during epidermal wound healing in pigs. J Invest Dermatol 77:240–243, 1981.

49. Clark RAF, Lanigan JM, DellaPelle P, et al: Fibronectin and fibrin provide a provisional matrix for epidermal cell migration during wound re-epithelialization. J Invest Dermatol 79:264–269, 1982.

50. Clark RAF, Winn HJ, Dvorak HF, et al: Fibronectin beneath re-epithelialization epidermis in vivo: Sources and significance. J Invest Dermatol (Suppl) 80:26S–30S, 1983.

51. Demarchez M, Desbas C, Prunieras M: Wound healing of human skin transplanted onto the nude mouse. Brit J Dermatol 113(Suppl 28):177–182, 1985.

52. Fine J-D, Redmar DA, Goodman AI, et al: Sequence of reconstitution of seven basement-membrane components following split-thickness wound induction in primate skin. Arch Dermatol 123:1174–1178, 1987.

53. Olerud JE, Gown AM, Bickenbach J, et al: An assessment of human epidermal repair in elderly normal subjects using immunohistochemical methods. J Invest Dermatol 90:845–850, 1988.

54. Dabelsteen E, Fejerskov O: Loss of epithelial blood group antigen A during wound healing in oral mucous membrane. J Pathol Microbiol Scand 82:431–434, 1974.

55. Donoff RB: Wound healing: Biochemical events and potential role of collagenase. J Oral Surg 28:356–363, 1970.

56. Woodley DT, Kalebec T, Banes RJ, et al: Adult human keratinocytes migrating over nonviable dermal collagen produce collagenolytic enzymes that degrade Type I and Type IV collagen. J Invest Dermatol 86:418–423, 1986.

57. Petersen MJ, Woodley DT, Stricklin GP, et al: Production of procollagenase by cultured human keratinocytes. J Biol Chem 262:835–840, 1987.

58. Morioka S, Lazarus GS, Baird JL et al: Migrating keratinocytes express urokinase-type plasminogen activator. J Invest Dermatol 88:418–423, 1987.

59. Grondahl-Hansen J, Lund LR, Ralfkiaer E, et al: Urokinase and tissue-type plasminogen activators in keratinocytes during wound re-epithelialization in vivo. J Invest Dermatol 90:790–795, 1988.

60. Bray D, White JG: Cortical flow in animal cells. Science 239:883–888, 1988.

61. Bretcher MS: Fibroblasts on the move. J Cell Biol 106:235–237, 1988.

62. Pierschbacher ND, Ruoslahti E: Cell attachment activity of fibronectin can be duplicated by small synthetic fragments of the molecule. Nature 309:30–33, 1984.

63. Donaldson DJ, Mahan JT, Hasty DL, et al: Location of a fibronectin domain involved in newt epidermal cell migration. J Cell Biol 101:73–78, 1985.

64. Donaldson DJ, Mahan JT, Smith GN: Newt epidermal cell migration in vitro and in vivo appears to involve Arg-Gly-Asp-Ser receptors. J Cell Sci 87:525–534, 1987.

65. Stenn KS: Coepibolin, the activity of human serum that enhances the cell spreading properties of epibolin, associates with albumin. J Invest Dermatol 89:59–63, 1987.

66. Stenn KS, Core NG, Halaban R: Phorbol ester serves as a coepibolin in the spreading of primary guinea pig epidermal cells. J Invest Dermatol 87:754–757, 1987.

67. Gilchrest BA, Nemore RE, Maciag T: Growth of human keratinocytes on fibronectin-coated plates. Cell Biol Int Reports 4:1009–1016, 1980.

68. Donaldson DJ, Smith GN, Kang AH: Epidermal cell migration on collagen and collagen-derived peptides. J Cell Sci 57:15–23, 1982.

69. Stenn KS, Madri JA, Tinghitella T, et al: Multiple mechanisms of disassociated epidermal cell spreading. J Cell Biol 96:63–67, 1983.

70. Donaldson DJ, Mahan JT: Fibrinogen and fibronectin on substrates from epidermal cell migration during wound closure. J Cell Sci 62:117–123, 1983.

71. Clark RAF, Folkvord JM, Wertz RL: Fibronectin, as well as other extracellular matrix proteins, mediates human keratinocyte adherence. J Invest Dermatol 84:378–383, 1985.

72. O'Keefe EJ, Payne RE, Russell N, et al: Spreading and enhanced motility of human keratinocytes on fibronectin. J Invest Dermatol 85:125–130, 1985.

73. Woodley DT, O'Keefe EJ, Prunieras M: Cutaneous wound healing: A model for cell-matrix interactions. J Am Dermatol 12:420–433, 1985.

74. McDonald JA: Fibronectin. A primitive matrix. In Clark RAF, Henson PM (eds): The Molecular and Cellular Biology of Wound Repair. New York, Plenum Press, 1988, pp 405–435.

75. Nishida T, Nakagawa S, Awata T, et al: Fibronectin promotes epithelial migration of cultured rabbit cornea in situ. J Cell Biol 39:139–151, 1983.

76. Martin GR, Timpl R: Laminin and other basement membrane components. Ann Rev Cell Biol 3:57–85, 1987.

77. Varani J, Nickoloff B, Riser B, et al: Regulation of keratinocyte motility and proliferation by extracellular matrix components and cytokines. FASEB J 2(6):A1821, 1988.

78. Suzuki S, Oldberg A, Hayman EVGV, et al: Complete amino acid sequence of human vitronectin deduced from cDNA. Similarity of cell attachment sites in vitronectin and fibronectin. EMBO J 4:2519–2524, 1984.

79. O'Keefe EJ, Chiu ML, Payne RE: Stimulation of growth of keratinocytes by basic fibroblast growth factor. J Invest Dermatol 90:767–769, 1988.

80. Halaban R, Langdon R, Birchall N, et al: Basic fibroblast growth factor from human keratinocytes is a natural mitogen for melanocytes. J Cell Biol 67:1611–1619, 1988.

81. Hennings H, Michael D, Cheng C, et al: Calcium regulation of growth and differentiation in mouse epidermal cells in culture. Cell 19:245–254, 1980.

82. Cohen S: The stimulation of epidermal proliferation by a specific protein (EGF). Develop Biol 12:394–407, 1965.

83. Franklin JD, Lynch JB: Effects of topical applications of epidermal growth factor on wound healing. Plast Reconstr Surg 64:766–770, 1979.

84. Brown GL, Curtsinger L, Brightwell JR, et al: Enhancement of epidermal regeneration by biosynthetic epidermal growth factor. J Exp Med 163:1319–1324, 1986.

85. Mertz PM, Davis SC, Arakawa Y, et al: Pulsed rhEGF treatment increased epithelialization of partial thickness wounds. J Invest Dermatol 90:588a, 1988.

86. Gilchrest BA, Marshall WL, Karassik RL, et al: Characterization and partial purification of keratinocyte growth factor from the hypothalamus. J Cell Physiol 120:377–383, 1984.

87. Mertz PM, Davis SC, Kilian P, et al: The effect of topical interleukin-1 on the epidermal healing rate of partial thickness wound. Clin Res 36:378A, 1988.

88. Martinet N, Harne LA, Grotendorst GR: Identification and characterization of chemoattractants for epidermal cells. J Invest Dermatol 90:122–126, 1988.

89. Lynch SE, Nixon JC, Colvin RB, et al: Role of platelet-

derived growth factor in wound healing: Synergistic effects with other growth factors. Proc Natl Acad Sci 84:7696–7700, 1987.

90. O'Keefe EJ, Payne RE, Russell N: Keratinocyte growth-promoting activity from human placenta. J Cell Physiol 124:439–445, 1985.

91. Stoker M, Gherardi E, Perryman M, et al: Scatter factor is a fibroblast-derived modulator of epithelial cell mobility. Nature 327:239–242, 1987.

92. Schultz GS, White R, Mitchell R, et al: Epidermal wound healing enhanced by transforming growth factor alpha and vaccinia growth factor. Science 235:350–352, 1987.

93. Barrandon Y, Green H: Cell migration is essential for sustained growth of keratinocyte colonies: The role of transforming growth factor-alpha and epidermal growth factor. Cell 50:1131–1137, 1987.

94. Tucker RF, Shipley GD, Moses HL, et al: Growth inhibition from BSC-1 cells closely related to platelet type beta transforming growth factor. Science 226:705–707, 1984.

95. Knabbe C, Lippman E, Wakefield LM, et al: Evidence that transforming growth factor beta is a hormonally regulated negative growth factor in human breast cancer cells. Cell 48:417–428, 1987.

96. Moses HL, Coffey RJ, Leof EB, et al: Transforming growth factor beta regulation of cell proliferation. J Cell Physiol (Suppl) 5:1–7, 1987.

97. Mansbridge JN, Hanawalt PC: Role of transforming growth factor beta in the maturation of human epidermal keratinocytes. J Invest Dermatol 90:336–341, 1988.

98. Barker AT, Jaffe LF, Vanable JW Jr: The glabrous epidermis of cavies contains a powerful battery. Am J Physiol 242:R358–R366, 1982.

99. Jaffe LF, Vanable JW: Electric fields and wound healing. Clin Dermatol 2:34–44, 1984.

100. Alvarez OM, Mertz PM, Smerbveck RV, et al: The healing of superficial skin wounds is stimulated by external electrical current. J Invest Dermatol 81:144–148, 1983.

101. Stenn KS, Milstone LM: Epidermal cell confluence and implications for a two step mechanism of wound closure. J Invest Dermatol 83:445–447, 1984.

102. Dunn GA, Ireland GW: New evidence that growth in 3T3 cell cultures is a diffusion limited process. Nature 312:63–65, 1984.

103. Grinnell F, Toda K-I, Takashima A: Activation of keratinocyte fibronectin receptor function during cutaneous wound healing. J Cell Sci (Suppl) 8:199–209, 1987.

104. O'Keefe EJ, Woodley D, Castillo G, et al: Production of soluble and cell associated fibronectin by cultured keratinocytes. J Invest Dermatol 82:150–155, 1984.

105. O'Keefe EJ, Woodley DT, Falk RJ, et al: Production of fibronectin by epithelium in a skin equivalent. J Invest Dermatol 88:634–639, 1987.

106. Takashima A, Billingham RE, Grinnell F: Activation of rabbit keratinocyte fibronectin receptor function in vivo during wound healing. J Invest Dermatol 86:585–590, 1986.

107. Toda K, Grinnell F: Activation of human keratinocyte fibronectin receptor function in relation to other ligand-receptor interactions. J Invest Dermatol 88:412–417, 1987.

II
STRUCTURAL AND REGULATORY COMPONENTS OF WOUND HEALING

8

COLLAGEN STRUCTURE AND FUNCTION

Edward J. Miller, Ph.D., and Steffen Gay, M.D.

Collagen is clearly the most prevalent protein in the animal kingdom. It appears to be an obligatory constituent of extracellular matrices and connective tissues from the most primitive multicellular organisms, the Porifera, to the most advanced and complex, the Vertebrata. In these organisms, aggregates of collagen molecules coursing through the tissues are responsible for establishing and maintaining the physical integrity of diverse extracellular structures, thereby contributing to the functional capabilities of the organism as a whole.

At the molecular level, collagen may be defined as a protein containing lengthy domain(s) of triple-helical conformation. The unique collagen fold is made possible by virtue of the repetitive Gly-X-Y sequence(s) in participating chains. In this type of sequence, glycine occurs in every third position along the chain, an absolute requirement for the triple helix in which there is no space for side chains at every third residue. Although the X and Y positions can be occupied by any amino acid, the conformation of individual chains is attained and stabilized by the presence of prolyl and hydroxyprolyl residues, respectively, in approximately one third of these positions in homoiothermic organisms. A second feature of the definition of collagen is that the protein participates in the formation of extracellular aggregates that function primarily as supporting elements. This second requirement is the more crucial one since it defines the protein on the basis of function. There are several known proteins that contain segments of triple-helical conformation but that apparently do not possess the capacity for self-assembly into extracellular aggregates. These are the circulating complement component, C1q,[1] the asymmetric or tailed form of the enzyme, acetylcholinesterase,[2] the apoprotein of pulmonary surfactant,[3, 4] and the serum and liver mannose-binding proteins.[5] In general, these proteins contain relatively short segments of triple helix and do not qualify for designation as a collagen on the basis of function. Nevertheless, their existence implies that the collagen fold (triple helix) may be considered as a generally useful conformation (or element of secondary structure) for many proteins similar to the α helix, the β pleated sheet, and the β turn.

Current information on collagen structure and function has been derived largely from studies on selected higher vertebrate species, including humans. To date, these studies have presented evidence for the existence of at least 13 distinct collagen types or systems that are collectively composed of as many as 25 unique polypeptide chains. The large number of chains in this family plus numerous post-translational modifications of the chains as well as alterations of the molecules derived from them creates an enormous diversity of chemical and structural features. The evolutionary pathway leading to this diversity remains obscure. It most probably arose, however, as a means of meeting the unique functional requirements of a variety of extracellular matrices in organisms of increasing complexity.

Several reviews appearing within the past two decades have chronicled the progress of investigations on the vertebrate collagens and have summarized extant data.[6–11] In spite of the indicated diversity, essentially all collagen molecules possess a common structural motif, i.e., a central core characterized by a high proportion of triple-helical conformation that is flanked at both ends by nontriple-helical or globular domains. This chapter surveys the various levels of structure for the vertebrate collagens. In addition, data on structural features as well as tissue distribution are used to evaluate functional parameters for each collagen system.

GENERAL CONSIDERATIONS

Table 8–1 summarizes pertinent information concerning the currently recognized vertebrate collagen types and provides a framework for the ensuing discussion. Several items noted in the table are worthy of comment. For the most part, the number of unique chains involved in forming molecules of each type of collagen has been fully documented. This is not the case, however, for type IV collagen, for which preliminary evidence suggests the presence of at least one[12] and possibly two[13] additional chains along with the more characterized α1(IV) and α2(IV) chains. Of extreme interest is the observation that the human Goodpasture epitope appears to reside in the COOH-terminal noncollagenous domain of one of the additional chains.[13] In addition, a chain designated α5(VI) has been identified on the basis of human cDNA clones coding for about one third of the chain. The chain is clearly homologous to α1(IV) and α2(IV), and its gene could be assigned to the X chromosome.[14] In view of the evidence presented in the latter studies, the table lists five unique chains for type IV collagen with the understanding that considerable future work will be necessary to fully document the prevalence of and molecular organization of α3(IV), α4(IV), and α5(IV).

There is also some uncertainty concerning the number of chains composing type VIII collagen. Recent work has described the isolation of two distinct 50,000 Da fragments that presumably represent pepsin-resistant portions of the primary constituents of a larger type VIII molecule.[15] In an alternate study, however, it was concluded that the type VIII collagen molecule was composed of three identical chains of 61,000 Da with a nonhelical domain at each end.[16] The latter view with respect to the size and domain structure of type VIII chains has been verified by sequence studies on overlapping cDNA clones encoding the entire primary structure of the α1(VIII) chain.[17] The studies did not, however, resolve the issue of the number of chains in type VIII molecules since the inferred sequence of α1(VIII) did not account for all of the sequences of cyanogen bromide peptide fragments derived from type VIII preparations. Thus, there appears to be at least two unique chains for type VIII collagen as listed in Table 8–1. An additional area of uncertainty involves the number of chains in type XIII collagen. The existence of this collagen has been inferred from data on a human cDNA clone encoding a unique collagen chain[18] as well as two overlapping genomic clones.[19] In spite of these reservations about the number of chains involved in forming molecular species of certain collagen types, it seems clear that the collagen family of proteins is a remarkably large one.

With respect to chromosomal localization, it is of interest to note that genes coding for 13 of the chains are distributed among 7 chromosomes in the human genome (see Table 8–1). This wide dispersion of the collagen genes was somewhat unexpected, particularly since coordinately expressed genes such as those coding for the α1(I) and α2(I) chains of the heteropolymeric type I collagen molecule are located on different chromosomes. In contrast, the genes for the coordinately expressed α1(IV) and α2(IV) chains of type IV collagen lie in close proximity on chromosome 13.[20] Similarly, the genes for two of the chains of type VI collagen, α1(VI) and α2(VI), are localized in band q 223 on chromosome 21. Nevertheless, the gene for α3(VI) is located in the distal region of the long arm of chromosome 2 where it is in relatively close proximity to the genes for chains of two other collagens, α1(III) and α2(V).

Although the data on chromosome localization are far from complete (only 13 of some 25 or more genes have been localized), they have profound implications for the mechanisms controlling evolutionary development and expression of the genes. Genes located close to each other or in clusters may have arisen through duplication of an ancestral gene. Coordinately expressed genes resident on different chromosomes may have evolved independently or may be products of a very early duplication event on the part of an ancestral gene. In any case, the data also suggest that coordinately expressed genes resident on different chromosomes have evolved in such a manner that they contain similar or identical regulatory sequences that can be recognized by one or more common sequence-specific regulatory proteins. Further investigations on the collagen genes and their respective protein products should provide significant insight into these matters.

For the sake of clarity, Table 8–1 lists only

Table 8–1. VERTEBRATE COLLAGEN TYPES

Type	Chain(s)	Locus of Human Gene (Chromosome)*	Major Molecular Species	Distribution	Function
I	$\alpha 1(I)$ $\alpha 2(I)$	17 7	$[\alpha 1(I)]_2 \alpha 2(I)$	All connective tissues except hyaline cartilage and basement membranes	Formation of striated supporting elements (fibers) of varying diameter
II	$\alpha 1(II)$	12	$[\alpha 1(II)]_3$	Hyaline cartilages and cartilage-like tissues, e.g., vitreous humor	Formation of striated supporting elements (fibrils) of generally smaller diameter than type I fibers
III	$\alpha 1(III)$	2	$[\alpha 1(III)]_3$	The more distensible connective tissues, e.g., blood vessels	Formation of small fibrous elements, similar to type II, but may also form cofibers with type I collagen molecules
IV	$\alpha 1(IV)$ $\alpha 2(IV)$ $\alpha 3(IV)$ $\alpha 4(IV)$ $\alpha 5(IV)$	13 13 X	$[\alpha 1(IV)]_2 \alpha 2(IV)$	Basement membranes Glomerular basement membrane	Formation of meshlike scaffold
V	$\alpha 1(V)$ $\alpha 2(V)$ $\alpha 3(V)$	 2	$[\alpha 1(V)]_2 \alpha 2(V)$	Essentially all tissues	Similar to type III collagen
VI	$\alpha 1(VI)$ $\alpha 2(VI)$ $\alpha 3(VI)$	21 21 2	$[\alpha 1(VI), \alpha 2(VI), \alpha 3(VI)]$	Essentially all tissues	Formation of microfibrillar elements
VII	$\alpha 1(VII)$		$[\alpha 1(VII)]_3$	Dermal-epidermal junctions	Anchoring fibrils
VIII	$\alpha 1(VIII)$ $\alpha 2(VIII)$		Unknown	Desçemet's membrane, produced by endothelial cells	Unknown
IX	$\alpha 1(IX)$ $\alpha 2(IX)$ $\alpha 3(IX)$	6	$[\alpha 1(IX), \alpha 2(IX), \alpha 3(IX)]$	Hyaline cartilage	Forms coaggregates with type II collagen
X	$\alpha 1(X)$		$[\alpha 1(X)]_3$	Hypertrophic cartilage	Unknown
XI	$\alpha 1(XI)$ $\alpha 2(XI)$ $\alpha 1(II)$	 6 12	$[\alpha 1(XI), \alpha 2(XI), \alpha 1(II)]$	Hyaline cartilage	Unknown, but may form cofibers with type II collagen molecules
XII	$\alpha 1(XII)$		$[\alpha 1(XII)]_3$	May be similar to type I collagen	Unknown, but may form coaggregates with type I collagen
XIII	$\alpha 1(XIII)$		Unknown	Synthesized by certain tumor cell lines	Unknown

*Data for type I-V collagen genes are from ref. 121; data for type VI collagen genes are from ref. 122; data for $\alpha 1(IX)$ are from ref. 123; data for $\alpha 5(IV)$ are from ref. 14; and data for $\alpha 2(XI)$ are from ref. 124.

the major molecular species known for each collagen type. In many cases, however, the chains associated with a given collagen type may be utilized to form more than one molecular species. Information concerning the multiple molecular species of type I and type V collagens has been delineated in previous reviews,[8, 11] and as noted previously, the presence of five unique chains in the type IV system would most certainly allow the formation of a number of molecular species. Therefore, there are many more triple-helical molecular species than collagen types and this phenomenon undoubtedly reflects unique regulatory mechanisms operative in certain cell types.

One of the more intriguing aspects of collagen molecular organization in higher vertebrates is that molecules may be homopolymeric, $(\alpha 1)_3$, or heteropolymeric, $(\alpha 1)_2\alpha 2$ and $\alpha 1\alpha 2\alpha 3$. Conventional wisdom would dictate that the simpler homopolymeric molecules constituted the initial evolutionary forms of collagen molecules and that the more complex heterotrimeric molecules represent structural refinements in the course of evolution. Since heteropolymeric molecules are found in a variety of invertebrate connective tissues,[21] it seems apparent that the tendency for formation of more complex molecules occurred at an early stage of evolution. At the moment, however, it is virtually impossible to trace the development of higher vertebrate collagens to their origins in more primitive species owing to a lack of data and the diversity of tissues involved. A recent study on lamprey fiber-forming collagens amply illustrates this point.[22] Using several criteria for identification of various collagens, the authors of the study were able to confirm that lamprey notochord collagen is composed largely of a molecular species clearly identifiable as type II collagen. They also demonstrated that a quantitatively smaller collagen fraction from the notochord is a type XI collagen. In addition, a small amount of body wall collagen could be identified as type V collagen. However, the major body wall collagen appeared to be a molecular species containing three unique chains, and the major dermis collagen was observed to be a homopolymer that lacked several of the chemical features of type III collagen. The lamprey is a contemporary descendant of one the most primitive vertebrate species. If it may be assumed that the modern organism is representative of the original species, these data suggest that type II, V, and XI collagens had already appeared at the time of the earliest vertebrates, but that type I and III collagens had not as yet achieved the form in which they exist in contemporary higher vertebrates. These data would appear to be at variance with the observation that the dermis of an octopus species, a member of the phyla of Protostomia, contains a molecular species of collagen characterized by the presence of $\alpha 1$ and $\alpha 2$ chains in a 2:1 ratio, similar to that in contemporary higher vertebrate type I collagen.[23] It is possible, however, that type I collagen evolved independently in different Eumetazoan groups, which further complicates the task of reconstructing the evolutionary history of collagen molecules.

STRUCTURAL FEATURES OF THE CHAINS

Figure 8–1 presents the general structural features of selected collagen chains. For the most part, the chains depicted are representative of the various known chain formats. With the exception of α chains of the fiber-forming collagens (Fig. 8–1B), the primary structure of the various chains is presented in terms of the initial biosynthetic product, excluding, however, the signal sequence that would not be expected to contribute to the ultimate extracellular structure of the chains or the molecules composed of them.

Proα(I, II, III, V, XI). Proα chains of type I, II, III, V, and XI collagens, the fiber-forming collagens,[24] constitute a set of unique but highly homologous chains. Although data on the chains composing type V and XI collagens are not as yet complete, sufficient information is available to warrant the inference that chains of the latter collagens exhibit the same general structural features as chains derived from the more well-characterized type I, II, and III collagens.[11] The nine proα chains of the fiber-forming collagens are therefore depicted in Figure 8–1A using data compiled for pro$\alpha 1$(I) in a previous review.[9] The chain is composed of a total of five alternating noncollagenous and repetitive triplet segments over a span of 1441 amino acids. The noncollagenous sequences are characterized by a relatively high proportion of acidic and hydrophobic residues. Depending on the chain, the two larger noncollagenous sequences located at the N- and C-termini contain several (7 to 10) cysteinyl residues. A portion of the cysteinyl residues in the C-terminal segment form interchain disulfide bonds at the time newly synthesized chains associate to form molecules. In general, cysteine is rarely observed in repetitive triplet sequences and the only additional cysteinyl residues of the fiber-forming collagens are confined to pro$\alpha 1$(III), where they occur in the C-terminal junction region between the two repetitive triplet segments and the following noncollagenous segments.

Using the pro$\alpha 1$(I) model, the nature and location of selected sequences in the proα chains of the fiber-forming collagens are also presented in Figure 8–1A. These are P-Q and A-D, the bonds cleaved by procollagen N- and C-proteinases, respectively, during the conversion of procollagen to collagen; E-K-S and E-K-A, nontriplet sequences each containing a lysyl (or hydroxylysyl) residue that is oxidatively deaminated to produce a highly reactive aldehyde function preparatory to covalent crosslinking; G-M-K*-G-H-R and G-I-K*-G-H-R, triplet sequences each containing a hydroxylysyl residue that reacts with one of the aforementioned aldehyde functions in a neighboring molecule to establish a covalent intermolecular

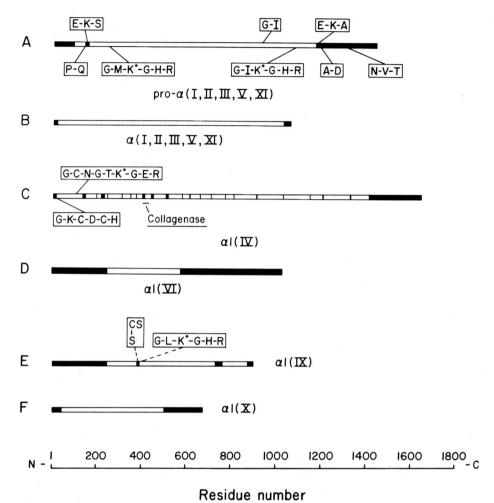

Figure 8–1. Schematic representation of selected collagen chains illustrating their length and the position of certain unique chemical features. Filled-in areas are regions of nontriplet sequence and open areas represent sequences of repetitive triplet structure. The positions of small interruptions in the repetitive triplet domains for α1(VI), α1(IX), and α1(X) are not shown. Amino acid sequences are presented using standard single-letter notation: A, alanine; R, arginine; N, asparagine; D, aspartic acid; C, cysteine; Q, glutamine; E, glutamic acid; G, glycine; H, histidine; I, isoleucine; L, leucine; K, lysine; K*, hydroxylysine; M, methionine; P, proline; S, serine; T, threonine; and V, valine. For α1(IX), the sequences depicted are from α2(IX) and their positions are therefore depicted by dashed lines. In addition, CS denotes a chondroitin sulfate chain attached to the polypeptide via a seryl (S) residue.

crosslink; G-I, the bond cleaved when native molecules are exposed to vertebrate collagenase; and N-V-T, a site for the attachment of an N-linked, mannose-rich oligosaccharide side chain. In general, proα chains of the fiber-forming collagens contain either one or two sites for attachment of this type of carbohydrate unit and these sites are located exclusively in nontriplet sequences. By far the most prevalent form of glycosylation for these chains (and all other collagen chains) is O-glycosidic linkage of galactosyl or glucosylgalactosyl moieties to hydroxylysine in repetitive triplet sequences. The number of hydroxylysyl residues per chain and the extent to which they are glycosylated may be quite variable, however, even among the closely related chains of the fiber-forming collagens.[9]

With respect to higher orders of structure and function, the proα chains of the fiber-forming collagens must be viewed in terms of three separate domains. The large central domain lying between the procollagen N- and C-proteinase cleavage sites is composed largely of repetitive triplets and is destined to constitute one of the chains of rodlike triple-helical molecules present in extracellular fibrous aggregates. In contrast, the C-terminal nontriplet domain assumes a globular conformation.[25] Analysis of the sequence of this domain from α1(I), α2(I), α1(II), α1(III), and α2(V) by methods predicting secondary structure potentials suggest a prevalence of α-helical segments in N-terminal portions of the domain while β-sheet structures are likely to be more prevalent in the C-terminal regions.[26] This analysis also suggests a periodic distribution of amino acid sequences with a high potential for β-turn conformation in the midrange of the domain. There is as yet, however, no information relevant to the three-dimensional organization of these potential elements of secondary structure. Nevertheless, there is good evidence indicating that the C-terminal globular domain plays a critical role in chain selection and assembly leading to the formation of various molecular species. In this regard, different molecular species of the fiber-forming collagens exhibit definitive chain compositions implying a mechanism for specifying the nature of the chains utilized in forming a given molecule. In addition, interchain disulfide bonding invariably precedes triple helix formation during biosynthesis of the fiber-forming collagens.[27] Since interchain disulfide bonding of proα chains of type I and II collagens occurs only through cysteinyl residues located in the C-terminal nontriplet domains, these observations clearly indicate that the proα chains are joined and aligned through interaction sites present in the C-terminal domain. Further evidence for the role of the C-terminal domain in chain assembly has been obtained in studies on collagen synthesized by an osteogenesis imperfecta patient. The proband synthesized a homopolymeric type I collagen, $[\alpha 1(I)]_3$, even though an apparently functional mRNA for proα2(I) was present. It was ultimately shown that the patient was homozygous for a small frameshift mutation in the proα2(I) gene and that the deletion radically altered the sequence of the last 33 amino acids in the proα2(I) chain.[28] The mutation created a much more hydrophobic sequence at the C-terminus of the patient's proα2(I) chain than is present when the chain is synthesized using the normal allele. Cumulatively, these results underscore the critical nature of the C-terminal propeptide domain of proα chains in facilitating chain recognition and assembly. They also strongly implicate the C-terminal portion of the domain as one of the sequences important for self-assembly.

At present, far less is known concerning the functional role of the N-terminal propeptide domain at the proα chain level. As noted in Figure 8–1A, approximately two thirds of this domain has a nontriplet primary structure that is likely to support conventional forms of secondary structure. The remainder of the domain is essentially composed of a relatively short repetitive triplet sequence that contributes to

the final segment of collagen fold as triple helix formation is propagated from the C-terminal regions of the chains. This domain, then, may play its most critical role at the molecular level in the extracellular matrix.

With respect to the latter possibility, there is some evidence that both the N- and C-terminal propeptides of the fiber-forming collagens have functional roles in the extracellular matrix. This potential arises from the fact that during the conversion of procollagen to collagen, the propeptides are released intact as independent entities. Recent studies leading to the isolation of the N-terminal propeptide of proα1(I) from bone[29] and the identification of the cartilage matrix component, chondrocalcin, as the C-terminal propeptide from proα1(II)[30] indicate that these domains have more than a transient existence in extracellular matrices. Their role in these locations may be regulatory in that preparations of N-terminal propeptides[31] as well as a fragment derived from the C-terminal propeptide of proα2(I)[32] inhibit procollagen synthesis when added to fibroblast cultures. The effect is somewhat specific for procollagen and perhaps other matrix components when evaluated in intact cell cultures,[32] but appears to be more generalized when evaluated in cell-free translation systems.[33] The results outlined previously indicated that control was exerted post-transcriptionally. Recent results, however, indicate that both N- and C-terminal type I propeptides are effective in specifically reducing procollagen mRNA levels in cultured human fibroblasts, underscoring a possible pretranslational regulation on the part of the peptides.[34] Although there are some discrepancies in the current findings, the results clearly establish that feedback inhibition may constitute at least one component of the mechanisms regulating procollagen synthesis. This role does not, however, exclude other potential regulatory or structural roles that are as yet undefined. In this regard, it is noteworthy that the name chondrocalcin was assigned originally on the basis of a presumed role in cartilage calcification,[35] yet chondrocalcin (the C-terminal propeptide derived from proα1(II)) accumulates in all developing cartilagenous tissues, including those with no potential for endochondral bone formation.[36]

The activity of the procollagen N- and C-proteinases also generates collagen molecules composed of chains depicted in Figure 8–1B. Although the repetitive triplet sequence of each chain is involved in triple-helical conformation, each chain begins and ends with a short nontriplet sequence. These "telopeptide" sequences are important for crosslinking (see further on) and have also been implicated in the linear as well as lateral growth of fibers.[37, 38] In this regard, selective degradation of the telopeptide sequences through limited proteolysis of native collagen molecules greatly diminishes their fiber-forming capacity in vitro. These observations support the notion that lateral aggregation of fiber-forming collagen molecules is dependent, at least in part, on conformation-dependent interactions between the telopeptide sequences and selected regions of triple-helical conformation in neighboring molecules. Attempts to evaluate conformational characteristics of the teleopeptide sequences by predictive methods have led to conflicting results. Thus, the N-terminal telopeptide of $\alpha 1(I)$ was predicted to have an antiparallel β-sheet conformation with the required turn in chain direction at residues surrounding the lysine crosslinking site.[39] The C-terminal telopeptide segment of several chains has been assessed as having short domains of α-helical structure separated by regions of β-turn or random coil.[26] However, an additional assessment of both N- and C-terminal telopeptide segments of several chains indicated the presence of little, if any, periodic conformation but did suggest the presence of β-turns in the vicinity of crosslinking sites.[40] The discrepancies in these results underscore the element of subjectivity inherent in predictions of secondary structure based solely on sequence data. Nevertheless, studies on the solution conformation of the C-terminal telopeptide segment of $\alpha 1(I)$ by circular dichroism and nuclear magnetic resonance spectroscopy tend to confirm the predictive analysis of Jones and Miller[40] in that the peptide was shown to have a nonrandom extended conformation with two regions of high mobility but no obvious periodic structure.[41] It must be noted that all of the studies on potential telopeptide conformation to date essentially ignore conformational characteristics that might be derived through mutual interactions of the telopeptides that lie in close proximity to each other at the ends of triple-helical molecules. Moreover, current data strongly suggest that in vivo the pN form of molecules (i.e., molecules retaining their N-terminal propeptide sequences) participate in fiber formation and that the propeptide sequences are removed following incorporation into fibrous elements (see later discussion). If this is the case, the N-terminal telopeptide segments are likely to be highly constrained with respect to secondary structure during the crucial stages of lateral aggregation due to their position between regions of triple-helical conformation.

$\alpha 1(IV)$. Figure 8–1C depicts the general structural features of the human $\alpha 1(IV)$ chain. The chain contains 1642 amino acid residues and its primary structure has been elucidated by a combination of protein sequencing and nucleotide sequencing of overlapping cDNA clones. Two recent publications have summarized these data.[42, 43] Comparably extensive data have been obtained for $\alpha 2(IV)$ and clearly show that $\alpha 2(IV)$ is highly homologous to $\alpha 1(IV)$ and that the two chains exhibit the same general structural features.[44, 45] The $\alpha 1(IV)$ chain may thus be considered as representative of the chains composing type IV molecules.

Chemical studies on type IV molecules extracted from tissues have shown that essentially the entire sequence depicted for $\alpha 1(IV)$ in Figure 8–1C is present in chains composing functional molecules deposited in basement membrane structures. In addition, nucleotide sequence data derived from overlapping cDNA clones indicate that the initial biosynthetic product for $\alpha 1(IV)$ is composed of the sequence depicted in Figure 8–1C plus a short N-terminal signal sequence of 27 amino acid residues. These data, then, corroborate those from several previous studies on the biosynthesis of type IV collagen indicating that type IV molecules undergo little, if any, processing prior to or following deposition in functional tissue aggregates. The distinction between proα chains and α chains in the type IV collagen system may therefore be a purely semantic one.

Interestingly, $\alpha 1(IV)$ begins (at the N-terminal end) in short nontriplet sequence similar in size to the N-terminal telopeptide segment in α chains of the fiber-forming collagens (compare Figure 8–1B and C). The N-terminal nontriplet segment of $\alpha 1(IV)$ also contains a lysyl residue and a cysteinyl residue near its C-terminal end. Following aggregate formation during which antiparallel molecules associate and overlap each other at their N-terminal regions, both of these residues may be involved in the formation of intermolecular crosslinks with comparable residues in the first triplet segment.[46, 47] The sequence surrounding these potential crosslinking sites are shown in Figure 8–1C. They bear little resemblance to the major crosslinking sites in chains of the fiber-forming collagens (Fig. 8–1A). The most striking difference is the presence of cysteinyl residues, suggesting the utilization of the more conventional protein crosslinking mechanism, disulfide bond formation, in addition to lysine-derived crosslinks in stabilizing aggregates of type IV collagen. In any event, the N-terminal nontriplet segment of $\alpha 1(IV)$ and other chains of the type IV system may therefore have the same general characteristics and function as previously described for the comparable segment in α chains of the fiber-forming collagens.

It is also noteworthy that α1(IV) as well as proα chains of the fiber-forming collagens contain a substantial C-terminal nontriplet segment (compare Fig. 8–1A and C). The α1(IV) sequence is, however, quite different from that in the C-terminal segment of proα chains and is characterized by the presence of two highly homologous sequences each constituting approximately one half of the total sequence.[48] Although direct evidence is lacking, it may be assumed that this segment of type IV collagen chains likewise serves as the site for chain recognition and alignment, allowing the proper chains to form triple-helical molecules. In addition, the oligomeric globular domain created on assembly of type IV chains provides important contact sites for the construction and stabilization of extracellular aggregates derived from type IV molecules (see further on). In this respect, then, the C-terminal nontriplet segment of type IV chains plays a broader role and at more levels of structure than the comparable segment in chains of the fiber-forming collagens.

The remainder of α1(IV) (i.e., the portion of the chain between the N- and C-terminal nontriplet segments) constitutes the repetitive triplet domain. In type IV chains, however, this domain is unique due to its relatively large size and the presence of numerous interruptions [21 for α1(IV)] in the triplet sequence. The latter are of varying size and tend to be larger and more numerous in the N-terminal half of the domain. This feature of type IV chains undoubtedly contributes to the high degree of flexibility observed for molecules composed of them. As might be expected from the unique characteristics of type IV chains, physiological degradation of type IV molecules apparently requires a distinct and specific collagenase. The sequence cleaved by type IV collagenase has not as yet been identified, although studies on the collagenase cleavage products of type IV collagen suggest the cleavage site lies in the region shown in Figure 8–1C.[49]

α1(VI). Complete data pertaining to the primary structure of the three chains of type VI collagen are currently available. Although the apparent molecular mass of α1(VI) and α2(VI) is 140 kDa,[50, 51] which is approximately the same as that for proα1(I) chains, amino acid sequences of these chains derived from cDNA sequencing as well as protein sequencing reveal that the human chains contain 1009 and 998

amino acids, respectively.[52] These data have been used in constructing the illustration of α1(VI) presented in Figure 8–1D, which shows an N-terminal globular domain of 238 residues, followed by a repetitive triplet domain of 336 residues and a C-terminal globular domain of 435 residues. The α2 chain has domains of similar size. The triple-helical domain in each chain has several interruptions in Gly-X-Y- repetitive structure as well as several R-G-D sequences potentially active in cell binding and attachment. Interestingly, the N-terminal globular domain in each chain exhibits a great deal of homology to the 200-amino acid collagen-binding regions in von Willebrand factor while the C-terminal globular domain in each chain is composed essentially of two of the collagen-binding domains. The illustration in Figure 8–1D is clearly not entirely applicable to α3(VI), which is synthesized as an apparent 260 kDa precursor chain and is subsequently modified to a 200 kDa chain constituent in type VI molecules resident in extracellular matrices.[53] Recent work on cDNA clones for α3(VI) shows that the chain has the same general domain structure as α1 and α2 but that the N-terminal globular domain contains an additional eight units homologous to the collagen-binding repeats of von Willebrand factor.[54, 55] Recent data indicate that this very large chain is truncated to different sizes in the processing from precursor to tissue form.[56]

These data underscore some of the unique features of type VI collagen. It is the only known collagen in which only one of the constituent chains is synthesized in precursor form. This situation is much different from that for the fiber-forming collagens and type IV collagen, in which all or none of the chains, respectively, are initially present as pro-chain forms. The amino acid sequence data strongly suggest that type VI molecules are particularly functional in cell attachment and collagen binding, and this has been confirmed in preliminary studies.[54] Lastly, it is likely that the central repetitive triplet domain of these chains contains a number of interruptions in triplet structure to allow the flexibility required for intertwining of antiparallel triple helices observed in aggregates of type VI collagen.[57]

α1(IX). The primary structure of chicken α1(IX) has been elucidated largely by studies on cDNA clones[58, 59] and is depicted in Figure 8–1E. It is characterized by seven alternating segments of nontriplet and repetitive triplet structure over a span approximating slightly less than 90 percent of the length of an α chain of the fiber-forming collagens. An identical domain structure has been demonstrated for α2(IX).[60] Thus, the general features illustrated in Figure 8–1E are likely to be valid for all type IX chains except that the N-terminal globular domain is significantly smaller in α2(IX) and α3(IX).[59] In addition, α1(IX) chains synthesized by avian corneal cells possess a much shorter (25 residue) N-terminal globular domain due to use of an alternate transcription start site downstream from the start site used in cartilage cells.[61]

Several characteristics of type IX chains are worthy of note. Although nontriplet segments of collagen chains are generally acidic, the N-terminal nontriplet segment of α1(IX) is highly basic (pI = 9.7), thereby providing numerous positive charges for potential interaction with anionic glycosaminoglycan chains in cartilagenous tissues. In addition, a slightly expanded second nontriplet segment in the α2(IX) chain contains a serine residue (S) to which a chondroitin sulfate chain (CS) is attached.[62, 63] This site is highlighted in Figure 8–1E and represents the only known example of attachment of a glycosaminoglycan moiety to a collagen chain. The α2(IX) chain also contains a lysyl (hydroxylysyl) residue in the N-terminal portion of the second triplet segment that is utilized to form crosslinks with oxidatively deaminated hydroxylysyl residues in the N-terminal telopeptides of type II molecules.[64] These data have been used to construct a model of the interaction of type IX collagen with fibrils derived from type II collagen (see further on). The sequence surrounding the α2(IX) crosslinking site is likewise highlighted in Figure 8–1E. The data show the helical crosslink region in α2(IX) to be highly homologous to helical crosslink regions in the chains of the fiber-forming collagens (Fig. 8–1A). Lastly, the C-terminal nontriplet segment of type IX chains is relatively small. By analogy with other collagen systems described above, it is likely that chain recognition and assembly in the type IX system depend on the capacity of these relatively short segments to associate. Delineation of the sequences important for chain association in the type IX system may be facilitated by the moderate size of these segments.

α1(X). The complete primary structure of chicken α1(X) has been derived from nucleotide sequences.[65] It is the shortest of the collagen chains for which complete sequence data are available. The domain structure likewise consists of a central triplet segment bracketed by nontriplet segments (Fig. 8–1F). Although not delineated in the figure, the central triplet segment contains eight interruptions in triplet structure that are more prevalent and closely spaced in the N-terminal half of the segment. This distribution of interruptions in triplet structure resembles that observed in α1(IV). The chain contains an unusually large number of methionyl residues and there are several tyrosyl residues located in the C-terminal nontriplet segment. The latter segment is also characterized by the presence of a highly hydrophobic 29-residue sequence near its C-terminus that could possibly serve as a transmembrane span.

Other Chains. α1(VII) chains are apparently the largest of the known vertebrate collagen chains. The pro form of these chains has an apparent molecular mass of 320 kDa and is characterized by a central triplet domain, which is about the same size as an entire α1(IV) chain, plus a large C-terminal globular domain and a smaller N-terminal globular segment.[66] Since the central triplet domain is likely to contain few interruptions in triplet structure,[67] the general format of proα1(VII) resembles that of the proα chains of the fiber-forming collagens. There is evidence that a portion, or perhaps all, of the N-terminal globular domain is removed by selective proteolysis from molecules composed of these chains subsequent to aggregate formation.[68] Thus, the distinction between proα chains and α chains in the type VII system appears to be valid, although the loss of chain mass is proportionally much smaller than is observed for the fiber-forming collagens.

It is of interest to note that recent data on α1(VIII) suggest a close evolutionary relationship between this chain and α1(X).[17] Also initial data on the chain of type XII collagen strongly suggested a chain format closely related to the chains of type IX collagen.[69] However, more recent data indicate that the α1(XII) chain is much larger than the chains of type IX collagen and that the chains of the two collagens are closely related only with respect to one relatively short repetitive triplet domain, i.e., the most C-terminal triplet domain.[70, 71] Lastly, the apparent size of the chain described for type XIII collagen (60,000 Da)[18] suggests a potential similarity to α1(X), although this possibility needs to be confirmed by further information detailing the primary structure of α1(XIII).

MOLECULAR STRUCTURE

The steps involved in the formation of molecular structure have been investigated most extensively for the fiber-forming collagens but are likely to be valid for all molecular species. The process is initiated in the endoplasmic reticulum following chain synthesis and involves association and alignment of individual chains. Figure 8–2 depicts these early events during the formation of a heterotrimeric molecule like the major molecular species of type I, IV, or V collagen in which two identical chains along with a different third chain constitute a molecule. Entry into the trimeric complexes is regulated by the chemical properties and conformation of the C-terminal nontriplet domain of each chain. Prior to propagation of triple-helical conformation (see further on), the trimeric complexes are stabilized through interchain disulfide bonds. Formation of the latter is likely to be catalyzed by the activity of a protein disulfide isomerase. In this regard, preparations of the enzyme added to reduced proα chains of type I or II procollagens in vitro diminish the time required to form interchain disulfide bonds and triple helices to times approximating those observed for the same phenomena in vivo.[72] Recent data indicate that the β subunit of prolyl 4-hydroxylase is in fact a disulfide isomerase and that isomerase activity is retained when the subunit is assembled in the tetrameric prolyl 4-hydroxylase complex.[73] These results strongly suggest that one and the same enzyme complex may be involved in prolyl hydroxylation of nascent collagen chains as well as the rearrangement of disulfide bonds in the C-terminal propeptides.

This mechanism of chain association and alignment requires that formation of the trimeric complexes be delayed until the entire primary structure of the individual chains is assembled since synthesis of any protein proceeds from the N- to the C-terminus of the chain. Although folding of a nascent polypeptide chain is likely to begin cotranslationally, it most certainly cannot be completed until the entire primary structure has been assembled and the chain is released from the ribosomal or polysomal complex.[74] The data described above with respect to protein disulfide isomerase strongly suggest that the native conformation of the C-terminal nontriplet domain of collagen chains is not attained until the chains associate and form a functional complex.

With respect to helix formation, studies on denatured fragments of type III collagen in which the chains were maintained in register by disulfide bonds at their C-terminal ends have shown that helix formation is initiated in the region adjacent to the disulfide bonds.[75] The observed rate of helix formation in these model systems was independent of the initial concentration of denatured fragments, indicating zero-order kinetics for the conversion of random coils to helix. This strongly suggests that the conversion occurs by a "zipperlike" mechanism in which the helix is propagated sequentially along the chain from the point of the original helix nucleation site. The process of helix formation was also shown to be temperature dependent with an activation energy consistent with the view that the rate limiting step in helix propagation is cis→trans isomerization of peptide bonds. Although the trans configuration of peptide bonds is energetically favored and virtually all peptide bonds in native proteins are trans, X-Pro bonds (where X is any amino acid) may adopt the cis configuration in a random coil owing to the cyclic five-membered ring structure of the prolyl side chain. Indeed, nuclear magnetic resonance studies on random coil (unfolded) collagen chains indicate that 16 percent of the X-Pro and 8 percent of the X-

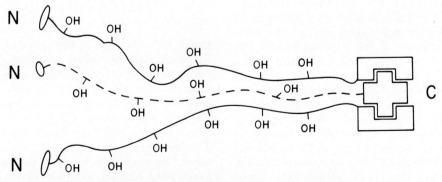

Figure 8–2. An intermediate step in the formation of a heterotrimeric molecule, i.e., the association of three individual chains at their C-terminal globular domains. The conformation of the globular domains specifies the nature of and the stoichiometry of the chains entering the trimer. As noted in the text, formation of appropriate interchain disulfide bonds in the globular complex is a prerequisite for the initiation of helix formation, and helical conformation is propagated from the C-terminal junctional region toward the N-termini of the participating chains.

Hyp bonds are cis.[76] Using these figures, it can be calculated that the typical random coil proα chain would contain 25 to 30 peptide bonds in the cis configuration, which is consistent with the observed energy requirements and temperature dependence of helix formation. Under physiological conditions, i.e., at temperatures of 37°C, helix formation is a spontaneous process due to a large decrease in enthalpy that more than adequately compensates for the loss of entropy generated by fixation of random coil chains in a moderately rigid helical structure.

The essential features of helix formation derived from the in vitro studies described previously have been verified in vivo in studies on collagen synthesized in cultured cells.[77] In vivo, the process of helix formation may also be facilitated by peptidyl-prolyl cis-trans isomerase, which has been shown to considerably accelerate the rate of folding of denatured type III collagen.[78]

On completion of helix formation, the collagen fold consists of three chains in slightly twisted, left-handed helical conformation similar to the helix formed by polyproline II chains in which all peptide bonds are in the trans configuration. The helix of the individual chains is termed the "minor" collagen helix and is a relatively open helix utilizing about three residues for one complete turn over an axial distance of 10 Å. This particular helical conformation is virtually the only periodic secondary structure in which prolyl residues can participate. Their presence, then, in collagen chains imparts rigidity and stability to the structure. In addition, the three chains are coiled about each other: this coil is right-handed and is referred to as the "major" coil since one complete turn spans some 30 residues over an axial distance of 100 Å.

The coiled-coil structure is stabilized by a series of interchain hydrogen bonds. The placement of these bonds is illustrated diagrammatically in Figure 8–3, which depicts the polypeptide backbone of three chains involved in forming a triple helix. The three-letter abbreviation for each amino acid is placed in the position of its α-carbon atom. Chains 1 and 2 and 2 and 3, respectively, are displaced relative to each other by one residue. This arrangement is required for the positioning of each glycyl residue along the central axis of the coiled-coil where it comes in close proximity to two other chains. The close packing of residues along the central axis of the triple helix is the basis for the requirement that glycine occupy every third position in the primary structure of a chain participating in the collagen fold. This

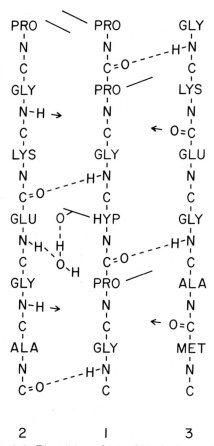

Figure 8–3. Disposition of interchain hydrogen bonds in a triple-helical collagen fold. Chain 1 should be considered as positioned above the plane of the page while chains 2 and 3 should be envisioned as lying slightly below the plane of the page in order to approximate their three-dimensional placement. As noted in the text, the α-amino hydrogen atom of each glycyl residue is in a position to form a hydrogen bond with a carbonyl oxygen in an adjacent chain. The side chain ring structure of prolyl residues is depicted as solid slanted lines. These ring structures actually project from the sides of the triple-helical structure. Thus, interchain hydrogen bond formation involving the γ-OH group in hydroxyproline requires the utilization of an intervening water molecule as depicted in the hydroxyproline–glutamic acid hydrogen bond between chains 1 and 2.

disposition of chains in the coiled-coil permits the chains to be linked by hydrogen bonds between the α-amino hydrogen atoms of glycyl residues and the carbonyl oxygen atoms of residues in the X position of alternate chains. These bonds between chains 1 and 2 and between chains 1 and 3 are depicted in the figure. The hydrogen bonds between chains 2 and 3 cannot be readily depicted in this two-dimensional view and are denoted by small arrows pointing in the direction of the bonds. This arrangement of hydrogen bonds provides one interchain link for each glycyl residue in the structure or one bond per repetitive triplet. It is now clear, however, that these hydrogen bonds are not sufficient to stabilize the structure at physiological temperatures and that additional hydrogen bonding is normally attained by the presence of hydroxyl groups on the prolyl side chains. This first became apparent in studies on collagen produced under conditions in which hydroxylation is inhibited.[27] The planes of prolyl side chains (denoted by solid lines in Fig. 8–3) lie on the surface of the triple-helical structure, and the formation of interchain hydrogen bonds utilizing the γ-OH group of hydroxyproline requires that one water molecule serve as an intermediary hydrogen-bonding agent per interchain bond.[79] This is illustrated in Figure 8–3 for the hydroxyprolyl residue in chain 1, which forms a link with the α-amino hydrogen atom of the glutamic acid residue in position X of chain 2 via a water molecule. Since a typical collagen α chain of the fiber-forming collagens contains 90 or more hydroxyprolyl residues, these types of bonds are theoretically capable of providing an additional 200 to 300 interchain links per molecule. In the collagen systems, then, post-translational modification of primary structure, specifically prolyl hydroxylation, plays a central role in the maintenance of molecular structure.

Since the chains in collagen molecules run colinearly throughout the length of the molecules, the general structural features of molecules are easily correlated with the primary structure of the individual chains. As noted, segments of triple-helical conformation are relatively rigid and rodlike by virtue of the coiled-coil conformation of the polyproline-like helices and interchain hydrogen bonding. However, considerable variation on this theme is introduced by interruptions in triple-helical conformation as well as by retention of sizable globular domains in the fully processed molecules.

The properties of the known collagens are consistent with the presence of three distinct forms of general molecular structure. The first of these is the lengthy and essentially linear structure assumed by molecules of the fiber-forming collagens (Fig. 8–4A). This structure is based on the presence of triple-helical conformation throughout the length of the molecules except at the short telopeptide sequences. Nevertheless, observations on rotary-shadowed molecules of the fiber-forming collagens as well as light scattering measurements on solutions of the molecules suggest they are capable of a limited degree of flexibility.[80, 81] The structural basis for flexibility in these molecules is not currently known but is likely to involve regions in which the individual chains lack or are relatively deficient in prolyl residues. The general structural features of type VII molecules are likely to be quite similar to those of the fiber-forming collagens with the exception that type VII molecules retain a large globular domain at the C-terminal end.

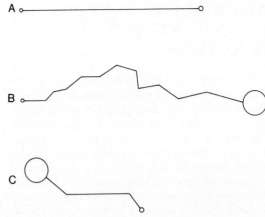

Figure 8–4. A schematic illustration of three general molecular conformations attained by collagen molecules. *A*, The rigid or, at most, semiflexible rod-shaped molecule of the fiber-forming collagens. *B*, The highly flexible type IV molecule in which several sites of bending are possible. *C*, The type IX molecule in which flexibility is confined to a small number of locations.

In contrast, type IV molecules exhibit a high degree of flexibility,[80, 82] which may be ascribed to the presence of numerous interruptions of helical conformation within the triple-helical domain. These molecules are also characterized by a substantial C-terminal globular domain. These features of type IV molecules are illustrated in Figure 8–4B and may also be applicable, albeit on a smaller scale, to type VIII, VI, and X molecules in which the helical domain is likewise characterized by several interruptions in helical conformation.

Type IX molecules provide the third example of general molecular structure, one that is intermediate between the semiflexible rods of the fiber-forming collagens and the highly flexible helical domain of type IV molecules. In this regard, the helical domain of type IX molecules appears to be capable of making a limited number of sharp bends as determined by observations on rotary-shadowed molecules.[83] This type of structure is made possible by the two major interruptions of helical conformation within the triple-helical domain of type IX molecules (Fig. 8–4C).

These three forms of molecular structure are of critical importance in determining the molecular architecture of the aggregates formed by the various molecular species of collagen.

AGGREGATE STRUCTURE AND FUNCTION

The major physiological functions of collagen are accomplished by extracellular aggregates of the molecules, and the structure of the aggregates is directly related to specific function. Therefore these two aspects of collagen systems are discussed together. Several unique modes of aggregation have been discerned. The most prevalent of these and the most well-characterized type of aggregate is the fiber. The capacity to form fibers is common to type I, II, III, V, and XI collagens. Type IX and perhaps type XII collagens are also involved in fiber formation, but only as surface adducts of previously formed fibers. In general, fiber formation involves lateral association and axial displacement of molecules arranged in parallel. All other known modes of aggregation involve associations of molecules allowing some degree of antiparallel orientation of individual molecules.

Fibers. Fiber formation is depicted in Figure 8–5A–C. It involves utilization of monomer molecules (Fig. 8–5A) to generate linear polymers in which individual molecules are staggered relative to one another by four D units (Fig. 8–5B). A single D unit comprises a distance of 67 nm along the axis of a fiber-forming molecule and the entire molecule has a length of 4.4 D units (Fig. 8–5A). The linear polymer appears to be a very stable mode of association[84] in which the N- and C-terminal telopeptide segments are placed next to helical crosslinking sites in neighboring molecules. Fibers and fibrils are then generated by lateral aggregation of linear polymers in which individual molecules are staggered relative to one another by one D unit (Fig. 8–5C). This alignment of molecules creates gap (G) and overlap (O) zones within as well as on the surface of fibers. These zones are responsible for the characteristic banding pattern of collagen fibers when they are observed in the electron microscope following negative staining. Data based on the ultrastructural staining pattern of fibers following exposure to antibodies specific for N-terminal propeptide segments strongly suggest that fi-

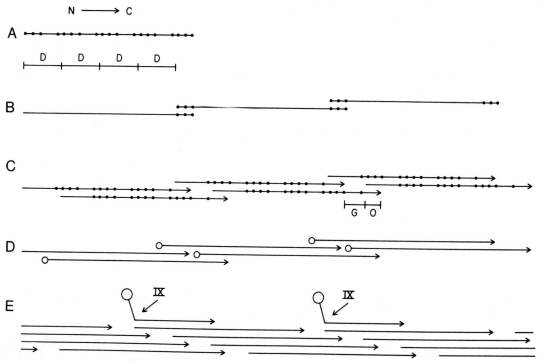

Figure 8–5. A model for the construction of collagen fibers. *A*, A monomer molecule accompanied by an illustration of the length and placement of its D units. The closed circles denote positions of regularly spaced hydrophobic amino acid clusters along the length of the molecule. N and C signify N-terminus and C-terminus, respectively. *B*, A linear polymer formed by head to tail association of monomers. *C*, Initial aggregate formed by lateral association and unit stagger of linear polymers. G and O signify the gap and overlap zones, respectively, created by the association of linear polymers. *D*, An illustration of gap zone obliteration, which occurs if molecules participating in the fiber retain their N-terminal propeptide sequences. *E*, An illustration of the site at which type IX molecules are attached to the surfaces of the fibrous aggregates in cartilage. Note that the N-terminal third of the type IX molecule slants away from the fiber surface. Open circles represent noncollagenous globular domains.

ber-forming molecules are initially incorporated into fibrous elements as pN-molecules, i.e., molecules retaining their N-terminal propeptide domain.[85, 86] These observations imply that the latter domain is, for the most part, excised from molecules resident in fibrous elements. If molecules retain their N-terminal propeptide sequences or if the sequences are removed over a lengthy time period, the gap zone between nonoverlapping molecules in the same plane is eliminated, as depicted in Figure 8–5D. Somewhat similar data have recently been acquired in studies involving antibody preparations specific for C-terminal propeptide sequences.[87–89] These studies revealed that the C-terminal propeptide domains may likewise be associated with newly formed fibrils in a periodic fashion suggesting retention of these sequences in molecules resident in fibers. These findings were somewhat unexpected since the size and shape of the C-terminal propeptide segments are such that they cannot generally be present in fibrous elements possessing the molecular architecture described above. It is possible, however, that these segments can be accommodated on surface regions of the growing fiber provided that the C-terminal globular domain protrudes toward the exterior of the fiber.

The mechanisms responsible for fiber formation and the factors controlling fiber placement and diameter are poorly understood. Recent studies on fiber formation utilizing type I collagen in an in vitro system have shown that the process is characterized by a net increase in enthalpy but is entropy-driven in the physiological temperature range.[90] These data are consistent with the notion that hydrophobic interactions play a predominant role in the lateral association and alignment of molecules during fiber formation. In this regard, the primary structure of $\alpha1(I)$ and $\alpha2(I)$ chains places clusters of hydrophobic residues at regular spacings within each D unit of the type I molecule.[91, 92] (The positions of these clusters are illustrated diagrammatically in Figure 8–5A by filled circles.) Thus it seems clear that both head-to-tail associations (Fig. 8–5B) and more lengthy lateral associations (Fig. 8–5C) can be specified by invoking the mechanism of hydrophobic cluster interaction. As already indicated, the energetics of fiber formation are consistent with this mechanism since loss of the water clathrate structure at each hydrophobic cluster and establishment of numerous hydrophobic interactions between clusters could lead to the positive enthalpy and entropy changes observed for fiber formation.

It would appear that fiber placement and orientation are ultimately controlled by cellular activity. Recent observations on fibrillogenesis in chick embryo tendons suggest that the process of fiber formation is initiated within deep, narrow cytoplasmic recesses formed as the result of alignment and fusion of several procollagen-containing intracellular vacuoles.[93] Subsequent fusion of the cytoplasmic recesses with the cell surface and retraction of the cytoplasmic boundaries results in placement of newly formed fibrils in the adjacent extracellular matrix in an orientation defined by the position of the cell and the direction of the cytoplasmic recess. These observations implicate direct cellular intervention in fibrillogenesis and orientation of the initial fibrous elements. The applicability of these findings to fibroblasts in general and to other collagen-producing cells remains to be established.

An additional area of uncertainty is the mechanism whereby discrete fiber size (diameter) is ultimately attained. The conversion of procollagen to collagen undoubtedly plays a role since retention of N-terminal and/or C-terminal propeptide sequences on the part of molecules entering a fibrous element would be expected to have an inhibitory effect on the addition of further molecules owing to distortions created at the surface of the growing fibril. Although in vitro studies indicate that each of the fiber-forming collagen types is capable of forming independent fibrous elements, there is a growing body of evidence suggesting that in vivo more than one collagen type is involved in forming individual fibers. Thus, ultrastructural immunolocalization studies have shown that the orthogonally placed fibers of chick cornea are composed of a mixture of type I and V collagens and that the type V collagen molecules are not visualized unless the fibers are swollen or partially disrupted.[94] Similar studies have shown that virtually all banded fibers in several human tissues are composed of type I and type III molecules.[95] Since a substantial proportion of type III as well as type V molecules retain their N-terminal propeptide sequences while resident in fibrous elements, it is tempting to speculate that fiber diameter is regulated at least in part by the proportion of participating molecules that retain their N-terminal propeptide sequences. Similarly, it is possible that fiber diameter in hyaline cartilages is regulated by the presence of varying proportions of type II and type XI collagen molecules with the latter collagen serving as the relatively minor component and retaining its N-terminal propeptide sequences. However, chemical data on the nature and location of covalent crosslinks between type IX and type II collagen (see preceding discussion)[64] as well as rotary shadowing and ultrastructural localization studies[96] indicate that type IX molecules are present on the surfaces of cartilage collagen fibers and are placed there in a periodic manner as depicted in Figure 8–5E. As noted in the figure, the relatively large N-terminal globular domain of the type IX molecule is directed away from the surface of the fiber by virtue of a distinct bend at a site of helix interruption in the collagenous domain. The presence of type IX adducts in the indicated locations would certainly inhibit the addition of further type II and type XI molecules and therefore serve to define and limit fiber diameter. It is also possible that type IX molecules are synthesized following attainment of the maximal fiber size and then placed at fiber surfaces for the purpose of facilitating interactions of the cartilage collagen fibers with other constituents of the extracellular matrix. Further work will be necessary to fully discern the nature of the potential roles played by type IX collagen. These considerations also apply to type XII collagen, which, as noted, is likely to have several structural features in common with type IX collagen and therefore serve similar functions in noncartilaginous tissues.

Although the foregoing discussion has underscored the limitations of current knowledge of fiber orientation and size regulation, these control mechanisms are of utmost importance in determining connective tissue integrity and function. In this regard, fiber orientation and diameter are, in large part, responsible for determining the mechanical properties of a given tissue.[97] The ability to withstand and recover from plastic deformation, for instance, can be correlated with a more or less random orientation of small diameter fibrils. In this situation, the area of contact between fibril surface and surrounding matrix is maximized. At the other extreme of the functional spectrum, the ability to resist high tensile stress can be correlated with the presence of large-diameter fibers running, for the most part, in the direction of the stress line. It seems apparent, then, that a wide variety of functional capabilities may be attained in a number of tissues by a judicious mixture of fiber sizes as well as appropriate orientation of the different fibers.

Aggregates of Type IV Collagen. Initial concepts concerning the nature of the aggregates formed by type IV collagen were formulated on the basis of ultrastructural observations on the protein extracted from a basement membrane–producing mouse tumor.[98] The model resulting from these studies proposed a basic tetrameric unit formed by association of four molecules at their N-terminal ends. Such tetrameric units were then envisioned to be linked via interaction sites in the noncollagenous globular domain at the ends of the tetramer arms. The model thus suggested that type IV molecules formed aggregates largely through end-to-end associations that resulted in the formation of an open meshlike network deemed suitable for structural support of basement membrane sheaths. Subsequent work has considerably refined this model of the molecular architecture of type IV collagen aggregates. In general, these studies have shown that end-to-end contacts are indeed crucial to the formation and maintenance of type IV aggregates but that lateral contacts between the molecules are quite prevalent. Thus, rotary-shadowed replicas of type IV collagen aggregates formed in vitro clearly show them to be composed largely of interconnected polygons, the sides of which are often more than one triple-helical strand thick and the vertices of which are commonly occupied by dimers of the C-terminal globular domains.[99] Subsequent studies in which the molecular architecture of type IV collagen aggregates was evaluated at the ultrastructural level in situ have shown the presence of an extensive irregular polygonal network similar to that observed in the earlier in vitro reconstitution experiments.[100] The precise manner in which these aggregates are formed is, as yet, unknown. However, recent studies demonstrating that the noncollagenous C-terminal globular domain of the type IV molecule binds specifically at distinct locations along the type IV molecule[101] suggests a scheme similar to that depicted in Figure 8–6A. In this model, dimers formed by union of two monomer type IV molecules at their C-terminal globular domains associate to form a tetramer. The latter is produced as the result of the tendency for globular domains to associate with discrete regions of the triple-helical domain, and this factor governs the axial displacement of the dimers relative to each other. It should be noted that this type of association also requires that, for a certain portion of their length, adjacent molecules are oriented in an antiparallel fashion. Eventually, addition of further dimers using the same principle of association could produce a polygonal structure exemplified by the hexagon depicted in Figure 8–6A. The hexagon has a dimer of C-terminal globular domains located at each of its vertices. Moreover, the N-terminal portion of each participating molecule protrudes from a vertex and is potentially available for complex formation with like segments from other polyg-

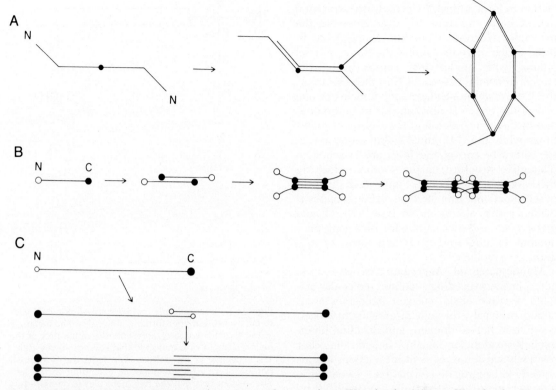

Figure 8–6. Proposed modes of aggregate formation on the part of type IV molecules *(A)*, type VI molecules *(B)*, and type VII molecules *(C)*. N and C denote N-terminus and C-terminus, respectively. Open circles represent N-terminal globular domains while closed circles represent C-terminal globular domains.

onal structures. In this fashion, then, three-dimensional networks of type IV molecules could be formed, fulfilling the structural and support requirements of basement membranes. In view of the complex nature of type IV collagen aggregates, it may be anticipated that several refinements in current information concerning these structures will be made in subsequent years.

Aggregates of Type VI Collagen. Data on the molecular architecture of aggregates formed by type VI molecules are also initially obtained through ultrastructural observations on rotary-shadowed preparations of the collagen.[57] These investigations indicated that the end product of type VI collagen polymerization was likely to be a microfibril formed by end-to-end association of tetrameric units. Formation of the microfibrils was envisioned to occur as depicted in Figure 8–6B. It involves assembly of monomers to dimers in which the triple-helical domains of participating molecules assume a staggered antiparallel alignment. Although not shown in this representation, the ultrastructural data indicated that molecules in each dimer were intertwined in the helical overlap zone. Lateral alignment of dimers produces tetramers

that are then polymerized through the formation of scissorlike structures involving crossover sites in the nonoverlapping positions of triple-helical domains. It is of interest that type VI molecules are apparently assembled as tetramers intracellularly and secreted in the latter form.[102] These findings again underscore the potential role of direct cellular involvement in the early events leading to the construction of extracellular collagenous aggregates.

The biological role of type VI collagen aggregates remains undefined. As a first approximation, it may be assumed that their structural or support role is similar, if not identical, to that of the smaller diameter fibrils formed from the fiber-forming collagens. In any event, the microfibrillar elements derived from type VI collagen molecules represent a highly significant proportion of the collagen in several connective tissues,[53] including cartilagenous structures.[103, 104]

Aggregates of Type VII Collagen. Type VII molecules aggregate in a unique manner to form relatively short polymers approximating the length of two monomer molecules as depicted in Figure 8–6C. In this case, antiparallel monomers overlap by about 60 nm at their N-terminal ends to form dimers that lose their N-terminal globular domains prior to lateral association to form a fibril.[68] Current ultrastructural data indicate that type VII aggregates are the principle structural elements of anchoring fibrils, which serve to stabilize the union of basal lamina with underlying connective tissue stroma in several tissues.[105, 106] In these locations the C-terminal noncollagenous domains at one end of the type VII fibril appear to be embedded in the lamina densa of the basement membrane while the C-terminal globular domains at the alternate end of the fibril are attached to plaquelike structures in the stroma underlying the basement membrane. Supporting this proposed functional role for type VII aggregates is evidence that alterations in type VII collagen metabolism are associated with blistering phenomena encountered in certain forms of epidermolysis bullosa.[107]

Maintenance of Aggregate Structure. As noted in the preceding sections, molecular stability of triple chain collagen molecules is attained primarily through interchain hydrogen bonding in helical domains and disulfide bonding in large globular domains. In addition, other relatively weak noncovalent interactions are involved in aggregate formation. Eventually, however, aggregate structures are stabilized by covalent bonding involving intermolecular lysine-derived crosslinks as well as disulfide bonds. Lysine-derived crosslinks constitute the most prevalent form of intermolecular linkage for the fiber-forming collagens.[9] These linkages are formed primarily in the locations illustrated in Figure 8–7, which presents a more detailed view of the head-to-tail contact sites between two molecules in a linear polymer (Fig. 8–5B) or in a growing fiber (Fig. 8–5C). The crosslinks shown here are (1) a Schiff base crosslink formed by condensation of an oxidatively deaminated lysyl residue in position 9 of an N-terminal telopeptide with a helical hydroxylysyl residue in position 930 in an adjacent molecule; and (2) a keto-amine crosslink formed by condensation of an oxidatively deaminated hydroxylysyl residue in position 16 of a C-terminal telopeptide with a helical hydroxylysyl residue in position 87. The initial condensation product in the latter type of crosslink is likewise a Schiff base, but it may undergo an internal oxidation-reduction reaction (Amadori rearrangement) to give the resultant keto-amine configuration shown in Figure 8–7. The system of crosslinks established by condensations of this nature ultimately serves to attach each molecule at both its head and tail region to neighboring molecules and thereby provides the physical stability required for fiber function. As noted above, other mole-

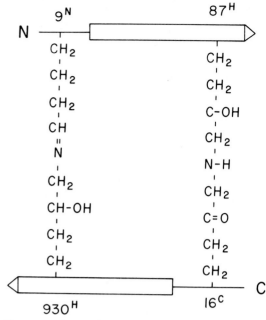

Figure 8–7. Intermolecular covalent crosslinking at head-to-tail overlaps of fiber-forming molecules. The rectangle at the top of the figure represents the initial part of the helical domain of a molecule that extends to the right. The rectangle at the bottom represents the C-terminal portion of an adjacent molecule extending to the left. The overlap between the two molecules juxtaposes two crosslink sites in each molecule and the crosslinks are formed as shown.

cules such as type IX collagen are apparently stabilized on the surfaces of fibers by similar types of linkages.

With respect to the other forms of aggregation, intermolecular disulfide bonding plays a major role. Thus, both lysine-derived crosslinks and disulfide bonds are likely to be involved in stabilizing N-terminal associations in type IV aggregates,[46] while interactions of the C-terminal globular domains of these molecules are apparently stabilized through disulfide linkages.[108] As far as is known, only disulfide bonding is utilized in stabilizing aggregates of type VI and VII collagens.

IMPLICATIONS FOR WOUND HEALING

As discussed previously, the collagenous scaffold of the extracellular matrix comprises at least 13 genetically distinct types of collagen. Most of the latter have just recently been discovered and the current literature concerning the role of the different collagen types in the pathophysiology of tissue repair is rather limited and confined to collagen types I through

V. Therefore, none of the available data on wound healing refer to the complex events involving all currently known collagens and associated noncollagenous matrix components. Those who have described the fibrillar components involved in wound healing have confined their attention either to the repair of interstitial stroma, such as types I and III collagen in dermis and type II collagen in cartilage, or to the remodeling of basement membrane in epidermal lesions.

With respect to collagen neosynthesis and deposition in normal wound repair, type III collagen was demonstrated at the earliest phase.[109] Immunologically detectable type III collagen and procollagen were detected 24 to 48 hours after surgical procedures in children. From 72 hours onward, a substantial increase in type I collagen was associated with the appearance of mature wound fibroblasts. Subsequent studies on the relative rates of collagen synthesis have extended these observations in a rat model by showing that the relative rate of type III collagen synthesis is increased (about 30 percent of the total) as early as 10 hours after the start of wound healing in skin.[110] By 24 hours, the percentage of type III collagen had returned to the normal value of 20 percent. In previous studies, it was reported that granulation tissue in rats contains significantly higher levels of type III collagen than normal skin.[111] The early appearance of collagen type III was further demonstrated to be associated with the deposition of fibronectin,[112, 113] which together may provide the initial scaffold for subsequent healing events. In other studies, an increase in the amount of type V collagen over the first 21 days was reported in experimental rat granulation tissue.[114] These authors concluded that the observed increase in type V collagen parallels the development of capillaries and suggest that type V collagen may be involved in the migration and movement of capillary endothelial cells during angiogenesis.

The early appearance of type III collagen in tissue repair was further documented in an experimental fracture healing model in rat bone.[115] The data show that during the first week of fracture repair, type III collagen mRNA is increased to the greatest extent, followed by type II collagen mRNA during the second week. The production of type II collagen in this type of wound repair appears to be associated with the presence of cartilaginous islets within the callus.[116] The latter is unique to bone healing in that only under the influence of certain bone growth factors does a transient deposition of type II collagen occur. On the other hand, a persistent deposition of type II collagen may occur under special circumstances such as in healing of certain surgically induced defects in hyaline articular cartilage.[117] In general, the connective tissue reaction to injury eventually leads to the appearance of increased numbers of fibroblasts and finally to the accumulation of numerous rather large fibrils derived from type I collagen molecules. Ultimately, the rather acellular but fiber-rich scar tissue contains predominantly fibrils derived from type I collagen molecules.[116]

With respect to the repair of epidermal basement membranes, it has been demonstrated in healing of primate skin that the sequence of deposition of collagen type IV and noncollagenous basement membrane components (i.e., laminin and lamina densa antigen (LDA-1)) followed that observed in the ontogeny of normal human skin.[118] Other studies concerning the reconstitution of skin basement membrane in swine have shown that noncollagenous matrix components such as bullous pemphigoid antigen reappear prior to collagen type IV.[119] Despite the fact that type IV collagen forms the scaffold of basement membranes and the reconstitution of the collagenous network composed of type IV collagen molecules represents a hallmark of normal epidermal wound healing, other collagenous matrix components are equally important. In this regard it has been emphasized that the synchronous appearance of collagen type VII containing anchoring fibrils and hemidesmosomes is essential for linking epithelium and underlying interstitial connective tissue.[120]

In light of the comprehensive reviews of the role of collagenous matrix in organ-specific tissue repair provided in subsequent chapters, the cited examples may only illustrate the pivotal structural role of collagens in all processes concerning wound healing and tissue repair. However, it is obvious that in view of the rapidly accumulating information on the nature and structure of the distinct collagen types, knowledge about the intricate interaction and regulation of the various components of connective tissue matrix is rather limited. Models of the design and construction of collagen-containing biomaterials should be based on the latest information concerning the biochemistry and nature of these matrix macromolecules. To this end, consideration should be made of the physiological proportions of "major" and "minor" collagens and noncollagenous matrix components in the native condition, and these factors should provide the basis for fabrication of biomaterials.

References

1. Kilcherr E, Hofmann H, Steigemann W, et al: Structural model of the collagen-like region of Clq comprising the kink region and the fibre-like packing of the six triple helices. J Mol Biol 186:403, 1985.
2. Mays C, Rosenberry TL: Characterization of pepsin-resistant collagen-like tail subunit fragments of 18S and 14S acetylcholinesterase from *Electrophorus electricus*. Biochemistry 20:2810, 1981.
3. Benson B, Hawgood S, Schilling J, et al: Structure of canine pulmonary surfactant apoprotein: cDNA and complete amino acid sequence. Proc Natl Acad Sci USA 82:6379, 1985.
4. Floros J, Steinbrink R, Jacobs K, et al: Isolation and characterization of cDNA clones for the 35-kDa pulmonary surfactant–associated protein. J Biol Chem 261:9029, 1986.
5. Drickamer K, Dordal MS, Reynolds L: Mannose-binding proteins isolated from rat liver contain carbohydrate-recognition domains linked to collagenous tails. J Biol Chem 261:6878, 1986.
6. Miller EJ: Biochemical characteristics and biological significance of the genetically-distinct collagens. Mol Cell Biochem 13:165, 1976.
7. Bornstein P, Sage H: Structurally distinct collagen types. Ann Rev Biochem 49:957, 1980.
8. Miller EJ, Gay S: Collagen: An overview. Methods Enzymol 82A:3, 1982.
9. Miller EJ: Chemistry of the collagens and their distribution. In Piez KA, Reddi AH (eds): Extracellular Matrix Biochemistry. New York, Elsevier, 1984, p 41.
10. Mayne R, Burgeson RE (eds): The structure and function of collagen types. Orlando, Academic Press, 1987.
11. Miller EJ, Gay S: The collagens: An overview/update. Methods Enzymol 144:3, 1987.
12. Dixit R, Harrison MW, Dixit SN: Isolation and partial characterization of a novel basement membrane collagen. Biochem Biophys Res Commun 130:1, 1985.
13. Butkowski RJ, Langeveld JPM, Wieslander J, et al: Localization of the Goodpasture epitope to a novel chain of basement membrane collagen. J Biol Chem 262:7874, 1987.
14. Hostikka SL, Eddy RL, Byers MG, et al: Identification of a distinct type IV collagen α chain with restricted kidney distribution and assignment of its gene to the locus of X chromosome-linked Alport syndrome. Proc Natl Acad Sci USA 87:1606, 1990.
15. Kapoor R, Bornstein P, Sage EH: Type VIII collagen from bovine Descemet's membrane: Structural characterization of a triple-helical domain. Biochemistry 25:3930, 1986.
16. Benya PD, Padilla SR: Isolation and characterization of type VIII collagen synthesized by cultured rabbit corneal endothelial cells. J Biol Chem 261:4160, 1986.
17. Yamaguchi N, Benya PD, van der Rest M, et al: The cloning and sequencing of α1(VIII) collagen cDNAs demonstrate that type VIII collagen is a short chain collagen and contains triple-helical and carboxyl-terminal non–triple-helical domains similar to those of type X collagen. J Biol Chem 264:16022, 1989.
18. Pihlajaniemi T, Myllylä R, Seyer J, et al: Partial characterization of a low molecular weight human collagen that undergoes alternative splicing. Proc Natl Acad Sci USA 84:940, 1987.
19. Tikka L, Pihlajaniemi T, Henttu P, et al: Gene structure for the α1 chain of a human short-chain collagen (type XIII) with alternatively spliced transcripts and translation termination codon at the 5′ end of the last exon. Proc Natl Acad Sci USA 85:7491, 1988.
20. Bowcock AM, Hebert JM, Wijsman E, et al: High recombination between two physically close human basement membrane collagen genes at the distal end of chromosome 13q. Proc Natl Acad Sci USA 85:2701, 1988.
21. Tanzer MA, Kimura S: Phylogenetic aspects of collagen structure and function. In Nimni ME (ed): Collagen, vol II. Boca Raton, FL, CRC Press, 1988, p 25.
22. Kelly J, Tanaka S, Hardt T, et al: Fibril-forming collagen in lamprey. J Biol Chem 263:980, 1988.
23. Kimura S, Takema Y, Kubota M: Octopus skin collagen. J Biol Chem 256:13230, 1981.
24. Miller EJ: The structure of fibril-forming collagens. Ann NY Acad Sci 406:1, 1985.
25. Doege KJ, Fessler JH: Folding of carboxyl domain and assembly of procollagen I. J Biol Chem 261:8924, 1986.
26. Dion AS, Myers JC: COOH-terminal propeptides of the major human procollagens. J Mol Biol 193:127, 1987.
27. Kivirikko KI, Myllylä R: Biosynthesis of the collagens. In Piez KA, Reddi AH (eds): Extracellular Matrix Biochemistry. New York, Elsevier, 1984, p 83.
28. Pihlajaniemi T, Dickson LA, Pope FM, et al: Osteogenesis imperfecta: Cloning of a pro-α2(I) collagen gene with a frameshift mutation. J Biol Chem 259:12941, 1984.
29. Fisher LW, Robey PG, Tuross N, et al: The M_r 24,000 phosphoprotein from developing bone is the NH$_2$-terminal propeptide of the α1 chain of type I collagen. J Biol Chem 262:13457, 1987.
30. Van der Rest M, Rosenberg LC, Olsen BR, et al: Chondrocalcin is identical with the C-propeptide of type II procollagen. Biochem J 237:923, 1986.
31. Wiestner M, Krieg T, Hörlein D, et al: Inhibiting effect of procollagen peptides on collagen biosynthesis in fibroblast cultures. J Biol Chem 254:7016, 1979.
32. Aycock RS, Raghow R, Stricklin GP, et al: Post-transcriptional inhibition of collagen and fibronectin synthesis by a synthetic homolog of a portion of the carboxyl-terminal propeptide of human type I collagen. J Biol Chem 261:14355, 1986.
33. Goldenberg R, Fine RE: Generalized inhibition of cell-free translation by the amino-terminal propeptide of chick type I procollagen. Biochim Biophys Acta 826:101, 1985.
34. Wu CH, Donovan CB, Wu GY: Evidence for pretranslational regulation of collagen synthesis by procollagen propeptides. J Biol Chem 261:10482, 1986.
35. Poole AR, Pidoux I, Reiner A, et al: Association of an extracellular protein (chondrocalcin) with the calcification of cartilage in endochondral bone formation. J Cell Biol 98:54, 1984.
36. Niyibizi C, Wu J-J, Eyre DR: The carboxypeptide trimer of type II collagen is a prominent component of immature cartilages and intervertebral-disc tissue. Biochim Biophys Acta 916:493, 1987.
37. Helseth DL Jr, Veis A: Collagen self-assembly *in vitro*. J Biol Chem 256:7118, 1981.
38. Capaldi MJ, Chapman JA: The C-terminal extrahelical peptide of type I collagen and its role in fibrillogenesis *in vitro*. Biopolymers 21:2291, 1982.
39. Helseth DL Jr, Lechner JH, Veis A: Role of the amino-terminal extrahelical region of type I collagen in directing the 4D overlap in fibrillogenesis. Biopolymers 18:3005, 1979.
40. Jones EY, Miller A: Structural models for the N- and C-terminal telopeptide regions of interstitial collagens. Biopolymers 26:463, 1987.

41. Otter A, Scott PG, Kotovych G: Type I collagen α-1 chain C-telopeptide: Solution structure determined by 600-MHz proton NMR spectroscopy and implications for its role in collagen fibrillogenesis. Biochemistry 27:3560, 1988.
42. Brazel D, Oberbäumer I, Dieringer H, et al: Completion of the amino acid sequence of the α1 chain of human basement membrane collagen (type IV) reveals 21 non-triplet interruptions located within the collagenous domain. Eur J Biochem 168:529, 1987.
43. Soininen R, Haka-Risku T, Prockop DJ, et al: Complete primary structure of the α1-chain of human basement membrane (type IV) collagen. FEB 225:188, 1987.
44. Brazel D, Pollner R, Oberbäumer I, Kühn K: Human basement membrane collagen (type IV). Eur J Biochem 172:35, 1988.
45. Hostikka SL, Tryggvason K: The complete primary structure of the α2 chain of human type IV collagen and comparison with the α1(IV) chain. J Biol Chem 263:19488, 1988.
46. Glanville RW, Qian R, Siebold B, et al: Amino acid sequence of the N-terminal aggregation and cross-linking region (7S domain) of the α1(IV) chain of human basement membrane collagen. Eur J Biochem 152:213, 1985.
47. Seibold B, Qian R, Glanville RW, et al: Construction of a model for the aggregation and cross-linking region (7S domain) of type IV collagen based upon an evaluation of the primary structure of the α1 and α2 chains in this region. Eur J Biochem 168:569, 1987.
48. Pihlajaniemi T, Tryggvason K, Myers JC, et al: cDNA clones coding for the pro-α1(IV) chain of human type IV procollagen reveal an unusual homology of amino acid sequences in two halves of the carboxyl-terminal domain. J Biol Chem 260:7681, 1985.
49. Fessler LI, Duncan KG, Fessler JH, et al: Characterization of the procollagen IV cleavage products produced by a specific tumor collagenase. J Biol Chem 259:9783, 1984.
50. Trüeb B, Winterhalter KH: Type VI collagen is composed of a 200 kd subunit and two 140 kd subunits. EMBO J 5:2815, 1986.
51. Schreier T, Winterhalter KH, Trüeb B: The tissue form of chicken type VI collagen. FEB 213:319, 1987.
52. Chu ML, Pan T, Conway D, et al: Sequence analysis of α1(VI) and α2(VI) chains of human type VI collagen reveals internal triplication of globular domains similar to the A domains of von Willebrand factor and two α2(VI) chain variants that differ in the carboxy terminus. EMBO J 8:1939, 1989.
53. Trüeb B, Schreier T, Bruckner P, et al: Type VI collagen represents a major fraction of connective tissue collagens. Eur J Biochem 166:699, 1987.
54. Bonaldo P, Russo V, Bucciotti F, et al: Structural and functional features of the α3 chain indicate a bridging role for chicken collagen VI in connective tissues. Biochemistry 29:1245, 1990.
55. Chu M-L, Zhang R-Z, Pan T, et al: Mosaic structure of globular domains in human type VI collagen α3 chain: Similarity to von Willebrand factor fibronectin, actin, salivary proteins and aprotinin type protease inhibitors. EMBO J 9:385, 1990.
56. Colombatti A, Ainger K, Colizzi F: Type VI collagen: High yields of a molecule with multiple forms of α3 chain from avian and human tissues. Matrix 9:177, 1989.
57. Furthmayr W, Wiedemann H, Timpl R, et al: Electron microscopical approach to a structural model of intima collagen. Biochem J 211:303, 1983.
58. Ninomiya Y, Olsen BR: Synthesis and characterization of cDNA encoding a cartilage-specific short collagen. Proc Natl Acad Sci USA 81:3014, 1984.
59. Vasios G, Nishimura I, Konomi H, et al: Cartilage type IX collagen-proteoglycan contains a large amino-terminal globular domain encoded by multiple exons. J Biol Chem 263:2324, 1988.
60. Ninomiya Y, van der Rest M, Mayne R, et al: Construction and characterization of cDNA encoding the α2 chain of chicken type IX collagen. Biochemistry 24:4223, 1985.
61. Nishimura I, Muragaki Y, Olsen BR: Tissue-specific forms of type IX collagen-proteoglycan arise from the use of two widely separated promoters. J Biol Chem 264:20033, 1989.
62. McCormick D, van der Rest M, Goodship J, et al: Structure of the glycosaminoglycan domain in the type IX collagen-proteoglycan. Proc Natl Acad Sci USA 84:4044, 1987.
63. Huber S, Winterhalter KH, Vaughan L: Isolation and sequence analysis of the glycosaminoglycan attachment site of type IX collagen. J Biol Chem 263:752, 1988.
64. Van der Rest M, Mayne R: Type IX collagen proteoglycan from cartilage is covalently cross-linked to type II collagen. J Biol Chem 263:1615, 1988.
65. Ninomiya Y, Gordon M, van der Rest M, et al: The developmentally regulated type X collagen gene contains a long open reading frame without introns. J Biol Chem 261:5041, 1986.
66. Lunstrum GP, Sakai LY, Keene DR, et al: Large complex globular domains of type VII procollagen contribute to the structure of anchoring fibrils. J Biol Chem 261:9042, 1986.
67. Bentz H, Morris NP, Murray LW, et al: Isolation and partial characterization of a new human collagen with an extended triple-helical structural domain. Proc Natl Acad Sci USA 80:3168, 1983.
68. Lunstrum GP, Kuo H-J, Rosenbaum LM, et al: Anchoring fibrils contain the carboxyl-terminal globular domain of type VII procollagen, but lack the amino-terminal globular domain. J Biol Chem 262:13706, 1987.
69. Gordon MK, Gerecke DR, Olsen BR: Type XII collagen: Distinct extracellular matrix component discovered by cDNA cloning. Proc Natl Acad Sci USA 84:6040, 1987.
70. Dublet B, Oh S, Sugrue SP, et al: The structure of avian type XII collagen. α1(XII) chains contain 190-kDa non-triple helical amino-terminal domains and form homotrimeric molecules. J Biol Chem 264:13150, 1989.
71. Gordon MK, Gerecke DR, Dublet B, et al: Type XII collagen. A large multidomain molecule with partial homology to type IX collagen. J Biol Chem 264:19772, 1989.
72. Koivu J, Myllylä R: Interchain disulfide bond formation in types I and II procollagen. J Biol Chem 262:6159, 1987.
73. Koivu J, Myllylä R, Helaakoski T, et al: A single polypeptide acts both as the β subunit of prolyl 4-hydroxylase and as a protein disulfide-isomerase. J Biol Chem 262:6447, 1987.
74. Tsou C-L: Folding of the nascent peptide chain into a biologically active protein. Biochemistry 27:1809, 1988.
75. Bächinger HP, Bruckner P, Timpl R, et al: Folding mechanism of the triple helix in type-III collagen and type-III pN-collagen. Eur J Biochem 106:619, 1980.
76. Sarkar SK, Young PE, Sullivan CE, et al: Detection of cis and trans X-Pro peptide bonds in proteins by ^{13}C NMR: Application to collagen. Proc Natl Acad Sci USA 81:4800, 1984.

77. Bruckner P, Eikenberry EF: Formation of the triple helix of type I procollagen in cellulo. Eur J Biochem 140:391, 1984.
78. Bächinger HP: The influence of peptidyl-prolyl cis-trans isomerase on the in vitro folding of type III collagen. J Biol Chem 262:17144, 1987.
79. Ramachandran GN: Stereochemistry of collagen. Int J Peptide Protein Res 31:1, 1988.
80. Hofmann H, Voss T, Kühn K, et al: Localization of flexible sites in thread-like molecules from electron micrographs. J Mol Biol 172:325, 1984.
81. Silver FH, Birk DE: Molecular structure of collagen in solution: Comparison of types I, II, III and V. Int J Biol Macromol 6:125, 1984.
82. Birk DE, Silver FH: Molecular structure and physical properties of type IV collagen in solution. Int J Biol Macromol 9:7, 1987.
83. Irwin MH, Silvers SH, Mayne R: Monoclonal antibody against chicken type IX collagen: Preparation, characterization, and recognition of the intact form of type IX collagen secreted by chondrocytes. J Cell Biol 101:814, 1985.
84. Silver FH, Langley KH, Trelstad RL: Type I collagen fibrillogenesis: Invitation via reversible linear and lateral growth steps. Biopolymers 18:2523, 1979.
85. Fleischmajer R, Timpl R, Tuderman L, et al: Ultrastructural identification of extension aminopropeptides of type I and III collagens in human skin. Proc Natl Acad Sci USA 78:7360, 1981.
86. Fleischmajer R, Olsen BR, Timpl R, et al: Collagen fibril formation during embryogenesis. Proc Natl Acad Sci USA 80:3354, 1983.
87. Fleischmajer R, Perlish JS, Olsen BR: Amino and carboxyl propeptides in bone collagen fibrils during embryogenesis. Cell Tissue Res 247:105, 1987.
88. Fleischmajer R, Perlish JS, Olsen BR: The carboxyl-propeptide of type I procollagen in skin fibrillogenesis. J Invest Dermatol 89:212, 1987.
89. Ruggiero F, Pfäffle M, von der Mark K, et al: Retention of carboxypropeptides in type-II collagen fibrils in chick embryo chondrocyte cultures. Cell Tissue Res 252:619, 1988.
90. Kadler KE, Hojima Y, Prockop DJ: Assembly of collagen fibrils de novo by cleavage of the type I pC-collagen with procollagen C-proteinase. J Biol Chem 262:15696, 1987.
91. Piez KA, Trus BL: Sequence regularities and packing of collagen molecules. J Mol Biol 122:419, 1978.
92. Hofmann H, Fietzek PP, Kühn K: The role of polar and hydrophobic interactions for the molecular packing of type I collagen: A three-dimensional evaluation of the amino acid sequence. J Mol Biol 125:137, 1978.
93. Birk DE, Trelstad RL: Extracellular compartments in tendon morphogenesis: Collagen fibril, bundle, and macroaggregate formation. J Cell Biol 103:231, 1986.
94. Birk DE, Fitch JM, Babiarz JP, et al: Collagen type I and type V are present in the same fibril in the avian corneal stroma. J Cell Biol 106:999, 1988.
95. Keene DR, Sakai LY, Bachinger H-P, et al: Type III collagen can be present on banded collagen fibrils regardless of fibril diameter. J Cell Biol 105:2393, 1987.
96. Vaughan L, Mendler M, Huber S, et al: D-periodic distribution of collagen type IX along cartilage fibrils. J Cell Biol 106:991, 1988.
97. Parry DAD: The molecular and fibrillar structure of collagen and its relationship to the mechanical properties of connective tissue. Biophys Chem 29:195, 1988.
98. Weber S, Engel J, Wiedemann H, et al: Subunit structure and assembly of the globular domain of basement-membrane collagen type IV. Eur J Biochem 139:401, 1984.
99. Yurchenco PD, Furthmayr H: Self-assembly of basement membrane collagen. Biochemistry 23:1839, 1984.
100. Yurchenco PD, Ruben GC: Basement membrane structure in situ: Evidence for lateral associations in the type IV collagen network. J Cell Biol 105:2559, 1987.
101. Tsilibary EC, Charonis AS: The role of the main noncollagenous domain (NC1) in type IV collagen self-assembly. J Cell Biol 103:2467, 1986.
102. Engvall E, Hessle H, Klier G: Molecular assembly, secretion, and matrix deposition of type VI collagen. J Cell Biol 102:703, 1986.
103. Wu J-J, Eyre DR, Slayter HS: Type VI collagen of the intervertebral disc. Biochem J 248:373, 1987.
104. Poole CA, Ayad S, Schofield JR: Chondrons from articular cartilage: I. Immunolocalization of type VI collagen in the pericellular capsule of isolated canine tibial chondrons. J Cell Sci 90:635, 1988.
105. Sakai LY, Keene DR, Morris NP, et al: Type VII collagen is a major structural component of anchoring fibrils. J Cell Biol 103:1577, 1986.
106. Keene DR, Sakai LY, Lunstrum GP, et al: Type VII collagen forms an extended network of anchoring fibrils. J Cell Biol 104:611, 1987.
107. Leigh IM, Eady RAJ, Heagerty AHM, et al: Type VII collagen is a normal component of epidermal basement membrane, which shows altered expression in recessive dystrophic epidermolysis bullosa. J Invest Dermatol 90:639, 1988.
108. Siebold B, Deutzmann R, Kühn K: The arrangement of intra- and intermolecular disulfide bonds in the carboxyterminal, non-collagenous aggregation and cross-linking domain of basement-membrane type IV collagen. Eur J Biochem 176:617, 1988.
109. Gay S, Viljanto J, Raekallio J, et al: Collagen types in early phases of wound healing in children. Acta Chir Scand 144:205, 1978.
110. Clore JN, Cohen IK, Diegelmann RF: Quantitation of the collagen types I and III during wound healing in rat skin (40548). Proc Soc Exp Biol Med 161:337, 1979.
111. Bailey AJ, Sims TJ, LeLous M, et al: Collagen polymorphism in experimental granulation tissue. Biochem Biophys Res Commun 66:1160, 1975.
112. Kurkinen M, Vaheri A, Roberts PJ, et al: Sequential appearance of fibronectin and collagen in experimental granulation tissue. Lab Invest 43:47, 1980.
113. Grinnell F, Billingham RE, Burgess L: Distribution of fibronectin during wound healing in vivo. J Invest Dermatol 76:181, 1981.
114. Hering TM, Marchant RE, Anderson JM: Type V collagen during granulation tissue development. Exp Mol Pathol 39:219, 1983.
115. Multimäki P, Aro H, Vuorio E: Differential expression of fibrillar collagen genes during callus formation. Biochem Biophys Res Commun 142:536, 1987.
116. Gay S, Miller EJ: Collagen in the Physiology and Pathology of Connective Tissue. Stuttgart-New York, Fischer, 1978, p 75.
117. Cheung HS, Lynch KL, Johnson RP, et al: In vitro synthesis of tissue-specific type II collagen by healing cartilage. Arthritis Rheum 23:211, 1980.
118. Fine J-D: Antigenic features and structural correlates of basement membranes. Arch Dermatol 124:713, 1988.
119. Stanley JR, Alvarez OM, Bere EW Jr, et al: Detection of basement membrane zone antigens during epidermal wound healing in pigs. J Invest Dermatol 77:240, 1981.

120. Gipson IK, Spurr-Michaud SJ, Tisdale AS: Hemidesmosomes and anchoring fibril collagen appear synchronously during development and wound healing. Develop Biol 126:253, 1988.

121. Myers JC, Emanuel BS: Chromosomal localization of human collagen genes. Collagen Rel Res 7:149, 1987.

122. Weil D, Mattei M-G, Passage E, et al: Cloning and chromosomal localization of human genes encoding the three chains of type VI collagen. Am J Hum Genet 42:435, 1988.

123. Kimura T, Mattei M-G, Stevens JW, et al: Molecular cloning of rat and human type IX collagen cDNA and localization of the $\alpha 1$(IX) gene on the human chromosome 6. Eur J Biochem 179:71, 1989.

124. Law ML, Chan SDH, Berger R, et al. The gene for the $\alpha 2$ chain of the human fibrillar collagen type XI (COL 11A2) assigned to the short arm of chromosome 6. Ann Hum Genet 54:23, 1990.

9

BIOSYNTHETIC AND GENETIC DISORDERS OF COLLAGEN

Charlotte Phillips, Ph.D., and Richard J. Wenstrup, M.D.

The previous chapter examined the structural features of collagen and how these may be related to its physiological functions. This chapter presents information on biochemical and molecular processes involved in collagen biosynthesis and how genetic alterations affect the expression of this protein.

COLLAGEN BIOSYNTHESIS

Collagen biosynthesis is remarkably complex, requiring coordinated transcription of genes on different chromosomes and several intracellular and extracellular post-translational modifications. Most of the modifications, such as the hydroxylations of proline and lysine residues, glycosylation of hydroxylysine, folding of the proα collagen chains into triple helical formation, and ordered aggregation into fibrils, are unique to collagen and collagen-like sequences. The following sections describe collagen biosynthesis beginning with gene transcription and proceeding through fibril formation (Fig. 9–1).

Nuclear Events

Collagen Gene Structure

Collagen genes (reviewed in reference 1), like most other eukaryotic genes, are not con-tinuous; the regions of the DNA that are ultimately translated into amino acids are called exons and are interrupted by intervening DNA sequences called introns. The organization of fibrillar collagen genes, that is, the size and number of exons, is quite similar and strongly suggests a common evolutionary origin (Fig. 9–2).[2] The standard nomenclature for the collagen genes is as follows: proα1(I), COL1A1; proα2(I), COL1A2; proα1(III), COL3A1; and so on. The type I collagen genes, COL1A1 and COL1A2, have 52 exons, of which 42 (7 through 48) comprise the triple helical domain. Exons 6 and 48 are transition exons, containing coding sequences for both triple helical and non–triple helical regions and containing coding sequences for the proteolytic cleavage sites of the amino- and carboxyl-terminal propeptides.[3,4] Exon sizes of the triple helical domain follow a very distinct pattern, either 54 or 54_n-9 base pairs (bp), with 45, 54, 99, and 108 being the most common sizes.[5] The repetitious pattern of the triple helical domain of collagen supports the theory that the triple helical domain evolved by tandem duplication of a 54 bp ancestor element.[2] The sizes of specific exons are highly conserved among types I, II, and III within a given species and across a broad spectrum of species. The differences in the sizes of the genes can be accounted for by differences in their intron sizes. COL1A1 and COL1A2 are 18 and 38 kilobases long, respectively, and both COL2A1 and COL3A1 are approximately 40 kilobases long.[5–9]

The nonfibrillar collagen genes are similar in

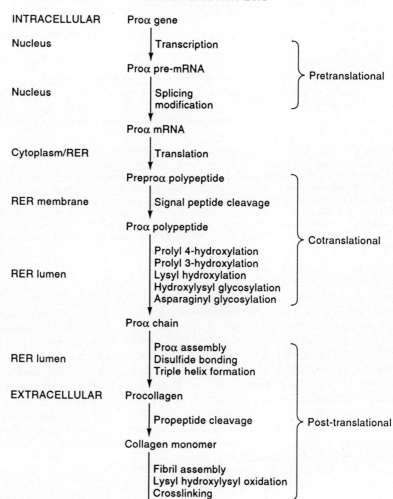

Figure 9–1. Steps in the biosynthesis of a collagen fiber and the location in the cell where they occur. RER = rough endoplasmic reticulum. (Adapted with permission from Wenstrup RJ, Murad S, Pinnell SR: Collagen. In Goldsmith LA (ed): Biochemistry and Physiology of the Skin, 2nd ed. New York, Oxford University Press (In Press)).

size to the fibrillar genes, but their organization is very different (reviewed in reference 1). The exons that encode the largely triple helical domain are far more variable in size. The genes for type IV chains, COL4A1 and COL4A2, lack the regular 54 bp exon pattern.[10, 11] Type IX collagen genes have only a few 54 bp exons, and in the chick type X collagen gene, the triple helical domain is coded by a single large exon.[12–14]

Transcription of collagen genes first results in synthesis of a large precursor RNA, termed heteronuclear RNA (hnRNA), that contains all the exonic and intronic sequences.[15] As with most eukaryotic genes, the hnRNA must undergo several post-transcriptional modifications to produce a single functional mRNA. The intervening sequences are removed, or "spliced out," and the exons are joined together.[16] α1(IX), α1(XIII), and α2(VI) procollagen chains

appear to demonstrate alternative splicing, which may be tissue specific.[13, 17–19] "Alternative splicing" refers to the joining of different exons in the processing of specific hnRNAs derived from the same gene. In the case of corneal α1(IX) mRNA, a different 5′ exon is alternatively spliced to exon 8 rather than exons 1 through 7, which are utilized by cartilage α1(IX) mRNA; the 5′ exon of corneal α1(IX) mRNA is identical to a sequence located in the intron between exons 6 and 7 of the α1(IX) gene (Fig. 9–3). The mRNAs for corneal and cartilage α1(IX) both code for the same triple helical domain.

The 5′ end of the mRNA is capped by 7-methylguanosine, which is linked to the first nucleotide of the mRNA by a 5′-5′ triphosphate bridge that both protects the 5′ end of the mRNA from phosphatases and nucleases and acts as a recognition signal for ribosomes during

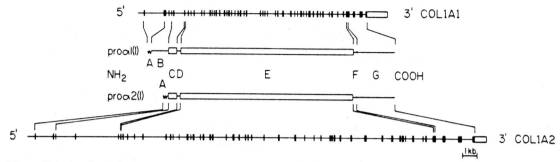

Figure 9–2. A schematic representation of the fibrillar collagen genes for type I procollagen. COL1A1 (*top*) and COL1A2 (*bottom*) encode proα1(I) collagen and proα2(I) collagen, respectively. The exons are indicated by solid boxes or vertical lines. The organization of the other fibrillar collagen genes is similar, and the intron-exon junctions and the exon sizes have been maintained. The domains of the procollagen polypeptides are also indicated: *A*, signal sequence; *B*, amino-terminal propeptide extension; *C*, minor triple helix of the amino-terminal propeptide extension; *D*, amino-terminal telopeptide; *E*, triple helix; *F*, carboxyl-terminal telopeptide; *G*, carboxyl-terminal propeptide extension. (Adapted with permission from Byers PH: Disorders of collagen biosynthesis and structure. In Scriver CR, Beaudet AL, Sly WS, Valle D (eds): The Metabolic Basis of Inherited Diseases, 6th ed. New York, McGraw-Hill, 1989, p 2807.)

protein synthesis.[20] The 3' end of the RNA is also modified by a stepwise addition of adenylate residues to the 3'OH end of the RNA to form the poly-A tail of approximately 150 to 200 nucleotides. The poly-A addition is believed to enhance the stability of the mRNA.[21, 22] The regions of the mRNA directly 5' and 3' to the coding sequences are not translated; they participate in initiation and termination of protein synthesis. The mature mRNA must be translocated across the nuclear membrane into the cytoplasm to be translated.

lagen mRNAs are translated into precursor forms, preprocollagens, that carry unique signal or leader sequences for each collagen type.[23] The nature of the signal sequence allows it to insert into the membrane of the RER.[24–26] The newly translated preprocollagen undergoes extensive post-translational modification including enzymatic cleavage of the signal sequence during elongation of the chains as they are transported through the membrane into the lumen of the RER.

Cytoplasmic Events

In the cytoplasm, the mature mRNA is translated on ribosomes that are attached to the rough endoplasmic reticulum (RER). The col-

Hydroxylation of Proline and Lysine Residues

As the newly synthesized procollagen chains enter into the lumen of the RER, some proline

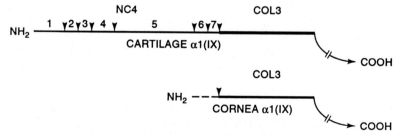

Figure 9–3. A schematic representation of the amino-terminal region of cartilage α1(IX) (*top*) and cornea α1(IX) (*bottom*) collagen chains. In cartilage, the nontriple helical sequence (NC4) is encoded by seven exons (indicated 1–7, arrow marks the intron/exon splice junction). In cornea, the nontriple helical sequence (NC4) is encoded by a single exon (*dashed line*) located in the intron between exons 6 and 7 utilized by cartilage. Both chains have identical triple helical domains (COL3). (Reprinted with permission from Nishimura I, Muragaki Y, Hayashi M, et al: Tissue specific expression of Type IX collagen. In Fleischmajer R, Olsen BR, Kuhn K (eds): Structure, Molecular Biology, and Pathology of Collagen. Ann NY Acad Sci 580:115, 1990.)

and lysine residues in the triple helical domain are hydroxylated (Fig. 9–4). Proline and lysine residues immediately amino-terminal to a glycine are hydroxylated by prolyl 4-hydroxylase and lysyl hydroxylase, respectively. In addition, some proline residues are hydroxylated by prolyl 3-hydroxylase.[27, 28]

Prolyl 4-hydroxylase converts proline residues to peptidyl *trans* 4-hydroxyproline and lysyl hydroxylase converts specific lysine residues to peptidyl *trans* 5-hydroxylysine.[28–30] The enzyme prolyl 3-hydroxylase has a minimum sequence requirement for -Pro-4-hydroxyPro-Gly- and converts a proline in the X position to a peptidyl *trans* 3-hydroxyproline.[29–31] All three of these enzymes require ferrous iron, α-ketoglutarate, ascorbic acid, and molecular oxygen as cofactors.[28, 29] These three enzymes are similar mechanistically in that their kinetic con-

stants for their substrates and cosubstrates are similar.[28, 30] Immunological studies suggest distinct structural similarities close to or at the catalytically active centers of prolyl 4-hydroxylase and lysyl hydroxylase.[32] The substrate for these enzymes is nascent unfolded procollagen chains and not free proline or lysine residues. The enzymes are sterically inhibited when chains are folded into a triple helix.

The function of prolyl 4-hydroxylation is to stabilize the triple helix under physiological conditions.[28, 33] Nonhydroxylated proα collagen chains can fold into a triple helix only at low temperatures; their transition temperature (Tm) for unfolding is only 24°C, a value approximately 15°C lower than the Tm for molecules consisting of hydroxylated proα collagen chains. Hence, the nonhydroxylated proα chains are unable to produce stable triple helical mole-

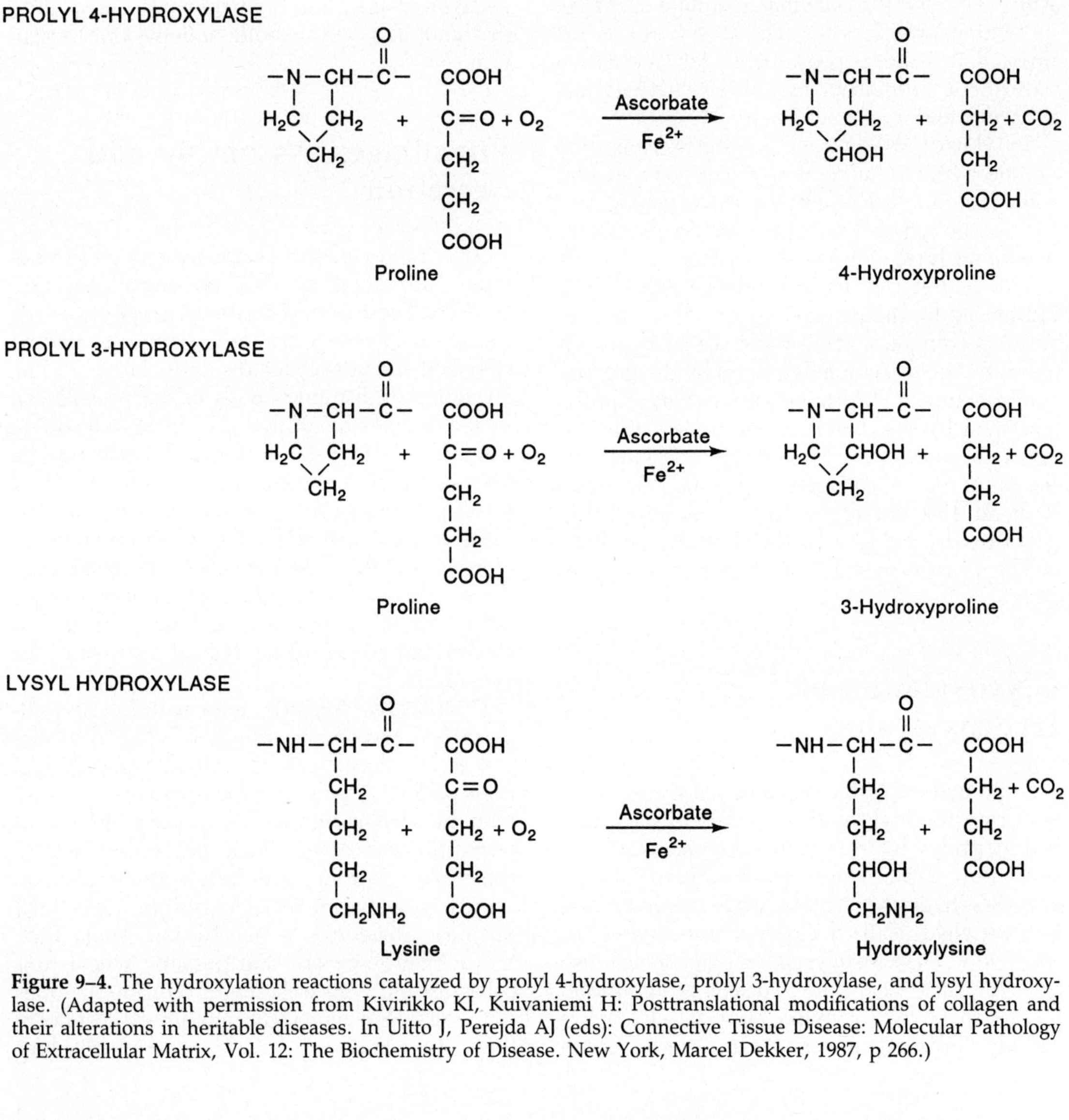

PROLYL 4-HYDROXYLASE

Proline → 4-Hydroxyproline

PROLYL 3-HYDROXYLASE

Proline → 3-Hydroxyproline

LYSYL HYDROXYLASE

Lysine → Hydroxylysine

Figure 9–4. The hydroxylation reactions catalyzed by prolyl 4-hydroxylase, prolyl 3-hydroxylase, and lysyl hydroxylase. (Adapted with permission from Kivirikko KI, Kuivaniemi H: Posttranslational modifications of collagen and their alterations in heritable diseases. In Uitto J, Perejda AJ (eds): Connective Tissue Disease: Molecular Pathology of Extracellular Matrix, Vol. 12: The Biochemistry of Disease. New York, Marcel Dekker, 1987, p 266.)

cules at the body temperature of 37°C. Almost complete 4-hydroxylation of all proline residues in Y positions of the triple helix is required for the formation of a molecule that is stable at 37°C. The function of prolyl 3-hydroxylation has not been defined.

The function of hydroxylation of lysyl residues is to provide substrates for glycosylation and for the formation of certain covalent intermolecular crosslinks, an important determinant of the collagen fibril's tensile strength.[33]

The molecular structure of prolyl 4-hydroxylase is a tetramer composed of two α and two β subunits.[28, 30, 34] The α and β subunits have molecular weights of 64 and 60 kilodaltons (kDa), respectively, and are the products of different genes. The cDNA for the β subunit has been isolated and from sequence analyses has proven to be structurally and functionally homologous to protein disulfide isomerase, whose function is to facilitate disulfide exchange in folding proteins.[35, 36] The β subunit is expressed in excess, presumably for association with the α subunit for hydroxylase activity and as free β for isomerase activity.[29]

Lysyl hydroxylase is a homodimer, consisting of one type of monomer which may exhibit some microheterogeneity in glycosylation.[32, 37] The carbohydrate residues are required for maximum lysyl hydroxylase activity.[37]

The activity of each of these enzymes is influenced by the primary structure of the substrate peptide at and near the site of hydroxylation, by the α chain length, and by the peptide conformation.[28, 33] Although the extent of prolyl and lysyl hydroxylation varies among different types of collagen, among different tissues for the same type of collagen, and among the same tissue at different ages, many observations suggest that the collagen hydroxylases do not have collagen type-specific or tissue-specific isozymes.[32, 38]

Glycosylation of Hydroxylysine

Some hydroxylysine residues are glycosylated to form peptidyl hydroxylysine-O-galactoside and peptidyl hydroxylysine-O-glucosylgalactoside (Fig. 9–5). These are catalyzed by the enzymes hydroxylysylgalactosyltransferase and galactosylhydroxylysyl glucosyl transferase, respectively.[39] Hydroxylysylgalactosyl transferase transfers galactose to the hydroxyl group on the 5′ carbon of hydroxylysine and galactosyl hydroxylysylglucosyl transferase transfers glucose

to galactosyl hydroxylysine. Both transferases use Mn^{+2} as the preferred divalent cation and require the free ε amino group of hydroxylysine.

The extent of glycosylation is determined primarily by the availability of the acceptor hydroxylysine and the conformation of the substrate.[39] The distribution of mono- and disaccharides is different in different collagen types, and the function of the carbohydrate moieties is unknown. They may influence fibril formation since there is an inverse relationship between collagen carbohydrate content and collagen fibril diameter.[39, 40]

Type I collagen has a single asparagine-linked carbohydrate group on the carboxyl-terminal propeptide of each procollagen chain (Fig. 9–6).[41, 42] This asparagine is N-glycosylated by a mechanism similar to that for other glycoproteins, which involves en bloc transfer of preformed oligosaccharides to intact nascent proα collagen chains, and is further processed within the rough and smooth endoplasmic reticulum.[43, 44]

Procollagen Assembly and Secretion

After proα collagen chains have been synthesized and modified, they are assembled into trimers. The carboxyl-terminal propeptides associate to form a trimeric structure that is stablized by interchain disulfide bonds.[45] The formation of disulfide bonds in the procollagen molecules may be catalyzed by protein disulfide isomerase. The disulfide-bonded trimer rapidly folds into helix conformation only after a critical level of hydroxyproline residues per chain has been reached and after cis-trans isomerization of approximately 20 per cent of prolyl residues.[46] Only after formation of the major triple helix will the amino-terminal propeptide, including its minor triple helical extension, be assembled.

Procollagen molecules appear to follow well-described secretory pathways.[47] The procollagen is translocated to the Golgi complex and then packaged into secretory vesicles that fuse with the cell membrane to release their contents into the extracellular environment.[48] In the Golgi complex the heterosaccharides on type I procollagen are cleaved to yield high mannose structures.[43] In addition, some type V, probably type III, and possibly type I procollagens undergo sulfation of tyrosine residues in the amino-terminal propeptide extensions in the Golgi complex.[49, 50] Certain serine residues

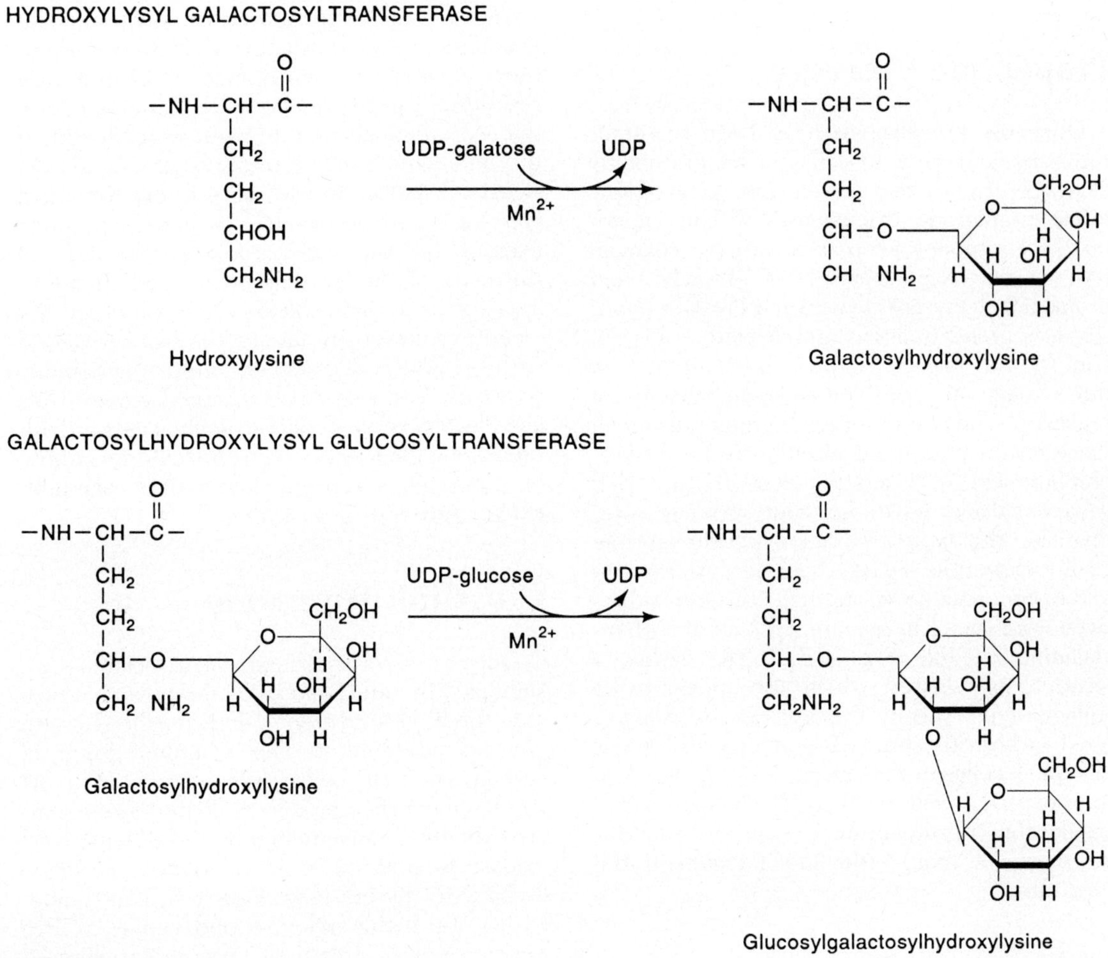

HYDROXYLYSYL GALACTOSYLTRANSFERASE

Hydroxylysine → Galactosylhydroxylysine

(UDP-galatose → UDP, Mn^{2+})

GALACTOSYLHYDROXYLYSYL GLUCOSYLTRANSFERASE

Galactosylhydroxylysine → Glucosylgalactosylhydroxylysine

(UDP-glucose → UDP, Mn^{2+})

Figure 9–5. The glycosylation reactions catalyzed by hydroxylysylgalactosyltransferase and galactosylhydroxylysyl-glucosyltransferase. (Adapted with permission from Kivirikko KI, Kuivaniemi H: Posttranslational modifications of collagen and their alterations in heritable diseases. In Uitto J, Perejda AJ (eds): Connective Tissue Disease: Molecular Pathology of Extracellular Matrix, Vol. 12: The Biochemistry of Disease. New York, Marcel Dekker, 1987, p 269.)

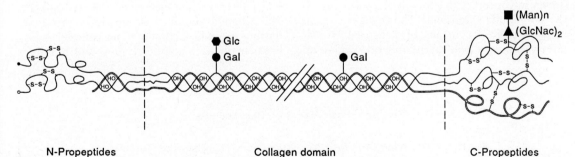

N-Propeptides   Collagen domain   C-Propeptides

Figure 9–6. A model of the type I procollagen molecule illustrating the location and the type of glycosylation. Glc = glucose; Gal = galactose; (Man)n = mannose; (GlcNac)$_2$ = N-acetylglucosamine. (Adapted with permission from Prockop DJ, Kivirikko KI, Tuderman L, Guzman NA: The biosynthesis of collagen and its disorders. N Engl J Med 301:16, 1979.)

of the type I procollagen extensions are phosphorylated in bone.[51] The function of sulfation, glycosylation, and phosphorylation is uncertain.

Propeptide Cleavage

Once the procollagens have been secreted, they are converted to collagen by proteolytic cleavage of both the amino- and carboxyl-terminal propeptide extensions.[52–54] The amino-terminal propeptide is cleaved by collagen type-specific N-proteinases.[53, 55] Proα1(I) and proα1(III) chains are cleaved at a Pro-Gln bond, whereas proα2(I) chains are cleaved at an Ala-Gln.[56–58] For maximal N-proteinase activity, all three chains of type I procollagen must be in register.[59] The amino-terminal glutamines in all three chains undergo cyclization to form pyroglutamic acid.[56, 57] Even though α1(III) and α1(I) collagen chains have the same cleavage site, Pro-Gln, the type I collagen-specific enzyme cannot cleave the α1(III) chain because there is a tyrosine residue in α1(III), three residues away from the cleavage site, instead of a phenylalanine residue (Fig. 9–7).[60] The carboxyl-terminal proteinases, which also appear to be collagen-type specific, cleave at an Ala-Asp bond in both the proα1(I) and proα2(I) chains of type I collagen and at an Arg-Asp bond in the proα1(III) chain of type III collagen.[58, 61, 62] Unlike the N-proteinases, the carboxy-proteinase does not require the intact trimer as the substrate.[62]

Fibril Formation

After removal of the propeptides the collagen monomers spontaneously assemble into fibrils by an entropy-driven process.[63] The assembly occurs in concert with proteolytic processing of the propeptide extensions. The collagen monomers associate by means of staggered lateral interactions in which the telopeptide region of one collagen monomer interacts with the triple helical region of adjacent molecules (Fig. 9–8).[64] The monomers are packed in a spiral five-stranded ropelike structure. The 300 nm collagen monomers are staggered with respect to their neighbor by a distance of 67 nm (234 residues). A gap exists between a monomer and the next monomer in line because the length of the monomer is not a multiple of 67 nm, the stagger distance. In each 67 nm unit there is a gap region and a region where there is complete overlap; the gap region contains four fifths of the mass of the overlap region and therefore appears as a light band when observed by electron microscopy; hence the classic banded pattern of the collagen fiber. Interactions among positively and negatively charged amino acids and clusters of hydrophobic amino acids distributed along the length of the molecule contribute to the precise staggered alignment of each molecule relative to its neighbor.[65]

Crosslink Formation

Once the fiber is formed, the associations are stabilized by intermolecular crosslinks that provide the fiber with tremendous tensile strength and insolubility.[56, 66] The ε amino group of certain lysyl or hydroxylysyl residues, most commonly in the nonhelical telopeptide region, are oxidatively deaminated by the enzyme lysyl oxidase to corresponding aldehydes, allysines, or hydroxyallysine (Fig. 9–9).[67, 68] These aldehydes are highly reactive and can form two major types of crosslinks, intramolecular and intermolecular. Intramolecular crosslinks are formed by the aldol condensation of two aldehydes within the same molecule, and aldol condensation with other lysine or hydroxylysine residues in the triple helical regions of adjacent molecules results in intermolecular crosslinks.[66, 69, 70] Although the divalent crosslinks form first, there is rapid formation of more complex crosslinks involving histidine, lysine, and hydroxy-

pN α1(I) —Gly—Gly—Asn—Phe—Ala—Pro—Gln—Leu—Ser—Tyr—Gly—Tyr—

pN α1(III)—Gln—Asn—Asn—Tyr—Ala—Pro—Gln—Tyr—Glu—Ala—Tyr—Asp—

Figure 9–7. The amino propeptide extension cleavage sites of proα1(I) and proα1(III) collagen. Even though the amino propeptide proteinases for proα1(I) and proα1(III) collagen cleave off the propeptide extensions at the same sites, Pro-Gln (*arrow*), these N-proteinases are collagen-type specific. The N-proteinase for proα1(I) collagen requires a phenylalanine residue to be present three amino acid residues amino-terminal to the cleavage site. The proα1(III) collagen has a tyrosine residue in this position. (Reprinted with permission from Kuhn K: The classical collagens: Type I, II, and III. In Mayne R, Burgeson RE (eds): Structure and Function of Collagen Types. (Biology of Extracellular Matrix: A Series). Orlando, Academic Press, 1987, p 24.)

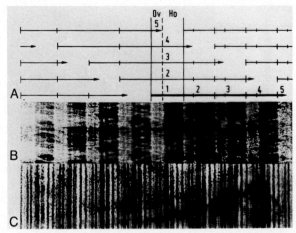

Figure 9–8. The alignment of the collagen molecules in a collagen fibril. *A,* Collagen molecules are packed in a 5-stranded ropelike structure. The 300 nm collagen molecules are staggered with respect to their neighbors by a distance of 67 nm. Since the length of a collagen molecule is not a multiple of 67, a gap exists between a collagen molecule and the next one in line. In a 67 nm unit, there is a gap or hole (Ho) region, and a region where there is complete overlap (Ov); the Ho contains four fifths the mass of the Ov region. *B,* The Ov region appears as a light band and the Ho region appears as a dark band when negatively stained with phosphotungstic acid. (Reproduced with permission from Kuhn K: The classical collagens: Type I, II, and III. In Mayne R, Burgeson RE (eds): Structure and Function of Collagen Types. (Biology of Extracellular Matrix: A Series). Orlando, Academic Press, 1987, p 8.)

lysine residues to form nonreducible crosslinks that later stabilize interactions among three adjacent molecules. As tissue ages there is further stabilization of collagen crosslinks: the divalent crosslinks are converted to more stable and complex crosslinks.[69] The crosslinks in young collagen fibrils can be reduced with sodium borohydride, but such reducible crosslinks gradually disappear from older collagen.[33, 69]

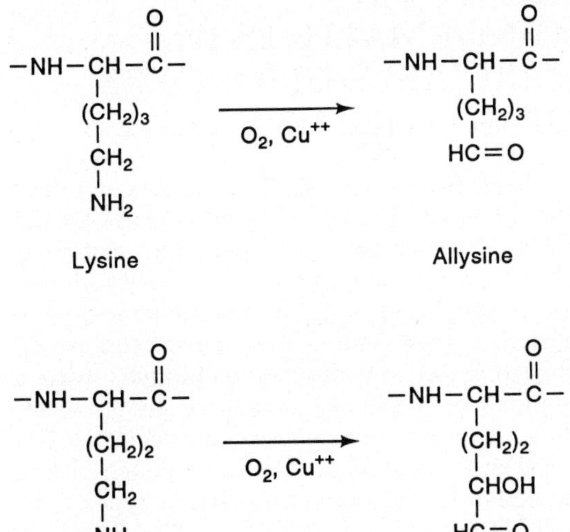

Collagen Degradation

Connective tissue is dynamic; the orderly degradation of interstitial and basement membrane collagens is the fundamental process governing growth, development, morphogenesis, remodeling, and repair under both normal and pathological conditions. The rate of collagen turnover can be increased under certain conditions, for example, during postpartum resorption of the uterus and following an injury. The triple helical nature of collagen has rendered it relatively resistant to most proteases. The degradation of collagen depends on a specific family of enzymes, collagenases, that recognize the collagenous sequences and cleave intact molecules.[71] The differing primary structures of the genetically distinct collagen types may require distinct enzymes. Collagen degradation occurs both extracellularly and intracellularly. While the majority of the newly synthesized collagen molecules are processed and secreted following the well-described route, 10 percent or more are degraded intracellularly under normal tissue culture conditions.[72, 73] Chapter 10 discusses collagen degradation in greater detail.

Figure 9–9. The reactions catalyzed by lysyl oxidase. (Reproduced with permission from Kivirikko KI, Kuivaniemi H: Posttranslational modifications of collagen and their alterations in heritable diseases. In Uitto J, Perejda AJ (eds): Connective Tissue Disease: Molecular Pathology of Extracellular Matrix, Vol. 12: The Biochemistry of Disease. New York, Marcel Dekker, 1987, p 276.)

REGULATION OF COLLAGEN BIOSYNTHESIS

Each step of the biosynthesis pathway of collagen, from initial transcription to the final fibril formation, is a potential regulatory step. The complexity of collagen biosynthesis is reflected not only by the series of post-translational modifications but also by the need for coordinated control of the collagen genes, many of which are on separate chromosomes (reviewed in reference 1). For example, the COL1A1 and COL1A2 genes of type I collagen are on chromosomes 17 and 7, respectively.[74–76] Both are present in one copy per haploid genome; however, the steady-state level of $\alpha1(I)$ mRNA is twice that of $\alpha2(I)$ mRNA. This is not due to differential RNA stability but rather to the fact that the two genes are coordinately transcribed at different efficiencies, which allows the expression of the $\alpha1(I)$ and $\alpha2(I)$ chains in a 2:1 ratio.[77]

Present in the 5′ flanking region of the collagen genes, the region upstream from the transcription start site that includes the promoter, are nucleotide sequences that provide positive transcriptional control.[78–82] There are additional nucleotide sequences present in the first intron that appear to act as enhancers and to direct tissue-specific expression.[83–86] In these regions there also appear to be some negative controlling sequences.[78, 86]

Collagen biosynthesis can also be regulated at the level of translation. Nucleotide sequences between the transcriptional start site and the first translated domain, the 5′ untranslated region, can form a stem-loop structure that appears to influence the efficiency of translation.[87, 88] Under certain culture conditions chondrocytes transcribe $pro\alpha2(I)$ collagen mRNAs that are inefficiently translated, apparently as the result of translational arrest.[89] The availability of certain charged tRNAs may also influence the efficiency of translation, but this appears not to be a general control mechanism.[90, 91] In addition, there is evidence that the synthesis of some procollagen mRNAs is controlled pretranslationally and translationally by the peptides derived from the cleavage of the amino- and carboxy-propeptides.[92–96]

Ascorbic acid has proven to be an important regulator of collagen biosynthesis. It is not only a necessary cofactor for prolyl and lysyl hydroxylases, but it also stimulates collagen biosynthesis and increases steady-state levels of procollagen mRNAs.[97, 98]

The expression of collagen genes can be altered by a variety of growth factors and cytokines, including transforming growth factor-β (TGF-β), insulin-like growth factors 1 and 2, interleukin-1, tumor necrosis factor-α (TNF-α), and interferon-γ. (Several chapters in this volume describe the influence of growth factors in fibroblasts and the resulting changes in collagen biosynthesis.) TGF-β stimulates collagen production by both transcriptional and post-transcriptional processes, but it appears not to be a collagen-specific effect since overall protein synthesis is also increased.[99–105] The general stimulation of matrix formation by TGF-β may be important to wound healing and fibrosis.[99, 106] The insulin-like growth factors also increase collagen synthesis along with general protein synthesis.[107, 108] Interleukin-1 has been reported to both increase and decrease collagen production.[109–111] Both TNF-α and interferon-γ inhibit collagen gene transcription, and when used in combination they can further inhibit this process, which suggests that they exert their effect by separate mechanisms.[112–116] The steroid hormones, such as glucocorticoids, have been shown to selectively inhibit procollagen gene transcription.[117–121] In addition, the steroid hormone $1,25(OH_2)D_3$ and the peptide hormone parathyroid hormone have been shown to decrease collagen synthesis.[122, 123]

COLLAGEN ABNORMALITIES IN HERITABLE DISORDERS OF CONNECTIVE TISSUE

There have been significant advances in the last 10 years in understanding the molecular basis of connective tissue disorders and their effects on collagen structure and biosynthesis. As collagen genes have been characterized, mutations in several of them have been associated through a variety of techniques with a number of heritable connective tissue disorders, including osteogenesis imperfecta and Ehlers-Danlos syndrome. Direct evidence of mutations in genes coding for collagen types I, II, and III have been identified in cells taken from individuals with connective tissue diseases, several of which involve dermal tissues.

The disorder for which the clinical and biochemical consequences of connective tissue gene mutations are best understood is osteogenesis imperfecta (OI), an autosomal dominant form of congenital osteopenia.[124] Studies have conclusively shown that virtually all cases of OI are due to mutations in the genes for type I collagen.[125, 126] It will be useful to review the molecular and biochemical findings in this disorder because it serves as a paradigm for other disorders of collagen.

Osteogenesis Imperfecta

There are at least two clinically and biochemically distinct forms of osteogenesis imperfecta. The first is a mild form characterized by blue sclerae and increased fracture rate in childhood with significant improvement after puberty.[124, 127] Most of these individuals also have presenile hearing loss. Careful clinical examination of the skin in these patients often demonstrates dermal thinning, and many report a mild propensity for increased bruising. Scarring is normal, however, and the skin is not hyperextensible. Virtually all of these patients fit into the clinical subtype of OI type I described by Sillence and co-workers (Table 9–1).[127] This form of OI is usually the result of mutations that produce a functional deletion of one proα1(I) allele and decreased biosynthesis of type I collagen.[128, 129] Willing and colleagues[130] recently showed that in one family with OI type I, affected members were heterozygous for a frameshift mutation that altered the carboxyl propeptide of proα1(I) chains, preventing their assembly into trimers and thereby decreasing the pool of proα1(I) chains available for biosynthesis of type I collagen molecules (Fig. 9–10).

The second class of mutations results in a more severe OI phenotype, characterized by greater osseous fragility, deformity of all bones, particularly long bones, and dentinogenesis im-

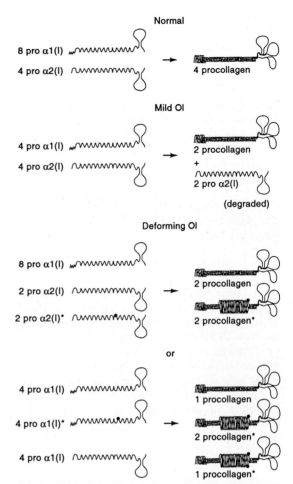

Figure 9–10. Stoichiometric relationship of normal and abnormal alpha chains of type I collagen resulting from dominant mutations in various forms of osteogenesis imperfecta (OI). Mild OI corresponds best to Sillence type I. Deforming OI corresponds to a wide range of clinical severities, from Sillence type IV to perinatal lethal. (Reproduced, with permission of the University of Chicago Press, from Wenstrup RJ, Willing MC, Starman BS, Byers PH: Distinct biochemical phenotypes predict clinical severity in nonlethal variants of osteogenesis imperfecta. Am J Hum Genet 46:981, 1990.)

perfecta. There is a wide range of severity, from mild osseous fragility and mild short stature to a severe, dwarfing form that is lethal in the perinatal period. This more severe form of OI is the result of heterozygous mutations in proα1(I) or proα2(I) chains that cause altered triple helical structure of some type I collagen molecules (Fig. 9–10).[131, 132] Many such mutations have been reported; a relatively small proportion are rearrangements involving insertions and deletions of the triple helical domain of proα1(I) or proα2(I) chains, but the great majority are due to a single amino acid substitution for a triple helical glycine residue in α1(I) or α2(I) chains that disrupts a Gly-X-Y repeat

Table 9–1. OSTEOGENESIS IMPERFECTA: CLINICAL AND GENETIC SUBTYPES

	Clinical Features	Inheritance
Type I	Mild osseous fragility, blue sclerae, ± presenile deafness, ± dentinogenesis imperfecta	Dominant
Type II	"Perinatal" lethal; several radiologic forms, usually with crumpled long bones, thin or beaded ribs, poorly calcified calvariae	Dominant
Type III	Progressively deforming; dozens or hundreds of fractures, early loss of ambulation	Dominant/recessive
Type IV	Mild to moderate osseous fragility, normal or grey sclerae, mild short stature, ± hearing loss, dentinogenesis imperfecta	Dominant

(reviewed in reference 125; see also references 133–145).

The consequences of glycine substitutions on type I collagen molecules incorporating one or more mutant proα chains may be quite dramatic, depending on the location of the mutations within the chain. A discussion of these consequences is worthwhile because they provide insight into type I collagen structure and because mutations in other collagen genes may result in similar biochemical findings.

Effects of Glycine Substitutions on Assembly of Type I Collagen Molecules

The most convincing evidence that even a single glycine substitution disrupts triple helical assembly is its effect on the extent and distribution of post-translational modifications. Lysyl hydroxylase catalyzes the hydroxylation of some but not all lysyl residues in the Y position of proα chains of type I collagen. The substrates for lysyl hydroxylase are unfolded proα chains; triple helical conformation of proα chains inhibits further lysyl hydroxylation, and experimental unfolding of the triple helix in vitro allows additional hydroxylation of α chains. Some proα and α chains of type I collagen molecules secreted from OI fibroblasts have altered migration in sodium dodecylsulfate (SDS)-polyacrylamide gels due to increased lysyl hydroxylation and hydroxylysyl glycosylation. The excessive post-translational modification is over the entire triple helical domain in some OI cell strains; in many others, it is present only in the amino-terminal portion of the helix.[146] In all OI cell strains in which both the distribution of overmodification and the sequence of the glycine substitution are known, the substitution is at the carboxyl end of the region of overmodification in the abnormal type I collagen molecules.[125] It appears likely that substitutions for glycine slow or disrupt winding of the helix at the site of the mutation, allowing continued modifications amino-terminal to the mutation before the molecule finally assumes a helical conformation (Fig. 9–11).

Glycine substitutions in α chains of type I collagen can serve as probes for determinants of triple helical stability, by examining the decrease in the Tm, the temperature of the helix-to-coil transition, in type I collagen molecules containing one or more mutant chains. Thermal stability of abnormal collagen made by OI cells has usually been tested by Bruckner and Prockop's method[147]: collagen molecules

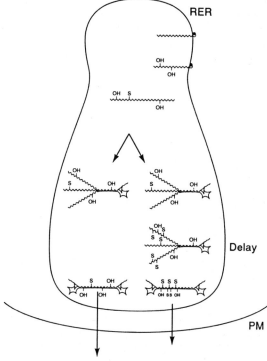

Figure 9–11. Assembly, modification, and secretion of normal and abnormal type I procollagens in cells of patients with osteogenesis imperfecta. Normally, type I procollagen chains are assembled and secreted from cells in 20 minutes (*left*). Incorporation of one or more proα chains with a mutation in the triple helical domain delays helix formation around the site of the mutation, rendering unwound portions of the chains amino-terminal to the mutation available for further modifications. PM = plasma membrane; RER = rough endoplasmic reticulum. (Reprinted with permission from Byers PH: Disorders of collagen biosynthesis and structure. In Scriver CR, Beaudet AL, Sly WS, Valle D (eds): The Metabolic Basis of Inherited Diseases, 6th ed. New York, McGraw-Hill, 1989, p 2819.)

dissolved in a buffered salt solution are subjected to steady increases in temperature, and aliquots are removed at different temperatures, cooled, and digested with proteases; resistance to digestion is taken as a measure of triple helical integrity. Nearly all glycine substitutions in the triple helical domain of type I collagen chains in OI cell strains result in decreased thermal stability of type I collagen molecules. The decrease in thermal stability of the abnormal type I collagen molecules from OI cell strains reflects the altered conformation of type I collagen and may correlate with rates of intracellular and extracellular degradation of abnormal type I collagen molecules in vivo. Differences in thermal stability between type I collagen molecules containing α chains with different glycine substitutions probably depend on which residue is substituted and the context of the mutation within an assembled type I collagen molecule.[141, 148]

Correlation Between Point Mutation Position and Severity of Associated Clinical Phenotype

Starman and co-workers[142] demonstrated that in three cell strains heterozygous for cysteine-for-glycine substitutions in $\alpha1(I)$ chains, the severity of the OI clinical phenotype correlated with the proximity of the substitution to the initiation of triple helix winding at the carboxyl end. Cysteine-for-glycine substitution at position 94 resulted in a very mild OI phenotype, at position 526 the substitution caused deforming OI type III, and at position 718 caused perinatal lethal OI type II (by convention, amino acid numbering in the triple helix begins at the amino-terminal end).

All cysteine-for-glycine substitutions carboxyl to glycine at position 718 in $\alpha1(I)$ chains have been associated with lethal OI, but this position effect does not hold for mutations in $\alpha2(I)$ chains. A relatively severe OI phenotype is associated with a cysteine-for-glycine substitution at position 259, but two different families with cysteine-for-glycine substitution at position 646 have very mild OI.[148a]

Ehlers-Danlos Syndrome

The Ehlers-Danlos syndromes (EDS) are a genetically, biochemically, and clinically distinct group of inherited disorders with common characteristics of joint laxity and skin hyperextensibility and fragility.[125, 149, 150] Ten distinct subtypes have been described (Table 9–2), but many individuals with some of these clinical features do not fit into a distinct subtype.

Table 9–2. EHLERS-DANLOS SYNDROMES: CLINICAL, GENETIC, AND BIOCHEMICAL CHARACTERISTICS

Type		Clinical Features	Inheritance*	Biochemical Defect
I	Gravis	Soft, hyperextensible skin; easy bruising; thin, atrophic scars; hypermobile joints; varicose veins; prematurity of affected newborns	AD	Not known
II	Mitis	Similar to EDS type I but less severe	AD	Not known
III	Familial hypermobility	Soft skin; large and small joint hypermobility	AD	Not known
IV	Arterial	Thin, translucent skin with visible veins; easy bruising; absence of skin and joint extensibility; arterial, bowel, and uterine rupture	AD	Abnormal type III collagen synthesis, secretion, or structure; deletions and point mutations in the gene
			(AR)	Not known
V	X-linked	Similar to EDS type II	XLR	Not known
VI		Soft, muscle hypotonia; scoliosis; joint laxity; hyperextensible skin	AR	Lysyl hydroxylase deficiency
VII	Arthrochalasis multiplex congenita	Congenital hip dislocation; severe joint hypermobility; soft skin with normal scarring	AD	Deletion of exons from type I collagen genes that encode the amino-terminal propeptide cleavage sites
VIII	Periodontal	Generalized periodontitis; soft hyperextensible skin	AD	Not known
IX		Soft, extensible, lax skin; bladder diverticulae and rupture; short arms, limited pronation and supination; broad clavicles; occipital horns	XLR	Abnormal copper utilization with defect in lysyl oxidase
X		Similar to EDS type II with abnormal clotting studies	AR	Possible defect in fibronectin

*AD = autosomal dominant; AR = autosomal recessive; XLR = X-linked recessive.

From Wenstrup RJ, Murad S, Pinnell SR: Collagen. In Goldsmith LA (ed): Biochemistry and Physiology of the Skin, 2nd ed. New York, Oxford University Press (In Press).

EDS Type I. Ehlers-Danlos syndrome type I is characterized by joint laxity, hyperextensibility of skin, poor wound healing, and autosomal dominant inheritance. The skin is soft and velvety and can be stretched easily. The dermis is fragile and there is marked bruisability. Scars after trauma or surgical procedures are thinned and atrophic and may stretch considerably after healing, having a characteristic "cigarette paper" appearance. About half of affected individuals with EDS type I are delivered prematurely as a result of premature rupture of fetal membranes, presumably due to abnormalities in fetal tissue structure. A significant number of individuals with EDS type I have cardiac defects, most commonly mitral valve prolapse; a few have dilatation and occasionally rupture of the ascending aorta or the proximal pulmonary artery. Musculoskeletal features include joint hyperextensibility in all patients and a high frequency of scoliosis and pes planus (flat feet). The joint hypermobility can be associated with osteoarthritis with onset in the third or fourth decade.

Disorders of collagen have long been suspected in EDS type I. Vogel and co-workers[151] found skin collagen fibrils to have an abnormally wide diameter in some EDS type I patients, and collagen fiber bundles were abnormally large (Fig. 9–12). However, there is no direct evidence for any specific collagen gene abnormality in EDS type I. Genetic linkage analysis of some EDS type I families has excluded linkage to genes for types I, II, and III collagen.

EDS Type II. Ehlers-Danlos syndrome type II is clinically similar to EDS type I except that the skin is less fragile and there is normal or near-normal scar formation. Inheritance is also autosomal dominant. Ultrastructural findings show thickened collagen fibrils in skin, similar to findings reported in dermis in patients with EDS type I.

EDS Type III. Ehlers-Danlos syndrome type III, also known as familial benign hypermobility syndrome, is characterized primarily by hyperextensibility of large and small joints and autosomal dominant inheritance. Individuals are at risk for premature onset of osteoarthritis in the third or fourth decade. There are no known collagen abnormalities associated with EDS type III.

EDS Type IV. Ehlers-Danlos syndrome type IV is characterized by thin, translucent skin with easy bruisability but normal scar formation. Affected individuals are at high risk for rupture of the large intestine, uterus, and medium-sized arteries. Arterial rupture is another life-threatening complication, the most common sites being the mesenteric arteries in the abdomen, the splenic artery, the renal arteries, and the descending aorta. There may also be an increased incidence of stroke in EDS type IV. A third potentially lethal complication is uterine rupture in the perinatal period.[152] EDS type IV is clinically distinct from other subtypes in that there is no skin hyperextensibility, scarring is usually normal, and joint hyperextensibility is not as prominent.

Although EDS type IV was initially thought to be autosomal recessive in inheritance,[153, 154] most individuals have family histories compatible with autosomal dominant inheritance, and linkage analysis has documented dominant inheritance in several families.[155]

Electron microscopic observations of the dermis in patients with EDS type IV have showed unusual variation in collagen fibrillar diameter and irregularly shaped collagen bundles.[156] The dermis is thinned, collagen bundles are small, and other structures, particularly elastin fibers, appear relatively abundant. Dermal fibroblasts from some EDS type IV patients show dilation of the rough endoplasmic reticulum (Fig. 9–13), suggesting that an abnormal protein product was synthesized but is retained within cells.[156]

Pope and colleagues[157] demonstrated an absence of type III collagen in skin and aortas of

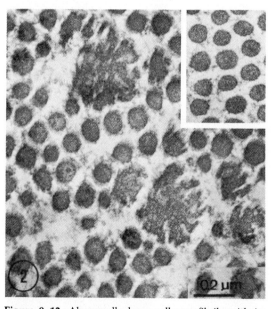

Figure 9–12. Abnormally large collagen fibrils with irregular outline from the skin of a patient with Ehlers-Danlos syndrome type I. Inset contains fibrils from a normal individual ($\times$ 60,000). (Adapted with permission from Vogel A, Holbrook KA, Steinman B, et al: Abnormal collagen fibril structure in the Gravis form (Type I) of Ehlers-Danlos syndrome. Lab Invest 40:202, 1979. © US & Canadian Academy of Pathology, Inc.)

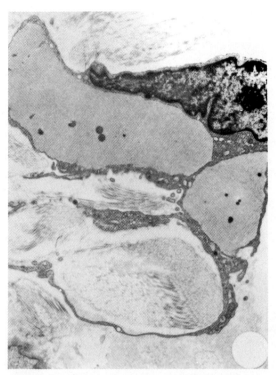

Figure 9–13. Electron micrograph (× 1450) of fibroblasts in the skin of an individual with Ehlers-Danlos syndrome type IV. There is marked dilation of the rough endoplasmic reticulum. (Adapted with permission from Holbrook KA, Byers PH: Ultrastructural characteristics of the skin in a form of Ehlers-Danlos syndrome type IV. Lab Invest 44:346, 1981. © US & Canadian Academy of Pathology, Inc.)

individuals with EDS type IV, as well as a decrease in type III collagen in fibroblast medium. Cells from another individual with EDS type IV secreted decreased amounts of type III collagen and made an abnormal, slow migrating population of proα1(III) collagen molecules (Fig. 9–14).[158] Cells from that patient had greatly increased immunofluorescence with an antibody to type III collagen, strongly suggesting that type III collagen had accumulated within the rough endoplasmic reticulum. Stolle and associates[159] demonstrated in another EDS type IV cell strain that the rates of secretion of type III collagen from cultured dermal fibroblasts was reduced dramatically (Fig. 9–15), and there was a structurally abnormal population of type III collagen with decreased thermal stability, similar to results seen with abnormal type I collagen synthesized by cells from patients with osteogenesis imperfecta.[125, 146]

The clinical phenotype of EDS type IV and the biochemical abnormalities in type III collagen in cultured dermal fibroblasts cosegregated with an *EcoRI* restriction fragment length polymorphism in the type III collagen gene

(COL3A1) in several families.[155] In one EDS type IV cell strain, Superti-Furga and colleagues showed that abnormal biochemical findings in type III collagen may be due to a structural rearrangement of the type III collagen gene that results in a peptidyl deletion.[160] Heterozygosity for a multi-exon deletion from the triple helical domain of COL3A1 was associated with intracellular retention and decreased thermal stability of molecules containing shortened proα1(III) chains.[160] More recently, DNA sequence analysis of cDNAs and genomic DNA from another family with EDS type IV showed an affected member to be heterozygous for a glycine-to-aspartate substitution at position 883 in the triple helical domain of COL3A1.[161] The effects of this substitution of a triple helical glycine were diminished secretion of type III collagen molecules into fibroblast medium and production of a population of type III collagen molecules with decreased thermal stability. Biochemical effects resulting from heterozygous mutations in type III collagen may be even more pronounced than those in type I collagen because random incorporation of mutant proα1(III) chains into homotrimeric type III collagen molecules results in seven eighths of the molecules having at least one mutant chain (Fig. 9–16).

EDS Type V. Ehlers-Danlos syndrome type V is a rare, X-linked disorder characterized by mild skin hyperelasticity, mildly abnormal scarring, and joint hyperextensibility. Female carriers are asymptomatic. There are only a few well-documented families with EDS type V in the literature.[162, 163] This rare disorder clinically resembles EDS type II except that the latter disorder has autosomal dominant inheritance. Thus in clinical situations in which EDS type V and EDS type II are both diagnostic possibilities, the more common EDS type II form should be considered unless family history clearly suggests X-linked inheritance. The molecular basis of EDS type V is unknown. Although lysyl oxidase activity in fibroblast medium from affected members in one family was found to be decreased,[164] the assay used in that study was later reported to give inconsistent results. In other families with EDS type V, lysyl oxidase activity from fibroblast medium was normal.

EDS Type VI. Type VI Ehlers-Danlos syndrome was the first of the EDS subtypes to have its biochemical and genetic basis understood: decreased hydroxylysine content of collagen in skin and other organs from affected individuals[165] and reduced activity of lysyl hydroxylase measured in cultured dermal fibro-

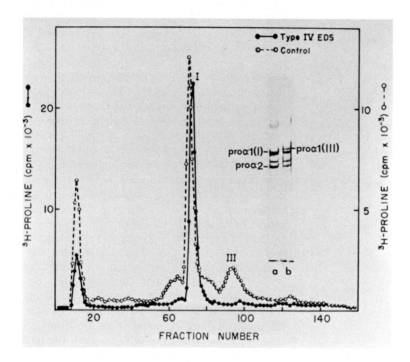

Figure 9–14. DEAE cellulose chromatography of ³H-proline–labeled proteins in medium of control cells (*open circles*) and a patient with Ehlers-Danlos syndrome (EDS) type IV (*closed circles*). There is very little material that elutes in the position of type III procollagen in the medium from affected cells. *Insets,* Fluorograms of ³H-proline–labeled proteins from EDS type IV (*a*) and normal (*b*) cells separated by SDS/polyacrylamide gel electrophoresis under reducing conditions. Only a small amount of proα1(III) is apparent in the medium from the affected cells. (Reprinted with permission from Byers PH, Holbrook KA, Barsch GS, et al: Altered secretion of type III procollagen in a form of type IV Ehlers-Danlos syndrome. Lab Invest 44:338, 1981. © US & Canadian Academy of Pathology, Inc.)

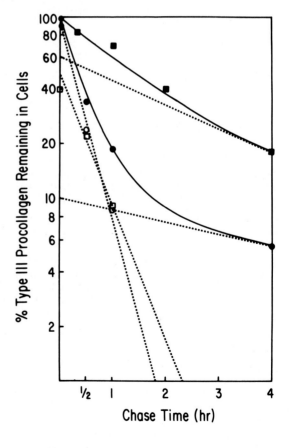

Figure 9–15. Secretion of type III procollagen from ³H-proline–labeled control (*closed circles*) and EDS type IV patient's (*closed squares*) fibroblasts, as determined by densitometric scanning of polyacrylamide gels. The rate constants for secretion were calculated using values obtained by exponential peeling of curves for control (*open circles*) and EDS type IV (*open squares*) fibroblasts. (Reprinted with permission from Stolle CA, Pyeritz RE, Myers JC, Prockop DJ: Synthesis of an altered type III procollagen in a patient with type IV Ehlers-Danlos syndrome. J Biol Chem 260:1942, 1985.)

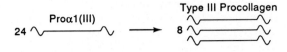

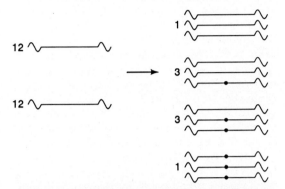

Figure 9–16. Stoichiometry of type III procollagen synthesis from an individual who is heterozygous for a structural mutation in one COL3A1 allele.

blasts.[166] A recent review of the clinical findings in ten patients with documented lysyl hydroxylase deficiency indicates that the cardinal features of lysyl hydroxylase deficiency are neonatal onset of joint laxity, kyphoscoliosis, and hypotonia.[167] Ocular fragility, which was noted in the original reports of lysyl hydroxylase deficiency,[165] was found in only a minority of patients. Skin fragility, easy bruisability, and dermal hyperextensibility were present to some extent in most EDS type VI patients. Three of ten affected individuals suffered a potentially catastrophic arterial rupture.

Hydroxylysine-deficient collagen is secreted efficiently from cultured fibroblasts of EDS type VI patients but does not undergo crosslinking as efficiently as collagen from controls.[168] Decreased hydroxylysine content of collagen from EDS type VI individuals varies not only among collagen types but also within the same collagen type isolated from different tissues. Collagens from skin (primarily types I and III) are deficient in hydroxylysine but collagen from cartilage (primarily type II) is not.[169] Although type I collagen is the predominant form of collagen in skin, tendon, and bone, collagen from skin and tendon was hydroxylysine deficient in one individual with EDS type VI while collagen in bone was not (Table 9–3). In cell culture experiments, types I, III, and V collagen isolated from the media of EDS type VI dermal fibroblasts were hydroxylysine deficient as compared to controls.[170] There is at present a reliable assay for lysyl hydroxylase from fibroblasts in which underhydroxylated skin collagen is used as a substrate and prolyl hydroxylase activity is used as a positive control.[171] Biochemical analysis suggests that more than one mutant lysyl hydroxylase allele may exist in humans; in one patient's fibroblasts, the enzyme had altered affinity for ascorbic acid and decreased thermal stability, and in another, lysyl hydroxylase had normal thermal stability and normal ascorbate affinity but decreased maximal activity.[172, 173] There are also individuals with clinical findings identical to those in documented lysyl hydroxylase deficiency who have normal lysyl hydroxylase activity but mildly decreased hydroxylysine content in the skin.[174] At present the protein structure, DNA sequence, and chromosomal location of the lysyl hydroxylase gene are unknown. Undoubtedly some of the apparent inconsistencies of expression in different tissues of EDS type VI individuals and apparent deficiency of hydroxylysine in individuals with normal enzyme activity will be resolved when genetic analysis of lysyl hydroxylase deficiency becomes possible.

EDS Type VII. Type VII Ehlers-Danlos syndrome (arthrochalasia multiplex) is characterized by extreme joint laxity, multiple joint

Table 9–3. HYDROXYLATION OF PROLINE AND LYSINE RESIDUES IN CLINICALLY AFFECTED TISSUES OF THE EDS PATIENT AND CONTROLS

	Skin		Tendon		Bone		Cartilage	
	Patient	*Controls*	*Patient*	*Controls*	*Patient*	*Controls*	*Patient*	*Controls*
$\dfrac{Hyp^*}{Hyp + Pro}$	40	40	41	40	41	40	45	41
$\dfrac{Hyl^*}{Hyl + Lys}$	0	7.7	6.7	23	6.4	6.2	39	35
Hyl/Hyp	0	0.04	0.05	0.09	0.04	0.04	0.19	0.14

*Expressed as per cent. Hyp = hydroxyproline; Pro = proline; Lys = lysine; Hyl = hydroxylysine.
Adapted from Ihme A, Kreig T, Nerlick A, et al: Ehlers-Danlos Type IV: Collagen type specificity of defective lysyl hydroxylation in various tissues. J Invest Dermatol 83:161–165, © Williams & Wilkins, 1984.

dislocations, and congenital hip dislocations that are difficult to repair surgically. The basic defect is failure of cleavage of the amino-terminal propeptide of type I procollagen chains by collagen aminopeptidase. Although it was originally thought that EDS type VII was due to an enzymatic abnormality in conversion of procollagen to collagen,[175] all known cases that have undergone molecular analysis are the result of heterozygosity for mutations in proα1(I) or proα2(I) chains of type I collagen that result in deletion or disruption of the aminopeptidase cleavage site rather than abnormalities of the procollagen aminopeptidase enzyme itself. Therefore, it appears that EDS type VII is usually an autosomal dominant disorder, although recessive forms due to deficiency of the enzyme are theoretically possible. Several cell strains from individuals with the clinical diagnosis of EDS type VII have undergone biochemical and molecular analysis. In one case, an individual with EDS type VII was heterozygous for a mutation that resulted in deletion of the 24 amino acid residues from proα1(I) chains that are coded for by exon 6 of COL1A1.[176] The deleted segment contained the aminopeptidase cleavage site, a short globular region, the amino-terminal telopeptide, and the first triplet at the amino-terminal end of the triple helix (Fig. 9–17). In another individual with EDS type VII, collagens prepared from dermis contained a PNα2(I) chain (produced by cleavage of the carboxyl-terminal propeptide from the proα2(I) collagen chain but not the amino-terminal propeptide) that was not seen in dermis from normal individuals.[177] Fibro-

blasts from that individual produced type I procollagen in which only one half of proα2(I) chains were cleaved with chick procollagen aminopeptidase. Weil and co-workers[178] showed that some proα2(I) mRNAs harvested from those cells contained a deletion of 54 bases coded for by exon 6 of COL1A2, containing the amino-terminal cleavage site of proα2(I) chains. This deletion was due to a single nucleotide substitution in the GT consensus sequence at the splice acceptor region immediately 3' to exon 6.[179] The mutation produced aberrant splicing in some mRNAs transcribed by the mutant allele and resulted in removal of exon 6 sequences during mRNA processing. Ultrastructural studies have shown that incorporation of molecules containing uncleaved proα1(I) chains distorts fibrillar structure (Fig. 9–18).[180]

EDS Type VIII. Ehlers-Danlos syndrome type VIII is a rare autosomal dominant condition characterized by soft, hyperextensible skin, abnormal scarring, easy bruising, hyperextensible joints, and generalized periodontitis.[181, 182] It resembles EDS type I but is clinically distinguished by the presence of periodontitis and by a characteristic purplish discoloration of scars, particularly those on the shins. The molecular basis of EDS type VIII is completely unknown.

EDS Type IX. Ehlers-Danlos syndrome type IX is a rare disorder characterized by lax, extremely soft skin at birth and by later development of skeletal deformities such as occipital horns, short humeri, and short broad clavicles.[183, 184] Inheritance is X-linked recessive.[185] Affected males may also have bladder diverticulae that can result in hydronephrosis, and may

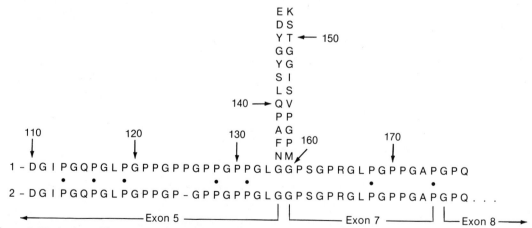

Figure 9–17. Amino acid sequences from the products of normal (*line 1*) and abnormal (*line 2*) COL1A1 alleles from an individual with Ehlers-Danlos syndrome type VII in the region of the amino-terminal propeptide cleavage site. The residues are numbered from the first residue of the proα1(I) chains at the amino-terminal end. The looped out region corresponds to the 24 amino acids coded for by exon 6 that are missing in the abnormal gene product. Closed circles above proline residues indicate hydroxyproline. (Adapted with permission from Cole WG, Chan D, Chambers GW, et al: Deletion of 24 amino acids from the proα1(I) chain of type I procollagen in a patient with the Ehlers-Danlos syndrome type VII. J Biol Chem 262:5500, 1986.)

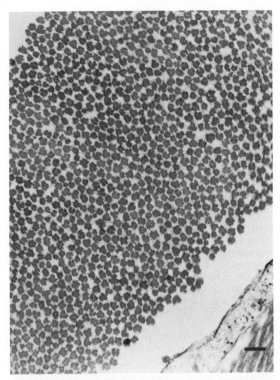

Figure 9–18. Transverse section of collagen fibrils of the skin of an individual with Ehlers-Danlos syndrome type VII who synthesized a population of proα1(I) chains missing 24 amino acids that contain the amino propeptide cleavage site (× 21,500) (see Fig. 9–17). (Adapted with permission from Cole WG, Evans R, Sillence DO: The clinical features of Ehlers-Danlos syndrome type VII due to a deletion of 24 amino acids from the proα1(I) chain of type I procollagen. J Med Genet 24:701, 1986.)

have a chronic diarrhea of unknown etiology.[184] Intellect is usually unaffected. The basic defect in EDS type IX is unknown, but it appears to be related to a defect in intracellular transport of copper.[186] This defect is shared with a related but far more severe condition, Menkes' syndrome, which is characterized by abnormalities of hair, arteries, and bones and by progressive cerebral degeneration that usually leads to death by 3 years of age. The result of the abnormal copper transport in both EDS type IX and Menkes' syndrome is a reduction in activity of the copper-dependent enzyme lysyl oxidase, which participates in the metabolism of crosslink precursors in both collagen and elastin.[187, 188] In cultured dermal fibroblasts from EDS type IX patients, copper in fibroblast medium is taken up normally into cells but accumulates intracellularly and is not released with lysyl oxidase into medium. In a series of individuals with either EDS type IX or Menkes' syndrome, intracellular concentration or uptake of ^{64}[Cu] was inversely related to lysyl oxidase activity.[188] It is likely that there are other af-

fected copper-dependent enzymes in both Menkes' syndrome and EDS type IX that account for some clinical manifestations of each. The diagnosis of EDS type IX is usually suspected by the clinical findings and by measurement of serum copper and ceruloplasmin, both of which are usually far below normal levels.

EDS Type X. In the case of Ehlers-Danlos syndrome type X, Arneson and co-workers[189] reported a single family in which two siblings of unaffected parents had joint hyperextensibility, mitral valve prolapse, easy bruisibility, and poor wound healing. Clotting studies performed to evaluate excessive bleeding at incision sites were normal except for a striking defect in platelet adhesion that is normally observed in response to exposure of platelets to collagen. Addition of purified fibronectin to the patients' plasma improved platelet adhesiveness. The authors suggested that this disorder may be due to a defect in fibronectin.

Unclassified EDS Variants

Sasaki and associates[190] described an individual with joint hypermobility, hyperextensible skin, and prolonged wound healing who developed dilation of the proximal aorta and consequent aortic valve insufficiency. Cultured dermal fibroblasts synthesized decreased amounts of type I collagen and did not synthesize proα2(I) chains. The family history was negative, and cells from the parents were not available for study. Cultured dermal fibroblasts from another EDS patient with similar skin and joint findings, easy bruising, and mitral valve prolapse but normal proximal aorta also failed to synthesize proα2(I) chains.[191] Steady-state proα2(I) mRNAs were greatly decreased but proα1(I) mRNAs were present in normal amounts. In the latter case, the authors postulated that the affected individual was homozygous for nonfunctional proα2(I) allele. At present it is not clear how deficiency of proα2(I) chains results in Ehlers-Danlos syndrome variants since previous data have clearly demonstrated that homozygosity for a mutation in the carboxyl propeptide of proα2(I) chains that completely prevents proα2(I) chains from being incorporated into type I collagen molecules results in osteogenesis imperfecta and not EDS.[192, 193]

Disorders Due to Mutations in Type II Collagen

Recent studies indicate that mutations in the type II collagen genes result in several disorders of cartilaginous tissue. Francomano and co-workers demonstrated linkage to COL2A1 with the Stickler syndrome (hereditary arthro-oph-thalmopathy),[194] an autosomal dominant disorder characterized by abnormal facies, large joints, marfanoid habitus, high myopia, retinal detachment, and cataracts. The nature of mutations at the COL2A1 locus have yet to be determined.

Two other chondrodysplasias, spondyloepi-physeal dysplasia (SED) and achondrogenesis type II, appear to also result from mutations in COL2A1. SED in one family was the result of heterozygosity for a tandem duplication of 45 bp in exon 48, which contains coding sequences for the carboxyl end of the triple helix.[195] In a second SED family, an affected individual was heterozygous for a deletion of exon 48.[196] An infant with lethal achondrogenesis type II was found to be heterozygous for a serine-for-gly-cine substitution at residue 943 in the triple helical domain of COL2A1.[197] Cultured chon-drocytes from individuals with either SED or achondrogenesis synthesized normal and over-modified populations of $\alpha1(II)$ chains (Fig. 9–19), similar to type I collagen synthesized by

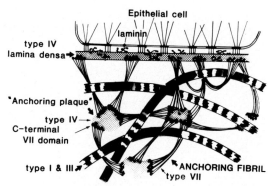

Figure 9–20. Proposed model of the anchoring fibril network. It has been proposed that the anchoring fibrils are composed of lateral aggregates of type VII procol-lagen aligned in a nonstaggered array. The anchoring fibrils most frequently originate within the lamina densa and extend perpendicularly to the basement membrane, inserting into anchoring plaques within the matrix. Additional anchoring plaques originate from these plaques and insert into other anchoring plaques farther into the matrix. The anchoring plaques contain both the carboxy-terminal of type VII procollagen and type IV collagen. (Reproduced from the *Journal of Cell Biology*, 1987, Vol. 104, p. 619, by copyright permission of the Rockefeller University Press.)

fibroblasts from individuals with osteogenesis imperfecta.

Disorders of Type VII Collagen

Several studies have shown that type VII collagen is the major component of anchoring fibrils of skin, which connect the lamina densa beneath the epidermis to anchoring plaques in the underlying dermis. (Fig. 9–20).[198] Using affinity-purified polyclonal antibodies to type VII collagen, Bruckner-Tuderman and co-work-ers showed complete absence of antibody stain-ing in the skin of patients with autosomal re-cessive dystrophic epidermolysis bullosa, a heritable skin disorder characterized by severe blistering between the basal layer of epidermal cells and the lamina densa.[199] Antibody staining of skin from patients with other forms of epi-dermolysis bullosa was normal as were the unaffected parents of patients with recessive dystrophic epidermolysis bullosa.

This chapter has reviewed the multiple, over-lapping mechanisms employed by cells to en-sure that only functional, triple helical collagen is deposited in the extracellular space. When-ever this control is lost owing to an environ-mental or genetic alteration, profound changes can occur in the capability of the synthesized collagen to perform its physiological functions.

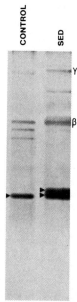

Figure 9–19. Separation by SDS/polyacrylamide gel elec-trophoresis of $\alpha1(II)$ collagen chains extracted from car-tilage from a patient with spondyloepiphyseal dysplasia (SED) and a normal fetal control. Arrowheads indicate slow-migrating and normally migrating populations of $\alpha1(II)$ chains from the patient. (Reprinted with permis-sion from Tiller GE, Rimoin DL, Murray LW, Cohn DH: Tandem duplication within a type II collagen gene (COL2A1 exon in an individual with spondyloepi-physeal dysplasia). Proc Natl Acad Sci USA 87:3890, 1990.)

As described, several variants of Ehlers-Danlos syndrome result in poor wound healing due to an inability to regain sufficient tensile strength at the wound site. Consequently, one needs to be cognizant of these possible alterations when considering the etiology of clinical problems of tissue repair.

References

1. Vuorio E, deCrombrugghe B: The family of collagen genes. Annu Rev Biochem. 59:837–872, 1990.
2. Yamada Y, Avvedimento VE, Mudryj M, et al: The collagen gene: Evidence for its evolutionary assembly by amplification of a DNA segment containing an exon of 54 bp. Cell 22:887–892, 1980.
3. De Wet W, Bernard M, Benson-Chanda V, et al: Organization of the human proα2(I) collagen. J Biol Chem 262:16032–16036, 1987.
4. Kuivaniemi H, Tromp G, Chu M-L, et al: Structure of a full-length cDNA for the preproα2(I) chain of human type I collagen. Biochem J 252:633–640, 1988.
5. Chu M-L, De Wet W, Bernard M, et al: Human proα1(I) collagen gene structure reveals evolutionary conservation of a pattern of introns and exons. Nature 310:337–340, 1984.
6. Myers JC, Dickson LA, De Wet WS, et al: Analysis of the 3' end of the human proα2(I) collagen gene. J Biol Chem 258:10128–10135, 1983.
7. Cheah KSE, Stoker NG, Griffin JR, et al: Identification and characterization of the human type II collagen gene (COL2A1). Proc Natl Acad Sci USA 82:2555–2559, 1985.
8. Sangiorgi FO, Benson-Chanda V, De Wet WJ, et al: Isolation and partial characterization of the entire human proα1(II) collagen gene. Nucleic Acids Res 13:2207–2225, 1985.
9. Chu M-L, Weil D, De Wet W, et al: Isolation of cDNA and genomic clones encoding human proα1(III) collagen. J Biol Chem 260:4357–4363, 1985.
10. Sakurai Y, Sullivan M, Yamada Y: α1 type IV collagen gene evolved differently from fibrillar collagen genes. J Biol Chem 261:6654–6657, 1986.
11. Kurkinem M, Bernard MP, Barlow DP, et al: Characterization of 64-, 123- and 182 base pair exons in the mouse α2(IV) collagen gene. Nature 317:177–179, 1985.
12. Lozano G, Ninomiya Y, Thompson H, et al: A distinct class of vertebrate collagen genes encodes chicken type IX collagen polypeptides. Proc Natl Acad Sci USA 82:4050–4054, 1985.
13. Nishimura I, Muragaki Y, Olsen BR: Tissue-specific forms of type IX collagen-proteoglycan arise from the use of two widely separated promoters. J Biol Chem 264:20033–20041, 1989.
14. Ninomiya Y, Gordon M, van der Rest M, et al: The developmentally regulated type X collagen gene contains a long open reading frame without introns. J Biol Chem 261:5041–5050, 1986.
15. Cheah KSE, Grant ME: Procollagen genes and messenger RNAs. In Weiss JB, Tayson MI (eds): Collagen in Health and Disease. Edinburgh, Churchill Livingstone, 1982, pp 73–100.
16. Avvedimento VE, Vogeli G, Yamada Y, et al: Correlation between splicing sites within an intron and their sequence complementarity with UI RNA. Cell 21:689–696, 1980.
17. Svoboda KK, Nishimura I, Sugrue SP, et al: Embryonic chicken cornea and cartilage synthesize type IX collagen molecules with different amino-terminal domains. Proc Natl Acad Sci USA 85:77496–7500, 1988.
18. Pihlajaniemi T, Tamminen M, Sandbert M, et al: The α1 chain of type XIII collagen polypeptide structure, alternative splicing, and tissue distribution. NY Acad Sci 580:440–443, 1990.
19. Chu M-L, Pan T, Conway D, et al: Sequence analysis of α1(VI) and α2(VI) chains of human type VI collagen reveals internal triplication of globular domains similar to the A domains of von Willebrand factor and two α2(VI) chain variants that differ in the carboxy terminus. EMBO J 8:1939–1946, 1989.
20. Paterson BM, Rosenberg M: Efficient translation of prokaryotic mRNAs in a eukaryotic cell free system requires addition of a cap structure. Nature 279:692–696, 1979.
21. Greenberg JR: Messenger RNA metabolism of animal cells. Possible involvement of untranslated sequences and mRNA-associated proteins. J Cell Biol 64:269–288, 1975.
22. Revel M, Groner Y: Post-transcriptional and translational controls of gene expression in eukaryotes. Annu Rev Biochem 47:1079–1126, 1978.
23. Liau G, Mudryi M, de Chrombrugghe B: Identification of the promoter and first exon of the mouse α1(III) collagen gene. J Biol Chem 260:3773–3777, 1985.
24. Kreil G: Transfer of proteins across membranes. Annu Rev Biochem 50:317–348, 1981.
25. Sabatini DD, Kreibich G, Morimoto T, et al: Mechanisms for the incorporation of proteins in membranes and organelles. J Cell Biol 92:1–22, 1982.
26. Gilmore R, Blobel G: Transient involvement of signal recognition particle and its receptor in the microsomal membrane prior to protein translocation. Cell 35:677–685, 1983.
27. Adams E, Frank L: Metabolism of proline and the hydroxyprolines. Annu Rev Biochem 49:1005–1061, 1980.
28. Kivirikko KI, Myllylä R: The hydroxylation of prolyl and lysyl residues. In Freedman RB, Hawkins HC (eds): The Enzymology of Post-translational Modification of Proteins. New York, Academic Press, 1980, pp 53–104.
29. Cardinale GJ, Udenfriend S: Prolyl hydroxylase. Adv Enzymol 41:245–300, 1974.
30. Kivirikko KI, Myllylä R: Post-translational enzymes in the biosynthesis of collagen: Intracellular enzymes. Meth Enzymol 82A:245–304, 1982.
31. Risteli J, Tryggvason K, Kivirikko KI: A rapid assay for prolyl 3-hydroxylase activity. Anal Biochem 84:423–431, 1978.
32. Turpeenniemi-Hujanen TM: Immunological characterization of lysyl hydroxylase, an enzyme of collagen biosynthesis. Biochem J 195:669–676, 1981.
33. Kivirikko KI, Kuivaniemi H: Post-translational modifications of collagen and their alterations in heritable diseases. In Uitto T, Perejola AT (eds): Diseases of Connective Tissue: The Molecular Pathology of the Extracellular Matrix. New York, Marcel Dekker, 1987, pp 263–292.
34. Berg RA, Kedersah NL, Guzman NA: Purification and partial characterization of the two nonidentical subunits of prolyl hydroxylase. J Biol Chem 254:3111–3118, 1979.
35. Koivu J, Myllylä R, Helaakoski T, et al: A single polypeptide acts both as the β subunit of prolyl 4-hydroxylase and as a protein disulfide-isomerase. J Biol Chem 262:6447–6449, 1987.

36. Pihlajaniemi T, Helaakoski T, Tasanen K, et al: Molecular cloning of the β-subunit of human prolyl 4-hydroxylase. This subunit and protein disulfide isomerase are products of the same gene. EMBO J 6:643–649, 1987.
37. Myllyla R, Pajunen L, Kivirikko KI: Polyclonal and monoclonal antibodies to human lysyl hydroxylase and studies on the molecular heterogeneity of the enzyme. Biochem J 253:489–496, 1988.
38. Puistola U: Catalytic properties of lysyl hydroxylase from cells synthesizing genetically different collagen types. Biochem J 201:215–219, 1982.
39. Kivirikko KI, Myllylä R: Collagen glycosyl-transferases. Int Rev Connect Tissue Res 8:23–72, 1979.
40. Harding JJ, Crabbe MJC, Panjwani NA: Collagen crosslinking. In Robert A-M, Robert L (eds): Biochemistry of Normal and Pathological Connective Tissues. Paris, Centre National de la Recherche Scientifique, 1980, pp 51–64.
41. Clark CC: The distribution and initial characterization of oligosaccharide units on the COOH-terminal propeptide extensions of the pro-α1 and pro-α2 chains of type I procollagen. J Biol Chem 254:10798–10802, 1979.
42. Anttinen H, Oikarinen A, Ryhänen L, et al: Evidence for the transfer of mannose to the extension peptides of procollagen within the cisternae of the rough endoplasmic reticulum. FEBS Lett 87:222–226, 1978.
43. Clark CC: Asparagine-linked glycosides. Methods Enzymol 82:346–360, 1982.
44. Kornfeld R, Kornfeld S: Assembly of asparagine-linked oligosaccharides. Annu Rev Biochem 54:631–664, 1985.
45. Koivu J: Identification of disulfide bonds in carboxy-terminal propeptides of human type I procollagen. FEBS Lett 212:229–232, 1987.
46. Bruckner P, Eikenberry EF, Prockop DJ: Formation of the triple helix of type I procollagen in cellulo. A kinetic model based on cis-trans isomerization of peptide bonds. Eur J Biochem 118:607–613, 1981.
47. Palade G: Intracellular aspects of the process of protein synthesis. Science 189:347–358, 1975.
48. Grant ME, Jackson DS: The biosynthesis of procollagen. Essays Biochem 12:77–113, 1976.
49. Fessler LI, Brosh S, Chapin S, et al: Tyrosine sulfation in precursors of collagen V. J Biol Chem 261:5034–5040, 1986.
50. Fessler LI, Chapin S, Brosh S, et al: Intracellular transport and tyrosine sulfation of procollagens V. Eur J Biochem 158:511–518, 1986.
51. Fisher LW, Robey PG, Tuross N, et al: The M_1 24,000 phosphoprotein from developing bone is the NH_2-terminal propeptide of the α1 chain of type I collagen. J Biol Chem 262:13457–13463, 1987.
52. Lapiere CM, Lenaers A, Kohn LD: Procollagen peptidase: An enzyme excising the coordination peptides of procollagen. Proc Natl Acad Sci USA 68:3054–3058, 1971.
53. Tuderman L, Prockop DJ: Procollagen N-proteinase: Properties of the enzyme purified from chick embryo tendons. Eur J Biochem 125:545–549, 1982.
54. Morris NP, Fessler LI, Fessler JH: Procollagen propeptide release by procollagen peptidases and bacterial collagenase. J Biol Chem 254:11014–11032, 1979.
55. Hailila R, Peltonen L: Neutral protease cleaving the N-terminal propeptide of type III procollagen: Partial purification and characterization of the enzyme from smooth muscle cells of bovine aorta. Biochemistry 23:1251–1256, 1984.
56. Heathcote JG, Grant ME: Extracellular modification of connective tissue proteins. In Freedman RB, Hawkins HC (eds): The Enzymology of Post-translational Modifications of Proteins. New York, Academic Press, 1980, pp 457–550.
57. Galloway D: The primary structure. In Weiss JB, Jayson MIV (eds): Collagen in Health and Disease. New York, Churchill Livingstone, 1982, pp 528–557.
58. Wozney J, Hanahan D, Tate V, et al: Structure of the proα2(I) collagen gene. Nature 294:129–135, 1981.
59. Tuderman L, Kivirikko KI, Prockop DJ: Partial purification and characterization of a neutral protease which cleaves the N-terminal propeptides from procollagen. Biochemistry 17:2948–2954, 1978.
60. Morikawa T, Tuderman L, Prockop DJ: Inhibitors of procollagen N-protease: Synthetic peptides with sequences similar to the cleavage site in the proα(I) chain. Biochemistry 19:2646–2650, 1980.
61. Hojima Y, van der Rest M, Prockop DJ: Type I procollagen carboxyl-terminal proteinase from chick embryo tendons: Purification and characterization. J Biol Chem 260:15996–16003, 1985.
62. Kivirikko KI, Myllylä R: Biosynthesis of the collagens. In Piez KA, Reddi AH (eds): Extracellular Matrix Biochemistry. New York, Elsevier, 1984, pp 83–118.
63. Helseth DL Jr, Veiss A: Collagen self-assembly in vitro: Differentiating specific telopeptide-dependent interactions using selective enzyme modification and the addition of free amino telopeptide. J Biol Chem 256:7118–7128, 1981.
64. Piez KA, Trus BL: A new model for packing of type I collagen molecules in the native fibril. Biosci Rep 1:801–810, 1981.
65. Piez KA, Trus BL: Sequence regularities and packing of collagen molecule. J Mol Biol 122:419–432, 1978.
66. Eyre D: Collagen cross-linking amino acids. Meth Enzymol 114:115–139, 1987.
67. Siegel RC: Lysyl oxidase. Int Rev Connect Tissue Res 8:73–118, 1979.
68. Kagan HM: Characterization and regulation of lysyl oxidase. In Mecham RP (ed): Regulation of Matrix Accumulation. New York, Academic Press, 1986, pp 322–389.
69. Robins SP: Turnover and cross-linking of collagen. In Weiss JB, Jayson MIV (eds): Collagen in Health and Disease. New York, Churchill Livingston, 1982, pp 160–178.
70. Pinnell SR, Murad S: Disorders of Collagen. In Stanbury JB, Wyngaarden JB, Fredrickson DS, et al (eds): The Metabolic Basis of Inherited Disease, 5th ed. New York, McGraw-Hill, 1983, pp 1425–1449.
71. Birkedahl-Hansen H: Catabolism and turnover of collagens-collagenases. Methods Enzymol 144D:140–171, 1987.
72. Bienkowski RS: Kinetics of intracellular degradation of newly synthesized collagen. Biochemistry 25:2455–2459, 1986.
73. Neblock DS, Berg RA: Intracellular degradation as a modulator of collagen production. In Uitto T, Perejola AT (eds): Diseases of Connective Tissue: The Molecular Pathology of the Extracellular Matrix. New York, Marcel Dekker, 1987, pp 233–246.
74. Solomon E, Hiorns L, Dalgleish R, et al: Regional localization of the human α2(I) collagen gene on chromosome 7 by molecular hybridization. Cytogenet Cell Genet 35:64–66, 1983.
75. Sunderraj CV, Church RL, Klobutcher LA, et al: Genetics of the connective tissue proteins: Assignment of the gene for human type I procollagen to chromosome 17 by analysis of cell hybrids and microcell hybrids. Proc Natl Acad Sci USA 74:4444–4448, 1977.
76. Huerre C, Junien C, Weil D, et al: Human type I procollagen genes are located on different chromosomes. Proc Natl Acad Sci USA 79:6627–6630, 1982.

77. De Wet WJ, Chu M-L, Prockop DJ: The mRNAs for the pro-α1(I) and pro-α2(I) chains of type I procollagen are translated at the same rate in normal human fibroblasts and in fibroblasts from two variants of osteogenesis imperfecta with altered steady state ratios of the two mRNAs. J Biol Chem 258:14385–14387, 1983.

78. Schmidt A, Rossi P, de Crombrugghe B: Transcriptional control of the mouse α2(I) collagen gene: Functional deletion analysis of the promoter and evidence for cell-specific expression. Mol Cell Biol 6:347–354, 1986.

79. Hatamochi A, Paterson B, de Crombrugghe B: Differential binding of a CCAAT DNA binding factor to the promoters of the mouse α2(I) and α1(III) collagen genes. J Biol Chem 24:11310–11314, 1986.

80. Liau G, Szapary D, Setoyama C, et al: Restriction enzyme digestions identify discrete domains in the chromatin around the promoter of the mouse α2(I) collagen gene. J Biol Chem 261:11362–11368, 1986.

81. Oikarinen H, Hatamochi A, de Crombrugghe B: Separate binding sites for nuclear factor 1 and a CCAAT DNA binding factor in the mouse α2(I) collagen promoter. J Biol Chem 262:11064–11070, 1987.

82. Ristiniemi J, Oikarinen J: Histone H1 binds to the putative nuclear factor I recognition sequence in the mouse α2(I) collagen promoter. J Biol Chem 264:2164–2174, 1989.

83. Bornstein P, McKay J, Morishima JK, et al: Regulatory elements in the first intron contribute to transcriptional control of the human α1(I) collagen gene. Proc Natl Acad Sci USA 84:8869–8873, 1987.

84. Rossi P, de Crombrugghe B: Identification of a cell-specific transcriptional enhancer in the first intron of the mouse α2(type I) collagen gene. Proc Natl Acad Sci USA 84:5590–5594, 1987.

85. Horton W, Miyashita T, Kohno K, et al: Identification of a phenotype-specific enhancer in the first intron of the rat collagen II gene. Proc Natl Acad Sci USA 84:8864–8868, 1987.

86. Bornstein P, McKay J: The first intron of the α1(I) collagen gene contains several transcriptional regulatory elements. J Biol Chem 263:1603–1606, 1988.

87. Yamada Y, Mudryj M, de Crombrugghe B: A uniquely conserved regulatory signal is found around the translational initiation site in three different collagen genes. J Biol Chem 258:14914–14919, 1983.

88. Schmidt A, Yamada Y, de Crombrugghe B: DNA sequence comparison of the regulatory signals at the 5′ end of the mouse and chick α2 type I collagen genes. J Biol Chem 259:7411–7415, 1984.

89. Bennett VC, Adams SL: Characterization of the translational control mechanism preventing synthesis of α2(I) collagen in chicken vertebral chondroblasts. J Biol Chem 262:14806–14814, 1987.

90. Carpousis A, Christner P, Rosenbloom J: Preferential usage of tRNA isoaccepting species in collagen synthesis. J Biol Chem 252:8023–8026, 1977.

91. Leboy PS, Uschmann BD, Lin D: Increased levels of glycine tRNA associated with collagen synthesis. Arch Biochem Biophys 259:558–566, 1987.

92. Paglia L, Wilczek J, de Leon LD, et al: Inhibition of procollagen cell-free synthesis by amino-terminal extension peptides. Biochemistry 18:5030–5034, 1979.

93. Wiestner M, Krieg T, Horlein D, et al: Inhibiting effect of procollagen peptides on collagen biosynthesis in fibroblast cultures. J Biol Chem 254:7016–7023, 1979.

94. Horlein D, McPherson J, Goh SH, et al: Regulation of protein synthesis: Translational control by procollagen-derived fragments. Proc Natl Acad Sci USA 78:6163–6167, 1981.

95. Aycock RS, Raghow R, Striklin GP, et al: Post-transcriptional inhibition of collagen and fibronectin synthesis by a synthetic homolog of a portion of the carboxyl-terminal propeptide of human type I collagen. J Biol Chem 261:14355–14360, 1986.

96. Wu CH, Donovan CD, Wu GY: Evidence for pretranslational regulation of collagen synthesis by procollagen propeptides. J Biol Chem 261:10482–10484, 1986.

97. Murad S, Grove D, Lindberg KA, et al: Regulation of collagen synthesis by ascorbic acid. Proc Natl Acad Sci USA 78:2879–2882, 1981.

98. Geesin JC, Darr D, Kaufman R, et al: Ascorbic acid specifically increases type I and type III procollagen messenger RNA levels in human skin fibroblasts. J Invest Dermatol 90:420–424, 1988.

99. Roberts AB, Sporn MB, Assoian RK, et al: Transforming growth factor type-β: Rapid induction of fibrosis and angiogenesis in vivo and stimulation of collagen formation in vitro. Proc Natl Acad Sci USA 83:4167–4171, 1986.

100. Varga J, Jimenez SA: Stimulation of normal human fibroblast collagen production and processing by transforming growth factor-β. Biochem Biophys Res Commun 138:974–980, 1986.

101. Varga J, Rosenbloom J, Jimenez SA: Transforming growth factor-β (TGFβ) causes a persistent increase in steady-state amounts of type I and type III collagen and fibronectin mRNAs in normal human dermal fibroblasts. Biochem J 247:597–604, 1987.

102. Ignotz RA, Endo T, Massague J: Regulation of fibronectin and type I collagen mRNA levels by transforming growth factor-β. J Biol Chem 262:6443–6446, 1987.

103. Rossi P, Karsenty G, Roberts AB, et al: A nuclear factor 1 binding site mediates the transcriptional activation of a type I collagen promoter by transforming growth factor-β. Cell 52:405–414, 1988.

104. Raghow R, Postlethwaite AE, Keski-Oja J, et al: Transforming growth factor-β increases steady state levels of type I procollagen and fibronectin messenger RNAs posttranscriptionally in cultured human dermal fibroblasts. J Clin Invest 79:1285–1288, 1987.

105. Penttinen RP, Kobayashi S, Bornstein P: Transforming growth factor-β increases mRNA for matrix proteins both in the presence and in the absence of changes in mRNA stability. Proc Natl Acad Sci USA 85:1105–1108, 1988.

106. Mustoe TA, Pierce GF, Thomason A, et al: Accelerated healing of incisional wounds in rats induced by transforming growth factor-β. Science 237:1333–1336, 1987.

107. Willis DH Jr, Liberti JP: Post-receptor actions of somatomedin on chondrocyte collagen biosynthesis. Biochim Biophys Acta 844:72–80, 1985.

108. McCarthy TL, Centrella M, Canalis E: Regulatory effects of insulin-like growth factors I and II on bone collagen synthesis in rat calvarial cultures. Endocrinology 124:301–309, 1989.

109. Canalis E: Interleukin-1 has independent effects on deoxyribonucleic acid and collagen synthesis in cultures of rat calvariae. Endocrinology 118:74–81, 1986.

110. Kahari V-M, Heino J, Vuorio E: Interleukin-1 increases collagen production and mRNA levels in cultured skin fibroblasts. Biochim Biophys Acta 929:142–147, 1987.

111. Bhatnagar R, Penfornis H, Mauviel A, et al: Interleukin-1 inhibits the synthesis of collagen by fibroblasts. Biochem Int 13:709–720, 1986.

112. Rosenbloom J, Feldman G, Freundlich B, et al: Inhibition of excessive scleroderma fibroblast collagen

production by recombinant τ interferon. Arthritis Rheum 29:851–856, 1986.

113. Granstein RD, Murphy GF, Margolis RJ, et al: Gamma-interferon inhibits collagen synthesis in vivo in the mouse. J Clin Invest 79:1254–1258, 1987.

114. Czaja MJ, Weiner FR, Eghbali M, et al: Differential effects of τ interferon on collagen and fibronectin gene expression. J Biol Chem 262:13348–13351, 1987.

115. Solis-Herruzo JA, Brenner DA, Chojkier M: Tumor necrosis factor inhibits collagen gene transcription and collagen synthesis in cultured human fibroblasts. J Biol Chem 263:5841–5845, 1988.

116. Nanes MS, McKoy WM, Marx SJ: Inhibitory effects of tumor necrosis factor-α and interferon τ on deoxyribonucleic acid and collagen synthesis by rat osteosarcoma cells (ROS 17/2.8). Endocrinology 124:339–345, 1989.

117. Raghow R, Gossage D, Kang AH: Pretranslational regulation of type I collagen, fibronectin, and a 50-kilodalton noncollagenous extracellular protein by dexamethasone in rat fibroblasts. J Biol Chem 261:4677–4684, 1986.

118. Cockayne D Jr, Sterling KM, Shull S, et al: Glucocorticoids decrease the synthesis of type I procollagen mRNAs. Biochemistry 25:3202–3209, 1986.

119. Cockayne D, Cutroneo KR: Glucocorticoid coordinate regulation of type I procollagen gene expression and procollagen DNA-binding proteins in chick skin fibroblasts. Biochemistry 27:2736–2745, 1988.

120. Weiner FR, Czaja MJ, Jefferson DM, et al: The effects of dexamethasone on in vitro collagen gene expression. J Biol Chem 262:6955–6958, 1987.

121. Oikarinen AI, Vuorio EI, Zaragoza EJ, et al: Modulation of collagen metabolism by glucocorticoids. Biochem Pharm 37:1451–1462, 1988.

122. Kream BE, Rowe D, Smith MD, et al: Hormonal regulation of collagen synthesis in a clonal rat osteosarcoma cell line. Endocrinology 119:1922–1928, 1986.

123. Kim HT, Chen TL: 1,25-Dihydroxyvitamin D3 interaction with dexamethasone and retinoic acid: Effects on procollagen messenger ribonucleic acid levels in rat osteoblast-like cells. Mol Endocrinol 3:97–104, 1989.

124. Smith R, Francis MJO, Houghton GR: The Brittle Bone Syndrome: Osteogenesis Imperfecta. London, Butterworths, 1983.

125. Byers PH: Disorders of collagen biosynthesis and structure. In Scriver CR, Beaudet AL, Sly WS, et al (eds): The Metabolic Basis of Inherited Diseases, 6th ed. New York, McGraw-Hill, 1989, pp 2805–2842.

126. Byers PH, Bonadio JF: The nature, characterization and phenotypic effects of mutations that affect collagen structure and processing. In Olsen BR, Nimni M (eds): Collagen: Biochemistry, Biotechnology, and Molecular Biology. Boca Raton, FL, CRC Press, 1988.

127. Sillence DO, Senn AS, Danks DM: Genetic heterogeneity in osteogenesis imperfecta. J Med Genet 16:101–116, 1979.

128. Barsh GS, David KE, Byers PH: Type I osteogenesis imperfecta: A nonfunctional allele for proα1(I) chains of type I procollagen. Proc Natl Acad Sci USA 79:3838–3842, 1982.

129. Rowe DW, Shapiro JR, Poirier M, et al: Diminished type I collagen synthesis and reduced α1(I) collagen messenger RNA in cultured fibroblasts from patients with dominantly inherited (type I) osteogenesis imperfecta. J Clin Invest 76:604–611, 1985.

130. Willing MC, Cohn DH, Byers PH: Frameshift mutation near the 3′ end of the COL1A1 gene of the type I collagen predicts an elongated proα1(I) chain

and results in osteogenesis imperfecta. J Clin Invest 85:282–290, 1990.

131. Byers PH, Tsipouras P, Bonadio JF, et al: Perinatal lethal osteogenesis imperfecta (OI type II): A biochemically heterogeneous disorder usually due to new mutations in the genes for type I collagen. Am J Hum Genet 42:237–248, 1988.

132. Wenstrup RJ, Willing MC, Starman BS, et al: Distinct biochemical phenotypes predict clinical severity in nonlethal variants of osteogenesis imperfecta. Am J Hum Genet 46:975–982, 1990.

133. Kuivaniemi H, Sabol C, Tromp G, et al: A 19-base pair deletion in the proα2(I) gene of type I procollagen that causes in-frame RNA splicing from exon 10 to exon 12 in a proband with atypical osteogenesis imperfecta and in his asymptomatic mother. J Biol Chem 263:11407–11413, 1988.

134. Tromp G, Prockop DJ: Single base mutation in the proα2(I) gene of type I procollagen that causes efficient splicing of RNA from exon 27 to exon 29 and synthesis of a shortened in-frame proα2(I) chain in a lethal variant of osteogenesis imperfecta. Proc Natl Acad Sci USA 85:5254–5258, 1988.

135. Bonadio JF, Ramirez F, Barr M: An intron mutation in the human α1(I) gene alters the efficiency of pre-mRNA splicing and is associated with osteogenesis imperfecta type II. J Biol Chem 265:2262–2268, 1990.

136. Wenstrup RJ, Shrago AW, Phillips CL, et al: Osteogenesis imperfecta (OI) type IV: Analysis for mutations in α2(I) chains of type I collagen by α2(I)-specific cDNA synthesis and polymerase chain reaction (PCR). Ann NY Acad Sci 580:500–561, 1990.

137. Patterson E, Smiley E, Bonadio J: RNA sequence analysis of a perinatal lethal osteogenesis imperfecta mutation. J Biol Chem 264:10083–10087, 1989.

138. Marini JC, Grange DK, Gotlesman GS, et al: Characterization of point mutations in Type I collagen detected with RNA/RNA hybrids. J Biol Chem 264:11893–11900, 1989.

139. Baldwin CT, Constantinou CD, Prockop DJ: A single base mutation that converts the codon for glycine 907 of the α2(I) chain of type I procollagen to aspartate. The single amino acid substitution in itself destabilizes the triple helix. J Biol Chem 264:3002–3006, 1989.

140. Constantinou CD, Neilsen KB, Prockop DJ: A lethal variant of osteogenesis imperfecta has a single base mutation that substitutes cysteine for glycine 904 in the triple helical domain of the α1(I) chain of type I procollagen. J Clin Invest 83:574–584, 1989.

141. Pack M, Constantinou CD, Kalia K, et al: Substitution of serine for glycine α1(I)-844 minimally destabilizes the triple helix of type I procollagen and causes a nonlethal variant of osteogenesis imperfecta. J Biol Chem 264:19694–19699, 1989.

142. Starman BJ, Eyre D, Charbonneau H, et al: Osteogenesis imperfecta: The position of a substitution for glycine in the triple helical domain of type I collagen determines the clinical phenotype. J Clin Invest 84:1206–1214, 1989.

143. Cohn DH, Byers PH, Steinmann B, et al: Lethal osteogenesis imperfecta resulting from a single nucleotide change in one human proα1(I) collagen allele. Proc Natl Acad Sci USA 83:6045–6047, 1986.

144. Vogel BE, Minor RR, Freund M, et al: A point mutation in a type I procollagen gene converts glycine 748 of the α1 chain to cysteine and destabilizes the triple helix in a lethal variant of osteogenesis imperfecta. J Biol Chem 262:14737–14744, 1987.

145. Bateman JF, Chan D, Walker ID, et al: Lethal perinatal osteogenesis imperfecta due to the substitution of arginine for glycine at residue 391 of the

α1(I) chains of type I collagen. J Biol Chem 262:7021–7027, 1987.

146. Bonadio JF, Byers PH: Subtle structural alterations in the chains of type I procollagen produce osteogenesis imperfecta type II. Nature 316:363–366, 1985.

147. Bruckner P, Prockop DJ: Proteolytic enzymes as probes for the triple helical conformation of collagen. Anal Biochem 110:360–368, 1981.

148. Privalov PL: Stability of proteins. Adv Protein Chem 35:1–104, 1982.

148a. Wenstrup RJ: Unpublished observations.

149. Beighton P: The Ehlers-Danlos Syndrome. London, Heinemann, 1970.

150. McKusick VA: Heritable Disorders of Connective Tissue. St. Louis, CV Mosby, 1972.

151. Vogel A, Holbrook KA, Steinmann B, et al: Abnormal collagen fibril structure in the gravis form type (I) of Ehlers-Danlos syndrome. Lab Invest 40:201–206, 1979.

152. Rudd NL, Nimrod C, Holbrook KA, et al: Pregnancy complications in type IV Ehlers-Danlos syndrome. Lancet 1:50–53, 1983.

153. Pope FM, Martin GR, McKusick VA: Inheritance of Ehlers-Danlos type IV syndrome. J Med Genet 14:200–204, 1977.

154. Sulh HMB, Steinmann B, Rao VH, et al: Ehlers-Danlos syndrome type IVD: An autosomal recessive disorder. Clin Genet 25:278–287, 1984.

155. Tsipouras P, Byers PH, Schwartz RC, et al: Ehlers-Danlos syndrome type IV: Cosegregation of the phenotype to a COL3A1 allele of type III procollagen. Hum Genet 74:41–46, 1986.

156. Byers PH, Holbrook KA, McGillivray B, et al: Clinical and ultrastructural heterogeneity of type IV Ehlers-Danlos syndrome. Hum Genet 47:141–150, 1979.

157. Pope FM, Martin GR, Lichtenstein JR, et al: Patients with Ehlers-Danlos syndrome type IV lack type III collagen. Proc Natl Acad Sci USA 72:1314–1316, 1975.

158. Byers PH, Holbrook KA, Barsh GS, et al: Altered secretion of type III procollagen in a form of type IV Ehlers-Danlos syndrome: Biochemical studies in cultured fibroblasts. Lab Invest 44:336–341, 1981.

159. Stolle CA, Pyeritz RE, Myers JC, et al: Synthesis of an altered type III procollagen in a patient with type IV Ehlers-Danlos syndrome. J Biol Chem 260:1937–1944, 1985.

160. Superti-Furga A, Gugler E, Gitzelmann R, et al: Ehlers-Danlos syndrome type IV: A multi-exon deletion in one of the two COL3A1 alleles affecting structure, stability and processing of type III procollagen. J Biol Chem 263:6226–6232, 1988.

161. Tromp G, Kuivaniemi H, Stolle C, et al: Single base mutation in the Type III procollagen gene that connects the codon for glycine 883 to aspartate in a mild variant of Ehlers-Danlos Syndrome IV. J Biol Chem 264:19313–19317, 1989.

162. Beighton P: X-linked recessive inheritance of the Ehlers-Danlos syndrome. Br Med J 2:9–11, 1968.

163. Beighton P, Curtis D: X-linked Ehlers-Danlos syndrome type V: The next generation. Clin Genet 27:472–478, 1985.

164. Almazan A: Lysyl oxidase deficiency in Ehlers-Danlos type V. Connect Tissue Res 3:49–53, 1975.

165. Pinnell SR, Krane SM, Kenzora JE, et al: A heritable disorder of connective tissue: Hydroxylysine-deficient collagen disease. N Engl J Med 286:1013–1020, 1972.

166. Krane SM, Pinnell SR, Erbe RW: Lysyl-protocollagen hydroxylase deficiency in fibroblasts from siblings with hydroxylysine deficient collagen. Proc Natl Acad Sci USA 69:2899–2903, 1972.

167. Wenstrup RJ, Murad S, Pinnell SR: Ehlers-Danlos syndrome type IV: Clinical manifestations of collagen lysyl hydroxylase deficiency. J Pediatr 115:405–409, 1989.

168. Eyre DR, Shapiro FD, Aldridge JF: Heterozygous collagen defect in a variant of the Ehlers-Danlos syndrome type VII: Evidence for a deleted amino telopeptide domain in the proαα2(I) chain. J Biol Chem 260:11322–11329, 1985.

169. Ihme A, Kreig T, Nerlick A, et al: Ehlers-Danlos syndrome type VI: Collagen type specificity of defective lysyl hydroxylation in various tissues. J Invest Dermatol 83:161–165, 1984.

170. Tajima S, Murad S, Pinnell SR: A comparison of lysyl hydroxylation in various types of collagen from Type VI Ehlers-Danlos syndrome fibroblasts. Collagen Rel Res 3:511–515, 1983.

171. Murad S, Pinnell SR: Suppression of fibroblast proliferation and lysyl hydroxylase activity by minoxidil. J Biol Chem 262:11973–11978, 1987.

172. Quinn RS, Krane SM: Abnormal properties of collagen lysyl hydroxylase from skin fibroblasts of siblings with hydroxylysine-deficient collagen. J Clin Invest 57:83–93, 1976.

173. Miller RL, Elsas LJ, Priest RE: Ascorbate action on normal and mutant human lysyl hydroxylases from cultured dermal fibroblasts. J Invest Dermatol 72:241–247, 1979.

174. Steinman B, Gitzelmann R, Vogel A, et al: Ehlers-Danlos syndrome in two siblings with deficient lysyl hydroxylase activity in childhood skin fibroblasts but only mild hydroxylysine deficiency in skin. Helv Pediatr Acta 30:255–274, 1975.

175. Lichtenstein JR, Martin GR, Kohn LD, et al: A defect in the conversion of procollagen to collagen in a form of Ehlers-Danlos syndrome. Science 182:298–300, 1973.

176. Cole WG, Evans R, Sillence DO: The clinical features of Ehlers-Danlos syndrome type VII due to a deletion of 24 amino acids from the proα1(I) chain of type I procollagen. J Med Genet 24:698–706, 1987.

177. Steinmann B, Tuderman L, Peltonen L, et al: Evidence for a structural mutation of procollagen type I in a patient with Ehlers-Danlos syndrome type VII. J Biol Chem 255:8887–8893, 1980.

178. Weil D, Bernard M, Combata N, et al: Identification of a mutation that causes exon-skipping during collagen pre-mRNA splicing in an Ehlers-Danlos syndrome variant. J Biol Chem 263:8561–8564, 1988.

179. Weil D, Allesio MD, Ramirez F, et al: A single base substitution in the exon of a collagen gene causes alternative splicing and generates a structurally abnormal polypeptide in a patient with Ehlers-Danlos syndrome type VII. EMBO J 8:1705–1710, 1989.

180. Cole WG, Chan D, Chambers GW, et al: Deletion of 24 amino acids from the proα1(I) chain of type I procollagen in a patient with the Ehlers-Danlos syndrome type VII. J Biol Chem 261:5496–5503, 1986.

181. Stewart RE, Hollister DW, Rimoin DL: A new variant of the Ehlers-Danlos syndrome: An autosomal dominant disorder of fragile skin, abnormal scarring, and generalized periodontis. Birth Defects 133B:85–93, 1977.

182. Linch DC, Acton CHC: Ehlers-Danlos syndrome presenting with juvenile destructive periodontis. Br Dent J 147:95–96, 1979.

183. Sartoris DJ, Luzzatti L, Weaver DD, et al: Type IX Ehlers-Danlos syndrome: A new variant with pathognomonic radiographic features. Radiology 152:665–670, 1984.

184. Lazoff SG, Rybak JJ, Parker BR, et al: Skeletal dysplasia, occipital horns, diarrhea and obstructive urop-

athy—a new hereditary syndrome. Birth Defects Orig Art Ser 112:71–82, 1975.

185. Blackston RD, Hirschhorn K, Elsas LJ: Ehlers-Danlos syndrome (EDS) type IX: Biochemical evidence for X-linkage. Am J Hum Genet 41:A49, 1987.

186. Byers PH, Siegel RC, Holbrook KA, et al: X-linked cutis laxa: Defective collagen crosslink formation due to decreased lysyl oxidase activity. N Engl J Med 303:61–65, 1980.

187. Kuivaniemi H, Peltonen L, Kivirikko KI: Type IX Ehlers-Danlos syndrome and Menkes syndrome: The decrease in lysyl oxidase activity is associated with a corresponding deficiency in the enzyme protein. Am J Hum Genet 37:798–808, 1985.

188. Peltonen L, Kuivaniemi H, Palotie A, et al: Alterations in copper and collagen metabolism in the Menkes syndrome and a new subtype of the Ehlers-Danlos syndrome. Biochemistry 22:6156–6163, 1983.

189. Arneson MA, Hammerschmidt DE, Furcht LT, et al: A new form of Ehlers-Danlos syndrome: Fibronectin corrects defective platelet function. JAMA 244:144–147, 1980.

190. Sasaki T, Arai K, Ono M, et al: Ehlers-Danlos syndrome: A variant characterized by the deficiency of proα2(I) chains of type I procollagen. Arch Dermatol 123:76–79, 1987.

191. Hata R, Kurata S, Shinkai H: Existence of malfunctioning proα2(I) collagen genes in a patient with a proα2(I)-chain–defective variant of Ehlers-Danlos syndrome. Eur J Biochem 174:231–237, 1988.

192. Nicholls AC, Osse G, Schloon HG, et al: The clinical features of homozygous α2(I) collagen deficient osteogenesis imperfecta. J Med Genet 21:257, 1984.

193. Pihlajaniemi T, Dickson LA, Pope FM, et al: Osteogenesis imperfecta: Cloning of a proα2(I) collagen gene with a frameshift mutation. J Biol Chem 259:12941–12944, 1984.

194. Francomano CA, Liberfarb RM, Hirose T, et al: The Stickler syndrome: Evidence for close linkage to the structural gene for type II collagen. Genomics 1:293–296, 1987.

195. Tiller GE, Rimoin DL, Murray LW, et al: Tandem duplication within a type II collagen gene (COL2A1) exon in an individual with spondyloepiphyseal dysplasia. Proc Natl Acad Sci USA 87:3889–3893, 1990.

196. Lee B, Vissing H: Identification of the molecular defect in a family with spondyloepiphyseal dysplasia. Science 244:978–980, 1989.

197. Vissing H, D'Alessio M, Lee B, et al: Glycine to serine substitution in the triple helical domain of proα1(II) collagen results in a lethal perinatal form of short-limb dwarfism. J Biol Chem 264:18265–18267, 1989.

198. Sakai LY, Keene DR, Morris NP, et al: Type VII collagen is a major structural component of the anchoring fibrils. J Cell Biol 103:1577–1586, 1986.

199. Bruckner-Tuderman L, Rüegger S, Odermatt B, et al: Lack of type VII collagen in unaffected skin of patients with severe recessive dystrophic epidermolysis bullosa. Dermatologica 176:57–64, 1988.

10

COLLAGEN DEGRADATION

John J. Jeffrey, Ph.D.

Nowhere in biology does there exist a more significant example of the need for carefully regulated, spatially organized degradation of collagen than in the process of wound healing. At the same time, it is perhaps also true that in no other biological system does there exist as great a dearth of data on the mechanisms by which this exquisitely regulated process is successfully engineered by the organism. As an example, after an extensive search of the literature, this reviewer has been unable to identify a single refereed publication specifically dealing with collagen degradation in wound healing since 1971.[1] In the face of this lengthy hiatus, the need for information is indeed great.

The goal of this chapter is to provide an up-to-date review of what is known about the specific nature of the physiologically relevant reagents involved in collagen degradation, how they act and interact and how they may be regulated. It will be the exciting task of future researchers to assess more precisely the role of these reagents as they act together to restore full physiological function to wounded tissue.

THE BIOCHEMISTRY OF COLLAGENOLYSIS

Until recently, the concept of collagen degradation was a relatively simple and altogether

elegant one.[2-6] In its essentials this picture remains intact; however, recent research has shown the process to be somewhat more complex. This chapter begins with the original notion and indicates, as appropriate, the modifications that have been made along the way.

To understand the enzymology of collagen degradation properly, it is useful to briefly review the nature of the substrate to be degraded: fibrillar collagen (for a detailed review see Chapter 8). The collagen fibril, formed as it is from the precisely ordered aggregation of collagen monomers, is an extraordinarily effective structural element for maintaining the integrity of the connective tissue. (Figure 10–1 illustrates the essential features of the pathway.) The resulting fibril on a weight basis has a greater tensile strength than steel. It is physically stable—disruption of fibrils begins to occur only at temperatures above 50°C—and chemically resistant—fibrillar collagen is essentially insoluble under physiological conditions. In its fibrillar form collagen is resistant to the degradative efforts of a wide range of naturally occurring proteolytic enzymes such as trypsin and chymotrypsin. In all these respects, the protein is ideally designed for biological permanency.

Nature, however, has provided an extremely effective way of allowing for removal of collagen from a tissue. As needed[7] cells produce specific enzymes—collagenases—that act primarily, if not exclusively, on collagen. These enzymes catalyze a single proteolytic cleavage in each of the three chains of the constituent monomers of collagen fibers, causing a massive change in the properties of collagen (Fig. 10–2).[8] The products of this cleavage, indicated as TC^A and

Support during the preparation of this chapter and for some of the studies described herein was provided by USPHS grants HD05291, AM12129, and AM02784. The author is grateful to Ms. Rosemarie Brannan and Ms. Ginger Roberts for their expert preparation of the manuscript.

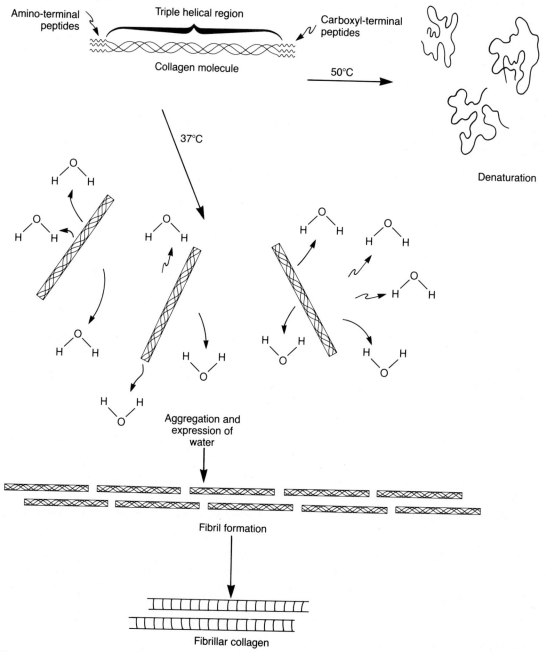

Figure 10–1. Temperature-dependent outcome for single triple helical molecules of collagen. At physiological temperatures, the molecules aggregate with a net removal of water associated with the individual collagen molecules to form fibrils. Individual native molecules of collagen will not denature until the temperature is raised to over 50°C.

TC[B] in Figure 10–2, are now freely soluble in physiological solvents and are thermally unstable at physiological temperatures.[9] The consequence of the action of collagenase on its substrate, then, is the rapid solubilization and the denaturation of the products, at which point they are degradable by any number of less specific proteases that may be present in the tissue. The existence and nature of proteases

that can act on the primary product of collagenase activity have attracted increasing attention and will be discussed later in this chapter.

Chemists use the term "rate limiting" to denote the slowest step in a series of reactions: the overall reaction can proceed no faster than the rate of this step. An even more restrictive terminology is reserved for a step such as that catalyzed by collagenase: "the committed

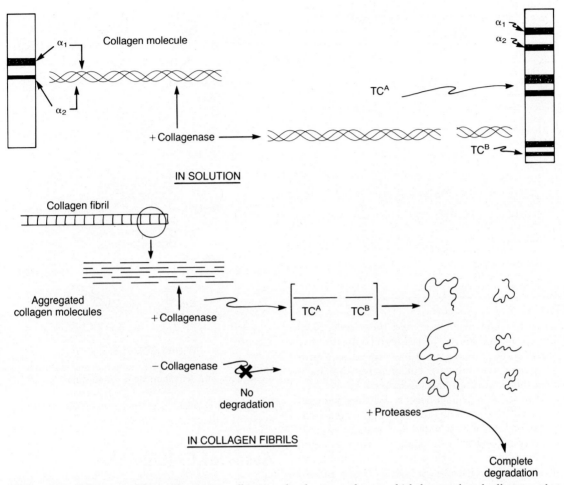

Figure 10–2. Collagenase cleaves the native collagen molecule at one locus, which has profound effects on the thermal stability of the resultant fragments.

step."[10] This is one that must occur before any other reaction in a series can take place. Thus, collagenase presides over the committed step in collagen degradation; no matter what concentrations exist of other enzymes necessary for the complete degradation of the protein, no degradation can occur until after the action of collagenase (Fig. 10–2). In physiology, then, the regulation of the activity of these enzymes is particularly crucial and one might expect that such regulation would be exceptionally complex. That such is the case is beginning to emerge from a variety of recent studies, and this area will be discussed further on. First, however, it will be useful to examine the properties of collagenases as they are now known in mammalian systems.

Historically, the first collagenase to be described was isolated from organ cultures of resorbing tadpole tail fin.[11, 12] During the transition of a tadpole to a frog, extensive connective tissue remodeling occurs; not only is the tail lost, but gills become lungs, legs emerge, the intestine is massively shortened, and changes occur in both the structure and the geography of oral and ocular tissues.[13] Thus, retrospectively, it is not surprising that collagenase plays a major role in metamorphosis. Nevertheless, given the then-confused state of the field, the identification of a true collagenolytic protease represented a major breakthrough. Since that time, collagenases have been identified in a wide variety of normal and pathological tissues; a representative, but by no means comprehensive, list appears in Table 10–1.[11-39]

For some time collagenases were studied only in enzymatic activities in crude culture media of one sort or another, and the effect of modulators on their activity could be studied only under impure conditions. The first collagenase to be purified and studied with standard chemical and enzymological techniques was that from human skin.[15, 40, 41] A variety of lines of human skin fibroblasts produce chemically significant

Table 10–1. SELECTED LIST OF TISSUES AND CELL SOURCES OF VERTEBRATE COLLAGENASE

Cell or Tissue Source	Key Reference
Tadpole tail fin	11, 12
Human skin	14, 15
Rheumatoid synovium	16, 17
Rat uterus	18
Human granulocytes	19
Rabbit cornea	20
Human cholesteatoma	21
Regenerating newt limb	22
Rat skin	23
Mouse bone	24
Guinea pig macrophages	25
Rat liver	26
Guinea pig pubic symphysis	27
Human gastric mucosa	28
Rat ovarian follicle	29
Rat smooth muscle cells	30
Rat osteoblasts	31
Human smooth muscle cells	32
Various tumors/tumor cells	33–39

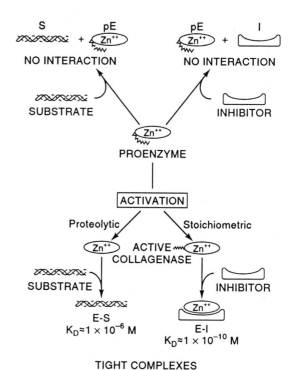

Figure 10–3. Schematic presentation of the multitude of interactions and activation steps for collagenase.

quantities of collagenase, and these cells have served as the source of crude enzyme for the purification. This enzyme has served as a prototype for a number of collagenases that have since been purified and characterized.

Human skin collagenase is synthesized and secreted by these cells in culture as a *zymogen*, a proenzyme, with a molecular mass of approximately 52,000 daltons (Da).[40, 41] The zymogen is incapable of catalytic activity or of binding to its eventual substrate, collagen.[42] The proenzyme can be activated by a variety of reagents of varying biological relevance,[43–47] after which the resultant active collagenase displays an avid affinity for its substrate;[48] these interactions are diagrammed in Figure 10–3. Thus, and this cannot be emphasized too strongly, the process of activation of procollagenase to the active enzyme is all-important in the biology of collagen degradation. This becomes even more significant when one considers the interaction of the enzyme with its naturally occurring inhibitors. In any event, in the absence of activation the molecule is incapable of interacting with substrate, and degradation cannot occur. Because of its importance, this aspect of collagenase biochemistry will be discussed in some detail later in this chapter.

Active collagenase can be produced from the zymogen by a process referred to as "limited trypsin activation"; this simply means exposing the zymogen to trypsin at room temperature for a short time, then inhibiting the trypsin with excess soybean trypsin inhibitor, after which the enzyme is ready for assay.[40] The result of this trypsin activation will be discussed

later; at this point a discussion of the accurate assay of collagenase is in order.

Assay of Collagenase

The assay of collagenase in a wide variety of biologically relevant solutions has been the topic of a number of studies over the years, and dozens of assay methodologies have now been published. In any study of collagenase activity in biologic systems, it is important to be able to properly assay the enzyme, and a large number of studies purporting to have measured the enzyme in both physiological and pathological situations have been flawed by having employed inadequate assay systems. The single most important requirement for any collagenase assay is that *the substrate must be native under the conditions of the assay system.* The original method used to ensure this was employed by Gross and Lapiere in their studies on the tadpole collagenase, and it remains useful to this day.[8, 11] Using native reconstituted type I collagen fibrils as substrate (Fig. 10–4), the collagen is radiolabeled in vivo by injecting animals (guinea pigs in this case) with 14-C glycine, allowing the amino acid to become incorporated into proteins, extracting the skin with neutral salt solution, and purifying the radioactive collagen from the extracts. For the purposes of the

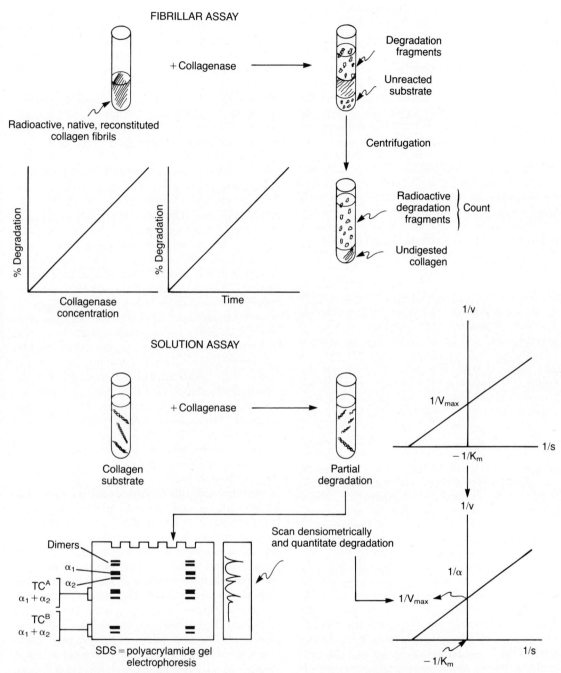

Figure 10–4. Methods to quantitate collagenolytic activity. *A,* Fibrillar or insoluble substrate method. *B,* Solution or soluble substrate assay.

assay, the collagen is allowed to form fibrils by incubation in small tubes at 37°C overnight; the fibrils thus formed are indistinguishable from those observed in vivo. In this form the substrate is degradable by no known protease other than collagenase.[11] Thus, solutions containing putative collagenase, after suitable activation as necessary, are added to the substrate and incubated at 37°C. The time of incubation, of

course, will depend upon the level of activity, the only caveat being that the reaction should not proceed to a point where substrate is rate limiting. After incubation, the reactions are terminated by the addition of EDTA, and the unreacted substrate is centrifuged down. The radioactivity in the supernatants, representing degraded collagen, is determined by liquid scintillation spectrometry, and the counts thus obtained are proportional to the concentration of collagenase in the test solution.[48] Typically in this assay a nonspecific protease "blank" is included in which a set of substrate gels is incubated with an amount of trypsin approximately equimolar to the amount of substrate collagen. In a good collagen preparation, the counts released by the trypsin will seldom be more than 10 percent of the total radioactivity of the substrate. Counts released above this level can then be attributed to collagenase. It should be noted that the use of large amounts of trypsin in the "blank" tubes represents a worst-case situation, so that collagenase activity may be somewhat underestimated in this assay. If the concentration of collagen in the substrate is known, a specific activity (μg collagen degraded per minute per μg protein) can be easily calculated.[48]

In this assay, the substrate is biologically labeled for the purposes of obtaining a suitable substrate. A disadvantage is that this method is relatively expensive: 14-C glycine is a costly reagent, and the yield of isotope in labeled collagen is low. For example, using 200 g guinea pigs injected with 200 μCi (1 μCi/g) of the radioactive amino acid, a typical yield is approximately 200 mg of collagen per animal, with a specific activity of from 35,000 to 60,000 cpm per mg. In practice this is sufficient for approximately 1000 assays. In the interest of economy, and occasionally sensitivity, several workers have modified the fibril-based assay by labeling the collagen by reacting certain amino acid side chains with radioactive reagents.[49–52] These modifications include formylation, acetylation, and reduction. In principle, such modifications are acceptable, but it is necessary to carefully establish the conditions for labeling the collagen. It is quite easy to overmodify the side chains of the molecule with consequences that range from partial or complete failure to obtain native fibril formation to complete dissolution of the substrate with the trypsin in the "blank" tubes. Thus, it is imperative to adhere to the original fundamental requirement: that the substrate be truly native. Several laboratories have successfully achieved this condition using chemically modified collagen substrates. One successful method is that of Cawston and Barrett,[52] which uses acetylated collagen. By way of summary, the biologically labeled substrate has the advantage of essentially guaranteeing fully native substrate, essentially identical to the in vivo situation, but it is expensive. The chemically modified substrate has the advantage of being less costly to prepare, but the disadvantage of not being fully native unless careful precautions and controls are used.

Collagenase activity can also be measured in solution; again, however, the substrate must remain native under the assay conditions. For solution assays, this means that the temperature (assuming mammalian collagens are used) must be kept below 30°C and preferably no higher than 28°C. In practice, solutions of type I collagen are incubated with appropriate aliquots of putative collagenase and incubated for time periods that are determined empirically, depending upon the amount of enzyme activity. The reactions are terminated with EDTA as discussed previously and subjected to polyacrylamide gel electrophoresis in sodium dodecyl sulfate (SDS). Under these conditions, the products of collagenase activity (TC^A and TC^B) appear as well-defined bands that can be scanned densitometrically.[53] The intensity of these bands is proportional to the collagenase activity. The principles of the solution assay are illustrated in Figure 10–4. The advantage of this kind of assay is that it is performed in homogeneous solution, rather than on a solid substrate, which allows for the determination of fundamental kinetic constants of the enzyme.[53] In addition, the gel confirms that the classical products of collagenase activity are indeed formed in the reaction. The disadvantage of the solution assay is that it is quite cumbersome if multiple samples, of potentially widely varying activity, are required to be assayed. Nevertheless, it is a valuable methodology to have at hand.

Another valuable technique for the detection of collagenase in biological solutions is that of zymography.[54, 55] This method involves the electrophoretic resolution of the collagenase present in impure solutions by a variation of SDS-polyacrylamide gel electrophoresis in which a protein substrate for collagenase is incorporated into the gel itself. Typically, gelatin or casein is employed. After electrophoresis, the SDS is removed by soaking the gel in the detergent Triton X-100 and allowed to incubate for a number of hours at 37°C or overnight at room temperature. After incubation, the gel is stained with Coomassie Blue, and the presence of unstained regions of the gel against the blue background of the incorporated protein is determined. This method is extremely sensitive in the detection of the enzyme, but because the region of clearing is only roughly proportional to the amount of enzyme present, it appears to be only marginally useful in its quantitation.

Finally, immunological methods have been developed for the detection of certain collagenases.[56–58] These take the form of enzyme-linked immunosorbent assays (ELISA) and are capable of detecting the enzyme in solutions in which inhibitors may make it difficult to measure it by the activity assays. Additionally, the immunological techniques make it possible to detect levels of collagenase that would stretch or exceed the limits of sensitivity of the activity-based assays. Developing such assays requires a considerable investment in purifying antigen, raising antibody, and setting up and verifying the assay. However, the rewards are worth the effort when detection of the enzyme would otherwise be extremely difficult and often impossible.

Before leaving the subject of the assay of collagenase, it is worth reiterating the primary requirement of all collagenase assays: the substrate must be verified as native and be maintained in that conformation throughout the assay. In the opinion of this reviewer, more false hopes have been raised as to the presence of collagenase in crude biological solutions because of improper assay conditions than for any other reason. As discussed later, denatured collagen (gelatin) is an excellent substrate for any number of proteases, and false positives can be (and have been) obtained very easily if the substrate is compromised. It is imperative that the use of non–triple helical collagenlike peptides be avoided in collagenase assays. These peptides, which are designed to mimic the sequence around the collagenase cleavage site in collagen, are useful *only* in studies with purified collagenases, and *not* in the assay of collagenase activity in crude samples.

The Nature of the Collagenases

Mammalian collagenase belongs to a family of extracellular metalloproteinases that are capable of degrading connective tissue components. This family of enzymes is composed of collagenase with specificity for the fibrillar collagens, gelatinase, which degrades denatured fibrillar collagens and type IV as well as type V collagen, and stromelysin, which has a wide specificity including fibronectin, laminin, type IV collagen, and cartilage proteoglycan.[59] Stromelysin has a homologue in the rat termed transin, which has been linked to oncogenic transformation in rat fibroblasts.[60] It has been proposed by Harris and associates that these enzymes be termed matrix metalloproteinase-1, 2, and 3, respectively, in order to indicate the related protease functionality.[60a]

As a class, all the collagenases examined to date possess a number of properties in common. They all require calcium for activity,[61] which can be easily removed from the enzyme by dialysis and re-added with no loss in activity. The concentration of calcium required for half-maximal collagenase activity is about 0.5 mM, some fourfold lower than the serum calcium concentration of about 2 mM. This suggests that under these circumstances the collagenase should be essentially completely active in vivo. If biological compartments exist in which the calcium concentration is markedly lower, however, calcium would be a significant regulator of collagenase activity. The exact role of calcium in the activity of collagenase remains unknown, but preliminary evidence, using impure enzyme preparations, suggests that calcium is required for conformational stability of these enzymes.[61] In the absence of the metal, collagenase appears to be less thermostable and more susceptible to proteolytic inactivation.

A second property of the collagenases is the requirement for zinc as a cofactor.[62–64] Unlike calcium, zinc is tightly bound within the protein and is not removed by dialysis. The presence of zinc near the active site in proteolytic enzymes is not uncommon. In the best defined example, that of carboxypeptidase A, zinc participates in the movement of electrons required for the hydrolysis of the peptide bond, and it very likely serves an analogous function in the collagenases. The presence of zinc in these proteases, coupled with the calcium requirement discussed previously, provides the basis for the consistent finding that the collagenases, as a group, are inhibited by metal chelating agents such as EDTA. This latter reagent is often used to terminate the action of collagenase in reaction mixtures; it is customarily added in concentrations in excess of the calcium in the reaction mixture.

In addition to these similarities in the collagenase molecules, all the enzymes so far examined catalyze the identical cleavage in the collagen molecule. This cleavage is at the peptide bond joining residues 775- and 776- in the three chains composing the collagen molecule.[65] The amino acids at this site—glycyl-isoleucine ($\alpha 1$ chains) and glycyl-leucine ($\alpha 2$ chains)—have been completely conserved throughout evolution and are the same in tadpole type I collagen as in type I human collagen. It should be noted that these bonds are completely different from those cleaved by the collagenase from the bacterium *Clostridium histolyticum*. The enzymes appear to have been highly conserved as well: the same bond is cleaved by both tadpole and human collagenase in the collagens from either species. This remarkable constancy over such a long period of evolutionary development argues for the importance of providing for appropriate degradation of the most common, and at the same time, toughest protein.

It should be noted that it is not *simply* the primary sequence around the peptide bond itself that specifies the cleavage site in collagen: numerous other glycyl-leucines and glycyl-isoleucines exist in both α chains of type I collagen, yet they are never cleaved by collagenase. Thus, some combination of the presence of the characteristic triple helix of collagen and the secondary sequence of the area around the cleavage site, specified in some unknown way by the amino acid side chains flanking that site, apparently allows for the binding and subsequent catalytic activity of the enzyme. Some direct indication that this is the case has been provided by studies that clearly show that trypsin is capable of cleaving type III collagen.[66] One of the numerous bonds that should be trypsin susceptible in type III collagen occurs just a few residues toward the carboxy terminus of the molecule from the collagenase cleavage site. This bond, and only this bond, is capable of being cleaved, albeit slowly, by trypsin. Thus, there appears to be something different about the region surrounding the cleavage site that allows access to proteolytic enzymes. The difference in structure must be very subtle indeed, since at least one type III collagen (chick) contains the susceptible bond, yet in this case the bond is *not* cleaved by trypsin.[67] The acquisition of new knowledge in this area has been limited by our inability to determine precisely the effect of amino acid side chains on the microstability of the collagen helix.

Of potentially more practical significance is the fact that the elastase produced by human neutrophils is capable of catalyzing the same cleavage in human type III collagen as does trypsin.[67] This cleavage by neutrophil elastase is relatively slow, but since neutrophils can be present in large numbers during inflammatory stages of wound healing, the enzyme concentration could be quite high. The likely consequence of the presence of this enzyme under these circumstances would be to interfere with the orderly process of collagen remodeling required for healing.

At a time when similarities between collagenases are being emphasized, it should be noted that there is one notable case in which the properties of collagenolytic enzymes are quite dissimilar. In humans, fibroblast collagenase and the analogous enzyme from the granulocyte appear to be quite different in terms of molecular properties and mutual antibody recognition.[68, 69] Furthermore, whereas the fibroblast clearly seems to synthesize its collagenase upon biological demand, the granulocyte seems just as clearly to store its collagenase in the neutral granules.[70] In spite of these differences, the two enzymes nevertheless do cleave the same peptide bond, albeit at very different rates from the fibroblast enzyme, depending upon the genetic type of collagen employed as substrates.[71, 72] The physiological significance of the differences between resident cell collagenase and the white cell enzyme, although not currently understood, could well be of great significance in wound healing.

Of considerable help to workers in this area are a variety of molecular biological reagents that have recently become available. Principal among them are complementary DNAs (cDNA) to collagenases from rabbit[73, 74] and human sources,[75] as well as to TIMP,[76, 77] the cell-derived inhibitor of connective tissue–related metalloproteinases from the human and mouse. Similar reagents should be forthcoming for these molecules in other species, where they will be invaluable for the study of the wide variety of collagen degradation systems available in nonhuman species.

Activation of Collagenase

The nature of the physiological mechanism(s) of procollagenase activation is one of the most important unanswered questions in the biology of the collagenases. To properly understand this concept it is necessary to understand the variety of pathways so far suggested or demonstrated to result in the conversion of procollagenase to active collagenase. In the original discovery of an inactive form of collagenase in human skin fibroblast culture medium,[15] limited trypsin activation was employed to activate the inactive form, whose nature was then unknown. The ambiguous term "limited trypsin activation" in this case denotes treating crude culture medium or other solutions containing inactive collagenase with trypsin, in empirically determined concentrations, at room temperature instead of at 37°C, as one would do for complete trypsin digestion of a protein. As was subsequently demonstrated, the use of trypsin in this way converted the procollagenase to active enzyme by the removal of a "pro-" piece of protein approximately 10,000 daltons in mass.[40] This conversion was very similar to the conversion of a large number of proproteins to their corresponding active molecules and provided a temporarily satisfying mechanism for the activation of procollagenase in vivo.

Indeed, it is quite possible that the activation of procollagenase in vivo does, at least in some circumstances, occur by the kind of proteolysis represented by limited trypsin activation. Over the years a variety of proteases known to occur in tissues and in biological fluids have been shown to activate the collagenase zymogen.[43–46] What has prevented the positive identification of such a process from occurring in vivo has been the fact that the chemical nature of the active form of collagenase in any tissue has never been firmly established. In other words, it is not known whether the active enzyme, operating in a tissue, does in fact correspond to a protein proteolytically derived from the zymogen. This is because the great bulk of collagenase present in a tissue undergoing degradation (and there never is very much enzyme, in chemical terms) is tightly bound to the collagen fibrils,[78, 79] and it has proven difficult to remove the enzyme from these tissue collagen fibrils, although such a dissociation has been reported to have been achieved, albeit under harsh conditions (60°C, 0.5 M CaCl$_2$), and with questionable yield.[80]

Information on this point is important because of the unusual behavior of procollagenase in solution. It was originally reported by Stricklin and colleagues that the zymogen could autoactivate after multiple freeze-thawings or upon prolonged incubation at 37°C. The product of this autoactivation appeared to be a molecule of the same molecular weight as the zymogen itself. This original observation has been extended, and a fascinating picture has emerged in which a variety of reagents (some of potential biological significance) are capable of promoting a conformational change in the zymogen molecule.[81] This change results in the originally observed "zymogen-sized" active enzyme; it appears that the propiece of the zymogen can be moved in space to provide the active and/or binding sites with access to the substrate. To further complicate the situation, the zymogen itself can display autocatalytic activity,[81, 82] most obviously after the conformational changes just described. The sequence of events appears to be as follows: the conformation changes, followed by an *intra*molecular cleavage of the propiece by the active site of the proenzyme itself. This latter cleavage seems to take place exclusively within the same molecule—one active zymogen molecule (or even an active collagenase molecule) appears unable

to produce this cleavage in another molecule. In fact, this ability of zymogen has been shown to be important even in the process of trypsin activation. Trypsin cleavage actually removes only about one half of the propiece (5000 daltons), while the subsequent activity of the procollagenase itself then catalyzes the removal of the remainder of the piece, to yield a molecule identical to that previously called the "trypsin-activated" collagenase. This admittedly confusing, yet important, set of interactions is illustrated in Figure 10–3.

This conformational change can be induced by a wide variety of reagents, the most important of which, from a historical standpoint, are members of a series of organomercurial compounds: phenyl mercuric chloride (PMC), 4-aminophenyl mercuric acetate (APMA), para-hydroxymercuribenzoate (PHMB), and mersalyl.[81, 83] How they effect the change in procollagenase conformation is unknown. Of interest, both from the standpoint of the biochemistry of these molecules and from a practical laboratory point of view, is the observation that not every batch of procollagenase is equally susceptible to activation by the organomercurial compounds.[83a] On occasion, preparations of enzyme can be encountered that are completely resistant to activation by APMA at any concentration but are fully activated by either trypsin or phenylmercuric chloride, the latter being by far the most effective activator of the series. This finding suggests the possibility that conformationally "tight" and "loose" forms of procollagenase can exist and that biology can modulate this conformation. The practical problem presented by this observation is that it is difficult to be sure of complete activation of collagenase by organomercurials especially in crude mixtures.

The potential biological significance of this conformation-dependent activation of procollagenase is to be found in the report of biologically derived molecules,[46] apparently proteins, that seem capable of producing the same sort of conformational activation of procollagenase as the rather more esoteric organomercurials described previously.[81, 82] One of the putative activators has been identified in the medium of organ cultures of human skin, the other in analogous cultures of rat uterus. When examined as semipurified preparations from tissue culture medium, both entities behave as though they were organomercurials: they produce full activity if added to pure proenzyme, and they do so in the absence of observable change in the molecular weight of the zymogen. In addition, the activation appears to take place very rapidly, within the time of mixing of the activator with the proenzyme; full enzymatic activity is observed at the earliest points at which measurements could be taken.

The existence of such entities in biological systems that are actively producing collagenase and concomitantly undergoing collagen degradation raises the possibility that, at least under some circumstances, physiological activation of collagenase can be caused by just such molecules—biological analogues of the chaotropes described previously. This is why it is important to know what the actual active species of collagenase is in a given tissue; in the absence of this knowledge, an assignment of the route of activation is all but impossible. This difficulty persists in spite of the circumstantial evidence provided by the existence of proteases in the system that can activate collagenase under laboratory conditions.

Parenthetically, in many studies of collagenase activation in a variety of biological systems, one or another of the above-mentioned organomercurials is added in order to activate the enzyme. The most commonly used reagent has been APMA. Usually only a single concentration of the compound (usually 1 mM) is added to the solution to be assayed. It must be emphasized that quantitation of collagenase by such a simple method is often extremely inaccurate for a number of reasons. First, the degree of activation of a given amount of procollagenase by a single concentration of APMA can vary widely, depending upon the total protein concentration of the solution and on whether the enzyme is uniformly susceptible to activation by APMA, as discussed before. Furthermore, if inhibitors are present in sufficient quantities in the solution, a variable and unknowable underestimate of the true levels of collagenase will result. All of these considerations argue once again for the need for caution on the part of investigators in examining relatively crude biological solutions for collagenase activity.

Once activated, collagenase binds avidly to its substrate (see Fig. 10–3). Reasonably extensive studies on the interaction of the enzyme with collagen have produced an intriguing glimpse into the nature of collagen degradation in vivo. One is the crucial role played by water in the process of collagenolysis.[84] The catalysis of the cleavage of any peptide bond by a proteolytic enzyme requires the participation of water, and water is even more crucial in collagenolysis. It seems clear that the aggregation of collagen molecules into fibrils is accompanied by a significant exclusion of water from between the molecules that make up the fibril. As a result of this scarcity of water, the rate of collagenase activity is slowed considerably, and collagen degradation becomes a very slow enzymatic process.[48] Furthermore, as the fibrils "age," or perfect their aggregated state, still more water is expressed from the interior of the fibril and the rate of collagenase activity slows even more, perhaps by fivefold or more.[84a] This exclusion of water as collagen fibrils age biologically suggests the presence of a formidable barrier to degradation in vivo. It is even conceivable that some collagen fibrils are essentially nondegradable for this reason alone. Although definitive proof for this notion is lacking, were it to be true the consequences for wound healing biology could be profound.

Perhaps the most unusual, and the most physiologically important, finding of these studies was that once bound to the molecules within a collagen fibril, the enzyme appears to move from molecule to molecule within that fibril without an intervening dissociation step.[48] This can be seen from the fact that collagenase bound to fibrillar collagen acts at essentially identical rates no matter in what volume the reaction takes place.[48] This finding flies in the face of conventional solution enzymology, in which rates of catalysis diminish linearly with dilution. It is as though (and it actually may be) the enzyme molecule does not undergo a discrete dissociation step after catalyzing cleavage in one molecule before binding to a second. Thus, like the Sorcerer's Apprentice, once collagenase has begun to attack the collagen of the extracellular space, if left to itself it will continue to act until the substrate has been completely degraded. Such a situation can easily be seen to be incompatible with the precise spatial control that biology exercises over its systems; clearly, other mechanisms must be invoked in order to ensure that the architecture of the extracellular matrix is properly maintained. One such mechanism of primary importance is the tissue-mediated inhibition of collagenase activity.

Biological Inhibition of Collagenase

An effective mechanism for the control of connective tissue degradation that has been identified and extensively studied in the past few years is the endogenous production of collagenase inhibitors by the resident cells of the matrix. The existence of such inhibitors was first suggested in the studies that indicated the production of collagenase by human fibroblasts. It appeared that the medium of the cultured cells that produced collagenase also contained an inhibitor of the enzyme[15] that has since been purified and characterized from a number of cell and tissue sources.[6] These studies show a collagenase inhibitor being produced by the same cells that synthesize collagenase itself. Indeed, individual cells in culture have been observed to produce both collagenase and inhibitor simultaneously,[85] and the existence of such an inhibitor has now been confirmed in a great many species and organs. As a class, these inhibitors are often referred to by the acronym TIMP (Tissue Inhibitor of Metallo Proteinases).[86] The best characterized of these inhibitors, that produced by the human skin fibroblast, is a glycoprotein about 30,000 daltons in mass, of which about one third is glycosaminoglycan[87] and that is broadly distributed in biological fluids.[88] The inhibitor is capable of forming extremely tight complexes with collagenase, characterized by a 1:1 stoichiometry[89] and dissociation constants of approximately 1×10^{-10} M.[90-92] The consequences of this tight binding are shown in Figure 10–5: the interaction of enzyme and inhibitor at this level resembles that of a strong acid and a strong base in a classical chemical titration. Until the two reagents are present in close to equimolar concentrations and in concentrations that are also close to the value specified by the dissociation constant ($\leqslant 1 \times 10^{-9}$ M), little or no reaction takes place. However, when these conditions are met, the tight binding described above occurs, and collagenase activity essentially ceases. As can be seen in Figure 10–5, a small change in either enzyme or inhibitor concentration can result in massive changes in the rate of tissue collagenolysis.

This property of enzyme-inhibitor binding allows the establishment of sharp geographical boundaries of collagenolytic activity and the protection of areas of connective tissue from the activity of the enzyme. In addition, it provides a mechanism for the cells of a tissue to *terminate* an ongoing process of collagenolysis in a tissue. In such a case the concentration of inhibitor (I) in the tissue can be envisioned as being increased to a level sufficiently high that previously active collagenase (E) is now drawn away from substrate (S) by the inhibitor, as suggested in the following simple equation:

$$(E-S) + I \rightarrow (E-I) + S$$

The fate of E-I complexes generated in this way is unknown but should be the subject of intense investigation in the next few years.

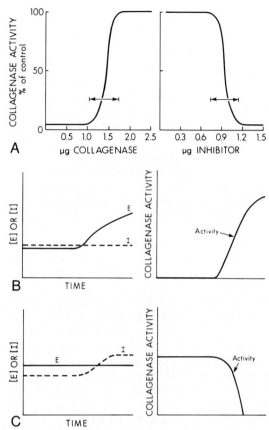

Figure 10–5. Interaction between collagenase and TIMP from human dermal fibroblasts. *A,* The collagenase activity is detected at a fixed concentration of inhibitor (I) and increasing amounts of collagenase (E) *(left)* or a fixed concentration of enzyme and increasing amounts of inhibitor *(right)*. *B* and *C,* Theoretical description of the collagenase activity in a situation in which the fractional change in either I or E produces orders of magnitude change in collagen degradation. This tight binding interaction allows for rapid and precisely localized modulation of degradative activity.

The chemical nature of the inhibitor has now been elucidated in a number of species,[86, 87, 93-98] and remarkable similarities appear to exist between them. The best characterized of the inhibitors is that of the human; the molecule consists of a protein core of approximately 20,000 daltons and a glycosylated domain of another 12,000 daltons. The protein portion of the molecule is tightly restrained conformationally by some 12 disulfide bonds. A cDNA clone of the molecule has been obtained,[76] and the recombinant protein has been refolded to the native conformation. The refolded molecule is fully active in inhibiting collagenase on the same 1:1 molar basis as observed in the biologically derived protein. Although the role of the glycosylated domain of the molecule is unclear at this time, it seems highly unlikely that such a major portion of a biological molecule should have no role in its activity. The elucidation of the function of the glycosylated moiety of the inhibitor will undoubtedly be a major research goal over the next few years. The amino acid sequence of the protein portion of the molecule has been obtained from several species, and it is clear that the sequence has been highly conserved throughout evolution. Very few differences exist in the first 25 amino terminal amino acids in the inhibitor molecules derived from mouse, rat, cow, and human. More differences seem to exist at the carboxy terminus of the molecule across species, as illustrated by the comparison of the molecules from mouse and man.[76, 77]

Several other significant features of the collagenase inhibitor should be mentioned. First, unlike the enzyme that it is designed to inhibit, the inhibitor has been shown to be secreted from the cell as a fully functional molecule.[76] Thus, there is *no* proinhibitor, and as a consequence there is no requirement for a zymogen-to-active-molecule conversion, as there is for the collagenase. No definitive data have been presented that bear on this, but it seems fair to suggest that the prevention or the termination of collagenolytic activity is of such significance to the organism that it is essential to have rapid access to fully functional inhibitory capability. The inhibitor has essentially no affinity for the zymogen form of collagenase; once the enzyme is activated, however, binding is rapid and efficient. Thus, somewhat anthropomorphically speaking, no inhibitor is "wasted" on inactive collagenase; rather, it is spared for interaction with only the biologically active form of the enzyme.

Another potentially important aspect of the action of this inhibitor is that it is not specific to collagenase. Instead, it has a spectrum of inhibitory activity against what now appears to be a set of proteases that are involved in the total management of the degradation of the various elements of the structural proteins of the connective tissue. One of these proteases is a gelatinolytic protease[98a] selective for proteins containing collagenous sequences in non–triple helical form. Interestingly, the gelatinolytic protease appears to be identical, at least in the human, to a substance previously referred to as "type IV collagenase"[98b] and appears to be the only protease in normal fibroblasts that is capable of degrading basement membrane collagen. Completing this group of noncollagenolytic proteases is stromelysin, originally identified in a variety of tissues as a proteoglycan-degrading proteinase.[59, 98c] Together, these proteases constitute a set of molecules that are capable of degrading the vast majority of the macromolecules making up the structural components of the extracellular matrix.

An extensive treatment of the biochemistry of these noncollagenolytic proteases is beyond the scope of this chapter; indeed, many of the salient facts are only now being elucidated in the laboratory. The story is indeed a fascinating one, in that all the proteases so far identified as playing a major role in the degradation of the components of the extracellular matrix appear to be members of a single gene family,[99, 100] all of which share significant sequence domains and possess extensive homology with one another, even across species fairly widely separated in evolution. At least two of the members of the family (collagenase and stromelysin) are secreted as zymogens that have very similar pathways of activation. As mentioned, all of these proteases are inhibited by the same inhibitor (TIMP); this may in part be the result of the particularly strong conservation of certain amino acid sequences at or near their active sites.[99] In any event, the biological consequence of these commonalities is that the vertebrate organism in general possesses a very effective mechanism for either preventing the onset or terminating the progress of massive degradative processes in the connective tissue by means of the appropriate deployment of a single reagent, TIMP. On the other hand, the requirement appears to exist for the specific activation of the zymogen form of each of the proteases, making the *onset* of connective tissue degradation difficult for the organism to effect, whereas the *termination* of the same processes is an easier task. In what specific ways this disjunction is put to use in physiology is not known at this time, but it will be fascinating to discover the "strategy" employed in regulating the activity of these enzymes.

Regulation of Collagenolysis

The regulation of these enzymes has been examined in a wide variety of systems and, as might be expected, a wide variety of potential mechanisms have been suggested.[6] This discussion will be restricted to those pathways indicated for the regulation of the activity of collagenase and TIMP in the human; the other members of the protease family have been only sparsely investigated, if at all, and so will not be dealt with here. Furthermore, no attempt will be made to list every agent, biological or pharmacological, that has been reported to modulate collagenase production in one or another system. Only those agents that appear to present a major and consistently active pathway of regulation in appropriate biological systems will be discussed.

The most consistently predictable regulators of collagenase production in human cell or organ culture systems are the glucocorticoids which, in general, have been found to be effective *inhibitors* of the production of collagenase.[101–106] In cultures of human fibroblasts, this inhibition has been suggested to take place at the level of mRNA transcription,[105] a mechanism consistent with that identified with steroid action in other enzyme systems. Steroid (e.g., hydrocortisone) concentrations of approximately 10^{-6} to 10^{-7} M are fully inhibitory in both cell and organ culture systems; overall protein synthesis is minimally affected at these hormone concentrations. By way of controls, high concentrations of estradiol, testosterone, or progesterone fail to effect the production of collagenase in these systems.

To demonstrate that regulation of collagenases can be cell- or tissue-specific, however, it should be noted that the glucocorticoids appear to be without effect in regulating the production of collagenase by human uterine myometrial smooth muscle cells.[32] These cells apparently produce the same enzyme as do the fibroblasts, but this regulatory pathway is seemingly not operative in the smooth muscle cell. Furthermore, in cultures of rat uterine explants or cultured rat myometrial smooth muscle cells, progesterone is an effective inhibitor of collagenase.[107–111] In this case, however, the glucocorticoids are similarly effective[103] and the pattern of steroid effect seems to mimic that of the interaction of these steroids with cytostolic steroid receptors. In the rat, progesterone and hydrocortisone appear to share affinity for cytostolic receptor molecules. In any event, it seems clear that steroid hormones, when effective, are *inhibitory* of collagenase production in the systems so far examined. The steroids that have been shown to inhibit collagenase production have no apparent effect upon the production of collagenase inhibitor (TIMP) in human fibroblasts.[106] Thus, the glucocorticoids appear to offer a mechanism whereby the ratio of enzyme to inhibitor can be effectively *decreased*.

Another class of compounds that appear to inhibit collagenase production in the systems so far studied are the retinoids. These pharmacologically active derivatives of vitamin A appear to selectively inhibit collagenase production. In contrast to the steroid hormones, the retinoids appear to concomitantly *augment* collagenase inhibitor (TIMP) production in human skin fibroblast cultures.[106] This class of compounds thus offers a different way to decrease the ratio of enzyme to inhibitor.

Phenytoin, a very effective antiepileptic drug, has been observed to produce gingival hyperplasia in about 20 percent of treated patients. Using an organ culture system, it was reported that this xenobiotic could increase collagen deposition, apparently by decreasing collagen degradation.[112] Subsequently, it was shown that phenytoin could decrease collagenolytic activity in human skin fibroblast cultures.[113] This compound has been used successfully in patients with recessive dystrophic epidermolysis bullosa,[114] a disorder characterized by a lack of anchoring fibrils attaching the epidermis to the underlying dermal stroma. Dermal fibroblasts from these individuals also show abnormal levels of collagenase activity in cultures, and this activity can be significantly reduced by phenytoin. Many patients treated with this compound have a lessening of the serious blistering that is associated with the disease, presumably due to a reduction in dermal collagenase at the epidermal-dermal junction. Currently, the mechanism of action of phenytoin on regulation of procollagenase synthesis is unknown.

Studies of growth factor biochemistry and physiology have demonstrated that these cell regulators can modulate collagenase expression by mesenchymal cells. Platelet-derived growth factor (PDGF) was shown by two groups to stimulate the de novo synthesis of procollagenase protein following addition to normal human skin fibroblasts.[115, 116] In addition, it was reported that both epidermal growth factor (EGF) and transforming growth factor-β (TGF-β) induced procollagenase synthesis.[116] However, more recent studies indicate that TGF-β can block EGF-stimulated procollagenase induction as well as directly inhibit synthesis of procollagenase.[117, 118] Simultaneously, TGF-β induces both TIMP synthesis and the production of another serine protease inhibitor that blocks the action of an enzyme capable of activating procollagenase in vivo.[118] Thus TGF-β is able to reduce new synthesis of collagenase by cells, enhance the ability of the cells to inhibit other sources of collagenolytic activity, and block the activation of procollagenase by serine proteases. All of these activities appear to enhance the deposition of collagen. With EGF, PDGF, and TGF-β all present within wounds, it remains to be determined how these factors, and possibly others, interact to result in the final expression of collagenase activity in the wound.

Another biologically significant reagent that has been shown to stimulate collagenase production in a variety of cell types is interleukin-1 (IL-1). A particularly important system, and the first in which this monokine was implicated, is in the rheumatoid synovium.[119, 120] In this pathological situation, the resident cells of the synovium produce the collagenase, the monocytes/macrophages produce the IL-1, and activated lymphocytes stimulate the latter cells to produce the monokine. The presence of IgG complexes as well as collagen in the lesion may serve to activate the lymphocytes, causing a virulent closed circle leading to continued production of collagenase and destruction of joint tissue.[121] Of additional interest in the rheumatoid synovium is a report that suggests that the resident cell of a tissue can produce autocrine products that regulate the subsequent synthesis of collagenase by the same cells.[122] Further details regarding the molecules and pathways involved are lacking at this time, and it will be of great interest to follow research into this potentially important mechanism for the modulation of collagen degradation.

Another apparently major regulatory pathway, in this case a stimulatory one, is produced by the tumor-promoting agent phorbol myristate acetate (PMA).[123-125] This component of coal tar invariably causes an increase in the ability of a given human fibroblast cell line to produce both collagenase and TIMP.[125] In some cells, such as human corneal fibroblasts, that produce no collagenase in culture, the tumor promoter acts essentially as a switch, turning on the synthesis of the enzyme in cells that are producing no detectable product. Whether PMA stimulation is mimicking the action of an in vivo hormone can only be a matter for speculation at this point. The phorbol esters have been shown to mimic the action of certain activators of the phosphoinositol pathway of hormonal transduction, and it is tempting to think that this is the case in the induction of collagenase production in these cells. Table 10–2 summarizes the effects of a variety of modulators on the levels of collagenase and TIMP in cultured human skin fibroblasts.

Another instance in which both enzyme and inhibitor are "up-regulated" in concert is that of the parathyroid hormone–induced increase in collagenase and TIMP production in the rat osteoblastlike cell line, UMR 106-01.[126] To the extent that it mimics the physiological activities of its ancestor the osteoblast, this cell line has

Table 10–2. REGULATION OF COLLAGENASE IN HUMAN SKIN

Compound	Enzyme Level	Inhibitor Level
Glucocorticoids	↓	Unchanged
Sex steroids	← Unchanged →	
Interleukin-1	↑	?
Phorbol esters (protein kinase C?)	↑	↑
Retinoids	↓	↑
TGF-β	↓	↑
Phenytoin	↓	?

classically been thought of as synthesizing the collagen required for bone turnover. In this case, however, parathyroid hormone induces the production of both collagenase and its inhibitor. While the reason for these hormonal effects is not presently clear, it is possible that the collagenase is required for the preparation of the mineralized bone surface to which osteoclasts specifically bind and begin the degradation of the substrate. This example of possible cellular cooperation within a given tissue is yet another area that must be fully elucidated before the natural history of collagen degradation can be completely described.

Returning at last to the wound healing process, it should be mentioned that this concept of cell-to-cell communication for the purpose of managing the metabolism of collagen in physiology was first suggested in 1967 by Grillo and Gross,[127] who were studying the healing guinea pig wound. These workers observed that in an in vitro organ culture system, both the dermis and the epidermis were required for the production of collagenase by the latter component at the margin of a healing wound. This finding clearly suggested the cooperation of epidermal and dermal cells in the induction of collagenolytic activity, but as mentioned, this relationship has remained largely unexamined since that time.

One system that has been utilized with some success to dissect this relationship has been the rabbit cornea. In this system, cultures of either epithelial or mesenchymal cells are unable, by themselves, to produce collagenase,[128] but cocultures of the two cell types together with cytochalasin B, a compound known to disrupt cytoskeletal structure, result in vigorous enzyme production. The production of enzyme was found to be proportional to the number of epithelial cells present in the culture. Subsequent studies have shown that epithelial cells, cultured with cytochalasin B, produced a macromolecule that induces the production of collagenase by cultured human fibroblasts.[129] The properties of this molecule bear a strong resemblance to those of interleukin-1, although the positive physiological significance of cytochalasin B in this system is unknown. Nevertheless, these observations clearly indicate the complex ways in which two cell types can interact in a tissue to produce collagenolysis. It is not far-fetched to imagine that the regulation of the turnover of collagen in the healing wound will require detailed analysis of a number of macromolecular products of a variety of cells present at one time or another during the healing process. This impression can only be reinforced by recent findings that growth factors such as PDGF and TGF-β have profound effects on wound healing.

Our understanding of the regulatory mechanisms invoked for the requisite precise control of proteases in wound healing remains fragmentary. Certainly, a great deal of phenomenology exists, but the integration of the various apparent pathways into a rational framework has not yet been achieved. This situation should improve dramatically in the next few years with the availability of a battery of molecular biological reagents for the analysis of the temporal and spatial regulation not only of collagenase but also of the other proteases of the extracellular matrix and their common inhibitor, TIMP.

References

1. Donoff RB, McLennan JE, Grillo HC: Preparation and properties of collagenases from epithelium and mesenchyme of healing mammalian wounds. Biochim Biophys Acta 227:639–653, 1971.
2. Gross J: Aspects of the animal collagenases. In Ramachandran GN, Reddi AH (eds): Biochemistry of Collagen. New York, Plenum Press, 1976, pp 275–310.
3. Gross J, Highberger JH, Johnson-Wint B, et al: Mode of action and regulation of tissue collagenase. In Woolley DE, Evanson JM: Collagenase in Normal and Pathological Connective Tissues. John Wiley & Sons, New York, 1980, pp 11–35.
4. Gross J: An essay on biological degradation of collagen. In Hay E (ed): Cell Biology of Extracellular Matrix. New York, Plenum Press, 1983, pp 217–253.
5. Woolley DE: Mammalian collagenases. In Piez KA, Reddi AH (eds): Extracellular Matrix Biochemistry. New York, Elsevier, 1984, pp 119–157.
6. Jeffrey JJ: The biological regulation of collagenase activity. In Mecham RP (ed): Regulation of Matrix Accumulation. New York, Academic Press, 1986, pp 53–78.
7. Gross J: How tadpoles lose their tails. J Invest Dermatol 47:274–277, 1966.
8. Nagai Y, Lapiere CM, Gross J: Tadpole collagenase. Preparation and purification. Biochemistry 5:3123–3130, 1966.
9. Sakai T, Gross J: Some properties of the products of reaction of tadpole collagenase with collagen. Biochemistry 6:518–528, 1967.
10. Stryer L: Glycolysis. In Biochemistry, 3rd ed. New York, WH Freeman, 1988, pp 361–362.
11. Gross J, Lapiere CM: Collagenolytic activity in amphibian tissues: A tissue culture assay. Proc Natl Acad Sci USA 48:1014–1022, 1962.
12. Gross J, Nagai Y: Specific degradation of the collagen molecule by tadpole collagenolytic enzyme. Proc Natl Acad Sci USA 54:1197–1204, 1965.
13. Gross J: Studies on the biology of connective tissues: Remodeling of collagen in metamorphosis. In Fitton S, Harkness RD, Partridge SM, et al: Structure and Function of Connective and Skeletal Tissue. London, Butterworths, 1964, pp 426–430.
14. Eisen AZ, Jeffrey JJ, Gross J: Human skin collagenase. Isolation and mechanism of attack on the collagen molecule. Biochem Biophys Acta 151:637–645, 1968.
15. Bauer EA, Stricklin GP, Jeffrey JJ, et al: Collagenase production by human skin fibroblasts. Biochem Biophys Res Commun 64:232–240, 1975.
16. Evanson JM, Jeffrey JJ, Krane SM: Human collagenase: Identification and characterization of an enzyme from rheumatoid synovium in culture. Science 158:499–502, 1967.
17. Evanson JM, Jeffrey JJ, Krane SM: Studies on collagenase from rheumatoid synovium in tissue culture. J Clin Invest 47:2639–2651, 1968.
18. Jeffrey JJ, Gross J: Collagenases from rat uterus. Isolation and partial characterization. Biochemistry 9:268–273, 1970.
19. Lazarus GS, Brown RS, Daniels JR, et al: Human granulocyte collagenase. Science 159:1483–1485, 1968.
20. Berman M, Dohlman CH, Gnadinger M, et al: Characterization of collagenolytic activity in the ulcerating cornea. Exp Eye Res 12:255–257, 1971.
21. Abramson M: Collagenolytic activity in middle ear cholesteatoma. Ann Otol Rhinol Laryngol 78:112–124, 1969.
22. Dresden MH, Gross J: The collagenolytic enzyme of the regenerating limb of the newt Triturus viridescens. Dev Biol 22:129–238, 1970.
23. Tokoro Y, Eisen AZ, Jeffrey JJ: Characterization of a collagenase from rat skin. Biochim Biophys Acta 258:289–303, 1972.
24. Vaes G: The release of collagenase as an inactive proenzyme by bone explants in culture. Biochem J 126:275–289, 1972.
25. Wahl LM, Wahl SM, Mergenhagen SE, et al: Collagenase production by endotoxin-activated macrophages. Proc Natl Acad Sci USA 71:3598–3601, 1974.
26. Fujiwara K, Sakai T, Oda T, et al: Presence of collagenases in Kupffer cells of the rat liver. Biochem Biophys Res Commun 54:531–537, 1973.
27. Wahl LM, Blandau RJ, Page RC: Effect of hormones on collagen metabolism and collagenase activity in pubic symphysis ligament of guinea pig. Endocrinology 100:571–579, 1977.
28. Woolley DE, Tucker JS, Green G, et al: Neutral collagenase from human gastric mucosa. Biochem J 153:119–126, 1976.
29. Morales TI, Woessner JF, Howell DS, et al: A microassay for the direct demonstration of collagenolytic activity in Graafian follicles of the rat. Biochim Biophys Acta 524:428–434, 1978.
30. Roswit WT, Halme J, Jeffrey JJ: Purification and properties of rat uterine procollagenase. Arch Biochem Biophys 225:285–295, 1983.
31. Partridge NC, Jeffrey JJ, Ehlich LS, et al: Hormonal regulation of the production of collagenase and a

collagenase inhibitor by rat osteogenic sarcoma cells. Endocrinology 120:1956–1962, 1987.

32. Roswit WT, Rifas L, Gast MJ, et al: Purification and characterization of human myometrial smooth muscle collagenase. Arch Biochem Biophys 262:67–75, 1988.

33. McCroskery PA, Richards JF, Harris ED Jr: Purification and characterization of collagenase extracted from rabbit tumours. Biochem J 152:131–142, 1975.

34. Steven FS, Itzhaki S: Evidence for a latent form of collagenase extracted from rabbit tumour cells. Biochim Biophys Acta 496:241–246, 1977.

35. Yamanishi Y, Dabbous MK, Hashimoto K: Effect of collagenolytic activity in basal cell epithelioma of the skin on reconstituted collagen and physical properties and kinetics of the crude enzyme. Cancer Res 32:2551–2560, 1972.

36. Yamanishi Y, Maeyens E, Dabbous MK, et al: Collagenolytic activity in malignant melanoma: Physicochemical studies. Cancer Res 33:2507–2512, 1973.

37. Biswas C, Moran WP, Bloch KJ, et al: Collagenolytic activity of rabbit V_2-carcinoma growing at multiple sites. Biochem Biophys Res Commun 80:33–38, 1978.

38. Fessler LI, Duncan KG, Fessler JH, et al: Characterization of the procollagen IV cleavage products produced by a specific tumor collagenase. J Biol Chem 259:9783–9789, 1984.

39. Kramer MD, Robinson P, Vlodavsky I, et al: Characterization of an extracellular matrix-degrading protease derived from a highly metastatic tumor cell line. Eur J Canc 21:307–316, 1985.

40. Stricklin GP, Bauer EA, Jeffrey JJ, et al: Human skin collagenase: Isolation of precursor and active forms from both fibroblast and organ cultures. Biochemistry 16:1607–1615, 1977.

41. Stricklin GP, Eisen AZ, Bauer EA, et al: Human skin fibroblast collagenase: Chemical properties of precursor and active forms. Biochemistry 17:2331–2337, 1978.

42. Welgus HG, Jeffrey JJ, Eisen AZ, et al: Human skin fibroblast collagenase. Interactions with substrate and inhibitor. Collagen Rel Res 5:167–179, 1985.

43. Birkedahl-Hansen H, Cobb CM, Taylor RE, et al: Activation of fibroblast procollagenase by mast cell proteases. Biochim Biophys Acta 438:273–286, 1976.

44. Eeckhout Y, Vaes G: Further studies on the activation of procollagenase, the latent precursor of bone collagenase. Effects of lysosomal cathepsin B, plasmin, and kallikrein, and spontaneous activation. Biochem J 166:21–31, 1977.

45. Horwitz AL, Crystal RG: Collagenase from rabbit pulmonary alveolar macrophages. Biochem Biophys Res Commun 69:296–303, 1976.

46. Tyree B, Seltzer JL, Halme J, et al: The stoichiometric activation of human skin fibroblast procollagenase by factors present in human skin and rat uterus. Arch Biochem Biophys 280:440–443, 1981.

47. Paranjape M, Engle L, Young N, et al: Activation of human breast carcinoma collagenase through plasminogen activator. Life Science 26:1223–1231, 1980.

48. Welgus HG, Jeffrey JJ, Stricklin GP, et al: Characteristics of the action of human skin fibroblast collagenase on fibrillar collagen. J Biol Chem 255:6806–6813, 1980.

49. Hu C-L, Crombie G, Franzblau C: New assay for collagenolytic activity. Anal Biochem 88:638–643, 1978.

50. Birkedahl-Hansen H, Dan K: A sensitive collagenase assay using ^{3}H-collagen labelled by reaction with pyridoxal phosphage and ^{3}H-borohydride. Anal Biochem 115:18–26, 1981.

51. Bhatnagar R, Decker K: A collagenase assay using ^{3}H-methyl-collagen. J Biochem Biophys Methods 5:147–152, 1981.

52. Cawston TE, Barrett AJ: A rapid and reproducible assay for collagenase using 1-^{14}C acetylated collagen. Anal Biochem 99:340–345, 1979.

53. Welgus HG, Jeffrey JJ, Eisen AZ: The collagen substrate specificity of human skin fibroblast collagenase. J Biol Chem 256:9511–9515, 1981.

54. Birkedahl-Hansen H, Taylor RE: Detergent activation of latent collagenase and resolution of its component molecules. Biochem Biophys Res Commun 107:1173–1178, 1982.

55. Murphy G, Reynolds JJ, Werb Z: Biosynthesis of tissue inhibitor of metalloproteases by human fibroblasts in culture—stimulation by 12-0-tetradecanolylphorbol, 13-acetate and interleukin-1 in parallel with collagenase. J Biol Chem 260:3079–3083, 1985.

56. Cooper TW, Bauer EA, Eisen AZ: Enzyme-linked immunosorbent assay for human skin collagenase. Collagen Rel Res 3:205–215, 1983.

57. Jeffrey JJ, Roswit WT, Ehlich LS, et al: Regulation of collagenase production by steroid in uterine smooth muscle cells: An enzymatic and immunologic study. J Cell Physiol 143:396–403, 1988.

58. Yoshioka H, Oyamada I, Usuku G: An assay of collagenase activity using enzyme-linked immunosorbent assay for mammalian collagenase. Anal Biochem 166:1–13, 1987.

59. Quinones S, Saus J, Otani Y, et al: Transcriptional regulation of human stromelysin. J Biol Chem 264:8339–8344, 1990.

60. Matrisian LM, Leroy P, Ruhlmann C, et al: Isolation of the oncogene and epidermal growth factor–induced transin gene: Complex control in rat fibroblasts. Mol Cell Biol 6:1679–1686, 1986.

60a. Okada Y, Nagase H, Harris ED Jr: A metalloproteinase from human rheumatoid synovial fibroblasts that digests connective tissue matrix components: Purification and characterization. J Biol Chem 261:14245–14255, 1986.

61. Seltzer JL, Jeffrey JJ, Eisen AZ: Evidence for mammalian collagenases as zinc ion metalloenzymes. Biochim Biophys Acta 484:179–187, 1977.

62. Berman MB, Manabe R: Corneal collagenases: Evidence for zinc metalloenzymes. Ann Ophthalmol 5:1193–1209, 1973.

63. Seltzer JL, Jeffrey JJ, Eisen AZ: Evidence for mammalian collagenases as zinc ion metalloproteases. Biochim Biophys Acta 484:179–187, 1977.

64. Swann JC, Reynolds JJ, Galloway WA: Zinc metalloenzyme properties of active and latent collagenase from rabbit bone. Biochem J 195:167–170, 1981.

65. Miller EJ, Harris ED Jr, Chung E, et al: Cleavage of type II and III collagens with mammalian collagenase: Site of cleavage and primary structure at the NH_2-terminal portion of the smaller fragment released from both collagens. Biochemistry 15:787–792, 1976.

66. Miller EJ, Finch JE Jr, Chung E, et al: Specific cleavage of the native type III collagen molecule with trypsin. Similarity of the cleavage products to collagenase-produced fragments and primary structure at the cleavage site. Arch Biochem Biophys 173:631–637, 1976.

67. Welgus HG, Burgeson RE, Wooton JAM, et al: Degradation of monomeric and fibrillar type III collagens by human skin collagenase: Kinetic constant using different animal substrates. J Biol Chem 260:1052–1059, 1985.

68. Hasty KA, Hibbs MS, Kang AH, et al: Heterogeneity among human collagenases demonstrated by monoclonal antibody that selectively recognizes and inhibits

human neutrophil collagenase. J Exp Med 159:1455–1463, 1984.

69. Hasty KA, Hibbs MS, Kang AH, et al: Secreted forms of human neutrophil collagenase. J Biol Chem 261:5645–5650, 1986.

70. Robertson PB, Ryel RB, Taylor RF, et al: Collagenase. Localization in polymorphonuclear leukocyte granules in the rabbit. Science 177:64–65, 1972.

71. Horwitz AL, Hance AJ, Crystal RG: Granulocyte collagenase: Selective digestion of type I relative to type III collagen. Proc Natl Acad Sci USA 74:897–901, 1977.

72. Hasty KA, Jeffrey JJ, Hills MS, et al: The collagen substrate specificity of human neutrophil collagenase. J Biol Chem 262:10048–10052, 1987.

73. Brinckerhoff C, Ruby PL, Austin SD, et al: Molecular cloning of human synovial cell collagenase and selection of a single gene from genomic DNA. J Clin Invest 79:542–546, 1987.

74. Fini, ME, Plucinski IM, Mayer AS, et al: A gene for rabbit synovial cell collagenase: Member of a family of metalloproteinases that degrade the connective tissue matrix. Biochemistry 26:6156–6161, 1987.

75. Goldberg GI, Wilhelm SM, Kronberger A, et al: Human fibroblast collagenase. Complete primary structure and homology to an oncogene transformation-induced rat protein. J Biol Chem 261:6600–6605, 1986.

76. Carmichael DF, Sommer A, Thompson RC, et al: Primary structure and cDNA cloning of human fibroblast collagenase inhibitor. Proc Natl Acad Sci USA 83:2407–2411, 1986.

77. Edwards DE, Waterhouse P, Holman ML, et al: A growth-responsive gene (16C8) in normal mouse fibroblasts homologous to a human collagenase inhibitor with erythroid-potentiating activity: Evidence for inducible and constitutive transcripts. Nucleic Acids Res 14:8863–8878, 1986.

78. Ryan JN, Woessner JF Jr: Mammalian collagenase: Direct demonstration in homogenates in involuting rat uterus. Biochem Biophys Res Commun 44:144–149, 1971.

79. Ryan JN, Woessner JF Jr: Oestradiol inhibition of collagenase role in uterine involution. Nature 248:526–528, 1974.

80. Weeks JG, Halme J, Woessner JF Jr: Extraction of collagenase from the involuting rat uterus. Biochim Biophys Acta 445:205–214, 1976.

81. Stricklin GP, Jeffrey JJ, Roswit WT, et al: Human skin fibroblast procollagenase: Mechanisms for activation by organomercurials and trypsin. Biochemistry 22:61–68, 1983.

82. Grant GA, Eisen AZ, Marmer BL, et al: The activation of human skin fibroblast procollagenase: Sequence identification of the major conversion products. J Biol Chem 262:5886–5889, 1987.

83. Sellers A, Cartwright E, Murphy G, et al: Evidence that latent collagenases are enzyme-inhibitor complexes. Biochem J 163:303–307, 1977.

83a. Jeffrey JJ, Roswit WT, Eisen AZ: Unpublished observations.

84. Jeffrey JJ, Welgus HG, Burgeson RA, et al: Activation energy and deuterium isotope effect of human skin collagenase using homologous collagen substrates. J Biol Chem 258:11123–11127, 1983.

84a. Welgus HG, Jeffrey JJ: Unpublished observations.

85. Hembry RM, Murphy G, Reynolds JJ: Immunolocalization of tissue inhibitor of metalloproteinases (TIMP) in human cells. J Cell Sci 73:105–119, 1985.

86. Murphy G, Sellers A: The extracellular regulation of collagenase activity. In Collagenase in Normal and Pathological Connective Tissues, New York, John Wiley & Sons, 1980, pp 65–104.

87. Stricklin GP, Welgus HG: Human skin fibroblast collagenase inhibitor. Purification and biochemical characterization. J Biol Chem 258:12252–12258, 1983.

88. Welgus HG, Stricklin GP: Human skin fibroblast collagenase inhibitor. Comparative studies in human connective tissue, serum, and amniotic fluid. J Biol Chem 258:12259–12264, 1983.

89. Welgus HG, Stricklin GP, Eisen AZ, et al: A specific inhibitor of vertebrate collagenase produced by human skin fibroblasts. J Biol Chem 254:1938–1943, 1979.

90. Vater CA, Mainardi CL, Harris ED: Inhibitor of human collagenase from cultures of human tendon. J Biol Chem 254:3045–3053, 1979.

91. Cawston TE, Murphy G, Mercer E, et al: The interaction of purified rabbit bone collagenase with purified rabbit bone metalloprotease inhibitor. Biochem J 211:313–318, 1983.

92. Welgus HG, Jeffrey JJ, Roswit WT, et al: Human skin fibroblast collagenase. Interactions with substrate and inhibitor. Collagen Rel Res 5:167–179, 1985.

93. Kerwar SS, Nolan JC, Ridge SC, et al: Properties of a collagenase inhibitor partially purified from cultures of smooth muscle cells. Biochim Biophys Acta 632:183–191, 1980.

94. Nolan JC, Ridge S, Oronsky AL, et al: Synthesis of a collagenase inhibitor by smooth muscle cells in culture. Biochem Biophys Res Commun 83:1183–1190, 1978.

95. Cawston TE, Galloway WA, Mercer E, et al: Purification of rabbit bone inhibitor of collagenase. Biochem J 195:159–165, 1981.

96. Cooper TW, Eisen AZ, Stricklin GP, et al: Platelet-derived collagenase inhibitor: Characterization and subcellular localization. Proc Natl Acad Sci USA 82:2779–2783, 1984.

97. Murray JB, Allison K, Sudhalter J, et al: Purification and partial amino acid sequence of a bovine cartilage-derived collagenase inhibitor. J Biol Chem 261:1454–1459, 1985.

98. Welgus HG, Campbell EJ, Bar-Shavit Z, et al: Human alveolar macrophages produce a fibroblast-like collagenase and collagenase inhibitor. J Clin Invest 76:219–224, 1985.

98a. Seltzer JL, Adams SA, Grant GG, et al: Purification and properties of a gelatin specific neutral protease from human skin. J Biol Chem 256:4662–4668, 1981.

98b. Liotta LA, Tryggvason K, Gerbisa S, et al: Partial purification and characterization of a neutral protease which cleaves type IV collagen. Biochemistry 20:100–104, 1981.

98c. Galloway WA, Murphy G, Sandy JD, et al: Purification and characterization of a rabbit bone metalloproteinase that degrades proteoglycan and other connective-tissue components. Biochem J 209:741–752, 1983.

99. Whitham SE, Murphy G, Angel P, et al: Comparison of human stromelysin and collagenase by cloning and sequence analysis. Biochem J 240:913–916, 1986.

100. Collier IE, Wilhelm SM, Eisen AZ, et al: H-ras oncogene transformed human bronchial epithelial cells (TBC-1) secrete a single metalloprotease capable of degrading basement membrane collagen. J Biol Chem 263:6579–6587, 1988.

101. Koob TJ, Jeffrey JJ, Eisen AZ: Regulation of human skin collagenase activity by hydrocortisone and dexamethasone in organ culture. Biochem Biophys Res Comm 61:1083–1088, 1974.

102. Werb Z: Biochemical actions of glucocorticoids on macrophages in culture. Specific inhibition of elastase,

collagenase and plasminogen activator secretion and effects in other metabolic function. J Exp Med 147:1695–1712, 1978.

103. Koob TJ, Jeffrey JJ, Eisen AZ: Hormonal interactions in mammalian collagenase regulation: Comparative studies in human skin and rat uterus. Biochim Biophys Acta 629:13–23, 1980.

104. Wahl LM, Winter CC: Regulation of guinea pig macrophage collagenase production by dexamethasone and colchicine. Arch Biochem Biophys 230:661–667, 1984.

105. Bauer EA, Kronberger A, Valle KJ, et al: Glucocorticoid modulation of collagenase expression in human skin fibroblast cultures. Evidence for pre-translational inhibition. Biochim Biophys Acta 825:227–235, 1985.

106. Clark SD, Kobayashi DK, Welgus HG: Regulation of the expression of tissue inhibitor of metalloprotease and collagenase by retinoids and glucocorticoids in human fibroblasts. J Clin Invest 80:1280–1288, 1987.

107. Jeffrey JJ, Coffey RJ, Eisen AZ: Studies on rat uterine collagenase in tissue culture. I. Relationship of enzyme production to collagen metabolism. Biochim Biophys Acta 252:136–142, 1971.

108. Jeffrey JJ, Coffey RJ, Eisen AZ: Studies on rat uterine collagenase in tissue culture. II. Effect of steroid hormones on enzyme production. Biochim Biophys Acta 252:143–149, 1971.

109. Koob TJ, Jeffrey JJ: Hormonal regulation of collagen degradation in the uterus. Inhibition of collagenase expression by progesterone and cyclic AMP. Biochim Biophys Acta 354:61–70, 1974.

110. Jeffrey JJ: Collagen synthesis and degradation in the uterine deciduoma. Regulation of collagenase activity by progesterone. Coll Rel Res 1:257–268, 1981.

111. Tyree B, Halme J, Jeffrey JJ: Latent and active forms of collagenase in rat uterine explants cultures. Regulation of conversion by progestational steroids. Arch Biochem Biophys 202:314–317, 1980.

112. Bergenholtz A, Hanstrom L: The effect of diphenylhydantoin upon the biosynthesis and degradation of collagen in cat palatal mucosa in organ culture. Biochem Pharmacol 28:2653–2659, 1979.

113. Moy LS, Tan EML, Holness R, et al: Phenytoin modulates connective tissue metabolism and cell proliferation in human skin fibroblast cultures. Arch Dermatol 121:79–83, 1985.

114. Bauer EA, Cooper TW, Tucker DR, et al: Phenytoin therapy of recessive dystrophic epidermolysis bullosa. Clinical trial and proposed mechanism of action on collagenase. New Engl J Med 303:776–781, 1980.

115. Bauer EA, Cooper TW, Huang JS, et al: Stimulation of in vitro human skin collagenase expression by platelet-derived growth factor. Proc Natl Acad Sci USA 82:4132–4136, 1985.

116. Chua CC, Geiman DE, Keller GH, et al: Induction of collagenase secretion in human fibroblast cultures by growth promoting factors. J Biol Chem 260:5213–5216, 1985.

117. Edwards DR, Murphy G, Reynolds JJ, et al: Transforming growth factor beta modulates the expression of collagenase and metalloproteinase inhibitor. EMBO J 6:1899–1904, 1987.

118. Overall CM, Wrana JL, Sodek J: Independent regulation of collagenase, 72-kDa progelatinase, and metalloendoproteinase inhibitor expression in human fibroblasts by transforming growth factor-β. J Biol Chem 264:1860–1869, 1989.

119. Dayer J-M, Breard J, Chess L, et al: Participation of monocyte-macrophages and lymphocytes in the production of a factor that stimulates collagenase and prostaglandin release by rheumatoid synovial cells. J Clin Invest 64:1386–1392, 1979.

120. Mizel SB, Dayer J-M, Krane SM, et al: Stimulation of rheumatoid synovial cell collagenase and prostaglandin production by partially purified. lymphocyte activating factor (interleukin 1). Proc Natl Acad Sci USA 78:2474–2477, 1981.

121. Krane SM, Amento EP: Cellular interactions and control of collagenase secretion in the synovium. J Rheumatol 10:7–12, 1983.

122. Brinckerhoff CE, Benoit MC, Culp WC: Auto-regulation of collagenase production by a protein synthesized and secreted by synovial fibroblasts—cellular mechanism for control of collagen degradation. Proc Natl Acad Sci USA 82:1916–1920, 1985.

123. Brinckerhoff CE, McMillan RM, Fahey JV, et al: Collagenase production by synovial fibroblasts treated with phorbol myristate acetate. Arthritis Rheum 22:1109–1116, 1979.

124. Moscatelli D, Jaffe E, Rifkin DB: Tetradecanoyl phorbol acetate stimulates latent collagenase production by cultured human endothelial cells. Cell 20:343–351, 1980.

125. Clark SD, Wilhelm SM, Stricklin GP, et al: Coregulation of collagenase and collagenase inhibitor by phorbol myristate acetate in human skin fibroblasts. Arch Biochem Biophys 241:36–44, 1985.

126. Partridge NC, Jeffrey JJ, Ehlich LS, et al: Hormonal regulation of the production of collagenase and a collagenase inhibitor of rat osteogenic sarcoma cells. Endocrinology 120:1956–1962, 1987.

127. Grillo HC, Gross J: Collagenolytic activity during mammalian wound repair. Develop Biol 15:300–317, 1967.

128. Johnson-Wint B: Regulation of stromal cell collagenase production in adult rabbit cornea: In vitro stimulation and inhibition by epithelial cell products. Proc Natl Acad Sci USA 77:5331–5335, 1980.

129. Johnson-Wint B, Gross J: Regulation of connective tissue collagenase production-stimulators from adult and fetal epidermal cells. J Cell Biol 98:90–96, 1984.

11

PROTEOGLYCAN GLYCOCONJUGATES

Michael Weitzhandler, Ph.D., and Merton R. Bernfield, M.D.

The most frequent and extensive post-translational modification of proteins is glycosylation of specific amino acids (serine, threonine, asparagine). The carbohydrate may be of various forms and may account for as little as 1 percent or as much as 90 percent of the mass of the glycosylated protein. Nearly all proteins at the cell surface or in the extracellular space are glycoproteins, a notable exception being serum albumin. The size and carbohydrate content of these glycoproteins vary widely, for example, fibronectin (2×10^5 Da, >4.5% carbohydrate), gastric mucus glycoprotein (2×10^6 Da, >80% carbohydrate), a large cartilage proteoglycan (>2×10^6 Da, >80% carbohydrate).

The carbohydrate modification can establish the function of the protein, but in many instances the role of the carbohydrate is unclear. Glycosylation may affect the orientation of the protein in the cell membrane, its solubility, half-life, and biological activity. Known functions include providing protective coatings (as on the intestinal epithelial lining), promoting cell adhesion (e.g., the cell adhesion molecules, or CAMs), acting as lubricants (as in the synovial fluid), dictating cell differentiation and intercellular recognition (as the discoidins of *Dictyostelium*), transporting metabolites across the cell membrane, and being part of the receptor sites for hormones and growth factors. They provide structure (as in the proteoglycans of cartilage) and act as antifreeze in the circulating fluids of certain fish and insects. Carbohydrate moieties on proteins participate in the sorting of proteins in the Golgi apparatus for transport to their final destinations and are implicated in the selective permeability of the glomerular filter as well as in immune function. Although the significance is unclear, changes in the glycosylation of proteins have been associated with neoplastic transformation.

The carbohydrate modifications of proteins in animal cells involve a limited number of sugars. These include N-acetylgalactosamine, N-acetylglucosamine, N-acetylneuraminic acid (or other acylated neuraminic acids), galactose, glucose, mannose, fucose, and glucuronic acid and its derivatives; these may be substituted with sulfate or, rarely, phosphate.

This chapter focuses on a subclass of glycoproteins, the proteoglycans. In general, proteoglycans have a greater carbohydrate content than other glycoproteins. Found in all tissues, proteoglycans support cells, provide tissue turgor, and mediate a variety of cellular interactions. The molecules are ubiquitous: all adherent vertebrate cells apparently have proteoglycans at their surfaces. Because they are grouped together solely on the basis of the presence of a glycosaminoglycan (GAG) chain, proteoglycan protein molecules have few structural features in common; this suggests a degree of functional versatility. The major functional element of the proteoglycans is the GAG chain, the nature of which will be discussed further on. The core proteins to which the chains are linked are apparently different although they may contain structurally similar domains. Indeed, from molecular cloning studies, certain proteoglycan structural motifs are becoming evident.

This chapter is organized into sections focusing on proteoglycan structure, metabolism, and function.

PROTEOGLYCAN STRUCTURE

A proteoglycan is a protein that contains one or more covalently bound polysaccharides known as glycosaminoglycans or GAGs. This section will review the structure of the various GAGs, the GAG attachment region, and finally the core proteins.

Glycosaminoglycans are polysaccharides composed of repeating disaccharide units in which one sugar is a hexosamine and the other is usually a uronic acid (Fig. 11–1). The hexosamine is either N^1-acetylated or N-sulfated, and both types of sugar may be O-sulfated. Hence, these polysaccharides are highly polyanionic. The GAGs are classified according to the type of hexosamine, whether they contain a uronic acid, and whether and where they are sulfated. With a single exception (hyaluronic acid), the GAGs are attached to a core protein in proteoglycans.

Hyaluronic acid (HA; also known as hyaluronan) is a large linear polysaccharide composed of alternating D-glucuronic acid and N-acetylglucosamine residues in $\beta 1 \rightarrow 3$ and $\beta 1 \rightarrow 4$ linkages. This GAG is exceptional in that it does not contain sulfate and does not exist as a proteoglycan; moreover, it is synthesized uniquely. Mammalian tissues with high HA concentrations are synovial fluid,[1] vitreous humor,[2] umbilical cord, and skin.[3] Nonmammalian sources include cockscomb and certain streptococci. HA is also the largest GAG with a molecular weight of 10^6 to 10^7 daltons.

The *heparan sulfates*, including the chemically related heparin, are composed of alternating N-substituted glucosamine and a uronic acid, in a $\beta 1 \rightarrow 4$ linkage.[4-6] The polymer of repeating disaccharides undergoes extensive enzymatic modification. The glucosamine residues are either N-acetylated (GlcNAc) or N-sulfated (GlcNSO$_3$), the latter substituent found only in heparan sulfate and heparin, and can be O-sulfated at C-6. The uronic acid residues are glucuronic acid and its C-5 epimer, iduronic acid, and the iduronate residues can be O-sulfated at C-2. Heparan sulfates are the only GAGs with continuous $1 \rightarrow 4$ linkages rather than alternating $1 \rightarrow 3$ and $1 \rightarrow 4$ linkages between sugars.

The variation in sulfation and uronic acid can yield several different possible disaccharides in the heparan sulfates. As larger forms of heparan sulfate chains may contain more than 100 disaccharides, extensive sequence variability can be generated by different arrangements of the dis-

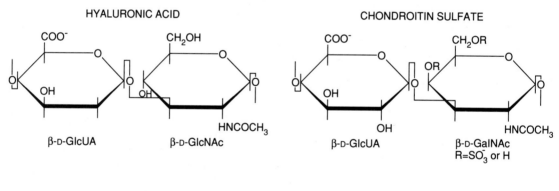

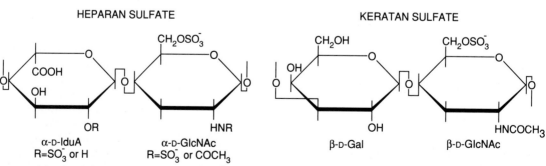

Figure 11–1. Structures of the glycosaminoglycans. The repeating disaccharides are shown. Chondroitin sulfate can be sulfated at the 4- or 6-position, and 4-sulfated chondroitin sulfate is often called dermatan sulfate when D-iduronate replaces a proportion of the D-glucuronate residue. Heparin resembles heparan sulfate except that the chain is more extensively sulfated.

tinct disaccharides. However, there are some restrictions on the sugar combinations that actually occur in the native polymer, so that the full potential for diversification is not fulfilled.[7-11]

Heparan sulfate and heparin contain identical sugar residues and linkages, but their proteoglycans represent separate families of molecules containing N-sulfated glycosaminoglycans.[12] Heparin is a mast cell product and is highly sulfated; it contains mostly N-sulfated hexosamines (more than 80 percent of GlcN units are N-sulfated) and there is always a molar excess of O-sulfates over N-sulfates.[13] In heparan sulfates, which are produced by all adherent mammalian cells, the GlcNSO$_3$ residues constitute about 50 percent of the total hexosamine, and there may be significant variation in the numbers of O-sulfate groups. The two species have a molecular mass ranging from 10,000 to 80,000 daltons.

Chondroitin sulfate consists of alternating residues of uronic acid and N-acetylgalactosamine and is sulfated at either C-4 or C-6 of the N-acetylgalactosamine. The repeating disaccharide of these galactosaminoglycans is also subject to a number of enzymatically catalyzed polymer modification reactions that may involve glucuronic acid epimerization to iduronate and O-sulfation of C-4 and C-6 of the galactosamine unit and C-2 of the iduronic acid component. When iduronic acid is present, this glycosaminoglycan is often referred to as dermatan sulfate. Chondroitin sulfates do not vary in sulfate content as much as heparan sulfates and usually have one sulfate group per repeating disaccharide, attached to either C-4 or C-6 of the galactosamine unit. Both oversulfated[14, 15] and undersulfated chondroitin sulfate chains occur in nature.[16, 17]

Keratan sulfate consists of alternating residues of glactose and N-acetylglucosamine and thus is unique among the glycosaminoglycans in not containing a uronic acid. Either sugar may be sulfated at the C-6 position. Keratan sulfate chains are bound to the core protein via a different linkage region than either heparan sulfates or chondroitin sulfates (discussed below) and typically have a lower molecular mass, 2000 to 20,000 daltons.

Attachment of Glycosaminoglycan Chains

The linkage between protein and polysaccharide for chondroitin sulfate and heparan sulfate chains consists of an O-glycosidic bond between D-xylose and a serine hydroxyl group. Adjacent to the xylose residue are two galactose residues, and it is this structure, gal-gal-xyl, that serves as a primer for addition of disaccharides in chondroitin sulfate and heparan sulfate. The xylose residue may be phosphorylated in heparan sulfate[18] and in chondroitin sulfate.[18, 19] Both Fransson and Oegema have speculated that the phosphoxylose residue could be a "recognition" signal for (1) primers that are going to acquire complex side chains or (2) interaction with other molecules in the extracellular environment.[18, 19]

Two additional types of carbohydrate-protein linkages are found in keratan sulfates. An O-glycosidic linkage can exist between N-acetylgalactosamine and the hydroxyl groups of threonine or serine, and the amide of asparagine can form a C-1-N bond to N-acetylglucosamine.

The recognition signal on the core protein for attachment of glycosaminoglycans to proteins in chondroitin and dermatan sulfate proteoglycans has been reported to consist of acidic amino acids closely followed by the tetrapeptide ser-gly-Xaa-gly, where Xaa is any amino acid.[20] A consensus core protein recognition signal has not as yet been identified for attachment of keratan sulfate or heparan sulfate to the core proteins of keratan or heparan sulfate proteoglycans. However, syndecan, a proteoglycan containing chondroitin sulfate and heparan sulfate, contains not only the expected chondroitin sulfate attachment sequence but also three sequences containing acidic amino acids, both N- and C-terminal to the ser-gly, presumably representing a heparan sulfate attachment site.[21] Studies with gene transfer and site-directed mutagenesis should answer questions regarding the similarity or dissimilarity of the core-protein recognition sequences for the attachment of chondroitin sulfate and heparan sulfate/heparin glycosaminoglycan chains.

Core Proteins

Classic protein chemistry and sequencing approaches are complicated by the large amounts of polysaccharide on the proteoglycan core proteins. Glycosaminoglycan side chains as well as O-linked oligosaccharides may be removed chemically from proteoglycans by treatment with hydrogen fluoride or trifluoromethane sulfonic acid. Alternatively, the bulk of the glycosaminoglycan side chains can be removed from proteoglycans by digestion with the appropriate enzyme(s) (chondroitinase, keratanase, heparitinase) to yield a core "preparation." Recently,

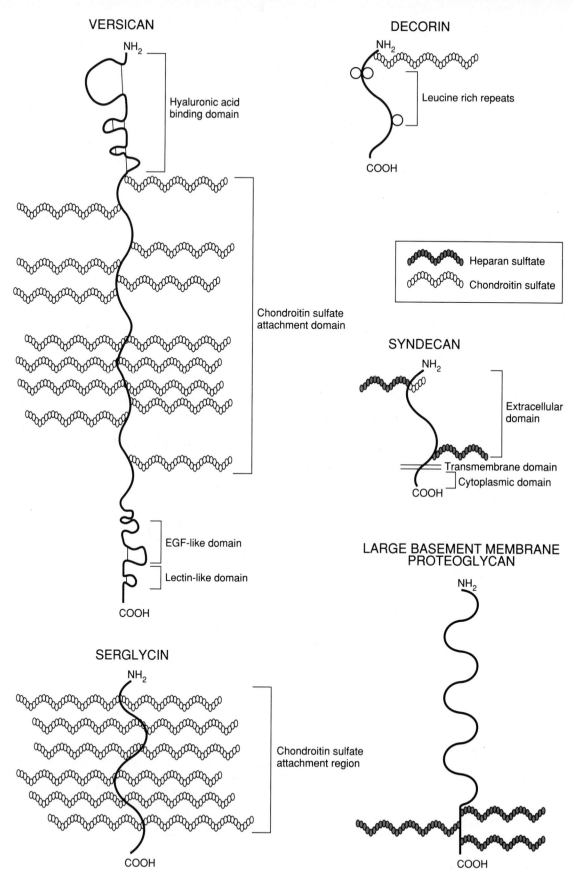

Figure 11–2 *See legend on opposite page*

molecular biology techniques have been used to determine the size and primary structure of several proteoglycan core proteins. These techniques have often shown that molecules from different sources previously thought to be distinct are the same or quite similar. Thus, designating these molecules with a descriptive name requires knowledge of their complete sequence.

The core protein of a yolk sac tumor proteoglycan[22, 23] was the first to be completely sequenced and is named serglycin. Serglycin is an unusual proteoglycan in that it contains a region of highly repetitive ser-gly sequences; more commonly, proteoglycans have one or a few ser-gly glycosaminoglycan attachment sites. It contains multiple chondroitin sulfate chains and is identical to the chondroitin sulfate proteoglycan found within mast cells.[24, 25]

The core protein of a small chondroitin sulfate proteoglycan[26] known as decorin is the major proteoglycan made by cultured human fibroblasts.[26] It has a single chondroitin sulfate chain and is apparently identical to various common connective tissue proteoglycans.[27]

The core proteins of proteoglycans from different sites may not be identical but may share identical or highly similar domains. Individual cell types appear to produce hydrophobic proteoglycans with several apparently distinct core proteins,[28, 29] some of which are translated from the same mRNA.[30] The large aggregating chondroitin sulfate proteoglycans of cartilage[31] and of fibroblasts (versican)[32] contain several similar domains, including a hyaluronic acid–binding region, an epidermal growth factor (EGF)–like domain, and a lectin-like domain. A domain containing EGF-like sequences is also present in the basement membrane heparan sulfate proteoglycan.[33] Two cell surface heparan sulfate/chondroitin sulfate proteoglycans—syndecan, a murine epithelial molecule,[21] and that from human fibroblasts[30]—contain very similar transmembrane and cytoplasmic domains but apparently distinct extracellular domains.

A variety of cell surface proteins are now known to have a portion of their complement substituted with glycosaminoglycan chains. These "part-time" proteoglycans include the transferrin receptor (heparan sulfate),[34] thrombomodulin (heparan sulfate),[23] the class II (Ia) histocompatibility antigen–associated invariant chain (chondroitin sulfate),[35] and the adhesive protein known by various names, including CD44, ECM receptor III, and the Hermes lymphocyte homing receptor (chondroitin sulfate).[36] The function of the glycosaminoglycans on these proteins is unclear.

The sequencing of proteoglycan core proteins and their cDNAs has provided a new view of proteoglycans. Previously these molecules were thought to be highly diverse, but it now appears that proteoglycan core proteins are multidomain molecules containing a common glycosaminoglycan attachment region in tandem with various functional regions common to several proteins (Fig. 11–2). Together, these domains constitute the complete core protein tailored by evolution for a specific function. Further work will likely reveal distinct core protein families, providing insight into the purpose of their covalently associated glycosaminoglycan chain.

PROTEOGLYCAN METABOLISM

Synthesis

Assembling a proteoglycan molecule requires the orchestration of a large number of post-translational processing reactions. Some of these are located in different regions of the cell. Other factors ensure that the different substituents are added to the core protein and modify the polysaccharide in the proper sequence. Moreover, additional controls govern the movement of the partially completed macromolecule through the intracellular compartments in an orderly fashion. Although mechanisms, organization, and control of protein biosynthesis have been elucidated in depth, analogous knowledge for glycosaminoglycans is lacking. Unlike protein biosynthesis, formation of the polysaccharide chain is not template directed. Instead, the nucleic acid template determines the sequence and properties of the biosynthetic enzymes, which in turn produce the polysaccharide. Consequently, the ultimate product typically displays structural heterogeneity.

With respect to proteoglycan biosynthesis, to be considered are formation of the polysaccharide-protein linkage region, polymerization of monosaccharide residues into polysaccharide

Figure 11–2. Structures of proteoglycans. The positions of the glycosaminoglycan chains and the structures of the protein cores are speculative.

chains, and modification of the polysaccharide chains.

Initial Glycosylation of Protein Core

Three types of carbohydrate-protein linkages are found in proteoglycans that involve the following monosaccharide-amino acid pairs: (1) xylose-serine; (2) N-acetylglucosamine-asparagine; and (3) N-acetylgalactosamine-threonine (or serine). The latter two types are presumably produced by the same biosynthetic pathways that have been well established for many glycoproteins, but details of these processes as they pertain to proteoglycans have not been fully established.

Initiation of polysaccharide chains joined by the xylose-serine linkage takes place by direct transfer of xylose from UDP-xylose to the hydroxyl groups of specific serine residues in the core proteins of the respective proteoglycans. The xylosyltransferase catalyzing these reactions has been detected in the rough endoplasmic reticulum of embryonic chick chondrocytes.[37, 38] The xylosyltransferase and two different galactosyl transferases involved in the biosynthesis of the xyl-gal-gal linkage region have been studied in heparin-synthesizing[39, 40] as well as in chondroitin sulfate–synthesizing systems.[15] Esko and co-workers described a Chinese hamster ovary cell mutant with a significantly decreased level of xylosyl transferase activity.[41] This mutant was defective in synthesis of both chondroitin sulfate and heparan sulfate, providing evidence that the same xylosyl transferase is responsible for the initiation of chondroitin sulfate and heparan sulfate chains. Additionally, the two galactose units of the linkage regions in different proteoglycans are synthesized by the same enzymes.[15] The linkage region is completed by transfer of glucuronic acid to the second galactose residue, catalyzed by a glucuronosyl transferase that differs from that involved in the formation of the polysaccharide chain proper.[42]

Although the natural substrates for xylose transfer are completed or nascent core proteins, a survey of potential exogenous substrates has shown that small peptides containing alternating serine and glycine residues may also serve as acceptors in this reaction.[43] Larger substrates, such as deglycosylated chondroitin sulfate proteoglycan or silk fibroin, which contains Ser-Gly pairs, were shown to be preferred substrates. Further evidence that Ser-Gly repeats may act as acceptors for chondroitin sulfate attachment comes from the molecular cloning of two different Ser-Gly pairs containing proteoglycan core proteins—the rat yolk sac tumor and the human fibroblast proteoglycan core proteins.[22, 32]

Assembly of N-linked high-mannose oligosaccharides commences when the core protein is within the endoplasmic reticulum.[44] The dolichol diphosphate intermediate oligosaccharide is then transferred intact via an N-glycosidic bond to asparagine on the core protein.[45, 46] Conversion of high-mannose oligosaccharide to the sialic acid–containing complex-type oligosaccharide occurs later in the Golgi apparatus.[47]

Formation of Glycosaminoglycan Chains

The structures of these polysaccharides result from the specific action of appropriate glycosyltransferases. Dorfman[48] summarized certain general characteristics of these glycosyltransferases:

1. They are specific for the monosaccharide unit transferred.
2. They are specific for the nonreducing terminal-accepting residue, including the configuration of its glycoside linkage.
3. They are not always specific for the penultimate sugar.

The key intermediates in GAG synthesis are UDP-glucose and UDP-N-acetylglucosamine. The former can be oxidized to form UDP-glucuronic acid, which can then be decarboxylated to form UDP-xylose. Both UDP-glucose and UDP-N-acetylglucosamine can undergo epimerization at the C-4 position to form UDP-galactose and UDP-N-acetylgalactosamine, respectively.[49]

Chondroitin Sulfate

Elongation of the chondroitin sulfate chains results from the alternate transfer of N-acetylgalactosamine and glucuronic acid residues from their respective nucleotides. The specificity of the two distinct transferases[50, 51] catalyzing these reactions provides the fidelity of the repeating disaccharide sequence.[52] The termination of chain elongation in chondroitin sulfate may be achieved by 4-sulfation of terminal hexosamine residues, since this, together with selective 4- and 6-sulfation, is a feature of newly synthesized chondroitin sulfate chains.[53] Chondroitin sulfate chains ending in N-acetylgalactosamine 4-sulfate are unable to accept a glucuronic acid.[52, 54, 55]

GAG sulfation, which occurs in the Golgi apparatus,[56, 57] is mediated by 3′-phosphoadenosine 5′-phosphosulfate[58] from which sulfate is transferred by different sulfotransferases to the specific sites on the GAG. Sulfation likely occurs simultaneously with chain polymerization.[59] The synthesis of oligosaccharides and the GAGs in the Golgi apparatus occurs rapidly; secretion from the Golgi may take as little as 5 minutes.[44]

Heparan Sulfate

Most of the information available pertaining to the biosynthesis of heparin and heparan sulfate has been obtained in experiments with cell-free systems, in particular, microsomal fractions from murine, heparin-producing mast cell tumors. Formation of the nonsulfated polysaccharide precursor, sometimes referred to as heparan, is the initial step in a sequence that results in the emergence of mature N-sulfated macromolecules. These modifications occur in particular regions of the GAG chains and are brought about by functionally integrated membrane-bound enzymes.[60] The process has been experimentally dissected in biosynthetically active microsomal preparations by restricting the availability of the sulfate precursor 3′-phosphoadenosine 5′-phosphosulfate in the incubation medium. The identification of a relatively discrete series of polysaccharide intermediates with increasing numbers of sulfate groups and iduronate residues has led to the concept of a stepwise mechanism of polymer level modifications.[61, 62]

In heparin, and to a lesser extent in heparan sulfate, there is N-sulfation, in contrast to the N-acetylation found in other GAGs. N-sulfation proceeds through the formation of a GAG containing N-acetylglucosamine,[63] which is then deacetylated with the replacement of the acetyl group by sulfate.[64, 65] After sulfation has occurred, epimerization of D-glucuronosyl takes place to produce L-iduronic acid in heparin and heparan sulfate.[66, 67]

Degradation

Proteoglycans can be found in various biosynthetic and degradative intracellular compartments and in the plasma membrane.[68] Thus, the disappearance of proteoglycans from the cell comprises exocytosis and shedding as well as intracellular degradation. Studies on proteoglycan turnover have been focused on the biochemical characterization of ^{35}[S]sulfate-labeled proteoglycan or glycosaminoglycan intermediates using pulse chase experiments or on the ultrastructural localization and intracellular movement of ^{35}S-labeled compounds using autoradiography.

Proteoglycans are degraded to their monomeric constituents within lysosomes. Partially degraded glycosaminoglycans are found within lysosomes in the genetic mucopolysaccharidoses, diseases in which one of the glycosaminoglycan-degrading enzymes has been rendered inactive by mutation.[69] These enzymes are exoglycosidases, with the exception of an endohexosaminidase (lysosomal hyaluronidase) found in various tissues but predominantly in testes. However, partial proteolytic or endoglycosidic degradation may occur extracellularly[70] or in a prelysosomal intracellular compartment.[71, 72] Nonlysosomal endoglycosidase activity against heparan sulfate has been implicated in rat ovarian granulosa cells.[73, 74] Nonlysosomal processing of cell-surface heparan sulfate proteoglycan has been reported in fibroblasts from patients with I-cell disease and NH_4Cl-treated normal skin fibroblasts.[75] A heparan sulfate–degrading endoglycosidase has been isolated from liver plasma membranes,[76] suggesting that some degradation of proteoglycans may occur at the cell surface. In cultured 3T3 cells, heparan sulfate proteoglycans are degraded in cell substratum adhesion sites.[77]

Heparan sulfate can be cleaved in extracellular sites by heparanases produced by platelets[78–80] and activated T lymphocytes.[81] The binding of heparan sulfate to type I collagen considerably reduces degradation of the proteoglycan in cultures of mammary epithelial cells.[82]

PROTEOGLYCAN FUNCTION

The functional role of the glycosaminoglycan chains on proteoglycans is primarily to act as a "glue"; binding interactions occur wherever proteoglycans are found, within intracellular granules, at the cell surface, or within the extracellular matrix. Overall characteristics of the proteoglycans are shown in Table 11–1.

Intracellular Proteoglycans

Secretory Granules. Proteoglycans are found within the secretory granules of a variety of

Table 11–1. CHARACTERISTICS OF PROTEOGLYCANS

GAG	Molecular Weight (daltons)	Attachment Sequence	Linkage to Protein	Distribution	Predominant Tissues
Hyaluronic acid	10^6–10^7	None	None	Cell surface, extracellular matrix	Skin fibroblasts, synovial fluid, vitreous humor, umbilical cord
Chondroitin sulfate	10,000–20,000	Asp(Glu)-Asp(Glu)-Xaa-(Ser-Gly)$_n$-Xaa-Gly	Ser-Xyl-gal-gal-GlcUA	Intracellular cell surface, extracellular matrix	Melanoma cells, cytolytic cells, cartilage
Heparan sulfate	10,000–80,000	Asp(Glu)-Asp(Glu)-Xaa-Ser-Gly-Asp-(Glu)	Ser-Xyl-gal-gal-GlcUA	Intracellular cell surface, extracellular matrix	Mast cells, epithelial cells, neurons, basement membrane
Keratan sulfate	2,000–20,000	—	(GlcNAc-gal)$_n$ | Ser(or Thr)-GalNAc-gal-NANA; man-(gal-GlcNAc)$_2$ \ Asn-GlcNAc-GlcNAc-man / man-(gal-GlcNAc)$_2$	Extracellular matrix	Cartilage, cornea

cells. Indeed, the presence of sulfated proteo-glycans is one of the few characteristics shared by almost all secretory vesicles, including those in exocrine and endocrine cells, neutrophils, mast cells, and polymorphonuclear leuko-cytes.[83] Because proteoglycans are present in substantial amounts in the secretory granules of cells involved in immune and inflammatory reactions, these macromolecules appear to play a role in the host response to diverse pathogens. Mast cell proteoglycans are unusual in the extent of their sulfation. In both rats and mice, heparin proteoglycan has ~4000 sulfate residues and ~2000 carboxylic acid residues per molecule, making it the most acidic macromolecule in the body.[84] Since both the serine proteases and the vasoactive amines of mast cells are positively charged at physiological pH, the proteoglycans may act like an ion-exchange resin to bind and concentrate these positively charged molecules within secretory granules. Once bound, the proteoglycan-protease-amine complexes may reversibly inactivate the intragranular proteases to prevent nonspecific enzymatic activity and unwarranted destruction of their microenvironments. Such bound proteases have substantially reduced enzymatic activity,[85] and this may be a mechanism for controlling the diffusion of the low molecular weight proteases into the surrounding connective tissue.

Neuronal Connections. Heparan sulfate proteoglycans are the major proteoglycans of the mammalian nervous system.[86] In general, reactivity with antibodies that recognize neural cell-surface proteoglycans shows a rapid increase during ganglionic growth and periods of rapid dendritic elaboration, reaching maximum levels in the young adult.[87, 88] Heparan sulfate proteoglycans are also the major antigenic components of cholinergic synaptic vesicles in many animal species.[89-91] Postsynaptic clusters of acetylcholine receptor (AChR) are tightly associated with a proteoglycan prior to synapse formation.[92] The nerve terminal also has the capacity to insert proteoglycan into its plasma membrane. Neuronal growth cones[93] and synaptic vesicles can fuse with the nerve terminal plasma membrane prior to contact with the target.[94, 95] Membrane-attached proteoglycans on both the nerve terminal and the AChR cluster are postulated to interact with the collagens and laminins of the basal lamina to "glue" the pre- and postsynaptic sides of the synapse to the basal lamina. Finally, neuronal cell-cell adhesion involves interactions of neural cell adhesion molecule (N-CAM) with cell-surface heparan sulfate proteoglycan.[96]

Cell-Surface Proteoglycans

Proteoglycans at the cell surface are either integral membrane proteins or proteoglycans that can be displaced from the surface by highly charged molecules, such as heparin. Additionally, heparan sulfate proteoglycan may be anchored to cell surfaces through a phosphoinositol linkage.[97] All adherent vertebrate cells have heparan sulfate at their surfaces. However, there also appear to be cell type-specific proteoglycans at cell surfaces, including those found primarily on epithelial cells[98] and melanoma cells.[99]

Cell-Matrix Interactions. Cell-matrix interactions involve heparan sulfate proteoglycans.[100, 101] Adhesion sites of newly attached fibroblasts are enriched in both fibronectin and cell-surface proteoglycan.[102-105] An association between both heparan sulfate proteoglycan[106] and a heparan sulfate–chondroitin sulfate hybrid proteoglycan[107] and the cytoskeleton has been described. Such an interaction would provide a mechanism for transmitting extracellular matrix reorganization directly into cytoskeletal organization. Additionally, the binding of a heparan sulfate–chondroitin sulfate hybrid proteoglycan to interstitial matrix, types I, III, and V collagen, fibronectin, and thrombospondin has been described.[108-110]

Antigen Presentation. The invariant chain Ii, a nonpolymorphic glycoprotein that associates with the immunoregulatory Ia proteins encoded by the major histocompatibility complex, has a form, Ii-CS, that bears a chondroitin sulfate glycosaminoglycan. The observations that Ii-CS is associated with Ia at the cell surface[35] and that interference with the synthesis of Ii-CS is accompanied by loss of antigen-presenting function[111, 112] suggest a role for Ii-CS in antigen presentation in helper T-cell recognition. Site-directed mutagenesis has distinguished the roles of Ii and Ii-CS in the immunobiology of Ia-antigen interactions and T-cell activation[113] and suggests that the GAG is used by the antigen-presenting cell. Moreover, xylosides, which inhibit proteoglycan synthesis,[114] diminish the capacity of spleen cells to serve as antigen-presenting cells.

Extracellular Proteoglycans

Basement Membrane Permeability. Basement membranes regulate the passage of cells, proteins, and ions between the lumenal spaces lined by epithelial and endothelial cells and the surrounding connective tissue stroma. Heparan sulfate proteoglycan is an important constituent of the glomerular basement membrane, a layer of matrix that separates the circulating blood from the urinary spaces. If treated with heparan sulfate–degrading enzymes, the glomerular membrane becomes permeable to ferritin[115] and albumin.[116] The charge-selectiveness of glomerular filtration owes its special properties to the heparan sulfate of this membrane.[117] A deficiency of this proteoglycan, as occurs in certain hereditary diseases, correlates with enhanced glomerular permeability, as seen in experimental diabetic nephropathy.[118]

Resistance to Compression. This property is critical for normal function of cartilage, such as the articular cartilage on the surfaces of bones that must act as cushions for variable, compressive loads. Proteoglycans have extended structures in solution and occupy very large hydrodynamic volumes relative to their molecular weights.[119–121] A proteoglycan monomer of 2.5×10^6 Da has a radius of gyration of about 60 nm. This dimension is defined primarily by the extended lengths of the chondroitin sulfate chains, about 50 nm for a chain of 20,000 Da. The molecules are reversibly compressible when subjected to a compressive load, but as solvent is displaced from the molecular domain, the intramolecular interactions between the GAG chains increase. When the load is removed, the molecular domains can once again expand.

Proteoglycans also are needed for normal growth and development of the skeleton. Alterations that cause a decrease in the amount of proteoglycan in the cartilage matrix or in the architecture of individual molecules, as occurs in such genetic anomalies as nanomelia in chickens,[122] cartilage matrix deficiency in mice,[123, 124] and 3'-phosphoadenosine-5'-phosphosulfate (PAPs) deficiency in brachymorphic mice result in foreshortened and malformed limbs.

PROTEOGLYCANS IN TISSUE REPAIR

GAGs and proteoglycans have been demonstrated to be an early, provisional extracellular matrix within injured tissue. In amphibious limb regeneration hyaluronic acid (HA) is the predominant matrix component following amputation as remaining cells dedifferentiate, migrate, and proliferate. A marked drop in the level of HA is coincident with cellular differentiation as collagen and proteoglycans, such as

chondroitin sulfate, are deposited in the matrix and the new extremity takes form.[125] It is felt that HA creates a large hydrated domain within the matrix that promotes migration and proliferation of the repair cells.[125] Similarly, the fetal wound, which grossly resembles regeneration without scar formation, is composed of a matrix rich in HA (see Chapter 21).

Proteoglycans and GAGs are also important in adult wound healing. The earliest matrix in these wounds results from the deposition of fibrin as a hemostatic response. It has been proposed that an interaction between HA and fibrin creates an initial scaffold on which cells involved in healing may migrate into the wound site.[126] Additionally, in vitro evaluation of burn scars suggests that HA may also interact with collagen.[127] Furthermore, a variety of proteoglycans enter the wound as acute inflammation ensues and vascular permeability increases.[128] Changes in the GAG or proteoglycan composition of open wounds also appear as healing proceeds. The edges of healing open wounds in rabbits seem to have an increased level of HA compared to the rest of the wound, and this is conjectured to facilitate epithelialization and movement of the wound edge. Granulation tissue formation in these wounds, which results from collagen deposition, was found to be correlated with the presence of dermatan sulfate.[129]

CONCLUSION

The proteoglycans are abundant glycoconjugates consisting of a protein core and covalently linked glycosaminoglycan chains. These chains are composed of monotonously repeating disaccharides except for the heparan sulfates and heparins, which show substantial compositional complexity due to varying extents of substitution of the sugars. The chains are linked to specific sequences on the protein cores. These attachment sequences are a common characteristic of the protein cores. Sequencing of the protein cores reveals that they are multidomain proteins that share sequences with a variety of other cellular proteins.

Proteoglycans are metabolized in a fashion analogous to that of other glycoproteins. Synthesis involves the production of the glycosaminoglycan chains from nucleotide sugars and extensive modifications of the chain by a variety of enzymes. The specificity of the biosynthetic enzymes and the fidelity with which they modify the polysaccharide are responsible for the unique characteristics of each of the glycosaminoglycan chains. Degradation of the proteoglycans follows a route analogous to that of other glycoproteins.

The functions of the proteoglycans are, in large part, due to their glycosaminoglycan chains. These are the most acidic molecules made by animal cells and they participate in a wide variety of binding interactions. Their highly polyanionic nature is responsible for their ability to concentrate secretory products within cells, to sequester a variety of extracellular proteins at cell surfaces, and finally, to bind water and cations extracellularly. Proteoglycans appear to have evolved to function where interactions via proteins were inadequate, but an explicit rationale for these molecules is not yet available.

References

1. Sundblad L: Studies on hyaluronic acid in synovial fluids. Acta Soc Med Uppsal 58:113–238, 1953.
2. Balazs EA: Amino sugar-containing macromolecules in the tissues of the eye and the ear. In Balazs EA, Jeanloz RW (eds): The Amino Sugars, vol IIA. New York, Academic Press, 1965, pp 444–445.
3. Pearce RH, Grimmer BJ, Mathieson JM: Fractionation of rat cutaneous glycosaminoglycans using an anion-exchange resin. Anal Biochem 50:63–72, 1972.
4. Lindahl U, Hook M: Glycosaminoglycans and their binding to biological macromolecules. Ann Rev Biochem 47:385–417, 1978.
5. Roden L: Structure and metabolism of connective tissue proteoglycans. In Lennarz WJ (ed): The Biochemistry of Glycoproteins and Proteoglycans. New York, Plenum Press, 1980, pp 267–371.
6. Comper WD: In Comper WD (ed): Heparin (and Related Polysaccharides). Structural and Functional Properties. New York, Gordon and Breach, 1981.
7. Bienkowski MJ, Conrad HE: Structural characterization of the oligosaccharides formed by depolymerization of heparin with nitrous acid. J Biol Chem 260:356–365, 1985.
8. Cifonelli JA, King JA: Structural characteristics of heparan sulfates with varying sulfate contents. Biochemistry 16:2137–2141, 1977.
9. Jacobsson I, Hook M, Pettersson I, et al: Identification of N-sulphated disaccharide units in heparin-like polysaccharides. Biochem J 179:77–87, 1979.
10. Sanderson PN, Huckerby TN, Nieduszynski IA: Very-high-field n.m.r. studies of bovine lung heparan sulphate tetrasaccharides produced by nitrous acid deaminative cleavage. Biochem J 223:495–505, 1984.
11. Linker A: Structure of heparan sulphate oligosaccharides and their degradation by exo-enzymes. Biochem J 183:711–720, 1979.
12. Gallagher JT, Walker A: Molecular distinctions between heparan sulphate and heparin. Analysis of sulphation patterns indicates that heparan sulphate and heparin are separate families of N-sulphated polysaccharides. Biochem J 230:665–674, 1985.
13. Taylor RL, Shively JE, Conrad HE, et al: Uronic acid composition of heparins and heparan sulfates. Biochemistry 12:3633–3637, 1973.
14. Razin E, Stevens RL, Akiyama F, et al: Culture of mouse bone marrow of a subclass of mast cells pos-

sessing a distinct chondroitin sulfate proteoglycan with glycosaminoglycans rich in N-acetylgalactosamine-4,6-disulfate. J Biol Chem 257:7229–7236, 1982.
15. Kolset SO, Kjellen L, Seljelid R, et al: Changes in glycosaminoglycan biosynthesis during differentiation in vitro of human monocytes. Biochem J 210:661–667, 1983.
16. Sobue M, Takeuchi J, Ito K, et al: Effect of environmental sulfate concentration on the synthesis of low and high sulfated chondroitin sulfates by chick embryo cartilage. J Biol Chem 253:6190–6196, 1978.
17. Ito K, Kimata K, Sobue M, et al: Altered proteoglycan synthesis by epiphyseal cartilages in culture at low SO_4^{2-} concentration. J Biol Chem 257:917–923, 1982.
18. Fransson LA, Silverberg I, Carlstedt I: Structure of the heparan sulfate–protein linkage region. Demonstration of the sequence galactosyl-galactosyl-xylose-2-phosphate. J Biol Chem 260:14722–14726, 1985.
19. Oegema TR Jr, Kraft EL, Jourdian GW: Phosphorylation of chondroitin sulfate in proteoglycans from the Swarm rat chondrosarcoma. J Biol Chem 259:1720–1726, 1984.
20. Bourdon MA, Shiga M, Ruoslahti E: Gene expression of chondroitin sulfate proteoglycan core protein PG19. Mol Cell Biol 7:33–40, 1987.
21. Saunders S, Jalkanen M, O'Farrell S, et al: Molecular cloning of syndecan, an integral membrane proteoglycan. J Cell Biol 108:1547–1556, 1989.
22. Bourdon MA, Oldberg A, Piersbacher M, et al: Molecular cloning and sequence analysis of a chondroitin sulfate proteoglycan cDNA. Proc Natl Acad Sci USA 82:1321–1325, 1985.
23. Bourin MC, Boffa MC, Bjork I, et al: Functional domains of rabbit thrombomodulin. Proc Natl Acad Sci USA 83:5924–5928, 1986.
24. Tantravahi RV, Stevens RL, Austen KF, et al: A single gene in mast cells encodes the core peptides of heparin and chondroitin sulfate proteoglycan. Proc Natl Acad Sci USA 83:9207–9210, 1986.
25. Alliel PM, Perin JP, Maillet P, et al: Complete amino acid sequence of a human platelet proteoglycan. FEBS Lett 236:123–126, 1988.
26. Krusius T, Ruoslahti E: Primary structure of an extracellular matrix proteoglycan core protein deduced from cloned cDNA. Proc Natl Acad Sci USA 83:7683–7687, 1986.
27. Vogel KG, Heinegard D: Characterization of proteoglycans from adult bovine tendon. J Biol Chem 260:9298–9306, 1985.
28. Lories V, De Boeck H, David G, et al: Heparan sulfate proteoglycans of human lung fibroblasts. Structural heterogeneity of the core proteins of the hydrophobic cell-associated forms. J Biol Chem 262:854–859, 1987.
29. David G, Van den Berghe H: Cell-surface heparan sulfate and heparan-sulfate chondroitin-sulfate hybrid proteoglycans of mouse mammary epithelial cells. Eur J Biochem 178:609–617, 1989.
30. Marynen P, Zhang J, Cassiman JJ, et al: Partial primary structure of the 48- and 90-kilodalton core proteins of cell surface–associated heparan sulfate proteoglycans of lung fibroblasts. Prediction of an integral membrane domain and evidence for multiple distinct core proteins at the cell surface of human lung fibroblasts. J Biol Chem 264:7017–7024, 1989.
31. Doege K, Sasaki M, Horigan E, et al: Complete primary structure of the rat cartilage proteoglycan core protein deduced from cDNA clones. J Biol Chem 262:17757–17767, 1987.
32. Krusius T, Gehlsen KR, Ruoslahti E: A fibroblast chondroitin sulfate proteoglycan core protein contains

lectin-like and growth factor–like sequences. J Biol Chem 262:13120–13125, 1987.

33. Noonan D, Horigan E, Ledbetter S, et al: Repetitive structure of the basement membrane proteoglycan deduced from cDNA clones. J Cell Biol 105:40a, 1987 (abstract).

34. Fransson LA: Structure and function of cell-associated proteoglycans. Trends Biochem Sci 12:406–411, 1987.

35. Sant AJ, Cullen SE, Giacoletto KS, et al: Invariant chain is the core protein of the Ia-associated chondroitin sulfate proteoglycan. J Exp Med 162:1916–1934, 1985.

36. Jalkanen S, Jalkanen M, Bargatze R, et al: Biochemical properties of glycoproteins involved in lymphocyte recognition of high endothelial venules in man. J Immunol 141:1615–1623, 1988.

37. Horowitz AL, Dorfman A: Subcellular sites for synthesis of chondromucoprotein of cartilage. J Cell Biol 38:358–369, 1968.

38. Hoffman HP, Schwartz NB, Roden L, et al: Location of xylosyltransferase in the cisternae of the rough endoplasmic reticulum of embryonic cartilage cells. Connect Tis Res 12:151–163, 1984.

39. Grebner EE, Hall CW, Neufeld EF: Incorporation of D-xylose-C^{14} into glycoprotein by particles from hen oviduct. Biochem Biophys Res Commun 22:672–677, 1966.

40. Helting T: Biosynthesis of heparin. Solubilization, partial separation, and purification of uridine diphosphate-galactose: Acceptor galactosyltransferases from mouse mastocytoma. J Biol Chem 246:815–822, 1971.

41. Esko JD, Stewart TE, Taylor WH: Animal cell mutants defective in glycosaminoglycan biosynthesis. Proc Natl Acad Sci USA 82:3197–3201, 1985.

42. Helting T, Lindahl U: Biosynthesis of heparin. I. Transfer of N-acetylglucosamine and glucuronic acid to low-molecular weight heparin fragments. Acta Chem Scand 26:3515–3523, 1972.

43. Roden L, Koerner T, Olson C, et al: Mechanisms of chain initiation in the biosynthesis of connective tissue polysaccharides. Fed Proc 44:373–380, 1985.

44. Kimura JH, Lohmander LS, Hassell VC: Studies on the biosynthesis of cartilage proteoglycan in a model system of cultured chondrocytes from the Swarm rat chondrosarcoma. J Cell Biochem 26:261–278, 1984.

45. Stow JL, Kjellen L, Unger E, et al: Heparan sulfate proteoglycans are concentrated on the sinusoidal plasmalemmal domain and in intracellular organelles of hepatocytes. J Cell Biol 100:975–980, 1985.

46. Waechter CJ, Lennarz WJ: The role of polyprenol-linked sugars in glycoprotein synthesis. Ann Rev Biochem 45:95–111, 1976.

47. Dunphy WG, Brands R, Rothman JE: Attachment of terminal N-acetylglucosamine to asparagine-linked oligosaccharides occurs in central cisternae of the Golgi stack. Cell 40:463–472, 1985.

48. Dorfman A: Proteoglycan biosynthesis. In Hay ED (ed): Cell Biology of the Extracellular Matrix. New York, Plenum Press, 1981, pp 115–138.

49. Silbert JE: Structure and metabolism of proteoglycans and glycosaminoglycans. J Invest Dermatol 79:31s–37s, 1982.

50. Perlman RL, Telser A, Dorfman A: The biosynthesis of chondroitin sulfate by a cell-free preparation. J Biol Chem 239:3623–3629, 1964.

51. Silbert JE: Incorporation of ^{14}C and ^{3}H from labeled nucleotide sugars into a polysaccharide in the presence of a cell-free preparation from cartilage. J Biol Chem 239:1310–1315, 1964.

52. Telser A, Robinson HC, Dorfman A: The biosynthesis of chondroitin sulfate. Arch Biochem 116:458–465, 1966.

53. Otsu K, Inoue H, Tsuzuki Y, et al: A distinct terminal structure in newly synthesized chondroitin sulphate chains. Biochem J 227:37–48, 1985.

54. Roden L, Baker JR, Helting T, et al: Biosynthesis of chondroitin sulfate. In Ginsburg V (ed): Methods in Enzymology. Complex Carbohydrates, vol 28. New York, Academic Press, 1972, pp 638–676.

55. Silbert JE: Biosynthesis of chondroitin sulfate. Chain termination. J Biol Chem 253:6888–6892, 1978.

56. Godman GC, Lane N: On the site of sulfation in the chondrocyte. J Cell Biol 21:353–356, 1964.

57. Peterson M, Leblond CP: Synthesis of complex carbohydrates in the Golgi region, as shown by radioautography after injection of labeled glucose. J Cell Biol 21:143–148, 1964.

58. Robbins PW, Lipmann F: Isolation and identification of active sulfate. J Biol Chem 229:837–851, 1957.

59. DeLuca S, Richmond ME, Silbert JE: Biosynthesis of chondroitin sulfate. Sulfation of the polysaccharide chain. Biochemistry 12:3911–3915, 1973.

60. Jacobsson I, Lindahl U: Biosynthesis of heparin. Concerted action of late polymer-modification reactions. J Biol Chem 255:5094–5100, 1980.

61. Riesenfeld J, Hook M, Lindahl U: Biosynthesis of heparin. Assay and properties of the microsomal N-acetyl-D-glucosaminyl N-deacetylase. J Biol Chem 255:922–928, 1980.

62. Jacobsson I, Lindahl U, Jensen JW, et al: Biosynthesis of heparin. Substrate specificity of heparosan N-sulfate D-glucuronosyl 5-epimerase. J Biol Chem 259:1056–1063, 1984.

63. Silbert JE: Incorporation of ^{14}C and ^{3}H from nucleotide sugars into a polysaccharide in the presence of a cell-free preparation from mouse mast cell tumors. J Biol Chem 238:3542–3546, 1963.

64. Lindahl U, Backstrom G, Jansson L, et al: Biosynthesis of heparin. II. Formation of sulfamino groups. J Biol Chem 248:7234–7241, 1973.

65. Silbert JE: Biosynthesis of heparin. IV. N-Deacetylation of a precursor glycosaminoglycan. J Biol Chem 242:5153–5157, 1967.

66. Hook M, Lindahl U, Backstrom G, et al: Biosynthesis of heparin. III. Formation of iduronic acid residues. J Biol Chem 249:3908–3915, 1974.

67. Malmstrom A, Fransson LA, Hook M, et al: Biosynthesis of dermatan sulfate. I. Formation of L-iduronic acid residues. J Biol Chem 250:3419–3425, 1975.

68. Hook M, Kjellen L, Johansson S, et al: Cell-surface glycosaminoglycans. Ann Rev Biochem 53:847–869, 1984.

69. McKusick VA, Neufeld EF: The mucopolysaccharide storage diseases. In Stanbury JB, Wyngaarden JB, Fredrickson DS (eds): The Metabolic Basis of Inherited Disease, 5th ed. New York, McGraw-Hill, 1983, pp 751–771.

70. Kresse H, Glossl J: Glycosaminoglycan degradation. In Meister A (ed): Advances in Enzymology, vol 60. New York, John Wiley & Sons, 1987, pp 217–311.

71. Diment S, Stahl P: Macrophage endosomes contain proteases which degrade endocytosed protein ligands. J Biol Chem 260:15311–15317, 1985.

72. Schaudies RF, Gorman RM, Savage CR Jr, et al: Proteolytic processing of epidermal growth factor within endosomes. Biochem Biophys Res Commun 143:710–715, 1987.

73. Yanagishita M, Hascall VC: Metabolism of proteoglycans in rat ovarian granulosa cell culture. Multiple intracellular degradative pathways and the effect of chloroquine. J Biol Chem 259:10270–10283, 1984.

74. Yanagishita M: Inhibition of intracellular degradation of proteoglycans by leupeptin in rat ovarian granulosa cells. J Biol Chem 260:11075–11082, 1985.

75. Brauker JH, Wang JL: Nonlysosomal processing of cell-surface heparan sulfate proteoglycans. Studies of I-cells and NH₄Cl-treated normal cells. J Biol Chem 262:13093–13101, 1987.

76. Gallagher JT, Walker A, Lyon M, et al: Heparan sulphate–degrading endoglycosidase in liver plasma membranes. Biochem J 250:719–726, 1988.

77. Lark MW, Culp LA: Turnover of heparan sulfate proteoglycans from substratum adhesion sites of murine fibroblasts. J Biol Chem 259:212–217, 1984.

78. Oosta GM, Favreau LV, Beeler DL, et al: Purification and properties of human platelet heparitinase. J Biol Chem 257:11249–11255, 1982.

79. Wasteson A, Hook M, Westermark B: Demonstration of a platelet enzyme, degrading heparan sulphate. FEBS Lett 64:218–221, 1976.

80. Yahalom J, Eldor A, Fuks Z, et al: Degradation of sulfated proteoglycans in the subendothelial extracellular matrix by human platelet heparitinase. J Clin Invest 74:1842–1849, 1984.

81. Naparstek Y, Cohen IR, Fuks Z, et al: Activated T lymphocytes produce a matrix-degrading heparan sulphate endoglycosidase. Nature 310:241–244, 1984.

82. David G, Bernfield MR: Collagen reduces glycosaminoglycan degradation by cultured mammary epithelial cells: Possible mechanism for basal lamina formation. Proc Natl Acad Sci USA 76:786–790, 1979.

83. Giannattasio G, Zanini A, Panerai AE, et al: Studies on rat pituitary homografts. II. Effects of thyrotropin-releasing hormone on in vitro biosynthesis and release of growth hormone and prolactin. Endocrinology 104:237–242, 1979.

84. Stevens RL, Otsu K, Austen KF: Purification and analysis of the core protein of the protease-resistant intracellular chondroitin sulfate E proteoglycan from the interleukin 3–dependent mouse mast cell. J Biol Chem 260:14194–14200, 1985.

85. Yurt R, Austen KF: Preparative purification of the rat mast cell chymase. J Exp Med 146:1405–1419, 1977.

86. Margolis RU, Margolis RK, Chang LB, et al: Glycosaminoglycans of brain during development. Biochemistry 14:85–88, 1975.

87. Greif KF, Reichardt LF: Appearance and distribution of neuronal cell surface and synaptic vesicle antigens in the developing rat superior cervical ganglion. J Neurosci 2:843–852, 1982.

88. Greif KF, Trenchard HI: Evidence for transsynaptic regulation of neuronal cell surface heparan sulfate proteoglycan in developing rat superior cervical ganglion. J Cell Biochem 26:127–133, 1984.

89. Kelly RB, Buckley KM, Burgess TL, et al: Membrane traffic in neurons and peptide-secreting cells. In: Molecular Neurobiology, vol. 48. Cold Spring Harbor Symposia on Quantitative Biology. Cold Spring Harbor Laboratory, New York, 1983, pp 697–705.

90. Stadler H, Dowe GHC: Identification of a heparan sulfate containing proteoglycan as a specific core component of cholinergic synaptic vesicles from Torpedo marmorata. EMBO J 1:1381–1384, 1982.

91. Jones RT, Walker JH, Stadler H, et al: Further evidence that glycosaminoglycan specific to cholinergic synaptic vesicles recycles during electrical stimulation of the electric organ of Torpedo marmorata. Cell Tissue Res 224:685–688, 1982.

92. Bayne EK, Anderson MJ, Fambrough DM: Extracellular matrix organization in developing muscle: Correlation with acetylcholine receptor aggregates. J Cell Biol 99:1486–1501, 1984.

93. Culp LA, Ansbacher R, Domen C: Adhesion sites of neural tumor cells: Biochemical composition. Biochemistry 19:5899–5907, 1980.

94. Young SH, Poo M: Spontaneous release of transmitter from growth cones of embryonic neurones. Nature 305:634–635, 1983.

95. Hume RI, Role LW, Fischbach GD: Acetylcholine release from growth cones detected with patches of acetylcholine receptor–rich membranes. Nature 305:632–634, 1983.

96. Cole GJ, Loewy A, Glaser L: Neuronal cell-cell adhesion depends on interactions of N-CAM with heparin-like molecules. Nature 320:445–447, 1986.

97. Ishihara M, Fedarko NS, Conrad HE: Involvement of phosphatidylinositol and insulin in the coordinate regulation of proteoheparan sulfate metabolism and hepatocyte growth. J Biol Chem 262:4708–4716, 1987.

98. Hayashi K, Hayashi M, Jalkanen M, et al: Immunocytochemistry of cell surface heparan sulfate proteoglycan in mouse tissues. A light and electron microscopic study. J Histochem Cytochem 35:1079–1088, 1987.

99. Bumol TF, Walker LE, Reisfeld RA: Biosynthetic studies of proteoglycans in human melanoma cells with a monoclonal antibody to a core glycoprotein of chondroitin sulfate proteoglycans. J Biol Chem 259:12733–12741, 1984.

100. Culp LA, Murray BA, Rollins BJ: Fibronectin and proteoglycans as determinants of cell-substratum adhesion. J Supramol Struc 11:401–427, 1979.

101. Schubert D, LaCorbiere M: Isolation of a cell-surface receptor for chick neural retina adherons. J Cell Biol 100:56–63, 1982.

102. Woods A, Hook M, Kjellen L, et al: Relationship of heparan sulfate proteoglycans to the cytoskeleton and extracellular matrix of cultured fibroblasts. J Cell Biol 99:1743–1753, 1984.

103. Laterra J, Ansbacher R, Culp LA: Glycosaminoglycans that bind cold-insoluble globulin in cell-substratum adhesion sites of murine fibroblasts. Proc Natl Acad Sci USA 77:6662–6666, 1980.

104. Culp LA, Rollins BJ, Buniel J, et al: Two functionally distinct pools of glycosaminoglycan in the substrate adhesion site of murine cells. J Cell Biol 79:788–801, 1978.

105. Rollins BJ, Culp LA: Glycosaminoglycans in the substrate adhesion sites of normal and virus-transformed murine cells. Biochemistry 18:141–148, 1979.

106. Woods A, Couchman JR, Hook M: Heparan sulfate proteoglycans of rat embryo fibroblasts. A hydrophobic form may link cytoskeleton and matrix components. J Biol Chem 260:10872–10879, 1985.

107. Rapraeger A, Jalkanen M, Bernfield M: Cell surface proteoglycan associates with the cytoskeleton at the basolateral cell surface of mouse mammary epithelial cells. J Cell Biol 103:2683–2696, 1986.

108. Koda JE, Bernfield M: Heparan sulfate proteoglycans from mouse mammary epithelial cells. Basal extracellular proteoglycan binds specifically to native type I collagen fibrils. J Biol Chem 259:11763–11770, 1984.

109. Koda JE, Rapraeger A, Bernfield M: Heparan sulfate proteoglycans from mouse mammary epithelial cells. Cell surface proteoglycan as a receptor for interstitial collagens. J Biol Chem 260:8157–8162, 1985.

110. Saunders S, Bernfield M: Cell surface proteoglycan binds mouse mammary epithelial cells to fibronectin and behaves as a receptor for interstitial matrix. J Cell Biol 106:423–430, 1988.

111. Sivak LE, Harris MR, Kindle C, et al: Inhibition of proteoglycan synthesis eliminates the proteoglycan form of Ia-associated invariant chain and depresses antigen presentation. J Immunol 138:1319–1321, 1987.

112. Rosamond S, Brown L, Gomez C, et al: Xyloside

inhibits synthesis of the class II-associated chondroitin sulfate proteoglycan and antigen presentation events. J Immunol 139:1946–1951, 1987.

113. Miller J, Hatch JA, Simons S, et al: Identification of the glycosaminoglycan-attachment site of mouse invariant-chain proteoglycan core protein by site-directed mutagenesis. Proc Natl Acad Sci USA 85:1359–1363, 1988.

114. Schwartz NB: Regulation of chondroitin sulfate synthesis. Effect of β-xylosides on synthesis of chondroitin sulfate proteoglycan, chondroitin sulfate chains, and core protein. J Biol Chem 252:6316–6321, 1977.

115. Kanwar YS, Linker A, Farquhar MG: Increased permeability of the glomerular basement membrane to ferritin after removal of glycosaminoglycans (heparan sulfate) by enzyme digestion. J Cell Biol 86:688–693, 1980.

116. Rosenzweig LJ, Kanwar YS: Removal of sulfated (heparan sulfate) or nonsulfated (hyaluronic acid) glycosaminoglycans results in increased permeability of the glomerular basement membrane to ^{125}I-bovine serum albumin. Lab Invest 47:177–184, 1982.

117. Kanwar YS, Farquhar MG: Presence of heparan sulfate in the glomerular basement membrane. Proc Natl Acad Sci USA 76:1303–1307, 1979.

118. Carrie BJ, Myers BD, Golbetz H: Proteinuria and functional characteristics of the glomerular barrier in diabetic nephropathy. Kidney Int 17:669–676, 1980.

119. Hascall VC, Sajdera SW: Physical properties and polydispersity of proteoglycan from bovine nasal cartilage. J Biol Chem 245:4920–4930, 1970.

120. Pasternack SG, Veis A, Breen M: Solvent-dependent changes in proteoglycan subunit conformation in aqueous guanidine hydrochloride solutions. J Biol Chem 249:2206–2211, 1974.

121. Reihanian H, Jamieson AM, Tang LH, et al: Hydrodynamic properties of proteoglycan subunit from bovine nasal cartilage. Self-association behavior and interaction with hyaluronate studied by laser light scattering. Biopolymers 18:1727–1747, 1979.

122. Pennypacker JP, Goetinck PF: Biochemical and ultrastructural studies of collagen and proteochondroitin sulfate in normal and nanomelic cartilage. Dev Biol 50:35–47, 1976.

123. Kimata K, Barrach H-J, Brown KS, et al: Absence of proteoglycan core protein in cartilage from the cmd/cmd (cartilage matrix deficiency) mouse. J Biol Chem 256:6961–6968, 1981.

124. Kochhar DM, Penner JD: Chondrogenic differentiation and limb morphogenesis in mutant mice homozygous for cartilage matrix deficiency (cmd). Anat Rec 196:101, 1980 (abstract).

125. Toole BP, Gross J: The extracellular matrix of the regenerating newt limb: Synthesis and removal of hyaluronate prior to differentiation. Dev Biol 25:57–77, 1971.

126. Weigel PH, Fuller GM, LeBoeuf RD: A model for the role of hyaluronic acid and fibrin in the early events during the inflammatory response and wound healing. J Theor Biol 119:219–234, 1986.

127. Burd DAR, Siebert JW, Ehrlich HP, et al: Human skin and post-burn scar hyaluronan: Demonstration of the association with collagen and other proteins. Matrix 9:322–327, 1989.

128. Schilling JA: Wound healing. Surg Clin N Amer 56:859–874, 1976.

129. Alexander SA, Donoff RB: The glycosaminoglycans of open wounds. J Surg Res 29:422–429, 1980.

12

CELL ADHESION

Frederick Grinnell, Ph.D.

During cutaneous wound repair, the extracellular matrix undergoes a series of transitions. Initially, a blood clot fills the physical defect caused by the wound. The clot contains high levels of plasma fibronectin in contrast to the adjacent dermal tissue, which contains low levels of connective tissue fibronectin. Figure 12–1 shows the resulting fibronectin-rich wound interface.[1, 2] Eventually, the blood clot is degraded and replaced with another transient matrix, that of granulation tissue. Unlike surrounding normal tissue, granulation tissue contains high levels of locally synthesized fibronectin, collagen, and residual fibrin and fibronectin from plasma.[1-4] Subsequent remodeling of the granulation tissue matrix results in scar tissue. The chemical composition of scar is similar to that of dermis, including low levels of fibronectin, but the arrangement of extracellular matrix components in scar is disorganized.[3-5]

The changes that occur after wounding result in changes in the extracellular matrix molecules with which cells interact (Table 12–1).[6-9] In dermis, for instance, fibroblasts usually are surrounded by a matrix that contains predominantly type I collagen and little fibronectin. During wound repair, however, fibroblasts are enmeshed in fibronectin-rich granulation tissue. In epidermis, basal keratinocytes normally rest on a laminin/type IV collagen–containing base-

ment membrane, but during wound repair these cells migrate along granulation tissue. The ability of tissue cells to respond to changes in the extracellular matrix is indicative of their dynamic, adhesive versatility.

To understand the normal and pathological features of wound repair, it is necessary to understand how cells interact with their extracellular matrices, including the regulation of these interactions and their influence on cell behavior and cell responsiveness to other wound factors. Extracellular matrix can influence cell behavior both directly through adhesive interactions and indirectly by serving as a reservoir for growth factors.[10, 11] Complex relationships exist among matrix, cells, and growth factors. For instance, transforming growth factor-β (TGF-β) acts on fibroblasts to promote synthesis of extracellular matrix,[12, 13] expression of cell adhesion receptors,[14, 15] and contraction of collagen gels.[16] After contraction, however, cells within collagen gels become unresponsive to TGF-β.[17]

One reason that studies on cell adhesion ligands and wound repair have focused on fibronectin is the transiently high levels of fibronectin in the matrix during wound repair. In addition, elevated fibronectin levels occur in a variety of inflammatory conditions including scleroderma,[18, 19] hypertrophic scars and keloids,[20] delayed-type hypersensitivity,[21] arthritis,[22, 23] hepatic fibrosis,[24, 25] and lung fibrosis.[26, 27] The roles of other adhesion proteins in wound repair are not so well understood.

This chapter focuses on some of the important features of cell adhesion ligands and receptors. It also summarizes recent evidence on the activation of keratinocyte adhesion function during wound healing and on enhancement of wound healing by fibronectin.

This research was supported by NIH grants CA14609 and GM31321. Studies on wound repair and keratinocyte adhesion were performed by Drs. Akira Takashima, Ken-Ichi Toda, and Tai-Lan Tuan. Clinical studies with fibronectin were performed in collaboration with Drs. Annette Wysocki, Paul Bergstresser, and Charles Baxter of University of Texas Southwestern and with Drs. Marilyn and Bernard Horowitz of the New York Blood Center. Drs. William Snell and Annette Wysocki made many useful suggestions regarding this manuscript.

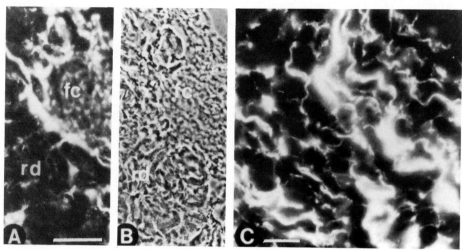

Figure 12–1. Fibronectin distribution in excisional cutaneous wounds observed by indirect immunofluorescence analysis. Frozen sections were prepared from samples taken 5 hours after wounding. *A*, Region of the fibrin clot (fc) and adjacent reticular dermis (rd) showing high levels of fibronectin in the clot. *B*, Corresponding phase contrast image. *C*, Higher magnification of fibrin clot showing fibronectin staining of individual fibrin fibrils. *A*, *B*, bar = 20 μm; *C*, bar = 10 μm. (From Grinnell F, Billingham RE, Burgess L: Distribution of fibronectin during wound healing in vivo. J Invest Dermatol 76:181–189, © by Williams & Wilkins, 1981.)

CELL-SUBSTRATUM ADHESION

Figure 12–2 illustrates the general events in cell-substratum adhesion. Initial interactions between cell surface receptors and adhesion ligands on the substratum trigger cytoskeletal changes leading to cytoplasmic reorganization.[28, 29] Adhesion of cells to large substrata results in cell spreading, while adhesion to small substrata results in phagocytosis. The relationship between cell spreading and phagocytosis can be illustrated by challenging cells with a series of particles of diverse sizes (Fig. 12–3).[30] Regarding wound repair, it is important to recognize that both cell migration through intact extracellular matrix and phagocytosis of fragmented matrix are likely to be important.

Fibroblasts that spread on substrata develop two major types of cell adhesion structures. "Close" adhesions have broad regions of ~30 nm space between the cell and substratum and an actin filament meshwork.[31, 32] These adhesions participate in cell motility.[33, 34] "Focal" adhesions have discrete plaques of ~10 nm space between the cell and substratum and actin filament bundles.[31, 32] These adhesions mediate cell resistance to tension[35, 36] and are found between fibroblasts and granulation tissue matrix components.[37]

Cell Adhesion Ligands

Table 12–2 lists several extracellular matrix molecules that have been shown to function in vitro as adhesion ligands for fibroblasts and for keratinocytes. Each cell type can attach and spread on several different matrix molecules. Moreover, these two different cell types recognize similar sets of matrix molecules. To learn

Table 12–1. CHANGES IN THE ADHESION SUBSTRATUM DURING REPAIR OF EXCISIONAL CUTANEOUS WOUNDS

Cell Type	Usual Substratum	Repair Process	Wound Substratum
Platelets	Endothelium (luminal surface)	Thrombosis	Subendothelium and dermis
Leukocytes, monocytes, lymphocytes	Endothelium (luminal surface)	Inflammation	Blood clot and granulation tissue
Endothelium	Basement membrane	Angiogenesis	Blood clot and granulation tissue
Fibroblasts	Dermis	Fibroplasia	Blood clot and granulation tissue
Keratinocytes	Basement membrane	Re-epithelialization	Granulation tissue

CELL ADHESION

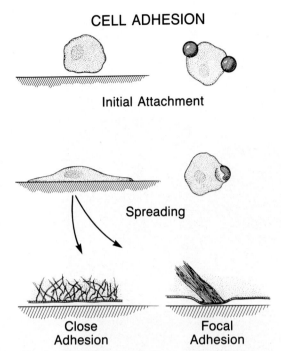

Initial Attachment

Spreading

Close
Adhesion

Focal
Adhesion

Figure 12–2. Model of cell adhesion. The model shows cell attachment and spreading on a large substratum or around small substrata. Close and focal adhesions are shown beneath spread cells.

which of the adhesion ligands cells actually use in vivo will require studies of the topographical distribution of the ligands and their temporal expression.

Of the molecules listed in Table 12–2, collagen and fibrin play the major structural roles. There are many different types of collagen, both fibrillar and nonfibrillar, as described in Chapter 8. Depending on the cell type, collagen and fibrin promote adhesion directly or in combination with other adhesion ligands such as fibronectin, laminin, thrombospondin, and vitronectin (Table 12–3). For instance, fibroblasts can attach directly to fibrillar type I collagen molecules,[38, 39] but adhesion to nonfibrillar or denatured type I collagen molecules requires fibronectin.[40, 41]

While the adhesion ligands summarized in Table 12–3 are diverse in size and subunit organization, they all contain domains specific for binding to collagen or fibrin.[42, 43] As a result, the extracellular matrix contains an exceedingly complex combination of different ligands, and it is possible for cells to interact simultaneously with more than one type.

Some adhesion ligands (e.g., fibronectin, vitronectin) can be found in tissue fluids and bound to extracellular matrix. The presence of an adhesion ligand in the fluid phase can potentially result in occupancy of cell surface receptors and inhibition of cell interactions with matrix-bound ligands. Under normal conditions, however, such competition does not occur. The lack of competition can be explained in part by the low affinity for cells of monomolecular ligands as compared to multimolecular forms.[28, 29] For instance, monomolecular fibronectin has a dissociation constant of 0.8 μM with baby hamster kidney (BHK) cells,[44] while multimolecular fibronectin-coated beads (~100 molecules/bead) have a dissociation constant of 4 nM.[45] Therefore, the affinity of multimolecular fibronectin-coated beads for cells is 200-fold greater than that of monomolecular fibronectin.

The activity of adhesion ligands can be regulated by other extracellular matrix molecules. The glycoprotein tenascin, which occurs in granulation tissue and beneath migrating epidermis,[46] may promote cell migration[47] by inhibiting cell adhesion to fibronectin.[48] Several proteoglycans (and glycosaminoglycans) also modify cell adhesion.[49] In particular, hyaluronic acid, a very large molecular weight glycosaminoglycan, may enhance cell migration during wound repair[8, 50] analogously to hyaluronate during embryogenesis.[51] As with tenascin, hyaluronate may promote cell migration by reducing the strength of cell adhesion or, alternatively, by expanding the extracellular matrix physically, thereby increasing the available space through which cells can move.

Fibronectin

Of the various glycoprotein adhesion ligands, fibronectin has been studied most thoroughly; its molecular biology and biochemistry have been described in detail in several recent reviews.[43, 52–54] The molecule is the product of a single gene and is composed of two almost identical polypeptide chains, M_r ~230 to 250 kDa. Three types of homologous repeating units designated type I (~45 amino acids), type II (~60 amino acids), and type III (~90 amino acids) make up most of the polypeptide chain. Figure 12–4 shows the arrangement of these repeating units and the corresponding matrix and cell binding domains.

Because of variations in splicing, several different forms of fibronectin are possible. Depending upon exon skipping mechanisms, fibronectin molecules occur with or without the type III repeats designated ED-B and ED-A (Fig. 12–4). The difference between plasma and cellular fibronectin may depend on the absence or presence of the ED-A domain.[43] The type III repeat designated IIICS is incorporated into

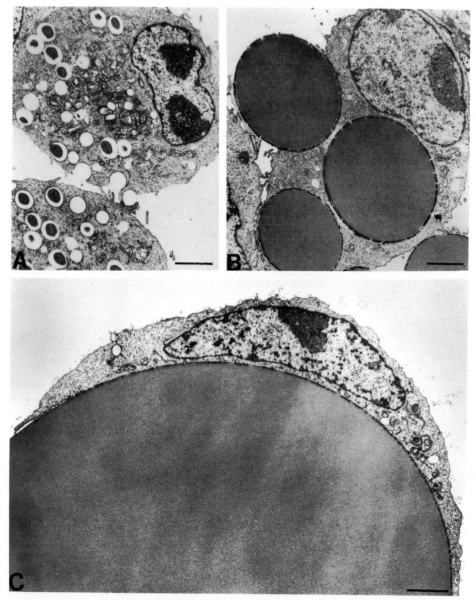

Figure 12–3. Adhesion of baby hamster kidney (BHK) fibroblasts to fibronectin-coated particles. BHK cells phagocytose 1 μm *(A)* or 6 μm *(B)* diameter particles but spread on the surface of 26 μm *(C)* diameter particles. Bar = 2 μm. (From Grinnell F: Fibroblast spreading and phagocytosis: Similar cell responses to different sized substrata. J Cell Physiol 119:58–64, 1984.)

Table 12–2. EXTRACELLULAR MATRIX ADHESION LIGANDS FOR FIBROBLASTS AND KERATINOCYTES

Cell Type	Adhesion Ligand	Selected References
Fibroblasts	Fibronectin	28, 139
	Laminin	140
	Collagen types I–V	38, 39, 141
	Fibrin(ogen)	142, 143
	Vitronectin	144, 145
	Thrombospondin	146
Keratinocytes	Fibronectin	97, 98
	Laminin	94, 147
	Collagen types I–IV	148–150
	Fibrin(ogen)	151
	Vitronectin	97
	Thrombospondin	152

the molecule to different extents depending upon exon subdivision. The biological significance of the different forms of fibronectin is not understood. By most criteria, even cellular and plasma fibronectin are difficult to distinguish from each other. There are some differences, however; of the two forms, cellular fibronectin is the less soluble and the more active in reversing the transformed cell phenotype.[42]

The precise mechanism by which fibronectin and other adhesion ligands interact with cell surface receptors is still being clarified. One important feature of fibronectin is an arg-gly-asp-ser (RGDS) sequence[55, 56] that is located in a type III repeat that forms part of the active site of fibronectin's cell binding domain (Fig. 12–4, *arrow*). Recent molecular studies using site-directed mutagenesis identified a second, functional region of the cell binding domain (Fig. 12–4, *asterisk*).[57]

RGD-containing sequences occur in a variety of adhesion proteins.[58] However, similar sequences are also found in proteins that probably play no role in cell adhesion. Indeed, 3 percent of the proteins whose sequences are known contain RGD.[54] Probably, the surrounding polypeptide sequences, not the RGD sequence, determine the specificity and affinity of adhe-

sion proteins. For instance, binding of RGDS to BHK cells occurred with a dissociation constant of ~100 μM compared to 0.4 μM for binding of the 75 kDa fibronectin fragment that contains the RGDS sequence.[59] Therefore, the 75 kDa fragment binds to the cell receptors 250-fold more tightly than the tetrapeptide.

Cell Adhesion Receptors

Recently, much has been learned about the cell surface receptors that mediate cell-matrix interactions. The high affinity of laminin for its receptor (Kd = 2 nM) simplified isolation of a ~70 kDa laminin receptor by affinity chromatography.[60–62] Fibronectin receptors were more difficult to isolate; nevertheless, several laboratories obtained monoclonal antibodies against fibronectin receptors and found them to contain an oligomeric complex of ~140 kDa molecules.[63, 64] Affinity chromatography experiments with a cell binding domain peptide as the eluant also resulted in isolation of fibronectin receptors.[65]

The amino acid sequences for one of the subunits of the chick fibronectin receptor[66] and the complete human fibronectin receptor[67] were determined from cDNAs. The sequences of the chick receptor and β (smaller) subunit of the dimeric human receptor are homologous based on their sequence similarity (85%). Comparison of these sequences with each other and with other adhesion-related molecules has led to the conclusion that fibronectin receptors are part of a superfamily of cell surface components, the integrins.[68, 69] Cell receptors that are part of the integrin family have related β subunits but distinct α subunits. Both α and β subunits are transmembrane glycoproteins.

Within the integrin superfamily, at least three families of adhesion receptors can be distinguished based on their β subunits. Table 12–4 lists some members of these families.

Table 12–3. MOLECULAR FEATURES OF SELECTED CELL ADHESION PROTEINS

Adhesion Protein	Molecular Weight (M_r)	Matrix Binding Domains
Fibronectin	Dimer: a, b subunits almost identical, 230,000–250,000 each	Fibrin, collagen, heparin
Laminin	Trimer: A subunit = 440,000 B1 subunit = 225,000 B2 subunit = 205,000	Collagen, heparin
Thrombospondin	Trimer: subunits = 127,400	Fibrinogen, collagen, heparin, fibronectin, laminin
Vitronectin (S-protein)	Monomer: mixture of subunits, ~65,000 and ~75,000	Collagen, heparin, thrombin/anti-thrombin III

Details can be found in references 42 and 43.

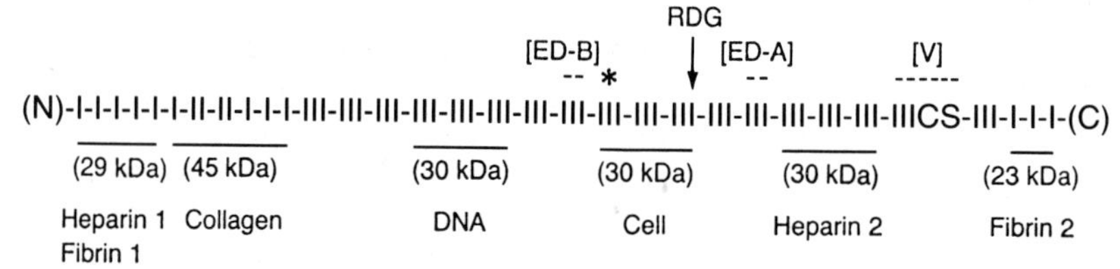

RDG

[ED-B] | [ED-A]   [V]

-- *   ↓ --   ------

(N)-I-I-I-I-I-I-II-II-I-I-I-III-III-III-III-III-III-III-III-III-III-III-III-III-III-III-III-IIICS-III-I-I-I-(C)

| (29 kDa) | (45 kDa) | (30 kDa) | (30 kDa) | (30 kDa) | (23 kDa) |

Heparin 1   Collagen   DNA   Cell   Heparin 2   Fibrin 2
Fibrin 1

Figure 12–4. Fibronectin. Model showing the arrangement of homologous repeating units (I, II, and III) and their relationship to the matrix and cell binding domains. Also shown are the positions of alternative splicing, ED-A, ED-B, and IIICS.

Receptors such as the avian 140 kDa complex and platelet IIb/IIIa have been shown to interact with more than one type of adhesion ligand.[70, 71] Also, many cell types express more than one type of receptor for the same adhesion ligand.[72] Thus, the cell adhesion system is potentially redundant not only in adhesion ligands (Table 12–2) but also in adhesion receptors (Table 12–4). The biological significance of this redundancy is unknown.

The current molecular model for cell adhesion suggests that cells interact with adhesion ligands by their specific receptors. This interaction theoretically causes a change in the cytoplasmic domain of the receptors that triggers the cytoskeleton to reorganize.[73] Consistent with this model are morphological and biochemical studies showing the association of fibronectin and laminin receptors with cytoskeletal components.[74–76] Another possibility, however, is that cell attachment results in osmotic changes leading to myosin-independent reorganization of the cytoskeleton and the actin cytoplasm.[77] This possibility would be consistent with the observation that myosin-deficient cells can spread and move.[78, 79] It may be, therefore, that the cytoplasmic domain of cell adhesion receptors is important in stabilizing receptor interactions with cytoskeletal components rather than causing their reorganization.

Although integrin receptors play a major role in diverse aspects of cell adhesion and motility, other cell surface components are also important in cell-matrix interactions. For instance, the ~70 kDa laminin receptor already described is not part of the integrin superfamily. Also, formation of focal adhesions by fibroblasts has been shown to require cell surface heparan sulfate in addition to integrin receptors.[80–82] Finally, assembly of fibronectin matrices around cells involves the participation of cell surface sialogangliosides.[83, 84]

Collagen Gels

Three-dimensional substrata are a recent innovation in studies on cell adhesion and wound repair. Fibroblasts cultured in hydrated collagen gels, unlike fibroblasts in monolayer culture, have morphological features similar to those of fibroblasts in vivo.[85–87] Moreover, collagen gels can be physically reorganized by fibroblasts. This extracellular matrix remodeling process was not appreciated from studies of cells in monolayer culture. Reorganization results in gel contraction[88–90] and has been likened to the in vivo process of wound contraction.[91, 92] The force of contraction results from cell motility[93] and depends on the actin cytoskeleton, since contraction can be inhibited by cytochalasins.[88, 94]

The consequences of collagen gel contraction depend upon whether gels are attached to a support or float during contraction.[17] In attached collagen gels, tension develops, collagen fibrils become aligned in the plane of cell spreading, and fibroblasts spread with an elongated, bipolar morphology (Fig. 12–5A and B). In floating gels, no tension develops, collagen fibrils remain randomly arranged, and fibroblasts spread with a stellate morphology (Fig. 12–5C and D). DNA synthesis and collagen synthesis occur to a much greater extent in attached gels compared to floating gels.[95, 96] Moreover, fibroblasts in floating collagen gels are generally unresponsive to TGF-β or other growth factors.[17] Therefore, extracellular matrix organization can influence not only cell growth and biosynthetic activity but also cell responsiveness to growth factors.

ACTIVATION OF KERATINOCYTE ADHESIVENESS DURING WOUND REPAIR

In previous sections, some of the in vitro features of cell adhesion were reviewed, and attention focused on the changing composition of the extracellular matrix with which cells interact during wound repair. In this section, evidence is presented regarding changes in cell

Table 12–4. SPECIFICITIES OF SELECTED CELL ADHESION RECEPTORS
IN THE INTEGRIN SUPERFAMILY

Receptor Family	Receptor Designation	Ligands Bound
Fibronectin receptor	Avian 140-kDa complex (integrin, CSAT, JG22)	Fibronectin, laminin
	VLA-2, ECM-2	Collagen
	VLA-3, ECM-1	Collagen, fibronectin, laminin
	VLA-5, Platelet Ic/IIa	Fibronectin
	Fibronectin receptor	
Platelet glycoprotein IIb/IIIa receptor	IIb/IIIa	Fibronectin, fibrinogen, von Willebrand factor
	Vitronectin receptor	Vitronectin
Leukocyte antigen	LFA-I	ICAM-1
	Mac-1	Complement iC3b
	p150, 95	?

Details can be found in references 54, 68, and 69.

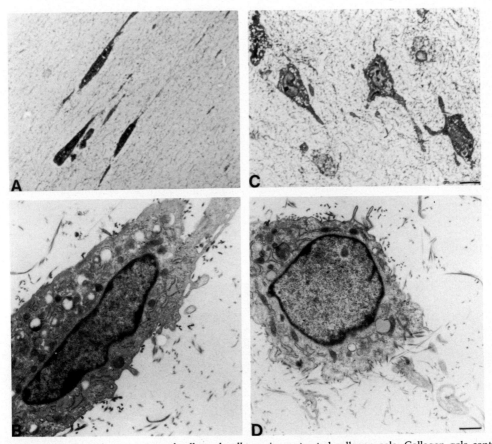

Figure 12–5. Morphological appearance of cells and collagen in contracted collagen gels. Collagen gels containing fibroblasts were attached to culture dishes *(A, B)* or floating in medium *(C, D)* for 24 hours. *A, B,* After contraction, cells in attached gels were elongated parallel to the surface of the culture dishes and collagen fibrils were aligned similarly. The cell nuclei were fusiform and collagen fibrils were bound individually and in small clusters all over the cell surface. *C, D,* After 24 hours of contraction in floating gels, the cells had a stellate morphology and collagen fibrils were randomly organized. Collagen fibrils were bound individually and in small clusters all over the cell surface. *A, C,* bar = 10 μm; *B, D,* bar = 1 μm. (From Nakagawa S, Pawelek P, Grinnell F: Extracellular matrix organization modulates fibroblast growth and growth factor responsiveness. Exp Cell Res 182:572–582, 1989.)

adhesiveness, particularly of epidermal cells, that occur during wound repair.

Fibronectin promotes the attachment and spreading of cultured keratinocytes on culture dishes[97-100] and phagocytosis of latex beads by keratinocytes.[98] Moreover, fibronectin promotes keratinocyte motility,[99, 101] whereas laminin inhibits motility.[102] The ability of fibronectin to promote phagocytosis and motility of keratinocytes may be particularly important for the movement of these cells through granulation tissue. Unlike cultured cells, epidermal cells freshly isolated from human skin do not attach to fibronectin or spread on any substrata in short-term assays. During cell culture, however, epidermal cell adhesion and spreading activity increase dramatically.[101, 103] Perhaps related to these findings, TGF-β promotes keratinocyte secretion of fibronectin and motility.[104, 105]

Activation of keratinocyte adhesiveness also occurs during wound repair in vivo. Rabbit ear epidermal cells were transplanted onto full-thickness wound beds on the backs of rabbits, and the cells were harvested and tested for adhesion to fibronectin after varying periods of time. Quantitative measurements showed an increase in keratinocyte adhesiveness toward fibronectin that reached a maximum in cells isolated from the graft bed after 3 days. Subsequently, around the time that the epidermis was reconstituted and the basement membrane resynthesized, keratinocyte adhesiveness toward fibronectin returned toward basal levels.[106]

To understand more about the mechanism underlying activation of keratinocyte adhesion to fibronectin, keratinocyte fibronectin receptors were analyzed. Initial experiments showed that these cells recognize the same cell binding domain of fibronectin as that recognized by fibroblasts. Moreover, polyclonal antibodies against 140 kDa fibronectin receptors inhibited the attachment and spreading of human keratinocytes on fibronectin substrata but not on collagen substrata.[107] Based on biochemical studies using these antibodies, fibronectin receptor expression apparently is greater on the surfaces of cultured keratinocytes than on keratinocytes freshly isolated from skin. The distribution of fibronectin receptors was observed in an epidermal sheet migrating out of explant cultures. Frozen sections stained with antibodies to 140 kDa fibronectin receptors showed a gradient with the highest concentration of receptors at the edge of migration (Fig. 12–6, *asterisk*).[153]

USE OF FIBRONECTIN TO PROMOTE HEALING

Fibronectin Deficiency

The first clinical application of fibronectin therapy was anticipated to be in the treatment of trauma patients who had markedly decreased plasma fibronectin levels.[108] Decreased circulating fibronectin after trauma may occur because plasma fibronectin is sequestered in damaged tissues.[109, 110] Since fibronectin functions as a nonimmune opsonin for phagocytosis, it seemed likely that decreased circulating fibronectin resulted in depressed mononuclear phagocyte function and the related development of sepsis.[108] Fibronectin levels can be reconstituted in trauma patients, reversing the opsonic deficiency.[111] Unfortunately, restoration of opsonic

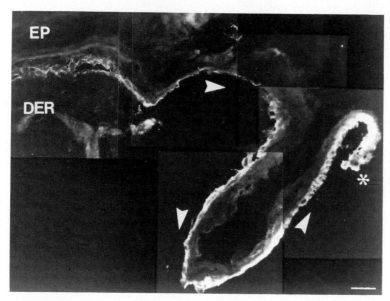

Figure 12–6. Distribution of fibronectin receptors in migrating epidermal cells. Epidermal explants composed of epidermis (EP) and dermis (DER) were placed in tissue culture. An epidermal sheet migrated *(arrows)* out of the explants along the culture dish surfaces. Samples were removed from the culture dishes (during which time the migrating epidermal sheet compressed), and frozen sections were prepared. Fibronectin receptors were expressed in a gradient with the highest concentration at the migratory edge *(asterisk)*. Bar = 20 μm.

activity does not appear to improve organ function or patient survival.[112, 113]

Periodontal Disease

In treatment of periodontal disease, fibronectin might promote attachment of connective tissue to exposed root surfaces, thereby limiting epithelial downgrowth along the tooth.[114] Experiments to test this procedure with cats, monkeys, and dogs have been encouraging.[115–117] Moreover, initial clinical trials of autologous fibronectin treatment with periodontal patients have been successful.[118]

Corneal Ulcers

Corneal wounds exhibit a fibronectin distribution similar to that found in cutaneous wounds; that is, shortly after wounding of the rabbit corneal epithelium, a thin layer of fibronectin and fibrin appears on the denuded corneal surface.[119, 120] Subsequent re-epithelialization of the cornea occurs over the fibronectin-coated matrix in the absence of basement membrane proteins to which the epithelium normally is attached. After re-epithelialization and resynthesis of the basement membrane, the level of fibronectin in the corneal stroma rapidly decreases to normal levels.[120, 121] In vitro, fibronectin promotes migration of corneal epithelial cells.[122]

Topical application of fibronectin enhanced healing of corneal ulcers prepared in rabbits.[123, 124] Also, autologous fibronectin eyedrops promoted healing in two patients with persistent corneal defects that had been unresponsive to conventional therapy.[125] Subsequent studies have confirmed these findings, and fibronectin eyedrops have been effective in treating a variety of epithelial defects.[126–130] In part, corneal ulceration may be caused by proteolytic degradation of the fibronectin/fibrin wound matrix by plasmin.[130, 131] Recently, the Food and Drug Administration has designated fibronectin as an orphan drug under the sponsorship of the New York Blood Center for the treatment of nonhealing corneal ulcers and epithelial defects.

Cutaneous Ulcers

The effects of fibronectin on cutaneous repair have been measured in several different experimental models. Insertion of precipitated fibronectin into rat incisional wounds modestly increased wound strength during the first 2 weeks after surgery.[132] Topical application of fibronectin resulted in increased wound closure and increased wound strength in rat excisional wounds.[133, 134] With rat burn wounds, added fibronectin did not promote wound closure, but decreased levels of circulating fibronectin resulted in slower healing.[135] Therapeutically, the combination of autologous fibronectin with heparin benefited several patients with chronic ulcers.[136]

Based on in vitro and in vivo studies, we believed that fibronectin might be useful in promoting re-epithelialization of cutaneous ulcers. In preliminary clinical trials, we have treated nonhealing venous stasis ulcers with topical fibronectin[137] that was treated with organic solvents and detergents to inactivate viruses.[138] Eleven individuals participated in the preliminary study (Table 12–5). The treatment period was 3 weeks with fibronectin solution containing human fibronectin (1 mg/ml) and human serum albumin (1 mg/ml) in 0.9% sterile NaCl or with placebo solution containing human serum albumin (2 mg/ml) in 0.9% sterile NaCl. The test or placebo solutions were used to saturate nonadhesive dressing material (Telfa) that were placed over the ulcers and covered by 4 × 4″ gauze sponges and secured in place with a roll of stretch gauze. Dressings were changed twice daily. Ulcer size was calculated based on quantitative measurements of ulcer width and length. While there was a wide variation in ulcer size and response to treatment, there was generally a more pronounced

Table 12–5. TREATMENT OF STASIS ULCERS WITH TOPICAL FIBRONECTIN

Parameter	Placebo Group (2 mg/ml HSA*)	Fibronectin Group (1 mg/ml FN† + 1 mg/ml HSA)
Number of patients	6	7
Number of ulcers	7	6
Range in ulcer size	0.9–97 cm²	1.1–126 cm²
Average ulcer size	26.9 cm²	25.6 cm²
Average % closure	19.7 ± 15.4	51.8 ± 27.9

*HSA = human serum albumin.
†FN = fibronectin.

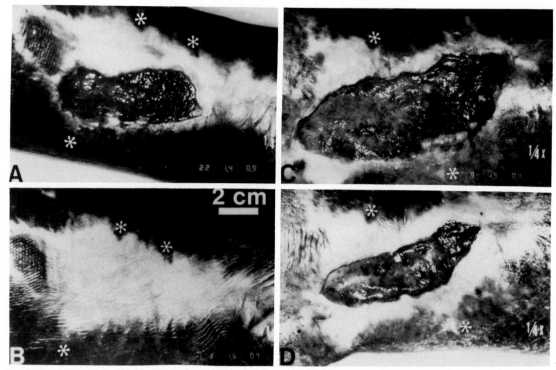

Figure 12–7. Photographic record of bilateral stasis ulcers during fibronectin treatment. *A,* Wound on left leg 9/22/86. *B,* Wound on left leg healed by 5/21/87. *C,* Wound on right leg 11/13/86. *D,* Wound on right leg markedly improved by 10/29/87. Distances between skin markings *(asterisks)* did not change during the treatment period, indicating that healing was by re-epithelialization and not by contraction. (From Wysocki A, Bergstresser PR, Baxter CR, et al: Topical fibronectin therapy for treatment of a patient with chronic stasis ulcers. Arch Dermatol 124:175–177. Copyright 1988, American Medical Association.)

wound closure in fibronectin-treated than in placebo-treated ulcers.

One patient in the study was a 69-year-old woman with bilateral ulcers who had been under treatment for more than 5 years. In her case, fibronectin therapy extended beyond the 3 week protocol. The ulcer on her left leg, which was 18.9 cm² at the beginning of treatment (Fig. 12–7A) healed after 8 months (Fig. 12–7B). The ulcer on her right leg, which was 26.8 cm² at the beginning of treatment (Fig. 12–7C), decreased in size to 13.1 cm² after 11 months (Fig. 12–7D). The distances between selected skin markings, labeled with asterisks in the photographs, did not change during treatment (Fig. 12–A vs. B and C vs. D). It can be concluded, therefore, that fibronectin promoted wound re-epithelialization, not wound contraction.

CONCLUSION

This chapter reviewed selected aspects of the current model of cell adhesion and its relationship to wound repair. Of particular importance are the dynamic changes in the extracellular matrix and cell-matrix interactions that occur after wounding. In adult organisms, such dramatic changes are unique to the wound repair process.

Fibronectin is the first of the well-characterized adhesion ligands. Interest in the role of fibronectin in wound repair arose because of the distribution of this molecule in the wound matrix. Also, keratinocyte adhesion and fibronectin receptor expression increased dramatically during wound healing, which may be important features of re-epithelialization. Initial clinical trials using fibronectin to promote healing of corneal ulcers and venous stasis ulcers have been encouraging.

References

1. Grinnell F, Billingham RE, Burgess L: Distribution of fibronectin during wound healing in vivo. J Invest Dermatol 76:181–189, 1981.
2. Clark RAF, Lanigan JM, DellaPelle P, et al: Fibronectin and fibrin provide a provisional matrix for epidermal cell migration during wound reepithelialization. J Invest Dermatol 79:264–269, 1982.
3. Kurkinen M, Vaheri A, Roberts PJ, et al: Sequential appearance of fibronectin and collagen in experimental granulation tissue. Lab Invest 43:47–51, 1980.

4. Viljanto J, Penttinen R, Raekallio J: Fibronectin in early phases of wound healing in children. Acta Chir Scand 147:7–13, 1981.

5. Peacock EE: Wound Repair, 3rd ed. Philadelphia, WB Saunders, 1984.

6. Grinnell F: Fibronectin and wound healing. J Cell Biochem 26:107–116, 1984.

7. Woodley DT, O'Keefe EJ, Prunieras M: Cutaneous wound healing: A model for cell-matrix interactions. J Am Acad Dermatol 12:420–433, 1985.

8. Clark, RAF: Cutaneous tissue repair: Basic biological considerations. J Am Acad Dermatol 13:701–725, 1985.

9. Dvorak HF: Wounds that do not heal. Similarities between tumor stroma generation and wound healing. N Engl J Med 315:1650–1659, 1986.

10. Bitterman PB, Rennard SI, Adelberg S, et al: Role of fibronectin as a growth factor for fibroblasts. J Cell Biol 97:1925–1932, 1983.

11. Fava RA, McClure DB: Fibronectin-associated transforming growth factor. J Cell Physiol 131:184–189, 1987.

12. Sporn MB, Roberts AB, Shull JH, et al: Polypeptide transforming growth factors isolated from bovine sources and used for wound healing in vivo. Science 219:1329–1331, 1983.

13. Ignotz RA, Massague J: Transforming growth factor-β stimulates the expression of fibronectin and collagen and their incorporation into the extracellular matrix. J Biol Chem 261:4337–4345, 1986.

14. Roberts CJ, Birkenmeier TM, McQuillan JJ, et al: Transforming growth factor-β stimulates the expression of fibronectin and of both subunits of the human fibronectin receptor by cultured human lung fibroblasts. J Biol Chem 263:4586–4592, 1988.

15. Heino J, Ignotz RA, Hemler ME, et al: Regulation of cell adhesion receptors by transforming growth factor-β. J Biol Chem 264:380–388, 1989.

16. Montesano R, Orci L: Transforming growth factor β stimulates collagen-matrix contraction by fibroblasts: Implications for wound healing. Proc Natl Acad Sci USA 85:4894–4897, 1988.

17. Nakagawa S, Pawelek P, Grinnell F: Extracellular matrix organization modulates fibroblast growth and growth factor responsiveness. Exp Cell Res 182:572–582, 1989.

18. Cooper SM, Keyser AJ, Beaulieu AD, et al: Increase in fibronectin in the deep dermis of involved skin in progressive systemic sclerosis. Arthritis Rheum 22:983–987, 1979.

19. Fleischmajer R, Dessau W, Timpl R, et al: Immunofluorescence analysis of collagen, fibronectin, and basement membrane protein in scleroderma skin. J Invest Dermatol 75:270–274, 1980.

20. Kischer CW, Shetlar MR, Chvapil M: Hypertrophic scars and keloids. A review and new concept concerning their origin. Scand Elec Micro 4:1699–1713, 1982.

21. Clark RAF, Dvorak HF, Colvin RB: Fibronectin in delayed-type hypersensitivity skin reactions. Associations with vessel permeability and endothelial cell activation. J Immunol 126:787–793, 1981.

22. Vartio T, Vaheri A, Von Essen R, et al: Fibronectin in synovial fluid and tissue in rheumatoid arthritis. Eur J Clin Invest 11:207–212, 1981.

23. Scott DL, Delamere JP, Walton KW: The distribution of fibronectin in the pannus in rheumatoid arthritis. Br J Exp Pathol 62:362–368, 1981.

24. Hahn E, Wick G, Pencer D, et al: Distribution of basement membrane proteins in normal and fibrotic liver: Collagen type IV, laminin, and fibronectin. Gut 21:63–71, 1980.

25. Kojima N, Isemura M, Yosizawa Z, et al: Distribution of fibronectin in fibrotic human livers at various states. Tohoku J Exp Med 135:403–412, 1981.

26. Biot N, Gindre D, Harf D, et al: Alveolar fibronectin and interstitial lung disease. In Arnold P (ed): Marker Proteins in Inflammation, vol 2. Berlin, Walter de Gruyter, 1984, pp 243–246.

27. Torikata C, Villiger B, Kuhn C III, et al: Ultrastructural distribution of fibronectin in normal and fibrotic human lung. Lab Invest 52:399–408, 1985.

28. Grinnell F: Cellular adhesiveness and extracellular substrata. Internat Rev Cytol 53:65–144, 1978.

29. Grinnell, F: Cell adhesion and spreading factors. In Guroff G (ed): Growth and Maturation Factors. New York, John Wiley & Sons, 1983, pp 454–486.

30. Grinnell F: Fibroblast spreading and phagocytosis: Similar cell responses to different sized substrata. J Cell Physiol 119:58–64, 1984.

31. Izzard CS, Lochner LR: Cell-to-substrate contacts in living fibroblasts: An interference reflexion study with an evaluation of the technique. J Cell Sci 21:129–159, 1976.

32. Heath JP, Dunn GA: Cell to substratum contacts of chick embryo fibroblasts and their relation to the microfilament system. A correlated interference-reflexion and high voltage electron microscopic study. J Cell Sci 29:197–212, 1978.

33. Couchman JR, Rees DA: The behavior of fibroblasts migrating from chick heart explants: Changes in adhesion, locomotion, and growth, and in the distribution of actomyosin and fibronectin. J Cell Sci 39:149–165, 1979.

34. Kolega J, Shure MS, Chen WT: Rapid cellular translocation is related to close contacts formed between various cultured cells and their substrata. J Cell Sci 54:23–34, 1982.

35. Byers HR, White GE, Fujiwara K: Organization and function of stress fibers in cells in vitro and in situ: A review. Cell Musc Motil 5:83–137, 1984.

36. Norton EK, Izzard CS: Fibronectin promotes formation of the close cell-to-substrata contact in cultured cells. Exp Cell Res 139:463–467, 1982.

37. Singer II, Kawka DW, Kazazis DM, et al: The in vivo codistribution of fibronectin and actin fibers in granulation tissue: Immunofluorescence and electron microscopic studies of the fibronexus at the myofibroblast surface. J Cell Biol 98:2091–2106, 1984.

38. Grinnell F, Minter D: Attachment and spreading of baby hamster kidney cells to collagen substrata: Effects of cold-insoluble globulin. Proc Natl Acad Sci USA 75:4408–4412, 1978.

39. Schor SL, Court J: Different mechanisms in the attachment of cells to native and denatured collagen. J Cell Sci 38:267–281, 1979.

40. Linsenmayer TF, Gibney E, Toole BP, et al: Cellular adhesion to collagen. Exp Cell Res 116:470–474, 1978.

41. Kleinman HK, Klebe RJ, Martin GR: Role of collagenous matrices in the adhesion and growth of cells. J Cell Biol 88:473–485, 1981.

42. Yamada KM, Akiyama SK: Cell surface interactions with extracellular materials. Ann Rev Biochem 52:761–799, 1983.

43. Kornblihtt AR, Gutman A: Molecular biology of the extracellular matrix proteins. Biol Rev 63:465–507, 1988.

44. Akiyama SK, Yamada KM: The interaction of plasma fibronectin with fibroblastic cells in suspension. J Biol Chem 260:4492–4500, 1985.

45. McAbee DD, Grinnell F: Fibronectin-mediated binding and phagocytosis of polystyrene latex beads by baby hamster kidney cells. J Cell Biol 97:1515–1523, 1983.

46. Mackie EJ, Halfter W, Liverani D: Induction of tenascin in healing wounds. J Cell Biol 107:2757–2767, 1988.

47. Mackie EJ, Tucker RP, Halfter W, et al: The distribution of tenascin coincides with pathways of neural crest cell migration. Development 102:237–250, 1988.

48. Chiquet-Ehrismann R, Kalla P, Pearson CA, et al: Tenascin interferes with fibronectin action. Cell 53:383–390, 1988.

49. Turley EA: Proteoglycans and cell adhesion. Cancer Metast 3:325–339, 1984.

50. Weigel PH, Fuller GM, LeBoeuf RD: A model for the role of hyaluronic acid and fibrin in the early events during the inflammatory response and wound healing. J Theor Biol 119:219–234, 1986.

51. Toole BP: Developmental role of hyaluronate. Conn Tiss Res 10:93–100, 1982.

52. Hynes RO: Molecular biology of fibronectin. Ann Rev Cell Biol 1:67–90, 1985.

53. Petersen TE, Skorstengaard K, Vibe-Pedersen K: Primary structure of fibronectin. In Mosher D (ed): Fibronectin. New York, Academic Press, 1989, pp 1–24.

54. Yamada KM: Fibronectin domains and receptors, In Mosher D (ed): Fibronectin. New York, Academic Press, 1989, pp 48–122.

55. Pierschbacher MD, Ruoslahti E: Cell attachment activity of fibronectin can be duplicated by small synthetic fragments of the molecule. Nature 309:30–33, 1984.

56. Yamada KM, Kennedy DW: Dualistic nature of adhesive protein function: Fibronectin and its biologically active peptide fragments can autoinhibit fibronectin function. J Cell Biol 99:29–36, 1984.

57. Obara M, Kang MS, Yamada KM: Site-directed mutagenesis of the cell-binding domain of human fibronectin: Separable, synergistic sites mediate adhesive function. Cell 53:649–657, 1988.

58. Ruoslahti E, Pierschbacher MD: Arg-Gly-Asp: A versatile cell recognition signal. Cell 44:517–518, 1986.

59. Akiyama SK, Hasegawa E, Hasegawa T, et al: The interaction of fibronectin fragments with fibroblastic cells. J Biol Chem 260:13256–13260, 1985.

60. Terranova VP, Rao CN, Kalebic T, et al: Laminin receptor on human breast carcinoma cells. Proc Natl Acad Sci 80:444–448, 1983.

61. Malinoff HL, Wicha MS: Isolation of a cell surface receptor protein for laminin from murine fibrosarcoma cells. J Cell Biol 96:1475–1479, 1983.

62. Lesot H, Kuhl U, Von der Mark K: Isolation of a laminin-binding protein from muscle cell membrane. EMBO J 2:861–865, 1983.

63. Neff NT, Lowrey C, Decker C, et al: A monoclonal antibody detaches embryonic skeletal muscle cells from extracellular matrices. J Cell Biol 95:654–666, 1983.

64. Brown PJ, Juliano RL: Selective inhibition of fibronectin-mediated cell adhesion by monoclonal antibodies to a cell surface glycoprotein. Science 228:1448–1451, 1985.

65. Pytela R, Pierschbacher M, Ruoslahti E: Identification and isolation of a 140 kd cell surface glycoprotein with properties expected of a fibronectin receptor. Cell 40:191–198, 1985.

66. Tamkun JW, DeSimone DW, Fonda D, et al: Structure of integrin, a glycoprotein involved in the transmembrane linkage between fibroblasts and actin. Cell 46:271–282, 1986.

67. Argraves WS, Suzuki S, Thompson K, et al: Amino acid sequence of the human fibronectin receptor. J Cell Biol 105:1183–1190, 1987.

68. Hynes RO: Integrins: A family of cell surface receptors. Cell 48:549–554, 1987.

69. Ruoslahti E, Pierschbacher MD: New perspectives in cell adhesion: RGD and integrins. Science 238:491–497, 1987.

70. Plow EF, Pierschbacher MD, Ruoslahti E, et al: The effect of Arg-Gly-Asp–containing peptides on fibrinogen and von Willebrand factor binding to platelets. Proc Natl Acad Sci USA 82:8057–8061, 1985.

71. Horowitz A, Duggan K, Greggs R, et al: The cell substrate attachment (CSAT) antigen has properties of a receptor for laminin and fibronectin. J Cell Biol 101:2134–2144, 1985.

72. Wayner EA, Carter WG, Piotrowicz RS, et al: The function of multiple extracellular matrix receptors in mediating cell adhesion to extracellular matrix. J Cell Biol 107:1881–1891, 1988.

73. Burridge K, Molony L, Kelly T: Adhesion plaques: Sites of transmembrane interaction between the extracellular matrix and the actin cytoskeleton. J Cell Sci 8(Suppl):211–230, 1987.

74. Chen WT, Hasegawa E, Hasegawa T, et al: Development of cell surface linkage complexes in cultured fibroblasts. J Cell Biol 100:1103–1114, 1985.

75. Cody RL, Wicha MS: Clustering of cell surface laminin enhances its association with the cytoskeleton. Exp Cell Res 165:107–116, 1986.

76. Horowitz A, Duggan K, Buck C, et al: Interaction of plasma membrane fibronectin receptor with talin, a transmembrane linkage. Nature 320:531–533, 1986.

77. Oster GF, Perelson AS: The physics of cell motility. J Cell Sci 8(Suppl):35–54, 1987.

78. Knecht DA, Loomis WF: Antisense RNA inactivation of myosin heavy chain gene expression in *Dictyostelium discoideum*. Science 236:1081–1085, 1987.

79. DeLozonne A, Spudich JA: Disruption of the *Dictyostelium* myosin heavy chain gene by homologous recombination. Science 236:1086–1091, 1987.

80. Lark MW, Laterra J, Culp LA: Close and focal adhesions of fibroblasts to a fibronectin-containing matrix. Fed Proc 44:394–403, 1985.

81. Izzard CS, Radinsky R, Culp LA: Substratum contacts and cytoskeletal reorganization of BALB/c 3T3 cells on a cell-binding fragment and heparin-binding fragments of plasma fibronectin. Exp Cell Res 165:320–336, 1986.

82. Woods A, Couchman JR, Johansson S, et al: Adhesion and cytoskeletal organization of fibroblasts in response to fibronectin fragments. EMBO J 5:665–670, 1986.

83. Spiegel S, Yamada KM, Hom BE, et al: Fluorescent gangliosides as probes for the retention and organization of fibronectin by ganglioside-deficient mouse cells. J Cell Biol 100:721–726, 1985.

84. Spiegel S, Yamada KM, Hom BE, et al: Fibrillar organization of fibronectin is expressed coordinately with cell surface gangliosides in a variant murine fibroblast. J Cell Biol 102:1898–1906, 1986.

85. Elsdale TR, Bard JBL: Collagen substrata for studies on cell behavior. J Cell Biol 41:298–311, 1972.

86. Grinnell F, Bennett MH: Fibroblast adhesion on collagen substrata in the presence and absence of plasma fibronectin. J Cell Sci 48:19–34, 1981.

87. Tomasek JJ, Hay ED, Fujiwara K: Collagen modulates cell shape and cytoskeleton of embryonic corneal and fibroma fibroblasts: Distribution of actin, α-actinin, and myosin. Dev Biol 92:107–122, 1982.

88. Bell E, Ivarsson B, Merrill C: Production of a tissue-like structure by contraction of collagen lattices by human fibroblasts of different proliferative potential in vitro. Proc Natl Acad Sci USA 76:1274–1278, 1979.

89. Bellows CG, Melcher AH, Aubin JE: Contraction and

organization of collagen gels by cell cultured from periodontal ligament, gingiva, and bone suggest functional differences between cell types. J Cell Sci 50:299–314, 1981.

90. Grinnell F, Lamke FR: Reorganization of hydrated collagen lattices by human skin fibroblasts. J Cell Sci 66:51–63, 1984.

91. Bellows CG, Melcher AH, Bhargava U, et al: Fibroblasts contracting three-dimensional collagen gels exhibit ultrastructure consistent with either contraction or protein secretion. J Ultrastruct Res 78:178–192, 1982.

92. Ehrlich HP, Wyler DW: Fibroblast contraction of collagen lattices in vitro: Inhibition by chronic inflammatory cell mediators. J Cell Physiol 116:345–351, 1983.

93. Harris AK, Stopak D, Wild P: Fibroblast traction as a mechanism for collagen morphogenesis. Nature 290:249–251, 1981.

94. Guidry C, Grinnell F: Studies on the mechanism of hydrated collagen gel reorganization by human skin fibroblasts. J Cell Sci 79:67–81, 1985.

95. Sarber R, Hull B, Merrill C, et al: Regulation of proliferation of fibroblasts of low and high population doubling levels grown in collagen lattices. Mech Ageing Devel 17:107–117, 1981.

96. Van Bockxmeer FM, Martin CE, Constable IJ: Effect of cyclic AMP on cellular contractility and DNA synthesis in chorioretinal fibroblasts maintained in collagen matrices. Exp Cell Res 155:413–421, 1984.

97. Stenn KS, Madri JA, Tinghitella T, et al: Multiple mechanisms of dissociated epidermal cell spreading. J Cell Biol 96:63–67, 1983.

98. Takashima A, Grinnell F: Human keratinocyte adhesion and phagocytosis promoted by fibronectin. J Invest Dermatol 83:352–358, 1984.

99. O'Keefe EJ, Payne RE, Russell N, et al: Spreading and enhanced motility of human keratinocytes on fibronectin. J Invest Dermatol 85:125–130, 1985.

100. Clark RAF, Folkvord JM, Wertz RL: Fibronectins, as well as other extracellular matrix proteins, mediate human keratinocyte adherence. J Invest Dermatol 84:378–383, 1985.

101. Takashima A, Grinnell F: Fibronectin-mediated keratinocyte migration and initiation of fibronectin receptor function in vitro. J Invest Dermatol 85:304–308, 1985.

102. Woodley DT, Bachmann PM, O'Keefe EJ: Laminin inhibits human keratinocyte migration. J Cell Physiol 136:140–146, 1988.

103. Toda K-I, Grinnell F: Activation of human keratinocyte fibronectin receptor function in relation to other ligand-receptor interactions. J Invest Dermatol 88:412–417, 1987.

104. Wikner NE, Persichitte KA, Baskin JB, et al: Transforming growth factor-β stimulates the expression of fibronectin by human keratinocytes. J Invest Dermatol 91:207–212, 1988.

105. Nickoloff BJ, Mitra RS, Riser BL, et al: Modulation of keratinocyte motility. Am J Pathol 132:543–551, 1988.

106. Takashima A, Billingham RE, Grinnell F: Activation of rabbit keratinocyte fibronectin receptor function in vivo during wound healing. J Invest Dermatol 86:585–590, 1986.

107. Toda K-I, Tuan T-L, Brown PJ, et al: Fibronectin receptors of human keratinocytes and their expression during cell culture. J Cell Biol 105:3097–3104, 1987.

108. Saba TM, Jaffe E: Plasma fibronectin (opsonic glycoprotein): Its synthesis by vascular endothelial cells and role in cardiopulmonary integrity after trauma as related to reticuloendothelial function. Am J Med 68:577–594, 1980.

109. Reese AC, Doran JE, Callaway BD, et al: Sequestration of fibronectin at the site of an injury. Adv Shock Res 8:119–127, 1982.

110. Gauperaa T, Seljelid R: Plasma fibronectin is sequestered into tissue damaged by inflammation and trauma. Acta Chir Scand 152:85–90, 1986.

111. Saba TM, Blumenstock FA, Shah DM, et al: Reversal of opsonic deficiency in surgical, trauma, and burn patients by infusion of purified human plasma fibronectin. Am J Med 80:229–240, 1986.

112. Grossman JE: Plasma fibronectin and fibronectin therapy in sepsis and critical illness. Rev Infect Dis 9:S420–S430, 1987.

113. Hesselvik F, Brodin B, Carlsson C, et al: Cryoprecipitate infusion fails to improve organ function in septic shock. Crit Care Med 15:475–483, 1987.

114. Fernyhough W, Page RC: Attachment, growth and synthesis by human gingival fibroblasts on demineralized or fibronectin-treated normal and diseased tooth roots. J Periodont Res 54:133–140, 1987.

115. Ryan PC, Waring CJ, Seymour GJ: Periodontal healing with citric acid and fibronectin treatment in cats. Aust Dent J 32:99–103, 1987.

116. Nasjleti C, Caffesse RG, Odont D, et al: Effect of fibronectin on healing of replanted teeth in monkeys: A histological and autoradiographic study. Oral Surg Oral Med Oral Pathol 63:291–299, 1987.

117. Caffesse RG, Holden MJ, Kon S, et al: The effect of citric acid and fibronectin application on healing following surgical treatment of naturally occurring periodontal disease in beagle dogs. J Clin Periodontol 12:578–580, 1985.

118. Thompson EW, Seymour GJ, Whyte GJ: The preparation of autologous fibronectin for use in periodontal surgery. Aust Dent J 32:34–38, 1987.

119. Fujikawa LS, Foster S, Harrist TJ, et al: Fibronectin in healing corneal wounds. Lab Invest 45:120–129, 1981.

120. Suda T, Nishida T, Ohashi Y, et al: Fibronectin appears at the site of corneal stromal wound in rabbits. Curr Eye Res 1:553–556, 1981.

121. Fujikawa LS, Foster CS, Gipson IK, et al: Basement membrane components in healing rabbit corneal epithelial wounds: Immunofluorescence and ultrastructural studies. J Cell Biol 98:128–138, 1984.

122. Nishida T, Nakagawa S, Awata T, et al: Fibronectin promotes epithelial migration of cultured rabbit cornea in situ. J Cell Biol 97:1653–1657, 1983.

123. Nishida T, Nakagawa S, Nishibayashi C, et al: Fibronectin enhancement of corneal epithelial wound healing of rabbits in vivo. Arch Ophthalmol 102:455–456, 1984.

124. Spigelman AV, Vernot JA, Deutsch TA: Fibronectin in alkali burns of the rabbit cornea. Cornea 4:169–172, 1985.

125. Nishida T, Ohashi Y, Awata T, et al: Fibronectin: A new therapy for corneal trophic ulcer. Arch Ophthalmol 101:1046–1048, 1983.

126. Nishida T, Nakagawa S, Manabe R: Clinical evaluation of fibronectin eyedrops on epithelial disorders after herpetic keratitis. Ophthalmology 92:213–216, 1985.

127. Kono I, Matsumoto Y, Kano K, et al: Beneficial effect of topical fibronectin in patients with keratoconjunctivitis sicca of Sjögren's syndrome. J Rheumatol 12:487–489, 1985.

128. Spigelman AV, Deutsch TA, Sugar J: Application of homologous fibronectin to persistent human corneal epithelial defects. Cornea 6:128–130, 1987.

129. Berman M, Manseau E, Law M, et al: Ulceration is

correlated with degradation of fibrin and fibronectin at the corneal surface. Invest Ophthalmol Vis Sci 24:1358–1366, 1983.

130. Phan T-M, Foster CS, Boruchoff SA, et al: Topical fibronectin in the treatment of persistent corneal epithelial defects and trophic ulcers. Am J Ophthalmol 104:494–501, 1987.

131. Salonen E-M, Tervo T, Torma E, et al: Plasmin in tear fluid of patients with corneal ulcers: Basis for new therapy. Acta Ophthalmol 65:3–12, 1987.

132. Falcone PA, Bonaventura M, Turner DC, et al: The effect of exogenous fibronectin on wound breaking strength. Plast Reconst Surg 74:809–812, 1984.

133. Litvinov RI, Izmailov SG, Zinkevich OD, et al: Effect of exogenous fibronectin on the healing of skin wounds as measured by tensiometry. Bull Exp Biol Med 12:727–730, 1987.

134. Cheng CY, Martin DE, Leggett CG, et al: Fibronectin enhances healing of excised wounds in rats. Arch Dermatol 124:221–225, 1988.

135. Nagelschmidt M, Becker D, Bonninghoff N, et al: Effect of fibronectin therapy and fibronectin deficiency on wound healing: A study in rats. J Trauma 27:1267–1271, 1987.

136. Pospasilov J, Riebelov V: Fibronectin—Its significance in wound epithelialization. Acta Chir Plast 28:96–102, 1986.

137. Wysocki A, Bergstresser PR, Baxter CR, et al: Topical fibronectin therapy for treatment of a patient with chronic stasis ulcers. Arch Dermatol 124:175–177, 1988.

138. Edwards CA, Piet MPJ, Horowitz B: Tri(n-butyl) phosphate/detergent treatment of licensed therapeutic and experimental blood derivatives. Vox Sang 52:53–59, 1986.

139. Yamada KM, Olden K: Adhesive glycoproteins of cell surface and blood. Nature 275:179–184, 1978.

140. Couchman JR, Hook M, Rees DA, et al: Adhesion, growth, and matrix production by fibroblasts on laminin substrates. J Cell Biol 96:177–183, 1983.

141. Farsi JMA, Sodek J, Aubin JE: Fibronectin-independent attachment of human gingival fibroblasts to in-terstitial and basement membrane collagens. Exp Cell Res 161:473–483, 1985.

142. Knox P, Crooks S, Rimmer CS: Role of fibronectin in the migration of fibroblasts into plasma clots. J Cell Biol 102:2318–2323, 1986.

143. Grinnell F, Feld M, Minter D: Fibroblast adhesion to fibrinogen and fibrin substrata: Requirement for cold-insoluble globulin (plasma fibronectin). Cell 19:517–525, 1980.

144. Barnes D, Wolfe R, Serrero G, et al: Effects of a serum spreading factor on growth and morphology of cells in serum-free medium. J Supramol Struct 14:47–63, 1980.

145. Knox P, Griffiths S: The distribution of cell-spreading activities in sera: A quantitative approach. J Cell Sci 46:97–112, 1980.

146. Tuszynski GP, Rothman V, Murphy A, et al: Thrombospondin promotes cell-substratum attachment. Science 236:1570–1573, 1987.

147. Terranova VP, Rohrbach DH, Martin GR: Role of laminin in the attachment of PAM212 (epithelial) cells to basement membrane collagen. Cell 22:719–726, 1980.

148. Karasek MA, Charlton ME: Growth of postembryonic skin epithelial cells on collagen gels. J Invest Dermatol 56:205–210, 1971.

149. Murray JC, Stingl G, Kleinman HK, et al: Epidermal cells adhere preferentially to type IV basement membrane collagen. J Cell Biol 80:197–202, 1979.

150. Donaldson DJ, Smith GN, Kang AH: Epidermal cell migration on collagen and collagen-derived peptides. J Cell Sci 57:15–23, 1982.

151. Donaldson DJ, Mahan JT: Fibrinogen and fibronectin as substrates for epidermal cell migration during wound closure. J Cell Sci 62:117–127, 1983.

152. Varani J, Dixit VM, Fligiel SEG, et al: Thrombospondin-induced attachment and spreading of human squamous carcinoma cells. Exp Cell Res 167:376–390, 1986.

153. Guo M, Toda KI, Grinnell F: Activation of human keratinocyte migration on type I collagen and fibronectin. J Cell Sci 96:197–205, 1990.

13

ELASTIN REPAIR

Jeffrey M. Davidson, Ph.D, M. Gabriella Giro, Ph.D,
and Daniela Quaglino, Jr., Ph.D.

An authoritative book on wound healing, published only seven years ago, devoted but three pages to the subject of repair of elastic tissue,[1] in part reflecting the rather poor state of knowledge of the protein and its biology at that time. Nevertheless, Dr. Peacock's review included the few examples of authentic repair of elastic tissue. As this chapter hopes to convey, much has been learned about this unique protein in the intervening years, including its complete primary structure as deduced from molecular cloning of elastin mRNA and the elastin gene. Several recent comprehensive reviews cover much of what has been learned about the basic chemistry and biology of the elastic fiber in general and elastin in particular,[2-5] and this chapter summarizes those findings. The major goal of this chapter is to emphasize the areas of incomplete knowledge of elastin biology that have an impact on wound repair.

CHEMISTRY AND BIOLOGY OF ELASTIC FIBERS

Elastin is the most insoluble protein in the vertebrate body. It is readily purified to near homogeneity by exhaustive extraction of any elastin-containing tissue with 0.1 N NaOH at 98°C[6] or by a combination of proteolysis of collagen with purified collagenase followed by guanidinium hydrochloride extraction under reducing conditions. Although elastin is often codistributed with collagen in connective tissue and its amino acid composition is somewhat similar, it is a completely distinct protein in

terms of primary structure and function. The elastic fiber functions as a nearly perfect rubber material in an aqueous environment, depending upon hydrophobic interactions for the bulk of its elasticity, and its only known physiological role is to provide elastic recoil in a variety of tissues. Elastic fibers, as they are visualized with the electron microscope (Fig. 13–1), are actually composed of two substances: (1) amorphous elastin, an electron-lucent component of the extracellular matrix of many tissues including skin, blood vessels, several specialized ligaments, and the interstitium of the lung, and (2) the elastic fiber microfibril, usually associated with elastin and more prominent during fibrillogenesis and whose structure and composition are clearly distinct from that of elastin.

Protein Structure and Function

The amino acid composition of elastin is distinctive (Table 13–1), regardless of the method of purification. Insoluble elastin from all species of warm-blooded vertebrates lacks methionine, histidine, and tryptophan, and cysteine is present at only 2 to 3 residues per molecule. Although secreted through usual pathways for matrix proteins, elastin is not known to be glycosylated. The most distinctive feature of the protein at the compositional level is the presence of two heterocylic crosslinks, desmosine and isodesmosine (Fig. 13–2), which are formed by the condensation of three oxidatively deaminated lysyl residues with a fourth ε-amino group of lysine to produce a stable condensation product that is resistant to acid hydrolysis and

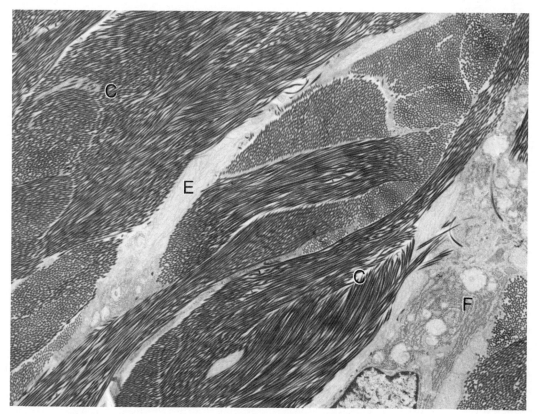

Figure 13–1. Normal arrangement of collagen (C) and elastic fibers (E) in rat skin. Elastin takes up conventional electron-dense stains poorly, and this specimen has been postfixed with tannic acid to improve contrast. Fine microfibrils can be seen coursing through the amorphous material ($\times$6500). F = fibroblast.

reduction. In general, the desmosine-isodesmosine content of a tissue can be converted to its elastin (desmosines $\approx$1.5 percent of elastin); however, this is probably not the case for tissues undergoing rapid synthesis or remodeling of newly formed elastin, as discussed later.

Based on sequence analysis of tryptic peptides of the biosynthetic precursor (discussed further on), Gray, Foster, and Sandberg proposed that elastin functions as an elastomer because of two domains in the protein: rigid α-helical regions with the typical sequence AAKAAAK(A/Y) and flexible hydrophobic repeat units, the prototypical sequence being a polypentapeptide $(PGVGV)_n$.[7] Pairing of the lysyl residues from adjacent chains provides the desmosine formation sites, and the extended sequences of small, hydrophobic amino acids give elasticity by their tendency to condense to reduce the number of contacts with water. The biophysical interpretation of elastic mechanisms in this protein are still in dispute. There are arguments in favor of a purely random arrangement of polypeptide chains in the folded protein[8–10] based on the physical behavior of purified elastin and its lack of regular structure

as revealed by x-ray diffraction and other physical methods. A second interpretation, based on studies of synthetic homopolymers, predicts a β-spiral conformation in which a series of β-turn elements are stabilized into a vibrating, coil-like structure.[11] Although highly polymerized elastin gives no evidence of ordered structure in its relaxed state, alignment of fibrils or chains occurs on stretching, and crossbanded intermediates have been reported.[12]

Biosynthesis of Elastin

Elastin is secreted from cells as a soluble precursor, tropoelastin (64,000 to 72,000 Da depending on species). The intracellular aspects of tropoelastin synthesis are not remarkable (hydroxylation excepted), but there are polymorphisms of the protein due to alternative splicing.[13–15] Assembly of tropoelastin may be driven in part by hydrophobic interactions. Upon warming in physiological solutions, tropoelastin and solubilized elastin peptides spontaneously coacervate into aggregates. Crosslinking is retarded below the temperature (15°C) at

Table 13–1. AMINO ACID COMPOSITION OF SOLUBLE (TROPOELASTIN) AND MATURE (INSOLUBLE) ELASTIN FROM THE PIG* BASED ON AMINO ACID ANALYSIS

Amino Acid	Soluble Elastin	Mature Elastin
	Number of Residues†	
Glycine	245	256
Alanine	187	181
Proline	91	90
Hydroxyproline	7	8
Valine	103	92
Isoleucine	14	14
Leucine	41	41
Tyrosine	14	12
Phenylalanine	24	25
Arginine	4	5
Lysine	37	5‡
Desmosines§	Very low	3
Aspartic acid and asparagine	3	5
Threonine	10	11
Serine	8	11
Glutamic acid and glutamine	12	16
Cysteine	2	2
Methionine, tryptophan, and histidine	0–1	1

*Human elastin has a similar composition.

†Based on an assumed chain length of 800 residues; conceptual translation of human elastin cDNA yields up to 768 residues, but composition will vary depending upon alternate splicing (see reference 31).

‡Seven lysine residues are unaccounted for in mature elastin (see footnote below).

§Lysine equivalents would be 12; if intermediates are included, the lysine equivalents total 25.

which the coacervation process occurs. Tropoelastin can be purified by organic solvent extraction, emphasizing its extreme hydrophobicity. Under normal circumstances, tropoelastin is rapidly assembled into insoluble elastic fibers followed by the oxidative deamination of lysyl residues. Crosslinking can be inhibited by lathyritic agents (β-aminopropionitrile or α-aminoacetonitrile) or dietary copper deficiency, both of which inhibit action of the metalloenzyme lysyl oxidase. Although there are 12 to 13 potential crosslink sites in each tropoelastin molecule, only 1 to 2 lysine tetrads form the mature desmosine crosslinks.

The other morphological element of the elastic fiber, at least during growth and development, is the microfibril.[16] This structure has also been identified, apparently independent of elastin, in structures such as the vitreous humor[17] and the ciliary zonule of the eye.[18] Several laboratories have identified cysteine-rich glycoproteins of varying molecular weights[19–22] that are likely to represent one or more components of the microfibril. Greenlee and co-workers proposed on morphological grounds that microfibrils provide a framework upon which elastin condenses to form elastic fibers.[23] Workers in the field have not yet been able to demonstrate a specific biochemical interaction between the two moieties, but antibodies to microfibrillar proteins (MFPs) localize to elastic fibers in a variety of locations. Little information is available on the biosynthesis of MFP or the primary structure of the protein components.

One perplexing aspect of elastin synthesis is the role of prolyl hydroxylation. Elastin has a low (about 10 residues per molecule) but significant level of hydroxyproline, reflecting the presence of suitable hydroxylation sites recognized by the enzyme prolyl hydroxylase. Unlike collagen, this modification serves no known function in elastin. Mammalian elastin is totally resistant to bacterial collagenase, but the avian protein appears to contain some (Gly-X-Y) peptide triplets recognized by the protease. There is no evidence for triple helicity in any elastin. Indeed, inhibition of prolyl hydroxylation by ascorbate deficiency or hypoxia has no effect on elastin production.[24, 25] Conversely, excessive ascorbate, usually used to promote maximal collagen synthesis in cell culture, dramatically reduces elastin accumulation[26, 27] into extracellular matrix and inhibits tropoelastin production as well as reducing steady-state levels of elastin mRNA.[28] These findings imply that conditions favoring collagen accumulation may oppose formation of functional elastin fibers.

The elastin genes[29, 30] and mRNAs[13–15, 31, 32] have been cloned, permitting a determination of elastin primary structure. In all species examined, the protein consists of an alternating series of hydrophobic and crosslink domains. Within the gene, these domains are widely separated by intervening sequences into separate exon structures, suggesting a selective pressure to reduce intradomain recombination events. A small amount of cysteine has been detected in biosynthetic experiments,[33] and DNA sequence analysis established that these two cysteinyl residues are part of a small, hydrophilic COOH-terminal tail.[34] This heretofore undetected region of the molecule could potentially be involved in either interactions among tropoelastin monomers in early phases of fiber assembly or interactions between tropoelastin and the MFP components.

Protein polymorphism (i.e., multiple sizes) of tropoelastin[35] appears to result from alternate splicing of the transcript from a single gene.[13–15] There is some evidence for selective expression of tropoelastin isoforms in development,[36] but no function can yet be assigned to

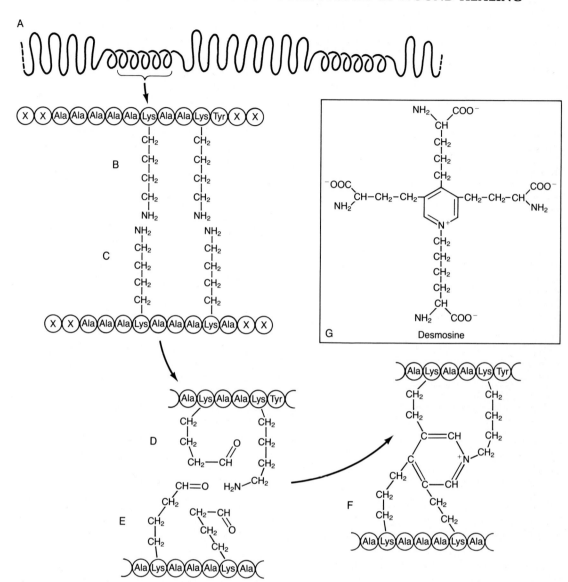

Figure 13–2. Details of the formation of the desmosine crosslink during the formation of insoluble elastin from tropoelastin. *B* and *C* show the apposition of two crosslinking sites on different chains with the probable positions of the lysine side chains before the oxidative removal of the ε-amino groups. In *B*, two alanine residues separate the two lysine residues and a tyrosine follows the second lysine. In *C*, there are three alanine residues between the lysines. In *D* and *E*, aldehydes have replaced three of the four ε-amino groups of the lysine side chains. The chains are folded to indicate their probable contribution to the desmosine ring structure. In *F*, the pyridinium ring of desmosine has been formed with its resonating double bonds. *G* shows a desmosine molecule free from the peptide linkages to the elastin chains. With isodesmosine, the lysine-derived side chain opposite the nitrogen (para) is moved to the ortho position. (From Sandberg LB, Soskel NT, Leslie JG: Elastin structure, biosynthesis, and relation to disease states. Reprinted by permission of the New England Journal of Medicine, Vol. 304, page 566, 1981.)

these numerous alternate forms. An alternative hypothesis is that multiple forms of the protein may favor a random arrangement of chains within the forming elastin polymer.

Elastin-Associated Components

As mentioned previously, the elastic fiber consists of several components. In the dermis, for example, there is a varying proportion of elastin and MFP, amorphous elastin being predominant in the deeper reticular dermis and microfibrils becoming more prominent in the papillary dermis in structures termed elaunin and oxytalan fibers. In solar elastosis and aging of dermis, these fine elastic fibers of the upper dermis are degraded and subsequently displaced by elastotic material derived from the reticular dermis. Proteoglycans are also associated with elastic fibers, although their abundance usually indicates pathology. One would not expect there to be any direct interaction between the highly anionic hydrophilic glycosaminoglycan side chains and the hydrophobic elastin core. In cases in which lysyl oxidation is inhibited, numerous ϵ-amino groups in tropoelastin could remain available for electrostatic interaction, and accumulation of proteoglycan has been observed in both experimental lathyrism[37] and copper deficiency.[38, 39]

Distribution of Elastin During Growth and Development

Elastin and elastic fibers appear relatively late in the course of connective tissue development. In the dermis, elastic fibers are not apparent until week 20 to 22 of gestation,[40] long after most other cutaneous structures have appeared. In the lung, elastin synthesis does not become prominent until the process of alveolarization is complete (during the perinatal period in large mammals).[41] In blood vessels, elastin begins to accumulate in conjunction with increased cardiovascular flow and pressure, but deposition of new elastic lamellae continues well into the postnatal phase, the region of its maximal rate of accumulation gradually shifting from the heart to more distal parts of the circulatory system.[42] In humans, the richest source of elastic fibers is the thoracic aorta, but elastin plays a critical functional role in the pulmonary interstitium, peripheral arterioles, skin, vocal cords, and the pregnant uterus. A specialized elastic ligament, the ligamentum nuchae, has evolved into a massive tendinous structure in grazing animals to counterbalance the head and neck of these creatures. Humans retain only a vestigial form of this structure. Elastin content approaches 80 percent of total protein in elastic ligaments.

The majority of elastin is accumulated by the end of juvenile growth, and the protein is remarkably stable thereafter. Estimates of turnover in the rat and human are equal to or greater than the lifespan of the individual.[43, 44] Thus in healthy individuals, the bulk of elastin at various sites is a permanent entity. As discussed below, elastin destruction and resynthesis can occur as a result of a variety of injuries. Nevertheless, it has evolved into a nearly indestructible protein. The major exception regarding lack of elastin turnover is in the uterine wall, where pregnancy initiates a rapid accumulation of both vascular and interstitial elastin, which is then rapidly resorbed at birth.

Cellular Sources of Elastin

Mesenchymal cells are the principal source of elastin. Both vascular smooth muscle cells[45–48] and nuchal ligament fibroblasts[49, 50] have been clearly identified as sources of the protein from cell culture studies. Studies from this laboratory have shown that dermal fibroblasts also produce significant amounts of elastin in culture.[51] That the former cells produce elastin is expected, since they are isolated from tissues undergoing rapid accumulation of elastin (>40 percent of mRNA in neonatal nuchal ligament codes for elastin),[52] but neosynthesis of elastin in dermis is rarely evident in the absence of injury. The stable expression of elastin by skin cells is likely to reflect the woundlike environment of the cell culture system (i.e., lack of a three-dimensional extracellular matrix, presence of platelet degranulation products, and absence of other cell types such as epidermal cells).

The stability of elastin expression in vitro is problematic. Although ligamentum nuchae cells from the fetus can express or be induced to express high levels of elastin, and vascular smooth muscle cells initially reflect the relative expression of elastin found in situ, these cells rapidly dedifferentiate in vitro; i.e., they lose the ability to synthesize elastin after 2 to 3 subcultivations.[48, 49] Dermal fibroblasts are much more stable with respect to elastin expression, although they exhibit an in vitro aging phenomenon at about 30 population doublings.[51] Skin cells from aged skin have a reduced capacity for elastin synthesis,[51] and several cutaneous elastin disorders can be diagnosed in cultured cells.[53–55]

Elastin is also synthesized by certain epithelial cells. Pleural mesothelium shows this capacity, which could be relevant to the restoration of pleural integrity after injury.[56] Aortic endothelial cells also produce elastin, at least in vitro,[57] possibly indicating a role in the synthesis or repair of the internal elastic lamina of muscular arteries.

Turnover of Elastic Tissue: Elastin Degradation

Since elastin is replaced extremely slowly under normal conditions,[43, 44] and since resynthesis is often delayed relative to other regenerative processes, degradation of elastic tissue can produce irreversible damage. The most clinically important aspect of elastin destruction is in pulmonary emphysema, where loss of interstitial elastin leads to irreversible loss of lung function. Although resynthesis of elastin occurs in models of lung injury and elastin content of emphysematous lungs is near normal, the sites of elastin deposition are not appropriate to lung function; i.e., new alveolar septae are not regenerated.[58]

Loss or fragmentation of elastic fibers is also characteristic of aging skin, cystic medial necrosis of large vessels, and a number of cutaneous diseases. Elastin is degraded by enzymes operationally termed elastases. This is a generic term, since all enzymes that can degrade elastin show a broad range of substrates. Elastases can be of either the serine or metalloprotease class.[59, 60] Best characterized are the serine elastases from the neutrophil and the two related enzymes (elastase I and II) from the pancreas. Both have the ability to cleave large and small substrates COOH-terminal to hydrophobic residues, and they are physiologically inhibited by the serum protein α_1-antiprotease. Metalloenzymes with the capacity to degrade elastin are produced by a variety of mesenchymal cells (smooth muscle, skin fibroblast), and mononuclear cells, and at least a portion of these activities are associated with the cell surface. Inhibitors of metalloenzymes are likely to be either α_2-macroglobulin or the tissue inhibitor of metalloproteinase (TIMP), but this is not clearly established.

Under normal circumstances, elastin degradation occurs very slowly, as estimated from desmosine excretion rates. However, in experimental lung injury or pulmonary hypertension there is evidence for increased elastin turnover expressed as either urinary desmosine or elastin peptides present in lavage fluid, pulmonary lymph drainage, or plasma.[61] Interestingly, such injuries do not necessarily result in a net loss of elastin. Studies in the lung show that elastin is redistributed by neosynthesis to other lung structures. What is evident is loss of functional elasticity because of inappropriate fiber distribution.[62] This theme is evident in dermal injury by ultraviolet irradiation, as discussed previously.

Three factors assure the longevity of elastic fibers: (1) the protein is extremely hydrophobic so that the interior of the fiber is rather inaccessible to the usual mechanisms of protein destruction or remodeling; (2) only a limited number of proteases can degrade the unusual primary structure of elastin; and (3) elastin exists in vivo as an extensively crosslinked three-dimensional polymer, and cleavage of individual segments between crosslinks must reach a very high level before functional loss of elastic behavior occurs. In contrast to elastin, tropoelastin is highly susceptible to proteolysis. It is possible that substantial turnover of tropoelastin occurs during the development of elastic fibers, but a distinctive marker for tropoelastin degradation (as opposed to desmosines as markers of mature elastin degradation) is lacking. A distinct marker peptide, PGVGV, is released from elastin or tropoelastin by thermolysin digestion.[63] It is conceivable that this property could be used to diagnose tropoelastin degradation independent of the crosslinking process.

Regulation of Elastin Accumulation

This topic has been dealt with in a number of recent reviews;[2, 64, 65] however, recent findings may shed more light on the control of elastin deposition during wound repair. The predominant systems used for studying regulation of elastin accumulation have been elastic tissues: lung, aorta, and nuchal ligament. Rates of synthesis of elastin are largely governed by steady-state levels of elastin mRNA. In ligament in particular, production of elastin continues at high levels in cell cultures explanted from the tissue, suggesting that there are either endogenous factors or persistent nuclear changes that favor the expression of the elastin gene. Vascular smooth muscle cells from the aorta produce high levels initially, but rapidly dedifferentiate into a nonelastogenic phenotype. Possible causes for this change are manifold: the loss of a surrounding extracellular matrix, the absence of pulsatile mechanical forces, or the removal of soluble factors present in interstitial fluid that support or promote elastogenesis during elastic tissue development. Skin fibroblasts readily produce elastin when grown under standard culture conditions; whether this is due to an intrinsically high capacity to express elastin, which is normally suppressed in situ, or an unusually sensitive response to the conditions of standard cell culture is not known.

A number of mediators have been shown to be involved in enhancing elastin expression, at least in cell culture. Injury brings about a complex pattern of expression of these mediators, undoubtedly altering elastin expression at some time during the repair process. Glucocorticoids stimulate fetal tissues to produce elastin[66, 67] but reduce its production in cells from adult skin.[68] Insulin-like growth factor-1 has elastogenic properties,[69] and an elastogenic factor has also been reported to be present in culture supernatant from hypertensive smooth muscle cells of the pulmonary artery.[70] Growth factors (or cytokines) are found in the circulation, attached to matrix macromolecules, released by mononuclear cells and platelets, and also endogenously produced by resident tissue cells. Our laboratory has recently found that transforming growth factor-β has very potent elastogenic properties,[71] increasing elastin production four to fivefold in vascular smooth muscle cells and skin fibroblasts.[72] Interestingly, these effects are antagonized by another potent growth factor: basic fibroblast growth factor.[73] One of the elements that could determine the efficiency of elastin replacement in a variety of injured tissues is the balance between these various hormonal influences.

The oxidative environment of the elastin-synthesizing cell may also have a role in regulating repair of elastic tissue. Hydroxyproline is normally present at low concentrations in elastin, but its role is uncertain since inhibitors of prolyl hydroxylation have no effect on elastin accumulation.[24, 25] On the other hand, ascorbic acid, a requirement for efficient hydroxylation of collagen chains and their helical stability, actually reduces the accumulation, synthesis, and even gene expression of elastic tissues in vascular smooth muscle cell cultures.[27, 28] It is presumed that the defects in accumulation result from production of an overhydroxylated form of tropoelastin that is less hydrophobic and fails to crosslink properly. Defects in synthesis could be the result of altered intracellular conformation of the protein, leading to reduced secretion and a form of feedback regulation that specifically represses elastin gene expression.[74] It is conceivable that highly vascularized sites of tissue repair possess an oxygen tension that is unfavorable to elastin accumulation, and hyperoxic conditions would be potentially inhibitory to effective repair of elastic tissue.

REPAIR OF ELASTIC TISSUE

There is scant literature describing the repair of elastic tissue, but replacement of elastic fibers is documented to occur after a variety of traumatic injuries. Compared to that of other matrix components, the rate of elastin accumulation is very slow, probably leading to the conclusion that there is no elastin in scar tissue.

Elastic Ligaments

The best evidence for elastic tissue repair has been presented by Bhangoo and Church[75] from a study of transected elastic ligaments in bat wings. Cut fibers initially retracted from the wound, and there was a gradual regrowth of new, smaller fibers within the wound site beginning after 4 weeks and finally spanning the original gap at the end of 10 to 12 weeks. The authors concluded that mechanical stress was not a factor in the induction of elastogenesis, since immobilized wings appeared to regenerate elastic fibers in the correct orientation. This paper also provides a good review of the earlier literature, which tended to dismiss elastic fiber repair, at least in cutaneous wounds.

The ligamentum nuchae of many large animals represents the largest and most specialized elastic tissue. Running from the vertebral processes to the base of the skull, it provides a resilient mechanical support for the head. An experimental study by Mills and associates provides clear evidence of elastic tissue regeneration. Ligaments were partially transected in dogs, with repair followed by morphological and other ultrastructural observations out to 52 weeks postsurgery.[76] These studies emphasized the slow rate of replacement of elastic tissue: by light microscopy, fibers were not seen until 14 weeks postinjury and were much finer than those of the surrounding, mature ligament. This phenomenon was preceded by an apparently typical granulation phase with deposition of fine collagen fibrils at 8 weeks and a dense meshwork of collagen by 10 weeks. The diameter and number of newly formed elastic fibers increased very gradually, being 50 percent of normal at 30 weeks and little increased after 52 weeks. Thus replacement of elastin was somewhat incomplete. Functional aspects were not discussed, but the authors felt that mechanical forces did not play an intrinsic role in the development of new ligament elastic tissue.

At the cellular level, fibroblasts were identified as the principal source of new elastic fibers. Regeneration appeared to recapitulate fetal elastogenesis, in that microfibrils preceded amorphous elastin in the developing fibers. Elastin-producing cells were not distinguished from those producing collagen; that is, there was no evidence for an "elastoblast" in this elastin-rich tissue.

Cutaneous Elastic Tissue Repair

The early literature on skin wounds and elastin appears to be biased toward the absence of this structure from granulation or scar tissue. As reviewed by Bhangoo and Church,[75] numerous studies had failed to identify elastic fibers in scars,[77] healed ulcers in the rabbit,[78] rat skin wounds,[79] rat granulation tissue,[80] or mouse skin.

Comprehensive studies by both Levenson and colleagues[81] and Van Winkle[82] concluded that elastin is markedly absent from skin wounds, consistent with the relative rigidity or inflexibility of scar tissue. These conclusions notwithstanding, a study by Schwartz[83] provides ample evidence of elastogenesis in healing skin wounds of rats and mice as early as 1 week postwounding, appearing first in the deeper portions of the wound site and in the regenerating dermis by 20 days. Fiber abundance appeared to be elevated above normal for at least 4 months, the number of fibers gradually diminishing but fiber diameter showing an increase. Elastic fibers were detected with several conventional stains as well as with toluidine blue and azure B in epoxy (Epon) embedded material. Electron microscopy confirmed the identity of the elastic fiber components and suggested that condensation of elastin often occurred on a previously secreted framework of microfibrillar components. The cells producing elastic fibers did not appear to have any unique features but became increasingly attenuated by the third month after injury. It is surprising that a number of previous studies had not identified repair of dermal elastic fibers. It should be noted that it took at least 3 weeks to observe dermal elastic tissue, and other studies may have preferentially focused on either earlier time points or deposition of collagen. This cited study suggests that elastin, at least in rodent skin, could play a significant role in dermal wound healing.

Our recent studies on the influence of TGF-β on wound repair have shown clear evidence of elastogenesis and elastin gene expression in wound sites of both pig and rat skin. Figure 13–3 shows the ultrastructural appearance of small elastic fibers in incisional granulation tissue of rat skin. Elastin gene expression has been visualized by in situ hybridization in several types of wounds: excisional pig dermal wounds,[84] incisional porcine wounds,[85] and rat granulation tissue (Fig. 13–4). These findings emphasize the fact that elastin expression occurs relatively early in the repair process (by 1 week) and that elastin expression is markedly enhanced by the topical administration or local injection of TGF-β. Studies in porcine skin[84] suggest that only a limited subset of dermal fibroblasts, found in the deeper, reticular dermis, have a high capacity for elastin expression. This observation contrasts with findings from similar in situ hybridization analysis of cultured fibroblasts, in which more homogeneous expression of elastin and other matrix macromolecules was observed.[86]

Two further morphological studies on the appearance of elastin in human cutaneous scar tissue put to rest the belief that elastin is absent in healed skin, although these studies do not show the formation of the typical, presumably more functional, elastic fibers. Both normal and hypertrophic dermal scars demonstrate the formation of very fine elastic fibrils, intermingled with abundant collagen, according to Tsuji and Sawabe.[87] Elastin was definitively identified by transmission electron microscopy and was found to be notably less abundant in hypertrophic scar specimens. As in the studies with rodent skin, elastic fibers were more prominent in the deeper (reticular) parts of scar tissue. These investigators found that a conventional stain for elastin, such as Weigert's resorcein-fuchsin, poorly revealed these new elastic fibers, and they suggested improved detection with a method developed by Humberstone and Humberstone.[88] In another study of elastin in scars, Bhangoo and associates[89] reported the evolution of fine elastic fibers. Scanning electron microscopy of autoclave-insoluble matrix (i.e., partially purified elastin) also revealed finely arranged elastic fibers in the deeper dermis of atrophic and hypertrophic scar tissue.

These studies did not indicate the biochemical concentration of elastin in normal versus scar tissue, and there has been no evidence that the fine meshworks that appear in human scar tissue would perform their biomechanical role in the same way as undisturbed dermal matrix.

Repair of Lung Elastic Tissue

Although pulmonary connective tissue is not commonly subjected to traumatic injury, chronic or acute inflammation can have an adverse effect on lung elastin. Elastic fibers serve important functions not only in the afferent vascular circulation but also as part of the bron-

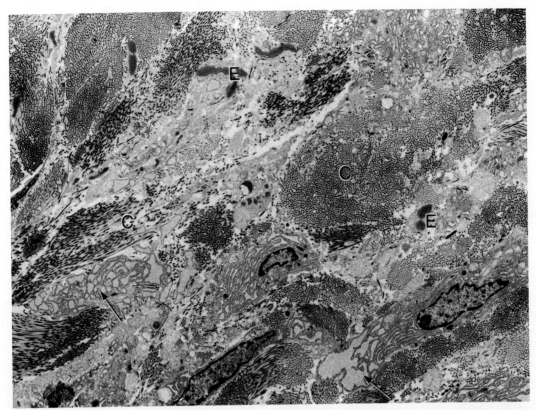

Figure 13–3. Electron micrograph of granulation tissue in the incisional wound of a rat at 7 days after injury. To enhance the expression of matrix proteins, this wound was treated with 2 μg of recombinant TGF-β1 3 days after injury. This treatment enhanced fibroplasia and the appearance of elastin. Under these conditions, small elastic fibers (E) can be seen in several parts of the section. Arrows indicate swollen endoplasmic reticulum of activated fibroblasts in granulation tissue (× 6500). C = collagen.

chial and bronchiolar walls, the alveolar walls, and the pleura. Alveolar elastin destruction, usually attributed to an imbalance between (neutrophil) elastase elaboration and the action of α_1-antiprotease (α_1-antitrypsin), manifests as pulmonary emphysema, an important clinical entity. Traumatic or inflammatory injuries may bring about destruction of the other elastic elements of the lung.[58, 61]

Models of emphysema have used instillation of papain[90] or elastase[91] to produce acute lung injury and follow the course of elastic tissue repair. Interstitial elastin is rapidly destroyed in these models, leading to loss of pulmonary function. Destruction of elastin has been quantitatively monitored by urinary excretion of desmosine and isodesmosine,[92] and our laboratory has found a correlation between lung destruction and the appearance of elastin peptides in lavage fluid, circulating plasma, and urine.[93] Although lung function is reportedly not recovered in experimental models of emphysema, elastin content of injured lungs returned within about 6 weeks. Emphysematous lungs in humans do not have reduced elastin content,

suggesting that despite the capacity for compensatory elastin accumulation, the alveolar units themselves cannot be regenerated (by an appropriate developmental sequence) during adult life.

Williams has provided a detailed description of the pleural response to injury.[94, 95] In guinea pig pleura subjected to burn, repair was followed in both pleura and overlying thoracic wall for 84 days. The thermal injury appeared to produce a fairly deep area of necrosis in the lung parenchyma, which was rapidly replaced by granulation tissue. The role of mesothelial cells, now known to produce elastin,[96] was not addressed in this study. The author divided the repair process into 3 phases: (1) granulation tissue maturation up to 28 days; (2) collagen accumulation by synthetically active, endoplasmic reticulum–filled fibroblasts during the period between 28 and 58 days; and (3) attenuation of fibroblast cytoplasm, appearance of secretory vacuoles ("acanthosomes"), and elaboration of elastic fibers composed of peripheral microfibrils and central amorphous elastin during the last period of observation (56–84 days).

ELASTIN

CONTROL   TGF−β

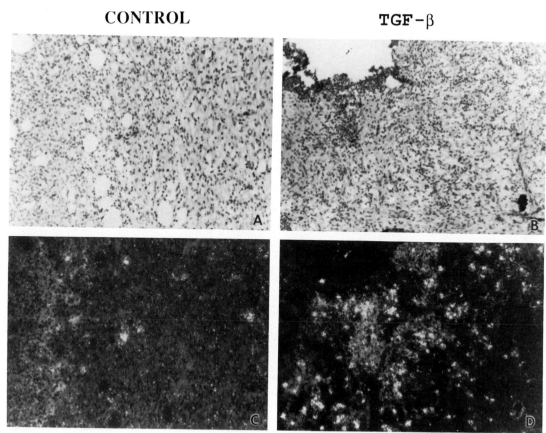

Figure 13–4. In situ hybridization of rat granulation tissue to detect elastin gene expression: enhancement by TGF-β1 treatment. Experimental granulation tissue was produced by the subcutaneous implantation of polyvinyl alcohol sponges in Sprague-Dawley rats, with some receiving a single injection of recombinant TGF-β1 (2 μg) on day 3 after implantation. On day 7, animals were euthanized, and sponges were fixed in paraformaldehyde in preparation for in situ hybridization with an elastin genomic DNA probe corresponding to the 3′ untranslated region of elastin mRNA. Upper panels show hematoxylin and eosin staining patterns of control (A) and treated (B) sponges, while lower panels (C and D) are darkfield photomicrographs of the hybridization results. While elastin expression is present in a few cells of the control, TGF-β1 markedly enhanced the number and intensity of cells expressing elastin mRNA. This finding is also consistent with the ultrastructural evidence of elastin deposition shown in Figure 13–3.

A similar sequence of events was found in the overlying incisional wounds. Elastic fiber accumulation occurred late in the repair process. New elastin consisted of fine fibers detected with the Victoria Blue stain,[88] and elastin appeared to be associated with cells having attenuated cytoplasm ("fibrocytes") rather than the more robust cell form associated with collagen production. Functionality of elastic fibers was not assessed.

Vascular Elastin Repair

In contrast to all the preceding examples, the arterial wall shows rapid elaboration of new elastin and elastic lamellae after many types of injury, including ligation,[97] surgery,[98, 99] and grafting[100–103] of arterial segments. Not all arterial injuries lead to elastin accumulation, however.[104] It appears that the so-called arterialization of venous grafts (of the coronary artery) is a clear example of the stress-induced formation of new elastin in vessel walls.[105] Hypertension can be characterized as a form of vascular injury,[106] and atherosclerosis appears to be a pathological response to intimal damage.[107] Both of these pathologies are accompanied by accumulation of elastin, leading to impaired vascular function through increased vessel wall stiffness, luminal stenosis, or occlusion.

Several authors have speculated on the basis for the relatively strong elastogenic response of vascular tissue, the pulsatile forces in the arterial wall being one likely explanation. This possibility has been explored by a number of investigators.[108–110] It is also likely that the vascular smooth muscle cell phenotype is predisposed to elastin production. Vascular smooth muscle cells in conventional, static cell culture show initially high levels of elastin production, from 20,000 to 60,000 molecules per cell per hour. Vascular smooth muscle cells rapidly lose their capacity to express elastin in cell culture, perhaps reflecting the vastly different mechanical or biochemical environments they encounter in monolayers on a culture dish. Only rat smooth muscle cells continue to grow in an aortalike fashion in vitro.[25, 101] Static stress on smooth muscle cells can increase elastin production;[111] however, dynamic models may be more relevant to vascular development, response to injury, and medial hypertrophy in hypertension.

Other Elastogenic Responses to Injury

Elastogenic responses in a variety of tissues can also involve the excessive accumulation of elastic fibers (elastosis). The most obvious and prevalent form of pathological elastogenesis is actinic elastosis, the response of dermis to chronic ultraviolet exposure. The condition is characterized by destruction or fragmentation of the fine elastic fibers in the papillary dermis accompanied by excessive accumulation of large, distorted elastic fibers in the deeper reticular dermis. Elastosis is also a characteristic of several kinds of cirrhotic liver disease, seen as trace periportal accumulations of new elastin. The cellular source of elastin in fibrotic liver disease is not known. Certain tumors are associated with a desmoplastic response in surrounding, apparently normal, connective tissue. In particular, some, but not all, breast tumors are characterized by the periductal deposition of elastic fibers, suggesting that soluble mediators from the tumor cells elicit a response in normal tissue. Whether this is a defensive reaction to wall off the tumor or actually provides the tumor with a selective advantage is unsettled. Evidence from our laboratory suggests that transforming growth factor-β could act as an intercellular signal in many of these elastoses, since this molecule can increase elastin production as much as fourfold in culture fibroblasts and smooth muscle.[71] The fact that other desmoplastic responses do not necessarily involve elastin suggests that something of the "seed and soil" concept works here as well: only certain types of tissues can mount an elastogenic response to injury or tumor invasion.

CONCLUSION

Repair of elastic tissue is not widely recognized, but many examples of the resynthesis and accumulation of new elastic fibers populate the literature. Not all neosynthesis of elastin produces new functional elastic tissue, and elastic fibers are often among the last structures to reappear morphologically at sites of injury. In the several cases in which elastin has been reported to be absent during the repair process, one must consider whether the investigation was of sufficient duration to detect the late appearance of elastic fibers. Possibly the biomechanical properties of repairing tissue injuries place elastin deposition at a low priority, the exception being the blood vessel wall.

There is still considerable uncertainty over the precise composition of the elastic fiber, and clues to its organization may depend on the more thorough characterization of the nonelastin components of the system. Since destruction of elastin is a complication not only of mechanical trauma but also of acute and chronic inflammation, ultraviolet irradiation, and the "aging process," factors that regulate or enhance the appropriate deposition of functional elastic fibers in connective tissue could play an important role in medicine and surgery.

References

1. Peacock EE: Wound Repair, 3rd ed. Philadelphia, WB Saunders, 1984, pp 97–99.
2. Davidson JM, Giro MB: Control of elastin synthesis: Molecular and cellular aspects. In Mecham RP (ed): Regulation of Matrix Accumulation. New York, Academic Press, 1986, pp 177–216.
3. Franzblau C, Faris B: Elastin. In Hay ED (ed): Cell Biology of Extracellular Matrix. New York, Plenum Press, 1985, pp 65–94.
4. Robert L, Hornebeck W: Elastin and Elastases, vols 1 and 2. Boca Raton, FL, CRC Press, 1989.
5. Tamburro AM, Davidson JM (eds): Elastin: Chemical and Biological Aspects. Galatina, Italy, Congedo Editore, 1990.
6. Lansing AL, Rosenthal TB, Alex M, et al: The structure and characterization of elastic fibers as revealed by elastase and electron microscopy. Anat Rec 114:555–575, 1952.
7. Gray WR, Sandberg LB, Foster JA: Molecular model for elastin structure and function. Nature 246:461–466, 1973.
8. Hoeve CAJ, Florey PJ: The elastic properties of elastin. J Am Chem Soc 80:6523–6526, 1958.
9. Aaron BB, Gosline JM: Optical properties of single elastin fibres indicate random protein conformation. Nature 287:865–867, 1980.
10. Torchia DA, Piez KA: Mobility of elastin chains as determined by 13C nuclear magnetic resonance. J Mol Biol 76:419–424, 1973.
11. Urry DW, Venkatachalam CM, Long MM, et al:

Dynamic β-spirals and a librational entropy mechanism of elasticity. In Srinivasan R, Sarma RH (eds): Conformation in Biology. New York, Adenine Press, 1982, pp 11–27.

12. Bressan GM, Castellani I, Giro MG, et al: Banded fibers in tropoelastin coacervates at physiological temperatures. J Ultrastruct Res 82:335–340, 1983.

13. Raju K, Anwar RA: Primary structures of bovine elastin a, b, and c deduced from the sequences of cDNA clones. J Biol Chem 262:5755–5762, 1987.

14. Yeh H, Ornstein-Goldstein N, Indik Z, et al: Sequence variation of bovine elastin messenger RNA due to alternative splicing. Coll Rel Res 7:235–247, 1987.

15. Fazio MJ, Olsen DR, Kuivaniemi H, et al: Isolation and characterization of human elastin cDNAs and age-associated variation in elastin gene expression in cultured skin fibroblasts. Lab Invest 58:270–277, 1988.

16. Cleary EG, Gibson MA: Elastin-associated microfibrils and microfibrillar proteins. Int Rev Connect Tiss Res 10:97–209, 1983.

17. Wright DW, Mayne R: Vitreous humor of chicken contains two fibrillar systems: An analysis of their structure. J Ultrastruct Mol Struct Res 100:224–234, 1988.

18. Streeten BW, Licari PA: The zonules and the elastic microfibril system in the ciliary body. Invest Ophthalmol Vis Sci 24:667–681, 1983.

19. Gibson MA, Cleary EG: The immunohistochemical localization of microfibril-associated glycoprotein (MAGP) in elastic and nonelastic tissues. Immunol Cell Biol 65:345–356, 1987.

20. Gibson MA, Hughes JL, Fanning JC, et al: The major antigen of elastin-associated microfibrils is a 31-kDa glycoprotein. J Biol Chem 261:11429–11436, 1986.

21. Sakai LY, Keene DA, Engvall E: Fibrillin, a new 350-kD glycoprotein, is a component of extracellular microfibrils. J Cell Biol 103:2499–2509, 1986.

22. Colombatti A, Poletti A, Bressan GM, et al: Widespread codistribution of glycoprotein gp115 and elastin in chick eye and other tissues. Coll Rel Res 7:259–275, 1987.

23. Greenlee TK Jr, Ross R, Hartman JL: The fine structure of elastin fibers. J Cell Biol 30:59–71, 1975.

24. Rosenbloom J, Cywinski A: Inhibition of proline hydroxylation does not inhibit secretion of tropoelastin by chick aorta cells. FEBS Lett 65:246–250, 1976.

25. Uitto J, Hoffman HP, Prockop DS: Synthesis of elastin and procollagen by cells of the embryonic aorta. Differences in the role of hydroxyproline and the effects of proline analysis on the secretion of the two proteins. Arch Biochem Biophys 173:187–200, 1976.

26. De Clerck YA, Jones PA: The effect of ascorbic acid on the nature and production of collagen and elastin by rat smooth-muscle cells. Biochem J 186:217–225, 1980.

27. Dunn DM, Franzblau C: Effects of ascorbate on insoluble elastin accumulation and cross-link formation in rabbit pulmonary artery smooth muscle cultures. Biochemistry 21:4195–4202, 1982.

28. LuValle PA, Quaglino D Jr, Davidson JM: Submitted for publication.

29. Sandberg LB, Davidson JM: Elastin and its gene. In Hearn MTW (ed): Peptide and Protein Reviews. New York, Marcel Dekker, 1984, pp 169–226.

30. Rosenbloom J: Molecular cloning and gene structure of elastins. Meth Enzymol 144:259–288, 1987.

31. Bressan GM: Repeating structure of chick tropoelastin revealed by complementary DNA cloning. Biochemistry 26:1497–1503, 1987.

32. Indik Z, Yeh H, Orstein-Goldstein N, et al: Alternative splicing of human elastin mRNA indicated by sequence analysis of cloned genomic and complementary DNA. Proc Natl Acad Sci USA 84:5680–5684, 1987.

33. Yoon K, Davidson JM, Boyd C, et al: Analysis of the 3′ region of the sheep elastin gene. Arch Biochem Biophys 241:684–691, 1988.

34. Davidson JM: Unpublished observations.

35. Wrenn DS, Parks WC, Whitehouse LA, et al: Identification of multiple tropoelastins secreted by bovine cells. J Biol Chem 262:2244–2249, 1987.

36. Rich CB, Foster JA: Evidence for the existence of three chick lung tropoelastins. Biochem Biophys Res Commun 146:1291–1295, 1987.

37. Pasquali-Ronchetti I, Bressan GM, Fornieri C, et al: Elastin fiber-associated glycosaminoglycans in β-aminopropionitrile-induced lathyrism. Exp Mol Pathol 40:235–245, 1984.

38. Shields S, Coulson WF, Kimball DA, et al: Studies on copper metabolism. XXXII. Cardiovascular lesions in copper deficient swine. Am J Pathol 41:603–617, 1962.

39. Hill KE, Davidson JM: Induction of increased collagen and elastin biosynthesis in the copper-deficient porcine aorta. Arteriosclerosis 6:98–104, 1985.

40. Smith LT, Holbrook KA: Development of dermal connective tissue in human embryonic and fetal skin. Scanning Electron Microsc 4:1745–1751, 1982.

41. Shibahara S, Davidson JM, Smith K, et al: Modulation of tropoelastin production and elastin messenger ribonucleic acid activity in developing sheep lung. Biochemistry 20:6577–6584, 1981.

42. Davidson JM, Hill KE, Mason MC, et al: Longitudinal gradients of elastin gene expression in the porcine aorta. J Biol Chem 260:1901–1908, 1987.

43. Slack HGB: Metabolism of elastin in the adult rat. Nature 174:512–513, 1954.

44. Lefevre M, Rucker RB: Aorta elastin turnover in normal and hypercholesterolemic Japanese quail. Biochim Biophys Acta 630:519–529, 1980.

45. Abraham PA, Hart ML, Winge AR, et al: The biosynthesis of elastin by an aortic medial cell culture. Adv Exp Med Biol 79:397–403, 1977.

46. Naranayan AS, Sandberg LB, Ross R, et al: The smooth muscle cell. VI. Elastin synthesis in arterial smooth muscle cell culture. J Cell Biol 68:411–419, 1976.

47. Faris B, Salcedo LL, Cook B, et al: The synthesis of connective tissue protein in smooth muscle cells. Biochim Biophys Acta 418:93–103, 1976.

48. Giro MG, Hill KE, Sandberg L, et al: Quantitation of elastin production in vascular smooth muscle cells by a sensitive and specific enzyme-linked immunoassay. Coll Rel Res 4:24–34, 1984.

49. Mecham RP, Lange G, Madaras J, et al: Elastic synthesis by ligamentum nuchae fibroblasts: Effects of culture conditions and extracellular matrix on elastin production. J Cell Biol 90:332–338, 1981.

50. Sear CHJ, Kewley MA, Jones CJP, et al: The identification of glycoproteins associated with elastic tissue microfibrils. Biochem J 170:715–718, 1978.

51. Sephel GC, Davidson JM: Elastin production in human skin fibroblasts and its decline with in vitro age. J Invest Dermatol 86:279–285, 1986.

52. Davidson JM, Smith K, Shibahara S, et al: Regulation of elastin synthesis in developing the sheep nuchal ligament by elastin mRNA levels. J Biol Chem 217:797–754, 1981.

53. Olsen DA, Fazio JJ, Shamban AT, et al: Cutis laxa–reduced elastin gene expression in skin fibroblast cultures as determined by hybridization with an ho-

mologous cDNA and an exon 1-specific oligonucleo-tide. J Biol Chem 263:6465–6468, 1988.

54. Sephel GC, Byers PH, Holbrook KA, et al: Heterogeneity of elastin expression in cutis laxa fibroblast strains. J Invest Dermatol 93:147–153, 1989.

55. Giro MG, Oikarinen AI, Oikarinen H, et al: Demonstration of elastin gene expression in human skin fibroblast cultures and reduced tropoelastin production by cells from a patient with atrophodermia. J Clin Invest 75:672–678, 1985.

56. Rennard SJ, Jaurand MC, Bignon J, et al: Role of pleural mesothelial cells in the production of subendothelial connective tissue matrix of lung. Am Rev Resp Dis 130:231–236, 1984.

57. Mecham RP, Madaras J, McDonald JB, et al: Elastin production by cultured calf pulmonary artery endothelial cells. J Cell Physiol 116:282–288, 1983.

58. Davidson JM: Biochemistry and turnover of lung interstitium. Eur Resp J 3:1048–1068, 1990.

59. Mainardi CL: The role of connective tissue degrading enzymes in human pathology. In Uitto J, Perejda A (eds): Connective Tissue Disease: Molecular Pathology of the Extracellular Matrix. New York, Marcel Dekker, 1987, pp 523–547.

60. Banda MJ, Werb A, McKerrow JH: Elastin degradation. Meth Enzymol 144:288–305, 1987.

61. Davidson JM: Elastin and the lung. Curr Top Rehab In press.

62. Soskel NT, Sandberg LB: Pulmonary emphysema: From animal models to human diseases. In Uitto J, Perejda A (eds): Connective Tissue Disease: Molecular Pathology of the Extracellular Matrix. New York, Marcel Dekker, 1987, pp 423–453.

63. Sandberg LB, Wolt TB, Leslie JG: Quantitation of elastin through measurement of its pentapeptide content. Biochem Biophys Res Commun 136:672–678, 1986.

64. Davidson JM: Regulation of elastin gene expression. In Robert L, Hornebeck W (eds): Elastin and Elastases, vol 1. Boca Raton, FL, CRC Press, 1989, pp 83–90.

65. Davidson JM, Giro MG, Sutcliffe M, et al: Regulation of elastin synthesis. In Tamburro AM, Davidson JM (eds): Elastin: Chemical and Biological Aspects. Galatina, Italy, Congedo Editore, 1990, pp 395–405.

66. Mecham RP, Morris SL, Levy BD, et al: Glucocorticoids stimulate elastin production in differentiated bovine ligament fibroblasts but do not induce elastin synthesis in undifferentiated cells. J Biol Chem 259:12414–12418, 1984.

67. Eichner R, Rosenbloom J: Collagen and elastin synthesis in the developing chick aorta. Arch Biochem Biophys 198:414–423, 1979.

68. Russell SB, Trupin JS, Davidson JM: Regulation of elastin synthesis by hydrocortisone in human dermal fibroblasts: Abnormal response of fibroblasts from keloids. Coll Rel Res 8:537, 1988 (abstract).

69. Foster J, Rich CB, Florini JR: Insulin-like growth factor 1, somatomedin C, induces the synthesis of tropoelastin in aortic tissue. Collag Rel Res 7:161–169, 1987.

70. Mecham RP, Whitehouse LA, Wrenn DS, et al: Smooth muscle–mediated connective tissue remodeling in pulmonary hypertension. Science 237:423–426, 1987.

71. Liu J-M, Davidson JM: The elastogenic effect of recombinant transforming growth factor-β on porcine aortic smooth muscle cells. Biochem Biophys Res Commun 154:895–901, 1988.

72. Giro MG, Duvic M, Kennedy RZ, et al: Increased elastin production in Buschke-Ollendorf fibroblasts is further augmented by TGF-β. J Cell Biol 107:49, 1989 (abstract).

73. Davidson JM, Zoia O: Basic fibroblast growth factor and transforming growth factor-α antagonize the stimulation of elastin production by transforming growth factor-β$_1$ in fibroblasts and smooth muscle cells. Matrix 10:254–255, 1990 (abstract).

74. Frisch S, Davidson JM, Werb Z: Blockage of tropoelastin secretion in rat smooth muscle cells by monensin represses its synthesis at pre-translational level. Mol Cell Biol 5:253–258, 1985.

75. Bhangoo KS, Church JC: Elastogenesis in healing wounds in bats. Plast Reconstr Surg 57:245–257, 1976.

76. Mills K, Takeda M, Read SE, et al: Regeneration of elastin in the ligamentum nuchae of the dog. Can J Surg 12:476–484, 1969.

77. Tammann H, Blubbel P, Roese R: Chemische und morphologische untersuchungen uber den stoffwechel in transplantaten. Arch Klin Chir 172:81, 1933.

78. Bunting CH: New formation of elastic tissue in adhesion between serous surfaces and myocardial scars. Arch Pathol 28:306, 1939.

79. Dann L, Glucksmann A, Tansley K: The healing of untreated experimental wounds. Br J Exp Pathol 22:1, 1941.

80. Lindquist G: The healing of skin defects—experimental study in the white rat. Acta Chir Scand 107(Suppl):7, 1946.

81. Levenson SM, Geever EF, Crowley LV, et al: The healing of rat skin wounds. Ann Surg 161:293–308, 1965.

82. Van Winkle W: Fibroblasts in wound healing. Surg Gynecol Obstet 124:369–386, 1967.

83. Schwartz D: The proliferation of elastic fibers after skin incisions in albino mice and rats: A light and electron microscopic study. J Anat 124:401–411, 1977.

84. Quaglino D Jr, Nanney LB, Kennedy RZ, et al: Localized effects of transforming growth factor-beta on extracellular matrix gene expression during wound healing. II. Incisional wound model. Lab Invest 63:307–319, 1990.

85. Quaglino D Jr, Nanney LB, Ditesheim JT, et al: Transforming growth factor-beta stimulates wound healing and modulates extracellular matrix gene expression in pig skin. II. Incisional wound model. J Invest Dermatol. In press.

86. Quaglino D Jr, Giro MG, Davidson JM: Unpublished observations.

87. Tsuji T, Sawabe M: Elastic fibers in scar tissue: Scanning and transmission electron microscopic studies. J Cutan Pathol 14:106–113, 1987.

88. Humberstone GCW, Humberstone FD: An elastic tissue stain. J Med Lab Tech 26:99–101, 1969.

89. Bhangoo KS, Quinlivan JK, Connelly JR: Elastic fibers in scar tissue. Plast Reconstr Surg 57:308–313, 1976.

90. Snider GC, Hayes JA, Franzblau C, et al: Relationship between elastolytic activity and experimental emphysema-induced properties of papain preparation. Am Rev Resp Dis 110:254–262, 1974.

91. Kaplan PD, Kuhn C, Pierce JA: The induction of emphysema with elastase. I. The evolution of the lesion and the influence of serum. J Lab Clin Med 82:349–356, 1973.

92. Kuhn C, Engelman W, Charaplyvy M, et al: Degradation of elastin in experimental elastase-induced emphysema measured by radioimmune assay for desmosine. Exp Lung Res 5:115–123, 1983.

93. Schriver EE, Bernard GR, Swindell BB, et al: Elastin fragment levels in human plasma, urine, and bronchoalveolar lavage fluid (BALF). Chest 96:1535, 1989 (abstract).

94. Williams G: The late phases of wound healing: Histological and ultrastructural studies on collagen and elastic-tissue formation. J Pathol 102:61–68, 1970.

95. Willams G: The pleural reaction to injury: A histological and electron-optical study with special reference to elastic tissue formation. J Pathol 100:1–7, 1970.

96. Rennard SJ, Jaurand MD, Bignon J, et al: Role of pleural mesothelial cells in the production of connective tissue matrix of the lung. Am Rev Resp Dis 130:231–236, 1984.

97. Glagov S, Tsao CH: Restitution of aortic wall after sustained necrotizing transmural ligation injury. Role of blood cells and artery cells. Am J Pathol 79:7–30, 1975.

98. Bjorkerud S: Reaction of the aortic wall of the rabbit after superficial, longitudinal, mechanical trauma. Virchows Arch Pathol Anat 347:197–210, 1969.

99. Oakes BW, North I, Rosen P, et al: A study of the development of arterial elastin in the dog and rabbit, following vascular surgery, and in the neonatal rat. J Anat 110:503, 1971.

100. Bowald S, Busch C, Eriksson I: Arterial regeneration following polyglactin 910 suture mesh grafting. Surgery 86:722–729, 1979.

101. Bowald S, Busch C, Eriksson I, et al: Repair of cardiac defects with absorbable material. Scand J Thorac Cardiovasc Surg 15:91–94, 1981.

102. Robert AM, Moczar M, Godeau G, et al: Biochemical studies on Dacron arterial prostheses. Pathol Biol (Paris) 24(Suppl):42–47, 1976.

103. Klima G, Papp C: New formation of elastic fiber material in aortic defects covered with muscle flaps. Anat Anz 160:227–228, 1985.

104. Camilleri JP, Phat VN, Bruneval P, et al: Surface healing and histologic maturation of patent polytetrafluorethylene grafts implanted in patients for up to 60 months. Arch Pathol Lab Med 109:833–837, 1985.

105. Moczar M, Allard R, Robert L, et al: Biosynthesis of elastin and other matrix-macromolecules in venous arterial prosthesis. Pathol Biol (Paris) 24(Suppl):37–41, 1976.

106. Clark JM, Glagov S: Transmural organization of the arterial media. The lamellar unit revisited. Arteriosclerosis 5:19–34, 1985.

107. Ross R: The pathogenesis of atherosclerosis. N Engl J Med 314:488–500, 1986.

108. Leung DY, Glagov S, Mathews MB, et al: Cyclic stretching stimulates synthesis of matrix components by arterial smooth muscle cells in vitro. Science 191:475–477, 1976.

109. Oakes BW, Batty AC, Handley CJ, et al: The synthesis of elastin, collagen, and glycosaminoglycans by high density primary cultures of neonatal rat aortic smooth muscle. An ultrastructural and biochemical study. Eur J Cell Biol 27:34–46, 1982.

110. Van der Lei B, Wilderour CR, Nieuwenhuis P: Compliance and biodegradation of vascular grafts stimulate the regeneration of elastic luminae in neoarterial tissue: An experimental study in rats. Surgery 99:45–52, 1986.

111. Sutcliffe MS, Davidson JM: Effect of static stretching on elastin production by porcine aortic smooth muscle cells. Matrix 10:148–153, 1990.

14

CHEMOATTRACTANTS AND GROWTH FACTORS

Gary R. Grotendorst, Ph.D.

Cellular migration and proliferation within an organism play an important role in its embryonic development and response to injury and infection. These events are controlled in large part by specific polypeptides that act as chemoattractants, mitogens, or both. This chapter focuses on the role of specific peptide factors that act to stimulate the directed cellular movement (chemotaxis) and proliferation of both connective tissue cells and endothelial cells during wound repair. It is likely that similar peptides function in an analogous manner to control early embryonic development and to regulate connective tissue formation and tissue reorganization during fibrotic diseases.

The chapter is divided into several parts, the first of which discusses chemotaxis and the biochemical events that regulate this process. The second section considers the relationship of some chemoattractants to mitogens, for example, platelet-derived growth factor, fibroblast growth factor, and epidermal growth factor, which can act as both chemotactic factors and mitogens for their target cells. The last section discusses the actions of these factors in wound healing, presents the evidence for the presence of such factors at sites of tissue regeneration and repair, and considers how the addition of these factors to wound sites could be used to accelerate or modify the repair response.

CHEMOTAXIS

During chemotaxis, cells respond to a chemical factor (chemoattractant) and move in the direction of an increasing concentration of that factor. The best characterized chemotactic response of mammalian cells is the directed migration of phagocytic cells, primarily macrophages and polymorphonuclear neutrophils, to sites of infection or trauma. Phagocytic cells recognize factors secreted by the infecting organism as well as those generated in the traumatized areas and migrate toward their source. However, chemotaxis is not limited to phagocytic cells and has been observed in other cell types, including fibroblasts, smooth muscle cells, and endothelial cells.[1-5]

There are a multitude of chemotactic factors (chemoattractants) and there is considerable specificity in the ability of cells to respond to a given attractant. The presence of cell surface receptors for a factor is required for a cell to respond to a specific chemical and determines the specificity of responding cells. Due to this requirement, most chemotactic factors recruit a single class of cells, such as inflammatory cells, connective tissue cells, or endothelial cells. Distinct chemoattractants arise in a wound at different times and coordinate the influx of cells and blood vessels (Fig. 14–1). A lack of a chemotactic factor for connective tissue cells may impair the rate of repair, whereas overproduction of a chemoattractant could result in excessive repair or scarring (e.g., fibrosis).

Assays for Chemotaxis

Our understanding of chemotaxis is based largely on in vitro systems used to assess the migratory response of cells. The Boyden cham-

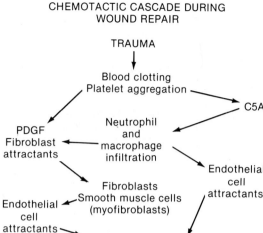

Figure 14–1. Schematic diagram of a cascade of chemotactic factors produced during wound repair. PDGF = platelet-derived growth factor. (From Grotendorst GR: Can collagen metabolism be controlled? J Trauma 24:S49–S52, © by Williams & Wilkins, 1984.)

ber assay is most commonly used (Fig. 14–2).[4] The assay is carried out in a specially designed chamber consisting of two compartments separated by a porous filter. Surfaces coated with collagen or fibronectin for cell adherence are used for fibroblast chemotaxis.[1] Cells in medium are placed in the top compartment and an attractant is added to the solution in the chamber beneath the filter. As the attractant diffuses across the filter, a stable concentration gradient is formed and maintained for the 1 to 4 hours required for the assay.[5] The number of cells that have migrated to the bottom surface of the filter is used as a measure of a substance's chemotactic activity and the cell's ability to respond. The number of cells passing from the top to the bottom surface increases with time

and with the concentration of the attractant (Fig. 14–3).

Most chemoattractants increase both directed and random motility of responding cells as measured by the checkerboard assay.[6] Here, the concentration of the putative attractant is varied in the upper and lower compartments of Boyden chambers. Chemicals that stimulate migration equally when placed in equal concentrations below and above the filter are characterized as affecting random motility. Attractants that are much more potent when placed below the filter are judged to elicit true directed motility.

Biochemical Events in Chemotaxis

Although it has not been shown in all systems, the first event in chemotaxis is detection of the chemoattractant by specific cell surface receptors.[7] Cells lacking such receptors are unresponsive. Responding cells are able to detect nanogram quantities of certain attractants, indicating that high affinity receptors on the cell surface are coupled to mechanisms that amplify the signal and activate the cells' motility. Both spatial and temporal mechanisms have been proposed in the detection of the concentration gradient of chemoattractant and the establishment of the direction of movement. As will be discussed, biochemical reactions initiated by the binding of the attractant to its receptor would be critical in either mechanism.

It is known that the interaction of an attractant with the cell receptor sets off diverse reactions and that these reactions occur even without a concentration gradient. Thus, it is unlikely that the intracellular reactions required for directed motion differ from those required

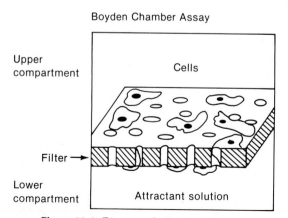

Figure 14–2. Diagram of a Boyden chamber.

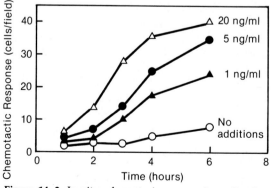

Figure 14–3. In vitro chemotaxis assay using a Boyden chamber shows effects of time and chemotactic factor concentration on cell response.

for random motion. In the case of a chemoat-tractant, a gradient across the cell body would be expected to cause a differential receptor occupancy along the cell surface. Presumably, the degree of receptor occupancy is propor-tional to the magnitude of the chemical reac-tions it triggers, and the rate of these reactions would be greatest in those portions of the cell exposed to the highest concentrations of attrac-tant. This would give rise to an internal gradient in the cell whose polarity could establish direc-tion and whose magnitude could establish the rate of cell movement.

Chemoattractants stimulate a pleiotropic re-sponse in target cells once bound to the cell surface receptor. Specifically, all chemoattrac-tants stimulate both sodium and calcium ion fluxes and changes in lipid metabolism, such as phosphoinositol metabolism and phosphoryl-ation of many membrane proteins as well as cytoplasmic proteins. These events occur within seconds to minutes after the binding of the attractant by the cell surface receptor.

At present the biochemical mechanisms that regulate the chemotactic response are unclear. In bacterial systems the attractant binds to a specific receptor and stimulates flagellar rota-tion, events that are controlled in part by meth-ylation reactions of protein components of both the receptor and the flagellum. However, in higher organisms, the mechanism is much less well understood. The schematic model shown in Figure 14–4 represents a potential mecha-nism for fibroblasts responding to the chemoat-tractant platelet-derived growth factor (PDGF). Once the hormone binds to the receptor, changes in both sodium and calcium flux occur that are stimulated in part by rapid turnover of inositol phospholipids on the cytoplasmic side of the plasma membrane. This turnover, in which phospholipase C removes the inositol head group, generates diphosphoinositol, which mobilizes calcium, and diacylglycerol, both of which are potent activators of protein kinase C. The C-kinase family is known to phosphorylate peptide hormone receptors and the light chain of myosin, among other substrates. The phos-phorylation of the epidermal growth factor (EGF) receptor by C-kinase alters the receptor affinity[8] and causes the hormone to dissociate from the bound receptor. Similar effects have also been seen with the PDGF receptor.[9] Ad-ditionally, since C-kinase can phosphorylate the light chain of myosin, it is an ideal candidate for the transducer element that links the bind-ing of a chemoattractant such as PDGF to the

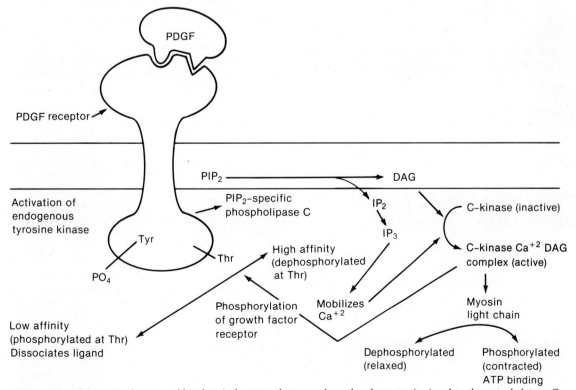

Figure 14–4. Schematic diagram of biochemical events that transduce the chemotactic signal to the cytoskeleton. C-kinase = protein kinase-C; DAG = diacylglycerol; IP_3 = inositol 1,4,5-trisphosphate; PIP_2 = phosphatidylinositol 4,5-bisphosphate; Thr = threonine; Tyr = tyrosine.

cytoskeleton. As discussed before, the gradient that exists outside the cell can now be transduced to a gradient of phosphorylated cytoskeletal proteins, along with other changes occurring simultaneously within the cell, resulting in directed cellular migration. In order for these events to occur continuously and for a gradient to be detected, the reactions must be capable of rapid termination and reversibility. Thus, phosphatases should be very active in the cell, removing the added phosphate from both the receptor and the light chain of myosin and resetting the mechanism so that the signals can be transduced again. In addition to potential changes in the phosphorylation of actin, there are alterations in the polymerization state of actin filaments and the distribution of these filaments in the cell. Modifications of other proteins that constitute the cytoskeleton and contractile elements of the cells by phosphorylation or methylation by specific kinases and methyltransferases are likely to be involved in this process.

The specificity of the chemotactic response is ultimately governed by the presence of particular cell surface receptors. Without the appropriate receptor, no attractant signal can be initiated. Furthermore, biochemical evidence supports the concept that the biochemical events that regulate cell motility are very similar within a variety of cells types, including endothelial cells, fibroblasts, smooth muscle cells, and even leukocytes. Therefore, whether a fibroblast or an endothelial cell is responding to its attractant, virtually the same internal biochemical mechanisms are at work. The specificity of the chemotactic response is then governed by the presence of unique receptors that confer the ability to respond to a particular attractant.

CHEMOATTRACTANTS IN WOUND HEALING

The cellular events that occur sequentially after trauma have been best described for skin wounds.[10] Polymorphonuclear neutrophils accumulate in the wound during the first 16 to 24 hours but subsequently decrease in number. Macrophages arrive soon after the neutrophils and persist in the wound for several days. Fibroblasts and smooth muscle cells appear by day 3 to 4, and endothelial cells in newly sprouted capillaries arrive shortly thereafter.

A number of chemotactic factors have been found in wounds, and others are known to be produced as a result of blood clotting and tissue breakdown (Table 14–1). Presumably, these attractants regulate the order and number of cells that enter the wound, with each cell type responding only to specific attractants. Chemoattractants show an enormous range in their effective doses in vitro, suggesting different functions in vivo. For example, low potency materials, such as collagen and elastin fragments, could create a low and prolonged signal in the presence of tissue debris and bring in phagocytic cells for continuing cleanup without eliciting a major inflammatory response in the tissue. Smaller molecules such as C_{5A} and PDGF would be expected to diffuse more thoroughly into the surrounding tissue than collagen or fibronectin and thus reach their cellular target more efficiently.

Various chemotactic factors have been identified for phagocytic cells from in vitro assays and it is likely that these factors work in vivo. Complement-related products such as C_{5A} are potent attractants for phagocytic cells and appear to be generated almost immediately in the wound.[11] Formylmethionine-like peptides, byproducts of protein synthesis in bacteria, are potent chemoattractants whose presence would be expected to be directly correlated with the degree of bacterial contamination in the wound.[12] Receptors for these peptides are present predominantly on phagocytic cells, which would account for the lack of a response of connective tissue cells or endothelial cells to such materials. The response elicited by the materials can vary with higher concentrations of these peptides stimulating degranulation.[7] Functionally, this dual action allows the neutrophils to find the bacteria and then secrete their bactericidal substances, such as H_2O_2 and lysozymes.

Connective tissue cells respond to a different set of chemotactic factors including collagen alpha chains, collagen fragments,[13] fibronectin,[14, 15] and PDGF.[2, 16] Collagen is almost insoluble under physiological conditions, and the rather high concentration required for chemotactic activity suggests that it is not an important chemoattractant for these cells. Fibronectin occurs in high amounts in plasma (300 μg/ml) and is introduced into the wound with the influx of blood. However, since fibronectin (440,000 Da) is large and binds to collagen, other matrix components, and fibrin, it is not likely that the intact molecule penetrates into the tissue around the wound. However, proteolytic fragments derived from fibronectin show equal or greater chemotactic activity and would be expected to diffuse more readily than the intact molecule.[14, 17]

Table 14–1. CHEMOATTRACTANTS AT WOUND SITES

Attractant	Target Cells	Active Concentration	References
Complement peptide (C_{5A})	Leukocytes	10^{-10}M	7, 11
f-Met peptides	Leukocytes	10^{-10}M	7, 12
Platelet-derived growth factor	Connective tissue cells	10^{-10}M	2, 9, 16, 25
Epidermal growth factor	Endothelial cells	10^{-9}M	3
Collagen and related peptides	Fibroblasts	10^{-6}M 10^{-8}–10^{-5}M	13
Fibronectin and related peptides	Fibroblasts, endothelial cells	10^{-8}–10^{-7}M 10^{-8}–10^{-6}M	14, 15, 17

Platelet-Derived Growth Factor

When platelets aggregate in the wound clot, they release platelet-derived growth factor (PDGF), a potent mitogen stored in the alpha granules of the platelets. PDGF (31,000 Da) is mitogenic for fibroblasts, smooth muscle cells, and glial cells but not endothelial, epithelial, or fibroblastic cells.[18–21] PDGF stimulates cell replication by synergistic action with other factors in serum, such as insulin and somatomedins (see Chapter 4).[22–24] PDGF is released from platelets into the blood only when they aggregate in response to injury or when they adhere to the surface of blood vessels where endothelial cells are denuded.

In searching for chemotactic factors for smooth muscle cells, it was observed that lysates of platelets contained a potent chemoattractant,[2] which was subsequently identified as PDGF.[2, 9, 16] PDGF is chemotactic for smooth muscle cells and for fibroblasts at 0.1 to 5 ng per milliliter. Endothelial and epithelial cells, which show no mitogenic response to PDGF, are not attracted to PDGF. Leukocytes do not respond to PDGF as an attractant and appear to lack PDGF receptors. Furthermore, of all the growth factors tested in our laboratory, including epidermal growth factor (EGF), fibroblast growth factor (FGF), tumor growth factor (TGF)-α and β, and insulin, only PDGF and PDGF-related factors exhibited chemotactic activity for connective tissue cells.

The migratory response of cells to PDGF is distinct from and does not require cell proliferation. Chemotaxis to PDGF occurs prior to an increase in DNA synthesis (Fig. 14–5) and in the presence of inhibitors of DNA synthesis.[16, 25] Insulin and the somatomedins that are required for DNA synthesis are not required nor do they enhance the cell's migratory response to PDGF.[25] PDGF appears to be more potent than other known fibroblast chemoat-

tractants. Interestingly, the concentrations of PDGF that are active in the Boyden chamber chemotaxis assay are less than those required for mitogenesis (Fig. 14–6). Furthermore, since the attractant is added to the lower chamber and forms a gradient in the filter, the actual amount of PDGF in contact with cells in the

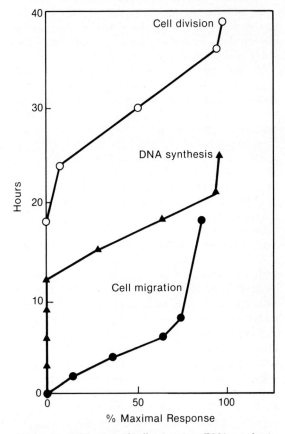

Figure 14–5. Kinetics of cell migration, DNA synthesis, and cell division. PDGF = platelet-derived growth factor. (From Grotendorst GR, Kang T, Seppa ATJ, et al: Platelet-derived growth factor is a chemoattractant for vascular smooth muscle. J Cell Physiol 113:261–266, Copyright © 1982. Reprinted by permission of Wiley-Liss, a division of John Wiley and Sons, Inc.)

upper chamber may be only one fifth to one tenth of that added to the lower chamber.[5] Since chemotaxis occurs at a lower concentration of PDGF than required for mitogenesis, it is likely that fibroblastic cells migrate into the wound site and do not proliferate until they encounter concentrations of PDGF that are sufficient to induce this response. This phenomenon would be important in increasing the penetration of responding cells into the injured area when there are no viable cells.

Endothelial Cell Chemotaxis and Vascularization

New capillaries appear in the wound soon after the influx of fibroblastic cells.[10] This process of neovascularization and angiogenesis appears to involve the sprouting of endothelial cells from capillaries in the surrounding tissue, the directed movement of organized endothelial cells into the wound, and the proliferation of the endothelial cells. Such vascularization is observed in wound healing in development, inflammation, and tumor growth.

Various soluble factors have been observed that increase the endothelial cell movement and growth[26] and that induce neovascularization when implanted in the cornea or on the chorioallantoic membrane.[27] Conditioned media from tumor cells[28] and from certain 3T3-derived cells[29, 30] induce neovascularization, increase the proliferation of endothelial cells, and direct their migration through chemotaxis. Banda and co-workers have reported the isolation of a nonmitogenic chemoattractant for endothelial cells from wound fluid possibly derived from macrophages.[31] Laminin and fibronectin have also been reported to show chemotactic activity with endothelial cells. However, as suggested by McCarthy and colleagues, these latter factors would be expected to function in situ by haptotaxis or contact guidance since they are large and bind strongly to other matrix components.[32] Different endothelial cells may respond to different factors as do primary cultures of vascular smooth muscle cells and certain fibroblasts.

Recently we have shown that both EGF and TGF-α, both of which act through the EGF receptor, can act as potent chemoattractants for a rat heart endothelial cell line.[3] These data support observations made by Schreiber and colleagues that indicated that both EGF and TGF-α act as angiogenic factors when injected

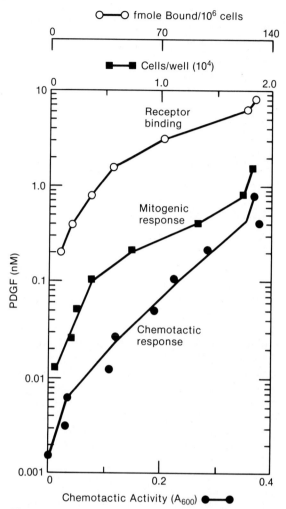

Figure 14–6. Comparison of response curves of chemotactic, mitogenic, and receptor binding actions of platelet-derived growth factor (PDGF) on connective tissue cells.

into the cornea.[33] Other growth factors, including PDGF, TGF-β, FGF, and insulin-like growth factor, are not active as chemoattractants for these endothelial cells. As with PDGF and fibroblasts, EGF and TGF-α stimulate both a chemotactic and a mitogenic response in rat heart endothelial cells. Thus, both PDGF and EGF can be classified as mitoattractants; i.e., factors that stimulate both directed cell migration and proliferation of target cells.

In summary, it is clear that endothelial cells respond to a variety of factors that could guide capillaries to specific sites during wound repair. The use of such factors to accelerate wound healing or to repair damaged tissue, particularly after coronary thrombosis, may have tremendous clinical relevance.

IN VIVO STUDIES ON CHEMOATTRACTANTS AND GROWTH FACTORS DURING WOUND REPAIR

A great deal of information has been accumulated concerning the growth properties, growth factor requirements, and chemotactic properties of various peptides on connective tissue cells and other cell types in vitro. Considerably less is known about the actions of these same factors in vivo. One reason for this is the difficulty of quantitating the repair process in vivo and the lack of control of the types of factors and cells present at the experimental sites. For example, while linear incision wounds or full-thickness skin wounds offer accurate models of naturally occurring wounds, it is nearly impossible to quantitate the formation of new tissue in these systems using biochemical or cellular assay systems, because once the healing process begins it is difficult to distinguish newly formed tissue from pre-existing surrounding tissue. Healing in these wound systems is normally quantitated either by increases in the tensile strength (incision) or by decreases in open surface area (full thickness), both of which represent the culmination of the repair process.

Another approach for studying tissue repair in vivo is to measure the growth of tissue into implants. A variety of systems have been developed along this line, including Silastic sponges, empty chambers, and porous Silastic and Gore-Tex implants. All these systems are more useful for the biochemical analysis of the repair process, since uniform samples can be removed for comparison between experimental and control groups. These systems permit the investigator to analyze various biochemical parameters of the repair process, which can be used to study its components.

Wound Chambers as a Model for Tissue Repair

Initial work from this laboratory on chemotaxis led to the identification of PDGF as a potent chemoattractant for connective tissue cells. Because of the involvement of platelets in wound repair, it was thought that PDGF might act in vivo to stimulate connective tissue formation. Consequently, a modified system for studying wound repair based on the one developed by Schilling[34] and Hunt[35] was used. In this method, stainless steel mesh chambers are implanted subcutaneously in rats to induce a wound repair response; these chambers fill initially with fluid (wound fluid) and subsequently with tissue. Histological studies of the chamber contents indicate that the healing process within these chambers progresses through the classic stages of inflammation, fibroblast infiltration, blood vessel formation, and collagen deposition.[34] Since these chambers are rigid and maintain a constant volume, one can easily quantitate new matrix, cells, or biological activity present within the chamber and compare it directly to that in other chambers. Additionally, this system can be used to isolate cells that can be grown in culture or to extract RNA to study gene expression during the repair process.

This system can also be used to study the levels of both chemotactic factors and growth factors present in wound fluid.[36] Empty chambers are implanted subcutaneously in rats, and at different times after the implantation, fluid is removed from the chamber and tested in biological assays for various growth factors. PDGF, TGF-β, and EGF related activities have been assayed in the wound chambers. The amount of activity present varies during the time course of the repair response, with peak levels present on different days depending on the particular activity measured.

The levels of growth factor and chemotactic factor activity present in wound fluid collected from animals that have healing impairments have also been investigated. The model system chosen was one in which the animals have been treated with the chemotherapeutic agent Adriamycin (doxorubicin). Most chemotherapeutic agents have an inhibitory effect on wound healing. Historically, this effect has been ascribed to the inhibitory action of the drug on fibroblast proliferation. However, it now seems that these agents act via an indirect mechanism through their cytotoxic action on bone marrow stem cells. Because the source of the growth factor activities present at sites of wound repair is inflammatory cells, such as platelets, macrophages, and neutrophils, the cytotoxic action of drugs such as Adriamycin on the bone marrow lowers the circulating levels of platelets and other leukocytes.

We and others have shown that administration of Adriamycin prior to implantation of the Schilling chambers results in an 80 percent reduction in the amount of new collagen deposited in the wound chamber. These results are comparable to those of Devereux and co-workers, who demonstrated a similar decrease in wound tensile strength after Adriamycin treatment.[37] Wound fluid collected from these chambers shows greatly reduced levels of PDGF, TGF-β and EGF–like activities,[36] making it likely that the impairment in healing caused by Adriamycin is due to the pharmacological effects on bone marrow and the subsequent reduction in growth factor and chemotactic factor activity at wound sites. Administration of the same level of Adriamycin after surgery or implantation of the wound chamber had little if any effect on the amount of connective tissue deposited in the wound.

Modulation of Healing by Addition of Chemotactic Factors and Growth Factors

At present there is considerable interest in the biotechnology, pharmaceutical, and medical communities in the potential usefulness of both chemotactic factors and growth factors in controlling tissue regeneration and repair. Applications in both soft and hard connective tissues have been examined in experimental models.

Several laboratories have investigated the effects of exogenously added growth factors on connective tissue formation in in vivo models, normally using rats. Addition of factors such as EGF or FGF to sponges by injection[38] or repeated injection of TGF-α or β into the Schilling chambers[39] stimulates an increase in the amount of collagen deposited at these sites. Schilling chambers filled with a gel composed of type I collagen have been used to study the effects of growth factors in vivo. Addition of this matrix to the chamber appears to have no effect on the healing process.[40] The gel formed within the chamber has a collagen concentration of 3 mg per milliliter, and does not appear to interfere with the biochemical analysis of the chamber contents, such as total protein, DNA, or total collagen. Our studies indicate that the total collagen content of the chamber gives the best measure of the extent of repair that has taken place. Analysis of DNA or total protein does not show a good correlation with the formation of new connective tissue. This is apparently due to the contribution of nonconnective tissue cells to the total DNA content and plasma and interstitial fluid proteins to the total protein content.

Another advantage of this system is that the added matrix acts as a time-release agent for the growth factors that are being studied. In addition, the matrix itself can be manipulated

so that various types of collagen attachment proteins or other matrix components can be added or subtracted from the chamber and the effects on the formation of new connective tissue evaluated. It has been demonstrated that the addition of concentrations of 50 to 100 ng per milliliter of PDGF to the collagen gel matrix causes an increase in the amount of connective tissue within the chambers.[40] These studies were done both in normal animals and in animals that had been made diabetic by streptozotocin injection.[40] Other growth factors, such as FGF or EGF, were less effective when used in this manner.

We have extended these studies to Adriamycin-impaired animals. In this situation the addition of single growth factors such as PDGF, EGF, or TGF-β had little effect on the amount of new connective tissue formed within the chamber. However, combinations of the factors were much more effective in stimulating new connective tissue formation, with a combination of TGF-β, EGF, and PDGF essentially overcoming the healing deficit seen in the Adriamycin-treated animal.[41]

These data suggest that a combination of factors is more effective than any individual factor by itself. This is not surprising, since in vitro studies have clearly demonstrated that more than one growth factor is required for anchorage-dependent growth of connective tissue cells[22-24] and that the same combination of PDGF, TGF-β, and EGF is required for anchorage-independent growth of connective tissue cells.[42] Perhaps because of the similarity in growth factor requirements for cell proliferation, the anchorage-independent growth of connective tissue cells in vitro may be a more accurate model of the growth of cells in vivo in wound sites.

It can be expected that research into the application of growth factors to enhance the rate of wound healing will continue and accelerate. With the advent of recombinant DNA technology and multiple bacterial, yeast, and mammalian cell protein expression systems, the different growth factors have become available in gram quantities. With the high biological activity exhibited by these compounds in affecting cell migration and proliferation, they are prime candidates for the pharmacological manipulation of wound healing. However, as is readily apparent from the Adriamycin studies, much work must be performed to determine the optimal growth factor to use, as well as the appropriate combination, dose, and timing of delivery of these agents.

References

1. Postlethwaite AE, Snyderman R, Kang AH: Chemotactic attraction of human fibroblast through a lymphocyte-derived factor. J Exp Med 144:1188–1203, 1976.
2. Grotendorst GR, Seppa HEJ, Kleinman HK, et al: Attachment of smooth muscle cells to collagen and their migration towards platelet-derived growth factor. Proc Natl Acad Sci USA 78:3669–3672, 1981.
3. Grotendorst GR, Soma Y, Takehara K, et al: EGF and TGF-alpha are potent chemoattractants for endothelial cells and EGF-like peptides are present at sites of tissue regeneration. J Cell Physiol 139:617–623, 1989.
4. Boyden SV: The chemotactic effect of mixtures of antibody and antigen on polymorphonuclear leukocytes. J Exp Med 115:453–466, 1962.
5. Lauffenberger PA, Zigmond SH: Chemotactic factor concentration gradient in chemotaxis assay systems. J Immunol Meth 49:45–60, 1981.
6. Zigmond S, Hirsch JG: Leukocyte locomotion and chemotaxis: New methods for evaluation and demonstration of cell drive chemotactic factor. J Exp Med 137:387–410, 1973.
7. Schiffman E, Gallin JI: Biochemistry of phagocyte chemotaxis. In Harker B, Statmen ER (eds): Current Topics in Cellular Regulation, vol 15. New York, Academic Press, 1979, pp 203–261.
8. Fearn JC, King AC: EGF receptor affinity is regulated by intracellular calcium and protein kinase-C. Cell 40:991–1000, 1985.
9. Grotendorst GR: Alteration of the NIH/3T3 cell chemotactic response to PDGF by transformation growth factors and tumor promoters. Cell 36:279–285, 1984.
10. Ross R, Benditt EP: Wound healing and collagen formation. I. Sequential changes in components of guinea pig skin wounds observed in the electron microscope. J Biophys Biochem Cytol 11:677–700, 1961.
11. Snyderman R, Phillips J, Mergenhagen SE: Polymorphonuclear leukocyte chemotactic activity in rabbit serum and guinea pig serum treated with immune complexes: Evidence for C_{5A} as the major chemotactic factor. Infect Immun 1:521–525, 1970.
12. Schiffman E, Showell HP, Corcoran BA, et al: The isolation and partial characterization of neutrophil chemotactic factors from Escherichia coli. J Immunol 114:1831–1387, 1975.
13. Postlethwaite AE, Seyer JM, Kang AH: Chemotactic attraction of human fibroblast to type I, II, and III collagen in collagen derived peptides. Proc Natl Acad Sci USA 75:871–875, 1978.
14. Postlethwaite AE, Keski-Oja J, Balian G, et al: Induction of fibroblast chemotaxis by fibronectin. Localization of the chemotactic region to a 140,000 molecular weight non-gelatin binding fragment. J Exp Med 153:494–499, 1981.
15. Gauss-Muller B, Kleinman HK, Martin GR, et al: Role of attachment factors and attractants in fibroblast chemotaxis. J Lab Clin Med 96:1071–1080, 1980.
16. Seppa ATJ, Grotendorst GR, Seppa SI, et al: The platelet derived growth factor is a chemoattractant for fibroblasts. J Cell Biol 92:584–588, 1982.
17. Seppa ATJ, Yamada KM, Seppa SI, et al: Cell binding fragment of fibronectin is chemotactic for fibroblasts. Cell Biol Int Rep 5:813–819, 1981.
18. Ross R, Glomset J, Kariya B, et al: The platelet dependent serum factor that stimulates the proliferation of arterial smooth muscle cell in vitro. Proc Natl Acad Sci USA 71:1207–1210, 1974.
19. Kohler N, Lipton A: Platelets as a source of fibroblast growth promoting activity. Exp Cell Res 87:297–301, 1974.
20. Antoniades HN, Scher CD, Stiles CM: Purification of human platelet derived growth factor. Proc Natl Acad Sci USA 76:1809–1813, 1979.
21. Westermark B, Wasterson A: A platelet factor stimulating human normal glial cells. Exp Cell Res 98:170–174, 1976.
22. Pledger WJ, Stiles CD, Antoniades HN, et al: Induction of DNA synthesis in BALB/c 3T3 cells by serum components: Re-evaluation of the commitment process. Proc Natl Acad Sci USA 74:4481–4485, 1977.
23. Vogel A, Raines E, Kariya B, et al: Coordinate control of 3T3 cell proliferation by platelet-derived growth factor and plasma components. Proc Natl Acad Sci USA 75:2810–2814, 1978.
24. Stiles CD, Pledger WJ, Tuclah RW, et al: Regulation of the BALB 3T3 cell cycle effects of growth factors. J Supramol Struct 13:489–499, 1980.
25. Grotendorst GR, Kang T, Seppa ATJ, et al: Platelet-derived growth factor is a chemoattractant for vascular smooth muscle cells. J Cell Physiol 113:261–266, 1982.
26. Folkman J: Tumor angiogenesis factor. Cancer Res 34:2109–2113, 1974.
27. Gimbrone MA, Cotran RS, Leapman SB, et al: Tumor growth and neovascularization in experimental models using the rabbit cornea. J Natl Cancer Inst 52:413–427, 1974.
28. Zetter BR: Migration of capillary endothelial cells is stimulated by tumor derived factors. Nature 285:41–43, 1980.
29. Seppa SI, Seppa H, Liotta LA, et al: Cultured tumor cells produce chemotactic factors specific for endothelial cells, a possible mechanism for tumor induced angiogenesis. Invasion Metathesis 3:139–150, 1983.
30. Castelollot JJ, Karnowski MJ, Speigelman BM: Differentiation-dependent stimulation of neovascularization and endothelial cell chemotaxis by 3T3 adipocytes. Proc Natl Acad Sci USA 79:5597–5601, 1982.
31. Banda MJ, Knighton DR, Hunt TK, et al: Isolation of a nonmitogenic angiogenesis factor from wound fluid. Proc Natl Acad Sci USA 79:7773–7777, 1982.
32. McCarthy JB, Pom SL, Furcht LT: Migration by haptotaxis of a Schwann cell tumor line to the basement membrane glycoprotein laminin. J Cell Biol 97:772–777, 1983.
33. Schreiber AB, Linkler ME, Derynck R: Transforming growth factor alpha: A more potent angiogenic mediator than epidermal growth factor. Science 232:1250–1253, 1986.
34. Schilling JA, Joel W, Shurley HM: Wound healing: A comparative study of the histochemical changes in granulation tissue contained in stainless steel wire mesh and polyvinyl sponge cylinders. Surgery 46:702–710, 1959.
35. Hunt TK, Twomey P, Zederfeldt B, et al: Respiratory gas tension and pH in healing wounds. Am J Surg 114:302–307, 1967.
36. Grotendorst GR, Grotendorst CA, Gilman T: Production of growth factors (PDGF & TGFβ) at the site of tissue repair. In Hunt TK, Pines E, Barbul A, et al (eds): Biological and Clinical Aspects of Tissue Repair. New York, Alan R. Liss, 1988, pp 47–54.
37. Devereux DF, Kent H, Vernon MF: Time dependent effects of adriamycin in X-ray therapy on wound healing in the rat. Cancer 45:2805–2810, 1980.
38. Davidson JM, Klagsbrun N, Hill KE, et al: Accelerated wound repair, cell proliferation, and collagen accumulation are produced by a cartilage derived growth factor. J Cell Biol 100:1219–1227, 1985.
39. Sporn MB, Roberts AB, Shull JH, et al: Polypeptide

transforming growth factors isolated from bovine sources and used for wound healing *in vivo*. Science 219:1329–1331, 1983.

40. Grotendorst GR, Martin GR, Pencev D, et al: Stimulation of granulation tissue formation by platelet-derived growth factor in normal and diabetic rats. J Clin Invest 76:2323–2329, 1985.

41. Lawrence WT, Norton JA, Sporn MB, et al: The reversal of an Adriamycin induced healing impairment with chemoattractant and growth factors. Ann Surg 203:142–147, 1986.

42. Assoian RK, Grotendorst GR, Miller DM, et al: Cellular transformation by coordinated action of three peptide growth factors from human platelets. Nature 309:804–806, 1984.

III
FACTORS AFFECTING TISSUE REPAIR

15

METABOLIC FACTORS

Stanley M. Levenson, M.D.,
and Achilles A. Demetriou, M.D., Ph.D.

Wound healing may be considered as a specific biological process related to the general phenomenon of growth and regeneration. It is a dynamic process involving complex mechanisms that manifest themselves through a spectacular progression of biochemical, physiological, and morphological changes. The various stages from blood clotting through inflammation, cellular proliferation, new blood vessel and lymphatic formation, and reconstitution of the extracellular matrix progress in a way that indicates that the entire process is an orderly one, showing a high degree of integration and organization characteristic of processes in which control mechanisms are operative. The various stages are not sharply separated: since wound healing is an integrated process, factors that stimulate or inhibit one phase have an effect on the overall process. The magnitude of a specific effect depends in part on how rate-limiting is the facet of healing being affected.

Some of the key steps in the healing processes are affected by the metabolic and nutritional status of the wounded patient. Like the infant, who has the most rapid growth and the highest metabolic and nutritional requirements, the patient with extensive wounds is most vulnerable to metabolic and nutritional derangements, and it is these same patients who are most apt to demonstrate disturbances in metabolism and nutrition after injury.

Clinicians have long noted that overtly malnourished patients often have delayed wound healing. But malnutrition need not be overt to

be physiologically significant. Thus, certain nutritional abnormalities occurring acutely may not be accompanied by specific, readily recognizable symptoms or physical signs and may be detectable only by biochemical, physiological, and immunological measurements. Physicians then, must be aware of which metabolic and nutritional changes are apt to complicate their patients' courses so that appropriate preventive and corrective measures can be taken.

Metabolic and nutritional factors can influence wound healing in dramatic ways, and these effects vary considerably because of the different influences of nutrients on mammalian metabolism and physiology and the complexity of systemic and local factors involved in the healing process. The illness or injury is often so severe as to give rise to a host of physiological, metabolic, and nutritional disorders which themselves influence wound repair. In addition, the nutritional condition of the patient prior to illness, injury, or operation has profound effects. Finally, the wounds may be inordinately complex, involving a number of different tissues and organs, and superimposed on these are problems of microbial contamination, foreign material, devitalized tissue, and compromised blood supply.

It should be emphasized that the problems of wound healing and wound infection are interrelated and what affects one affects the other. Thus, resistance to infection is affected by metabolic and nutritional factors in ways roughly parallel to the effects of wound healing on them. When wound healing is impaired, infection is a frequent complication; when clinically apparent wound infection is present, healing is delayed.

The preparation of this chapter as well as some of the studies cited therein was supported in part by NIH grant GM35768.

METABOLIC CHANGES AFTER INJURY

During the past 50 years, many studies have shown that following injury, changes occur in energy, protein, carbohydrate, fat, water, vitamin, and mineral metabolism. Alterations in activity and interactions of neuroendocrines and cytokines, including interleukin-1 and tumor necrosis factor, play key roles, including stimulation of skeletal muscle proteolysis. The responses are dynamic, parallel the severity of the injury, and follow a generally predictable pattern but are still incompletely understood. These are reviewed in many publications.[1-8]

A multiplicity of factors modify these metabolic changes, including age, sex, and prior nutritional status, nature and severity of the injury, nutrient intake, immobilization, and environmental temperature and relative humidity. These metabolic changes have profound effects on nutrition, wound healing, and defense mechanisms.

The view had been advanced by Hunter in 1794 and later in 1954 by Cuthbertson[9] that from the teleological point of view a major function of the disturbed metabolism after injury is to provide nutrients (e.g., amino acids) to the healing wounds at a time when the injured animal is unable to search for food. Later, Moore[10] pointed out that wounds heal to "tensile integrity" during the period of negative nitrogen balance after injury. This was interpreted by many to mean that wounds following severe injury heal normally. However, Levenson and associates showed that wound healing in burned rats,[11] guinea pigs,[12] and rats with femoral fracture[13] is significantly slower than in uninjured controls. In contrast, liver regeneration proceeds faster in burned rats than in unburned controls.[14]

The findings are independent of hemodynamic, respiratory, or renal problems; rather, they reflect some of the metabolic disturbances that follow serious injury. The findings are consistent with ^{15}N-glycine metabolic studies,[15] which showed that anabolism and catabolism remain accelerated after thermal injury, that organs do not react in a uniform way, and that changes in protein metabolism in the different organs result in variable physiological effects. Thus, the protein content of metabolically very active organs, such as the liver, increases in burned rats (i.e., anabolism predominates) despite markedly increased protein turnover rates. In contrast, the protein content of the carcass decreases (i.e., catabolism predominates), and indeed, the decrease in carcass protein accounts mathematically for almost the entire extraurinary nitrogen loss. This suggests that the integrity of certain vital organs is maintained at the expense of other tissues, such as skeletal muscle and skin.

There is little objective, quantitative information on how severe injury affects wound healing in patients; what data are available suggest that wound healing is impaired.

EFFECT OF SPECIFIC NUTRIENTS ON WOUND HEALING

Changes in metabolism of one metabolite may cause functional or quantitative changes in other metabolites and affect the responses of certain target organs and tissues, including healing wounds. Although the various metabolites and nutrients will be discussed separately, all metabolites are interrelated, and in the final analysis all must be considered together.

Protein

That abnormal protein metabolism and nutrition may interfere with wound healing in important ways has been recognized clinically almost since proteins were first discovered, and especially once techniques for measuring and assessing protein metabolism and nutrition became available. Among the early experimental studies were those of Howes and colleagues in 1933,[16] which showed a prolongation of the so-called lag period (i.e., the early days after wounding before intrinsic wound strength increased measurably) in the healing of gastric incisional wounds in acutely partially starved rats. Several years later, Thompson and associates in a series of papers[17-19] reported finding remarkably impaired fibroplasia and a high incidence of dehiscence (72%) in laparotomy wounds in chronically protein-depleted dogs. These dogs were hypoproteinemic and their wounds were very edematous. Transfusions of plasma or gum acacia, a nonmetabolizable colloid, begun at operation and continued postoperatively largely obviated the edema and impaired wound healing. Recently, Felcher and colleagues[20] found wound healing to be normal in genetically analbuminemic rats as assessed by strength gain in skin incisions and accumulations of reparative collagen in subcutaneous implanted polyvinyl alcohol sponges. These results suggest that hypoalbuminemia per se is not the direct cause of impaired wound healing in protein deficiency; rather, the associated decrease in plasma oncotic pressure and consequent tissue edema, especially at wounded and injured sites, may be a causative factor. But it should be pointed out that in rats, chronic protein deficiency and hypoproteinemia are generally not accompanied by obvious edema, and yet the lag period of healing of laparotomy wounds is slowed significantly as shown by Kobak and associates.[21] However, after the lag period, healing progressed at a seemingly normal rate in that study.

Other studies, however, have shown that chronic protein deficiency in animals leads to impairment of angiogenesis, of fibroblastic proliferation, and of reparative collagen synthesis, accumulation, and remodeling in healing wounds. This is as expected because normal protein synthesis and cell multiplication cannot occur unless adequate proteins and amino acids are available. Protein-depleted rats also exhibit decreased rates of wound contraction; however, protein repletion immediately following wounding prevents this effect.[22]

Studies by Delany and associates suggest that changes in wound healing reflect nutritional status more accurately than has been appreciated previously.[23] They demonstrated that 3 days of post-trauma, postoperative nutrient deprivation in preoperatively normally nourished rats altered nitrogen balance, weight loss pattern, and colon anastomotic wound strength without changes in cutaneous wound strength or in hydroxyproline content of polyvinyl alcohol sponge implants. Therefore, the healing of the colon anastomosis was more sensitive to nutritional depletion than the healing of the skin incision and the formation of the reparative tissue in the subcutaneous polyvinyl alcohol sponges.

Protein synthesis must be increased at the wound site during the repair process if normal healing is to occur. A deficiency or imbalance of some amino acids has singular effects on protein synthesis and healing, just as it does on growth. The effects of specific amino acids vary both quantitatively and qualitatively. All amino acids are essential physiologically, whether or not there is a dietary requirement for them; for example, glycine makes up about one third of the collagen molecule. When there is a dietary requirement for amino acids (the so-called dietary essential amino acids), this is generally not because the body cannot synthesize them, but rather because they are synthesized too slowly to meet the body's needs. The quantities syn-

thesized can be increased by providing appropriate precursors, such as keto- and hydroxy-acid analogues, and this may be useful in the care of patients with renal or hepatic dysfunction to lessen the rates of urea and ammonia formation.[24] Only lysine and threonine cannot be synthesized, as far as we know.

Edwards and colleagues,[25] Williamson and associates,[26] and Localio and colleagues[27] reported many years ago that administration of the sulfur-containing amino acids methionine or cyst(e)ine to protein-deficient rats largely corrected their impaired healing, as judged in part by fibroblastic proliferation and reparative collagen accumulation. They did not, however, test the effect of other single amino acids. In later studies, Caldwell and co-workers did not find similar ameliorating effects when methionine was given to protein-depleted rats.[28] Cyst(e)ine may be required for fibroblast proliferation and is a critical component of the terminal peptide of the intracellular procollagen molecule. We think it unlikely that when biologically significant protein depletion is present, administration of a single amino acid alone will correct the impaired healing.

After injury the requirement for certain amino acids, which are normally synthesized at adequate rates for maintenance of the adult steady-state, may increase, so that a dietary supply must be provided. This was shown for arginine in a series of studies by Barbul and colleagues.[29-31] When rats ingesting an arginine-free chemically defined diet (which supports the growth of unwounded rats) are wounded, weight loss is excessive and the rate of healing of skin incisions is slowed.

In subsequent experiments, it was shown that when a commercial rat chow containing 1.8 percent arginine that supports normal growth, reproduction, and longevity was supplemented by an additional 1 percent arginine, wound strength and accumulation of reparative collagen in subcutaneous polyvinyl alcohol sponges were accelerated over normal control rates. It appears that the arginine effect requires an intact hypothalamic-pituitary-adrenal axis, because the effect of supplemental arginine was not seen in hypophysectomized rats receiving growth hormone, thyroxin, testosterone propionate, and ACTH.[31] Supplemental arginine also prevented the thymic involution and adrenal weight gain following wounding; it is possible that this is a factor underlying arginine's effect on wound healing. Barbul and colleagues have demonstrated that intravenous alimentation with an amino acid mixture modified to contain arginine in increased concentration improved wound healing in rats.[32] Very recently, Barbul and colleagues have shown stimulation of reparative tissue formation in subcutaneous implanted polytetrafluoroethylene (PTFE) tubes in healthy humans ingesting substantial amounts of supplemental arginine.[33]

Nagai and co-workers showed that carnosine, β-alanine, and histidine together, but not β-alanine alone, mitigated the otherwise impaired wound healing of animals treated with hydrocortisone.[34] Exogenous carnosine is degraded in the body by carnosinase and histidine decarboxylase to yield histamine. They suggested that the increased availability of histamine enhances the inflammatory process and results in increased wound strength. In earlier studies, Fitzpatrick and Fisher suggested that carnosine serves as a histidine reserve and showed that rats fed histidine-deficient diets had decreased growth rates and impaired wound healing.[35] Thus, it appears that several amino acids may provide necessary metabolites involved in the inflammatory process and other early phases of wound healing. It is possible that certain amino acids may have specific trophic effects on various cell types involved in the inflammatory reaction.

Niinikoski and associates examined the effect of "local hyperalimentation" on open wound granulation tissue in rats and were able to demonstrate increased collagen and cells in the wounds of treated animals.[36] Kaufman and colleagues found that applying a mixture of 19 amino acids to burns of guinea pigs enhanced formation of granulation and scar tissue, decreased epithelialization, and had no effect on contraction.[37] Other studies utilizing specific amino acids (L-cysteine, glycine, DL-threonine) showed mixed results.[38]

The effect of protein malnutrition and enteral hyperalimentation on wound healing was examined by Irvin in rats with colon anastomoses and incisional skin wounds.[39] He noted progressive weight loss and impaired wound healing in rats placed on a protein-free diet for 7 weeks. When such malnourished rats were given oral supplements of amino acids for 7 days before and after operation there was significant improvement in the healing of skin wounds and colon anastomoses.

Haydock and Hill examined the relationship between nutritional status and wound healing in 66 adult surgical patients by measuring the hydroxyproline content of subcutaneously implanted Gore-Tex (expanded PTFE) tubes.[40] They showed that the reparative tissue within the implanted tubes at 7 days in normally nourished patients had higher hydroxyproline content than those of patients with mild to moderate protein-calorie malnutrition. In another study by the same investigators, preoperative total parenteral nutrition (TPN) produced a faster wound healing response as measured by accumulation of hydroxyproline at 7 days in subcutaneous PTFE Gore-Tex catheters than was observed when only postoperative nutritional support was given.[41]

Kay and associates examined healing of lower extremity amputation sites prospectively in 41 consecutive patients and found that 15 of 16 patients in good nutritional state healed their wounds well whereas 11 of 25 patients with abnormal nutritional parameters developed wound and systemic complications.[42]

Protein deficiency inhibits certain antibody responses, as was shown in the 1940s by Cannon and associates.[43] Presumably, this reflects in part the general impairment of protein synthesis when there is inadequate protein. Protein-calorie undernutrition also appears to interfere with certain cell-mediated responses and white blood cell functions, including phagocytosis and intracellular killing of bacteria.[44, 45] The bactericidal activity of the leukocytes isolated from children with protein-calorie malnutrition is considerably less than normal. This has been demonstrated in vitro by the fact that the number of viable bacteria in the white cells following incubation is higher in the leukocytes of these children than in leukocytes of well-nourished children, and by the finding that the clearance from the serum of injected viable bacteria is delayed in undernourished animals. The lymphocytes are altered in protein-calorie malnutrition, as reflected in atrophy of the thymus gland and altered functions of T and B lymphocytes.

Thus, protein deficiency is associated with impaired wound healing and decreased resistance to infection; correction of the deficit is associated with improvement of wound healing and host defense. Clinically, protein deficiency is most often associated with calorie deficiency, and deficiencies of other nutrients, such as vitamins and trace minerals, may be present. These, too, have to be corrected to help assure good wound healing and effective host defense.

Carbohydrates

Disturbances in carbohydrate and fat metabolism have both direct and indirect effects on wound healing. The indirect effects are the result of excessive oxidation of amino acids for caloric needs when inadequate amounts of carbohydrate and fat are available. If this continues, progressive amino acid and protein depletion occurs and the already described adverse effects on wound healing follow.

As for direct effects, unless glucose is present in adequate amounts (including its derivation as the result of glycogenolysis and gluconeogenesis) and metabolized normally, the energy requirement of cells such as leukocytes and fibroblasts cannot be met. Coulton[46] has shown that pentose shunt metabolic activity is involved in biosynthetic processes needed for cell proliferation, which suggests that regulation of carbohydrate metabolism at the wound site may be important in controlling proliferation of various cells in the wound. A possible special role for lactate in wound healing is discussed in Chapter 16.

Diabetes Mellitus

The serious impairment of healing and decreased resistance to infection that occurs in diabetics with inadequately controlled and/or longstanding disease have long been recognized clinically. This is a major public health problem, since there are about ten million diabetics in the United States and about half undergo one or more operations at some time during their life. The mechanisms underlying the impairment in healing are multiple and are not understood completely.

In animals with acute experimental diabetes (most commonly induced by streptozotocin), the early inflammatory response after wounding is impaired and fibroblast and endothelial cell proliferation is reduced, as is the accumulation of reparative collagen and gain in wound breaking strength. Using C57-BL ob/ob mice as a model for type II adult-onset diabetes, Goodson and Hunt demonstrated delayed epithelialization of open skin wounds and decreased collagen accumulation in subcutaneous stainless steel mesh cylinder implants.[47] Barr and Joyce have recently reported that re-endothelialization of an experimental microarterial anastomosis is slowed in streptozotocin diabetic rats[48] and was not alleviated by treatment with insulin starting at operation and continuing postoperatively. This is in contrast to earlier findings of Goodson and Hunt regarding the healing of skin incisions and accumulation of reparative collagen in subcutaneous stainless steel mesh cylinders in streptozotocin-induced diabetes in rats.[49] They had found that early treatment of the streptozotocin diabetic rats with insulin (beginning on day 1 postoperatively and continuing to day 11) corrected the hyperglycemia

and alleviated the impaired healing assessed on postoperative day 21. If insulin administration was not begun until day 11 postoperatively and was continued thereafter, the impaired healing (day 21) was not corrected.

On the basis of results of experiments in which some streptozotocin-induced diabetic mice with dermal ear wounds were treated with antisera to insulin or 2-deoxyglucose or rendered hypoglycemic by starvation, Weringer and associates concluded that hyperglycemia per se did not inhibit wound healing but that lack of insulin was critical.[50–52] Supporting this view are the findings of Hanam and colleagues,[53] who showed improved healing following topical application of insulin to infected skin wounds of diabetic mice. Similarly, topical application of insulin was shown by Saragas and associates to partially prevent the inhibitory effect of corticosteroid therapy on corneal wound healing.[54]

Wound epithelialization was not found to be impaired in the diabetic state by other investigators. Snip and co-workers[55] observed similar epithelialization rates in corneal wounds of diabetic and nondiabetic patients, and similar findings were obtained in rabbits with corneal epithelial wounds by Hatchell and colleagues.[56]

Additional evidence that wound healing may proceed at a near normal rate in the presence of marked hyperglycemia, glycosuria, polydipsia, and polyuria and without insulin administration is afforded by the findings of Seifter and colleagues.[57] They found that supplemental vitamin A given to streptozotocin-induced diabetic rats alleviated the impaired healing (gain of skin wound breaking strength and accumulation of reparative collagen in subcutaneous polyvinyl alcohol sponges) without affecting the hyperglycemia (>400 mg/100 ml blood), glycosuria, polydipsia, and polyuria.

It should be noted that high levels of glucose interfere with cellular transport of ascorbic acid into various cells, including fibroblasts and leukocytes[58] and cause decreased leukocyte chemotaxis. That competitive inhibition in membrane transport by glucose for ascorbic acid might exist was suggested to Mann by the structural similarity between glucose and ascorbic acid.[58, 59] Pecoraro and Chen have suggested that "these results are consistent with the hypothesis that chronic hyperglycemia may be associated with intracellular deficits of leukocyte ascorbic acid, an impaired acute inflammatory response, and altered susceptibility to infection and impaired wound repair in patients with diabetes."[60] In this regard, Schneir and associates have shown that daily dietary intake of very large amounts of ascorbic acid (about 3.5 g/kg body weight) increases nascent collagen production in the skin of streptozotocin-induced diabetic rats by partially reversing procollagen underhydroxylation and intracellular degradation and by normalizing the depressed ribosomal efficiency for collagen production.[61]

Several reports have shown that some of the growth-promoting cytokines ameliorate the impaired healing in diabetic rats. One of the first such demonstrations was by Grotendorst and colleagues, using subcutaneous Hunt-Schilling stainless steel mesh chambers in rats with diabetes induced 5 days earlier by streptozotocin. They found that platelet-derived growth factor (PDGF) added to the chamber caused an earlier influx of connective tissue cells, a marked increase in DNA synthesis, and increased collagen accumulation in the chamber during the first 2 weeks after implantation, but by 3 weeks, the levels of collagen were similar in the treated and untreated groups.[62] Combinations of insulin and PDGF caused an even more rapid collagen deposition in the diabetic rats. No data on the influence of PDGF on blood sugar are provided but one infers that it was not affected. Also, very recently Taubol and Rifkin have shown that recombinant basic fibroblast growth factor (FGF) stimulates wound healing (open skin wounds and skin incisions) in healing-impaired db/db mice,[63] and Hennessey and co-workers found that epidermal growth factor (EGF) and insulin act synergistically to improve wound healing (collagen accumulation in subcutaneously implanted PTFE tubing) in diabetic rats; neither EGF nor insulin alone had an ameliorating effect.[64]

Zimbler and colleagues collected "wound" fluid from subcutaneous Silastic wound chambers in normal and streptozotocin-induced diabetic rats. They found a substance of more than 400 kDa in the fluid from the diabetic rats that inhibited ^{3}H-thymidine uptake by fibroblasts in microcultures.[65]

Indirect effects of severe acute lack of insulin and hyperglycemia on wound healing are hyperosmolarity, dehydration, metabolic acidosis, and inadequate tissue perfusion, which may slow healing.

If diabetes has been present for a long time, healing is interfered with by the neuropathy and vascular abnormalities, particularly of the small vessels, that have developed. Severe renal disease, a common complication in such diabetics, with its abundant metabolic and physiological abnormalities, and serious cardiac dysfunction also contributes to impaired healing. Brownlee and associates have concluded from in vitro and in vivo studies with rats that "age associated increases in collagen crosslinking and accumulation of advanced glycosylation products are both accelerated by diabetes, suggesting that glucose derived crosslink formation may contribute to development of chronic diabetic complications as well as certain physical changes of aging."[66] They found that administration of aminoguanidine mitigated the formation of diabetes-induced glycosylation products and crosslinking of arterial wall connective tissue protein without affecting normal developmental collagen. Manner and co-workers have found that aminoguanidine does not interfere with the crosslinking of reparative collagen in normal wounded rats.[67]

The metabolism of the diabetic patient is often deranged following severe injury or infection, requiring increased insulin administration to control the blood sugar and prevent ketoacidosis. In addition, the various metabolic and physiological changes that follow serious injury affect wound healing. This may occur to a lesser extent following major elective surgery.

The decreased host resistance (local and systemic) of diabetic patients, especially those inadequately controlled, may lead to serious wound infection. Penn[68] recently summarized the current information regarding the susceptibility of diabetics to infection.

Maintaining glucose levels in diabetic patients is particularly important during injury, operation, infection, and illness. Blood sugar is regulated by diet, insulin, and certain oral hypoglycemic agents. Efforts to improve prophylactic and therapeutic regimens (including pancreatic and pancreatic islet cell transplantation) are intensifying because current regimens do not prevent certain deleterious major complications, such as vascular abnormalities.

Fats

The role of fats in wound healing has not been studied as extensively as that of carbohydrates or proteins. Certain key unsaturated fatty acids must be supplied exogenously; that is, they are dietary essentials. Linoleic acid cannot be synthesized by mammals, and evidence suggests that the biosynthesis of linolenic acid and arachidonic acid from linoleic acid does not proceed at a rate adequate for the growing animal. These fatty acids are critical constituents of the triglycerides and phospholipids that are part of subcellular membranes. The unsaturated fatty acids are also essential building blocks for the prostaglandins that regulate many aspects of cellular metabolism and inflammation.

Deficiencies in dietary essential unsaturated fatty acid were rarely detected clinically until seriously ill or injured patients were maintained on prolonged parenteral feedings not containing fat. Infants, especially newborns and prematures, are particularly vulnerable, since they have not built up a body store of these essential fatty acids. Evidence also suggests that requirements for dietary essential fatty acids may be increased after severe injury.[69]

Clinical reports have suggested that essential fatty acid deficiency causes impaired wound healing. In an extensive study that examined the effect of essential fatty acid deficiency, Hulsey and associates[70] demonstrated significant impairment of wound healing in rats. They examined skin and fascial incisions, small and large bowel anastomoses, and burn wounds and showed that the main effect of essential fatty acid deficiency was on skin wound healing; a lesser effect was seen in colon anastomosis healing. Rolandelli and colleagues found that intraluminal infusion of short-chain fatty acids enhanced rat colon anastomotic strength[71] and that the addition of pectin to an elemental diet led to the development of greater colon anastomotic bursting strength.[72] Intracolonic pH was decreased in the pectin-supplemented animals; the authors speculate that this is consistent with a local increase in the concentration of short-chain fatty acids as a result of pectin fermentation.

Water-Soluble Vitamins

Ascorbic Acid. Descriptions of markedly abnormal wound healing in sailors suffering from scurvy appear in the writings of explorers and physicians as early as the 16th century and continuing through much of the 18th century. "The whole body, and more especially the legs, were subject to ulcers of the worst kind attended with rotten bones and such a luxuriancy of fungus flesh as yielded to no remedy." This vivid description appeared in *An Account of the Ravages of Scurvy in Lord Anson's Fleet During a Voyage Around the World, 1740–44*.[73] It was not long thereafter that Lind demonstrated the curative properties of citrus for scurvy in what may have been the first prospective clinical research trial to determine efficacy of a treatment regimen.[74] However, it was not until 1928 that the active citrus compound (hexuronic acid) was isolated by Szent-Gyorgyi. In 1932 it was identified as ascorbic acid by Svirbely and Szent-Gyorgyi and by King and Waugh, and in 1933 its chemical structure was determined by Hirst and Haworth and its synthesis accomplished by Reichstein.

Just prior to those discoveries, Wolbach and Howe published their pioneering study showing the failure of production of intercellular substances by scorbutic guinea pigs and the prompt production of the intercellular substances by fibroblasts when ascorbic acid was given (Fig. 15–1).[75] Since then numerous studies have detailed the gross, histological, histochemical, and mechanical features of healing wounds in vitamin C–deficient guinea pigs. The healing of laparotomy wounds and skin incisions is seriously impaired with considerable hemorrhage, very little reparative collagen formation, and markedly slowed gain in wound strength (Figs. 15–2 and 3).[76–79] Angiogenesis is decreased and the capillaries formed are abnormal and rupture

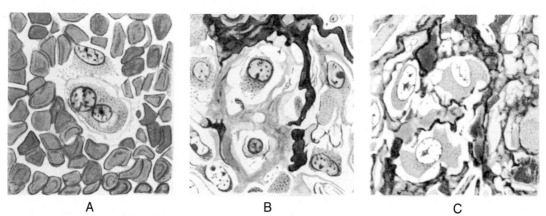

A   B   C

Figure 15–1. Effect of ascorbic acid on collagen synthesis. (Mallory's connective tissue stain, ×1000.) *A*, Fibroblast in center of hemorrhagic area (blood clot in extensor thigh muscle) in scorbutic guinea pig. Note minimal staining material (collagen) at periphery of fibroblast. *B* and *C*, Forty-eight and 72 hours after ascorbic acid administration. Note resorption of hemorrhage and progressive collagen formation. (From Wolbach SB: Controlled formation of collagen and reticulum. A study of the source of intercellular substance in recovery from experimental scorbutus. Am J Pathol (Suppl) IX:689–700, 1933.)

Figure 15–2. *A*, Healed wound, 14 days old, in a guinea pig on adequate doses of vitamin C. Arrows indicate upper and lower poles of wound. *B*, Rinehart stained section, ×396, same wound as in *A*. Area just under epidermis shows many collagen fibers. *C*, Guinea pig wound, 14 days postoperative, in an animal deprived of vitamin C during that time. Note hemorrhage and compare with *A*. *D*, Rinehart stained section, ×396, same wound as in *C*. Area just under epidermis shows lack of collagen fibers. *E*, Same normal animal as in *A* on adequate doses of vitamin C. Skin reflected from two of the 14 day polyvinyl alcohol sponge implants infiltrated by moderately hyperemic granulation tissue. *F*, Rinehart stained section (×396) of polyvinyl alcohol sponge from right upper quadrant, same animal as in *A* and *E*. Note bundle of collagen fibers. *G*, Same scorbutic guinea pig as in *C*. Skin reflected from two of the polyvinyl sponge implants floating in pools of fluid blood. Delicate muscle seal about one sponge has been broken and blood has escaped and stained adjacent skin and fur. Compare with *E*. *H*, Rinehart stained section (×396) of polyvinyl sponge from right upper quadrant, same animal as in *C* and *G*. Note absence of collagen fibers. (From Levenson SM, Crowley LV, Geever ER, et al: Some studies on wound healing: Experimental methods, effect of ascorbic acid, and effect of deuterium oxide. J Trauma 4:543–566, © by Williams & Wilkins, 1964.)

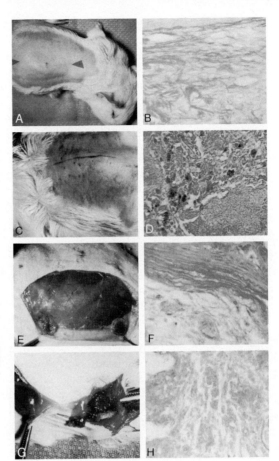

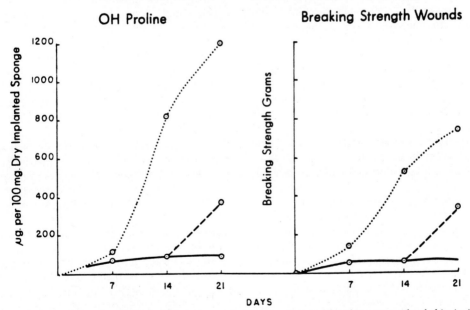

NORMAL, SCORBUTIC AND REPLETED GUINEA PIGS

OH Proline

Breaking Strength Wounds

Figure 15–3. Relationships of polyvinyl alcohol sponge hydroxyproline and breaking strength of skin incisions. In both graphs, the dotted lines represent normal guinea pigs fed ascorbic acid 2 mg per day; the solid lines denote animals fed no ascorbic acid; the dashed lines represent animals repleted with ascorbic acid 2 mg per day at the noted time. (From Levenson SM, Crowley LV, Geever ER, et al: Some studies on wound healing: Experimental methods, effect of ascorbic acid, and effect of deuterium oxide. J Trauma 4:543–566, © by Williams & Wilkins, 1964.)

easily, as do capillaries elsewhere in the body when traumatized, because capillary basement membrane formation and maintenance are interfered with in scurvy.

While the healing of incisions is remarkably impaired in ascorbic acid–deficient guinea pigs, some investigators have reported that uncomplicated, uninfected open skin wounds contract at a normal rate in these guinea pigs,[80, 81] while others have found the rate of contraction to be slowed.[82] This may reflect differences in the degree and duration of ascorbic acid deficiency suffered by the guinea pigs.

Although impaired wound healing in humans has for centuries been associated with scurvy, it is only relatively recently that the problem has been studied systemically in vivo. The pioneering experimental observations of controlled vitamin C deficiency in an otherwise healthy young man were reported by Crandon and associates in 1940.[83] Crandon ate a diet essentially free of ascorbic acid, but otherwise nutritionally complete, for a period of 6 months. Forty-two days later, his plasma vitamin C level had dropped to zero, but the white blood cell ascorbic acid did not sink to that level until day 122. Crandon at that time was clinically well except for a moderate loss of weight and drop in basal metabolic rate. A 2 inch experimental skin incision made 3 months after the start of the experiment appeared to heal normally, the criteria used being those of gross appearance and histological findings from a wound biopsy. At 161 days, petechiae were noted on his limbs. A second skin incision made at the end of 6 months revealed faulty healing as evidenced by gross failure of the wound edges to unite below the skin. A lack of formation of intercellular substances and vascular elements was apparent on histological examination of a 10-day biopsy specimen of the wound. After this biopsy, Crandon was given a daily supplement of 1 g of ascorbic acid. A second biopsy 10 days later revealed "good healing, the sections showing ample intercellular substance and capillary formation."

Wolfer and associates reported later (1947) that the efficiency of wound healing in experimental vitamin C–deficient human subjects as estimated by breaking strength measurements, as well as histological appearance, was markedly impaired.[84]

What Wolbach and Crandon called intercellular substances has been determined to be collagen and it is in the synthesis of this substance that ascorbic acid plays its key role in wound healing. (See Chapters 8 and 9 for an in-depth discussion of collagen biosynthesis and its essential cofactors.) Fibroblastic proliferation is either unaltered or is delayed to only a limited extent, but fibroblast maturation is remarkably impaired.

What is the specific role of ascorbic acid in collagen synthesis? Ross and Benditt[85] found an orderly rowlike arrangement of the ribosomes along the rough endoplasmic reticulum (ER) and some polysome arrangement in the fibroblasts of healing wounds in normal guinea pigs. In contrast, in ascorbic acid–deficient animals, the ribosomes were irregularly arranged, with little if any polysome arrangement. In studies with tritium-labeled proline, Ross and Benditt found that in fibroblasts of wounds of normal guinea pigs, the label progressed from the ER to the cysternae of the ER, then to the Golgi complex and finally appeared in extracellular collagen fibers, the entire process taking about 8 hours. In contrast, in ascorbic acid–deficient guinea pigs, the progression of the labeled proline was much slower and no label appeared in the extracellular collagen fibers; the label seen extracellularly was thought to be due to an influx of serum. Within hours after the administration of ascorbic acid to such guinea pigs, the ribosomes assumed their normal orderly arrangement along the rough ER, some polysome arrangement occurred, and the progression of the labeled proline and its appearance in extracellular collagen fibrils proceeded in a normal fashion (Figs. 15–4 to 15–7).

Others had shown that the hydroxylation of proline and lysine require molecular O_2, α-ketoglutarate, Fe^{++}, and ascorbate. It has been suggested that ascorbic acid may act as an electron transport substance between Fe^{++} and O_2 in the hydroxylation reaction and in the activation of propyl hydroxylase and lysyl hydroxylase, the enzymes catalyzing these reactions. The view has been put forth that these enzymes apparently exist in an inactive subunit form in vitamin C deficiency; when ascorbic acid is present, the enzymes polymerize into active configuration. However, Englard and Seifter have pointed out in a recent comprehensive review of the biochemical functions of ascorbic acid that the precise roles of ascorbic acid, and those for which it is specifically (absolutely) required, are not at all clear.[87] However, Kivirikko and colleagues, who have contributed so much to this field, have stated that ascorbate is a highly specific requirement for prolyl 4-hydroxylase, which is not consumed stoichiometrically.[88] They indicate that the reaction requiring ascorbate is probably an uncoupled decarboxylation of 2-oxoglutarate; therefore the principal function of ascorbate in the

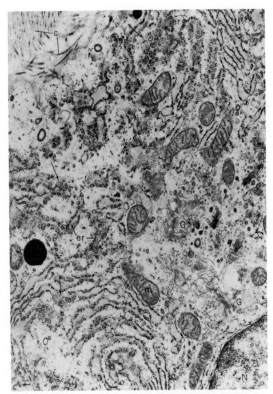

Figure 15–4. An electron micrograph of part of a fibroblast from a 7-day-old wound in a nondeficient animal. The nucleus (N), mitochondria (m), and Golgi complex (G) of this cell are apparent. A characteristic feature of this cell is the extensive, well-developed rough endoplasmic reticulum (er) that is arranged in the form of flat sacs often interconnecting with each other. When the membranes of the ergastroplasm are sectioned tangentially, the ribosomes attached to their surface appear to be arranged in characteristic patterns *(arrows)*, not visible when the membranes are sectioned normally. Collagen fibrils (c) are seen in the extracellular space (×20,000). (Reproduced from the *Journal of Cell Biology*, 1964, Vol. 22, pp. 365–389, by copyright permission of the Rockefeller University Press.)

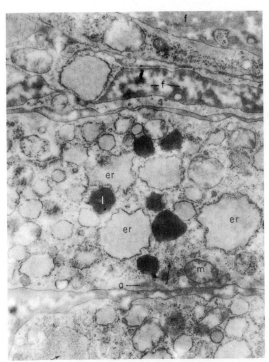

Figure 15–5. An electron micrograph of a portion of a 7-day-old scorbutic wound. The cisternae of endoplasmic reticulum (er) appear as rounded, separate profiles that contain somewhat dense, amorphous material. The surfaces of these wounded cisternae often appear ruffled and irregular. Lipid deposits (l) are evident as are large mitochondria (m). Numerous free ribosomes *(arrows)* and peripheral cytoplasmic, filamentous aggregates (a) can be seen. The extracellular spaces contain the nonbanded filamentous material (f) characteristic of scorbutic wounds (×21,000). (Reproduced from the *Journal of Cell Biology*, 1964, Vol. 22, pp. 365–389, by copyright permission of the Rockefeller University Press.)

prolyl 4-hydroxylase reaction is to act as an alternative oxygen acceptor in the uncoupled catalytic cycles (Fig. 15–8).

Englard and Seifter have offered the view that the primary defect in ascorbic acid–deficient animals is a decrease in collagen synthesis per se, citing among many others the experiments of Chojkier and colleagues[89] and Schwarz and co-workers.[90] We suggest that this view is in keeping with the findings of Ross and Benditt dealing with the disorganized arrangement of ribosomes on the rough endoplasmic reticulum and absence of polysomes in fibroblasts of ascorbic acid–deficient guinea pigs and the prompt reorganization of the ribosomes and polysomes when ascorbic acid is given. The biochemical basis for this abnormality in ribo-

somal arrangement in the ascorbic acid–deficient animal and how it is corrected by ascorbic acid are not known.

There appears to be an abnormal accumulation of one or more substances within scorbutic wound fibroblasts, the specific nature of which is still not known. Many years ago, Klemperer using light microscopy described what he thought were fat bodies within the fibroblasts. Some have postulated that unhydroxylated protein accumulates intracellularly in the fibroblasts of scorbutic animals and that it is subject to rapid proteolysis. However, no accumulation of significant amounts of proline-rich protein was found in carrageenin granulomas by Robertson,[91] in uninjured tissue or reparative tissue (implanted polyvinyl alcohol sponges) in ascorbic acid–deficient guinea pigs by Gould,[92] or in ascorbic acid–deficient media in tissue culture.

Robertson has reported that in guinea pigs placed on an ascorbic acid–free diet at the time

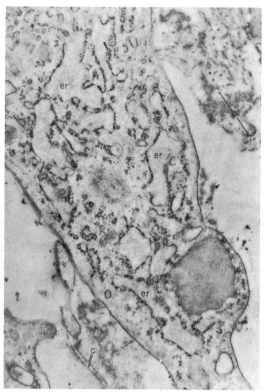

Figure 15–6. An electron micrograph of part of a wound in a scorbutic animal 12 hours after administration of ascorbic acid, showing parts of two cells. The profiles of endoplasmic reticulum (er) of the cell in the center appear to be more intercommunicating. Here again, collagen fibrils (c) cut both longitudinally and transversely can be seen in the extracellular regions, as well as numerous fine filaments (×33,000). (Reproduced from the *Journal of Cell Biology,* 1964, Vol. 22, pp. 365–389, by copyright permission of the Rockefeller University Press.)

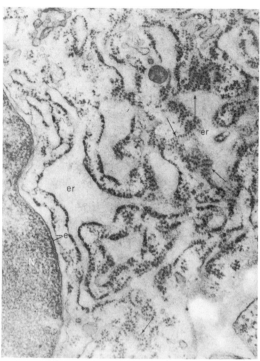

Figure 15–7. An electron micrograph from part of a fibroblast in a wound in a scorbutic guinea pig 24 hours after ascorbic acid administration. Part of the nucleus (N), nuclear envelope (e), and endoplasmic reticulum (er) are visible. The endoplasmic reticulum membranes have been cut tangentially in several regions, and the ribosomal orientation on the membranes is observable. By this time, the typical paired rows are routinely present (*arrows*) and can be seen to take curved forms (×54,000). (Reproduced from the *Journal of Cell Biology,* 1964, Vol. 22, pp. 365–389, by copyright permission of the Rockefeller University Press.)

of subcutaneous injection of carrageenin, there is an accumulation of acid mucopolysaccharide (hyaluronic acid) five to seven times the amount found in the reparative tissue from normal animals.[93] Catchpole found that the increase in mucoproteins in the wounds of scorbutic guinea pigs was paralleled by and probably accounted for by an increase in plasma mucoprotein concentration.[94]

Metabolic utilization of vitamin E appears decreased when large amounts of ascorbic acid are given and in such instances plasma vitamin E levels may be elevated,[95, 96] but there may be an increased vitamin E requirement during high vitamin C intakes.[97, 98]

Hollingshead and co-workers have found that administration of very large amounts of ascorbic acid to mice 30 minutes after burning or freezing their tails decreases the severity of the injuries dramatically.[99, 100] Others have shown that additional agents (e.g., chlorpromazine[101])

also show protective effects for burned rodents, so the response is not unique to ascorbic acid supplementation, although the underlying mechanisms may well be the same for the various agents.

Because wounds are metabolically more active than normal connective tissue for long periods (years in humans), more vitamin C is required to maintain wound integrity than to maintain developmental collagen. Pirani and Levenson showed in guinea pig laparotomy wounds that had healed normally for 6 weeks that when dietary ascorbic acid was withheld the dynamic relationship between collagen synthesis and collagenolysis was disrupted, with failure of adequate synthesis.[102] As a result, there was gradual and progressive loss of the reparative collagen, capillaries became defective, hemorrhage occurred, and the wound reverted to an immature state, with resultant weakness and hernia development. The adverse

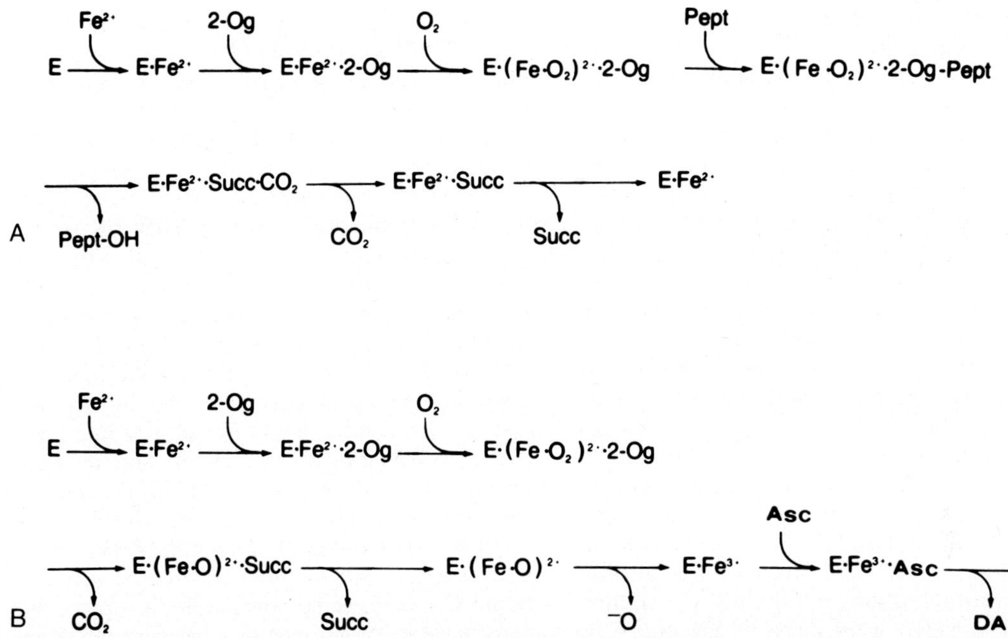

Scheme A:

$$E \xrightarrow{Fe^{2+}} E\cdot Fe^{2+} \xrightarrow{2\text{-Og}} E\cdot Fe^{2+}\cdot 2\text{-Og} \xrightarrow{O_2} E\cdot (Fe\cdot O_2)^{2+}\cdot 2\text{-Og} \xrightarrow{Pept} E\cdot (Fe\cdot O_2)^{2+}\cdot 2\text{-Og}\cdot Pept$$

$$\xrightarrow{Pept\text{-OH}} E\cdot Fe^{2+}\cdot Succ\cdot CO_2 \xrightarrow{CO_2} E\cdot Fe^{2+}\cdot Succ \xrightarrow{Succ} E\cdot Fe^{2+}$$

A

Scheme B:

$$E \xrightarrow{Fe^{2+}} E\cdot Fe^{2+} \xrightarrow{2\text{-Og}} E\cdot Fe^{2+}\cdot 2\text{-Og} \xrightarrow{O_2} E\cdot (Fe\cdot O_2)^{2+}\cdot 2\text{-Og}$$

$$\xrightarrow{CO_2} E\cdot (Fe\cdot O)^{2+}\cdot Succ \xrightarrow{Succ} E\cdot (Fe\cdot O)^{2+} \xrightarrow{^-O} E\cdot Fe^{3+} \xrightarrow{Asc} E\cdot Fe^{3+}\cdot Asc \xrightarrow{DA} E\cdot Fe^{2+}$$

B

Figure 15–8. Schematic representation proposed by Kivirikko and Myllyla of the mechanism for the prolyl 4-hydroxylase and lysyl hydroxylase reactions. The complete hydroxylation reaction is thought to proceed according to scheme A, in which the order of binding of O_2 and the peptide substrate and the order of release of the hydroxylated peptide and CO_2 are uncertain. In the absence of the peptide, the enzymes catalyze uncoupled decarboxylation of 2-oxoglutarate ($-$ ketoglutarate) (scheme B). Certain peptides that do not become hydroxylated are known to increase the rate of the uncoupled decarboxylation. In the uncoupled reaction the reactive iron-oxo complex is probably converted to Fe^{3+} and O_2, and ascorbate is needed to reactivate the enzyme by reducing the Fe^{3+} to Fe^{2+} (scheme B). E = enzyme; 2-Og = oxoglutarate; Pept = peptide; Pept-OH = hydroxylated peptide; Succ = succinate; Asc = ascorbate; DA = dehydroascorbate. (Reproduced, with permission, from the Annual Review of Nutrition, Vol. 6, © 1986 by Annual Reviews Inc.)

effect of ascorbic acid deficiency on previously healed wounds and fractures was recognized clinically centuries ago as illustrated by the following passage describing Lord Anson's circumnavigation of the world on the HMS *Centurion* beginning in 1740.[73]

But a most extraordinary circumstance, and what would be scarcely credible upon any single evidence, is that the scars of wounds which had been for many years healed were forced open again by this virulent distemper. Of this there was a remarkable instance in one of the invalids on board the "Centurion," who had been wounded about fifty years before at the battle of the Boyne, for though he was cured soon after, and had continued well for a great number of years past, yet on his being attacked by the scurvy, his wounds, in the progress of his disease, broke out afresh and appeared as if they had never been healed; nay, what is still more astonishing, the callus of a broken bone, which had been completely formed for a long time, was found to be hereby dissolved, and the fracture seemed as if it had never been consolidated.

In addition to impaired wound healing, vitamin C–deficient animals are more susceptible to wound infection, and infection is apt to be more severe. Studies of experimental abscesses following subcutaneous innoculation of *Staphylococcus aureus* have revealed less localization and more diffusion of the inflammatory reaction and infecting organisms in vitamin C–deficient guinea pigs.[103] In another study, when virulent organisms were injected at a point distant from a wound, the same organism was found later at the operative site in a higher percentage of scorbutic animals than in controls. Among the reasons for this increased susceptibility to infection are (1) impairment of collagen synthesis interferes with the walling-off process localizing an infection; (2) there is impairment of neutrophil antibacterial function because ascorbic acid is involved in the reduction of oxygen to superoxide, which acts as an antibacterial substance and helps generate other bactericidal agents; (3) complement-dependent immune reactions are depressed because ascorbic acid is necessary for the synthesis of some components of complement; and (4) ascorbic acid may play a role in the synthesis of some gamma globulins.

Humans, other primates, and guinea pigs cannot synthesize ascorbic acid because they lack the enzyme L-gulonolactone oxidase needed for the final step, the conversion of L-gulonic acid to ascorbic acid. Humans metabolize ascorbic acid to dehydroascorbic acid (the reversibly oxidized form, still biologically active as an antiscorbutic), diketogulonic acid (the irreversibly oxidized form, which is biologically inactive as an antiscorbutic), oxalate, and ascorbate sulfates. Healthy young men have a total body pool of about 2.3 g of ascorbate, a level they can maintain by ingesting 10 to 20 mg of ascorbic acid per day. Healthy elderly humans, men to a greater extent than women, appear to require more ascorbic acid, perhaps 60 to 70 mg per day, to maintain such levels.

Clinical studies of how wound healing is affected by the vitamin C nutriture of patients are limited. In 1942, Bartlett and associates showed in a patient undergoing a two-stage bilateral herniorrhaphy that wound healing, as measured by breaking strength measurements, was inferior when the plasma and tissue vitamin C levels were low, and that normal healing followed postoperative oral vitamin C administration (1 g daily for 10 days).[104] Vitamin C is concentrated in wounds, reaching substantially higher levels than in unwounded adjacent areas.

There have been reports showing that a number of surgical patients (especially the elderly) enter the hospital with relatively low plasma vitamin C levels. Some have inferred that such patients are deficient in vitamin C and thus, presumably, would have impaired wound healing unless supplemented with vitamin C. However, interpretation of plasma vitamin C concentrations alone is difficult; a low plasma concentration does not necessarily indicate tissue vitamin C deficiency. White blood cell ascorbic acid and ascorbic acid tissue saturation tests are better indices.

Interest has been aroused in the possible abnormalities of vitamin C metabolism following acute trauma. Levenson and associates demonstrated that following injury there is a fall in plasma ascorbic acid concentration, a decrease in urinary ascorbic acid excretion, and a decreased response to ascorbic and "load" tests, indicating decreased ascorbic acid body saturation in previously well-nourished patients.[105, 106]

For example, the plasma vitamin C concentration fell to close to zero within a few days in patients with extensive third degree burns, despite their receiving as much as 1 g per day of vitamin C intramuscularly. At the same time, urinary ascorbic acid was low and tissue saturation tests showed marked depletion. The patients, previously well and in good nutritional states, had become "biochemical scorbutics": they acted biochemically like uninjured patients who became scorbutic as the result of prolonged inadequate intake. It was only after 2 g per day

were given to the severely burned patients that the various biochemical indices approached normal. This same type of response, though not as severe, was demonstrated in patients with burns of lesser severity and in those with other serious injuries, hemorrhages, or infections.

Does this "biochemical scurvy" after injury mean "physiological scurvy"? That this is the case was demonstrated in guinea pigs by Levenson and colleagues.[107] When normal guinea pigs receiving enough vitamin C daily (2 mg) to maintain normal growth and plasma levels of vitamin C were wounded (dorsal skin incision), healing progressed normally, and by the seventh postoperative day there were ample fibroblasts, substantial new collagen, and no hemorrhage. In contrast, when comparable incisions were made in guinea pigs with third degree scald burns of the back involving 30 percent of body surface and maintained on that same vitamin C intake, there was ample fibroplasia but considerable hemorrhage, increased ground substance, and failure of accumulation of reparative collagen. These same findings were seen in unburned guinea pigs deprived of vitamin C starting at the time of wounding. Giving the burned guinea pigs additional vitamin C (100 mg daily postoperatively) prevented the abnormal healing.

It should be noted that the biochemical changes in ascorbic acid metabolism after injury in patients may go on for long periods. The mechanisms underlying the disturbances in ascorbic acid metabolism following injury have not been established, but one theory suggests that the rate of metabolism of ascorbic acid may be increased and that ascorbic acid accumulates in the injured area.

There is no evidence that wound healing can be accelerated by administration of more vitamin C than is required to maintain normal tissue levels. However, since vitamin C is not stored to any great extent in the body, seriously ill and injured patients may rapidly develop physiologically significant deficiency unless ascorbic acid supplementation is given. We recommend that seriously ill and injured patients be given 1 to 2 g of ascorbic acid daily starting promptly and continuing until convalescence is well advanced (e.g., until skin coverage is almost complete in burn patients). No significant adverse consequences are associated with the ingestion of large quantities of this vitamin.[108] It should be noted that the higher amount (2 g) recommended is equivalent *each day* to almost the *total* amount of ascorbic acid present in the healthy adult!

Vitamin B Complex. There are few data

regarding the specific influences of the B-complex vitamins on wound healing. It is to be expected, however, that serious deficiencies of some of these vitamins will interfere with healing, since the B vitamins serve as cofactors in a wide variety of enzyme systems, and in their absence disturbances in protein, carbohydrate, and fat metabolism occur. Deficiencies of the B-complex vitamins, notably pyridoxine, pantothenic acid, and folic acid, decrease resistance to infection in part because antibody formation and some white blood cell functions are impaired.

Certain drugs, such as isonicotinic acid, hydrazide, and estrogens, increase the requirement for pyridoxine; estrogens also increase the need for folic acid. Following severe injury or acute illness, there is a reduction in the urinary excretion of thiamine, riboflavin, and nicotinamide, and tissue saturation tests suggest that the body content of these vitamins is decreased.[101, 102] We recommend intakes of B-complex vitamins of 5 to 10 times normal for severely injured and seriously ill patients.

Fat-Soluble Vitamins

Vitamin A. It was known for centuries that the ingestion of liver as well as the local applications of liver oil or liver juice to the eyes would cure night blindness and prevent (or reverse) xerophthalmia, but it was not until 1915 that McCollum and Davis and Osborne and Mendel discovered the dietary essential factor vitamin A. Its structure was determined in 1930 by Karrer and his associates, and it was synthesized in 1937. Vitamin A does not occur as such in plants but is derived from plants by mammals from its precursor, β-carotene.

In 1925, Wolbach and Howe demonstrated the special role vitamin A plays in cell differentiation and the epithelial keratinization that occurs in vitamin A deficiency.[109] This offered some explanation for the use of liver oil as a folk remedy. Its efficacy was shown experimentally in 1941 by Brandaleone and Papper,[110] who found that the local and oral administration of cod liver oil mitigated the poor healing (delayed epithelialization and closure of open wounds) that occurred in vitamin A–deficient rats.

A quarter of a century later, Ehrlich, Hunt, and associates showed in studies in rats and humans that supplemental vitamin A prevents or reverses the impaired healing due to excess cortisone.[111-113] Lee and Tong demonstrated not long thereafter that the retardation of healing by salicylates, hydrocortisone, and prednisone is reversed by applying retinoic acid, a metabolite of vitamin A, to the wound.[114]

In the last 20 years, a number of studies of the role of vitamin A in wound healing have been made by Seifter, Levenson, Rettura, Demetriou and others,[115-126] the findings of which may be summarized as follows. Rats on a diet containing a marginal level of vitamin A, sufficient to maintain near normal growth, lost weight after minor wounding, became hypoglycemic, and had poorly healing wounds. Less reparative collagen accumulated and it had fewer crosslinks than normal. About half of the rats on marginal vitamin A intake died, while none of the wounded controls died. Administration of vitamin A postoperatively to such rats mitigated these effects.

Supplemental vitamin A given to healthy wounded (skin incisions, subcutaneous implantation of polyvinyl alcohol sponges) rats eating a commercial standard rat chow that supports normal growth, reproduction, and longevity promotes the early inflammatory reaction to wounding and increases angiogenesis, reparative collagen accumulation, and the incidence and severity of intra-abdominal postoperative adhesions following ligation of a small fold of peritoneum in mice. In contrast, citral, a vitamin A antagonist, decreases the adhesions. Supplemental vitamin A also increases the hydroxyproline content of both normal colon and colon anastomotic sites, prevents the decrease in gastrointestinal tract collagen after injury, and increases the bursting strength both of the anastomotic site and of normal colon. It also increases the breaking strength and accumulation of reparative collagen of rat aortic anastomosis and the collagen concentration of adjacent unwounded aorta. This occurs without affecting collagenase activity at either location, indicating that the effect is largely on synthesis of reparative collagen.

Supplemental vitamin A also mitigates the impaired healing that occurs following serious injury and in a number of associated pathological states. It ameliorates the otherwise impaired wound healing of rats with unilateral or bilateral femoral fractures by increasing the rate of strength gain in skin incisions and accumulation of reparative collagen in subcutaneously implanted sponges. It increases the peripheral blood monocyte count and the influx of monocytes/macrophages into the wound site adjacent to a femoral fracture.

Supplemental vitamin A prevents impaired wound healing and thymic involution and lessens the weight loss, adrenal and kidney enlargement, and lymphopenia of streptozotocin-induced diabetic rats without affecting the hyperglycemia, polydipsia, glycosuria, and polyuria. The beneficial effects on wound healing are considered to be the result of correcting the otherwise impaired early inflammatory response after wounding in the diabetic rat.

Supplemental vitamin A also prevents the impaired wound healing, thymic involution, adrenal enlargement, hemorrhage, and weight loss seen in rats given cyclophosphamide without interfering with its antitumor action, and in fact increasing it.[117] The resistance of rats to whole body gamma irradiation is increased and the impaired wound healing, thymic involution, adrenal enlargement, leukopenia, thrombocytopenia, and gastric ulceration are prevented by supplemental vitamin A. Chernov and associates found that supplemental vitamin A prevents or minimizes stress ulcers.[127] Additionally, Mahmood and colleagues reported that chemically induced ulcerations of the stomach and duodenum were minimized by supplemental vitamin A.[123] Also, the poor wound healing, thymic involution, increased adrenal weight, leukopenia, and thrombocytopenia of tumor-bearing mice are mitigated.[124]

Mechanisms of the Effect of Vitamin A on Wound Healing. The specific mechanisms underlying the effects of vitamin A on wound healing are not known. We believe the improved wound healing to be due to an early increase in the inflammatory response. This includes an increase in the influx of macrophages and most likely their activation with release of growth-promoting factors and an increase in the rates of fibroblast differentiation and collagen synthesis. Demetriou and colleagues have shown that vitamin A added to the culture medium of 3T3 fibroblasts speeded fibroblast maturation and increased the fibroblast layer collagen (hydroxyproline) content, without affecting collagenase activity.[125] An increase in crosslinking of reparative collagen in healing skin incisions is suggested by some experiments, but this has not been established with certainty.

Chytil and Omori believe that vitamin A influences cellular phenotype by directly affecting gene expression, and that the cellular binding proteins for retinol and retinoic acid are essential factors.[128, 129] Their hypothesis is outlined in Figure 15–9 as depicted by Olson.[130] Olson has also pointed out that vitamin A affects cell surface glycoproteins involved in cellular adhesion, intracellular communication, and interaction with hormones and growth factors.

In culture, vitamin A increases the fibroblast receptors for epidermal growth factor and increases fibroblast multiplication.[131] The mechanism by which retinol affects glycoproteins has been studied by DeLuca and colleagues.[132]

Of possible importance are some other effects of vitamin A on cellular membranes. The labilizing effect of excess vitamin A on lysosomal membranes was demonstrated by Fell and Thomas when they showed that feeding excessive amounts of vitamin A to rabbits led to the "floppy ear" syndrome.[133] Vitamin A may enter cell membranes because of its lipid solubility; the alternating double bonds in its structure may facilitate electron transport across the membrane. As mentioned, Ehrlich and Hunt

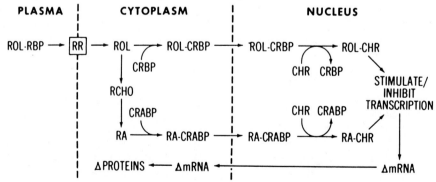

Figure 15–9. Chytil and Ong's direct interaction genome hypothesis (see text for details). ROL-RBP = holo-RBP; RR = cell surface receptor for holo-RBP on the target cell membrane; ROL = retinol; RCHO = retinal; RA = retinoic acid; CRBP = cellular retinol-binding protein; CRABP = cellular retinoic acid-binding protein; ROL-CRBP = a complex of ROL with CRBP; RA-CRABP = a complex of RA with CRABP; CHR = chromatin; ROL-CHR = a complex between ROL and a specific site on CHR; RA-CHR = a complex between RA and a specific site on CHR; mRNA = new mRNA molecules produced as a result of ROL and RA interactions with CHR; PROTEINS = new proteins produced from the new mRNA. (From Olson JA: Vitamin A, retinoids, and carotenoids. In Shils ME, Young VR (eds): Modern Nutrition in Health and Disease. Philadelphia, Lea and Febiger, 1988.)

and their associates[111-113] have shown that vitamin A antagonizes the inhibitory effects of glucocorticoids on wound healing. They have suggested that the differential effects of vitamin A and glucocorticoids on membrane stabilization (glucocorticoids stabilize cell membrane) may be the basis for their antagonistic effects on wound healing, but to date no experiments to explore this hypothesis have been reported.

There is some evidence that the synthesis of the sulfated proteoglycans in healing wounds is depressed in vitamin A deficiency. The significance of these glycoproteins in healing is described in Chapter 11.

Vitamin A Metabolism After Injury. Frank vitamin A deficiency is frequent in developing countries but uncommon in developed countries. However, subclinical deficiencies are widespread in the United States. Following serious injury, there is evidence for an increased requirement for vitamin A.

Decreases in serum vitamin A, retinol binding protein, prealbumin, retinyl esters, and β-carotene occur following burns, fractures, and elective surgery.[134-137] In the latter patients, urinary excretion of vitamin A and retinol binding protein are increased. Liver vitamin A was also found to be low at autopsy in patients dying from burns or other injuries.[138] Serum vitamin A levels fell in psychiatric patients during short-term hyperpyrexia induced by external heat.[139]

Kagan and Kaiser found that rats with subcutaneous abscesses induced by repeated injections of turpentine and sweet almond oil demonstrated sustained decreases in serum vitamin A concentration and in liver vitamin A concentration and content.[140] Gastrointestinal absorption of vitamin A was not altered, but its urinary excretion increased, and the kidney concentration of vitamin A was elevated. Rettura and associates showed that intermittent daily immobilization of rats led to decreases in serum, liver, testes, and kidney vitamin A, and the wearing of partial body casts by rats lowered the vitamin A content of tissues, especially in the thymus where the level fell to 1 percent of the control value.[141]

Large doses of cortisone resulted in the rapid depletion of vitamin A from the rat liver and kidneys,[142] and large doses of corticosterone (the natural glucocorticoid of rats) led to rapid loss of vitamin A from plasma, liver, adrenals, and thymus.[143] These decreases were prevented when supplemental vitamin A was given with the corticosterone.

Adrenal enlargement and thymic involution occurring during stress are obviated by feeding supplemental vitamin A. This effect may be attributed in part to vitamin A's antagonism of glucocorticoids released during stress.[144] Similar effects of vitamin A have been found by Atukorala and colleagues in rats injected with corticosterone[143] and by Seifter and associates in mice injected with epinephrine or norepinephrine.[145]

It was mentioned earlier that injured rats have an increased requirement for dietary arginine. Levenson and co-workers have shown that this is evidenced in part by an increase in urinary orotic acid excretion after injury (increases in urinary orotic acid are well documented in dietary arginine deficiency).[146, 147] It was predicted and observed by Levenson and colleagues that the orotic aciduria following severe burns of rats could be prevented by supplemental dietary vitamin A, just as it is by feeding supplemental arginine.[141] This was interpreted to mean that vitamin A modulated the metabolic response to injury.

Vitamin A and Infection. It has long been known that nutritional vitamin A deficiency increases the incidence of infections.[143] During the past 15 to 20 years, it has been repeatedly shown that supplemental vitamin A improves various host defense responses when given to uninjured rodents, to immobilized and fasting animals, or to those with neoplasms.

Supplemental vitamin A increases cell-mediated immune responses in normal, injured, and tumor-bearing animals.[148-152] It is thyrotropic, prevents or lessens the thymic involution and adrenal enlargement that follows fracture, neoplasia, and radiation, hastens skin allograft rejection, interferes with induction of neonatal tolerance, and increases resistance of mice to a variety of experimental neoplasms. The basis of these effects is immunological, largely thymic dependent, and a reflection of alterations in T lymphocyte subsets. Kalimi and colleagues have shown that supplemental vitamin A prevents stress-induced increase in glucocorticoid receptors in the rat liver.[153]

Vitamin A also plays an important role in humoral defense mechanisms. Several groups of investigators have found a decrease in the number of antibody-producing cells and in antibody production following various antigenic and microbial challenges in vitamin A–deficient rats.[154, 155] In contrast, others have shown that these responses are increased in normally nourished rats given supplemental vitamin A.[156-158] Supplemental vitamin A also increased the ability of alveolar macrophages to phagocytize opsonized sheep red blood cells and increased the in vitro tumoricidal activity of the macrophages.[159]

There are limited data to show how supplemental vitamin A affects host resistance following injury. Cohen and Elin have shown that the severity of *Pseudomonas aeruginosa* infections in burned animals is lessened when supplemental vitamin A is given intraperitoneally.[160] Levine and associates have shown that death is prevented when burned mice challenged with Moloney sarcoma virus are fed supplemental vitamin A.[161] Seifter and associates found that supplemental vitamin A reduces the severity of experimental vaccinia infections in mice,[162] while Demetriou and colleagues found that the severity of peritonitis in rats following perforation of the ligated cecum is lessened by supplemental vitamin A.[163] In addition, Fusi and coworkers have shown that supplemental vitamin A mitigates the depression of the one-way mixed lymphocyte reaction in burned mice,[164] and Cohen and colleagues found that supplemental vitamin A given to patients undergoing elective abdominal operations lessens the early postoperative depression in lymphocyte reactivity.[165]

Recommendations for Vitamin A Intake.
Since large amounts of vitamin A are stored in the liver of healthy individuals, it is unlikely that they will develop a deficiency following ordinary uncomplicated elective surgical procedures. (This will depend, of course, on the nutritional status of the patient prior to surgery.) Deficiencies of vitamin A may occur when there is prolonged interference with food intake and gastrointestinal digestion or absorption. Vitamin E appears to protect vitamin A from oxidation in food and in the gut and increases its absorption, utilization, and storage by mechanisms not yet fully elucidated. Zinc may be necessary for the transport of vitamin A from the liver and maintenance of normal concentrations of vitamin A in the plasma.[166] In this regard, it should be noted that following severe acute stress there is an abrupt increase in urinary zinc excretion, a fall in serum zinc, and an apparent increase in zinc requirements.[167]

The authors believe that malnourished patients with gastrointestinal tract dysfunction should receive supplemental vitamin A (25,000 IU daily) prior to and after elective surgery. Previously satisfactorily nourished patients undergoing operations that interfere with alimentation for long periods of time or who develop gut complications postoperatively also require vitamin A supplementation.

Only the most minimal data are available regarding the "requirement" for vitamin A for seriously injured patients. The word requirement is in quotes because the criteria for assessing it are not established. The few papers dealing with injured or ill patients have dealt largely with measurements of serum vitamin A and retinol-binding protein levels. This is an inadequate approach; for example, serum vitamin A levels may be in the normal range for considerable periods of time while the individual is becoming progressively depleted of vitamin A. Because of lack of information, there is considerable variation in the amounts of vitamin A given to seriously injured patients. The AMA Nutrition Advisory Group Guidelines for Multivitamin Preparations for Parenteral Use adopted in 1975 recommends 3300 IU of vitamin A.[168] No specific mention is made of patients with serious injury, but many surgeons follow that recommendation for their injured patients; some give less[169] and others, including ourselves, give considerably more.[170]

We recommend that supplemental vitamin A be given to all patients with severe injury beginning as soon as possible, in an amount of 25,000 IU per day. This is about seven and one half times the recommended daily allowance for the healthy uninjured adult. This recommendation is based on the following rationale: The amount of supplemental vitamin A required by the seriously injured animal or patient to modulate ("correct") the metabolic host defense and wound healing changes is much greater than that needed for the prevention of the classic signs of vitamin A deficiency (e.g., impaired dark adaptation, failure of epithelial cell differentiation, and weight loss) in uninjured individuals. In fact, the amounts of vitamin A required by the severely injured may well be in the "pharmacological" range, a view also expressed by Malkovsky and associates regarding the effect of supplemental vitamin A on neoplasia.[171] It should be noted that very large doses of vitamin A (100,000 IU) per day have been given for as long as a year to cancer patients with only a few isolated instances of mild toxicity.[172] Also, supplemental β-carotene, which in some experimental studies of neoplasia, radiation, stress ulcer, and healing of skin incisions has shown effects similar to those of supplemental vitamin A, has minimal toxicity.[173]

Available data strongly suggest that administration of supplemental vitamin A to seriously injured patients will lower morbidity, speed convalescence, and decrease mortality, although this remains to be established experimentally. Considerably more data are needed to establish how vitamin A is metabolized after injury and how supplemental vitamin A affects the metabolic reactions to injury. In addition, such questions as how serious injury affects wound healing in patients, what mechanism(s) underline its effects on wound healing, and how it affects host defense mechanism following injury must be answered. It is important to determine whether the effects of supplemental β-carotene, which has minimal toxicity even in very large doses, are similar to, less than, or greater than those of supplemental vitamin A.

Vitamin K. Vitamin K is involved in the synthesis of prothrombin and clotting factors VII, IX, and X. A special role for vitamin K in bone metabolism has been described by Gallop and colleagues,[174] who found that it is required for the synthesis of a calcium-binding protein. Also, if vitamin K deficiency exists, excessive bleeding can occur in wounds, impairing healing and predisposing to infection. Parenteral vitamin K is indicated for obstructive jaundice, severe chronic pancreatitis, and other disorders of fat digestion and absorption. However, patients with serious liver disease may not be able to synthesize adequate amounts of prothrombin even when vitamin K is absorbed and available; in those instances, transfusion of fresh frozen plasma and/or specific blood coagulation component factors may be required.

Vitamin E. There is no clear-cut evidence for a special role for vitamin E in normal wound healing or alteration in vitamin E metabolism or requirements after injury. Vitamin E deficiency in humans has been described in premature infants, particularly those on a diet high in polyunsaturated fats and lacking vitamin E. It is possible that vitamin E deficiency may occur in patients with severe prolonged impairment of fat absorption. Also, because fatty acid deficiency has been reported in patients receiving long-term parenteral nutrition without lipids, seriously ill and injured patients may develop vitamin E deficiency if parenteral vitamin E is not given during a prolonged illness requiring such nutritional therapy. The parenteral vitamin E available commercially is contained in multivitamin preparations, usually providing 25 mg vitamin E in the commonly used daily dose. Whether severe injury affects vitamin E metabolism and requirements has not been reported.

When excess dietary vitamin E is given, wound healing is delayed,[126, 175] formation of experimental postoperative adhesions is lessened,[176] allograft rejection is slowed,[177] and the salutary effects of vitamin A on wound healing are interfered with.[175] Vitamin E also affects various host defense functions, stimulating some and inhibiting others.

Trace Elements

The body stores of most trace minerals are not large but the bodily economy of trace minerals in healthy individuals is high. Until recently little attention was paid to the trace mineral requirements of surgical patients, other than that for iron. However, recognition of trace mineral deficiency became increasingly frequent with the introduction of long-term parenteral feeding of highly purified nutrients. It has also become evident that serious injury, severe infections, alcoholism, diabetes, and disorders of the digestive system may induce trace mineral deficiencies, especially when dietary intake of these minerals is marginal. Associating a specific deficit in wound healing in patients with a deficiency of a specific trace mineral is complicated by the fact that metabolic and nutritional deficiencies in patients are almost always multiple.

Zinc. Solomons[178] has pointed out that although zinc had been known since the early 16th century, it was not until 1923 that its role as an essential nutrient for rats was shown,[179] and only in the 1950s was a zinc deficiency syndrome described in humans.[180] Chronic dietary zinc deficiency is characterized by a failure of normal growth, low plasma zinc levels, hypogonadism, mild anemia, and impaired wound healing.

If zinc levels in the body are low, wound healing is slowed; when the deficiency is corrected, normal healing follows provided there are no other associated nutritional deficiencies.[181] The metabolic roles of zinc have been described by Solomons:[178] Zinc is an essential component of many metalloenzymes (e.g., DNA polymerase, RNA polymerase, and reverse transcriptase) and is involved in polysome conformation during protein synthesis. As a result, DNA synthesis, protein synthesis, mitosis, and cell proliferation are interfered with in zinc deficiency. Lysyl oxidase activity is decreased in animals on a very high zinc diet; lysyl oxidase is a copper-containing enzyme and in the presence of high zinc levels, copper may be displaced from the enzyme or be unavailable for its synthesis. Zinc also stabilizes cell membranes, probably through an inhibition of lipid peroxidases. In its effect on the stability of cell membranes, zinc acts like the glucocorticoids (although probably through different mechanisms) and counter to vitamin A. The possible role of zinc in the hepatic storage and transport of vitamin A has been mentioned earlier.

In zinc deficiency a number of host defense

mechanisms (e.g., phagocytosis, bactericidal activity, cellular and humoral immune functions) are impaired. Accordingly, the zinc-deficient individual is more susceptible to wound and other infections, which may then interfere with healing.

Zinc is excreted mainly in the feces, and gastrointestinal tract dysfunction can cause increased excretion, especially if diarrhea is present, along with decreased absorption of dietary zinc. Urinary excretion of zinc is normally modest, but it is increased after severe injury. There is also a sharp decrease in plasma zinc concentration during the acute phase response to injury, likely due in part to accumulation of zinc in the liver.[167, 182]

Giving zinc to a patient who is *not* zinc deficient will *not* improve wound healing, and may be detrimental if excessive amounts are taken. The National Regulatory Commission (NRC) recommended daily allowance (RDA) of zinc for healthy adults is 15 mg. The AMA Food and Nutrition Board has recommended that stable adult patients on TPN (with no enteral feeding) be given 2.5 to 4.0 mg zinc daily; adults in an acute "catabolic" state (e.g., after severe injury) should receive 4.5 to 6.0 mg; and stable adults with extensive intestinal losses should get an additional 12.2 mg per liter of upper small bowel fluid losses and 17.1 mg per kilogram of stool or ileostomy output.[164]

Excess zinc can interfere with copper metabolism and consequently with wound healing because of copper's special role as a constituent of lysyl oxidase.

Iron. The necessity of Fe^{++} for the hydroxylation of lysine and proline has already been discussed. It is only when iron deficiency anemia is severe and acute that it may have an adverse effect on oxygen transport and thus secondarily on wound healing. Iron deficiency may interfere with leukocyte functions, specifically their bactericidal activity; however, this may be balanced by the slower bacterial growth (demonstrated in vitro) in sera of iron-deficient animals. If iron metabolism is disturbed (beyond low body levels because of inadequate intake), the underlying disorder must be corrected before adequate restoration of the red blood cell mass can be achieved. When the hemoglobin of a seriously ill or injured patient is low enough to be functionally disabling, red blood cells should be transfused.

Copper. Copper is essential for normal erythropoiesis. As in the case of zinc deficiency, clinicians became more aware of copper deficiency when it developed in patients who received long-term TPN without the inclusion of copper in the solutions.

Copper is excreted chiefly in the bile and hence in the feces. This excretion is increased in patients with gastrointestinal tract dysfunction, especially if diarrhea is present and copper absorption is decreased. Urinary copper excretion is normally small. As the major transport protein for copper, ceruloplasmin catalyzes the oxidation of ferrous ions, ascorbic acid, and aromatic amines by molecular oxygen. During the acute phase response, serum ceruloplasmin rises sharply to levels 2 to 3 times normal.

Copper is a component of a number of metalloenzymes of direct importance in wound healing, specifically lysyl oxidase, the enzyme catalyzing collagen crosslink formation, and Zn-Cu superoxide dismutase.

Administration of penicillamine to patients with Wilson's disease and to experimental animals caused impaired wound healing due to decreased copper stores.[184, 185] As mentioned, patients on long-term intravenous alimentation have developed copper deficiency when supplemental copper was not provided, but as far as we know no impairment of healing specifically attributable to this has been reported in such patients. This may be because the copper deficiency was accompanied by other nutritional deficiencies which themselves influence wound healing. In any case, copper should be included in the dietary regimen of seriously injured patients. This is accomplished "automatically" when a mix of ordinary foods are fed to patients with good gastrointestinal tract function, but when gut function is impaired and/or prolonged parenteral feeding is required, supplementation is required.

The daily copper requirement for healthy adults is not known. Accordingly, the NRC has not published an RDA for copper, but instead has recommended a Safe and Adequate Daily Dietary Intake (SADDI) for copper, namely 2.0 to 3.0 mg. For patients receiving TPN and no enteral feeding, the AMA Food and Nutrition Board has recommended 0.5 to 1.5 mg daily for stable adults; no specific recommendations were made for adults in acute "catabolic" states or those with intestinal losses. Serum copper levels are an imperfect guide to copper needs; the entire clinical setting must be considered when calculating appropriate levels of copper administration.

HORMONES
Glucocorticoids

An increase in plasma glucocorticoids brought about by various means, including the administration of ACTH and glucocorticoids, significantly modifies inflammatory reactions and affects wound healing.[186–189] The effects vary according to the specific glucocorticoid involved and the timing, level, and duration of the increase in glucocorticoids in relation to wounding. The glucocorticoid effects are modified by the individual's overall nutritional state; for example, concomitant protein deficiency potentiates the effects of glucocorticoids on wound healing.

The adverse effects of glucocorticoids on wound healing are observed principally when they are present in excess at the time of and in the early days after wounding. When cortisone administration to rats was delayed for several days after wounding, little effect on healing was noted by Ragan and Howes, who were among the first to study the wound healing effects of glucocorticoids (cortisone given to rats).[186] The inflammatory response to wounding is lessened dramatically and there is a significant delay in angiogenesis, fibroblastic proliferation, and the synthesis of proteoglycans and collagen. Wound strength is impaired, as well as epithelialization and closure of open wounds. These effects are seen in wounds of various tissues (e.g., skin, subcutaneous tissue, tendon, gut, bone) regardless of whether the glucocorticoids are given systemically or locally.

The specific mechanisms underlying these effects have not been fully elucidated. Lattes and co-workers suggested in 1954 that one effect of cortisone was to prevent the release of chemical substances by the wounded tissue that are necessary for the initiation and completion of repair.[190]

Glucocorticoid effects on protein metabolism may also be involved; that is, there is an apparent decrease in protein synthesis with a lesser effect on protein catabolism in many tissues (but not the liver where anabolism predominates). As a result, there may be an inhibitory effect on cell proliferation and proteoglycan and collagen synthesis. The glucocorticoids may also act systemically, by antagonizing insulin or growth hormone, or locally, perhaps by interfering with the production, secretion, or action of one or more growth-promoting cytokines or by retarding cell growth directly. In regard to the last two possibilities, Baker and Whitaker showed a number of years ago that the local application of cortisone, in amounts too small to induce measurable systemic effects, delays healing at the site of application.[191] It is possible also that the stabilizing effect of the glucocorticoids on lysosomal membranes may play a role. Additionally, excess glucocorticoids may decrease host resistance and thereby increase susceptibility to wound and other infections, and these infections, in turn, impair wound healing.

Thyroid and Parathyroid Hormones

Clinical observations suggest that hypothyroidism is associated with impaired wound healing. Alexander and colleagues demonstrated an increased incidence of fistula formation in patients treated for cancer of the larynx in the presence of hypothyroidism (secondary to surgery and irradiation).[192] Prompt healing of the fistula tracts occurred following thyroid replacement.

The role of calcitonin on wound healing is not clear. Synthetic salmon calcitonin stimulates protein synthesis, keratinogenesis, and collagen formation in epidermal cells and fibroblasts during wound healing in rabbit experimental wounds.[193] However, in examining the results of calcitonin administration on the rate of bone fracture healing in rabbits, Schatzker and colleagues demonstrated no apparent effect of the hormone.[194]

It has been suggested that parathyroid hormone, a primary regulator of calcium metabolism, affects wound healing. Stanisstreet[195] examined the role of calcium in healing wounds made in the ectoderm of Xenopus early embryos. It was demonstrated that lanthanum, which competes with calcium for calcium channels, and EDTA, a calcium chelator, inhibit wound healing. He hypothesized that wound healing in the amphibian early embryo is initiated by a local influx of calcium ions. The role of calcium and parathyroid hormone on mammalian soft tissue wound healing remains unclear.

Fracture healing is impaired in male adult rats with closed tibial fractures following parathyroidectomy.[196] The effect of nutritional secondary hyperparathyroidism and dietary calcium supplementation on bone healing in dogs was examined by Hubbard and colleagues who were unable to detect any effects on bone healing.[197]

Growth Hormone

Prudden and associates reported in 1958 that growth hormone given to rats increased wound breaking strength and postoperative anabolism.[198] Growth hormone was also shown to

ameliorate the corticosteroid-decreased collagen synthesis in granulation tissue of rats.[199]
Interest in the effect of growth hormone in
wound healing has been stimulated by several
recent developments. The first is the recent
availability of recombinant human growth hormone. Secondly, the demonstration by Wilmore and colleagues that nitrogen balance in
burned patients undergoing major elective abdominal surgery receiving hypocaloric alimentation is improved when they receive growth
hormone. Finally, there is the anecdotal report
of Wilmore that wound healing is accelerated
in burn patients receiving growth hormone.[200, 201]

It has recently been reported that perioperative treatment (3 days preoperatively and 5
days postoperatively) of seriously protein-depleted rats (dietary protein restriction) with rat
growth hormone increased the early laparotomy
wound bursting strength (6 days) to levels
higher than that in the well-nourished controls.
When the growth hormone was given only
postoperatively (5 days) to the protein-depleted
rats, bursting strength was also increased
though not to the same extent. Allowing protein-depleted rats to eat the nutritionally complete commercial rat chow for 3 days preoperatively increased wound bursting strength to a
greater extent than did growth hormone
alone.[202, 203]

Belcher and Ellis found that the administra-
tions of biosynthetic *human* growth hormone
(somatropin) increased the early (6 day) gain of
laparotomy wound breaking strength in normal
rats but did not affect the impaired healing in
burned rats.[204] They concluded that the limited
anabolic activity of somatropin in rats with
normal pituitary function is abolished by injury.
One wonders what would have been found had
rat growth hormone been used.

In a prospective, randomized, double-
blinded study recently reported by Herndon
and colleagues,[206] daily administration of recombinant human growth hormone to severely
burned children shortened hospital stay and
accelerated healing of donor sites when compared to administration of placebo (saline).

Kirkeby and Ekeland found no effect of systemic administration of human recombinant somatomedin C on the early repair of a femoral
osteotomy in rats.[205] Again, would this be the
case were rat somatomedin to be used?

Investigations into the role of growth hormone in wound healing and the effect of its
administration are many and active and these
matters should be clarified soon.

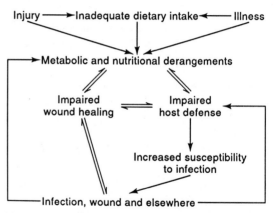

Figure 15–10. Interrelationship of injury, metabolic changes, resistance to infection, impaired wound healing, and sepsis.

CONCLUSION

It is clear that wound healing and infection
are affected by a wide variety of metabolic and
nutritional factors. Their effects on the patient's
reparative and defense systems are complex,
additive, and at times synergistic. The interrelationships among injury, metabolic changes,
resistance to infection, impaired wound healing,
and the development of local and systemic
sepsis are depicted in Figure 15–10.

Only by lessening the severity of the injury
by modifying an individual's local and systemic
resistance to injury and by preventing or correcting the accompanying metabolic, nutritional, and physiological alterations can we set
the stage for uncomplicated wound healing.

References

1. Cuthbertson DP: Nutrition in relation to trauma and surgery. Prog Food Nutr Sci 1:263–287, 1975.
2. Moore FD: Metabolic care of the surgical patient. Philadelphia, WB Saunders, 1959.
3. Levenson SM, Pulaski EJ, Del Guercio LRM: Metabolic changes associated with injury. In Zimmerman LM, Levine R (eds): Physiologic Principles of Surgery. Philadelphia, WB Saunders, 1964, pp 1–44.
4. Wilmore DW: Metabolic Management of the Critically Ill. New York, Plenum Press, 1978.
5. Bessey PQ: Metabolic response to critical illness. In Wilmore DW, Brennan MF, Harken AH, et al (eds): Care of the Surgical Patient. Critical Care, Vol 1. New York, Scientific American, 1989, pp 11-1—11-30.
6. Clowes GHA Jr: Trauma, Sepsis and Shock. The Physiological Basis of Therapy. New York, Marcel Dekker, 1988.
7. Kinney JM, Jeejeebhoy KN, Hill GL, et al: Nutrition and Metabolism in Patient Care. Philadelphia, WB Saunders, 1988.
8. Michie HR, Spriggs DR, Manogue KR, et al: Tumor

necrosis factor and endotoxin induce similar metabolic responses in human beings. Surgery 104:280–286, 1988.

9. Cuthbertson DP: Interrelationships of metabolic changes consequent to injury. Br Med Bull 10:33–37, 1954.

10. Moore FD: Getting well. The biology of surgical convalescence. Ann NY Acad Sci 73:387–400, 1958.

11. Levenson SM, Pirani CL, Braasch JW, et al: The effect of thermal burns on wound healing. Surg Gynecol Obstet 99:74–82, 1954.

12. Levenson SM, Upjohn HL, Preston JA, et al: Effect of thermal burns on wound healing. Ann Surg 146:357–368, 1957.

13. Crowley LV, Seifter E, Kriss P, et al: Effects of environmental temperature and femoral fracture on wound healing in rats. J Trauma 17:436–445, 1977.

14. Levenson SM, Crowley LV, Oates JF, et al: Effect of severe burn on liver regeneration. Surg Forum 9:493–500, 1959.

15. Levenson SM, Crowley LV, Oates JF, et al: Injury, wound healing and liver regeneration. Proc Second Army Sci Conf 2:109–122, 1959.

16. Howes EL, Briggs H, Shea R, et al: Effect of complete and partial starvation on the rate of fibroplasia in the healing wound. Arch Surg 27:846–858, 1933.

17. Thompson WD, Ravdin IS, Frank IL: Effect of hypoproteinemia on wound disruption. Arch Surg 26:500–508, 1938.

18. Thompson W, Ravdin IS, Rhoads JE, et al: The use of lyophile plasma in correction of hypoproteinemia and prevention of wound disruption. Arch Surg 26:509–518, 1938.

19. Rhoads JE, Fliegelman MT, Panzer LM: The mechanism of delayed wound healing in the presence of hypoproteinemia. JAMA 118:21–25, 1942.

20. Felcher A, Schwartz J, Schechter C, et al: Wound healing in normal and analbuminemic (NAR) rats. J Surg Res 43:546–549, 1987.

21. Kobak MW, Benditt EP, Wissler RW, et al: The relation of protein deficiency to experimental wound healing. Surg Gynecol Obstet 85:751–756, 1947.

22. Modolin M, Vevilaoqua RG, Margarido NF, et al: Effects of protein depletion and repletion on experimental open wound contraction. Ann Plast Surg 15:123–126, 1985.

23. Delany HM, Demetriou AA, Teh E, et al: Effect of early postoperative nutritional support on skin wound and colon anastomosis healing. J Parent Enter Nutr 14:357–361, 1990.

24. Walser M, Williamson JR: Metabolism and Clinical Implications of Branched Chain Amino and Keto Acids. Amsterdam, Elsevier, 1981.

25. Edwards LC, Dunphy JE: Methionine in wound healing during protein starvation. In Williamson MB: The Healing of Wounds. London, McGraw-Hill, 1957, pp 1–27.

26. Williamson MB, Fromm HJ: The incorporation of sulphur amino acids into proteins of regenerating wound tissue. J Biol Chem 212:705–712, 1955.

27. Localio SA, Morgan ME, Hinton JW: The biological chemistry of wound healing. The effect of methionine on the healing of wounds in protein-depleted animals. Surg Gynecol Obstet 86:582–589, 1948.

28. Caldwell FT, Rosenberg IK, Rosenberg BF, et al: Effect of single amino-acid supplementation upon the gain of tensile strength of wounds in protein-depleted rats. Surg Gynecol Obstet 119:823–830, 1964.

29. Barbul A, Rettura G, Levenson SM, et al: Arginine: A thymotropic and wound healing promoting agent. Surg Forum 28:101–103, 1977.

30. Seifter E, Rettura G, Barbul A, et al: Arginine: An essential amino acid for injured rats. Surgery 84:224–230, 1978.

31. Barbul A, Rettura G, Levenson SM, et al: Wound healing and thymotropic effects of arginine: A pituitary mechanism of action. Am J Clin Nutr 37:786–794, 1983.

32. Barbul A, Fishel RS, Shimazu S, et al: Intravenous hyperalimentation with high arginine levels improves wound healing and immune function. J Surg Res 38:328–334, 1985.

33. Barbul A, Lazarou S, Efron BA, et al: Arginine enhances wound healing and lymphocyte immune responses in humans. Surgery 108:331–337, 1990.

34. Nagai K, Suda T, Kawasaki K, et al: Action of carnosine and beta-alanine on wound healing. Surgery 100:815–821, 1986.

35. Fitzpatrick DW, Fisher H: Carnosine, histidine, and wound healing. Surgery 91:56–60, 1982.

36. Niinikoski J, Kivisaari J, Viljanto J: Local hyperalimentation of experimental granulation tissue. Acta Chir Scand 143:201–206, 1977.

37. Kaufman T, Levin M, Hurwitz DJ: The effect of topical hyperalimentation on wound healing rate and granulation tissue formation of experimental deep second degree burns in guinea-pigs. Burns Incl Therm Inj 10:252–256, 1984.

38. Harvey SG, Gibson JR: The effects on wound healing of three amino acids—a comparison of two models. Br J Dermatol 111(Suppl):171–173, 1984.

39. Irvin TT: Effects of malnutrition and hyperalimentation on wound healing. Surg Gynecol Obstet 146:33–37, 1978.

40. Haydock DA, Hill GL: Impaired wound healing in surgical patients with varying degrees of malnutrition. J Parent Enter Nutr 10:550–554, 1986.

41. Haydock DA, Hill GL: Improved wound healing response in surgical patients receiving intravenous nutrition. Br J Surg 74:320–323, 1987.

42. Kay SP, Moreland JR, Schmitter E: Nutritional status and wound healing in lower extremity amputations. Clin Orthop 217:253–256, 1987.

43. Cannon PR: Recent advances in nutrition with particular reference to protein metabolism. Kansas University Press (No. 14 of the Porter Lecture Series), 1950.

44. Smythe PM, Brereton-Stiles GG, Grace HJ, et al: Thymolymphatic deficiency and depression of cell-mediated immunity in protein-calorie malnutrition. Lancet 2:939–943, 1971.

45. Daly JM, Reynolds S, Sigal RK, et al: Effect of dietary protein and amino acids on immune function. Crit Care Med 18(Suppl)586–593, 1990.

46. Coulton LA: Temporal relationship between glucose 6-phosphate dehydrogenase activity and DNA-synthesis. Histochemistry 50:207–215, 1977.

47. Goodson WH III, Hunt TK: Wound collagen accumulation in obese hyperglycemic mice. Diabetes 35:491–495, 1986.

48. Barr LC, Joyce AD: Microvascular anastamoses in diabetes: An experimental study. Br J Plast Surg 42:50–53, 1989.

49. Goodson WH, Hunt TK: Studies of wound healing in experimental diabetes mellitus. J Surg Res 22:221–227, 1977.

50. Weringer EJ, Kelso JM, Tamai IY, et al: Effects of insulin on wound healing in diabetic mice. Acta Endocrinol 99:101–108, 1982.

51. Weringer EJ, Arquilla ER: Wound healing in normal and diabetic Chinese hamsters. Diabetologia 4:394–401, 1981.

52. Weringer EJ, Kelso JM, Tamai IY, et al: The effect

of antisera to insulin, 2-deoxyglucose–induced hyperglycemia, and starvation on wound healing in normal mice. Diabetes 30:407–410, 1981.

53. Hanam SR, Singleton CE, Rudek W: The effect of topical insulin on infected cutaneous ulcerations in diabetic and nondiabetic mice. J Foot Surg 22:298–301, 1983.
54. Saragas S, Arffa R, Rabin B, et al: Reversal of wound strength retardation by addition of insulin to corticosteroid therapy. Ann Ophthalmol 17:428–430, 1985.
55. Snip RC, Thoft RA, Tolentino FI: Similar epithelial healing rates of the corneas of diabetic and nondiabetic patients. Am J Ophthalmol 90:463–468, 1980.
56. Hatchell DL, Ubels JL, Stekiel T, et al: Corneal epithelial wound healing in normal and diabetic rabbits treated with tretinoin. Arch Ophthalmol 103:98–100, 1985.
57. Seifter E, Rettura G, Padawer J, et al: Impaired wound healing in streptozotocin diabetes: Prevention by supplemental vitamin A. Ann Surg 194:42–50, 1981.
58. Mann GV: The impairment of transport of amino acid by monosaccharides. Fed Proc 33:251, 1974 (abstract).
59. Mann GV, Newton P: The membrane transport of ascorbic acid. Ann NY Acad Sci 258:243–252, 1975.
60. Pecoraro RE, Chen MS: Ascorbic acid in diabetes mellitus. Ann NY Acad Sci 498:248–258, 1987.
61. Schneir M, Imberman M, Golub L, et al: Dietary ascorbic acid increases collagen production in skin of streptozotocin induced diabetic rats by normalizing ribosomal efficiency. Ann NY Acad Sci 498:514–516, 1987.
62. Grotendorst GR, Martin GR, Pencev D, et al: Stimulation of granulation tissue formation by platelet-derived growth factor in normal and diabetic rats. J Clin Invest 76:2323–2329, 1985.
63. Taubol R, Rifkin DB: Recombinant basic fibroblast growth factor stimulates wound healing in healing-impaired db/db mice. J Exp Med 172:245–251, 1990.
64. Hennessey PJ, Black CT, Audressy RJ: Epidermal growth factor and insulin act synergistically during diabetic healing. Arch Surg 125:926–929, 1990.
65. Zimbler AG, Mills CD, Caldwell MD: Effect of diabetic rat wound fluid on fibroblast growth. Surg Forum 39:629–632, 1988.
66. Brownlee M, Vlassara H, Kooney A, et al: Aminoguanidine prevents diabetes induced arterial wall protein cross-linking. Science 232:1629–1632, 1986.
67. Manner P, Chang TH, Levenson SM: Unpublished observations.
68. Penn I: Diabetes mellitus and the surgeon. Curr Prob Surg 24:537–603, 1987.
69. Nordenstrom J, Carpentier YA, Askanazi S, et al: Free fatty acid mobilization and oxidation during total parenteral nutrition in trauma and infection. Ann Surg 198:725–735, 1983.
70. Hulsey TK, O'Neill JA, Neblett WR, et al: Experimental wound healing in essential fatty acid deficiency. J Pediatr Surg 15:505–508, 1980.
71. Rolandelli RH, Koruda MJ, Settle RG, et al: Effects of intraluminal infusion of short-chain fatty acids on the healing of colonic anastomosis in the rat. Surgery 100:198–204, 1986.
72. Rolandelli RH, Koruda MJ, Settle RG, et al: The effect of enteral feedings supplemented with pectin on the healing of colonic anastomoses in the rat. Surgery 99:703–707, 1986.
73. Faunholt A: An Account of the Ravages of Scurvy in Lord Anson's Fleet During a Voyage Around the World, 1740–44, and Some Notes Concerning British Naval Hygiene at the Time. Mil Surg 25:38–47, 1909.

74. Lind J: Treatise on Scurvy. Containing a Reprint of the First Edition of A Treatise of the Scurvy with Additional Notes. In Stewart CP, Guthrie D (eds): A Bicentenary Volume. Edinburgh, The University Press, 1953.
75. Wolbach SB, Howe PR: Intercellular substances in experimental scorbutis. Arch Pathol Lab Med 1:1–24, 1926.
76. Bourne GH: Effect of vitamin C deficiency on experimental wounds. Tensile strength and histology. Lancet 1:688–692, 1944.
77. Lanman TH, Ingalls TH: Vitamin C deficiency and wound healing (experimental and clinical study). Ann Surg 105:616–625, 1937.
78. Bartlett MK, Jones CM, Ryan AE: Vitamin C and wound healing. I. Experimental wounds in guinea pigs. N Engl J Med 226:469–473, 1942.
79. Hunt AH: The role of vitamin C in wound healing. Br J Surg 28:436–461, 1940.
80. Abercrombie M, Flint MH, James DW: Wound contraction in scorbutic guinea pigs. J Embryol Exp Morphol 4:167–175, 1956.
81. Grillo HC, Gross J: Studies in wound healing. III. Contraction in vitamin C deficiency. Proc Soc Exp Biol Med 101:268–270, 1959.
82. Woessner JF: Collagen formation in living systems. Doctoral thesis, Massachusetts Institute of Technology, Cambridge, Massachusetts, 1956.
83. Crandon JH, Lund CC, Dill DB: Experimental human scurvy. N Engl J Med 223:353–369, 1940.
84. Wolfer JA, Farmer CJ, Carroll WW, et al: Experimental study of wound healing in vitamin C depleted human subjects. Surg Gynecol Obstet 84:1–15, 1947.
85. Ross R, Benditt EP: Wound healing and collagen formation. II. Fine structure in experimental scurvy. J Cell Biol 12:533–551, 1962.
86. Ross R, Benditt EP: Wound healing and collagen formation. V. Quantitative electron microscope radioautographic observations of proline-II^3 utilization by fibroblasts. J Cell Biol 27:83–106, 1965.
87. Englard S, Seifter E: The biochemical functions of ascorbic acid. Ann Rev Nutr 6:365–406, 1986.
88. Kivirikko KI, Helaakoski T, Tasanen K, et al: Molecular biology of prolyl 4-hydroxylase. Ann NY Acad Sci 580:132–142, 1990.
89. Chojkier M, Spanheimer R, Peterkofsky B: Specifically decreased collagen biosynthesis in scurvy dissociated from an effect on proline hydroxylation and correlated with body weight loss. In vitro studies in guinea pig calvarial bones. J Clin Invest 72:826–835, 1983.
90. Schwarz RI, Mandell RB, Bissell MJ: Ascorbate induction of collagen synthesis as a mean for elucidating mechanism for quantitative control of tissue-specific function. Mol Cell Biol 1:843–853, 1981.
91. Robertson WV, Schwartz B: Ascorbic acid and formation of collagen. J Biol Chem 201:689–696, 1953.
92. Gould BS: Collagen biosynthesis. In Levenson SM, Stein JM, Grossblatt N (eds): Wound Healing—Proceedings of a Workshop. Washington, DC, National Academy of Sciences—National Research Council, 1966, pp 99–106.
93. Robertson W, Van B: Carrageenin granuloma. In Levenson SM, Stein JM, Grossblatt N (eds): Wound Healing—Proceedings of a Workshop. Washington DC, National Academy of Sciences—National Research Council, 1966, pp 296–306.
94. Catchpole HR: Changes in ground substance. In Levenson SM, Stein JM, Grossblatt N (eds): Wound Healing—Proceedings of a Workshop. Washington, DC, National Academy of Sciences—National Research Council, 1966, pp 107–113.

95. Chen LH, Lee MS, Hsing WF, et al: Effect of vitamin C on tissue antioxidant status of vitamin E deficient rats. Int J Vitam Nutr Res 50:156–162, 1980.
96. Packer JE, Slater TF, Wilson RL: Direct observation of a free radical interaction between vitamin E and vitamin C. Nature 278:737–738, 1979.
97. Chen LH, Chang HH: Effects of high level of vitamin C on tissue antioxidant status of guinea pigs. Int J Vitam Nutr Res 49:87–91, 1979.
98. Chen LH: An increase in vitamin E requirement induced by high supplementation of vitamin C in rats. Am J Clin Nutr 34:1036–1401, 1981.
99. Hollingshead MB, Spillert CR, Lazaro EJ: The beneficial effects of ascorbic acid on murine burns. J Burn Care Res 6:50–54, 1985.
100. Spillert CR, Hollingshead MB, Lazaro EJ: Protective effects of ascorbic acid in murine frostbite. Ann NY Acad Sci 498:517–518, 1987.
101. Bibi RR, Babyatsky M, Levenson SM: Acquired local resistance to burns: Prevention of its acquisition by chlorpromazine. Burns 9:387–393, 1983.
102. Pirani CL, Levenson SM: Effect of vitamin C deficiency on healed wounds. Proc Soc Exp Biol Med 82:95–99, 1953.
103. Meyer E, Meyer MB: The pathology of staphylococcus abscesses in vitamin C deficient guinea pigs. Johns Hopkins Hosp Bull 74:98–110, 1944.
104. Bartlett MK, Jones CM, Ryan AE: Vitamin C and wound healing. II. Ascorbic acid content and tensile strength of healing wounds in human beings. N Engl J Med 226:474–481, 1942.
105. Lund CC, Levenson SM, Green RW, et al: Ascorbic acid, thiamine, riboflavin, and nicotinic acid in relation to acute burns in man. Arch Surg 55:557–583, 1947.
106. Levenson SM, Green RW, Taylor FHL, et al: Ascorbic acid, riboflavin, thiamin and nicotinic acid in relation to severe injury, hemorrhage and infection in the human. Ann Surg 124:840–856, 1946.
107. Levenson SM, Upjohn HL, Preston JA, et al: Effect of thermal burns on wound healing. Ann Surg 146:357–368, 1957.
108. Rivers JM: Safety of high-level vitamin C injection. Ann NY Acad Sci 498:445–454, 1987.
109. Wolbach SB, Howe PR: Tissue changes following deprivation of fat-soluble A vitamin. J Exp Med 42:753–757, 1925.
110. Brandaleone H, Papper E: The effect of the local and oral administration of cod liver oil on the rate of wound healing in vitamin A deficient and normal animals. Ann Surg 114:791–798, 1941.
111. Ehrlich HP, Hunt TK: Effects of cortisone and vitamin A on wound healing. Ann Surg 167:324–328, 1968.
112. Ehrlich HP, Tarvet H, Hunt TK: Effects of vitamin A and glucocorticoids upon inflammation and collagen synthesis. Ann Surg 177:222–227, 1973.
113. Hunt TK: Control of wound healing with cortisone and vitamin A. In Longacre JJ (ed): The Ultrastructure of Collagen. Springfield, IL, Charles C Thomas, 1976, pp 497–503.
114. Lee KH, Tong TG: Studies on the mechanism of action of salicylates. VI. Effect of topical application of retinoic acid on wound-healing retardation action of salicylic acid. J Pharmacol Sci 58:773–774, 1969.
115. Demetriou AA, Seifter E, Levenson SM: Effect of vitamin A and citral on peritoneal adhesion formation. J Surg Res 17:325–329, 1974.
116. Seifter E, Crowley LV, Rettura G, et al: Influence of vitamin A on wound healing in rats with femoral fracture. Ann Surg 181:836–841, 1975.
117. Niu XT, Cushin B, Reisner A, et al: Effect of dietary supplementation with vitamin A on arterial healing in rats. J Surg Res 42:61–65, 1987.
118. Barbul A, Thysen B, Rettura G, et al: White cells' involvement in the inflammatory, wound healing, and immune actions of vitamin A. J Parent Enter Nutr 2:129–140, 1978.
119. Seifter E, Rettura G, Padawer J, et al: Impaired wound healing in streptozotocin diabetes: Prevention by supplemental vitamin A. Ann Surg 194:42–50, 1981.
120. Seifter E, Rettura G, Stratford F, et al: Vitamin A inhibits some aspects of systemic disease due to local X-radiation. J Parent Enter Nutr 5:288–294, 1981.
121. Levenson SM, Gruber CA, Rettura G, et al: Supplemental vitamin A prevents the acute radiation-induced defect in wound healing. Ann Surg 200:494–512, 1984.
122. Seifter E, Rettura G, Padawer J, et al: Morbidity and mortality reduction by supplemental vitamin A or beta carotene in CBA mice given total-body gamma radiation. J Natl Cancer Inst 73:1167–1177, 1984.
123. Mahmood T, Tenenbaum S, Niu XT, et al: Prevention of duodenal ulcer formation in the rat by dietary vitamin A supplementation. J Parent Enter Nutr 10:74–77, 1986.
124. Weinzweig J, Levenson SM, Weinzweig B, et al: Supplemental vitamin A prevents the tumor induced defect in wound healing. Ann Surg 211:269–276, 1990.
125. Demetriou AA, Levenson SM, Rettura G, et al: Vitamin A and retinoic acid: Induced fibroblast differentiation in vitro. Surgery 98:931–934, 1985.
126. Greenwald DP, Sharzer LA, Padawer J, et al: Zone II flexor tendon repair: Effects of vitamins A, E, beta-carotene. J Surg Res 49:98–102, 1990.
127. Chernov MS, Hale HW, Wood M: Prevention of stress ulcers. Am J Surg 122:674–677, 1971.
128. Chytil F, Ong DE: Cellular retinol- and retinoic acid–binding proteins in vitamin A action. Fed Proc 38:2510–2514, 1979.
129. Omori M, Chytil F: Mechanism of vitamin A action: Gene expression in retinol-deficient rats. J Biol Chem 257:14370–14374, 1982.
130. Olson JA: Vitamin A, retinoids, and carotenoids. In Shils ME, Young VR (eds): Modern nutrition in health and disease. Philadelphia, Lea & Febiger, 1988, pp 328–339.
131. Jetten AM: Modulation of cell growth by retinoids and their possible mechanisms of action. Fed Proc 43:134–139, 1984.
132. DeLuca LM, Bhat PV, Sasak W, et al: Biosynthesis of phosphoryl and glycosyl phosphoryl derivatives of vitamin A in biological membranes. Fed Proc 38:2535–2539, 1979.
133. Fell HB, Thomas L: Comparison of the effects of papain and vitamin A on cartilage. J Exp Med 111:719–744, 1940.
134. Rai K, Courtemanche AJ: Vitamin A assay in burned patients. J Trauma 15:419–424, 1975.
135. Moody BJ: Changes in the serum concentrations of thyroxine-binding pre-albumin and retinol binding protein following burn injury. Clin Chim Acta 118:87–92, 1982.
136. Ramsden DB, Prince HP, Burr WA, et al: The interrelationship of thyroid hormones, vitamin A, and their binding proteins following acute stress. Clin Endocrinol 8:109–122, 1978.
137. Kuroiwa K, Trocki O, Alexander JW, et al: Effect of vitamin A in enteral formulae for burned guinea pigs. Burns 16:265–272, 1990.
138. Underwood BA, Siegel H, Wzisell RC, et al: Liver stores of vitamin A in normal population dying suddenly or rapidly from unnatural causes in New York City. Am J Clin Nutr 23:1037–1042, 1970.
139. Mendez J, Scrimshaw NS, Salvado C, et al: Effects of

artificially induced fever on serum protein, vitamin levels, and hematological values in human subjects. J Appl Physiol 14:768–770, 1959.

140. Kagan BM, Kaiser E: Vitamin A metabolism in infections. Effect of sterile abscesses in rat on serum and tissue vitamin A. J Nutr 57:277–286, 1955.

141. Rettura G, Smoke R, Schitteck A, et al: Stress depletes thymic vitamin A. Am Chem Soc 172nd Nat Meeting, Sept. 1976, AGFD #67.

142. Clark I, Colburn RW: A relationship between vitamin A metabolism and cortisone. Endocrinology 56:232–238, 1955.

143. Atukorala TMS, Basu TK, Dickerson JWT: Effect of corticosterone on the plasma and tissue concentrations of vitamin A in rats. Ann Nutr Metab 25:234–238, 1981.

144. Seifter E, Rettura G, Seifter J, et al: Thymotropic action of vitamin A. Fed Proc 32:947, 1973 (abstract).

145. Seifter E, Rettura G, Makman L, et al: Supplemental vitamin A moderates catecholamine toxicity. Soc Parent Enter Nutr, Las Vegas, Jan 29–Feb 1, 1984.

146. Levenson SM, Rettura G, Seifter E, et al: Unpublished observations.

147. Milner JA, Visek WJ: Orotic aciduria and arginine deficiency. Nature 245:211–213, 1973.

148. Barbul A, Thysen B, Rettura G, et al: White cell involvement in the inflammatory wound healing and immune actions of vitamin A. J Parent Enter Nutr 2:129–138, 1978.

149. Jurin M, Tannock IF: Influence of vitamin A on immunologic response. Immunology 23:283–287, 1972.

150. Medawar PB, Hunt R: Anti-cancer action of retinoids. Immunology 42:349–353, 1981.

151. Malkovsky M, Medawar PB, Hunt R, et al: A diet enriched in vitamin A acetate or in vivo administration of interleukin-2 can counteract a toleragenic stimulus. Proc R Soc Lond Biol 220:439–445, 1984.

152. Seifter E, Rettura G, Levenson SM, et al: A mechanism of action of vitamin A in immunogenic tumor systems. Curr Chemother Proc, 10th Int Cong Chemother, vol II, 1290–1291, 1978.

153. Kalimi M, Rettura G, Barbul A, et al: Stress increases glucocorticoid receptor proteins in rats—vitamin A prevents this. Fed Proc 37:708, 1978 (abstract).

154. Faruque SM, Bashar SA: Effect of vitamin-A deficiency on plaque forming response of antibody producing spleen cells against Salmonella typhimurium in rats. Bangladesh Med Res Counc Bull 9:37–42, 1983.

155. Parent G, Rousseaux-Prevost R, Carlier Y, et al: Influence of vitamin A on the immune response of Schistosoma mansoni–infected rats. Trans R Soc Trop Med Hyg 78:380–383, 1984.

156. Cohen BE, Cohen IK: Vitamin A: Adjuvant and steroid antagonist in the immune response. J Immunol 111:1376–1380, 1973.

157. Athanassiades TJ: Adjuvant effect of vitamin A palmitate and analogs on cell-mediated immunity. J Natl Cancer Inst 67:1153–1156, 1981.

158. Pletsityvi KD, Askerov MA: Ovliianii vitamina A na immunogenez (Effect of vitamin A on immunogenesis). Vopr Pitan 11:38–40, 1982 (English abstract).

159. Tachibana K, Sone S, Tsubura E, et al: Stimulatory effect of vitamin A on tumoricidal activity of rat alveolar macrophages. Br J Cancer 49:343–348, 1984.

160. Cohen BE, Elin RJ: Enhanced resistance to certain infections in vitamin A treated mice. J Plast Reconstr Surg 54:192–194, 1974.

161. Levine NS, Salisbury RE, Seifter E, et al: Effects of vitamin A on tumor development in burned, un-

burned and glucocorticoid treated mice inoculated with an oncogene virus. Experientia 31:1309–1312, 1975.

162. Seifter E, Rettura G, Padawer J, et al: Anti-pyretic and anti-viral action of vitamin A in Moloney sarcoma and pox-virus-inoculated mice. J Natl Cancer Inst 57:355–359, 1976.

163. Demetriou AA, Franco I, Rettura G, et al: Effect of vitamin A and beta-carotene on intraabdominal sepsis. Arch Surg 119:161–165, 1984.

164. Fusi S, Kupper TS, Green DR: Reversal of postburn immunosuppression by administration of vitamin A. Surgery 96:330–335, 1984.

165. Cohen BE, Gill G, Cullen PR, et al: Reversal of postoperative immunosuppression in man by vitamin A. Surg Gynecol Obstet 149:658–662, 1979.

166. Smith JC, Brown EI, McDaniel EG, et al: Alterations in vitamin A metabolism during zinc deficiency and food and growth restriction. J Nutr 106:569–574, 1976.

167. Beisel WR, Pekarek RS, Wannemacher RW Jr: Homeostatic mechanics affecting plasma zinc levels in acute stress. In Prasad AS (ed): Trace Elements in Human Health and Disease. Zinc and Copper, vol I. New York, Academic Press, 1976.

168. Multivitamin preparation for parenteral use. A statement by the Nutrition Advisory Group, American Medical Association, Department of Foods and Nutrition. J Parent Enter Nutr 3:258–262, 1979.

169. Jeppson B, Fischer JE: Nutritional support of the burn patient. In Hummel RP (ed): Clinical Burn Therapy. A Management and Prevention Guide. John Wright, PSG, Inc, Boston, 1982, Chapter 14, pp 321–334.

170. Levenson SM, Hopkins BS, Waldron M, et al: Vitamin requirements of seriously injured patients with and without sepsis. In Fischer JE (ed): Relevance of Nutrition to Sepsis. Ross Laboratories, Columbus, Ohio, 1982, pp 111–116.

171. Malkovsky M, Hunt R, Palmer L, et al: Retinyl acetate–mediated augmentation of resistance to a transplantable 3-methylcholenthrene–induced fibrosarcoma. Transplantation 38:158–161, 1984.

172. Meyskens FJ Jr: Vitamin A and synthetic derivatives (retinoids) in the prevention and treatment of human cancer. In Butterworth CB, Hutchinson ML (eds): Nutritional Factors in the Induction and Maintenance of Malignancy. Academic Press, New York, 1983, pp 206–216.

173. Seifter E, Rettura G, Padawer J, et al: Vitamin A and beta carotene as adjunctive therapy to tumor excision, radiation therapy, and chemotherapy. In Prasad KN (ed): Vitamins, Nutrition and Cancer. Basel, Karger Press, 1984, pp 1–19.

174. Gallop PM, Lian JB, Hawschka PV: Carboxylated and calcium-binding protein and vitamin K. N Engl J Med 302:1460–1466, 1980.

175. Ehrlich HP, Tarver H, Hunt TK: Inhibitory effects of vitamin E on collagen synthesis and wound repair. Ann Surg 175:235–240, 1972.

176. Kagoma P, Burger SN, Seifter E, et al: The effect of vitamin E on experimentally induced peritoneal adhesions in mice. Arch Surg 120:949–951, 1985.

177. Bark S, Rettura G, Seifter E, et al: Effect of supplemental vitamin E on skin allograft survival in mice. Fed Proc 42:811–812, 1983.

178. Solomons NW: Zinc and Copper. In Shills ME, Young VR (eds): Modern Nutrition in Health and Disease. Philadelphia, Lea & Febiger, 1988, pp 238–262.

179. Todd WR, Elvehjem CA, Hart EB: Zinc in nutrition of rat. Am J Physiol 107:146–156, 1934.

180. Vallee BL: Metabolic role of zinc. Report of Council on Foods and Nutrition. JAMA 162:1053–1057, 1956.

181. Chvapil M: Zinc and Wound Healing. In Zederfeldt B (ed): Symposium on Zinc. Lund, Sweden, AB Tika, 1974.
182. Sobocinski PZ, Canterbury WJ Jr, Mapes CA, et al: Involvement of hepatic metallothionines in hypozincemia associated with bacterial infection. Am J Physiol 234:E399–E406, 1978.
183. Sternlieb I, Fisher M, Scheinberg IH: Penicillamine induced skin lesions. J Rheumatol 8(suppl):149–154, 1981.
184. Nimni ME: Mechanism of collagen cross-linking by penicillamine. Proc R Soc Med 70(suppl):65–72, 1977.
185. Geever EF, Youssef SA, Seifter E, et al: Penicillamine and wound healing in young guinea pigs. J Surg Res 6:160–166, 1967.
186. Ragan C, Howes EL, Plotz CM, et al: The effect of ACTH and cortisone on connective tissue. Bull NY Acad Med 26:251–259, 1950.
187. Sandberg N: Time relationship between administration of cortisone and wound healing in rats. Acta Chir Scand 127:446–455, 1964.
188. Peacock EE Jr: Wound Repair, 3rd ed. Philadelphia, WB Saunders, 1984, pp 130–133.
189. Aszodi A, Ponsky JL: Effects of corticosteroid on the healing bowel anastomosis. Am Surg 50:546–548, 1984.
190. Lattes R, Martin JR, Ragan C: Suppression of cortisone effect on repair in the presence of local bacterial infection. Am J Pathol 30:901–911, 1954.
191. Baker BL, Whitaker WL: Interference with wound healing by the local actions of adrenocortical steroids. Endocrinology 46:544–551, 1950.
192. Alexander MV, Zajtchuk JT, Henderson RL: Hypothyroidism and wound healing: Occurrence after head and neck radiation and surgery. Arch Otolaryngol 108:289–291, 1982.
193. Lupulescu A, Habowsky J: Effects of calcitonin on epidermal regeneration and collagen synthesis in rabbits with experimental wounds. Exp Pathol 16:291–302, 1978.
194. Schatzker J, Chapman M, Ha'Eri GB, et al: The effect of calcitonin on fracture healing. Clin Orthop 141:303–306, 1979.
195. Stanisstreet M: Calcium and wound healing in Xenopus early embryos. J Embryol Exp Morphol 67:195–205, 1982.
196. Andreen O, Larsson SE: Effects of parathyroidectomy and vitamin D on fracture healing. Acta Orthop Scand 54:805–809, 1983.
197. Hubbard GB, Schmidt RE, Gleiser CA, et al: Effects of hyperparathyroidism and dietary calcium supplementation on bone healing. Am J Vet Res 40:288–293, 1979.
198. Prudden JF, Nishihara G, Ocampo L: Studies on growth hormone. III. The effect on wound tensile strength of marked postoperative anabolism induced with growth hormone. Surg Gynec Obstet 107:481–482, 1958.
199. Mikkonan L, Lampiaho K, Kuloneu E: Effect of thyroid hormones, somatotropin, insulin and corticosteroids on synthesis of collagen in granulation tissue both in vivo and in vitro. Acta Endocrinol 51:23–26, 1966.
200. Jiang Z, He G, Zhang S, et al: Low-dose growth hormone and hypocaloric nutrition. Ann Surg 210:513–525, 1989.
201. Wilmore DW: Unpublished observations.
202. Zaizen Y, Ford EG, Costin G, et al: The effect of postoperative exogenous growth hormone on wound bursting strength in normal and malnourished rats. J Pediatr Surg 25:70–74, 1990.
203. Zaizen Y, Ford EG, Costin G, et al: Stimulation of wound bursting strength during protein malnutrition. J Surg Res 49:333–336, 1990.
204. Belcher HJ, Ellis H: Somatotropin and wound healing after injury. J Clin Endocrinol Metab 70:939–943, 1990.
205. Kirkeby OJ, Ekeland A: No effect of systemic administration of somatomedin C on bone repair in rats. Acta Orthop Scand 61:335–338, 1990.
206. Herndon DN, Barrow RE, Kunkel KR, et al: Effect of recombinant human growth hormone on donor-site healing in severely burned children. Ann Surg 212:424–429, 1990.

16

WOUND MICROENVIRONMENT

Thomas K. Hunt, M.D., and Zamir Hussain, Ph.D.

Each normal tissue has a characteristic microenvironment in which the metabolic needs of its cells are met and through which functional signals may be sent. Although most tissues can retain their essential form despite a variety of insults, certain kinds of environmental change initiate a healing, fibrotic process.

Surgery provides two major examples of this phenomenon. Epithelial surface injury removes a protective cell layer, exposes underlying tissue to desiccation, and incites a regenerative process in the residual epithelium. Equally important, and more common, is the general category of microvascular injury, which includes injury and infarct. This injury severely changes the local environment, which leads to regeneration of the microvasculature. This reconstitution of the microvasculature is but one component of the wound healing response that also includes the deposition of new connective tissue leading to a "scar."

When microvessels are divided or flow is stopped due to thrombosis or proximal vascular injury, a metabolic crisis ensues in which hypoxia and acidosis are prominent. This may lead to death of severely affected cells and to profound metabolic changes in others. In addition, both cell death and local mechanical injury activate a variety of chemoattractant signals. Leukocytes then marginate on injured endothelial cells and subsequently migrate into this already deprived environment, accentuating the metabolic problem.

At first, coagulation, with its mixture of fibrin, trapped erythrocytes, platelets, and assorted components of the coagulation cascade, dominates the environment and becomes the first signal to repair. Fibrin degradation products are chemoattractants for tissue macrophages, and fibrin itself subsequently "activates" them. For instance, injection of fibrin into poorly vascularized tissues such as the cornea is sufficient in itself to produce a monocytic inflammation and subsequent "wound healing," with angiogenesis and scar formation.[1]

CELLULAR ACTIVITY IN THE WOUND ENVIRONMENT

The first reparative "cells" to appear in most wounds are platelets, which release a number of substances that are capable of initiating a repair process. These include platelet-derived growth factor (PDGF),[2] platelet factor IV,[3] insulin-like growth factor-1 (IGF-1),[4] transforming growth factor-β (TGF-β),[5] and an uncharacterized chemoattractant to endothelial cells.[6] (Numerous chapters in this book discuss the biological effects of these growth factors, particularly Chapter 14.) Since hemorrhage is limited by coagulation, the supply of platelet substances may be limited to a few days following injury. Nevertheless, it seems fair to assume that repair starts as platelets release their granules. How much longer the platelets may contribute to the healing process is not clear.

The second set of cells, polymorphonuclear leukocytes, migrate into wounds largely under the direction of complement factors. As shown by Stein and Levenson, however, elimination of granulocytes does not materially affect wound repair except insofar as it detracts from local immunity and increases susceptibility to infection.[7]

The third wave of cells consists of monocytes, particularly macrophages, which are attracted to injured tissue by platelet factors, complement, and fibrinopeptides. These multipotent cells appear to be the major directors of subsequent repair and remain dominant in wounds until repair stops.[8] Macrophages are multipotential cells that release a large number of substances, including growth factors, in response to external stimuli.[9] Inasmuch as they are mobile, characteristically present in wounds, react to disturbed environmental conditions, and secrete a variety of growth factors, chemoattractants, and proteolytic enzymes, macrophages appear to have the capacities to detect and interpret environmental changes and to elicit repair phenomena in response.

If macrophages are as important to repair as they seem, it should be possible to determine "specific" stimuli that elicit reparative behavior. Their absence or inaction might also lead to the cessation of repair. Macrophages exposed to fibrin elicit components of repair when injected into rabbit corneas.[8] However, repair persists past the initial deposition of fibrin in wounds, and therefore it seems realistic to postulate that other environmental factors also stimulate macrophages. Likely candidates are the hypoxia and high lactate levels that characterize the wound environment, and exposure to them does in fact elicit a growth factor response as will be detailed later. This construct is appealing because, if true, it can explain why empty spaces in wounds continue to heal until they are filled despite the fact that injured tissue and products of coagulation are removed long before healing is complete.

STUDIES OF THE WOUND ENVIRONMENT

Measurements of wound extracellular fluid taken soon after injury show decreasing P_{O_2}, increasing P_{CO_2}, and decreasing pH. These approach 10 torr, 80 torr, and 6.8, respectively, and then slowly return toward normal blood values as the wound space closes. Lactate concentration rises from 1 mM blood levels to 5 to 15 mM. While wound fluid electrolytes remain approximately the same as blood,[10] the protein electrophoretic pattern changes somewhat with an increase in α_1-globulins. Glucose levels are lower than serum, reaching 1 or 2 mM in focal areas.[11]

The type of cells floating in the extracellular fluid that collect in wounds change quickly from fat and cell debris to granulocytes and then more slowly to macrophages, which predominate after about a week or so, and then to lymphocytes. The granulocytes are "primed" in the sense that their capacity to generate superoxide radicals in response to a single new stimulus is increased.[12] Wound macrophages are also clearly "activated" and release a number of substances including angiogenesis factor, large amounts of lactate, collagenase, interleukin-1, a PDGF-like substance, TGF-β and probably numerous other substances.

The wound microenvironment has been shown to contain a number of growth promoters, including TGF-β,[13] interleukins (IL-6 and perhaps others),[14] IGF-1, and insulin.[15] Epidermal growth factor (EGF), IL-2, and fibroblast growth factor (FGF) have not been detected in wounds, but it is probably safe to assume that they, or active fragments thereof, pass through them.

Questions obviously arise about how growth substances arrive there. Even though macrophages release many of them, the full answer is far from clear. Obviously, PDGF can be deposited in wounds by platelets, but the nature of the PDGF-like activity that persists in wound fluid has only partially been characterized.[16] (Other chapters will develop this topic.) IGF-1 probably derives from blood and fibroblasts as well as from platelets.

Insulin levels in wounds are very low, while IGF-1 levels approximate those of plasma.[15] The low insulin level obviously indicates that insulin (and IGF-1 as well) is actively destroyed in the healing tissue and probably that IGF-1 is actively released there.

The amino acid content of wound fluid reflects, and may to some extent influence, metabolic events. At first, amino acid concentrations are close to those of serum. Thereafter, they approach the amino acid content of inflammatory cells, perhaps as a result of rapid leukocyte turnover. Though little is known of the details, the fluid also contains lysosomal enzymes, superoxide dismutase, and some superoxide. There is clearly some traffic between phagosomes, lysosomes, and the extracellular space. In time, the concentration of most amino acids, in particular glutamine and glutamate, rises well over that of serum. However, arginine concentration falls to very low levels because it is rapidly consumed; some is converted to ornithine by arginase and some to citrulline by nitric oxide synthetase with the release of nitric oxide. This is intriguing because nitric oxide is a powerful vasodilator and also influences mitochondrial function. Ingestion of large amounts of arginine increases collagen deposition in human wounds[17] without influencing arginine levels in wound fluid. The effect, therefore, might theoretically involve growth hormone and IGF-1, various aspects of immune function, mitochondrial respiration, and local blood perfusion, or it may merely reflect the increased availability of arginine for protein synthesis and cell cycling. Low arginine levels appear to activate macrophages.[18]

It should be emphasized that wounds contain a number of microenvironments. However, there can be little doubt that their sum is conducive to the replication of fibroblasts and endothelial cells since many cells grow faster in wound fluid than in serum.[19]

To explore the significance of the local environment, a useful method is to limit the thickness of the wound space. This is easily done in rabbit ear chambers (Fig. 16–1) in which healing tissue is displayed in a transparent chamber that can be mounted on a microscope and thus examined in the intact animal. The thinnest space that will allow healing is about 50 μ, only enough for one or two cells to pass at one time. This size requires that wound cells progress

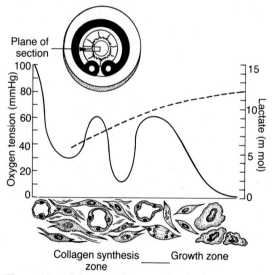

Figure 16–1. Schematic diagram of cell relationships in rabbit ear chamber wounds. The cells to the right next to the wound space are always macrophages. Fibroblasts replicate (apparently) in the "growth zone," with the young cells "pushed" toward the wound space. Collagen in the growth zone is amorphous. Visible collagen fibers separate the fibroblasts in the "collagen synthesis zone." Note that most collagen seems to be made in fairly high levels of P_{O_2} and lactate. (From Hunt TK, van Winkle W Jr: Normal repair. In Hunt TK, Dunphy JE (eds): Fundamentals of Wound Management. New York, Appleton-Century-Crofts, 1979, p 55.)

into the space in a coherent order, leaders first, and reparative cells do in fact align themselves in a characteristic order in these chambers. Figure 16–1 indicates that order and shows the characteristic oxygen tensions and lactate concentrations measured by microprobes.[20] Cells normally respond to a "pull" rather than a "push," and this implies that the first cells in that order, macrophages, actively lead the others. It further implies that the spatial arrangement of cells somehow creates an environment that is favorable to angiogenesis and collagen deposition. Granulocytes, red cells, and fibrin appear first in the wound space. Macrophages soon follow, and in a few days fibroblasts and collagenous reparative tissue appear, led by a thin layer of macrophages followed by fibroblasts lying in a gelatinous (nonfibrillar) extracellular matrix. Just behind this layer are a few youthful fibroblasts, some in mitosis. Regenerating vessels follow and are quite dense, forming a 1 to 2 mm hyperemic layer. Back from the zone of dense angiogenesis, blood vessels become larger and less dense, apparently as a result of enlargement or coalescence of a few channels, with the remainder having dropped out of the flow patterns. Between these vessels lie mature fibroblasts and new fibrillar collagen.

The few dividing fibroblasts always occupy the same location, just ahead of the regenerating vessel, where the P_{O_2} is optimal for replication (about 40 torr). It seems logical to deduce that the mitotic zone behaves as a growth point and that new fibroblasts that are generated at that spot remain there, to be overtaken by the advancing neovasculature and incorporated into the zone of fibrillar collagen. In other words, fibroblasts seem to be born in one environment and eventually deposit mature collagen in another. Macrophages, on the other hand, seem to remain as leaders just ahead of all other cells.

This progression, first noted 20 years ago, suggested certain hitherto unsuspected roles for the various cells as well as certain functions for their environment. For instance, macrophages are facultative cells that seem in their many roles to flourish in impoverished surroundings. Their position in this procession suggested that they release large amounts of lactate, and in vitro testing demonstrated that they do so almost regardless of oxygen tension. They also appear to lead angiogenesis. When isolated and placed in environments equally hypoxic and/or hyperlactated as wound extracellular fluid, macrophages release a substance that is a chemoattractant for vascular endothelial cells and a stimulant for angiogenesis when implanted into normal corneas.[21, 22] The mechanism responsible for this stimulation is not fully understood; however, lactate alone causes macrophages to release the angiogenic substance, and the lactate effect is blocked by oxamate, which inhibits lactate dehydrogenase and thus prevents conversion of nicotinamide adenine dinucleotide (NAD^+) to reduced NAD^+ or NADH. One consequence of the lowered NAD^+ in wound macrophages exposed to lactate is a decrease in its metabolite, adenosine diphosphoribose (ADPR) and its polymers (PADPR), which are known to control the activities of a number of enzymes and nuclear transcriptional events.[23] Therefore, angiogenesis may be regulated by ADPR in a manner similar to the regulation of collagen synthesis, as will be outlined below.

Macrophages both release large amounts of lactate and respond to high concentrations of it. A logical extension of this observation is that having made their way into the wound environment, macrophages continue the initial momentum of wound healing by stimulating angiogenesis, and the resultant restoration of tissue perfusion may provide a means to clear lactate and provide oxygen, thus down-regulating macrophage activity and thereby contributing to the suppression of repair when healing approaches completion.

CONTROL OF COLLAGEN SYNTHESIS

The combination of gradients of both oxygen tension and lactate is also a fortuitous environment for collagen synthesis and deposition. The ear chamber studies show that fibroblasts replicate in one environment and make collagen in a different one.[11] The optimum PO_2 for replication is 30 to 40 torr, while that for collagen synthesis may be far higher, probably about 200 torr (see below).

Several groups of investigators, starting with Green and Goldberg in 1964, noted that periods of hypoxia or exposure to high lactate concentrations increase the capacity of fibroblasts to synthesize collagen when they are subsequently placed in oxygenated environments.[24-26] Investigations from our laboratory led us to suggest that lactate stimulates collagen synthesis via at least two separate mechanisms. First, recent experiments suggest that lactate induces an increase in procollagen mRNAs (unpublished observations). We hypothesize that collagen gene transcription in fibroblasts is normally down-regulated by polyADP-ribose (PADPR) in the resting state and that accumulation of

lactate decreases PADPR levels by depleting intracellular NAD^+, the source of ADPR. In support of this hypothesis, inhibitors of PADPR synthetase also increase collagen gene transcription (Fig. 16–2). Additionally, the effect of lactate is blocked by oxamate, which binds the active site of lactate dehydrogenase and prevents the reduction of NAD^+.[27]

Independent of its stimulatory action on procollagen mRNA levels, lactate also increases the activity of prolyl hydroxylase, a crucial enzyme in collagen biosynthesis. This activation effect appears to be mediated by removal of an inhibitor of the enzyme, ADPR or its metabolite.[27] As shown in Figure 16–2, these observations suggest an interesting scenario for the lactate effect on collagen synthesis. A high concentration of lactate lowers the normal intracellular NAD^+ level, decreasing the level of ADP-ribosylation products. Thus, lower levels of PADPR in the nucleus result in enhanced production of transcriptional products (procollagen mRNAs) that are translated into an increased level of unhydroxylated collagen peptides. Concurrently, lower levels of ADP-ribose in the cytoplasm activate prolyl hydroxylase, thereby ensuring full hydroxylation of these collagen peptides. Thus, by modulating ADP-ribosylation, lactate may act as a dual signal to "turn on" collagen synthesis for wound repair. Activation also increases the need for higher oxygen and ascorbate concentrations. If they are supplied, collagen deposition proceeds at higher rates, as will be explained later.

Lactate concentration in test wounds is greatest in the central space and persists well into the zone of fibrillar collagen synthesis (see Figure 16–1). Presumably, therefore, as the new vessels overtake the immature fibroblasts and change their environment from high lactate and low PO_2 to high lactate and high PO_2, they increase both their collagen synthesis and their deposition. Once the integrity of the vascular system reaches the point at which lactate can be removed as rapidly as it is produced, the impetus to neovascularization and collagen synthesis should also diminish, as it seems to do.

Other aspects of the extracellular environment may also perpetuate repair and may be seen either as alternative hypotheses or as additional mechanisms. For instance, numerous studies have shown that regenerating vasculature is more than normally permeable to large molecules. This may lead to local accumulation of fibrin and thus assure continued stimulation of macrophages, lactate production, and "programming" of newly generated fibroblasts in the hypoxic and lactated extracellular fluid.

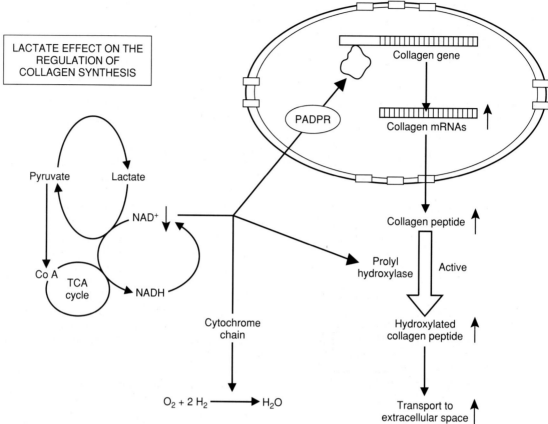

LACTATE EFFECT ON THE
REGULATION OF
COLLAGEN SYNTHESIS

Collagen gene

PADPR

Collagen mRNAs

Pyruvate   Lactate

NAD^+ ↓

Co A

TCA
cycle

NADH

Collagen peptide ↑

Prolyl
hydroxylase   Active

Cytochrome
chain

Hydroxylated
collagen peptide ↑

$O_2 + 2 H_2 \longrightarrow H_2O$

Transport to
extracellular space ↑

Figure 16–2. Lactate effect on the regulation of collagen synthesis. Normally, PADPR enables a putative nuclear protein to bind to a collagen transcription component as well as inhibits prolyl hydroxylase. Lactate lowers PADPR, releases these inhibitions, and thus allows stimulated mRNA synthesis and prolyl hydroxylase activation.

In summary, a variety of studies have outlined the changing extracellular environment of healing wounds. The responses of isolated fibroblasts and macrophages with respect to the presence or absence of fibrin, oxygen, lactate, amino acids, and growth factors are, at least in theory, congruent with the behavior of these cells during wound healing.

OXYGEN TENSION IN WOUNDS

In addition to the data indicating that hypoxia, lactate, and "energy metabolism" play an important role in the assembly of the "module" of wound cells, there is considerable information that the partial pressure at which oxygen is delivered to the wound governs the rate of collagen deposition and development of tensile strength, even in normal adult wounds.[28–31] This at first seems contradictory to the idea that high lactate levels enhance collagen synthesis; however, lactate and oxygen concentrations in

wounds are essentially independent of one another. When the oxygen tension in the wound space is raised by allowing animals with wire mesh cylinders implanted subcutaneously to breathe 40% oxygen, their arterial PO_2 almost doubles, while wound space PO_2 rises only a few torr and lactate concentration falls only slightly.[10] Breathing an enriched oxygen mixture markedly steepens the oxygen gradient into the wound spaces.[32] It is axiomatic, therefore, that the added oxygen is consumed, i.e., oxygen consumption rises. Lactate concentration falls only slightly, presumably because the lead macrophages produce lactate aerobically as well as anaerobically. These oxygen and collagen data, developed in animals, have now been duplicated in surgical patients.[29, 33]

In wound healing, oxygen tension and oxygen supply must be considered as separate concepts. Collagenous tissue deposition in wounds is largely independent of the oxygen content of arterial blood; that is, it is unaffected by large changes in hematocrit and oxygen delivery.[33, 34]

This distinction between oxygen tension and

oxygen supply causes considerable confusion to clinicians who do not have a full understanding of the physiology of oxygen once it leaves blood and enters tissue. Contrary to the usual notion, the rate of a number of enzymes is dependent upon the concentration (i.e., the partial pressure) of oxygen. Several of these enzymes, such as (collagen) prolyl hydroxylase and (collagen) lysyl hydroxylase, are prominent in wound healing.

Prolyl hydroxylase is felt to be one of the rate-limiting enzymes in collagen synthesis. It hydroxylates prolines that are already incorporated into collagen (a similar enzyme hydroxylates collagen lysine) via a reaction involving the bivalent reduction of molecular oxygen. The rate of hydroxylation is dependent upon oxygen tension even at fairly high physiological levels. The Km (half maximal rate) of this enzyme with regard to oxygen tension is variously estimated at between 20 and 100 torr.[35, 36] This implies that hydroxylation is influenced by PO_2 in this range. When prolyl hydroxylase is deinhibited by falling concentrations of PADPR (see above), the effect of increasing local PO_2 intensifies. As mentioned, increased lactate decreases the level of nuclear PADPR and may enhance collagen gene transcription, with the sum of the lactate effect and high oxygen tension equaling increased collagen synthesis.

Oxygen tension in human as well as animal wounds depends on a variety of influences.[37] At normal rates of blood perfusion, wounds extract only about 1 ml of oxygen from each 100 ml of perfusing blood.[38] In contrast, working heart muscle extracts as much as 6 to 10 ml. The hemoglobin reservoir of oxygen in blood with a hematocrit as low as 20 is entirely adequate to maintain a high PO_2 as blood perfuses the *wound* capillaries. If only 1 volume of oxygen is removed from blood entering a tissue at a PO_2 of 100 and a hematocrit of 45, the PO_2 of venous blood draining from the wound will be above 75 torr. The PO_2 will fall to only 55 or 60 if hematocrit is lowered to 20 and the normal flow is maintained. However, the decreased viscosity of blood at low hematocrit and the well-known increased cardiac output that compensates for anemia can easily increase flow in wounds, thus preventing a drop in the PO_2 of venous blood.

On the other hand, when blood perfusion falls as a consequence of poor cardiac output, obstruction of regional blood supply, vasoconstriction, or any other reason, such as polycythemia, local oxygen tension will fall with it. When perfusion is critically impaired, the tissue oxygen tension will depend totally on oxygen delivery. Thus, while moderate anemia does not ordinarily interfere with the normal transfer of oxygen to wounds, impaired perfusion does. If perfusion is sufficiently impaired, no amount of arterial hyperoxia short of hyperbaric delivery will support PO_2 in wounds at adequate levels for healing or resistance to infection.

These concepts are powerful, and they demand a wider view of effects that have other more traditional explanations. For instance, as noted, high doses of arginine increase collagen deposition in test wounds in humans.[17] One can postulate various mechanisms (e.g., nutritional, immunological, endocrine), but one interesting possibility is that nitric oxide, thought to be the endothelial relaxing factor (ERF), is generated from arginine. One result of increased arginine might well be an increase in wound blood flow and therefore PO_2 but this idea has not yet been tested.

OXYGEN REGULATES RESISTANCE TO INFECTION

Oxygen in the wound extracellular environment is also vital to another critical process in wounds: the intracellular killing of bacteria by granulocytes. Leukocytes marginate, migrate, attach to and ingest bacteria, apparently without need for oxygen. However, many and perhaps most of the important wound pathogens are killed, at least in major part, by a mechanism that requires molecular oxygen.

Phagocytosis activates a membrane-bound enzyme that reduces extracellular molecular oxygen to superoxide, which it inserts into phagosomes. Within phagosomes, an enzyme system converts superoxide to a number of high energy, bactericidal oxygen radicals without which bacterial killing is less than optimal. This system has been summarized in a number of publications[39, 40] and is diagrammed in Figure 16–3.

Numerous studies in normovolemic animals show that they clear bacteria from wounds in proportion to the fraction of oxygen in their breathing mixture. Infections become less invasive or fail to develop at all in hyperoxygenated guinea pigs when bacteria are injected into skin.[40] Infectious skin lesions in dogs are invasive in tissue with a mean extracellular fluid PO_2 of less than 60 torr, while they remain localized in better oxygenated tissue.[39]

Experience in humans tends to support these findings. Ironically, basic clinical observations

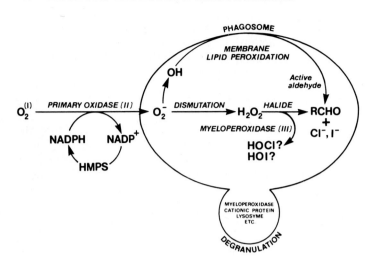

Figure 16–3. Schema of the oxidative bacteria-killing mechanism and its relation to the nonoxidative mechanism. Note that the first step is reduction of dissolved molecular oxygen. This step is rate-limiting if Po_2 falls below 30 torr. (From Hunt TK, van Winkle W Jr: Normal repair. In Hunt TK, Dunphy JE (eds): Fundamentals of Wound Management. New York, Appleton-Century-Crofts, 1979, p 85.)

that attest to the importance of this system have gone almost unnoticed by surgeons for hundreds of years. The capacity for well circulated and oxygenated tissues such as tongue, heart, and anus to resist wound infections is astounding when compared to that of less perfused tissues such as bone and the skin of the hands and feet.

CONCLUSION

Practicing surgeons depend heavily on the adequacy of the wound environment, and fortunately have a great deal of control over it. Studies of wounds in human patients have confirmed the essential hypoxia and high lactate in the wound space. The oxygen tension in test needle wounds in patients is a function of blood perfusion and of arterial Po_2.[33] These studies also show that repairing fluid deficits, correcting excessive autonomic nervous activity, and warming profoundly effect wound Po_2.

Arterial Po_2 is often measured in patients, but perfusion of connective tissue has not been a concern of most surgeons. Recent investigation has shown, however, that perfusion of connective tissue is highly sensitive to autonomic activity and is therefore severely impaired by hypovolemia, cold, pain, and fear. The result is that next to poor surgical technique and excessive bacterial contamination, impaired oxygen supply is probably the most frequent contributory cause of infection and defective repair in surgical patients. Simple clinical measures such as assuring pulmonary function, aggressively replacing fluids, and providing oxygen therapy, pain relief, and warmth can all be expected to add to the rate of repair and resistance of wounds to infection.

At the present time, the oxygen concentration in the wound environment is the only component that can be easily regulated on a clinical scale. New technology with respect to growth factors and stimulants to macrophages may provide other means of controlling repair. While this seems to promise new horizons, it is sobering to realize that surgical practice has not yet exhausted the potential that the recent findings in support of the wound environment have made possible.

References

1. Knighton DR, Hunt TK, Thakral K: Role of platelets and fibrin in the healing sequence. Ann Surg 196:379–388, 1982.
2. Deuel TF, Senior RM, Huang JS, et al: Chemotaxis of monocytes and neutrophils to platelet-derived growth factor. J Clin Invest 69:1046–1049, 1987.
3. Deuel TF, Senior RM, Chang D, et al: Platelet factor 4 is chemotactic for neutrophils and monocytes. Proc Nat Acad Sci USA 78:4584–4587, 1981.
4. Karey PK, Sirbasku DA: Human platelet-derived mitogens. II. Localization of insulin-like growth factor I to the alpha-granule and release in response to thrombin. Blood 74:1093–1100, 1989.
5. Assoian RK, Komoriya A, Myers CA, et al: Transforming growth factor-beta in human platelets. J Biol Chem 258:7155–7160, 1983.
6. Folkman J, Klagsbrun M: Angiogenesis factors. Science 235:442–447, 1987.
7. Stein JM, Levenson SM: Effect of the inflammatory reaction on subsequent wound healing. Surg Forum 17:484–485, 1966.
8. Hunt TK, Knighton DR, Thakral KK: Studies on inflammation and wound healing. Angiogenesis and collagen synthesis stimulated in vivo by resident and activated wound macrophages. Surgery 96:48–54, 1984.
9. Werb Z, Chin JR, Takemura R, et al: The cell and molecular biology of apolipropsoten E synthesis by macrophages. In Evered D, Nugent J, O'Connor M (eds): Biochemistry of Macrophages. Ciba Foundation Symposium 118, London, Pitman, 1986, pp 155–171.
10. Hunt TK, Conolly WB, Aronson SB: Anaerobic metabolism and wound healing. An hypothesis for the initi-

WOUND MICROENVIRONMENT 281

ation and cessation of collagen synthesis in wounds. Am J Surg 135:328–332, 1978.

11. Hunt TK, Banda MJ, Silver IA: Cell interactions in post-traumatic fibrosis. In Evered D, Whelan J (eds): Fibrosis. Ciba Foundation Symposium 114, London, Pitman, 1985, pp 127–129.

12. Paty PB, Graeff RW, Mathes FJ, et al: Superoxide production by wound neutrophils. Arch Surg 125:65–69, 1990.

13. Grotendorst GR, Grotendorst CA, Gilman T: Production of growth factors (PDGF and TGF-β) at the site of tissue repair. In Hunt TK, Pines E, Barbul A, et al (eds): Growth Factors and Other Aspects of Wound Healing. Biological and Clinical Implications. New York, Alan R. Liss, 1988, pp 1–17.

14. Ford HR, Hoffman RA, Wing EJ, et al: Characterization of wound cytokines in the sponge matrix model. Arch Surg 124:1422–1428, 1989.

15. Spencer EM, Skover G, Hunt TK: Somatomedins: Do they play a pivotal role in wound healing? In Hunt TK, Pines E, Barbul A, et al (eds): Growth Factors and Other Aspects of Wound Healing. Biological and Clinical Implications. New York, Alan R. Liss, 1988, pp 103–116.

16. Matsuoka J, Grotendorst GR: Two peptides related to platelet derived growth factor are found in human wound fluid. Proc Natl Acad Sci USA 86:4416–4420, 1989.

17. Barbul A, Lazarou SA, Efron DT, et al: Arginine enhances wound healing and lymphocyte immune responses in humans. Surgery 108:331–337, 1990.

18. Albina JE, Caldwell MD, Henry WL, et al: Regulation of macrophage functions by L-arginine. J Trauma 29:842–846, 1989.

19. Greenburg GB, Hunt TK: The proliferative response in vitro of vascular endothelial and smooth muscle cells exposed to wound fluids and macrophages. J Cell Physiol 97:353–360, 1978.

20. Silver IA: The physiology of wound healing. In Hunt TK (ed): Wound Healing and Wound Infection: Theory and Surgical Practice. New York, Appleton-Century-Crofts, 1980, pp 11–31.

21. Jensen JA, Hunt TK, Scheuenstuhl H: Effect of lactate, pyruvate and pH on secretion of angiogenesis and mitogenesis factors by macrophages. Lab Invest 54:574–578, 1986.

22. Banda MJ, Knighton DR, Hunt TK: Isolation of a nonmitogenic angiogenesis factor from wound fluid. Proc Nat Acad Sci USA 79:7773–7777, 1983.

23. Althaus FR, Richter C: ADP-ribosylation of proteins. Enzymology and biological significance. Mol Biol Biochem Biophys 37:3–230, 1987.

24. Green H, Goldberg B: Collagen and cell protein syn-thesis by an established mammalian fibroblast line. Nature 204:347–349, 1964.

25. Comstock JP, Udenfriend S: Effect of lactate on collagen proline hydroxylase activity in cultured L-929 fibroblasts. Proc Nat Acad Sci USA 66:552–557, 1970.

26. Levene CI, Bates CJ: The effect of hypoxia on collagen synthesis in cultured 3T6 fibroblasts and its relationship to the mode of action of ascorbate. Biochim Biophys Acta 444:446–452, 1976.

27. Hussain MZ, Ghani QP, Hunt TK: Inhibition of prolyl hydroxylase by poly(ADP-ribose) and phosphoribosyl-AMP. J Biol Chem 264:7850–7855, 1989.

28. Pai MP, Hunt TK: Effect of varying ambient oxygen tensions on wound metabolism and collagen synthesis. Surg Gynecol Obst 135:561–567, 1972.

29. Jonsson K, Jensen JA, Goodson WH, et al: Wound healing in subcutaneous tissue in surgical patients in relation to oxygen availability. Surg Forum 37:86–88, 1986.

30. Stephens FO, Hunt TK: Effects of changes in inspired oxygen and carbon dioxide tensions on wound tensile strength. Ann Surg 173:515–519, 1971.

31. Shandall A, Lowndes R, Young HL: Colonic anastomotic healing and oxygen tension. Brit J Surg 72:606–609, 1985.

32. Ehrlich HP, Grislis G, Hunt TK: Metabolic and circulatory contributions to oxygen gradients in wounds. Surgery 72:578–583, 1972.

33. Chang N, Goodson WH III, Gottrup F, et al: Direct measurement of wound and tissue oxygen tension in postoperative patients. Ann Surg 197:470–478, 1983.

34. Jensen JA, Goodson WH III, Vasconez LO, et al: Wound healing in anemia. West J Med 144:465–466, 1986.

35. Hutton JJ, Tappel AL, Udenfriend S: Cofactor and substrate requirements of collagen proline hydroxylase. Arch Biochem Biophys 118:239–240, 1967.

36. Myllyla R, Tuderman L, Kivirikko KI: Mechanism of the prolyl hydroxylase reaction. Kinetic analysis of the reaction sequences. Eur J Biochem 80:349–357, 1977.

37. Jonsson K, Jensen JA, Goodson WH III, et al: Assessment of perfusion in postoperative patients using tissue oxygen measurements. Brit J Surg 74:263–267, 1987.

38. Gottrup F, Firmin R, Rabkin J, et al: Directly measured tissue oxygen tension and arterial oxygen tension assess tissue perfusion. Crit Care Med 15:1030–1036, 1988.

39. Jonsson K, Hunt TK, Mathes SJ: Effect of environmental oxygen on bacterial induced tissue necrosis in flaps. Surg Forum 35:589–591, 1984.

40. Knighton DR, Halliday B, Hunt TK: Oxygen as an antibiotic: The effect of inspired oxygen on infection. Arch Surg 119:199–204, 1984.

17

ROLE OF THE IMMUNE SYSTEM

Adrian Barbul, M.D.

The immune system permits the host to recognize and eliminate foreign materials including bacteria and viruses, soluble proteins, and neoplastically altered autologous cells. It comprises a cellular compartment (neutrophils, monocytes/macrophages, lymphocytes) and a humoral component (immunoglobulins). The thymus, a lymphoepithelial organ containing both lymphocytes (thymocytes) and epithelial cells, regulates the development of T lymphocytes (thymus-dependent lymphocytes). It is the first lymphoid organ to develop during ontogeny and reaches its maximum size at puberty, after which there is continued involution and atrophy. It is organized into two compartments: The cortex, the larger of the two, contains numerous thymocytes, some epithelial cells, and a few macrophages. Through progressive migration from the cortex to the medulla, lymphocytes become differentiated into mature, immunocompetent cells. The medulla constitutes the other thymic compartment and contains small thymocytes that are considered mature and are in the process of leaving the gland. Maturation within the thymus is thought to be regulated by locally synthesized proteins or thymic hormones that are synthesized by the epithelial cells.

B lymphocytes (bone marrow–dependent lymphocytes), which maintain humoral immunity by synthesizing immunoglobulins, mature in avians in the bursa of Fabricius; no mammalian equivalent of this bursa has been defined. Recent evidence would suggest that B

lymphocyte maturation may occur within the fetal liver and bone marrow. The mature B cell does not secrete antibodies constitutively, but it can readily do so upon antigenic stimulation. During ontogeny both B and T lymphocytes populate peripheral lymphoid tissue such as spleen, lymph nodes, and the intestinal Peyer's patches.

T-cell populations are divided into multiple subsets depending upon the presence of differentiating surface antigens and their functional characteristics. It thus includes inducer cells, helper cells, cytotoxic cells, suppressor cells, and many other types. Functionally, T-helper cells are defined as those cells that facilitate B-cell responses to antigen or cytoxic lymphocyte development. Macrophages, but also other antigen-presenting cells such as endothelial cells, fibroblasts, or dendritic cells, present antigen to T-helper lymphocytes in association with class II MHC (major histocompatibility) antigens, which leads to activation and clonal expansion of this lymphocyte subset. T-suppressor cells have been defined by their ability to inhibit antibody production by B cells. T-suppressor cells are activated by antigen-presenting cells expressing class I MHC molecules. T-cell subpopulations are also involved in cell-mediated responses such as delayed-type hypersensitivity, contact sensitivity, and resistance to certain bacterial and viral infections. The activation and clonal expansion of T lymphocytes are dependent upon endogenous synthesis and release of effector molecules and proteins (lymphokines)[1] and also upon elaboration of macrophage-derived effector proteins (monokines). (A thorough description of these proteins is presented in Chapter 3).

This chapter was supported in part by NIH grant 1R29GM38650.

282

IMMUNE CELLS IN WOUNDS

Migration and Activation

Macrophages appear at the site of injury within 48 to 96 hours after wounding. Their first function is to participate in the inflammatory phase of wound healing that has to precede the fibroblastic phase. Macrophages then become the predominant cell prior to fibroblast migration and replication. It is during these phases of wound healing that macrophages play a major role in the events that lead to successful wound repair. There is evidence that macrophages become activated at the site of healing. Using electron microscopic criteria (presence of branching cytoplasmic processes and multilobulated nuclei or increased numbers of mitochondria, vacuoles and phagosomes), approximately 10 percent of wound-infiltrating macrophages were noted to be activated.[2] Using the simple yet elegant technique of polymerase chain reaction and amplification, Rappolee has shown that wound macrophages express messenger RNA (mRNA) for a variety of cytokines including transforming growth factor-α (TGF-α), TGF-β, and interleukin-1α (IL-1α).[3] Resting macrophages do not express mRNA for these cytokines, suggesting that wound macrophages become activated. However, more recent evidence indicates that enhanced mRNA induction does not always result in increased protein translation,[4] which is one limitation of this experimental approach. The other limitation of the polymerase chain reaction technique is that it provides qualitative data and does not yield much information regarding actual secretion or bioactivity of monokines at the wound site.

T lymphocytes migrate into wounds following the influx of inflammatory cells and macrophages. The ratio of T-helper to T-suppressor lymphocytes at the wound site is less than 1, much decreased in comparison to peripheral blood and lymph node subpopulation ratios.[5] Currently, there is no information regarding T-cell activation at the site of normal repair, with available evidence suggesting that T lymphocytes are actually down-regulated and suppressed at the wound site (see below).

Presence of Monokines and Lymphokines in Wounds

Another approach to the understanding of the role of immune cells in wound healing has been the direct study of the wound environment for the presence of monokines and lymphokines. Ford has demonstrated that biologically active IL-1, tumor necrosis factor/cachectin (TNF-α), and IL-6 are present at various times after injury in murine wound fluid.[6] Interestingly, the cytokines were present in the highest concentration in the early phase of wound healing (i.e., within the first three days), at a time when neutrophils are the predominant cell population. On the other hand, we have not been able to detect biologically active TNF-α or interferon-γ (IFN-γ) in 10 day old rat wound fluid.[7]

An IL-2 inhibitory factor[6, 8] has also been described that could play a role in down-regulating the exuberant cell proliferation and activity that characterizes the early phases of wound healing. Wound fluid also contains TGF-β, although the biological activity of the cytokine and its cellular origin (platelets, macrophage, or lymphocyte) have not been determined.[9]

ROLE OF MACROPHAGES IN WOUND HEALING

The crucial role of macrophages in wound healing was first demonstrated in vivo. Leibovich and Ross showed that guinea pigs treated with antimacrophage serum plus steroids (to remove circulating monocytes) had impaired wound debridement and fibroplasia.[10] Subsequently, injection of wound macrophages into rabbit corneas was shown to induce angiogenesis and scar formation,[11] while intradermal injections increased collagen synthesis and breaking strength in 8 day rat skin wounds.[12]

The major monokines released by activated macrophages are IL-1 and TNF-α. These monokines have a broad spectrum of biological effects on endothelial cells in vitro (Table 17–1) and thus may influence one of the earliest phases of wound healing, angiogenesis. Recently, it has been reported that TNF-α is the angiogenic factor secreted by wound macrophages.[29, 30] However, TNF-α has also been shown to be cytostatic for endothelial cells in vitro,[30, 32] so perhaps its angiogenic properties are more closely related to its proinflammatory effect.[46] This points out some of the difficulties in translating in vitro data to the in vivo situation. Nevertheless, the in vitro activities of IL-1 and TNF-α on endothelial cells are so diverse that it is likely that they play a role in modulating the angiogenic phase of wound healing.

Induce synthesis and surface expression of an
   adhesion molecule for leukocytes (IL-1, TNF-α)[13–18]†
Induce release of leukocyte adhesion inhibitor protein
   (IL-1, TNF-α)[19]
Induce synthesis and release of neutrophil chemotactic
   factor (IL-1, TNF-α)[20]
Induce synthesis and release of hematopoietic growth
   factors (IL-1, TNF-α)[21–23]
Induce synthesis and release of endogenous IL-1 (TNF-
   α)[24, 25]
Induce release of IL-6 (IL-1)[26]
Induce synthesis and expression of class I MHC
   antigens (TNF-α)[27]
Induce synthesis and surface expression of a
   neoantigen (IL-1, TNF-α)[28]
Stimulate chemotaxis (TNF-α)[29]
Inhibit proliferation (IL-1, TNF-α)[30–32]
Induce synthesis of platelet-activating factor and
   prostacyclin (IL-1, TNF-α)[33–35]
Induce release of platelet-derived growth factor (IL-1,
   TNF-α)[36, 37]
Induce synthesis and surface expression of tissue factor
   (IL-1, TNF-α)[38, 39]
Induce synthesis and release of tissue plasminogen
   activator-inhibitor (IL-1)[40–42]
Suppress cell surface–dependent activation of protein
   C (IL-1, TNF-α)[39, 43]
Reorganize endothelial cytoskeleton (IL-1, TNF-α)[32, 44]
Increase superoxide release (IL-1)[45]

*Adapted from Harlan JA: Consequences of leukocyte–vessel
wall interactions in inflammatory and immune reactions. Semin
Thrombosis Hemostasis 13:434–444, 1987.
   †Superscript numbers refer to references.

Macrophage secretory products have also
been shown to influence in vitro fibroblast
chemotaxis, proliferation, and collagen synthesis (Table 17–2). Most of these monokines have
not been fully characterized or sequenced, although some evidence suggests that macrophage-derived growth factor may be a PDGF-
like molecule.[55] More recently, the proliferative
effects of IL-1 on fibroblast have been shown
to be secondary to induction of platelet-derived
growth factor synthesis and release from the
fibroblast,[67] highlighting the interdependent relationship between monokines/lymphokines and
other growth factors on cells involved in wound
healing. Antagonistic effects have been ascribed
to IL-1 and TNF-α, which have been shown to
both stimulate and inhibit collagen synthesis in
fibroblast cultures. In vivo, IL-1 has been found
to enhance collagen deposition using a stainless
steel chamber model,[68] and conversely, to inhibit collagen synthesis in subcutaneously implanted sponges in rats.[69] The conditions under
which one or the other effect may predominate
are not known. TNF-α decreases wound collagen deposition in subcutaneously implanted
polyvinyl alcohol sponges, while anti–TNF-α
increases fibroplasia.[70] Furthermore, TNF-α

can inhibit the positive effects of TGF-β on
wound collagen synthesis without affecting
PDGF treatment.[71] This is an example of the
difficulty in applying in vitro data to in vivo
situations without a full understanding of the
interplay among these various factors.

LYMPHOCYTES AND WOUND HEALING

Lymphokines, products of activated lymphocytes, have varied effects on vascular endothelial cells (Table 17–3). Two lymphokines with
significant effects on endothelial cell behavior
are interferon-γ and TGF-β. INF-γ has primarily an immune modulatory effect on endothelial
cells, affecting MHC antigen expression of both
class I and II type, although it can inhibit
proliferation. Interestingly, while TGF-β has
been shown to have in vivo angiogenic properties,[85] both it and IFN-γ, inhibit in vitro endothelial cell proliferation. This is similar to the
action of TNF-α described previously. It appears that either angiogenic stimulation may
somehow require a concomitant growth inhibitory signal (which seems unlikely) or, more
probably, that the angiogenic effects of these
cytokines may be secondary to other activities,
such as macrophage stimulation and activation.[86]

A variety of lymphokines have been shown
to affect fibroblast recruitment at the healing
site (Table 17–4). TGF-β is a potent fibroblast
chemotactic molecule.[87] In addition, it induces
monocyte chemotaxis and secretion of fibroblast
growth factors, including IL-1.[97] TGF-β, which
is also secreted by platelets and monocytes, is
present in large quantities at the wound site[9]
and, as stated previously, can modulate fibroblast activity directly or via its effect on monocyte function and growth factor secretion.

Following recruitment of fibroblasts, lymphokines can lead to expansion of the fibroblasts
present by inducing proliferation. Fibroblast-
activating factor (FAF), which stimulates fibroblast proliferation, has been described in humans and in guinea pigs and is a product of
activated T lymphocytes. On the other hand,
IFN-γ is a potent inhibitor of fibroblast proliferation. Once fibroblasts have been recruited
and their numbers increased, synthesis of collagenous protein can be stimulated by lymphokines, such as TGF-β and lymphotoxin. Lymphokines that inhibit collagen synthesis have
also been described, most notably IFN-γ, which
blocks constitutive as well as growth factor–

Table 17–2. MONOKINES THAT REGULATE FIBROBLAST GROWTH AND FUNCTION*

Fibroblast Function	Monokine (M_r)	References
Chemotaxis	Fibronectin	47
	MDCF-F mu (<10,000)†	48
Proliferation		
Stimulation	IL-1 hu (10–15,000)	49
	AMDGF hu (18,000)	50
	MDGF mu (56,000)	51
	mu (≥100,000)	52
	mu (46–57,000)	53
	mu (10–16,000)	53
	FAF gp (40–60,000)	54
	PDGF	55
	TNF-α	56
Inhibition	IFN-β	57, 58
Collagen synthesis		
Stimulation	†	54
	IL-1 hu	59
	TNF-α	60
Inhibition	†	61
	IL-1 hu	62
	TNF-α	63, 64
Collagenase and PGE₂ synthesis	IL-1	65
	TNF-α	66

*Adapted from Wahl SM: Host immune factors regulating fibrosis. In Fibrosis. Ciba Foundation Symposium 114, London, Pitman, 1985, pp 175–195.
†Not characterized.
‡AMDGF = alveolar macrophage–derived growth factor; PDGF = platelet-derived growth factor; MDCF-F = macrophage-derived chemotactic factor for fibroblasts; MDGF = macrophage-derived growth factor; FAF = fibroblast-activating factor; IL-1 = interleukin-1; TNF-α = tumor necrosis factor-α; IFN-β = interferon-β; hu = human; mu = murine; gp = guinea pig; PGE₂ = prostaglandin.

induced collagen synthesis.[96] It is evident that lymphokines can exert both stimulatory and inhibitory signals on all aspects of fibroblast activity, and there seems to be a well-defined balance between these effects. Our knowledge is scant regarding how this balance is achieved in vivo; however, it is clear that an imbalance could result in wound failure or, conversely, in excessive fibrosis. This has been elegantly demonstrated by Wahl,[98] who showed that the continued presence of antigenic stimulus at the healing site leads to excessive fibrosis, presumably because of continued activation of T lymphocytes with unchecked production of fibroblast-activating factor (FAF).

The only lymphokines used in vivo thus far have been TGF-β, IFN-γ, and IL-2. Subcutaneous injection of 800 ng of TGF-β into newborn mice resulted in increased formation of granulation tissue.[85] Application of TGF-β to linear incisions in rats led to increased wound breaking strength and collagen deposition with a concomitant rise in mononuclear cell and fibroblast infiltration.[99] On the other hand, implantation of subcutaneous osmotic pumps containing IFN-γ into mice resulted in decreased thickness and collagen content of the fibrous capsule that forms around the pumps.[100] In vivo administration of human recombinant IL-2

(60,000 and 140,000 units per day) to rats significantly augmented wound breaking strengths (fresh and fixed) with a parallel increase in collagen deposition as assessed by the hydroxy-L-proline content of subcutaneously implanted polyvinyl alcohol sponges.[101]

Role of the Thymus in Repair

A strong correlation exists between the thymus gland and the healing wound. Agents that enhance thymic function have a stimulatory effect on wound healing, while those that depress it impair wound healing.[102] However, neither neonatal[103] nor intrauterine[104] thymectomy has an influence on the healing of incisional wounds in rats and on fibroplasia in guinea pigs, respectively. It should be pointed out that neonatal thymectomy causes global host perturbations, including generalized T-cell dysmaturation and wasting disease, which makes the interpretation of wound healing data difficult.

Rats thymectomized as young adults (4 to 8 weeks of age) and wounded 8 weeks later demonstrate increased wound tensile strength with-

Table 17–3. EFFECTS OF LYMPHOKINES ON CULTURED ENDOTHELIAL CELLS*

Interferon-γ
  Increases class I and induces class II MHC antigen expression[72, 73]†
  Confers antigen-presenting capability on EC[74]
  Induces neoantigen expression[75]
  Increases adhesivity for lymphocytes[76, 77]
  Reorganizes cytoskeleton[32]
  Increases superoxide anion release[45]
  Inhibits proliferation[32]

Transforming growth factor-β
  Inhibits proliferation[79, 80]

Lymphokine-containing supernatants
  Enhance plasminogen activator synthesis[81]
  Enhance proliferation and motility[82, 83]
  Inhibit migration[84]

---

*Adapted from Harlan JA: Consequences of leukocyte–vessel wall interactions in inflammatory and immune reactions. Semin Thrombosis Hemostasis 13:434–444, 1987.
†Superscript numbers refer to references.

---

out increased collagen synthesis. This effect is reversible by the intraperitoneal placement of autologous thymic grafts contained within Millipore chambers,[105] suggesting that thymic humoral products (thymic hormones) modulate the thymic inhibitory effect on wound maturation. Administration of thymic hormones to thymus-

Table 17–4. LYMPHOKINES THAT REGULATE *IN VITRO* FIBROBLAST GROWTH AND FUNCTION*

Fibroblast Function	Lymphokine (M$_r$)	Reference
Migration		
Stimulation	TGF-β†	85, 87
Inhibition	FIF (28–34,000)	88
Proliferation		
Stimulation	FAF gp (40,000)	89
	gp (50,000)	90
	hu (40,000)	91
	gp (10–15,000)	90
	IFN-γ	92
	LT	93
Inhibition	IF	90
	IFN-γ	57
Collagen synthesis		
Stimulation	CPF (100–170,000)	94
	TGF-β hu	85, 95
	FAF	95
	LT	60
Inhibition	—(55,000)	90
	IFN-α and γ	96

---

*Adapted from Wahl SM: Host immune factors regulating fibrosis. In Fibrosis. Ciba Foundation Symposium 114. London, Pitman, 1985, pp 175–195.
†FIF = fibroblast migration inhibitory factor; FAF = fibroblast-activating factor; CPF = collagen production factor; IF = inhibitor of fibroblast proliferation; IFN = interferon; LT = lymphotoxin; TGF = transforming growth factor; gp = guinea pig; hu = human.

bearing mice and rats or to congenitally athymic nude mice leads to impaired wound healing as assessed by wound breaking strength and collagen synthesis (Fig. 17–1).[106, 107] Thus, the thymus normally exerts an inhibitory effect on wound fibroplasia; this can be accentuated by administering thymic hormones to thymus-bearing animals or reversed by adult thymectomy. Since adult thymectomy abrogates T-suppressor cell induction and thymic hormones induce T-suppressor differentiation,[108, 109] this is indirect evidence that T-suppressor lymphocytes may play a role in inhibiting wound healing, a phenomenon that is discussed in the next section.

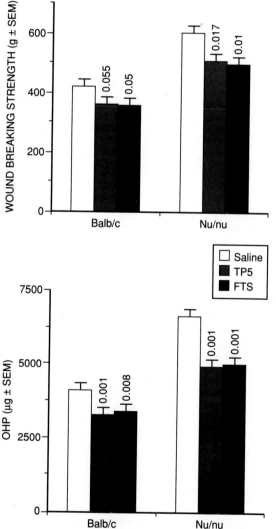

Figure 17–1. Impairment of wound breaking strength and wound collagen synthesis by thymic hormones in both euthymic and athymic nude (nu/nu) mice. OHP = hydroxy-L-proline; TP5 = thymopentin; FTS = facteur thymique serique. (From Barbul A, Shawe T, Frankel H, et al: Inhibition of wound repair by thymic hormones. Surgery 106:373–377, 1989.)

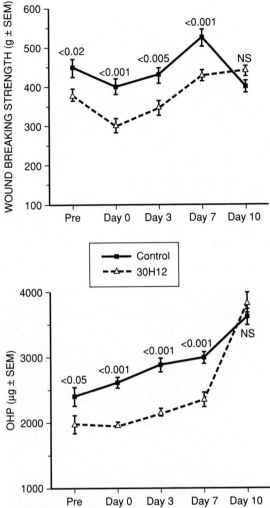

Figure 17–2. Depletion of T lymphocytes using the 30H12 monoclonal antibody (against the Thy1.2 marker) impairs wound breaking strength and collagen synthesis in 4-week-old wounds in mice. Times on the abscissa refer to the start of the monoclonal treatments in relation to the time of wounding. (From Barbul A, Beslin RJ, Woodyard JP, et al: The effect of in vivo T-helper and T-suppressor lymphocyte depletion on wound healing. Am Surg 209:479–483, 1989.)

Role of T Lymphocytes

We have studied the effect of T-lymphocyte depletion on wound healing in vivo. Using the monoclonal antibody 30H12, a rat antimouse antibody, against the Thy1.2 determinant (present on all T cells) [IgG2b type (cytotoxic in vivo)], it was observed that mice depleted of T lymphocytes prior to wounding have decreased wound breaking strength and decreased collagen synthesis.[110] Starting T-lymphocyte depletion even 1 week postwounding results in impaired wound healing and collagen deposition, as assessed 4 weeks postwounding. T-cell

depletion started later (10 days postwounding) does not affect wound fibroplasia (Fig. 17–2).[111]

Depletion of the T helper/effector subset (CD4) using the Gk1.5 (anti L3T4 monoclonal antibody)[112, 113] had no effect on wound breaking strength or collagen synthesis, whether the treatment was started prior to or up to 14 days after wounding.[114] Conversely, depletion of T suppressor/cytotoxic lymphocytes (CD8) (2.43 against the Lyt 2.1 antigen)[115] significantly enhanced all wound healing parameters studied.[114] This enhancement was noted when the depletion was carried out prewounding or starting up to day 14 postwounding. These studies indicate that there are at least two populations of T cells involved in wound healing (Fig. 17–3). One population, bearing the all–T-cell marker, appears to be required for successful repair, as shown by the impairment caused by their depletion. The T-suppressor/cytotoxic subset appears to have a counter-regulatory effect on wound healing since their depletion enhances wound breaking strength and collagen synthesis.

Role of B Lymphocytes

There is no evidence that the humoral immune system or B lymphocytes participate in wound healing. Severe burn injuries are associated with the appearance of circulating autoantibodies to collagen,[116] of rheumatoid factors, and of antinuclear and antiepithelial antibodies.[117] In addition it has been suggested that burn hypertrophic scar results from an autoimmune response.[118] However it is likely that the generation of these antibodies is related to

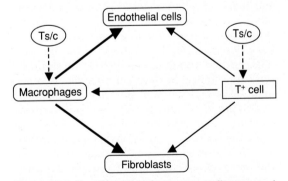

Figure 17–3. Postulated role for immune cells in wound healing. Macrophages exert direct stimulatory effect on endothelial cells and fibroblasts. A T-cell marker–positive subset (T+), which is not fully characterized, has direct action on endothelial cells and fibroblast and acts indirectly by stimulating macrophages. T suppressor/cytotoxic cells (Ts/c) down regulate wound healing by direct action on macrophages and T cells.

massive tissue destruction with exposure of self-antigens to the immune system rather than to wound healing per se. Perhaps a function of the anti–IL-2 factor described in wounds is to limit the possible clonal expansion of lymphocytes exposed to autoantigens at the wound site.

ROLE OF THE WOUND ON HOST IMMUNITY

As previously mentioned wound fluid contains an anti–IL-2 factor that is effective in abrogating IL-2–mediated immune events. This factor, which is not cytotoxic and whose action can be partially reversed by exogenous IL-2, appears 7 to 10 days postwounding. The factor appears to be a heavily glycosylated protein that is constitutively secreted by wound mononuclear cells.[111] Systemic administration of 10 day old wound fluid obtained from rats results in impaired host immune responses as reflected by prolongation of allograft survival[118] and increased mortality following a septic challenge.[7] Such a factor may participate in down-regulating the activated mononuclear cells that play such a critical role in the successful completion of wound healing. It is conceivable that the effects of this local immunosuppressive factor may become systemic if the tissue injury is extensive and/or severe, but this hypothesis remains as yet unproven.

CONCLUSION

Mononuclear cells that infiltrate wounded tissue prior to fibroblast migration play a major role in the expansion of the fibroblast population and their subsequent synthesis of collagen and other extracellular matrix proteins. More recently both a positive and a negative role have been described for T lymphocytes and the thymus, further strengthening the case for immune system–wound healing interaction. Since monokines and lymphokines that stimulate or inhibit fibroblast function have been described, a balance must exist that leads to regulated and successful tissue repair. Conversely, an imbalance in the production and/or activity of these factors could lead to wound failure or abnormal fibrosis. Therefore, an understanding of the role of these cytokines in normal wound healing would provide a biochemical tool for correcting disorders of repair. However, direct in vivo application of in vitro findings awaits a clearer understanding of the interplay among these various cells and their secretory products.

References

1. O'Garra A. Interleukins and the immune system Lancet 1:943–949, 1989.
2. Diegelmann RF, Kim JC, Lindblad WJ, et al: Collection of leukocytes, fibroblasts and collagen within an implantable reservoir tube during tissue repair. J Leukocyte Biol 42:667–672, 1987.
3. Rappolee DA, Mark D, Banda MJ, et al: Wound macrophages express TGF-α and other growth factors in vivo: Analysis by mRNA phenotyping. Science 241:708–712, 1988.
4. Chantry D, Turner M, Abney E, et al: Modulation of cytokine production by transforming growth factor-β. J Immunol 142:4295–4300, 1989.
5. Fishel RS, Barbul A, Beschorner WE, et al: Lymphocyte participation in wound healing. Morphologic assessment using monoclonal antibodies. Ann Surg 206:25–29, 1989.
6. Ford HR, Wing EJ, Hoffman RA, et al: Characterization of wound cytokines in the sponge matrix model. Arch Surg 124:1422–1428, 1989.
7. Lazarou SA, Barbul A, Wasserkrug HL, et al: The wound is a possible source of post-traumatic immunosuppression. Arch Surg 124:1429–1431, 1989.
8. Breslin RJ, Barbul A, Kupper T, et al: Generation of an anti-IL2 factor in healing wounds. Arch Surg 123:305–308, 1988.
9. Cromack DT, Sporn MB, Roberts AB, et al: Transforming growth factor-β levels in rat wound chambers. J Surg Res 42:622–628, 1987.
10. Leibovich SJ, Ross R: The role of the macrophage in wound repair. A study with hydrocortisone and anti-macrophage serum. Am J Pathol 78:71–91, 1975.
11. Clark RA, Stone RD, Leung DYK, et al: Role of macrophages in wound healing. Surg Forum 27:16–18, 1976.
12. Casey WJ, Peacock EE Jr, Chvapil M: Induction of collagen synthesis in rats by transplantation of allogenic macrophages. Surg Forum 27:53–55, 1976.
13. Bevilacqua MP, Pober JS, Wheeler ME, et al: Interleukin-1 acts on cultured human vascular endothelium to increase the adhesion of polymorphonuclear leukocytes, monocytes, and related leukocyte cell lines. J Clin Invest 76:2003–2011, 1986.
14. Cavender D, Haskard DO, Joseph B, et al: Interleukin 1 increases the binding of human B and T lymphocytes to endothelial cell monolayers. J Immunol 136:203–207, 1986.
15. Cavender D, Saegusa Y, Ziff M: Stimulation of endothelial cell binding of lymphocytes by tumor necrosis factor. J Immunol 139:1855–1860, 1987.
16. Gamble JR, Harlan JM, Klebanoff SJ, et al: Stimulation of the adherence of neutrophils to umbilical vein endothelium by human recombinant tumor necrosis factor. Proc Natl Acad Sci USA 82:8667–8671, 1985.
17. Pohlman TH, Stanness KA, Beatty PG, et al: An endothelial cell surface factor(s) induced in vitro by lipopolysaccharide, interleukin-1, and tumor necrosis factor-α increases neutrophil adherence by a CDw18-dependent mechanism. J Immunol 136:4548–4553, 1986.
18. Schleimer RP, Rutledge BR: Cultured human vascular endothelial cells acquire adhesiveness for neutrophils after stimulation with interleukin 1, endotoxin and tumor-promoting phorbol diesters. J Immunol 136:649–654, 1986.
19. Wheeler ME, Luscinskas FW, Bevilacqua MP, et al: Cultures of human endothelial cells stimulated with

cytokines or endotoxin produce an inhibitor of leukocyte adhesion. J Clin Invest 82:1211–1218, 1988.

20. Strieter RM, Kunkel SL, Showell HJ, et al: Endothelial cell gene expression of a neutrophil chemotactic factor by TNF-α, LPS and IL-1β. Science 243:1467–1469, 1989.

21. Asherson GL, Zembala M, Mayhew B, et al: Adult thymectomy prevention of the appearance of suppressor T cells which depress contact sensitivity to picryl chloride and reversal of adult thymectomy effect by thymus extract. Eur J Immunol 6:669–703, 1976.

22. Broudy VC, Kaushansky K, Segal GM, et al: Tumor necrosis factor-α stimulates human endothelial cells to produce granulocyte/macrophage colony-stimulating factor. Proc Natl Acad Sci USA 83:7467–7471, 1986.

23. Munker R, Gasson J, Ogawa M, et al: Recombinant human tumor necrosis factor induces production of granulocyte-monocyte colony-stimulating factor. Nature 323:79–82, 1986.

24. Libby P, Ordovas JM, Auger KR, et al: Endotoxin and tumor necrosis factor induce interleukin-1 gene expression in adult human vascular endothelial cells. Am J Pathol 124:179–185, 1986.

25. Nawroth PP, Bank I, Handley D, et al: Tumor necrosis factor/cachectin interacts with endothelial cell receptors to induce release of interleukin 1. J Exp Med 163:1363–1323, 1986.

26. Sironi M, Breviario F, Proserpio P, et al: IL-1 stimulates IL-6 production in endothelial cells. J Immunol 142:549–553, 1989.

27. Collins T, Capierrer LA, Fiers W, et al: Recombinant human tumor necrosis factor increases mRNA levels and surface expression of HLA-A,B antigens in vascular endothelial cells and dermal fibroblasts in vitro. Proc Natl Acad Sci USA 83:446–450, 1986.

28. Pober JS, Bevilacqua MP, Mendrick DL, et al: Two distinct monokines, interleukin 1 and tumor necrosis factor, each independently induce biosynthesis and transient expression of the same antigen on the surface of cultured human vascular endothelial cells. J Immunol 136:1680–1687, 1986.

29. Leibovich SJ, Polverini PJ, Shepard MH, et al: Macrophage-induced angiogenesis is mediated by tumour necrosis factor-α. Nature 328:630–632, 1987.

30. Frater-Scroder M, Risau W, Hallmann R, et al: Tumor necrosis factor type α, a potent inhibitor of endothelial cell growth in vitro, is angiogenic in vivo. Proc Natl Acad Sci USA 84:5277–5281, 1987.

31. Norioka K, Hara M, Kitani A, et al: Inhibitory effect of human recombinant interleukin-1 α and β on growth of human vascular endothelial cells. Biochem Biophys Res Comm 145:969–975, 1987.

32. Stolpen AH, Guinan EC, Fiers W, et al: Recombinant TNF and immune interferon act singly and in combination to reorganize human vascular endothelial cell monolayers. Am J Pathol 123:16–24, 1986.

33. Bussolino F, Breviario F, Tetta C, et al: Interleukin 1 stimulates platelet-activating factor production in cultured human endothelial cells. J Clin Invest 77:2027–2033, 1986.

34. Kawakami M, Ishibashi S, Ogawa H, et al: Cachectin/TNF as well as interleukin-1 induces prostacyclin synthesis in cultured vascular endothelial cells. Biochem Biophys Res Comm 141:482–487, 1986.

35. Rossi V, Breviario F, Ghezzi P, et al: Prostacyclin synthesis induced in vascular cells by interleukin-1. Science 229:174–176, 1984.

36. Hajjar KA, Hajjar DP, Silverstein RL, et al: Tumor necrosis factor–mediated release of platelet-derived growth factor from cultured endothelial cells. J Exp Med 166:235–245, 1987.

37. Libby P, Janicka MW, Dinarello CA: Interleukin 1 promotes production by human endothelial cells of activity that stimulates the growth of arterial smooth muscle cells. Fed Proc 44:1908a (abstr), 1985.

38. Bevilacqua MP, Pober JS, Majeau GR, et al: Interleukin 1 (IL-1) induces biosynthesis and cell surface expression of procoagulant activity in human vascular endothelial cells. J Exp Med 160:618–623, 1984.

39. Nawroth PP, Stern DM: Modulation of endothelial cell hemostatic properties by tumor necrosis factor. J Exp Med 163:740–745, 1986.

40. Bevilacqua MP, Schleef RR, Gimbrone MA Jr, et al: Regulation of the fibrinolytic system of cultured human vascular endothelium by interleukin 1. J Clin Invest 78:587–591, 1986.

41. Emeis JJ, Kooistra T: Interleukin 1 and lipopolysaccharide induce an inhibitor of tissue-type plasminogen activator in vivo and in cultured endothelial cells. J Exp Med 163:1260–1266, 1986.

42. Nachman RL, Hajjar KA, Silverstein RL, et al: Interleukin-1 induces endothelial cell synthesis of plasminogen activator inhibitor. J Exp Med 163:1595–1600, 1986.

43. Nawroth PP, Handley DA, Esmon CT, et al: Interleukin 1 induces endothelial cell procoagulant while suppressing cell-surface anticoagulant activity. Proc Natl Acad Sci USA 83:3460–3464, 1986.

44. Montesano R, Orci L, Vassalli P: Human endothelial cell cultures. Phenotypic modulation by leukocyte interleukins. J Cell Physiol 122:424–434, 1985.

45. Matsubara T, Ziff M: Increased superoxide anion release from human endothelial cells in response to cytokines. J Immunol 137:3295–3298, 1986.

46. Sharpe RJ, Margolis RJ, Askari M, et al: Induction of dermal and subcutaneous inflammation by recombinant cachectin/tumor necrosis factor (TNF-α) in the mouse. J Invest Dermatol 91:353–357, 1988.

47. Tsukamoto Y, Helsel WE, Wahl SM. Macrophage production of fibronectin, a chemoattractant for fibroblasts. J Immunol 127:673–678, 1982.

48. Diegelmann RF, Schuller-Levis G, Cohen IK, et al: Identification of a low molecular weight, macrophage-derived chemotactic factor for fibroblasts. Clin Immunol Immunopathol 41:331–341, 1986.

49. Schmidt JA, Mizel SB, Cohen D, et al: Interleukin 1, a potential regulator of fibroblast proliferation. J Immunol 128:2177–2182, 1982.

50. Bitterman PB, Rennard SI, Hunninghake GW, et al: Human alveolar macrophage growth factor for fibroblasts: Regulation and partial characterization. J Clin Invest 70:806–822, 1982.

51. Estes JE, Pledger WJ, Gillespie GY. Macrophage-derived growth factor for fibroblasts and interleukin-1 are distinct entities. J Leuk Biol 35:115–129, 1984.

52. Martin BM, Gimbrone MA Jr, Unanue ER, et al: Stimulation of nonlymphoid mesenchymal cell proliferation by a macrophage-derived growth factor. J Immunol 126:1510–1515, 1981.

53. Wyler DJ, Stadecker MJ, Dinarello CA, et al: Fibroblast stimulation in schistosomiasis. V. Egg granuloma macrophages spontaneously secrete a fibroblast-stimulating factor. J Immunol 132:3142–3148, 1984.

54. Wahl SM, Wahl LM, McCarthy JB, et al: Macrophage activation by mycobacterial water soluble compounds and synthetic muramyl dipeptide. J Immunol 122:2226–2231, 1979.

55. Shimokado K, Raines EW, Madtes DK, et al: A significant part of macrophage-derived growth factor consists of at least two forms of PDGF. Cell 43:277–286, 1985.

56. Palombella VJ, Mendelsohn J, Vilcek J: Mitogenic

action of tumor necrosis factor in human fibroblasts: Interaction with epidermal growth factor and platelet-derived growth factor. J Cell Physiol 135:23–31, 1988.

57. Duncan MR, Berman B: γ-Interferon is the lymphokine and β-interferon is the monokine responsible for inhibition of fibroblast collagen production and late but not early fibroblast proliferation. J Exp Med 162:516–527, 1985.

58. Kohase M, Henriksen-DeStefano D, May LT, et al: Induction of beta-2-interferon by tumor necrosis factor: A homeostatic mechanism in the control of cell proliferation. Cell 45:659–666, 1986.

59. Kahari V-M, Heino J, Vuorio E: Interleukin-1 increases collagen production and mRNA levels in cultured skin fibroblasts. Biochem Biophys Acta 929:142–147, 1987.

60. Amento EP, Granstein RD: Effects of immune cytokines (IL1, TNF, LT and IFN-γ) on fibroblasts. Presented at the 2nd International Symposium on Tissue Repair, May 13–17, 1987, Tarpon Springs, FL.

61. Jimenez SA, McArthur W, Rosenbloom J: Inhibition of collagen synthesis by mononuclear cell supernates. J Exp Med 150:1421–1431, 1979.

62. Bhatnagar R, Penfornis H, Mauviel A, et al: Interleukin-1 inhibits the synthesis of collagen by fibroblasts. Biochem Int 13:709–720, 1986.

63. Mauviel A, Daireaux M, Redini F, et al: Tumor necrosis factor inhibits collagen and fibronectin synthesis in human dermal fibroblasts. FEBS Lett 236:47–52, 1988.

64. Solis-Heruzzo JA, Brenner DA, Chojkier M: Tumor necrosis factor α inhibits collagen gene transcription and collagen synthesis in cultured human fibroblasts. J Biol Chem 263:5841–5845, 1988.

65. Mizel SB, Dayer JM, Krane SM, et al: Stimulation of rheumatoid synovial cell collagenase and prostaglandin production by partially purified lymphocyte activating factor (interleukin 1). Proc Natl Acad Sci USA 78:2474–2477, 1980.

66. Dayer JM, Beutler B, Cerami A: Cachectin/tumor necrosis factor stimulates collagenase and prostaglandin E₂ production by human synovial cells and dermal fibroblasts. J Exp Med 162:2163–2168, 1985.

67. Raines EW, Dower SK, Ross R: Interleukin-1 mitogenic activity for fibroblasts and smooth muscle cells is due to PDGF-AA. Science 243:393–396, 1989.

68. Hunt TK: Personal communication.

69. Laato M, Heino J: Interleukin 1 modulates collagen synthesis by rat granulation tissue cells both in vivo and in vitro. Experientia 44:32–34, 1988.

70. Barbul A, et al: Unpublished observations.

71. Steenfos H, Hunt TK, Goodson WH III: Selective effects of tumor necrosis factor alpha on wound healing in rats. Surgery 106:171–176, 1989.

72. Collins T, Korman AJ, Wake CT, et al: Immune interferon activates multiple class II major histocompatibility complex genes and the associated invariant chain gene in human endothelial cells and dermal fibroblasts. Proc Natl Acad Sci USA 81:4917–4921, 1984.

73. Pober JS, Gimbrone MA, Cotran KS, et al: Ia expression by vascular endothelium is inducible by activated T cells and by human gamma-interferon. J Exp Med 157:1339–1353, 1983.

74. Geppert ID, Lipsky PE: Antigen presentation by interferon-gamma–treated endothelial cells and fibroblasts: Differential ability to function as antigen presenting cells despite comparable Ia expression. J Immunol 135:3750–3762, 1985.

75. Duijvestijn AM, Schreiber AB, Butcher EC: Interferon-gamma regulates an antigen specific for endothelial cells involved in lymphocyte traffic. Proc Natl Acad Sci USA 83:9114–9118, 1986.

76. Masuyama JI, Minato N, Kano S: Mechanisms of lymphocyte adhesions to human vascular endothelial cells in culture. T lymphocyte adhesion to endothelial cells through endothelial HLA-DR antigens induced by gamma interferon. J Clin Invest 77:1596–1605, 1986.

77. Yu CL, Haskard DO, Cavender D, et al: Human gamma interferon increases the binding of T lymphocytes to endothelial cells. Clin Exp Immunol 62:554–560, 1985.

78. Bagby GC, Dinarello CA, Wallis P, et al: Interleukin-1 stimulates granulocyte and macrophage colony stimulating activity release by vascular endothelial cells. J Clin Invest 78:1316–1323, 1986.

79. Frater-Schroder M, Muller G, Birchmeier W, et al: Transforming growth factor-beta inhibits endothelial cell proliferation. Biochem Biophys Res Commun 137:295–302, 1986.

80. Heimark RL, Twardzik DR, Schwartz SM: Inhibition of endothelial regeneration by type-beta transforming growth factor from platelets. Science 233:1078–1980, 1986.

81. Tiku M, Tomasi TB: Enhancement of endothelial plasminogen activator synthesis by lymphokines. Transplantation 40:293–298, 1985.

82. Groenewegen G, Buurman WA, van der Linden CJ: Lymphokines induce changes in morphology and enhanced motility of endothelial cells. Clin Immunol Immunopathol 36:378–385, 1985.

83. Watt SL, Auerbach R: A mitogenic factor for endothelial cells obtained from mouse secondary mixed leukocyte cultures. J Immunol 136:197–202, 1986.

84. Cohen MC, Picciano PT, Douglas WJ, et al: Migration inhibition of endothelial cells by lymphokine-containing supernatants. Science 215:301–303, 1982.

85. Roberts AB, Sporn MB, Assoian RK, et al: Transforming growth factor type β: Rapid induction of fibrosis and angiogenesis in vivo and stimulation of collagen formation in vitro. Proc Natl Acad Sci USA 83:4167–4171, 1986.

86. Fiegel VD, Knighton DR: Transforming growth factor-β causes indirect angiogenesis by recruiting monocytes. FASEB 2:1601 (abstr) 1988.

87. Postlethwaite AE, Keski-Oja J, Moses HL, et al: Stimulation of the chemotactic migration of human fibroblasts by transforming growth factor β. J Exp Med 165:251–256, 1987.

88. Rola-Pleszczynski M, Lieu H, Hamel J, et al: Stimulated human lymphocytes produce a soluble factor which inhibits fibroblast migration. Cell Immunol 74:104–110, 1982.

89. Wahl SM, Wahl LM, McCarthy JB: Lymphocyte mediated activation of fibroblast proliferation and collagen production. J Immunol 121:942–946, 1978.

90. Neilson EG, Phillips SM, Jimenez S: Lymphokine modulation of fibroblast proliferation. J Immunol 128:1484–1486, 1982.

91. Wahl SM, Gately CL: Modulation of fibroblast growth by a lymphokine of human T cell and continuous T cell line origin. J Immunol 130:1226–1230, 1983.

92. Brinckerhoff CE, Guyre PM: Increased proliferation of human synovial fibroblasts treated with recombinant immune interferon. J Immunol 134:3142–3146, 1985.

93. Hofsli E, Austgulen R, Nissen-Meyer J: Lymphotoxin-induced growth stimulation of diploid human fibroblasts in the presence and absence of gamma interferon. Scand J Immunol 26:585–588, 1987.

94. Postlethwaite AE, Smith GN, Mainardi CL, et al:

Lymphocyte modulation of fibroblast function *in vitro:* Stimulation and inhibition of collagen production by different effector molecules. J Immunol 132:2470–2477, 1984.

95. Agelli M, Sobel ME, Wahl SM: Mononuclear cell modulation of fibroblast collagen synthesis. Fed Proc 46:924, 1987 (abstract).

96. Jimenez SA, Freundlich B, Rosenbloom J: Selective inhibition of human diploid fibroblast collagen synthesis by interferons. J Clin Invest 74:1112–1116, 1984.

97. Wahl SM, Hunt DA, Wakefield LM, et al: Transforming growth factor type β induces monocyte chemotaxis and growth factor production. Proc Natl Acad Sci USA 84:5788–5792, 1987.

98. Wahl SM: Host immune factors regulating fibrosis. In Evered D, Whelan J (eds): Fibrosis. Ciba Foundation Symposium 114, London, Pitman, 1985, pp 175–195.

99. Mustoe TA, Pierce GF, Thomason A, et al: Accelerated healing of incisional wounds in rats induced by transforming growth factor-β. Science 237:1333–1336, 1987.

100. Granstein RD, Murphy GF, Margolis RJ, et al: Gamma-interferon inhibits collagen synthesis in vivo in the mouse. J Clin Invest 79:1254–1258, 1987.

101. Barbul A, Knud-Hansen J, Wasserkrug HL, et al: Interleukin 2 enhances wound healing in rats. J Surg Res 40:315–319, 1986.

102. Barbul A: Role of T cell–dependent immune system in wound healing. In Hunt TK, Pines E, Barbul A, et al. (eds): Growth Factors and Other Aspects of Wound Healing. Biological and Clinical Implications. New York, Alan R. Liss, Progress in Clinical and Biological Research, 266:161–175, 1988.

103. Fisher ER, Fisher B: Lack of thymic effect on wound healing. Proc Soc Exp Biol Med 119:61–63, 1965.

104. Savunan T, Merikanto J, Viljanto J, et al: Intrauterine thymectomy induced T-lymphocyte suppression and wound healing. Acta Chir Scand Suppl 493:120–146, 1979.

105. Barbul A, Sisto D, Rettura G, et al: Thymic inhibition of wound healing: Abrogation by adult thymectomy. J Surg Res 32:338–342, 1982.

106. Barbul A, Knud-Hansen JP, Wasserkrug HL, et al: Thymic hormones inhibit wound healing. Surg Forum 38:34–36, 1987.

107. Barbul A, Shawe T, Frankel H, et al: Inhibition of wound repair by thymic hormones. Surgery 106:373–377, 1989.

108. Katz MM, Oliver J, Goldstein AL, et al: Suppressor cell responses in patients with rheumatoid arthritis: The effect of thymosin. Thymus 6:205–218, 1984.

109. Kaufman DB. Maturational effects of thymic hormones on human helper and suppressor T cells. Effects of FTS (facteur thymique serique) and thymosin. Clin Exp Immunol 39:722–727, 1980.

110. Peterson JM, Barbul A, Breslin RJ, et al: Significance of T lymphocytes in wound healing. Surgery 102:300–305, 1987.

111. Breslin RJ, Barbul A, Woodyard JP, et al: T-lymphocytes are required for wound healing. Surg Forum 40:634–636, 1989.

112. Dialynas DP, Wilde DB, Marrack P, et al: Characterization of the murine antigenic determinant designated L3T4a, recognized by monoclonal antibody GK1.5: Expression of L3T4a by functional T cell clones appears to correlate primarily with class II MHC antigen reactivity. Immunol Rev 74:29–56, 1983.

113. Wilde DB, Marrack P, Kappler J, et al: Evidence implicating L3T4 in class II MHC antigen reactivity; monoclonal antibody GK1.5 (anti-L3T4a) blocks class II MHC antigen-specific proliferation, release of lymphokines and binding of cloned murine helper T lymphocyte lines. J Immunol 131:2178–2183, 1983.

114. Barbul A, Breslin RJ, Woodyard JP, et al: The effect of in vivo T helper and T suppressor lymphocyte depletion on wound healing. Ann Surg 209:479–483, 1989.

115. Sarmiento M, Dialynas DP, Lancki DW, et al: Cloned T lymphocytes and monoclonal antibodies as probes for cell surface molecules active in T cell–mediated cytolysis. Immunol Rev 68:135–169, 1982.

116. Bray JP, Estess F, Bass JA: Anticollagen antibodies following thermal trauma. Proc Soc Exp Biol Med 130:394–398, 1969.

117. Quismorio FP, Bland SL, Friou GJ. Autoimmunity in thermal injury: Occurrence of rheumatoid factors, antinuclear antibodies and antiepithelial antibodies. Clin Exp Immunol 8:701–711, 1971.

118. Barbul A, Fishel RS, Shimazu S, et al: Inhibition of host immunity by fluid and mononuclear cells from healing wounds. Surgery 96:315–320, 1984.

18

EICOSANOIDS, CYTOKINES, AND FREE RADICALS

Martin C. Robson, M.D., and John P. Heggers, Ph.D.

The physiological process of wound healing or tissue repair has been arbitrarily divided into three basic phases: the inflammatory phase, the proliferative phase, and the remodeling phase. Physiological and biochemical events can be correlated with macroscopic and microscopic changes in the wound (Fig. 18–1).[1, 2] The first, or inflammatory phase of wound repair is initiated by a sequence of biochemical and cellular events that begins once the integrity and homeostasis of the tissue membranes are disrupted.[1, 3] Among the biochemical and humoral events are release or activation of messengers that seem to orchestrate cell-cell interaction and cell-matrix interaction in wound repair. There appear to be two sets of such mediators,

primary and secondary. This chapter presents evidence suggesting that the eicosanoids, metabolites of arachidonic acid, function as primary mediators in the wound healing scheme and cytokines as secondary mediators.

Wound healing activities begin almost simultaneously with the wounding event. Penneys has shown that there is local activation of phospholipase A whenever the cell membrane is disrupted in any kind of wound.[4] This activation of phospholipase A cleaves phospholipids that are usually bound to cholesterol and triglycerides in the cell membrane. Once phospholipase A is activated, it begins the metabolism of arachidonic acid to the various eicosanoids. As will be seen, the initial events following wound-

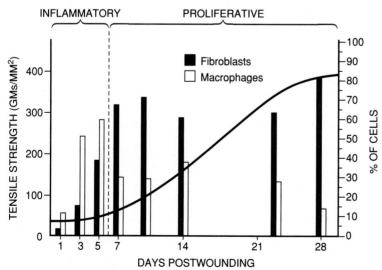

Figure 18–1. Interrelationship between tensile strength and cell types during the early stages of wound healing.

ing (activation of platelets with release of their granules, activation and granule release of mast cells, and activation and respiratory burst of leukocytes) all release additional eicosanoids.[5] For this reason, it is suggested that these soluble mediators play a major role in wound healing.

Any mechanism that disturbs cellular homeostasis triggers eicosanoid biosynthesis (Fig. 18–2).[1-7] The first compound made from the phospholipids by phospholipase A is arachidonate. Once released, it can be reincorporated into a phospholipid or metabolized by one of the pathways of the arachidonic acid cascade, the cyclo-oxygenase or lipoxygenase pathway. Alternatively, arachidonate can be produced nonenzymatically from chemotactic lipids via the oxygen-derived free radical–generating systems or through stimulation by ultraviolet irradiation (Fig. 18–2).

Eicosanoids are formed from essential fatty acids and contain 20 carbon atoms with a cyclopentane ring. They are present throughout the body and consist of the prostanoids (formed via the cyclo-oxygenase pathway) and the leukotrienes (hydroperoxy or hydroxy fatty acids) produced via the lipoxygenase pathway. Although the prostanoids are the best studied, one cannot discuss them without also examining the role of leukotrienes and oxygen-derived free radicals in wound repair, since any disruption of the cell membrane will trigger the formation of both.

CYCLO-OXYGENASE PATHWAY PRODUCTION OF PROSTANOIDS

Before exploring the role of the various metabolites of the cyclo-oxygenase pathway (i.e., the prostaglandins and thromboxanes) in wound healing, one must briefly review the pathway. Once the arachidonate is released following injury to the cell membrane, it combines with oxygen, converting the arachidonate to the intermediates of the cascade PGG_2 and PGH_2 with the aid of tryptophan and heme (Fig. 18–2). PGH_2 is the parental form from which all other eicosanoids of the cyclo-oxygenase pathway are synthesized (PGD_2, PGE_2, $PGF_{2\alpha}$, PGI_2, and TxA_2).

Prostacyclin (PGI_2) is a potent stimulator of cAMP and is regarded as the key to maintaining platelet homeostasis through inhibition of platelet aggregation. Since, as will be seen, thromboxane A_2 (TxA_2) is a potent platelet aggregator, there seems to be a unique relationship (resembling the yin and yang of Oriental philosophy) between the platelet effects of these eicosanoids. Similarly, there is a relationship between the vasodilatory action of PGI_2 and the vasoconstrictive nature of TxA_2 that appears to arise from the interaction of the endothelial lining of the blood vessel and the platelet. Keeping this relationship in balance, or homeostasis, is important for wound blood flow and function; an imbalance toward excess TxA_2 occurs after injury in an attempt to shut down the microvasculature.[6, 8]

Another bidirectional intracellular control system exists between PGE_2 and $PGF_{2\alpha}$ that is initiated in the presence of cofactor nicotinamide adenine dinucleotide phosphate ($NADP^+$ or NADPH) by the enzyme PGE_2 9-keto-reductase. While only one enzyme pathway exists from the parental PGH_2 to PGE_2, there are two pathways by which $PGF_{2\alpha}$ can be synthesized. These two bidirectional activities appear to affect the initial platelet plug of wound healing since the platelet is activated by eicosanoids of the PGE_2 sequence.

PGE_2 and $PGF_{2\alpha}$ are stable and active byproducts of arachidonate, whereas PGI_2 and TxA_2 are highly active but unstable byproducts of the endoperoxide PGH_2 (see Figure 18–2). Prostacyclin (PGI_2) is a potent vasodilator as described previously, and a potent endogenous inhibitor of platelet aggregation. Therefore, it may contribute to the nonthrombogenicity of the endothelial lining of the vessel wall and to the regulation of the local blood flow. This may be particularly important at the time of injury. However, PGI_2 has a half-life of only 3 minutes and is produced in small amounts. This production increases under pulsatile conditions; consequently, venular PGI_2 concentrations may be lower than arterial concentrations.[9, 10] This is important in evaluating wound healing data such as in pedicle flaps.

Thromboxane A_2 is a potent vasoconstrictor that is also synthesized from the endoperoxide PGH_2. It is a facilitator of platelet aggregation and is considered the major mediator of progressive dermal ischemia after wounding.[6, 8] This has been shown to be particularly important in wounds that demonstrate delayed or progressive tissue necrosis such as burns, frostbite, electrical injuries, and crush injuries.[6] The half-life of TxA_2 is even shorter than that of PGI_2, but it can be continuously produced by ischemic tissue.

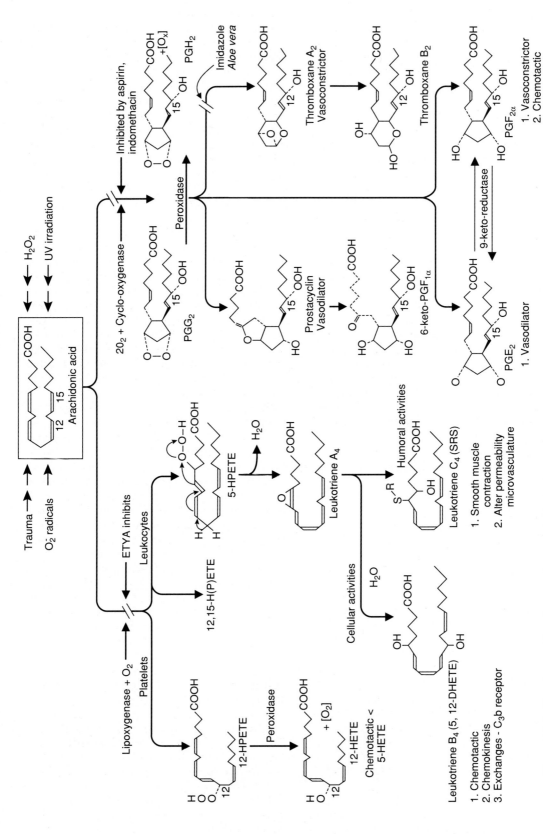

Figure 18–2. The eicosanoid pathways, depicting both the lipoxygenase and cyclo-oxygenase pathways. ETYA = 5,8,11,14-eicosatetraynoic acid. (Modified from Robson MC, Heggers JP: Quantitative bacteriology and inflammatory mediators in soft tissue. In Hunt TK, Heppenstall RB, Pines E, et al (eds): Tissue Repair: Biological and Clinical Aspects of Soft and Hard Tissue Repair. New York, Praeger, 1984, pp 483–507.)

PROSTANOIDS AND THEIR ROLE IN INFLAMMATION

Although it is felt that the eicosanoids function mainly as messengers in wound healing, they appear to have a more central role in the first stage. The inflammatory phase has both humoral and cellular components, with the signs and symptoms of inflammation due largely to the action of prostanoids. The inflammatory response to wounding is classically described as rubor, tumor, calor, dolor, and functio laesa.

The first response observed during inflammation is *redness*, or rubor, probably initially as a result of the vasodilator PGI_2.[11] However, because of its short half-life, it may only initiate this cardinal sign of inflammation, whereas, the stable prostaglandins A, D, and E, which also cause vasodilation, may continue to provoke rubor. The endoperoxides PGG_2 and PGH_2 initially cause vasoconstriction but eventually result in a secondary vasodilation. Those cyclo-oxygenase metabolites with counteractive activities of vasoconstriction are TxA_2, the most potent and unstable, and $PGF_{2\alpha}$, which is stable but of limited potency (Table 18–1).[3, 7–9]

Swelling, or tumor, the second sign of inflammation, is due to the influx of plasma proteins into the vascular endothelium. While the eicosanoids do not directly provoke edema, arachidonate and PGE potentiate carrageenan edema, and PGI_2, PGG_2, and PGH_2 all potentiate bradykinin and carrageenan edema.[11] The stable prostanoids, PGE_2 and $PGF_{2\alpha}$, have been implicated in provoking edema; however, they do so only at low doses, not at high concentrations, which suggests that they are not the chief mediators of edema and that edema occurs during the release of the prostanoid metabolites that precede the production of PGE_2 and $PGF_{2\alpha}$ (Table 18–1).[3, 7–10] It has been suggested that other noneicosanoid mediators, specifically histamine and bradykinin, are more potent stimulators of edema formation. However, the eicosanoids, especially PGE_1, PGE_2, PGA, and $PGF_{2\alpha}$, appear to potentiate their action, and this seems to be more than simply additive effects.[3, 8, 9, 11]

Fever, or calor, the third sign of inflammation, is more difficult to correlate directly with the release of the eicosanoids of the cyclo-oxygenase pathway. Whereas experimental evidence implicates the role of injected arachidonate, PGE_1, and PGE_2, antiprostanoic acid metabolites have no effect on endogenously pyrogen-provoked fever.[3, 7–10]

The fourth sign, *pain* (dolor) is easier to correlate with eicosanoid metabolism. Under experimental conditions, arachidonate can provoke severe pain whereas the remaining metabolites of the cyclo-oxygenase pathway provoke varying lesser degrees of hyperalgesia.[11] The endoperoxides PGH_2 and PGG_2 produce a mild hyperalgesia. Alone, PGI_2 can provoke hyperalgesia for short periods of time, but in conjunction with bradykinin or histamine it can produce more severe pain. PGE_1 and PGE_2 both provoke a longer lasting hyperalgesia that is also synergistic with bradykinin and histamine.[3, 7–10] In addition, PGE_2 is known to stimulate cyclic AMP, which in turn induces pain. The best argument for the involvement of cyclo-oxygenase metabolites in the pathogenesis of pain is that inhibitors of this pathway, aspirin, indomethacin, and ibuprofen, are effective analgesics. Additionally, agents that stimulate the

Table 18–1. PHYSIOLOGICAL EFFECTS OF THE EICOSANOIDS

Activity	Pathways		
	Cyclo-oxygenase	*Lipoxygenase*	*Others*
Constriction	PGG_2, PGH_2, TxA_2, $PGF_{2\alpha}$	LTC_4, LTD_4, LTE	
CMA	PGE_2	LTD_4, LTE_2	
Clot production	TxA_2		
Chemotactic	TxA_2, $PGF_{2\alpha}$	12-HETE, LTB_4	
Vascular permeability	PGE_2	12-HETE, LTC_4, LTD_4	Histamine, bradykinin, carrageenan
Platelet aggregation	TxA_2, $PGF_{2\alpha}$	12-HETE	
Eicosanoid biosynthesis	Trauma, LTC_4, LTD_4, IL-1, catalase, UV light	12-HPETE, IL-1, LTD_4, catalase, UV light	
PMN aggregation		LTB_4	
NK suppression		LTD_4	

CMA = cell-mediated activity; PMN = polymorphonuclear leukocytes; NK = natural killer cells; PG = prostaglandins; TxA_2 = thromboxane A_2; LT = leukotrienes; 12-HETE = 12-hydroxyeicosatetraenoic acid; 12-HPETE = 12-hydroperoxyeicosatetraenoic acid.

production of cyclic GMP, such as $PGF_{2\alpha}$, antagonize the pain-provoking effect of PGE_2.[11]

The last sign of inflammation is *loss of function* (functio laesa). Anything that mediates the edema of injury will decrease function and inhibit wound healing. Hunt has recently shown that mediators of pain decrease local perfusion to the wound and decrease oxygen,[12] both of which are detrimental to normal healing.

Mast cells, which originate from undifferentiated mesenchymal cells, are found mainly in loose connective tissue. The mast cell is activated by degradation products of the complement cascade such as C_{5A} and the proteases released at the time of injury.[6] Once activated, it releases its granules, which contain factors such as histamine, serotonin, eicosanoids, and polysaccharides. All of these factors play major roles in establishing the inflammatory response at the site of injury. Histamine, serotonin, and eicosanoids released by the mast cell are vaso-

active substances that induce vascular permeability and chemotaxis of the leukocytes.

The humoral responses are followed by the cellular response of inflammation. The main cells involved in this process are polymorphonuclear leukocytes (PMNs) and macrophages. The PMN remains the predominant cell for approximately 48 hours, followed by the monocytes,[1, 5] which reach maximum numbers 24 hours later. The latter cells quickly evolve into macrophages, the main cell involved in wound debridement. While the neutrophil is not necessary for normal wound healing, the macrophage is.[13] Each of these cells involved in the inflammatory process can transform arachidonate into its biologically active metabolites (Fig. 18–3).

Mediators released by the infiltrating cells of the inflammatory response interact with cells and structures of the skin. The cellular exudate that initially develops contains PGE_2 and $PGF_{2\alpha}$

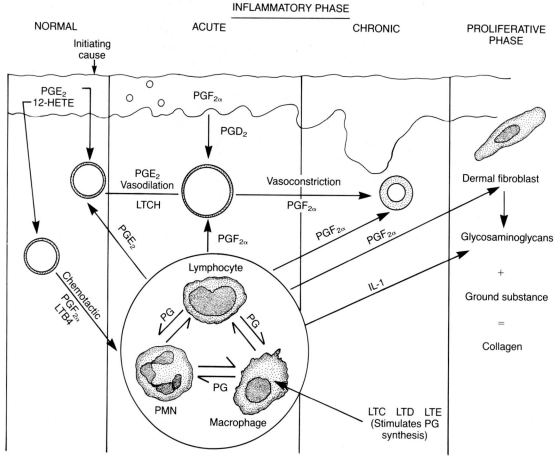

Figure 18–3. Probable effects of the eicosanoids on cells and tissues during the different stages of wound repair. These include the acute and chronic inflammatory phases and the proliferative phase. (Modified from Penneys NS: Prostaglandins and the Skin. Current Concepts/Scope Publication. Kalamazoo, MI, Upjohn Company, 1980, pp 1–28.)

at a 1:2 ratio during the first 6 hours; however, within 24 hours the ratio changes to 1:6, and by 48 hours it is 1:40 as the amount of PGE_2 decreases.[4] This decrease in PGE_2 and increase in $PGF_{2\alpha}$ indicate a waning of the inflammatory response.[4] As $PGF_{2\alpha}$ increases in relation to PGE_2, the cellular population changes to a mononuclear type; therefore, $PGF_{2\alpha}$ could be considered an endogenous agent that initiates repair or restitution of the damaged tissue.[11] Since the repair and reconstitution of the damaged tissue is initiated as the ratio of the endogenous anti-inflammatory agent increases, the biosynthesis of $PGF_{2\alpha}$ has a profound effect on the fibroblast and the dermal reparative process.[4]

PROLIFERATIVE PHASE OF REPAIR

Both PGE_2 and $PGF_{2\alpha}$ stimulate the biosynthesis of collagen.[11] The reduction of PGE_2 and increase in $PGF_{2\alpha}$ toward the end of the inflammatory phase provide a stimulus for dermal fibroblasts to synthesize and release new ground substance. $PGF_{2\alpha}$ is the most potent stimulator of hexosamine production,[14] and it is also known to initiate fibroblast synthesis of hyaluronic synthetase, resulting in an increase in hyaluronic acid.[15] Most of the stimulating effect of $PGF_{2\alpha}$ is in production of glycosaminoglycans (80%), although $PGF_{2\alpha}$ increases glycoprotein production (20%).[11] PGE_1 also increases the concentration of hyaluronic acid in skin. Both PGE_2 and $PGF_{2\alpha}$ stimulate production of connective tissue–activating peptide.[11]

EPITHELIALIZATION AND EPIDERMAL MATURATION

While the deeper region of a wound is progressing from the inflammatory to the proliferative phase, the basal epithelium on the surface of an integumentary wound is flattening and beginning to migrate. The basal cells at the wound margin multiply in a horizontal direction, while the cells more distant from the wound edges assume a more vertical orientation. Normal skin maturation is a complex process involving eicosanoids, essential fatty acids, epidermal proliferation, and the maintenance of normal epidermal function. The development of skin and its adnexa is affected by the eicosanoid derivatives. PGE_2 is the key substrate in the process of epidermal maturation. When an individual ingests a normal diet containing the essential fatty acids, sufficient concentrations of PGE_2 are maintained, allowing for normal skin maturation. The adequate amount of PGE_2 suppresses abnormal sterol-ester formation and allows an increased level of intracellular cyclic AMP necessary for epidermal cell keratinization. Dietary fatty acid deficiency can result in decreased PGE_2 and increased sterol-ester formation and epidermal scaling.[4] (This condition can be seen after a major burn when an essential fatty acid deficiency can occur.) If cAMP accumulation were to be decreased or completely stopped, epidermal cells would remain in the proliferative pool.[3, 4, 6–9]

Arachidonate, the precursor to the eicosanoids, is one of the essential fatty acids, along with linoleic and linolenic acid, which can relieve essential fatty acid deficiency.[16] It then becomes clear that an essential fatty acid deficiency can lead to an eicosanoid deficiency and failure of normal epithelialization and epidermal maturation.

THE IMMUNE RESPONSE

Recently much has been reported about the interaction between wound healing and immunity. The regulation of cell-mediated immunity can occur through the pathways of the essential fatty acid metabolites (i.e., eicosanoids).[17] Immediate hypersensitivity results from the interaction between IgE and mast cells with resulting histamine release. The presence of PGE_2 can apparently effect the release of histamine. As discussed previously in regard to inflammation, prostanoids of the E and F class provoke edema in the presence of histamine and bradykinin. However, both PGE_1 and PGE_2 drastically inhibit antigen-induced IgE-mediated release of histamine from human mast cells.[17]

Current evidence suggests that the action of eicosanoids with respect to delayed-type hypersensitivity is limited to the cells and tissues in the immediate area of its production. Endogenous synthesis of prostaglandins following an antigenic or mitogenic stimulus represents a negative regulatory signal for the lymphocyte. For example, eicosanoids can prolong allograft survival and inhibit antibody secretion, lymphokine secretion, migration inhibition factor, and cellular cytotoxicity.[3, 8–10] Table 18–2 lists additional inhibitory activities of the eicosanoids.[18] Webb and colleagues have shown that inhibitors of eicosanoid synthesis can reverse this suppression.[18]

The eicosanoids of most importance in affect-

*Adapted from Webb DR, Rogers TJ, Nowowiejski I: Endogenous prostaglandin synthesis and the control of lymphocyte function. Ann NY Acad Sci 332:262–270, 1979.
†MIF = migration inhibition factor.

Table 18–2. INHIBITORY EFFECTS OF PROSTAGLANDINS*

Inhibition
Antibody secretion
Antibody dependent cytotoxicity
Cellular toxicity
Prolongation of graft survival
Lymphokine secretion
MIF† activity
Mixed lymphocyte culture activity
Mitogen stimulation
Monokine secretion

Suppression
Humoral responses

ing cell-mediated immunity are prostanoids of the E type, which are known to influence the activity of lymphocytes via stimulation of cAMP and cGMP activity. Two mechanisms for such prostanoid action can be suggested. In the first, soluble products of activated T cells stimulate macrophages to release PGE_2, which enhances cAMP production, consequently inhibiting further lymphocyte reaction. Alternatively, this prostanoid could trigger the release of a suppressor factor from a specific T-cell subgroup, preventing lymphocyte transformation. Either way, the availability of precursors can provide for increased PGE production, which could be the basis for essential fatty acid and metabolite immunosuppression.[17]

The spleen is a major site for synthesis of the immunologically active eicosanoids.[19] Therefore, the observation that suppression of cell-mediated immunity by essential fatty acids in skin allografts cannot be demonstrated in splenectomized animals is strong indirect evidence of an essential fatty acid–eicosanoid interrelationship.[19]

BACTERIAL INHIBITION OF WOUND HEALING

Robson and associates have recently reported on wound healing alterations caused by infection.[5] Eicosanoids such as PGE_2 and TxA_2 are produced by certain strains of bacteria.[7] The leukocyte response to the initial breach of the integumentary barrier will also result in an increase in arachidonic acid metabolites and free oxygen radicals,[20] and these increased levels of inflammatory mediators, especially the vasoconstrictive ones, have been shown experimentally to enhance bacterial proliferation and

microabscess formation.[21] This sets up a vicious cycle resulting in an imbalance of mediators normally useful in the repair process.

Release of lysozymes, hydrolases, and other proteases can be affected by eicosanoids. It has been well documented that when the stable prostanoids are added to human polymorphonuclear leukocytes, they inhibit the release of lysosomal hydrolases.[3] Consequently, when PMNs encounter these prostanoids in the presence of opsonized particles, chemotactic factors, or immune complexes, the release of lysosomal enzymes is significantly inhibited.[3, 9] These inhibitory effects also occur when these cells are stimulated by exogenous cAMP. Therefore, agents such as PGE_1, PGE_2, and PGI_2 have the ability to inhibit lysosomal enzyme release in direct proportion to their ability to enhance cAMP accumulation within the PMNs (Fig. 18–4). These inhibitory effects on the phagocytic activity and intracellular killing mechanism of leukocytes coupled with the direct bacterial production of prostanoids help explain why a wound must be in bacterial balance to proceed through the normal phases of wound healing.[5]

LIPOXYGENASE PATHWAY—THE ALTERNATE ROUTE FOR ARACHIDONATE METABOLISM TO LEUKOTRIENE SYNTHESIS

As previously stated, once arachidonate is released, it can either be reincorporated into phospholipid or metabolized via the cyclo-oxygenase pathway into prostaglandins or via the lipoxygenase pathway into the leukotrienes. When inhibitors of cyclo-oxygenase are employed, leukotriene synthesis is enhanced.[22]

There are two major biosynthetic pathways of the lipoxygenase system. The first is via leukocyte 5-lipoxygenase, a calcium-dependent enzyme that metabolizes arachidonate to 5-hydroperoxy, 6,8,11,14-eicosatetraenoic acid (5-HPETE), a component of the slow-reacting substance of anaphylaxis (SRS-A) (see Figure 18–2). 5-HPETE enhances the release of anaphylactic mediators in the lung and also inhibits the formation of PGI_2.[22] The next stage is to produce 5-hydroxyeicosatetraenoic acid (5-HETE). While the products of 5-lipoxygenase apparently have regulatory functions of their own, 5-HPETE has been reported to augment

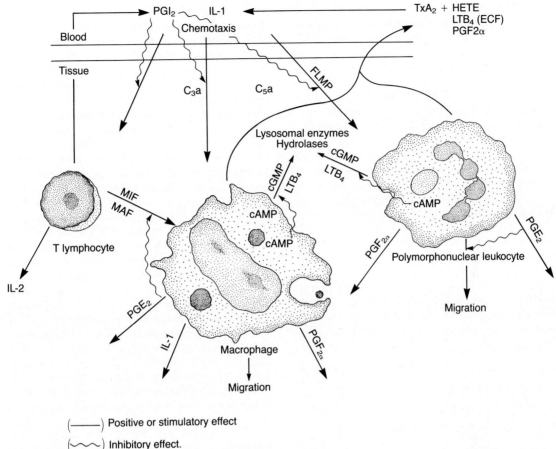

Figure 18–4. Probable effects of the eicosanoids on cellular events at an inflammatory site. Wavy lines indicate inhibitory responses; continuous lines indicate stimulatory responses.

the release of arachidonate while 5-HETE does not.[22] The release of preformed mediators such as histamine is stimulated by both 5-HETE and 5-HPETE. The end product of 5-HPETE (5-HETE) is a potent stimulator of the release of the gonadotropin-releasing hormone from pituitary cells.[22]

From 5-HETE, the next product is leukotriene A_4 (LTA_4) (see Figure 18–2). LTA_4 seems to be a pivotal point for other leukotriene production. LTB_4, LTC_4, and LTD_4 are all synthesized from LTA_4. However, there are other polyunsaturated fatty acids that can be converted into leukotrienes: for example, LTC_3, 8-9LTC_3, and LTC_5 are synthesized from 5,8,11-eicosatrienoic acid and 8,11,14-eicosatrienoic acid, and 5,8,11,14,17-eicosapentaenoic acid, respectively.[22]

The other pathway of the lipoxygenase system is via the platelet enzyme 12-lipoxygenase (see Figure 18–2). This results in 12-HPETE, which is metabolized to 12-HETE. Inhibition of PGI_2 formation is caused by 12-HPETE, which in turn results in a decrease in cAMP. Production

and release of anaphylactic mediators have been implicated in the negative modulation of cAMP production.

Leukotrienes have much fewer recognized effects on the wound healing process than other eicosanoids, and many of the effects seem to occur through the regulation of cyclo-oxygenase metabolites. Leukotrienes C_4 and D_4 cause increased microvascular permeability, and LTB_4 causes leukocytes to adhere to vessel walls.[23] However, Samuelson has stated that LTB_4 induces its effects via release of thromboxane.[24] Other leukotrienes can induce the synthesis of eicosanoids of the cyclo-oxygenase pathway from arachidonate, and LTC_4 and LTD_4 can cause almost a dose-dependent production of PGE_2 and PGI_2.[22]

This interrelationship among the eicosanoids of the lipoxygenase and cyclo-oxygenase pathways is best shown in wound repair by studying the regulation of hemostasis. Clot formation and maintenance are dependent on platelet aggregation, which is regulated through TxA_2 production. Thus, TxA_2 acts as a positive feedback mechanism in that, once released, it serves as a potent stimulus for more platelet aggregation. This eicosanoid, plus its intermediates PGG_2 and PGH_2, is a product of the arachidonate cyclo-oxygenase pathway. However, during platelet aggregation other arachidonate byproducts, primarily 12-HPETE and 12-HETE, are produced via the lipoxygenase pathway.

LTB_4 stimulates both chemotaxis and chemokinesis of PMNs, and it also induces degranulation and lysosomal enzyme release from human PMNs. This secretory action of LTB_4 is dependent on cytochalasin B and is enhanced by extracellular Ca^{++}. LTB_4 induces PMN aggregation and Ca^{++} mobilization and acts as a Ca^{++} ionophore in liposomes.[22] Leukotrienes of the C, D, and E groups have been reported to cause such diverse effects as negative inotropism on the heart, constriction of the coronary arteries, stimulation of macrophage eicosanoid synthesis, alteration in blood pressure, inhibition of mitogen-induced lymphocyte transformation, and lung excitation of cerebellar Purkinje neurons.[22]

CYTOKINES— SECONDARY MEDIATORS OF WOUND HEALING

If eicosanoids function as primary mediators of cell-cell and cell-matrix interactions, the various cytokines act as secondary mediators, functioning more as regulators or modulators. They are initially involved in many of the same wound healing stages as are the eicosanoids, and it is impossible to discuss the role of one class of mediators without discussing the other. Such substances produced by mononuclear phagocytes are called monokines, while those produced by lymphocytes are called lymphokines. Together these monocytic factors are classified as cytokines since they modulate inflammatory and immunological responses by regulating the mobility, differentiation, and growth of leukocytes and other cells including osteoclasts, chondrocytes, fibroblasts, and epithelial and endothelial cells. Some transformed cell lines such as the macrophage, keratinocyte, lymphocyte, and fibroblast continually release cytokines into the surrounding culture media. Several other chapters in this book describe individual cytokines in great detail. However, due to the relationship of these mediators with the eicosanoids, a brief overview of a selected number of cytokines is presented here to place these compounds into perspective.

Cytokines are glycoproteins having molecular weights ranging from 4000 to 60,000 daltons.[25] These extremely potent substances stimulate activity of each target cell at extremely minute concentrations from $10^{-10}M$ to $10^{-15}M$. Cytokines are classified according to their target activity, i.e., immunological or inflammatory cell response.[25] Those that modulate the lymphocyte activity with regard to enhancement or suppression of the immunological response are called afferent cytokines. They also are responsible for growth or differentiation of T and B lymphocytes. Those cytokines that modulate the cells that are responsible for degradative and reparative functions as well as bactericidal and cytocidal actions are called efferent cytokines. These cytokines can potentiate inflammatory reactions and normal wound healing through regulation of the mobility and metabolic functions of the nonlymphoid cell.[25]

Among the most well-studied cytokines are the monokine interleukin-1 (IL-1), the lymphokine interleukin-2 (IL-2), and the interferons. Monocytes constitute the major cell line that has been identified as the source of IL-1. However, macrophages from the peritoneal cavity, spleen, lung, and Kupffer cells from the liver can also produce IL-1.[25] Normal B lymphocytes, Langerhans cells, fibroblasts, a subset of large granular lymphocytes (LGL), neutrophils, and endothelial cells all produce an IL-1–like factor as well, which has been shown to act as a chemotactic agent for the neutrophils.[25] The enhancement of PGE_2 production in monocytes appears to be stimulated by IL-1 and concomitantly acts as a chemoattractant,[25] suggesting that IL-1 might have autostimulatory effects.

IL-1 derived from macrophages promotes the growth or metabolic function of every nonlymphocytic cell type that responds to the cytokine. IL-1 can account for many of the signs and symptoms of both acute and chronic inflammation including fever, elevation of acute phase proteins, changes in concentration of circulating plasma metals, cartilage and bone resorption, cachexia, anorexia, leukocytosis, and leukocytic infiltration to inflammatory localities.[25] Stimulation of arachidonate metabolism and eicosanoid production by IL-1 plays a central role in fever induction, perhaps by initiating eicosanoid production by the endothelial cell lining of the blood vessels in the highly vascularized hypothalamus.[25]

IL-1 stimulates endothelial cell replication, fibrinogen production, and procoagulant activity. Consequently, it appears to play a role in the early inflammatory response in clot formation. Therefore, like the eicosanoids, IL-1 induces a wide variety of activities and functions like a hormone or other pleiotrophic mediator such as interferon, affecting not only cells of the leukocytic series but also those of the non-leukocyte type as well (Fig. 18–5).[25]

The origin of IL-2 rests solely with the T cell. IL-2 promotes several cellular and metabolic functions in activated T cells prior to the onset of proliferation. IL-2–activated T cells produce other cytokines, B-cell growth factor (BCGF), B-cell differentiation factors (BCDFs), and enhanced interferon activation of T-cell cytotoxicity. This latter effect occurs even in the presence of mitomycin C, which inhibits DNA synthesis.[25]

Human T-suppressor cells can inhibit stimulated or activated T cells from producing IL-2. Other immunosuppressive agents such as PGE_2, cyclosporine, and glucocorticosteroids also act as inhibitors of IL-2 production. While cyclosporine and steroids act directly on the T cells, PGE_2 probably inhibits accessory cell function in the production of IL-2.

Just as IL-1 functions more as a monokine and IL-2 as a lymphokine, the interferons possess functions that mimic those of both classes of cytokines. Interferons (IFNs) can be defined as peptides that are genetically restricted and that promote antiviral activity in treated cells. They have been classified into three different classes (α, β, γ) based on physiochemical and antigenic differences. Interferons also influence immune reactivity and inhibit cell proliferation, but promote cell differentiation.[25]

While IFN-α and IFN-β are both regulators of humoral immunity, IFN-α is the more potent. IFN augments immunity through many complex mechanisms such as induction of accessory cell Ia/DR antigen expression and IL-1 production on direct promotion of the maturation of B cells and selective inhibition of the proliferation of T-suppressor cells.[25] Interferon's

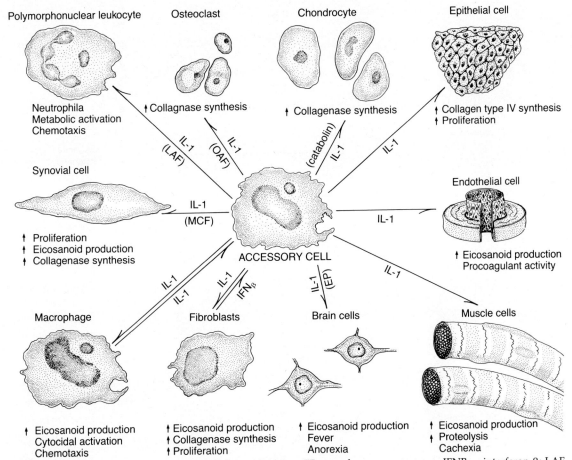

Figure 18–5. The effects of IL-1 on various cells and tissues. EP = endogenous pyrogens; IFNB = interferon-β; LAF = leukocyte activating factor; MCF = macrophage cytotoxicity factor; OAF = osteoclast activating factor. (Modified from Oppenheim JJ: Interleukins and Interferons in Inflammation. Current Concepts/Scope Publications. Kalamazoo, MI, Upjohn Company, 1980, pp 1–41.)

immunosuppressive effects may result from its antiproliferative effects or from activation of nonspecific T-suppressor cells.

This concise overview provides the evidence that interleukins and interferons regulate the inflammatory response and the immune systems as cytokines that control the cell responses. These responses alter cell proliferation and differentiation and can be either beneficial or detrimental to the process of wound healing.[25]

OXYGEN-DERIVED RADICALS AND RELATIONSHIP TO THE EICOSANOIDS

During the metabolism of a variety of lipids, including arachidonate, oxygen-derived free radicals are produced. Intermediates in mito-chondrial and microsomal electron-transport systems also generate free-radical compounds. Current evidence suggests that tissue damage associated with inflammatory responses and is-chemic injuries may be mediated by oxygen-derived free radicals (Fig. 18–6).[26, 27] As molecular O_2 accepts an electron from a reducing agent, it generates a superoxide (O_2^-) anion as a primary product. While O_2^- is relatively un-reactive, many of its derivative compounds, such as H_2O_2, have the capability of oxidizing organic molecules.[26, 27]

Several potential sources of free radicals exist within cell plasma membranes. Intermediate peroxy compounds and hydroxyl radicals $(OH\cdot)$ are produced by metabolites of arachidonate by both the cyclo-oxygenase and the lipoxygenase pathways. A potent oxidant, the $OH\cdot$ radical is produced from the peroxide PGG_2. This oxidant and PGG_2 regulate prostanoid production through a wide variety of mechanisms, which include deactivation of cyclo-oxygenase, pros-

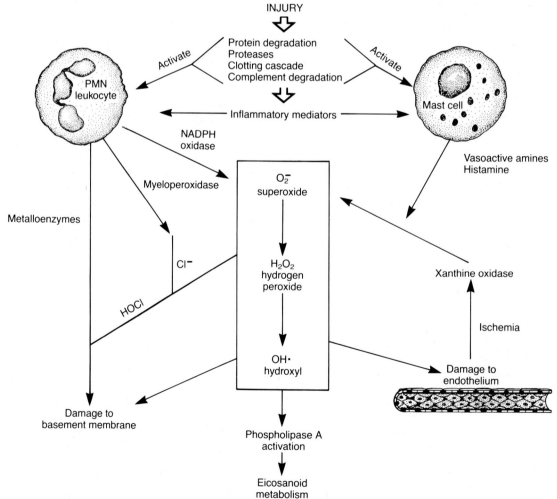

Figure 18–6. A possible scheme showing the production of oxygen-derived free radicals following injury.

tacyclin synthetase, and peroxidase. Conversion of the prostaglandin endoperoxides to form the stable prostanoids PGE_2 and $PGF_{2\alpha}$ and the labile PGI_2 and TxA_2 is modulated by free radical scavengers.[26, 27]

IgE-mediated degranulation of mast cells is inhibited by both PGI_2 and PGE_2. Both also inhibit functional responses of neutrophils such as chemotaxis, phagocytosis, O_2^- production and degranulation. Consequently, $OH\cdot$, a potent oxidant produced from the synthesis of PGH_2 via PGG_2, may in turn modulate the initiation and progressive phases of the inflammatory response. This sequence of events is important, since free radicals produced during phagocytosis are mediators of tissue injury.[26, 27]

An important source of free radicals in phagocytes is mediated by NADPH and NADH+. When a specific soluble inflammatory mediator stimulates a macrophage or PMN, it experiences a respiratory burst characterized by increased consumption of O_2 and the metabolism of glucose secondary to activation of the hexose monophosphate shunt.[26] After initiation of this respiratory burst in stimulated PMNs, more than 90 percent of the oxygen consumed can be accounted for by the generation of O_2^-.[26, 27] The majority of the H_2O_2 produced during stimulation of the phagocytic cell is directly derived from the dismutation of O_2^-. O_2 and H_2O_2 are the rate-limiting factor in the generation of O_2^- by phagocytes. $OH\cdot$ radicals are also formed.

Mediators of both acute and chronic inflammatory reactions include oxygen-derived free radicals and subsequent metabolites. Oxygen radicals generate chemotactic factors for phagocytes, directly, as a result of their reactions with unsaturated lipids, or indirectly, as intermediate metabolites in normal biochemical pathways of the cell. Phagocyte-mediated tissue injury and enhanced proteolysis of tissue substrates are potentiated by oxygen-derived free radicals and their subsequent metabolites.[26, 27] In addition, a variety of lysosomal enzymes are secreted into the extracellular milieu by phagocytes responding to a chemotactic stimuli. This proteolytic activity can synergistically enhance direct damage produced by oxygen-derived free radicals.

It appears that structural matrices of tissues at inflammatory sites can be altered with or without lysosomal proteases in the presence of oxygen metabolites. Cell injury through multiple mechanisms can be caused by O_2^- and its metabolites.[26, 27] Primary targets of oxygen-derived free radicals and their metabolites are polyunsaturated lipids (fatty acids). The oxidation of these lipids results in lipid hydroperoxide and concomitant alteration of the structural integrity and function of membranes. Consequently, those membranes damaged by free radicals are unable to maintain ionic gradients, which ultimately results in an influx of Ca^{++} and Na^+ ions and the efflux of intracellular K^+ ions.[26, 27]

Intracellular Ca^{++} accumulation has been noted when free-radical–induced cell injury occurs and is also associated with cytoskeletal function as well as activation of Ca^{++}-dependent phospholipases and protein kinases. As stated previously, phospholipases in the membrane, when activated, will cleave fatty acids from phospholipids, which causes changes in the physiological and chemical composition of the membrane.[4] Lipid peroxides and free radicals cause protein polymerization, and fragments of lipid oxidation products are incorporated into the protein structure. Free radicals are not only transferred to proteins but also cause damage to amino acid and carbohydrates by Fe^{++}-dependent mechanisms.[26, 27]

Free-radical–induced cell injury can occur by a more incipient mechanism.[26] Free radicals can induce breaks in both single- and double-stranded DNA. While O_2^- and H_2O_2 alone do not create any significant alterations in DNA structure, the $OH\cdot$ radicals and other peroxy-radical compounds can sever both single- as well as double-stranded DNA. Such alterations in the DNA structure can result in biochemical changes, changes in the maintenance of the cell's physiological state, and changes in the cell's ability to conserve its genetic constitution during subsequent division, thus leading to mutations.[26]

While tissue damage resulting from oxygen-derived free radicals can occur at the inflammatory site and involve many different cells, the cell most susceptible is the vascular endothelial cell.[26, 27] It is interesting that with all the evidence incriminating oxygen-derived free radicals as agents of tissue damage, all inflammatory foci do not cause multiple necrotic lesions throughout the body. Individuals with multiple injuries should eventually succumb because of the accumulation of these devastating products. In fact, since the vascular endothelial cell is most susceptible, anyone injured should suffer a major vascular collapse of the circulatory system almost immediately after injury. This, of course, does not happen. It is for this reason that the authors believe that many processes attributed directly to the effects of oxygen-derived free radicals are probably not direct effects but occur through the interactions of free radicals with the eicosanoids.

CONCLUSION

The ubiquitous eicosanoids initiate and modulate a myriad of biochemical, physiological, and pathophysiological reactions upon the host's cellular, tissue, and organ functions. While this chapter deals primarily with their role in wound healing, they have multiple functions as mediators of cell-cell and cell-matrix interaction. There is a fine line between the beneficial and detrimental role the eicosanoids play in normal or abnormal states. In some conditions, these ubiquitous compounds attenuate the disease process and in other instances they tend to exacerbate the process. In many of their activities they appear to be modulated or regulated by other mediators such as various cytokines or free radicals.

The difficulty in exactly defining the role of mediators such as eicosanoids in wound healing lies in the fact that the compounds are often bidirectional. While major efforts recently have been directed toward the development of global eicosanoid inhibitors as anti-inflammatory agents, it behooves researchers and clinicians to direct their efforts toward the development of a drug that acts at specific points along the eicosanoid pathway. Despite the scarcity of knowledge, it is obvious that the role of eicosanoids in wound healing is critical and requires further investigation. However, any attempt at this time to prematurely manipulate them pharmacologically could seriously upset the wound healing process. Only those specific pathways in which a single metabolite is known to cause a specific effect can be safely manipulated at this time.

References

1. Robson MC, Raine TJ, Smith DJ, et al: Principles of wound healing and repair. In James E, Corry RJ, Perry JF (eds): Principles of Basic Surgical Practice. Philadelphia, Hanley and Belfus, 1987, pp 61–72.
2. Timberlake GA: Wound healing. The physiology of scar formation. In McSwain NE (ed): Current Concepts in Wound Care. Chicago, Macmillan Professional Journals, 1986, pp 4–14.
3. Weissman G: Prostaglandins in Acute Inflammation. Kalamazoo, MI, Current Concepts/Scope Publication, Upjohn, 1980, pp 1–32.
4. Penneys NS: Prostaglandins and the Skin. Kalamazoo, MI, Current Concepts/Scope Publication, Upjohn, 1980, pp 1–28.
5. Robson MC, Stenberg BD, Heggers JP: Wound healing alterations caused by infections. Clin Plast Surg 17:485–492, 1990.
6. Robson MC: The immediate and delayed cellular damage following soft tissue trauma. In Zarins C (ed): Essays in Surgery. New York, Churchill Livingstone, 1989, pp 153–158.
7. Robson MC, Heggers JP: Quantitative bacteriology and inflammatory mediators in soft tissue. In Hunt TK, Pines E, Happenstall RB, et al (eds): Tissue Repair. Biological and Clinical Aspects of Soft and Hard Tissue Repair. New York, Praeger, 1984, pp 483–507.
8. Heggers JP, Robson MC: Prostaglandins and thromboxanes. In Ninnemann J (ed): Traumatic Injury Infection and Other Immunologic Sequelae. Baltimore, University Park Press, 1983, pp 79–102.
9. Heggers JP, Robson MC: Prostaglandins and thromboxane. In Wachtel T (ed): Critical Care Clinics. Philadelphia, WB Saunders, 1985, pp 59–77.
10. Bonta IL, Parnham MJ: Prostaglandins and chronic inflammation. Biochem Pharmacol 27:1611–1623, 1978.
11. Heggers JP, Robson MC: Eicosanoids in wound healing. In Watkins WD (ed): Prostaglandins in Clinical Practice. New York, Raven Press, 1989, pp 183–194.
12. Hunt TK: Personal communication.
13. Robson MC, Raine TJ, Smith DJ: Wounds and wound healing. In Lawrence PF, Bilbao M, Bell RM, et al (eds): Essentials of General Surgery. Baltimore, Williams & Wilkins, 1988, pp 107–114.
14. Murota S, Chang WC, Abe M, et al: The stimulatory effect of prostaglandins on production of hexosamine-containing substances by cultured fibroblasts. Prostaglandins 12:93–195, 1976.
15. Murota S, Abe M, Otsuka K, et al: Stimulative effect of prostaglandins on production of hexosamine-containing substances by cultured fibroblasts. III. Induction of hyaluronic acid synthetase prostaglandin $F_{2\alpha}$. Prostaglandins 14:983–991, 1977.
16. Alfin-Slater RB, Aftergood L: Essential fatty acids reinvestigated. Physiol Rev 48:758–784, 1968.
17. Mertin J: Essential fatty acids and cell mediated immunity. Prog Lipid Res 20:851–856, 1981.
18. Webb DR, Rogers TJ, Nowowiejski I: Endogenous prostaglandin synthesis and the control of lymphocyte function. Ann NY Acad Sci 332:262–270, 1979.
19. Mertin J, Stackpoole A: The spleen is required for the suppression of experimental allergic encephalomyelitis by prostaglandin precursors. Clin Exp Immunol 36:449–455, 1979.
20. Ward PA: Leukotaxis and leukotactic disorders. Am J Pathol 77:520–538, 1974.
21. Heggers JP, Robson MC, London MD: Prevention of microabscess formation following thermal injury. J Am Med Technol 44:215–218, 1982.
22. Bach MK: The Leukotrienes. Their Structure, Actions, and Role in Disease. Kalamazoo, MI, Current Concepts/Scope Publication, Upjohn, 1983, pp 1–52.
23. Robson MC, Smith DJ, Heggers JP: Innovations in burn wound management. Adv Plast Reconstr Surg 4:149–176, 1987.
24. Samuelson B: Leukotrienes: Mediators of immediate hypersensitivity reactions and inflammation. Science 220:568–575, 1983.
25. Oppenheim JJ: Interleukins and Interferons in Inflammation. Kalamazoo, MI, Current Concepts/Scope Publication, Upjohn, 1986, pp 1–45.
26. Fantone JC, Ward PA: Oxygen-derived Radicals and Their Relationship to Tissue Injury. Kalamazoo, MI, Current Concepts/Scope Publication, Upjohn, 1985, pp 1–51.
27. McCord JM: Oxygen-derived free radicals in postischemic tissue injury. N Engl J Med 312:159–163, 1985.
28. Ogburn PL, Brenner WE: Physiologic Actions and Effects of Prostaglandins. Kalamazoo, MI, Current Concepts/Scope Publication, Upjohn, 1981, pp 1–41.

19

PHARMACOLOGICAL INTERVENTIONS

George C. Fuller, Ph.D., and Kenneth R. Cutroneo, Ph.D.

As described in preceding chapters, mammals have evolved complex, multimediated, and coordinate processes for maintaining and restoring homeostasis in response to an injurious stimulus that impairs function. The processes needed to restore function after injury include removal of the injurious stimuli and the rapid restoration of structure consistent with the functional needs of the organ. When the functional need is supportive, immediate structural reinforcement in the form of a fibrotic response occurs that must later be remodeled and reorganized to achieve the final goal of re-establishment of normal architecture and specialized function. Since this spectrum of events and activities requires a multitude of endogenously mediated phased activities, it follows that wound repair is vulnerable to pharmacological manipulation by many different mechanistic approaches.

PHARMACOLOGICAL CONSIDERATIONS

The possible sites for pharmacological control can be conceptually defined in the context of the known responses of tissues to injury as simplified in Figure 19–1. When a tissue is injured (the cause may be mechanical, chemical, metabolic, or other), an acute inflammatory reaction occurs at the site that includes the release of various inflammatory mediators.

These provoke vascular permeability changes to permit extravasation of plasma constituents and the chemoattraction and migration of leukocytes to the tissue. This acute reaction is a defensive action by which the organism through humoral and cellular effectors destroys foreign material and initiates removal of damaged tissue components.

Early tissue response to injury also includes changes in cell composition and extracellular matrix formation. A fibroplastic process begins early with the establishment of cell populations responsible for increased synthesis of matrix. These fibroblasts or equivalent reparative cells are recruited by migration and subsequent proliferation of cells from the surrounding tissue and are responsible for the early and rapid repair needed for wound closure. The processes mediating this shift in cell populations have been studied with in vitro experiments on the actions of various factors derived from inflammatory cells on fibroblasts or equivalent reparative cells (e.g., smooth muscle cells). Growth factors from platelets, polymorphonuclear leukocytes, macrophages, and activated lymphocytes stimulate cell proliferation and synthesis of hyaluronate and collagen. These growth factors, discussed elsewhere in this book, offer a potential form of therapy to enhance both connective tissue formation and to stimulate re-epithelialization.

Early repair may be regarded as provisional, intended to rapidly restore the continuity of the tissue and to provide sufficient mechanical integrity. Slower processes in the organ decrease the wound volume and further improve the mechanical properties of the new tissue. This process requires the production and activation

This chapter was supported in part by NIH grant AR19808 awarded to KRC. The authors thank Linda Tepper for her assistance with the manuscript preparation.

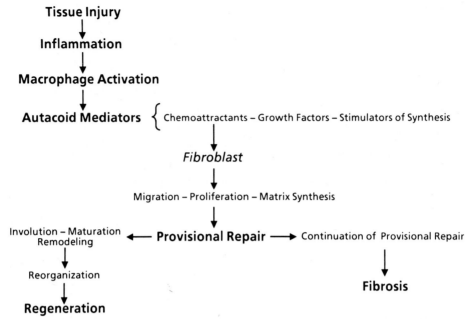

Figure 19–1. Tissue responses to injury needed for reconstitution of the extracellular matrix and regeneration.

of proteases, which are also potential therapeutic agents if applied during the correct phase of repair.

Although provisional repair should be self-limiting, this fibroplastic process may not subside, due to the failure to modify the early components of the repair process, to replace critical components of normal matrix (elastin, basement membrane), or to permit timely regeneration of an epithelial cell layer following injury. Tissue regeneration or scar tissue removal should occur promptly following withdrawal of the source of injury. In the absence of regeneration, the repair process will be followed by the excessive accumulation of collagen, leading eventually to irreversible fibrosis in the form of scar tissue. Because of the central role of collagen in this process, the pathway for collagen synthesis has been studied extensively in various settings of wound healing in experimental animals and in humans.

This oversimplified outline of the events occurring between injury and repair or eventual regeneration identifies a number of potential strategies for the pharmacological modulation of wound repair. The theoretical possibilities include

1. Modulation of cell populations with appropriate growth factors. This strategy includes the early application of factors that promote monocyte maturation to macrophages and fibroplasia to restore tissue integrity, followed by the specific growth factor necessary to promote epithelial regeneration and angiogenesis. Obviously, antiproliferative agents would have the opposite effect.

2. Modulation of matrix synthesis and accumulation. This strategy may include the early application of factors that will enhance matrix accumulation until tissue integrity is achieved but would be followed by pharmacological interventions to limit the fibrotic response with the expectation that connective tissue remodeling and regeneration would occur. The latter strategy could include agents that modulate connective tissue matrix synthesis, processing, or degradation.

Since earlier chapters focused on the role of various growth factors in wound repair settings, this chapter considers the array of agents and pharmacological strategies that influence matrix accumulation and turnover in settings of wound healing and regeneration. Pharmacological approaches to modulate collagen accumulation were discussed in a previous review.[1] Agents that impair collagen synthesis or processing include inhibitors of matrix crosslink formation that have been studied extensively as antifibrotic agents. Penicillamine has been tested as a potential antifibrotic agent because of its ability to block reactive aldehydes and, therefore, prevent collagen crosslinking. β-Aminopropionitrile (BAPN), used in short-term clinical trials for the past decade, inhibits lysyl oxidase and therefore decreases collagen crosslinking. Proline analogues have been used to control scar tissue formation because of their ability to decrease collagen synthesis and by their incorporation into peptides that inhibit prolyl hydroxylase. This results in the production of collagens deficient in hydroxyproline, which causes decreased thermal stability of the collagen triple helix and subsequent enhanced turnover of the matrix.

The best documented example of the clinical modulation of collagen production is the effect of glucocorticoids. Because these agents have been known for years to have a significant impact on wound repair, their effects on collagen production and accumulation and wound repair will be discussed extensively.

GLUCOCORTICOIDS

The rates of both collagen and noncollagen protein synthesis are increased in dermal wounds compared with normal skin. This increase in collagen synthesis is observed as early as 24 hours after wounding and continues over the next 5 days. Both natural and synthetic glucocorticoids alter collagen metabolism in normal skin and during wound healing, which may result in qualitative and quantitative changes in the extracellular matrix of skin and in the skin wound healing processes.[2] Since the tensile strength of a tissue is dependent on its collagen content, as expected, glucocorticoid treatment results in decreased wound tensile strength.[3, 4] However, Oxlund and co-workers[5] noted a biphasic effect of glucocorticoid treatment on rat skin: an initial increase in tensile strength associated with increased collagen crosslinking is followed by decreased collagen synthesis resulting in decreased collagen content and thinner skin. A similar biphasic effect was reported by Vogel.[6] In addition, topical corticosteroid treatment also results in a decrease in collagen synthesis and a delay in re-epithelialization in dermal wounds.[7]

Other tissues have also been found to have decreased breaking strength and breaking energy in healing wounds following corticosteroid treatment.[8, 9] For example, the restoration of mechanical strength and increase in collagen content in wounds in stomach and duodenum are both decreased by corticosteroid treatment. Glucocorticoid treatment at the site of tendon repair results in a dose-related response that ranges from a slight decrease to a total absence of fibroplasia.[9]

Corticosteroid treatment retards corneal epithelial wound healing,[10, 11] with this inhibitory effect dependent on the dose of corticosteroid and the time of onset of treatment.[12] These two parameters are important considerations in avoiding the toxic side effects of corticosteroid therapy. Concerns about the systemic toxicity of corticosteroids have led to many attempts to eliminate or control their adverse effects during the wound healing process. For example, zinc supplements have been used to treat corticosteroid-induced serum zinc deficiency and impaired wound healing.[13]

The first evidence that glucocorticoids could regulate granuloma growth and collagen content was the observation that adrenalectomy increased granuloma collagen content.[14] Replacement glucocorticoid treatment resulted in both an inhibition of granuloma growth and an involution of pre-existing granulomas. It is now known that glucocorticoids inhibit a spectrum of biochemical processes in growing granulomas.

Several investigators have shown that granuloma collagen content is decreased by glucocorticoid treatment.[15-17] The number of fibroblasts as well as the synthesis and secretion of collagen is decreased by glucocorticoids. This reduction in granuloma collagen content is associated with decreased collagen synthesis observed as a lessening in the incorporation of radioactive proline into both collagen and noncollagen protein.[18] In several studies, the inhibitory effect of glucocorticoids on collagen synthesis is reported to be selective;[19-21] that is, the inhibition of granuloma collagen synthesis is greater than the inhibition of total granuloma protein synthesis. The mechanism of this selective inhibition has not yet been elucidated. The glucocorticoid-mediated selective inhibition of collagen synthesis in granuloma is also associated with a decrease in prolyl hydroxylase activity,[15, 21, 22] but this does not result in decreased prolyl hydroxylation in the collagen that is synthesized.[21] Although granuloma formation is decreased to the same extent by equivalent anti-inflammatory doses of corticosteroids, at these same doses granuloma and skin collagen synthesis are decreased to different extents depending on the corticosteroid (Fig. 19–2).

For a number of years, retinoids have been associated with altered wound healing. The glucocorticoid-mediated inhibition of granuloma growth, collagen content, and collagen synthesis is reversed or retarded by co-administration of vitamin A.[23-26] Glucocorticoid-mediated reductions in inflammatory cell infiltration, fibroplasia, capillary budding, and deposition of collagen fibers are prevented by concurrent vitamin A therapy.[24] In addition, vitamin A blocks the inhibitory effects of glu-

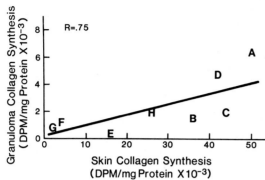

Figure 19–2. Correlation of corticosteroid-induced inhibition of granuloma and skin collagen synthesis. Twenty-four hours after polyvinyl sponge implantation in 200 g rats, corticosteroid treatment was initiated and continued for five daily injections. Neonatal rats received three daily injections. Twenty-four hours later all animals were given radioactive proline. Granuloma and skin collagen synthesis were determined using the bacterial collagenase digestion assay. The corticosteroids were injected at equivalent anti-inflammatory doses. The correlation coefficient R was determined. A = control; B = hydrocortisone; C = prednisolone; D = methyl-20-dihydroprednisolonate; E = triamcinolone; F = dexamethasone; G = betamethasone; H = dichlorisone.

cocorticoids on collagen, total protein, and DNA in granulomas.[15] Vitamin A has also been reported to overcome the inhibitory effects of glucocorticoids on tensile strength and collagen deposition during wound healing.[23, 27] While vitamin A deficiency slows repair, retinoids restore glucocorticoid-retarded repair of wounds.[28] Although the exact mechanism remains unknown, retinoids were proposed as important factors in macrophage activation, a critical cellular component of the successful wound healing process.

In other studies[29, 30] in which inhibition of wound healing by glucocorticoids is stabilized by vitamin A, the proposed mechanism is an antagonistic effect of corticosteroids and vitamin A on multiple inflammatory components. Vitamin A increases α_1- and α_2-globulin and decreases albumin in serum. In addition, leukocytes are decreased in glucocorticoid-treated animals, thereby decreasing the extent of tissue inflammation and possible damage to normal components. The effects cited above for vitamin A and glucocorticoids are dependent on the route of administration and the glucocorticoid employed. Golan and colleagues[31] demonstrated that although hydrocortisone did not delay wound healing, the longer acting corticosteroid Depo-Medrol (methylprednisolone) did. It is also possible that vitamin A may inhibit the effects of glucocorticoids on granuloma collagen content and wound healing by inhibiting collagenase production.[32]

As pointed out earlier, glucocorticoids have an antianabolic effect on skin collagen metabolism. Initial studies in skin demonstrated that glucocorticoids nonspecifically decrease skin collagen biosynthesis.[33–35] In all of these studies, various corticosteroids decreased collagen synthesis to the same extent as total proline incorporation. The most pronounced inhibition of collagen synthesis was noted with the fluorinated corticosteroids.[35] However, other studies using neonatal rat skin demonstrated that glucocorticoid treatment resulted in a selective reduction of collagen synthesis.[36, 37]

To elucidate the mechanisms involved in glucocorticoid suppression of collagen biosynthesis, the effect of steroid treatment on levels of translatable procollagen messenger RNA (mRNA) was determined. When polysomes isolated from skins of normal and glucocorticoid-treated neonatal rats were translated in the wheat germ lysate system, the synthesis of procollagen was decreased to a greater extent than total noncollagen protein synthesis.[38] This finding was substantiated by examining membrane-bound polysomes, the site of collagen translation versus free polysomes.[39] It is of interest that synthesis of prolyl hydroxylase directed by total skin polysomes was not affected by glucocorticoid treatment.

In more recent studies to determine whether glucocorticoids regulate procollagen gene expression, the synthesis of nuclear type I procollagen mRNA sequences was analyzed. Following glucocorticoid treatment, synthesis of procollagen mRNA sequences was decreased by 2, 4, and 24 hours (Fig. 19–3). These findings strongly suggest that glucocorticoids decrease procollagen gene expression. Accordingly, nuclei isolated from glucocorticoid-treated chick skin fibroblasts synthesized in vitro had fewer type I procollagen mRNA sequences than control nuclei.[40] This study also demonstrated that glucocorticoids coordinately regulated type I procollagen gene expression and procollagen DNA-binding proteins.

Another mechanism whereby glucocorticoids could decrease collagen biosynthesis is through destabilization of procollagen mRNA. While the degradation of total cellular RNA is stabilized by glucocorticoid treatment, the degradation of total procollagen mRNAs is not affected. These studies indicate that message destabilization is not responsible for the glucocorticoid-mediated decrease in procollagen synthesis in chick skin fibroblasts. In contrast, there are other reports in the literature that demonstrate a glucocorticoid-mediated destabilization of type I procollagen mRNAs in human skin fibroblasts and in

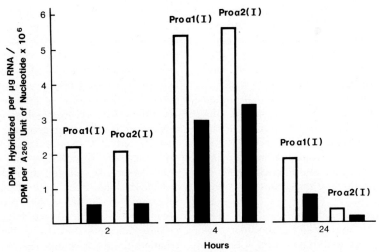

Figure 19–3. Glucocorticoid-mediated decrease of nuclear type I procollagen mRNA synthesis in cellulo. Chick skin fibroblasts were labeled with radioactive uridine in the presence or absence of glucocorticoid. Nuclear RNA was isolated and hybridized to unlabeled cDNA probes for proα1(I) and proα2(I). All incorporations were normalized for the total precursor pool specific radioactivities of CTP and UTP. Open bar = control; solid bar = dexamethasone. (Reprinted with permission from Cockayne D, Cutroneo KR: Glucocorticoid decreases the synthesis of type I procollagen in RNA. Biochemistry 25:3202–3209, 1986. Copyright 1986 American Chemical Society.)

rat dermal fibroblasts without an effect on procollagen gene expression.[41, 42] However, other reports demonstrate that glucocorticoids regulate procollagen gene expression.[43, 44] These latter studies determined glucocorticoid regulation of gene expression using in vitro nuclear runoff assays and transfection assays. These data in toto strongly suggest that glucocorticoids decrease procollagen synthesis at the level of gene expression.

The major structural collagens synthesized in skin are type I and type III. In neonatal rat skin, systemic glucocorticoid treatment results in a coordinate decrease in the synthesis of type I and type III procollagens, while fibronectin synthesis is increased (Fig. 19–4). This glucocorticoid-mediated inhibition of type I and type III procollagen synthesis is coordinated with respect to time and dose of glucocorticoid.[45] Whereas mouse fibroblasts treated with glucocorticoids demonstrate a decreased ratio of type III to type I procollagens,[46] further studies with rat dermal fibroblasts supported the concept that glucocorticoids coordinately regulate the suppression of type I and type III collagen biosynthesis.[47]

The selective glucocorticoid-mediated inhibition of collagen synthesis in skin is also associated with a reduction of several enzymes required for post-translational processing of collagen. The amount and activity of prolyl hydroxylase are decreased in skin.[36, 37, 48–50] Although activity of this enzyme is decreased, the degree of prolyl hydroxylation of total cellular procollagen[51] and procollagen nascent chains[37] is not altered. Lysyl hydroxylase, collagen glucosyltransferase, collagen galactosyltransferase,[49] and lysyl oxidase[50, 52] are also decreased by glucocorticoid treatment.

Interestingly, the selective inhibition of procollagen synthesis by human dermal fibroblasts is observed only in the presence of ascorbate.[53] The inhibitory effect on collagen synthesis in human fibroblasts is also associated with a decrease in translatable procollagen mRNAs[54] and in prolyl hydroxylase activity.[55]

Figure 19–4. Glucocorticoid-mediated coordinate decrease of type I and type III procollagen synthesis. Neonatal rats were treated for three consecutive days and given radioactive proline 20 minutes before sacrifice. For fibronectin synthesis radioactive leucine was used. Type I and type III procollagen synthesis and fibronectin synthesis in skin were determined using radioimmunoassays.

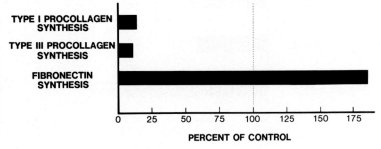

Skin collagen content depends upon the dynamic regulation of collagen synthesis and collagen degradation. Besides affecting skin collagen synthesis, corticosteroids may also alter collagen degradation in skin. Koob and associates[56] demonstrated that hydrocortisone and dexamethasone treatment of normal human skin explants decreased both collagen degradation and the appearance of collagenase in the media. However, Jeffrey and co-workers[57] demonstrated that collagen degradation and fibrillar collagenase activity remained unchanged in neonatal rat skin following triamcinolone treatment in vivo.

Glucocorticoids modulate many cellular metabolic processes by binding to intracellular proteinaceous receptors that have been localized within dermal cells.[58–60] Therefore, it is reasonable to suggest that glucocorticoids may selectively decrease procollagen synthesis through a glucocorticoid-receptor–mediated decrease of procollagen mRNAs. This assumption predicts that treatment with corticosteroids decreases procollagen mRNA levels by decreasing transcription. Consistent with this, glucocorticoids decrease the steady state levels of type I procollagen mRNAs in chick skin.[61] In neonatal rat skin, glucocorticoids also coordinately decrease the steady state amounts of type I and type III procollagen mRNAs (Fig. 19–5). However, it is also possible that the glucocorticoid-receptor complex does not bind directly to the promoter regions of procollagen genes. Instead, it may interact with the promoter of a regulatory gene that modulates procollagen gene expression through transacting factor(s).

One model of aberrant wound healing that has been studied extensively is the keloid, a fibrous lesion characterized by excessive synthesis and deposition of collagen. (This topic is dealt with in detail in Chapter 30.) Studies of the resident keloid fibroblasts have demonstrated an increased collagen biosynthetic rate[62] that is stable in vitro.[63] In addition, collagenase has been shown to be elevated in keloids.[64] However, while keloids contain high levels of this enzyme, the collagenase is probably incapable of breaking down collagen because collagenase-inhibiting α-globulins are increased in keloids.[65] These workers propose that the excessive accumulation of collagen in keloids is secondary to increased collagen synthesis and inhibition of collagen degradation. Macrophages may be activated to stimulate collagen synthesis and increase α-globulins in keloids, which would decrease collagen degradation.

Keloids have been treated with intralesional injections of corticosteroids for a number of years. It has been reported that although the keloids became softer and smaller following triamcinolone treatment, the normally high rate of collagen synthesis is not altered.[66] It is possible that corticosteroid treatment reduces plasma protease inhibitors, thus allowing collagenase to catabolize keloid collagen. In keloids that regress following intralesional triamcinolone treatment, there is a decrease of α_1-antitrypsin deposition in the treated lesions.[65] Russell and associates[67] demonstrated that glucocorticoid treatment resulted in different responses in normal and keloid-derived human fibroblasts. Although hydrocortisone decreased procollagen synthesis in normal skin fibroblasts, this glucocorticoid did not effectively decrease procollagen synthesis in keloid-derived fibroblasts. This disparity in response did not result from differences in glucocorticoid receptors in normal and keloid-derived fibroblasts.[68] However, differences were observed in the V_{max} of System A amino acid transport in normal and keloid-derived fibroblasts treated with glucocorticoids.[69] In contrast to these results, McCoy and colleagues[70] demonstrated that triamcinolone treatment of both normal and keloid-derived fibroblasts resulted in a selective decrease of procollagen synthesis. These differences may be explained by the dose and the type of corticosteroid used in the different studies.

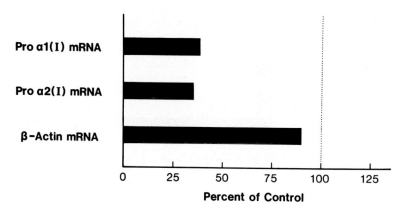

Figure 19–5. Glucocorticoids coordinately decrease the steady state levels of type I and type III procollagen mRNAs in neonatal rat skin. Neonatal rats were treated for 3 consecutive days with triamcinolone diacetate. Twenty-four hours after the last injection, total RNA was isolated from the skin and was hybridized with recombinant probes using the dot blot procedure.

PROLINE ANALOGUES

Interest in proline analogues as antifibrotic agents is based on observations that many of them are incorporated into protein in place of proline and that this substitution results in decreased accumulation of mature collagen.[71] Four of these analogues, azetidine-2-carboxylic acid (AZC), cis-4-fluroproline (CFP), cis-4-hydroxyproline (COP), and L-3,4-dehydroproline (DHP), have been shown to be incorporated into collagen at positions normally occupied by proline.[72] The results of these and other in vitro studies indicate that (1) proline analogues reduce the rate of collagen production and secretion; (2) the collagen produced lacks helical stability and is protease sensitive; and (3) DHP incorporation results in the formation of peptides that cannot be hydroxylated and become inhibitors of prolyl hydroxylase.[73] Since these analogues are incorporated into all proteins in place of proline, minor changes also occur in the function and conformation of noncollagen proteins as a result of this substitution. The clinical implications of inhibiting elastin secretion, and the impact of these analogues on noncollagen (in some cases regulatory) proteins will be a concern if this type of therapy is employed in clinical trials, especially if this problem remains unexplored in intact animal models. The specificity of proline analogues for the collagen pathway is imparted only by the relatively large requirement of this pathway for proline. In fact, a surprisingly high degree of replacement is achieved with COP or CFP.[74] It is thus not surprising that the reported whole animal toxicity of CFP[75] and DHP[76] reveal significant toxicity related to inhibition of total protein synthesis. Both studies also reported alterations in liver histology consisting of reversible lipid infiltration with DFP and disruption of rough endoplasmic reticulum with DHP.

Attempts to demonstrate the antifibrotic efficacy of proline analogues have met with varying degrees of success depending upon the animal model. COP and DHP prevent lung fibrosis resulting from hyperoxia or bleomycin.[77] The collagen content associated with neuronal scarring in rats[78] and with tendon adhesions in rats[79] was also reduced by COP. However, all of the active analogues have been used without effect in radiation fibrosis of skin and in dermal wounds with the exception of AZC, which reduced hydroxyproline content when applied topically to skin wounds on pigs.[80] In this study, 0.2 mg of AZC in water was applied topically to split-thickness wounds that were serially excised on days 2 through 10 after wounding. AZC decreased hydroxyproline content of the underlying dermis and decreased the rate of wound re-epithelialization in the absence of a significant effect on epidermal collagen. Based on these observations, the authors concluded that the migrating epithelium is dependent on the integrity of the collagenous matrix of the dermis. If so, the use of antifibrotic agents to influence scar tissue formation in this setting would be a seriously flawed strategy unless the impaired re-epithelialization can still be stimulated by the application of an appropriate growth factor (see Chapter 7).

In summary, the variable success achieved when using proline analogues to control collagen accumulation is likely to be related to local differences in the target organ where factors such as proline pool size and the availability of proline influence the amount of analogue required to evoke a significant change. The selection of one of these as an antifibrotic agent in this situation would require information on the relative effect of the analogue on elastogenesis and additional studies on the impact of this strategy on re-epithelialization.

INHIBITORS OF COLLAGEN CROSSLINKING

The use of inhibitors of matrix crosslink formation for reduction of scar formation has been studied more extensively than the proline analogues. Penicillamine is a potential antifibrotic agent because of its ability to block reactive aldehydes and therefore prevent crosslinking.[81] However, it is unlikely that penicillamine prevents crosslinking of matrix collagen at doses used systemically in clinical settings for treatment of arthritis or Wilson's disease. In a study of delayed surgical wound healing in rheumatoid arthritis, 600 mg of penicillamine per day as continuous therapy did not influence the rate of wound healing or increase the frequency of operative re-intervention compared with no therapy.[82] This is consistent with the conclusion that clinical penicillamine doses (300 to 600 mg/day) administered systemically are not sufficient to alter collagen maturation.

Unlike penicillamine, β-aminopropionitrile (BAPN), which has been used in short-term clinical trials for the past decade, specifically inhibits lysyl oxidase, making it possible to titrate the effect of this agent on crosslink formation. However, the prolonged systemic use of BAPN to prevent collagen deposition in chronic diseases carries the risk of producing a lathyritic syndrome. The cardiovascular damage observed with this syndrome is related to impaired crosslinking of collagen and elastin resulting in aneurysms when doses of 1 g per kilogram per day are given to weanlings. This problem may be manageable with acute use in adults since the same dose fails to produce fatal aortic aneurysms when given to mature animals.[83] In view of the dependence of elastic fiber formation on the crosslinking reactions mediated by lysyl oxidase, it is possible that the vascular aneurysm development induced by BAPN in growing animals is a result of impaired elastogenesis and that the mature animal is more resistant because of a reduced requirement for elastogenesis and new collagen formation to retain functional integrity in normal pressure-bearing organs. However, as expected because of its effect on crosslinking, systemic BAPN does impair healing of surgically induced periosteal wounds in rats.[84]

Increased lysyl oxidase activity has been reported in various forms of scar tissue; in some cases it persisted for up to 5 years. Collagen fibrils that are crosslinked through these reactions become at least ten times more resistant to degradation by mammalian collagenase.[85] This suggests that levels of lysyl oxidase may be important not only in determining or explaining differences in the rates of extracellular maturation of various collagen types but also in influencing the degree of reversibility of the fibrotic lesion. It would also follow that inhibition of lysyl oxidase would provide control of aggressive collagen deposition in scar tissue. Animal studies have established that subtoxic doses of BAPN reduce collagen deposition in animal models of scar tissue formation. Studies designed to evaluate the dose-response curve for BAPN as an antifibrotic agent revealed that single doses as low as 10 mg per kilogram inhibited lysyl oxidase for 6 hours in dermal wounds of rats, with the inhibition persisting for up to 48 hours when the larger doses (40 mg/kg) were used.[86] Reduction of scar tissue by systemic BAPN has been demonstrated in dermal wounds in rats[86] and in esophageal strictures in dogs.[87]

The healing strength and crosslinking of collagen (estimated from extractability) were also reduced by the topical administration of BAPN to rat incision wounds.[88] Thus, it is apparent that BAPN effects on matrix are also produced by topical administration, a dose form that would be expected to limit the toxicity to internal organs. However, at present there are no published studies that assess the effect of BAPN-induced alterations of wound matrix on re-epithelialization of dermal wounds.

The inhibition of collagen crosslinking by BAPN as a strategy to control ocular scarring has been explored in rabbit models of penetrating injury,[89] alkali-induced conjunctival scarring,[90] and keratotomy.[91] The topical application of BAPN in petrolatum three times a day reduced the degree of post-traumatic vitreous fibrous proliferation and also enhanced compliance and reduced refractive regression 6 to 8 weeks after radial keratotomy. However, Busin and colleagues[92] found no effect on keratometry readings when they used a similar keratotomy procedure followed by BAPN treatment for 6 weeks.

In clinical studies, purified preparations of BAPN have been administered in doses up to 1 g per day for 5 weeks without acute hypersensitivity reactions.[93] In view of the observation that 10 mg per kilogram is effective in dermal wounds in rats,[86] 1 g per day (or ~15 mg/kg) may exceed the dose required in humans and account for the fact that Peacock and Madden could detect no dose-related differences in the effect of 1, 3, and 5 g doses in their clinical studies.[93] Arguments for the safety of these BAPN doses in mature animals are supported by the lifetime studies conducted by LaBella and Vivian.[94] These investigators fed mice BAPN in drinking water (1 mg/ml, which is at least 100 mg/kg/day) for up to 18 months. In this and a previous study, they found that this dose increased longevity by 2 months, a difference that was statistically significant. However, the historical data base that BAPN is a lathyrigen argues that BAPN used for clinical concept testing should be restricted to local application.

BAPN is metabolized through oxidative deamination in liver.[95] The drug disappears rapidly from serum, with its metabolite appearing in urine several hours later. In rabbits, the liver radioactivity derived from ^{14}C-BAPN is two to three times the level found in lung tissue.[95] In view of the low levels of BAPN required to produce inhibition of lysyl oxidase, it should be possible to identify topical dose forms of BAPN that inhibit lysyl oxidase with minimal effects on the connective tissues of other organs because of the "first pass" effect of the liver. Studies pursuing this hypothesis are currently being conducted, predicated on the research of Chvapil and co-workers.[96, 97] These early animal studies demonstrated that the free-base form of BAPN would be absorbed through the rat dermis and could impair wound healing, presumably by altering collagen crosslinking.

Extrapolating from these results to the topical application of BAPN fumarate in an ointment in humans, several ongoing clinical trials are examining the efficacy of this drug in temporomandibular joint stiffness and tendon adhesions as well as in the treatment of keloids.

Preliminary results indicate that topical application of BAPN is useful in the treatment of fibrotic lesions accessible from the dermis. While some hypersensitivity reactions have been noted, the ointment is well tolerated, and subjective positive responses have been obtained. In addition, a surprising apparent anti-inflammatory effect has been observed. Although definitive conclusions are not possible, these initial results suggest that antifibrotic therapy with BAPN has significant potential, and work is progressing to enhance its efficacy.

CONCLUSION

This review focused on agents that modulate scar tissue development in the wound healing setting. It is apparent that the fibrotic response can be pharmacologically controlled with presently available therapy (e.g., glucocorticoids) or with experimental compounds with greater specificity for the collagen pathway. Additional forms of therapy in the latter category are likely to become available in the future if clinical concept testing with currently available probes demonstrates prevention of scar formation during wound healing. However, the clinical implications and consequences of pharmacologically modulating the processes leading to scar tissue formation are not clearly defined and remain as a challenge for clinical research. It is clear, for example, that future pharmacological strategies will include the use of growth factors to promote the reconstitution of the connective tissue matrix and re-epithelialization. However, there is no evidence that the impaired re-epithelialization associated with modified matrix formation in animal models can be obtained through the application of appropriate growth factors. As in many other clinical situations, a polypharmacy strategy will be used that calls for the rational application of agents directed at specific biochemical lesions to enhance the process of healing and regeneration and/or prevent scar formation. In this context, the role of modulators of matrix formation will vary depending on the specific setting and documentation of their use in other pharmacological strategies.

References

1. Fuller GC: Perspectives for the use of collagen inhibitors as antifibrotic agents. J Med Chem 24:651–658, 1981.
2. Goforth P, Gudas CJ: Effects of steroids on wound healing: A review of the literature. J Foot Surg 19:22–28, 1980.
3. Oxlund H, Fogdestam I, Viidik A: The influence of cortisol on wound healing of the skin and distant connective tissue response. Surg Gynecol Obstet 148:876–880, 1979.
4. Phillips K, Arffa R, Cintron C, et al: Effect of prednisolone and medroxyprogesterone on corneal wound healing, ulceration and neovascularization. Arch Ophthalmol 101:640–643, 1983.
5. Oxlund H, Sims T, Light ND: Changes in mechanical properties, thermal stability, reducible cross-links and glycosyl-lysines in rat skin induced by corticosteroid treatment. Acta Endocrinol 101:312–320, 1982.
6. Vogel HG: Correlation between tensile strength and collagen content in rat skin. Effect of age and cortisol treatment. Connect Tissue Res 2:177–182, 1974.
7. Alvarez OM, Levendorf KD, Smerbeck RV, et al: Effect of topically applied steroidal and nonsteroidal anti-inflammatory agents on skin repair and regeneration. Fed Proc 43:2793–2798, 1984.
8. Gottrup F, Oxlund H: Healing of incisional wounds in stomach and duodenum: The effect of long-term cortisol treatment. J Surg Res 31:165–171, 1981.
9. Ketchum LD: Effects of triamcinolone on tendon healing and function. Plast Reconstr Surg 47:471–482, 1971.
10. Sanchez J, Polack FM: Effect of topical steroids on the healing of corneal endothelium. Invest Ophthal 13:17–22, 1974.
11. Petroutsos G, Guimaraes R, Giraud JP, et al: Corticosteroids and corneal epithelial wound healing. Br J Ophthal 66:705–708, 1982.
12. Kara-Jose N, Lorenzetti DWC, McAuliffe R, et al: Time response effects of corticosteroids on corneal wound healing. Can J Ophthal 7:48–51, 1972.
13. Flynn A, Pories WJ, Strain WH, et al: Zinc deficiency with altered adrenocortical function and its relation to delayed healing. Lancet 1:789–791, 1973.
14. Robertson W, Van B, Sanborn EC: Hormonal effects on collagen formation in granulomas. Endocrinology 63:250–252, 1958.
15. Wehr RF, Smith JG Jr, Counts DF, et al: Vitamin A prevention of triamcinolone acetonide effects on granuloma growth: Lack of effect on prolyl hydroxylase. Proc Soc Exp Biol Med 152:411–414, 1976.
16. Salmela K: Comparison of the effects of methylprednisolone and hydrocortisone on granuloma tissue development. Scand J Plast Reconstr Surg 15:87–91, 1981.
17. Nocenti MR, Lederman GE, Furey CA, et al: Collagen synthesis and ^{14}C-labeled proline uptake and conversion to hydroxyproline in steroid-treated granulomas. Proc Soc Exp Biol Med 117:215–218, 1964.
18. Fukuhara M, Tsurufuji S: The effect of locally injected anti-inflammatory drugs on the synthesis of collagen and non-collagen protein of carrageenin granuloma in rats. Biochem Pharmacol 18:2409–2414, 1969.
19. Nakagawa H, Fukuhara M, Tsurufuji S: Effect of a single injection of betamethasone disodium phosphate on the synthesis of collagen and noncollagen protein of carrageenin granuloma in rats. Biochem Pharmacol 20:2253–2261, 1971.
20. Tsurufuji S, Nakagawa H: Metabolic study of the action mechanism of anti-inflammatory steroids. In Otaka Y

(ed): Biochemistry and Pathology of Connective Tissue. Tokyo, Igaku Shoin, 1974, pp 139–151.

21. Kruse NJ, Rowe DW, Fujimoto WY, et al: Inhibitory effects of glucocorticoids on collagen synthesis by mouse sponge granulomas and granuloma fibroblasts in culture. Biochim Biophys Acta 540:101–116, 1978.

22. Cutroneo KR, Costello D, Fuller GC: Alteration of proline hydroxylase activity by glucocorticoids. Biochem Pharmacol 20:2797–2804, 1971.

23. Ehrlich HP, Tarver H: Effects of beta-carotene vitamin A and glucocorticoids on collagen synthesis in wounds. Proc Soc Exp Biol Med 137:936–938, 1971.

24. Ehrlich HP, Tarver H, Hunt TK: Effects of vitamin A and glucocorticoids upon inflammation and collagen synthesis. Ann Surg 177:222–227, 1973.

25. Salmela K: The effect of methylprednisolone and vitamin A on wound healing. II. Acta Chir Scand 147:313–315, 1981.

26. Salmela K, Ahonen J: The effect of methylprednisolone and vitamin A on wound healing. I. Acta Chir Scand 147:307–312, 1981.

27. Hunt TK, Ehrlich HP, Garcia JA, et al: Effect of vitamin A on reversing the inhibitory effect of cortisone on healing of open wounds in animals and man. Ann Surg 170:633–641, 1969.

28. Hunt TK: Vitamin A and wound healing. J Am Acad Dermatol 15:817–821, 1986.

29. Kohnlein HE, Muckle B: Modification of cortisol-induced wound healing disorder by vitamin A. Z Exp Chir 8:373–378, 1975.

30. Seitz HD, Kohnlein HE, Buckle B: Animal experiment studies on the effect of vitamin A on cortisol-induced wound healing disorders. Langenbecks Arch Chir (Suppl):181–185, 1975.

31. Golan J, Mitelman S, Baruchin A, et al: Vitamin A and corticosteroid interaction in wound healing in rats. Isr J Med Sci 16:572–575, 1980.

32. Brinckerhoff CE, McMillan RM, Dayer J-M, et al: Inhibition by retinoic acid of collagenase production in rheumatoid synovial cells. N Engl J Med 303:432–436, 1980.

33. Kivirikko KI, Laitinen O, Aer J, et al: Studies with ^{14}C-proline on the action of cortisone on the metabolism of collagen in the rat. Biochem Pharmacol 14:1445–1451, 1965.

34. Smith QT, Allison DJ: Skin and femur collagens and urinary hydroxyproline of cortisone-treated rats. Endocrinology 77:785–791, 1965.

35. Uitto J, Teir H, Mustakallio KK: Corticosteroid-induced inhibition of the biosynthesis of human skin collagen. Biochem Pharmacol 21:2161–2167, 1972.

36. Cutroneo KR, Counts DF: Anti-inflammatory steroids and collagen metabolism: Glucocorticoid-mediated alterations of prolyl hydroxylase activity and collagen synthesis. Mol Pharmacol 11:632–639, 1975.

37. Newman RA, Cutroneo KR: Glucocorticoids selectively decrease the synthesis of hydroxylated collagen peptides. Mol Pharmacol 14:185–198, 1978.

38. McNelis B, Cutroneo KR: A selective decrease of collagen peptide synthesis by dermal polysomes isolated from glucocorticoid-treated newborn rats. Mol Pharmacol 14:1167–1175, 1978.

39. Rokowski RJ, Sheehy J, Cutroneo KR: Glucocorticoid-mediated selective reduction of functioning collagen messenger ribonucleic acid. Arch Biochem Biophys 210:74–81, 1981.

40. Cockayne D, Cutroneo KR: Glucocorticoid coordinate regulation of type I procollagen gene expression and procollagen DNA-binding proteins in chick skin fibroblasts. Biochemistry 27:2736–2745, 1988.

41. Hamalainen L, Oikarinen J, Kivirikko KI: Synthesis and degradation of type I procollagen mRNAs in cultured human skin fibroblasts and effect of cortisol. J Biol Chem 260:720–725, 1985.

42. Raghow R, Gossage D, Kang AH: Pretranslational regulation of type I collagen, fibronectin and a 50-kilodalton noncollagenous extracellular protein by dexamethasone in rat fibroblasts. J Biol Chem 261:4677–4684, 1986.

43. Walsh MJ, LeLeiko N, Sterling KM Jr: Regulation of Type I, III, and IV procollagen mRNA synthesis in glucocorticoid-mediated intestinal development. J Biol Chem 262:10814–10818, 1987.

44. Weiner FR, Czaja MJ, Jefferson DM, et al: The effects of dexamethasone on *in vitro* collagen gene expression. J Biol Chem 262:6955–6958, 1987.

45. Shull S, Cutroneo KR: Glucocorticoids coordinately regulate procollagens Type I and Type III synthesis. J Biol Chem 258:3364–3369, 1983.

46. Verbruggen LA, Abe S: Glucocorticoids alter the ratio of Type III/Type I collagen synthesis by mouse dermal fibroblasts. Biochem Pharmacol 31:1711–1715, 1982.

47. Shull S, Cutroneo KR: Glucocorticoids change the ratio of Type III to Type I procollagen extracellularly. Coll Rel Res 6:295–300, 1986.

48. Cutroneo KR, Stassen FLH, Cardinale GJ: Anti-inflammatory steroids and collagen metabolism: Glucocorticoid-mediated decrease of prolyl hydroxylase. Mol Pharmacol 11:44–51, 1975.

49. Risteli J: Effect of prednisolone on the activities of the intracellular enzymes of collagen biosynthesis in rat liver and skin. Biochem Pharmacol 26:1295–1298, 1977.

50. Benson SC, LuValle PA: Inhibition of lysyl oxidase and prolyl hydroxylase activity in glucocorticoid treated rats. Biochem Biophys Res Commun 99:557–562, 1981.

51. Counts DF, Rojas FJ, Cutroneo KR: Glucocorticoids decrease prolyl hydroxylase activity without the cellular accumulation of underhydroxylated collagen. Mol Pharmacol 15:99–107, 1979.

52. Counts DF, Shull S, Cutroneo KR: Skin lysyl oxidase activity is not rate limiting for collagen crosslinking in the glucocorticoid-treated rat. Connect Tissue Res 14:237–243, 1986.

53. Russell SB, Russell JD, Trupin KM: Collagen synthesis in human fibroblasts: Effects of ascorbic acid and regulation by hydrocortisone. J Cell Physiol 109:121–131, 1981.

54. Oikarinen J, Pihlajaniemi T, Hamalainen L, et al: Cortisol decreases the cellular concentration of translatable procollagen mRNA species in cultured human skin fibroblasts. Biochem Biophys Acta 741:297–302, 1983.

55. Trupin JS, Russell SB, Russell JD: Variation in prolyl hydroxylase activity of keloid-derived and normal human fibroblasts in response to hydrocortisone and ascorbic acid. Coll Rel Res 3:13–23, 1983.

56. Koob TJ, Jeffrey JJ, Eisen AZ: Regulation of human skin collagenase activity by hydrocortisone and dexamethasone in organ culture. Biochem Biophys Res Commun 61:1083–1088, 1974.

57. Jeffrey JJ, DiPetrillo T, Counts DF, et al: Collagen accumulation in the neonatal rat skin: Absence of fibrillar collagen degradation during normal growth. Coll Rel Res 5:157–165, 1985.

58. Epstein EH Jr, Munderloh NH: Glucocorticoid receptors of mouse epidermis and dermis. Endocrinology 108:703–711, 1981.

59. Epstein EH Jr: Hormone receptors. In Goldsmith LA (ed): Biochemistry and Physiology of the Skin, vol 2. New York, Oxford University Press, 1983, pp 1200–1209.

60. Smith K, Shuster S, Rawlins M: Characterization of glucocorticoid receptor in rat skin. J Endocrinol 96:229–239, 1983.

61. Sterling KM Jr, Harris MJ, Mitchell JJ, et al: Dexamethasone decreases the amounts of Type I procollagen mRNAs in vivo and in fibroblast cell cultures. J Biol Chem 258:7644–7647, 1983.

62. Abergel RP, Pizzurro D, Meeker CA, et al: Biochemical composition of the connective tissue in keloids and analysis of collagen metabolism in keloid fibroblast cultures. J Invest Dermatol 84:384–390, 1985.

63. Diegelmann RF, Cohen IK, McCoy BJ: Growth kinetics and collagen synthesis of normal skin, normal scar, and keloid fibroblasts in vitro. J Cell Physiol 98:341–346, 1979.

64. Cohen IK, Diegelmann RF, Keiser HR: Collagen metabolism in keloid and hypertrophic scar. In Longacre JJ (ed): Relation of the ultrastructure of collagen to the healing of wounds and to the surgical management of hypertrophic scar. Springfield, IL, Charles C Thomas, 1976, pp 199–212.

65. Diegelmann RF, Bryant CP, Cohen IK: Tissue alpha-globulins in keloid formation. Plast Reconstr Surg 59:418–423, 1977.

66. Cohen IK, Diegelmann RF, Johnson ML: Effect of corticosteroids on collagen synthesis. Surgery 82:15–20, 1977.

67. Russell JD, Russell SB, Trupin KM: Differential effects of hydrocortisone on bone growth and collagen metabolism of human fibroblasts from normal and keloid tissue. J Cell Physiol 97:221–230, 1978.

68. Gadson PF, Russell JD, Russell SB: Glucocorticoid receptors in human fibroblasts derived from normal dermis and keloid tissue. J Biol Chem 259:11236–11241, 1984.

69. Russell SB, Russell JD, Trupin JS: Hydrocortisone induction of System A amino acid transport in human fibroblasts from normal dermis and keloid. J Biol Chem 259:11464–11469, 1984.

70. McCoy BJ, Diegelmann RF, Cohen IK: In vitro inhibition of cell growth, collagen synthesis and prolyl hydroxylase activity by triamcinolone acetonide. Proc Soc Exp Biol Med 163:216–222, 1980.

71. Fuller GC: The pharmacology and toxicology of antifibrotic agents. In Gerlach V, Pott G, Rauterberg J (eds): Connective Tissue of the Normal and Fibrotic Human Liver. New York, G Thieme Verlag, 1982, pp 219–227.

72. Uitto J, Prockop DJ: Incorporation of proline analogues into collagen polypeptides. Biochem Biophys Acta 336:234–251, 1974.

73. Nolan JC, Ridge S, Oronsky AL, et al: Studies on the mechanism of reduction of prolyl hydroxylase activity by D-L-3,4-dehydroproline. Arch Biochem Biophys 189:448–453, 1978.

74. Uitto J, Prockop DJ: Incorporation of proline analogs into procollagen. Assay for replacement of amino acids by cis 4 hydroxy-L-proline and cis 4 fluoro-L-proline. Arch Biochem Biophys 181:293–299, 1977.

75. Bakerman S, Martin RL, Burgstahler AW, et al: In vivo studies with fluoroprolines. Nature 181:293–299, 1977.

76. Madden JW, Chvapil M, Carlson EC, et al: Toxicity and metabolic effects of 3,4 dehydroproline in mice. Toxicol Appl Pharmacol 26:426–437, 1973.

77. Riley DJ, Berg RA, Edelman NH, et al: Prevention of collagen deposition following pulmonary oxygen toxicity in the rat by cis-4-hydroxy-L-proline. J Clin Invest 65:643–651, 1980.

78. Lane JM, Bora FW Jr, Pleasure D: Neuroma scar formation in rats following peripheral nerve transection. J Bone Joint Surg 60A:197–203, 1978.

79. Lane JM, Bora FW Jr, Black J: Hydroxyproline limits work necessary to flex a digit after tendon injury. Clin Orthop 109:193–200, 1975.

80. Alvarez OM, Merta PM, Eaglestein WH: Effect of the proline analogue L-azetidine-2-carboxylic acid on epidermal and dermal wound repair. Plast Reconstr Surg 69:284–289, 1982.

81. Nimni M: The molecular organization of collagen and its role in determining the biophysical properties of connective tissues. Biorheology 17:51–82, 1980.

82. Bamert W, Stojan B, Wiedman V: D-penicillamine and wound healing in patients with rheumatoid arthritis. Z Rheumatol 39:9–13, 1980.

83. Julian M, Pieraggi MT, Bouissou H: Effect of beta-aminopropionitrile on the aortic wall in the adult rat. Pharmacol Res Commun 11:501–508, 1979.

84. Kuebel MA, Yeager VL, Taylor JJ: Effect of phenytoin and/or BAPN on a surgically induced periosteal wound. J Exp Pathol 2:99–109, 1985.

85. Vater CA, Harris ED, Siegel RC: Native cross-links in collagen fibrils induce resistance to human synovial collagenase. Biochem J 181:639–645, 1979.

86. Arem AJ, Misiorowski R, Chvapil M: Effects of low-dose BAPN on wound healing. J Surg Res 27:228–232, 1979.

87. Butler C, Madden JW, Davis WM, et al: Morphologic aspects of experimental esophageal lye strictures. II. Effect of steroid hormones, bougienage, and induced lathyrism on acute lye burns. Surgery 81:431–435, 1977.

88. Hoffman DL, Owen JA, Chvapil M: Healing of skin incision wounds treated with topically applied BAPN free base in the rat. Exp Mol Pathol 39:154–162, 1983.

89. Moorhead LC: Effect of BAPN after posterior penetrating injury in the rabbit. Am J Ophthalmol 95:97–109, 1983.

90. Moorhead LC: Inhibition of collagen cross-linking: A new approach to ocular scarring. Curr Eye Res 1:77–83, 1981.

91. Moorhead LC, Carroll J, Constance G, et al: Effects of topical treatment with BAPN after radial keratotomy in the rabbit. Arch Ophthalmol 102:304–307, 1984.

92. Busin M, Yau CW, Yamaguchi T, et al: The effect of collagen cross link inhibitors on rabbit corneas after radial keratotomy. Invest Ophthalmol Visual Sci 27:1001–1005, 1986.

93. Peacock EE, Madden JW: Administration of beta-aminopropionitrile to human beings with urethral strictures: A preliminary report. Am J Surg 136:500–505, 1978.

94. Labella F, Vivian S: Beta-aminopropionitrile promotes longevity in mice. Exp Gerontol 13:251–254, 1978.

95. Fleisher JH, Speer D, Brendel K, et al: Effect of pargyline on the metabolism of beta-aminopropionitrile (BAPN) by rabbits. Toxicol Appl Pharmacol 47:61–69, 1979.

96. Fleisher JH, Misiorowski R, Owen JA, et al: Topical application of β-aminopropionitrile. Life Sci 29:2553–2556, 1981.

97. Hoffman DL, Owen JA, Chvapil M: Healing of incision wounds treated with topically applied BAPN free base in the rat. Exp Mol Pathol 39:154–162, 1983.

20

TRAUMATIC INJURY

William H. Goodson III, M.D.

Accidental injury is generally called "trauma," but all surgery is traumatic in a sense. What sets accidental injury or trauma apart from surgery is the way in which it happens and its extent. The effects of trauma on wound healing have been poorly studied (specific studies are described in a short section at the end of this chapter). However, it is possible to review how trauma differs from elective surgery and to consider how the known aspects of trauma might influence healing.

Trauma differs from elective surgery in at least four general ways.

1. There are usually multiple injuries.
2. There is extensive preoperative stress, with concomitant catecholamine release and hormone changes.
3. Patients almost always experience some degree of shock.
4. There is depletion of body reserves resulting from the extent of injury and from shock.

Our apochryphal primordial ancestor had no hospital at which to seek care. If he suffered a minor injury he continued to forage and was likely to survive. If unable to continue to care for himself, his body was "designed" to try (though probably most often unsuccessfully) to find shelter and hide until some repair occurred. This system of repair presupposes decreased fluid and caloric intake and favors formation of scar and control of injury over regeneration of tissue, even at the expense of resources elsewhere in the body, especially muscle protein. With this system a person with good muscle mass and a moderate injury could survive on reduced intake and generally recover. From an evolutionary standpoint, this was an effective strategy.

Much of modern surgery and anesthesia attempts to undo or compensate for the destructive side effects of this inborn response to injury. Decontamination reduces the need to overcome infection, fluid management lessens vasoconstriction, which causes secondary injury in hypoperfused organs, and analgesia reduces centrally mediated responses to stress. For elective surgery, the response to injury is greatly modified from that experienced by patients as recently as a hundred years ago—a very short time relative to the 2.5 million years of hominid evolution.

Traumatic injury affects a number of physiological systems (Fig. 20–1) that can directly alter wound healing events. This chapter discusses the salient interactions thought to occur in trauma that can result in nonoptimal wound healing.

IMMUNE SYSTEM

The cornerstone of successful surgery is prevention of entry of bacteria into a wound. Classic works on asepsis by Semmelweis, on sterilization by Pasteur, and on the use of surgical gloves by Bloodgood have shown that reducing the bacterial content of wounds reduces infection. Although infection rates increase in trauma, the increase is proportional to contamination and not simply due to trauma itself.[1] For example, the infection rate in a series of 1436 trauma patients was 11.3 percent. For clean cases by usual definitions, the rates were 3.2 percent and 5.8 percent for abdominal and extremity injuries, respectively; for contaminated cases, however, the infection rates were 24.6 percent and 25.9 percent, respectively.

In experimental studies, some contamination

316

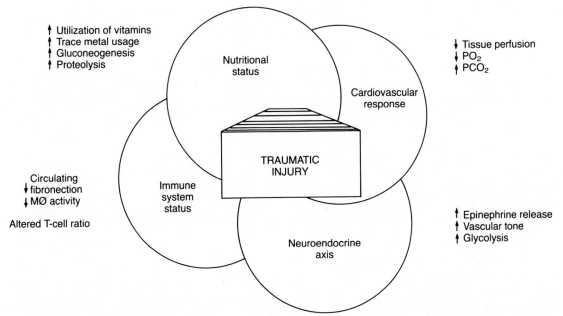

Figure 20–1. Influence of traumatic injury on physiologic systems that mediate the wound healing response. (Courtesy of William J. Lindblad, Ph.D.)

can enhance healing. However, this has been done in animals that are otherwise healthy and therefore is not analogous to the situation obtained in a debilitated patient following trauma and surgery. A more appropriate clinical evaluation is that by Marks and co-workers, who found that although staphylococcal wound infection, when accompanied by anaerobic infection, may be more injurious than staphylococcal infection alone, elimination of the staphylococcal infection clearly is associated with more rapid healing.[2]

CARDIOVASCULAR EFFECTS

Healing requires perfusion,[3] hypovolemia decreases perfusion,[4] and hemorrhagic shock is the extreme of hypovolemia. Several wars' worth of experience have illustrated the importance of resuscitation and intra- and postoperative fluid replacement. This is not the entire answer, however, since decreased perfusion appears also to be a cause of secondary injury that is not reversed simply by reperfusion. Hemorrhagic shock causes decreased tissue perfusion: the body attempts to protect oxygen-sensitive tissue by centralizing the residual circulatory volume. Blood flow to liver, kidney, heart, and lung is maintained as long as possible, while flow to skin, subcutaneous tissue, and bowel is decreased. When blood flow is

decreased there is a reduction in tissue oxygen and an increase in CO_2, with relative acidosis.[5]

Several authors have found that even after restoration of central perfusion pressure, tissue blood flow and oxygen delivery may not return to normal. In isolated adipose tissue, blood flow decreases during hemorrhagic shock but does not return to normal during resuscitation. This response is in part due to sympathetic tone, since phenoxybenzamine-treated dogs have less decrease in perfusion and a return of normal blood flow after resuscitation.[6] When perfusion is restricted in the limb of a canine model (with isolated vessels), there is a predictable decrease in blood flow and oxygen delivery, but this remains low even after the occlusion has been relieved and blood pressure is normal. Electron micrographs of the extremities postinjury showed interstitial and intracellular edema with swelling of mitochondria and microhemorrhages. These changes suggest a reperfusion injury. That the injury occurs during restoration of flow rather than during decreased flow is suggested by the observation that persistent low perfusion injury does not occur if mannitol is given just prior to reperfusion.[7]

These reperfusion effects are not due simply to hemodilution during resuscitation since a low hematocrit does not limit wound oxygen delivery. Measurements during stepwise hemodilution (by simultaneous withdrawal of blood and substitution of saline) led to a decrease in hematocrit, but kidney, gut, and whole body oxygen consumption remained constant. Only exercising muscle had a decrease in oxygen consumption, presumably because oxygen needs outstripped the hemoglobin-carrying capacity of the blood.[8] Wounds also have specific oxygen needs, which are greatly increased relative to skin, but these are not as great as those of exercising muscle, and even hematocrits as low as 17 can be tolerated without decreased oxygen delivery to the wound.[9]

Later, when wounds are established, they seem to have an autonomous circulation. Measurement of blood flow (by plethysmography of burned legs) found that perfusion is not responsive to sympathetic tone but is not usually maximal either since warming of the same extremity will increase blood flow even further.[10, 11] An interesting sidelight on this increasing perfusion is that it may be part of a process that aids healing: wounds made in the area of increased flow around an arteriovenous fistula heal with greater breaking strength than those in the distal part of the dog extremity. This is a reversal of the usual preeminence of distal healing, which suggests that local blood flow can enhance healing.[12]

As discussed in Chapter 16, oxygen delivery to wounds is also significantly decreased by trauma. Initially these results were interpreted with an emphasis placed solely on the importance of oxygen in the wound. However, it subsequently became apparent that in addition to the absolute requirement for oxygen, oxygen is a convenient marker to demonstrate blood flow. Thus the decrease in oxygen delivery to a wound in trauma patients reflects not only decreased oxygen but also decreased perfusion in general.

NEUROENDOCRINE AXIS

Metabolic responses to trauma are caricatures of those seen after any surgical procedure, but this is probably a simple extension in proportion to the magnitude of tissue disruption and stress. For example, there is no evidence that minor trauma such as a simple fracture causes major metabolic disruption other than an increase in hydroxyproline turnover. In major trauma, however, fractures are routinely combined with visceral, soft tissue, or cutaneous injuries. These combined disruptions of many different tissues are rarely encountered in planned surgery, so the greater metabolic response after trauma can be seen as a "punishment that fits the crime" rather than as an injury-specific event. (Note that there is decreased healing after very extensive elective surgery; see below.)

Metabolic response to injury can be divided into ebb and flow phases: the former lasting roughly a day and the latter most of the remainder of the healing process (Fig. 20–2). These stages have been reviewed extensively by Frayn.[13]

When danger is perceived there is activation and release of pituitary hormones even before injury. As soon as injury occurs there is pain, disruption and contusion of tissue with release of tissue and visceral content toxins (e.g., bacterial toxins), and loss of blood, which necessitates rapid redirection of blood flow. This redistribution is influenced by local factors and by some under central control, possibly in response to changes noted by the carotid body.[14]

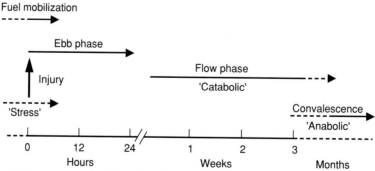

Figure 20–2. Phases of the response to injury. The duration of each phase is variable, and representative figures only are given. The first phase, that of fuel mobilization, may begin before injury occurs, initiated by "stress" or awareness of approaching danger. This is intimately merged, should injury occur, with the "ebb" or "shock" phase, which in turn—in survivors—merges into the more prolonged "flow" phase, often termed the catabolic response. Although wound healing may commence during the flow phase, general anabolism and true recovery do not begin until it has subsided. (From Frayn KN: Hormonal control of metabolism in trauma and sepsis. Clin Endocrinol 24:577–599, 1986.)

These latter factors certainly include vasoconstriction, changes in neurosympathetic tone, and adrenal release of epinephrine.

Along with redistribution of blood flow there is rapid mobilization of glucose. This occurs from breakdown of liver glycogen (which is rapidly depleted), followed quickly by breakdown of muscle glycogen. Only about 8 percent of glucose from muscle glycogen can be released from muscles to the circulation; the majority must be partially metabolized to lactate. This lactate release is stimulated by epinephrine and provides substrate to the liver for gluconeogenesis via the Cori cycle that will continue long into the flow phase.

Other responses, such as lipolysis and release of muscle amino acids, require a longer time to initiate and are not part of the early ebb phase. From the standpoint of wound healing, this early sympathetic response supplies substrate but also contributes to decreased circulation to many tissues and may initiate the apparent reperfusion injury that accompanies resuscitation (Fig. 20–3).

During the ebb phase there is significant hyperglycemia but no proportional insulin response. This may be due in part to inhibition of insulin release by epinephrine, but it may also be an indirect effect since pancreatic blood flow is decreased in shock. The hyperglycemia is perpetuated by insulin resistance (at least partly related to plasma cortisol levels, which rise less rapidly than epinephrine but still within several hours). At the same time there is stimulus for lipolysis, but adipose tissue is also hypoperfused, so that blood flow is inadequate to allow maximum egress of fatty acids, and other substances.

The flow phase of injury, which has been studied extensively, is associated with an increased metabolic rate and a massive breakdown of muscle protein (as evidenced by increased urinary nitrogen). There is continued rapid protein turnover and gluconeogenesis. Insulin is present in increased amounts, but the level is still low in proportion to glucose.[15] This insulin resistance is especially important in muscles, which do not respond with increased glucose utilization and amino acid uptake, but in fact continue to lyse protein to make amino acids for gluconeogenesis in the liver. Since muscles are usually the primary energy consumers, this seems an adaptation for conserving glucose for the brain and wound, while adapting other tissues to meet their energy needs with free fatty acids.[16]

The importance of glucose for wound metabolism is clear. Wounds consume glucose, and this seems to be independent of insulin.[17] Most wound glucose is metabolized to lactate, which circulates to the liver where it is used for gluconeogenesis. There is no direct proof, but this seems to preserve the three carbon fragments that can be rejoined to make glucose, whereas total oxidation to carbon dioxide and water would deprive the body of a carbon base for energy transport as glucose. Thus, the liver can be an energy supplier to the wound through the Cori cycle as long as there is a three-carbon chain available to resynthesize glucose. This mechanism was of great importance prior to the advent of intravenous dextrose and water.

In the wound, relatively high levels of lactate are maintained due to glucose metabolism.[18] Whereas this three-carbon compound is a substrate for gluconeogenesis, as mentioned, it may also play an additional role by directly modulating collagen biosynthesis. It has been known for quite some time that lactate can stimulate collagen biosynthesis in cell cultures of fibroblasts and myofibroblasts.[19, 20] In all of these studies there appeared to be a dose response between the level of lactate and the increase in collagen biosynthesis. Therefore, one might expect that the high levels of lactate in the wound could be a trigger for enhanced collagen expression by resident fibroblasts.

In addition to changes in substrate there is a general increase in metabolic rate, which seems to be fueled by the free fatty acids rather than glucose, since the overall use of glucose is decreased.[21] Recently, it was shown that there is increasing cycling of both glycolytic-glucogenic and triglyceride-fatty acid cycles.[22] The increase in metabolism is somewhat surprising since there is also good evidence of relative hypothyroidism in seriously ill patients.[23]

There is debate whether glucose is oxidized aerobically or anaerobically in wounds. Studies of isolated limb burn show consumption of glucose, formation of lactate, and apparent anaerobic glycolysis. Of note is that normal skin usually converts a high proportion of glucose only as far as lactate[24] so that formation of lactate anaerobically by a skin wound reflects an exaggeration of normal conditions. If, on the other hand, a granuloma is induced in muscle, there is more evidence of aerobic metabolism and, in fact, lactate and pyruvate are consumed in the wound.[25] This is probably due to at least two factors. Muscle has excellent circulation, prior-adapted to high blood flow to meet its energy needs during exercise. Thus, a granuloma in muscle has a greater blood supply than a skin wound. Second, muscle cells will be part of any such preparation, and therefore they may give

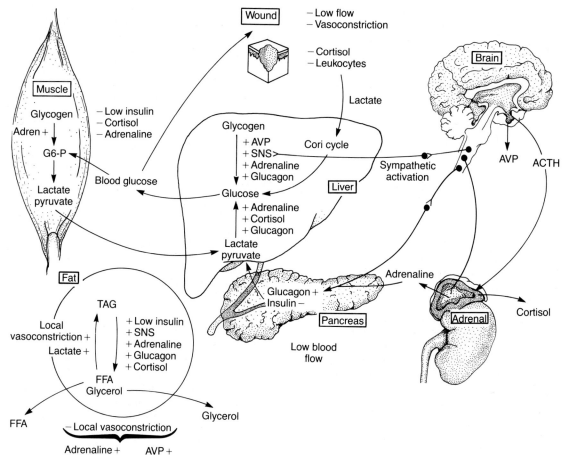

Figure 20–3. Central nervous control of metabolism in the ebb phase of the response to injury. Primary events are the activation of the sympathetic nervous system (SNS) and release of adrenaline from the adrenal medulla, with pituitary secretion of vasopression (AVP) and corticotropin (ACTH). The metabolic changes can all be viewed as stemming, directly or indirectly, from these central responses. Secondarily, the sympathoadrenal activation acts on the pancreas to stimulate secretion of glucagon and inhibit that of insulin, and ACTH promotes cortisol release from the adrenal cortex (+, stimulation of a process; –, inhibition). These changes result in stimulation of liver and muscle glycogenolysis; release of lactate and pyruvate from muscle, together with the hormonal changes, act to promote hepatic gluconeogenesis. Liver glucose release is thus massively stimulated. Glucose uptake by muscle is not, however, increased as it would normally be in hyperglycemia because of inhibition by adrenaline and cortisol, and because of the failure of insulin to respond to the hyperglycemia ("low insulin"). In adipose tissue several factors act to stimulate lipolysis, i.e., the breakdown of triacylglycerol (TAG) to free fatty acids (FFA) and glycerol; impaired insulin secretion ("low insulin") allows this to proceed unchecked. Release of FFA into the general circulation is not, however, as great as expected after severe injury. Local vasoconstriction—brought about by adrenaline and AVP—limits the availability of albumin to transport FFA out of adipose tissue, and local hypoxia, together with any rise in the systemic lactate concentration, acts to stimulate reesterification of FFA (through increased provision of glycerol 1-phosphate). Therefore, the wound is exposed to high glucose as part of the ebb phase, but low flow and vasoconstriction reduce oxygen delivery. Most metabolism is anaerobic, yielding lactate, which is recycled to glucose by the Cori cycle in the liver. Low flow is caused by sympathetic tone and restricts delivery of nutrients and leukocytes. (Modified from Frayn KN: Hormonal control of metabolism and trauma in sepsis. Clin Endocrinol 24:577–599, 1986.)

an appearance of aerobic metabolism that might not reflect the wound tissue itself.

Whatever the oxidative state of wound metabolism, it is clear that wounds consume glucose, independent of insulin concentration, and that much body metabolism is geared to provide this substrate primarily from muscles (via gluconeogenesis from amino acids). The severity of trauma determines how extreme the re-

sponses will be, so that the degree of lactate acidosis and hyperglycemia soon after injury are proportional to the severity of injury as measured by the injury severity score (Figs. 20–4 and 5).[26, 27]

The net flux of amino acids from muscle reaches a peak soon after injury and remains high for some time.[28] Why it does so is not clear since most of the acute-phase hormones

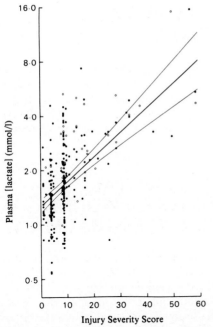

Figure 20–4. Plasma lactate is related to the Injury Severity Score, which assigns points for each aspect of a patient's injury so that with more points of anatomical injury the score is higher. (Reprinted by permission from Stoner HB, Frayn KN, Barton RN, et al: Clinical Science, vol 56, pp 563–573 copyright © 1979, The Biochemical Society, London.)

approach normal levels within a day or two.[13] These mechanisms seem to support healing, but at the expense of body muscle mass. The loss of muscle leads to decreased strength in respiratory and ambulatory muscles, which eventually is manifested in such long-term sequelae as respiratory failure. What is unclear is how these massive changes do or do not directly affect wounds. For instance, cortisol is the only one of the stress hormones known to have a direct influence on healing. However, after an initial sharp rise, it is only mildly elevated relatively soon after injury, and this is probably not in the pharmacological range known to inhibit healing. This is an area for further research.

NUTRITIONAL CONSIDERATIONS

Depletion of and/or failure to use body resources is a great problem in trauma. Blood coagulation factors, circulating blood cells, and nutrients (substrate, vitamins, and minerals) are affected.

Hypercoagulability is a fact of major trauma. Experimental studies in the 1960s found that partial thromboplastin time shortens by 1 hour after hemorrhage but then increases and continues to be abnormally increased.[29] During this time there is depletion of factors V, VII, IX, X, and XI, as well as fibrinogen, prothrombin, and platelets.[29] Human studies have shown decreased levels of antithrombin 3 (consumed during thrombus formation) in trauma patients in shock, which seems to be the extreme of the general activation seen by the same investigators in lesser trauma.[30] Since these events occur even with minor trauma, it is easy to see how acidosis, hypothermia, and transfusion of banked blood (which is deficient in factors V and VIII, platelets, and calcium) would decrease coagulation.[31] Platelets would possibly be missed most in early injury, not only because of bleeding problems but also due to the lack of the growth factors they release, such as platelet-derived growth factor and transforming growth factor-β (TGF-β).[32, 33] Thrombin and fibrin have also been implicated in healing, and consumption of them would also restrict healing.

Fibronectin, a high molecular weight glycoprotein that circulates in the blood is a protein whose depletion might cause deficient healing after trauma. It is involved in opsonization of bacteria and also has a role in cell adhesion to

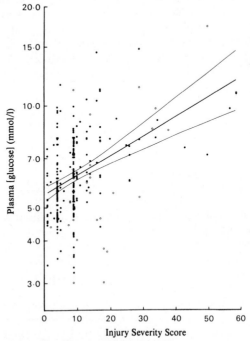

Figure 20–5. The elevation of glucose after trauma is related to the extent of injury as measured with the Injury Severity Score. (Reprinted by permission from Stoner HB, Frayn KN, Barton RN, et al: Clinical Science, vol 56, pp 563–573, copyright © 1979, The Biochemical Society, London.)

the extracellular matrix (see Chapter 12). Fibronectin accumulates in wounds and is significantly depleted following injury.[34] In experimental studies fibronectin deficiency is associated with decreased healing.[35]

Trauma decreases white cell function and availability. Polymorphonuclear leukocyte chemotaxis is greatly depressed after major trauma, and there is evidence that hormonal factors may be involved.[36] Skin-test anergy is common with severe injury, indicating a functional defect in host inflammatory cells.[36] Monocyte chemotaxis is also decreased after major trauma even if the patient survives.[37] Studies of lymphocytes (although the absolute need for lymphocytes in healing of uninfected wounds is unclear)[38] found evidence of decreased lymphocyte culture activity, possibly because of activation of T-suppressor cells.[39]

Because patients with multiple trauma, especially visceral injury, are unable to eat, nutrition becomes a major problem. The normal metabolic response to injury seems to be an evolutionary adaptation to this condition, but it is sufficient only for lesser injuries. Loss of protein in muscle mass is self-explanatory. In addition, wounds consume zinc. Stores of vitamin A, which is necessary for an adequate inflammatory response, drop rapidly after trauma; after severe trauma, up to 20,000 IU per day may be required. Vitamin C cannot be stored, and large amounts are needed to complete healing of anything more than minor injury. This results from the necessity for vitamin C in the formation of hydroxy-L-proline during collagen biosynthesis. After severe injury, patients may require 2 g or more of vitamin C. Since excess vitamin C is cleared by the kidneys, overdose is unlikely.

ALCOHOL

Alcohol is another major factor that influences the preoperative preparation of trauma patients.[40] Up to 60 percent of patients with multiple trauma have blood alcohol levels of greater than 1 g per liter,[41] which causes lactic acidosis and thus starts patients off in poor condition metabolically.[26, 42] In alcohol pretreated animals there is a negative base excess that is further exacerbated by trauma. In these same animals, pulmonary vascular resistance increases with a concurrent increase in pulmonary artery pressure. Such effects of alcohol may predispose patients to the pulmonary complications that are associated with trauma.[43]

NEUROHUMORAL FACTORS

Trauma is frequently associated with anxiety, fear, and pain. The initial insult occurs without medication (except for alcohol or drugs) and often elicits a severe neurohumoral response that starts the entire catabolic gluconeogenic mechanism even before surgery.

EXPERIMENTAL STUDIES OF WOUND HEALING IN TRAUMA

Of the few studies of trauma and healing, the most important is by Zederfeldt,[44] in which he found decreased tensile strength in experimental wounds made in animals that sustained trauma (a femur fracture) remote from the test wound. He also used blunt trauma and found the same decrease in healing in the test wound. The effect of trauma on healing of a wound at a different site seems to persist for about a month (Fig. 20–6). Zederfeldt was also the first to suggest the importance of reduced perfusion after injury when he observed a decrease in blood flow in conjunctival capillaries after trauma.

Very few of the methods used for the systematic study of healing are acceptable for human subjects. Wound cylinders are one of the most widely used methods in animals, while only a few techniques using small subcutaneous tubes as an acceptable human equivalent to a wound chamber have been reported. In one such report with human subjects, the authors observed decreased healing in two trauma patients who were hospitalized for several weeks after injury.[45] This is a clinical confirmation of the decrease seen after trauma, but its magnitude is similar to that seen in any group of severely ill patients who have undergone nontrauma surgery.[46]

There is a paucity of other studies, but it is possible to find some that relate poor healing to some of those factors that distinguish trauma patients from elective surgery patients, especially blood loss and preoperative stress. Unfortunately, experimental studies have not sought to relate wound healing defects to preoperative psychological stress, alcohol, or absence of visceral emptying.

The effect of shock on wound healing has been studied in several ways. Foster and coworkers[47] removed 10 percent of circulating

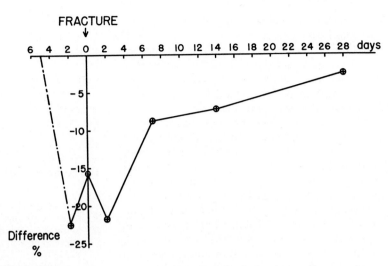

Figure 20–6. The decrease in tensile strength of a wound (as percent decrease compared to controls) is greatest if the wound is made at the time or just before or just after a remote injury (in this case, a femur fracture). As the time of second injury becomes more remote the effect is less but still evident. If the remote injury is a contusion there is a similar effect. (From Zederfeldt B: Studies on wound healing and trauma. Acta Chir Scand (Suppl 224) 1–85, 1957.)

blood volume during an experimental operative procedure. They found that there was significantly less collagen content in ileocolic and colocolic anastomoses on the third postoperative day. A study that is closer to the situation in trauma was conducted by McGinn,[48] who investigated the effects of acute hemorrhage after the induction of anesthesia for an experimental incision. If blood volume was removed for 4 minutes and then returned to the animals, there was no difference in wound strength compared to controls. If, however, the animals were bled and left hypotensive for 30 to 60 minutes, there was a significant reduction in wound strength. This suggests that there is some minimum time

during which hemorrhagic shock does not have an adverse effect on healing, but that the critical time is clearly less than 1 hour and probably less than 30 minutes (Fig. 20–7). Abraham and Chang[49] evaluated carrageenin-induced edema after 30 percent blood loss. They noted decreased inflammatory response even after blood had been reinfused, and this effect persisted even if carageenin was injected 24 hours after the reinfusion of blood. Initiation of inflammation was still suppressed 48 hours later, though not significantly.

A recent human study suggests that hypovolemia need not involve blood loss to affect healing.[50] Collagen formation in human test

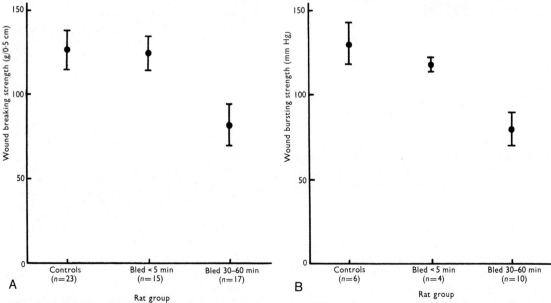

Figure 20–7. Breaking strength (A) and bursting strength (B) of abdominal incision, as influenced by hemorrhage. If blood is reperfused within 5 minutes there is no change in wound strength. If blood is reinfused 30 to 60 minutes later there is a significant decrease in wound strength. (From McGinn FP: Effects of haemorrhage upon surgical operations. Br J Surg 63:742–743, 1976.)

wounds was reduced after operations that were associated with preoperative emesis, decreased oral intake, and presumed mild dehydration. The decrease in collagen formation was proportional to the length of preoperative illness, suggesting that it was indeed this illness that caused the decrease in healing.

The metabolic stress of trauma has not been studied as an independent factor influencing wound healing. Failure of glucose utilization, as occurs in experimental diabetes, is associated with decreased healing,[51] but this is clearly different from the situation in trauma.

Hill and associates[52] studied healing in human subjects who were malnourished, as would be expected some time after the occurrence of trauma. They found that wound healing was decreased by malnutrition and that parenteral nutrition restored this deficit.

The effects of absence of inflammatory cells on wound healing have been studied independently in models of chemotherapy. It is particularly important to note that the effects of chemotherapeutic agents are most striking if the agents are given just before or at the time of wounding so that there is a decrease in white cell availability at the time healing is initiated. This corresponds well to the time of white cell defects seen in trauma patients and suggests that the depletion and/or malfunction of white cells may be a major factor in post-traumatic healing problems.

CONCLUSION

Patients heal poorly after trauma, but in many respects it seems that this is in proportion to the severity of the injury and presence of contamination at the time of trauma. The few available studies of trauma and wound healing suggest that remote trauma has an influence on test wounds. By observation, this seems to be related, in part at least, to hypovolemia associated with trauma. Other studies have shown that hypovolemia leads to hypoperfusion and that reperfusion leads to release of toxic substances. These have been studied primarily in relation to pulmonary complications, but it is also quite possible they have a general effect that impairs healing. Since factors such as fibronectin are depleted in trauma patients, it would be useful to determine whether repletion of these factors would be of benefit to trauma patients. This would lead to other studies of how nutritional support might best be tailored to the needs of trauma patients.

In improving our understanding of the degree to which trauma causes a decrease in overall healing ability, the most important need is for studies that determine whether the decrease in healing is related specifically to severity of injury as reflected by various severity of injury index scores or whether there are specific aspects of trauma that by themselves impair healing.

References

1. Weigett JA: Risk of wound infections in trauma patients. Am J Surg 150:782–784, 1985.
2. Marks J, Harding KG, Hughes LE: Staphylococcal infection of open granulating wounds. Br J Surg 74:95–97, 1987.
3. Jonsson K, Jensen JA, Goodson WH III, et al: Wound healing in subcutaneous tissue of surgical patients in relation to oxygen availability. Surg Forum 37:86–88, 1986.
4. Jensen JA, Goodson WH III, Omachi R, et al: Subcutaneous tissue oxygen tension falls during hemodialysis. Surgery 101:416–421, 1987.
5. Jussila EJ, Ninnikoski J, Vanttinen E: Intraoperative recording of tissue gas tensions in calf muscles of patients with peripheral arterial disease. J Surg Res 29:533–540, 1980.
6. Kovach AGB, Rosell S, Sandor P, et al: Blood flow, oxygen consumption, and free fatty acid release in subcutaneous adipose tissue during hemorrhagic shock in control and phenoxybenzamine-treated dogs. Circ Res 24:733–741, 1980.
7. Shah DM, Powers SR Jr, Stratton HH, et al: Effects of hypertonic mannitol on oxygen utilization in canine hind limbs following shock. J Surg Res 30:593–601, 1981.
8. Wright CJ: The effects of severe progressive hemodilution on regional blood flow and oxygen consumption. Surgery 79:299–305, 1976.
9. Jensen JA, Goodson WH III, Vasconez L, et al: Wound healing in anemia: A case report. West J Med 144:465–467, 1986.
10. Aulick LH, Wilmore DW, Mason AD Jr, et al: Influence of the burn wound on peripheral circulation in thermally injured patients. Am J Physiol 233:H520–526, 1977.
11. Rabkin J, Hunt TK: Local heat increases blood flow and oxygen tension in wounds. Arch Surg 122:221–225, 1987.
12. Takiff H, Owens ML, Williams RA: Effect of arteriovenous fistula on wound healing and skin blood flow. Br J Exp Pathol 65:677–681, 1984.
13. Frayn KN: Hormonal control of metabolism in trauma and sepsis. Clin Endocrinol 24:577–599, 1986.
14. Althoff M, Acker H: The influence of carotid body stimulation on oxygen tension and microcirculation of various organs of the cat. Int J Microcirc Clin Exp 4:379–396, 1985.
15. Neguid MM, Brennan MF, Asoki TT, et al: Hormone-substrate interrelationships following trauma. Arch Surg 109:776–783, 1974.
16. Wood CD, Bentz Y, Martin M, et al: The relationship of glucagon and insulin to sequential changes in metabolic fuel utilization in shock. J Surg Res 28:239–243, 1980.
17. Black PR, Brooks DC, Bessey PQ, et al: Mechanisms

of insulin resistance following injury. Ann Surg 196:420–435, 1982.

18. Green H, Goldberg B: Collagen and cell protein synthesis by an established mammalian fibroblast line. Nature 204:347–349, 1964.

19. Savolainen ER, Leo MA, Timpl R, et al: Acetaldehyde and lactate stimulate collagen synthesis of cultured baboon liver myofibroblasts. Gastroenterology 87:777–787, 1984.

20. Comstock JP, Udenfriend S: Effect of lactate on collagen proline hydroxylase activity in cultured L-929 fibroblasts. Proc Natl Acad Sci USA 66:552–557, 1970.

21. Little RA: Heat production after injury. Br Med Bull 41:226–231, 1985.

22. Wolfe RR, Herndon DN, Jahoor F, et al: Effect of severe burn injury on substrate cycling by glucose and fatty acids. N Engl J Med 317:403–408, 1987.

23. Baue AE, Gunther B, Hartl W, et al: Altered hormonal activity in severely ill patients after injury or sepsis. Arch Surg 119:1125–1132, 1984.

24. Im MJC, Hoopes JE: Energy metabolism in healing skin wounds. J Surg Res 10:459–465, 1970.

25. Caldwell MD, Shearer J, Morris A, et al: Evidence for aerobic glycolysis in alpha-carrageenin–wounded skeletal muscle. J Surg Res 37:63–68, 1984.

26. Stoner HB, Frayn KN, Barton RN, et al: The relationships between plasma substrates and hormones and the severity of injury in 277 recently injured patients. Clin Sci 56:563–573, 1979.

27. Oppenheim WL, Williamson DH, Smith R: Early biochemical changes and severity of injury in man. J Trauma 20:135–140, 1980.

28. Duke JH, Jorgensen SB, Broell JR, et al: Contribution of protein to caloric expenditure following injury. Surgery 68:168–174, 1970.

29. Rutherford RB, West RL, Hardaway RM: Coagulation changes during experimental hemorrhagic shock. Clotting activity, contribution of splanchnic circulation and acidosis as controlled by THAM. Ann Surg 164:203–214, 1966.

30. Risberg B, Medegard A, Heideman M, et al: Early activation of humoral proteolytic systems in patients with multiple trauma. Crit Care Med 14:917–925, 1986.

31. Silva R, Moore EE, Galloway WB: Reducing coagulopathy after trauma. Infect Surg 4:329–336, 1985.

32. Deuel TF, Huang JS: Platelet-derived growth factor. Structure, function, and roles in normal and transformed cells. J Clin Invest 74:669–676, 1984.

33. Sporn MB, Roberts AB: Transforming growth factor-β. Multiple actions and potential clinical applications. JAMA 262:938–941, 1989.

34. Rogers FB, Sheaff M, Nolan PJ, et al: Fibronectin depletion and microaggregate clearance following trauma. J Trauma 26:339–342, 1986.

35. Nagelschmidt M, Becker D, Bonninghoff N, et al: Effect of fibronectin therapy and fibronectin deficiency on wound healing: A study in rats. J Trauma 27:1267–1271, 1987.

36. Christou NV, McLean APH, Meakins JL: Host defense in blunt trauma: Interrelationships of kinetics of anergy and depressed neutrophil function, nutritional status, and sepsis. J Trauma 20:833–841, 1980.

37. Antrum RM, Solomkin JS: Monocyte dysfunction in severe trauma: Evidence for the role of C5a in deactivation. Surgery 100:29–37, 1986.

38. Peterson JM, Barbul A, Breslin RJ, et al: Significance of T-lymphocytes in wound healing. Surgery 102:300–304, 1987.

39. Baker CC: Immune mechanisms and host response in the trauma patient. Yale J Biol Med 59:387–393, 1986.

40. Trowbridge A, Giesecke AH Jr: Multiple injuries. In Giesecke AH Jr (ed): Anesthesia for the Surgery of Trauma, vol 11/2. Philadelphia, FA Davis, 1976, pp 79–84.

41. Herve C, Gaillard M, Roujas F, et al: Alcoholism in polytrauma. J Trauma 26:1123–1126, 1986.

42. Watson TD, Lee JF: Intoxication and trauma. In Giesecke AH Jr (ed): Anesthesia for the Surgery of Trauma, vol 11/2, Philadelphia, FA Davis, 1976, pp 31–38.

43. Blomquist S, Thorne J, Elmer O, et al: Early posttraumatic changes in hemodynamics and pulmonary ventilation in alcohol pretreated pigs. J Trauma 27:40–44, 1987.

44. Zederfeldt B: Studies on wound healing and trauma. Acta Chir Scand (Suppl 224):1–85, 1957.

45. Diegelmann RF, Lindblad WJ, Cohen IK: A subcutaneous implant for wound healing studies in humans. J Surg Res 40:229–237, 1986.

46. Goodson WH III, Hunt TK: Development of a new miniature method for the study of wound healing in human subjects. J Surg Res 33:394–401, 1982.

47. Foster ME, Laycock JRD, Silver IA, et al: Hypovolaemia and healing in colonic anastomoses. Br J Surg 72:831–834, 1985.

48. McGinn FP: Effects of haemorrhage upon surgical operations. Br J Surg 63:742–746, 1976.

49. Abraham E, Chang Y-H: Effects of hemorrhage on inflammatory response. Arch Surg 119:1154–1157, 1984.

50. Goodson WH III, Lopez-Sarmiento A, Jensen JA, et al: The influence of a brief preoperative illness on postoperative healing. Ann Surg 205:250–255, 1987.

51. Goodson WH, Hunt TK: Wound collagen accumulation in obese hyperglycemic mice. Diabetes 35:491–495, 1986.

52. Haydock DA, Hill GL: Improved wound healing in surgical patients receiving intravenous nutrition. Br J Surg 74:320–323, 1987.

21

TISSUE REPAIR IN THE MAMMALIAN FETUS

Bruce A. Mast, M.D., Jeffrey M. Nelson, M.D., and Thomas M. Krummel, M.D.

Tissue repair in the adult occurs as a consequence of well-documented, organized events that usually result in a collagenous scar. The healing process occurs via similar mechanisms in all postnatal animals, but is not uniform among various age groups. Clinical observations of neonates suggest that tissue repair occurs in an accelerated fashion with less scarring in this population. On the other hand, the healing response appears to be delayed and less efficient as aging progresses.[1]

This chapter discusses the current concepts of wound healing and tissue repair in the mammalian fetus. Prior to such a discussion it is important to understand the organism in which this process takes place. The fetus is a developing organism in which cellular migration, proliferation, and differentiation occur at an unparalleled magnitude. Since healing of damaged tissue is an adaptive process of cellular interaction, the mechanisms underlying fetal tissue repair cannot be fully understood without an awareness of the unique physiological and biochemical processes within the fetus. These aspects of fetal development, as well as the unique fetal environment as a tolerated "graft" within a maternal "host" supported by the placenta, are presented prior to a detailed discussion of fetal tissue repair. Although most fetal wound healing studies have been performed in animal models, the physiology and environment of the human fetus is discussed since the goal is to understand the processes of human fetal tissue repair.

THE HUMAN FETUS

Intrauterine life can be divided into an embryonic period and a fetal period. The twelfth week of gestation marks the end of the embryonic period, which is defined by the complete establishment of all major organ systems and an external form having the gross features of the developed organism. During this time, cellular proliferation and differentiation are the predominant processes. Following conception, the unicellular zygote divides into a cluster of cells called the morula, which subsequently differentiates into the trilaminar germ disc. The three layers of this structure each lead to the formation of different tissues. The ectoderm forms tissues involved in environmental interaction such as the nervous system, the skin and its appendages, and the pituitary, mammary, and sweat glands. The mesoderm gives rise to the supporting structures of the animal via individual somites. Each somite is further divided into three structures: the sclerotome forms bone and cartilage; the dermatome gives rise to dermis and subcutaneous tissue; and the myotome forms muscle. The third germ layer, the endoderm, forms the epithelial lining of the urinary bladder, respiratory and gastrointestinal tracts, as well as the parenchyma of the thyroid, parathyroid, thymus, liver, and pancreas.[2] The mortality of the organism is highest during this period, largely attributed to chromosomal and genetic abnormalities or maternal factors.[3]

The fetal period of intrauterine life occurs from the twelfth week of gestation to birth. This is a period of growth and development of the previously formed organ systems. The second trimester is characterized by rapid linear growth and functional acquisition as maturation proceeds. The third trimester, beginning at the 28th to 29th week is marked by further growth, particularly in muscle mass, and accumulation of subcutaneous tissue.[3] The lack of subcutaneous tissue is responsible for the red, wrinkled skin seen in premature infants born during the early third trimester.

Fetal Physiology

There are many physiological differences between the developing fetus and the postnatal animal which may affect the fetus' healing capabilities (Table 21–1). The physiologic processes of fetal energy requirements, endocrinology, immunology, tissue oxygen conditions, and hepatic metabolism will be discussed.

The fetus must have a source for the energy required to maintain the cellular activities necessary for development and maturation. The primary energy source is glucose, which along with amino acids and glycerol, is supplied by the maternal circulation through the placenta. Insulin does not cross the placenta, so that fetally derived insulin is responsible for glucose utilization. Insulin is also implicated as one of the main anabolic hormones of the fetus. Pancreatic endocrine function occurs early in the fetus; insulin-containing pancreatic granules are present at 8 weeks gestational age (GA), and the hormone can be detected in the fetal plasma at 12 weeks GA.[4] A generalized trophic effect of insulin can be inferred from the prevalence of large-for-GA infants born to diabetic mothers. These fetuses are thought to be hyperglycemic as result of the elevated maternal glucose, and therefore, are also hyperinsulinemic. Elevated insulin levels in the cord blood of such babies has been detected, whereas small-for-GA infants have been noted to have decreased levels.[5]

Table 21–1. ASPECTS OF FETAL DEVELOPMENT THAT MAY AFFECT HEALING

Functionally different endocrine system
Immunologic immaturity
Hypoxic tissue
Underdeveloped hepatic metabolism
Dependency on the placenta
Sterile environment
Presence of amniotic fluid

Interestingly, glucagon is detectable in the pancreas at 8 weeks GA, although maternally induced hypoglycemia fails to cause its secretion in the monkey fetus.[6] Therefore, this important adult hormone may function differently in the fetus.

The adrenal gland of the fetus is vastly different from that of the adult. The fetal adrenal gland is proportionately very large, probably second only to the liver in size. It is composed mostly of a fetal zone (85%), which quickly involutes after birth. An estimate of the daily steroid secretion of the fetal adrenal is 200 to 300 mg, approximately ten times the steroid production in the nonstressed adult. A significant proportion of these hormones are delivered to the placenta for estrogen production.[7]

Fetal adrenal development begins prior to vascularization of the pituitary by the hypothalamus. Therefore, corticotropin-releasing hormone and ACTH are not involved in regulation of the gland at this time. However, the adrenals are ultimately dependent on the pituitary as indicated by the scant fetal zone present when the pituitary is absent. Low-density lipoprotein (LDL)–cholesterol and fetal pituitary prolactin are probably additional mediators of adrenal function, the latter most likely late in pregnancy. Fetal plasma prolactin levels are high during the last 5 weeks of gestation, which correlates with the period of maximum adrenal growth.[8] The actual function of the adrenal hormones is not fully known. Cortisol production rises in the latter weeks of gestation and has been implicated in fetal lung maturation. Aldosterone is also elevated late in pregnancy with higher levels than in maternal blood. The renal tubules of the fetus are probably sensitive to this hormone.[7]

The fetal pituitary is able to synthesize and store the normal variety of hormones by the end of the first trimester. The role of these hormones, including growth hormone, which normally has high levels in cord blood, is unclear; anencephalic fetuses with little or no pituitary tissue are approximately the same size and weight as normal fetuses. Other active fetal hormones are the thyroid hormones, parathormone, testosterone, and estrogens. As with cortisol, thyroxine and estrogens have been implicated in fetal lung maturation.[7]

It is clear that the endocrine system of the human fetus is operationally different from that of the adult. The hormones are important trophic factors in fetal development. Indeed, the huge quantities of steroids produced by the adrenal gland that are subsequently converted to estrogen are vital for the maintenance of pregnancy. Cellular activities within the fetus are surely affected by the hormonal milieu of the organism, which, in turn, may affect the processes involved in tissue repair.

Components of the immune system are intimately involved in adult tissue repair. The fetus is immunologically immature and less competent than the adult such that a potential effect on fetal wound healing is plausible. Neutropenia and a lack of antigenic stimulation may be involved in this "incompetence."[9, 10] Additionally, chemotactic ability may be reduced, although phagocytosis appears to be normal.[11] Despite these deficits, the fetus can respond to intrauterine infections, such as cytomegalovirus, with an obvious cellular immune reaction.[12] Humoral immunity is composed mostly of IgG obtained passively from the maternal circulation, but the fetus is capable of producing IgM antibodies when provoked.[7] Components of the complement system are present but in lesser quantities than found in the adult; some components can be detected as early as 8 weeks GA.[13, 14]

The fetus and mother are not immunologically allogenic since half of the fetus' genome is derived from the father. In this sense, the fetus can be considered a tolerated "graft" transplanted to the uterus. Maternal tolerance of this graft continues as long as the circulations of the two organisms are separated by the intact structure of the placenta. If this separation is violated, maternal exposure to foreign fetal antigens may occur, leading to potentially disastrous immune reactions. Maternal immunoglobulins produced by such exposure can cross the placenta and attack fetal tissue. Erythroblastosis fetalis is a result of maternal isoimmunization against fetal Rh antigen, causing immunological destruction of fetal red blood cells.[15] Such immune reactions may lead to fetal demise.

Oxygen is essential to the maintenance of energy production and cellular function. The fetus is markedly hypoxemic compared to the postnatal animal with a Po_2 of about 20 torr. This reflects the oxygen content of maternal blood in the placental intervillous spaces, having a Po_2 of 30 to 35 torr.[7] The fetus compensates for hypoxemia in a number of ways. Fetal hemoglobin is primarily hemoglobin F, which has a much higher oxygen affinity than adult hemoglobin A as a consequence of a lower 2,3-diphosphoglycerate content. Second, the fetus has a higher hemoglobin concentration (16 mg/dl). This, combined with the greater oxygen affinity, facilitates oxygen transfer to the fetus. Another compensatory measure is the fetus' cardiac output per unit body weight, which is

greater than that of the adult. Evidence that the fetus compensates well for hypoxemia is provided indirectly by the observation that the lactic acid level (a product of anaerobic metabolism) of fetal blood is only slightly higher than in the mother.[7]

A final noteworthy aspect of fetal physiology is hepatic function. The liver is the metabolic guardian of the body with its multitude of degradative and synthetic enzyme systems. The neonatal liver is obviously not yet fully functional as evidenced by the prevalence of hyperbilirubinemia, which results from a deficiency in the conjugative enzyme glucuronyl transferase. In fact, many liver enzymes are present in the fetal liver but in diminished quantities. The fetus does not have difficulty with hyperbilirubinemia since the unconjugated form of bilirubin easily crosses the placenta. In any event, it is clear that the fetal liver is functionally immature.[7]

In summary, the fetus differs from the adult in many ways, undergoing simultaneous rapid growth and differentiation. Fetal endocrine control and function are different, the fetus is immunologically immature, its tissues are perfused in hypoxemic blood, and the liver is not fully functional. Clearly the intercellular milieu of the fetus differs greatly from that of the adult, and it is not unreasonable to presume that these differences affect the processes involved in tissue repair.

THE FETAL ENVIRONMENT

The environment of an organism has definite ramifications for its ability to repair injured tissue. Postnatal external conditions such as infection and repeated trauma may be deleterious to healing. The fetal environment is obviously unique. The existence of the placenta and the amniotic fluid surrounding the developing organism are aspects of the fetal environment that may affect the repair process (Table 21–1).

Placenta

The placenta is a structure unique to the gravid uterus, representing the symbiosis of mother and fetus (Fig. 21–1). The maternal portion of the organ consists of the uterine decidua basalis, and the fetal component consists of the chorionic villi. The latter arise from

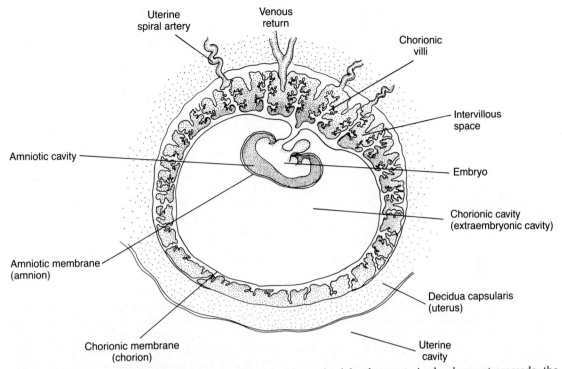

Figure 21–1. Human embryo at the beginning of the second month of development. As development proceeds, the decidua capsularis and its portion of the placenta recede such that the fetus and amniotic fluid contained within the fetal membranes fill the uterine cavity. Additionally, as the fetus enlarges the amniotic cavity also enlarges, and the extraembryonic cavity is obliterated as the amnion and chorion become apposed. (From Sadler TW: Langman's Medical Embryology, 5th ed. © 1985, The Williams & Wilkins Co., Baltimore.)

the chorion fondosum, a derivative of embryonic trophoblastic tissue. Implantation of the embryo occurs by the end of the first week of gestation, at which time the placenta forms as the uterine wall is invaded by trophoblasts. The cytotrophoblasts remain as the chorionic villi, which are intermingled with the intervillous spaces filled with maternal blood from uterine spiral arteries. The maternal and fetal circulations are separated by a syncytium of fetal cells covering the fetal endothelium, the so-called placental barrier.[2, 16] The placenta continues to grow throughout pregnancy in proportion to the growth of the fetus. The placenta is an active organ; it functions as a semipermeable membrane exchanging gases, nutrients, and metabolic wastes of the fetus, thereby acting as the surrogate lungs, intestinal tract, and kidneys. Additionally, the placenta is a prolific producer of hormones.

The placenta functions as a transfer or exchange organ without direct contact between maternal and fetal blood, as noted before. Most substances cross the placenta by passive or simple diffusion; examples are oxygen, carbon dioxide, glucose, water, most electrolytes, urea, unconjugated bilirubin, IgG, and drugs. Most anesthetic agents, with the exception of muscle relaxants such as succinylcholine and curare, are also readily diffusable. Selective, active, or facilitated diffusion is important in providing the fetus with key substances such as ascorbic acid and iron. It is important to note that most protein hormones in the maternal circulation do not cross the placenta. Thyroxine is an exception, although it is transferred in very small quantities. Infectious agents can also cross the placenta as evidenced by the intrauterine infections caused by rubella, cytomegalovirus, and toxoplasma.[7, 16]

Many variables may affect the diffusion of substances across the placenta. Because the area of the fetal villi is huge, ranging from 4 to 14 m^2, a loss of villi substantial enough to cause impaired diffusion is unlikely. The diffusion capacity of the placental barrier and the concentration of substances in each circulation remains relatively constant. Placental blood flow is susceptible to changes such that it is most apt to affect the transfer of substances to the fetus. In the normal fetus, blood flow to the placenta remains stable, therefore, most changes in placental blood flow result from changes in uterine perfusion. Decreased flow may be encountered in maternal hypertension and diabetes.[7, 16]

The role of the placenta as a synthesizer of hormones is crucial in maintaining pregnancy. Human chorionic gonadotropin (hCG), produced early in pregnancy, maintains the corpus luteum in early pregnancy until the placenta usurps the production of progesterone. It also acts on the fetus to promote testosterone synthesis prior to pituitary production of leutenizing hormone. It is, therefore, important in the sexual differentiation of the fetus.[7]

Human placental lactogen (hPL) is detectable in trophoblasts as early as 3 weeks GA. This protein hormone has an amino acid sequence very similar to that of growth hormone: the genes of each hormone are closely linked on chromosome 17, and it is speculated that the gene for hPL may have resulted from duplication of the growth hormone gene. HPL has both lactogenic and growth hormone–like activities. It represents 7 to 10 percent of protein synthesis in the placenta at term and its production is greater than any other human hormone.[7] Found primarily in the maternal blood and in amniotic fluid, hPL promotes lipolysis and inhibits glucose utilization so that the maternal energy source is mainly fatty acids. Thus, glucose, the primary energy source of the fetus, is made available for placental transfer. Although the production of hPL at term is immense, normal infants have resulted from pregnancies in which this hormone could not be detected. Therefore, it appears that its presence is not mandatory for normal development.[7]

The placenta is the only source of estrogens in the pregnant woman, producing amounts equivalent to that of 1000 premenopausal women in one day. The estrogens are derived from blood-borne precursors supplied primarily by the fetal adrenal gland. Normally more than 90 percent of these estrogens are secreted into the maternal circulation such that their direct effects on the fetus are minimal.[7] Despite this disproportionate allocation, estrogens may play a role in fetal lung maturation. It was found that higher than normal levels of steroid hormones were detectable in cord blood of newborns from pregnancies in which uteroplacental blood flow was diminished. Fetal lung maturation appears to be accelerated in fetuses exposed to such a change in uteroplacental flow.[7]

Progesterone is also produced by the placenta, but unlike estrogens, its precursors are maternally derived. LDL-cholesterol from the mother is used by the placenta to produce progesterone. In this process the protein component of LDL is hydrolyzed into amino acids, and the cholesterol ester is broken down to cholesterol (for progesterone) and fatty acids,

including the essential fatty acid linoleic acid. In this manner progesterone synthesis provides essential amino acids and fatty acids to the fetus. As with estrogen, most of the progesterone does not enter the fetal circulation.[7]

Evidence supports the presence of many other placental hormones, including chorionic thyrotropin, chorionic ACTH, and hypothalamic-like releasing hormones. The function of these hormones is speculative at this time. Additionally, there are many "pregnancy-specific" proteins that are under investigation.[7]

The placenta is the fetal link to life. It functions as the fetus' lungs, kidneys, and intestinal tract, providing substances required for survival and eliminating those that are toxic upon accumulation. It provides the necessary circulatory juxtaposition to maintain fetal existence, yet keeps the maternal and fetal cells separated so that potentially disastrous immune reactions are prevented. The placenta produces enormous quantities of hormones, some of which are functional in the mother, others in the fetus. Their effects are varied, but generally they play important roles in maintaining pregnancy, and regulating fetal growth and development. Certainly, conditions that adversely affect the function of the placenta may sacrifice the well-being of the fetus. In this manner, fetal functions may be altered, including those involved in repair of injured tissue.

Amniotic Fluid

The fetus is surrounded by amniotic fluid, which provides a bouyant, sterile, thermally stable environment that allows for unrestricted fetal movement while acting as a protective cushion. The amnion, or amniotic membrane, is composed of cells of trophoblastic or ectodermal derivation. As the amniotic cavity distends with fluid, the amnion obliterates the extraembryonic coelom, becoming apposed to the chorion, or chorionic membrane, without fusing to it (see Fig. 21–1). Although the amnion is avascular and without nervous tissue, enzyme activity is detectable in the forms of 5-α-reductase and phospholipase.[7]

Amniotic fluid accumulates throughout pregnancy. Early in pregnancy, this fluid is essentially a dialysate of maternal blood. The fetus begins to swallow amniotic fluid as early as 14 weeks GA.[3] As the urinary system becomes functional later in pregnancy, a significant portion of the fluid consists of fetal urine. This is mostly water, since most metabolic wastes are still transferred across the placenta.[2]

The function of amniotic fluid is probably not limited to its mechanical qualities. Substances in the fluid may have physiological effects by direct local action or via the fetal circulation following intestinal absorption. It has been suggested that amniotic fluid plays a role in the development of the gastrointestinal tract. In fact, amniotic fluid has been shown to have a trophic effect in supporting rabbit fetal gastric parietal cells in culture. Specific growth factors have not been identified but may include gastrin, epidermal growth factor, enteroglucagon, and cortisol.[17, 18] The nutrient-related activities of hPL have been discussed. Since this substance is found in amniotic fluid, a trophic role is conceivable.

An immunological component in amniotic fluid may exist as well. Alpha-fetoprotein, found in the fluid, has been shown to inhibit the expression of macrophage Ia antigens in mice.[19] Furthermore, injured tissue may be locally affected by this fluid in which it is bathed.[20]

The presence of amniotic fluid is certainly requisite for fetal well-being. An active role in the processes of tissue repair is likely, whether it is by biochemical or mechanical means.

OVERVIEW OF ADULT MAMMALIAN WOUND HEALING

Normal adult wound healing is considered the norm to which all other repair processes can be compared. Therefore, prior to a detailed discussion of fetal tissue repair a brief summary of adult wound healing will be presented.

Adult mammalian tissue repair occurs via a complex series of cellular and extracellular matrix (ECM) events initiated by the injury itself. (These events are described in detail throughout this book.) Regeneration is limited, while fibroblast proliferation predominates, culminating in the deposition of large amounts of collagen. Crosslinking and remodeling of the collagen ultimately results in a mature, fibrous scar. This integrated response occurs in continuum but for descriptive purposes can be divided into four biological periods,[21, 22] which are briefly discussed. The contraction of open wounds is also considered.

Wounding

At the time of injury, blood vessels are disrupted, causing local hemorrhage. Hemostatic mechanisms are initiated, including vasoconstriction, platelet aggregation with degranulation, and blood clotting with fibrin deposition. Thus, the initial ECM is composed of fibrin, which provides a scaffolding for the influx of acute and chronic inflammatory cells. This process may be orchestrated in part by polypeptide growth factors[23] released initially from platelets and subsequently from many of the cells recruited to the wound site. Bacterial contamination usually occurs at the time of injury and may contribute to initiation of the inflammatory response.

Inflammatory Phase

Initial vasoconstriction gives way to vasodilatation and increased capillary permeability. Chemotaxis of polymorphonuclear leukocytes (PMNs) to a wound site within 12 to 24 hours defines acute inflammation. These cells provide local control of bacteria but may not be mandatory for successful wound healing since neutropenic patients appear to heal normally.[24] Following acute inflammation, chronic inflammatory cells predominate, primarily macrophages and lymphocytes. These cells, especially macrophages, secrete various polypeptide growth factors that affect subsequent fibroblast activity.[25] Fibrin is then degraded and the ECM is largely replaced by proteoglycans.

Proliferative Phase

This is marked by proliferation of cells present at the wound site, rather than further extravascular migration into the wound. Fibroblast, endothelial, and epithelial cells may all be involved at this point. The proteoglycan matrix is replaced by collagen.[26]

Remodeling Phase

This final phase occurs over several months and completes the healing process with the continued synthesis, crosslinking and remodeling of collagen. Thus, a mature, collagenous scar is formed with the eventual tensile strength that approaches, but never reaches, that of normal tissue.[21, 22]

Contraction

A distinct feature of adult open wounds is their ability to concentrically decrease the area of lost tissue by a process called contraction. The forces generated for wound contraction are thought to arise from myofibroblasts. These specialized fibroblasts contain actin, the contractile protein found in muscle.[27] Additional features of these cells include intercellular connections by gap junctions and desmosomes.[28] Evidence also exists for fibroblast-collagen matrix interaction causing contraction without the presence of myofibroblasts.[29] By reducing the area of tissue defect, contraction facilitates repair of the injury with proliferating granulation tissue (fibroblasts and capillaries) and epithelialization. "Healing by secondary intention" is a term frequently used to describe the contraction of open wounds.

To summarize, adult mammalian wound healing proceeds through an orderly chain of events. Cellular events begin with acute inflammation (PMNs), followed by infiltration of chronic inflammatory cells (macrophages and lymphocytes), and then by fibroblast recruitment and proliferation. The ECM undergoes changes characterized by temporary depositions of fibrin, then proteoglycans, and finally collagen. Open wounds have the ability to contract.

TECHNIQUES FOR STUDYING WOUND HEALING IN THE FETUS

Many mammalian animals have been employed in the study of fetal wound healing, including sheep,[30] monkeys,[31] rats,[32–34] and rabbits;[10, 20, 35–38] specifics regarding the techniques of in utero surgery are discussed in each report. Generally, the maternal animal undergoes a laparotomy. A hysterotomy is made providing direct access to the fetus, which is wounded while contained in the uterus (Fig. 21–2). Most commonly, incisional or excisional wounds are created, although burning and freezing have also been performed. The hysterotomy is closed and the animal is sacrificed prior to delivery.

Many studies have performed gross and microscopic evaluation of the wounds by the use of observation and biopsy, respectively. Although useful data are obtained in this fashion, limitations arise by the inability to reliably define the boundary between wounded and uninjured tissue and to quantitate parameters of wound healing. Thus, a number of wound implant devices have been designed, including the Hunt-Shilling chamber,[39, 40] viscose cellulose (the Celstic device),[41] Goodson and Hunt's expanded polytetrafluoroethylene (Goretex)

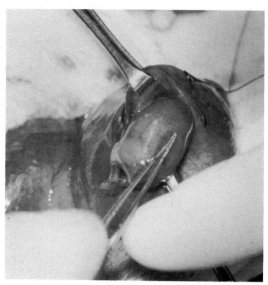

Figure 21–2. Placement of a polyvinyl alcohol (PVA) implant into a rabbit fetus.

tube,[42] and the polyvinyl alcohol (PVA) implant.[43] Each device has its proponents and opponents, as well as advantages and disadvantages. The ideal implant is inert in the wound so that the observed cellular and ECM events closely correlate, qualitatively and temporally, with those of wound biopsies. (For details of these devices, consult the pertinent references.)

CHARACTERISTICS OF MAMMALIAN FETAL WOUND HEALING

Fetal wounds differ markedly from adult wounds in several ways (Table 21–2). The processes involved in primarily closed wounds, open wounds, and burn wounds will be presented, as well as observations from the human fetus.

Primarily Closed Wounds

Gross Observations

Essentially all studies performed on fetal wounds have noted rapid healing. Linear

Table 21–2. UNIQUE FEATURES OF FETAL REPAIR

Rapid healing
No scarring
No acute inflammation
Minimal fibroblast proliferation
Matrix rich in hyaluronic acid
No excessive collagen
Open wounds do not contract in some species

wounds in the fetal rabbit appear to be grossly healed by 7 days following injury,[38] within 3 days in fetal sheep,[30] and within minutes for small wounds in rat embryos.[44] In addition to the rapidity with which these wounds heal, scarring is absent.[30, 31, 38, 45, 46]

Cellular Observations

While the first cellular event in adult wounds following thrombus and clot formation is the influx of acute inflammatory cells (PMNs), studies in several different animals have demonstrated an absence of this response in fetal wounds. Burlington incised fetal sheep skin and noted very few acute inflammatory cells.[30] Sopher made a similar observation using full-thickness incisional wounds in cynomolgus monkeys.[31] Vilijanto and colleagues,[37] Adzick and co-workers,[10] and Krummel and associates[38] noted the absence of PMNs in epidermal wounds in fetal rabbits. The lack of PMN infiltration does not appear to be limited to injury of the skin: studies in which full-thickness incisional wounds through oral muscle and/or mucosa in rats also demonstrated the absence of an acute inflammatory response.[32, 33, 47]

The reason for the absence of acute inflammation in fetal wounds is not understood, but it has been suggested that the sterile intrauterine environment of the fetus fails to provide antigenic stimulation for PMN infiltration. However, when presumedly sterile wounds from germ-free, adult guinea pigs were studied, acute inflammatory cells were present, albeit in lesser quantities than in control animals.[48] Immunological immaturity and neutropenia have also been implicated as causative.[30] This suggests that the fetus is unable to elicit an acute inflammatory response under varied circumstances, but evidence exists that this is not the case. In an experiment that examined biliary atresia, noxious substances were injected into the biliary tree of fetal dogs. Three days following injection of sodium morrhuate there was periportal necrosis and acute inflammation in the liver.[49]

Following the acute inflammatory phase in adults, chronic inflammatory cells enter the wound site. Lymphocytes and macrophages are noticeably absent or rare in experimental fetal wounds. Mononuclear cells and mesenchymal cells have been repeatedly observed in fetal rabbit wounds using PVA implants.[38] The mononuclear cells have thus far eluded specific identification, though Adzick and co-workers have shown nonspecific esterase staining characteristic of macrophages.[10]

In adults, fibroblast infiltration and proliferation follow the chronic inflammatory response. Observations regarding fibroplasia in fetal wounds are not as uniform as with inflammatory cells. Fetal sheep wounds were noted to have a plentitude of fibroblasts,[30] as was the healing amnion in monkeys[31] and rats.[34] The dermal wounds in fetal monkeys, however, lacked fibroblasts.[31] The data for rabbits are also conflicting. Wounds that were evaluated by simple biopsy[35] or PVA implant histology[38] contained only a scant presence of fibroblasts. However, when Goretex implants were used, fibroblastic encapsulation was observed.[10]

The process of epithelialization appears to occur rapidly in primarily closed fetal wounds. The epidermis of fetal rat cheek wounds was completely restored to its normal state within 24 hours of injury. The healing of the mucosal epithelium in these wounds seems to occur at a slower rate than in the epidermis; although continuity had been restored in 24 hours, complete normality had not been achieved such that the epithelium was only one cell thick in some areas. Healing in the underlying muscle occurred even more slowly.[33] Closed, linear wounds in rabbits had the gross appearance of complete healing by 7 days, but microscopically, epithelialization was not complete.[38] The neoepithelium in fetal wounds appears to originate from the wound margins rather than from within the wound itself. It was noted that the hair follicles on the perimeter of linear wounds in fetal sheep had proliferated and that these were apparently the source of the migrating epithelium.[30]

Endothelial proliferation in adult wounds leads to neovascularization within the granulation tissue. Most studies support the absence of adultlike granulation tissue and angiogenesis in fetal linear or primarily closed wounds. Studies that provide evidence for this finding include those in which wound biopsies were taken in sheep,[30] monkeys,[31] rabbits,[35] and rats.[32, 33] When PVA implants were used in rabbit wounds, similar findings were observed.[38] Once again, conflicting data exist from studies in which Goretex[10] or viscose cellulose[36, 37] implants were used in rabbits. In these cases granulation tissue containing capillary loop formations was seen infiltrating the implants.

Wound Matrix

The primary components of the extracellular matrix (ECM) of skin are proteoglycans, elastin, and collagen. The adult wound consists of sequential provisional matrices of fibrin and proteoglycan, but the final matrix is composed primarily of collagen. The gross absence of a scar in healed fetal wounds suggests a low collagen content. Fetal sheep wounds appear to be lacking in collagen,[30] as do wounds through muscle in rats.[32] Histological studies of PVA implants from fetal rabbit wounds following 7 days of healing showed no evidence of collagen in that there was no staining with trichrome blue. The implants were analyzed using high-pressure liquid chromatography and found to contain no collagen hydroxyproline (sensitivity of this assay is 40 picamoles). Tissue from these implants stained positively with alcian blue, which was eliminated following pretreatment with hyaluronidase, thus providing indirect evidence for the presence of the glycosaminoglycan (GAG) hyaluronic acid (HA).[38] Confirmation of the presence of HA and its quantitation was provided by analysis of the wound matrix within PVA implants. The HA content of the wounds progressively increased up to 5 days after wounding, the end of the study period (Fig. 21–3). Cellulose acetate membrane electrophoresis following selective enzymatic digestion of extracted GAGs demonstrated the primary component to be HA; a minor component of chondroitin sulfate-B (dermatan sulfate) was present beginning 5 days postwounding, and collagen was absent at all time periods studied.[50] Wounds in which either cellulose[37] or Goretex[10] implants were used contained collagen as evidenced by the accumulation of hydroxyproline. This is not an unexpected finding in view of the fibroblasia present in these wound models.

Although hyaluronic acid is the predominant component of the ECM in fetal rabbit wounds, fibronectin also appears to be present very early. Wound biopsies of fetal rabbits were evaluated using antibodies against the ECM components laminin, fibronectin, and collagen. Fibronectin was visualized 4 hours postwounding (the earliest time period studied), associated with fibrin clot. At 8 hours, fibronectin appeared at the wound edges, and at 24 hours, it was distributed throughout the wound. Fibronectin was first seen in adult wounds at 12 hours. A role for this protein in the rapid epithelialization observed with linear wounds was suggested by the investigators.[51]

It appears that the ECM of fetal wounds is primarily hyaluronic acid (HA). It might then be hypothesized that fibroblasts present in the wound preferentially produce this GAG, rather than collagen. Fetal sheep[52] and fetal bovine[53] serum have been demonstrated to stimulate HA production by rat fibrosarcoma cells in culture. Using similar in vitro techniques, urine[54] and wound fluid[55] from fetal sheep have been observed to have HA stimulating activity as well. Although these experiments do not provide conclusive evidence for the stimulation of GAG production by fetal fibroblasts, they do show that such stimulatory activity may exist within the fetus. Further investigation is required to determine if these findings have significance for the regulation of matrix events in the fetal wound.

Another hypothesis for the frequently observed relative lack of collagen in fetal wounds is that fetal fibroblasts have an intrinsic synthetic defect for this protein. To test this, adult and fetal rabbit fibroblasts were grown in cell culture and collagen synthesis was evaluated by the incorporation of tritiated proline. The fetal cells synthesized more collagen than their adult counterparts when they were grown in 21 and 2 percent oxygen.[56] Therefore, it appears that the low collagen content of fetal wounds is not secondary to an intrinsic inability of fibroblasts to produce this protein, nor is this capacity altered by a hypoxic environment.

Open Wounds

Studies of open wounds have been performed on guinea pigs, sheep, monkeys, and rabbits. Hess created wounds by transecting the vertebral column of guinea pigs.[57] He noted very rapid healing with granulation tissue in a process that appeared to be adultlike. Excisional wounds created in sheep by Burrington appeared histologically different than linear wounds; scant acute inflammation was present, but fibroblasts and mesenchymal cells were abundant.[30] Contrary to these observations, the repair of excisional wounds in monkeys[31] and rabbits[20, 38, 58, 59] appears to occur without acute inflammation, fibroplasia, neovascularization, and collagen deposition.

Contraction

Similar to adult wounds, fetal sheep open wounds contract, but more rapidly; there was extensive contraction and epithelialization within 72 hours of injury.[30] A lack of contraction has been observed in open wounds in fetal monkeys and rabbits. Interestingly, epithelialization did not occur in the noncontracted monkey and rabbit wounds, though epithelial proliferation was present at the margins of the open monkey wounds.[31, 58] Perhaps, epithelialization seen in open sheep wounds may occur because

Figure 21–3. There is a progressive deposition of glycosaminoglycan (GAG) in fetal rabbit wounds up to 6 days following injury. The GAG content of fetal wounds is significantly greater than that of adult rabbit wounds on postwound days 2 through 6. Note that total GAG deposition in fetal wounds is essentially the same as hyaluronic acid deposition since this is the only GAG detectable in these wounds until postwound day 6. (Reprinted by permission of VCH Publishers, Inc., 220 East 23rd St., New York, N.Y. 10010 from: *Matrix*, Vol. 9, pp. 224–231, 1989, *Characterization and Quantitation of Wound Matrix in the Fetal Rabbit*, R. Lawrence Depalma, Thomas M. Krummel, Lucian A. Durham III, Barbara A. Michna, Brian L. Thomas, Jeffrey M. Nelson, Robert F. Diegelmann; Figure 2 (Glycosaminoglycan deposition in adult and fetal wounds).)

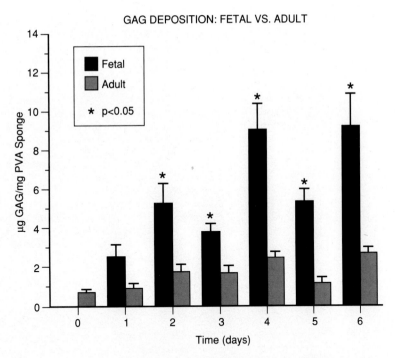

of the decreased area of the wounds as a result of contraction.

Excisional wounds in fetal rabbits not only fail to contract but actually enlarge.[58, 60] Studies have shown that the increase in size of these wounds was not due to rapid fetal growth, since wound expansion occurred more rapidly than the adjacent unwounded skin. In consideration of the theory of adult contraction resulting from forces created by fibroblast-matrix interaction, a study of the contractile capacity of fetal fibroblasts was performed. Fetal and adult rabbit fibroblasts were grown in culture, and their cell surface areas measured. Following the addition of medium containing adenosine triphosphate (ATP), the cell areas of the fetal and adult cells diminished by 70 to 80 percent, indicating that contraction occurred to the same extent in each. To quantitate contractile forces, fetal and adult fibroblast populated collagen lattices (FPCL) were utilized.[61] The lattice composed of fetal rabbit fibroblasts and fetal rabbit dermal collagen demonstrated a greater reduction of lattice area after 48 hours of incubation compared to the adult populated lattice. When a 40 percent concentration of amniotic fluid was added to the FPCL assay, the contraction of fetal and adult fibroblasts was inhibited.[58] Thus, in vitro evidence exists that fetal rabbit fibroblasts can exert contractile forces on an artificial collagen lattice and that amniotic fluid from this species may contain an inhibitor of contraction.

The effect of the fetal environment on the open wound has been studied in utero. Soma-

sundaram and Prathap covered open fetal rabbit wounds by suturing a Silastic sheet over them.[20] While other cellular events remained unchanged, the wounds appeared to contract. In a similar study of fetal rabbits, excisional wounds were observed to contract when covered with a latex patch. The wounds were evaluated using computerized morphometry and their decrease in size was determined to be 26 percent. These contracted wounds were also 97 percent re-epithelialized.[60] These studies raised the possibility of the presence of one or more factors within amniotic fluid that inhibit wound contraction. Furthermore, these two studies provide evidence of adultlike healing in newborn rabbits. Excisional wounds in the newborn animals contracted rapidly and healed by the infiltration of granulation tissue.[20, 60]

To further characterize the lack of contractility of open fetal rabbit wounds, histological and electron microscopic evaluations of open wound biopsies were done. Histologically, the wounds showed no migration of epithelium from the wound edges, no acute inflammation, no fibroblastic response, and no collagen deposition. To indirectly check for the presence of myofibroblasts, immunohistochemical evaluation was performed by staining the specimens with antiactin antibody. This procedure revealed staining of the subcutaneous panniculus carnosis muscle, but no staining of the wound tissue. Transmission electron micrographs provided detailed information on the cellular structure of the fibroblasts present (Fig. 21–4). Morpholog-

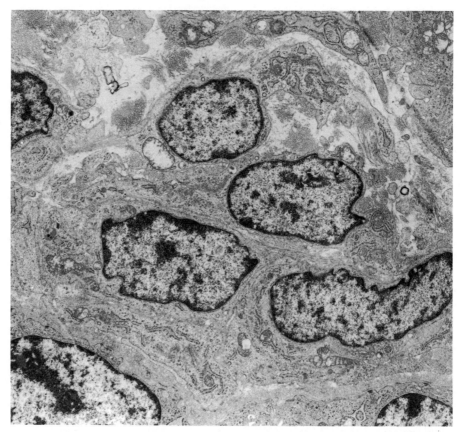

Figure 21–4. Transmission electron micrograph of fibroblasts from the edge of an open fetal rabbit wound (×8600). Their nuclear envelopes are smooth rather than multiply indented as in myofibroblasts. Other features typical of myofibroblasts, such as desmosomes, gap junctions, and cytoplasmic actin filaments, are absent on higher magnification. Myofibroblasts have not been identified in noncontracting, open fetal rabbit wounds. (Courtesy of Dr. Jeffrey Haynes.)

ical features of myofibroblasts such as multiply indented nuclear envelopes, desmosomes, gap junctions, and intermediate cytoplasmic filaments that can be identified as actin by immunohistochemistry were absent.[59]

In summary, open wounds in fetal sheep appear to heal by secondary intention, whereas those of monkeys and rabbits do not. Evidence exists that fetal rabbit fibroblasts are able to contract and transmit contractile forces to a collagen lattice. It appears that myofibroblasts are not present in fetal rabbit open wounds. Finally, amniotic fluid seems to have an inhibitory effect on open wound contraction, as demonstrated by in vitro and in vivo studies. The possible relationship between amniotic fluid and noncontraction of these wounds is an example of the influence the fetal environment may exert upon the processes of tissue repair.

Other Wounds

Dixon created electrical burn wounds in fetal rats at 16½ through 19½ days GA (term is 21 days).[62] The younger fetuses lacked an acute inflammatory response, although this was variably noted in the older fetuses. The lack of acute inflammation was attributed to poor capillary vasodilatation at the wound site and to neutropenia. The wounds appeared to heal by a mesenchymal cell "filling-in," while the older fetuses had more of an adultlike response within their wounds.

Evidence exists that results seen in surgically created simple wounds apply to repair of structural defects. Fetal cleft lip repair undertaken in mice and rhesus monkeys showed no gross or microscopic scarring.[45, 46]

Human Observations

Some data concerning wound healing in the human fetus do exist. Postmortem examination was undertaken on a spontaneously aborted infant of approximately 20 weeks gestational age. Trauma from amniotic bands was evident: many digits were missing, as well as an amputated distal third of the right leg. There was a large, full-thickness ulcer down to bone at the left knee felt to be secondary to friction from exposed bone of the contralateral lower extremity stump. Study of the amputation sites revealed the absence of acute inflammation, granulation tissue, and contraction. The ulcer also contained no acute inflammation. Healing appeared to have occurred by "coagulation" of exposed tissue and by a lesser degree of mesenchymal cell proliferation.[63] These observations corroborate many of the findings of the animal studies.

WOUND SITE MANIPULATION

One of the advantages of using wound implants is the ability to manipulate the wound site by the introduction of substances into the wound. In this manner, hypotheses regarding the mechanisms involved in fetal wound healing may be tested.

In an attempt to produce acute inflammation in fetal rabbit wounds, formyl-methionyl-leucyl-phenylalanine (F-MLP) was introduced into the wounds using PVA implants. This substance is a potent chemoattractant for PMNs. Histological examination of the implants confirmed the presence of an acute inflammatory response consisting of PMNs one day postwounding. At day 5, numerous fibroblasts were noted, as well as collagen deposition as indicated by trichrome staining. The magnitude of these responses was roughly dose dependent. This study provided evidence that an adultlike response was possible in fetal rabbit wounds.[64]

Transforming growth factor-β (TGF-β) is a peptide growth factor with important regulatory functions that is released by a number of cells involved in adult inflammation and healing.[65] It has been shown to increase total protein, collagen, and DNA content in wound chambers in vivo and to stimulate biosynthetic rates of collagen and fibronectin in cultured fibroblasts.[66, 67] Furthermore, the formation of granulation tissue was stimulated when TGF-β was injected subcutaneously into newborn mice.[68] To test whether the fetal rabbit is capable of responding to TGF-β, wound implants were impregnated with varying concentrations of lyophilized TGF-β and placed subcutaneously in fetal rabbits.[69] When implants were removed after 7 days they were encased in a fibrotic capsule in which fibroplasia and collagen deposition was evident. Some dose-dependent response did appear to be present.

To determine if this response was due to a direct effect on the fetal fibroblasts, TGF-β–fibroblast binding capacity was evaluated using flow cytometry.[70] The results revealed that rabbit embryonal fibroblasts contained the greatest density of receptors. There was a sequential reduction in receptor density as the cells became more differentiated (fetal density greater than adult). Additionally, the adult cells exhibited slower binding kinetics than the embryonal or fetal fibroblasts. These studies imply that the fetus is capable of responding to physiological doses of exogenously provided TGF-β, and that this response may be a result of a direct effect on fibroblasts via cell surface receptors. Thus, the observed normal fetal response to tissue injury may result from regulatory control of mediators rather than an intrinsic defect in fetal responsiveness.

Noting the results of the TGF-β experiment, a study was designed that attempted to introduce adult mediators into fetal wounds. Polyvinyl alcohol implants were placed subcutaneously into the backs of pregnant rabbits and removed 24 hours later. They were then immediately inserted into fetuses of the same doe from which they were removed. After 5 days the implants contained an abundance of PMNs. The number of acute inflammatory cells in the fetal implants was significantly greater than the number in 24 hour adult implants, indicating that fetal PMN infiltration had occurred. Despite this marked inflammatory response, fibroplasia and collagen deposition was absent.[71] This study demonstrated that acute inflammation can be elicited in fetal rabbit wounds given appropriate provocation. However, the presence of acute inflammatory cells and their mediators does not necessitate fibroblast proliferation and collagen deposition.

FETAL WOUND HEALING AND REGENERATION: A POSSIBLE ROLE FOR HYALURONIC ACID

Regeneration is the process by which animals repair injured tissue so that the premorbid state of that tissue is established or very nearly approximated.[72] Some lower vertebrates are quite adept at this as exemplified by the newt, which can regenerate an amputated extremity, but this process exists to a more limited extent in higher animals. For example, skeletal muscle regeneration has been demonstrated in rats, hamsters, and cats.[73] In humans, digits amputated distal to the distal interphalangeal joint in small children appear to regenerate. Although some feel that this may represent exuberant contraction and rapid wound healing, the healed digit appears nearly morphologically normal, complete with fingerprints.[74] It is also well recognized that following hepatic resection humans can regenerate a metabolically functional organ. This is not a uniform response to liver injury, as evidenced by the prevalence of a scarring response that results in cirrhosis. Furthermore, no other major human organ system appears to have this regenerative ability. The study of fetal wound healing has brought a new aspect to regeneration. Gross observations in the fetus have demonstrated healing without scarring and some microscopic studies have observed reconstitution of normal tissue.

Studies in regeneration have often used the newt as a model.[75–77] Following the amputation of an extremity in this animal an epithelial cap forms over the injury. Dedifferentiation of the underlying tissue into a collection of embryonal-like cells called the blastema ensues. This is followed by cellular proliferation, migration, and differentiation. The formation of the blastema is temporally correlated with changes in the extracellular matrix. Collagenase activity increases and hyaluronic acid (HA) is synthesized, yielding a glycosaminoglycan (GAG)-enriched, collagen-poor extracellular matrix. HA synthesis continues throughout the period of cellular dedifferentiation and proliferation. As the level of HA falls, hyaluronidase activity increases, corresponding to cellular differentiation. Accumulation of HA was also found in the regenerating lens of a newt iris.[78] It appears from these observations that HA is associated with cellular dedifferentiation, proliferation, and migration. The absence of HA and the presence of hyaluronidase or the degradation products of HA are associated with differentiation.

The formation of a blastema with subsequent cellular migration and proliferation is similar to processes of normal development. Chick embryos have been used as models in the study of development.[79–81] As in the above-mentioned regeneration studies, HA appears to have an important role. During lens development in the chick, HA accumulates within the cornea during the period in which mesenchymal cell invasion and stromal swelling occur. Its level subsequently decreases, at which time hyaluronidase activity is present. This correlates with corneal dehydration prior to acquisition of transparency.[79] HA seems to have an effect on the developing vascular system in chick embryos as well. When epithelial tissues that synthesize relatively large amounts of HA were implanted into normally vascular regions that are devoid of HA, angiogenesis was inhibited.[80] HA is also present in the chick chorioallantoic membrane during the period of vessel formation. It is felt that depletion of HA and a concomitant increase in HA degradation products may be important in vessel migration and proliferation.[81, 82]

Hyaluronic acid is a GAG that is a linear polymer of repeating disaccharide units. The actual size and molecular weight of each GAG vary depending upon the number of repeating units it contains. Due to the disaccharide content of the GAGs, they are highly negatively charged. HA is the largest GAG, having a molecular weight as high as several million. It differs from other GAGs in that it is nonsulfated and has disaccharide units consisting of glucuronic acid and N-acetylglucosamine. Additionally, unlike most GAGs, HA probably does not covalently bind to proteins to form proteoglycans.[83] It is felt that the presence of HA provides for a malleable matrix highly permissable of cellular movement.[75] Furthermore, by virtue of its large mass, cellular contact is blocked and thus so is inhibition of movement and growth. Consequently, circumstances for cell proliferation and migration are optimized. It is possible that the removal of HA from the wound allows for cellular contact inhibition, thereby causing migration and proliferation to cease and differentiation to proceed.

Fetal wounds have an abundance of HA, yet the wounds are hypocellular in relation to their adult counterparts. This seems to be contradictory to the previous discussion. One may hypothesize that HA provides a suitable environment for mesenchymal cell invasion. However, the abundance of this GAG may prevent their differentiation into mature fibroblasts so that collagen deposition is prevented. Another possible role for HA in the fetal wound may relate to angiogenesis. Most studies of these wounds have observed a lack of granulation tissue and neovascularization. As noted, evidence exists supporting HA, or its degradation products, as a mediator in blood vessel formation and migration.

The actual source of HA in the fetal wound is not known. One possibility is that this GAG is synthesized by the cells present within the wound or by fibroblasts on the periphery of the wound. Alternatively, HA may diffuse into the wound from the surrounding normal skin. Accumulation of HA may be a result of preferential deposition with increased synthesis or decreased degradation.

CONCLUSION

Tissue repair in the mammalian fetus differs greatly from that in the developed animal. Primarily closed wounds heal rapidly without scarring. There appears to be no acute inflammation and only a mild chronic inflammatory response with minimal fibroblast or endothelial cell proliferation. The extracellular matrix of these wounds is lacking in excessive collagen; rather it is rich in hyaluronic acid. Open wounds in rabbits and monkeys do not contract, although this process does occur in sheep. Lastly, gross, microscopic, and biochemical similarities exist among fetal tissue repair, regeneration, and developmental systems.

The mechanisms underlying these observations are beginning to be understood. The fetus is able to mount an inflammatory response given provocation. Thus, the absence of acute inflammation is not secondary to a fetal inability to produce such a reaction. Fibroplasia is not dependent merely on an acute inflammatory reaction since fibrosis does not necessarily follow PMN infiltration. Furthermore, the lack of collagen in the wounds does not seem to be due to an intrinsic synthetic defect of fibroblasts. The abundance of hyaluronic acid in fetal wounds may have great importance in the regenerative qualities of these wounds. Lastly, the local supply of or response to growth factors in the fetus may be different than that in adult wounds and may account for some of the unique healing events.

The cellular and matrix responses in fetal wounds are undoubtedly affected by the milieu of this developing organism. Physiological circumstances that may be important are (1) an endocrine system greatly different than the adult; (2) lack of antigenic stimulation; (3) immunological immaturity; (4) tissue hypoxemia; and (5) a metabolically underdeveloped liver. The environment of the fetus is also vital: maternal and placental dependency is obvious; amniotic fluid has local effects on the injured tissue which it bathes and possible systemic effects as well.

Perhaps the greatest potential benefit of understanding tissue repair in the mammalian fetus is the possible application of its mechanisms to abnormal postnatal wound healing. If the mechanisms responsible for a lack of wound contraction and scarring can be uncovered, it may be possible to manipulate pediatric or adult

wounds to improve healing, with potential benefits to anastomotic strictures, burn contractures, pressure sores, and poorly healing diabetic wounds. Support for such applications exists: when open wounds in diabetic mice were topically treated with hyaluronic acid, the rate of healing was enhanced.[84]

Finally, the study of tissue repair in the mammalian fetus may provide an easily accessible model that approximates mammalian tissue regeneration. Regeneration can be considered a recapitulation of development[73] as tissue proceeds from a blastema into a differentiated state. Therefore, insight into regeneration and development may be achieved by studying the response of injured tissue in the fetus. An enhanced knowledge of these fields may have implications for the in utero prevention and treatment of developmental defects.

References

1. Goodson WH, Hunt TK: Wound healing and aging. J Invest Dermatol 73:88–91, 1979.
2. Sadler TW: Langman's Medical Embryology, 5th ed. Baltimore, Williams & Wilkins, 1985, pp 19–108.
3. Behrman RE, Vaughan VC: Fetal growth and development. In Behrman RE, Vaughan VC, Nelson WE (eds): Nelson's Textbook of Pediatrics, 12th ed., Philadelphia, WB Saunders, 1983, pp 11–12.
4. Adam PAJ, Teramo K, Raiha N, et al: Human fetal insulin metabolism early in gestation. Response to acute elevation of the fetal glucose concentration and placental transfer of human insulin I-131. Diabetes 18:409–416, 1969.
5. Brinsmead MW, Liggins GC: Somatomedin-like activity, prolactin, growth hormone and insulin in human cord blood. Aust NZ Obstet Gynaecol 19:129–134, 1979.
6. Chez RA, Mintz DH, Reynolds WA, et al: Maternal-fetal plasma glucose relationships in late monkey pregnancy. Am J Obstet Gynecol 121:938–940, 1975.
7. Pritchard JA, MacDonald PC, Gant NF: Williams' Obstetrics. Norwalk CT, Appleton-Century-Crofts, Norwalk, 1985, pp 119–137, 145–180.
8. Winters AJ, Colston C, MacDonald PC, et al: Fetal plasma prolactin levels. J Clin Endocrinol Metab 41:626–629, 1974.
9. Playfair JHL, Wolfendalen MR, Kay HEM: The leukocytes of peripheral blood in the human fetus. Br J Haematol 9:336–344, 1966.
10. Adzick NS, Harrison MR, Glick PL, et al: Comparison of fetal, newborn and adult wound healing by histologic enzyme-histochemical and hydroxyproline determination. J Pediatr Surg 20:315–319, 1985.
11. Nelson NM: Respiration and circulation before birth. In Smith CA, Nelson NM (eds): The Physiology of the Newborn Infant, 4th ed. Springfield, IL, Charles C Thomas, 1976, pp 15–16.
12. Altshuler G: Immunologic competence of the immature human fetus: Morphologic evidence from intrauterine cytomegalovirus infection. Obstet Gynecol 43:811–816, 1974.
13. Kohler PF: Maturation of the human complement

system. I. Onset, time and sites of fetal C1q, C4, C3 and C5 synthesis. J Clin Invest 52:671–677, 1973.

14. Adinolfi M: Human complement: Onset and site of synthesis during fetal life. Am J Dis Child 131:1015–1023, 1977.

15. Moore KL: The Developing Human. Clinically Oriented Embryology, 4th ed. Philadelphia, WB Saunders, 1988, pp 112–113.

16. Moore KL: The Developing Human. Clinically Oriented Embryology, 4th ed. Philadelphia, WB Saunders, 1988, pp 65–129.

17. Mulvihill SJ, Stone MM, Fonkalsrud EW: Trophic effects of amniotic fluid on fetal gastrointestinal development. J Surg Res 40:291–296, 1986.

18. Mulvihill SJ, Halden G, Debas HT: Trophic effect of amniotic fluid on cultured fetal gastric mucosal cells. J Surg Res 46:327–329, 1989.

19. Lu CY, Changelian PS, Unanue ER: Alpha-fetoprotein inhibits macrophage expression of Ia antigens. J Immunol 132:1722–1727, 1984.

20. Somasundaram K, Prathap K: The effect of exclusion of amniotic fluid on intrauterine healing of skin wounds in rabbit fetuses. J Pathol 107:127–130, 1972.

21. Schilling JA: Wound healing. Physiol Rev 48:374–423, 1968.

22. Schilling JA: Wound healing. Surg Clin North Am 56:859–874, 1976.

23. Pessa ME, Blank KI, Copeland EM III: Growth factors and determinants of wound repair. J Surg Res 42:207–217, 1987.

24. Simpson DM, Ross R: The neutrophilic leukocyte in wound repair. A study with antineutrophilic serum. J Clin Invest 51:2009–2023, 1972.

25. Diegelmann RF, Cohen IK, Kaplan AM: The role of macrophages in wound repair: A review. Plast Reconstr Surg 68:107–113, 1981.

26. Ross R: The fibroblast and wound repair. Biol Rev 43:51–95, 1968.

27. Gabbiani G, Hirschel BJ, Ryan B, et al: Granulation tissue as a contractile organ. J Exp Med 135:719–734, 1972.

28. Gabbiani G, Rungger-Brandle E: The fibroblast. In Glynn LE (ed): Tissue Repair and Regeneration. Amsterdam, Elsevier/North-Holland, 1981, pp 22–29.

29. Ehrlich HP: Wound closure: Evidence of cooperation between fibroblasts and collagen matrix. Eye 2:149–157, 1988.

30. Burrington JD: Wound healing in the fetal lamb. J Pediatr Surg 6:523–528, 1971.

31. Sopher D: A study of wound healing in the foetal tissues of the cynomolgus monkey. Lab Anim Handbooks 6:327–335, 1975.

32. Rowsell AR: The intra-uterine healing of foetal muscle wounds: Experimental study in the rat. Br J Pediatr Surg 37:635–642, 1984.

33. Robinson BW, Goss AN: Intra-uterine healing of fetal rat cheek wounds. Cleft Palate J 18:251–255, 1981.

34. Sopher D: The response of rat fetal membranes to injury. Ann Roy Coll Surg 51:240–249, 1972.

35. Chignier E, Baguet J, Dessapt B, et al: Skin healing and fibrin stabilizing factor blood levels in the rabbit fetus. J Surg Res 31:415–432, 1981.

36. Thomasson B, Vilijanto J, Jaakelainen A, et al: Enzyme histochemical observations on the formation of granulation tissue in rabbit fetuses and does. Acta Chir Scand 139:327–333, 1973.

37. Vilijanto J, Thomasson B, Pikkarainen J, et al: Enzyme foetal connective tissue regeneration: A biochemical study in rabbits. Acta Chir Scand 141:85–89, 1975.

38. Krummel TM, Nelson JM, Diegelmann RF, et al: Fetal response to injury in the rabbit. J Pediatr Surg 22:640–644, 1987.

39. Schilling JA, Joel W, Shurley HM: Wound healing: A comparative study of the histochemical changes in granulation tissue contained in stainless steel wire mesh and polyvinyl sponge cylinders. Surgery 48:702–710, 1959.

40. Hunt TK, Twomey P, Zederfeldt B, et al: Respiratory gas tensions and pH in healing wounds. Am J Surg 114:302–307, 1967.

41. Vilijanto J: Celstic: A device for wound healing studies in man: Description of method. J Surg Res 20:115–118, 1976.

42. Goodson WH III, Hunt TK: Development of a new miniature method for the study of wound healing in human subjects. J Surg Res 33:394–401, 1982.

43. Diegelmann RF, Lindblad WJ, Cohen IK: A subcutaneous implant for wound healing studies in human subjects. J Surg Res 41:229–237, 1986.

44. Smedley MJ, Stanisstreet M: Scanning electron microscopy of wound healing in rat embryos. J Embryol Exp Morph 83:109–117, 1984.

45. Hallock GG: In utero cleft lip repair in A/J mice. Plast Reconstr Surg 75:785–788, 1985.

46. Hallock GG, Rice DC, McClure HM: In utero lip repair in the rhesus monkey: An update. Plast Reconstr Surg 80:855–858, 1987.

47. Goss AN: Intra-uterine healing of fetal rat oral mucosal skin and cartilage wounds. J Oral Pathol 6:35–43, 1977.

48. Tipton JB, Dingman RO: Some aspects of wound healing in the germ-free animal. Plast Reconstr Surg 38:499–506, 1966.

49. Holder TM, Ashcroft KW: The effects of bile duct ligation and inflammation in the fetus. J Pediatr Surg 2:35–40, 1967.

50. DePalma RL, Krummel TM, Durham LA III, et al: Characterization and quantitation of wound matrix in the fetal rabbit. Matrix 9:224–231, 1989.

51. Longaker MT, Whitby DJ, Ferguson MWJ, et al: Studies in fetal wound healing. III. Early deposition of fibronectin distinguishes fetal from adult wound fluid. J Pediatr Surg 24:799–805, 1989.

52. Longaker MT, Harrison MR, Crombleholme TM, et al: Studies in fetal wound healing. I. A factor in fetal serum that stimulates deposition of hyaluronic acid. J Pediatr Surg 24:789–792, 1989.

53. Decker M, Chiu ES, Dollbaum C, et al: Hyaluronic acid–stimulating activity in sera from the bovine fetus and from breast cancer patients. Cancer Res 49:3499–3505, 1989.

54. Williams SI, Longaker MT, Harrison MR, et al: A factor in fetal urine stimulates deposition of hyaluronic acid. Fetal Ther. In press.

55. Longaker MT, Chiu ES, Harrison MR, et al: Studies in fetal wound healing. IV. Hyaluronic acid stimulating activity distinguishes fetal wound fluid from adult wound fluid. Ann Surgery 210:667–672, 1989.

56. Thomas BL, Krummel TM, Melany M, et al: Collagen synthesis and type expression by fetal fibroblasts in vitro. Surg Forum 39:642–644, 1988.

57. Hess A: Reactions of mammalian fetal tissues to injury. II. Skin. Skin Anat Res 119:435–448, 1958.

58. Krummel TM, Ehrlich HP, Nelson JM, et al: Fetal wounds do not contract in utero. Surg Forum 40:613–615, 1989.

59. Haynes JH, Krummel TM, Schatzki PF, et al: Histology of the open fetal rabbit wound. Surg Forum, 40:558–560, 1989.

60. Ditesheim JA, Delozier JB, Rees RS, et al: Covered fetal excisional wounds heal by tissue regeneration. Surg Forum 40:615–617, 1989.

61. Bell E, Ivarsson B, Merrill C: Production of tissue-like structures by contraction of collagen lattices by human

fibroblasts of different proliferative potential *in vitro*. Cell Biol 76:1274–1278, 1979.

62. Dixon JB: Inflammation in the foetal and neonatal rat: The local reactions to skin burns. J Pathol Biol 80:73–82, 1960.

63. Rowlatt U: Intrauterine wound healing in a 20 week human fetus. Virchows Arch 381:353–361, 1979.

64. Thomas BL, Krummel TM, Diegelmann RF, et al: Unpublished observations.

65. Sporn MB, Roberts AB, Wakefield LM, et al: Transforming growth factor beta: Biological function and chemical structure. Science 233:532–534, 1986.

66. Sporn MB, Roberts AB, Shull JH, et al: Polypeptide transforming growth factor beta isolated from bovine sources and used for wound healing in vivo. Science 219:1329–1331, 1983.

67. Ignotz RA, Massague J: Transforming growth factor beta stimulates the expression of fibronectin and collagen and their incorporation into the extracellular matrix. J Biol Chem 261:4337–4345, 1986.

68. Roberts AB, Sporn MB, Assoian RK, et al: Transforming growth factor type-beta: Rapid induction of fibrosis and angiogenesis in vivo and stimulation of collagen formation in vivo. Proc Natl Acad Sci USA 83:4167–4171, 1986.

69. Krummel TM, Michna BA, Thomas BL, et al: Transforming growth factor-β induces fibrosis in a fetal wound model. J Pediatr Surg 23:647–652, 1988.

70. Durham LA III, Krummel TM, Cawthorn JW, et al: Analysis of transforming growth factor-beta receptor binding in embryonic, fetal and adult rabbit fibroblasts. J Pediatr Surg 24:784–788, 1989.

71. Borchelt BD, Krummel TM, Cawthorn JW, et al: Transposition of an early adult wound to a fetal rabbit wound does not result in recruitment of fibroblasts. Surgical Forum 40:555–557, 1989.

72. Goss RJ: Prospects for regeneration in man. Clin Orthop Rel Res 151:270–282, 1980.

73. Carlson BM: Regeneration of entire skeletal muscles. Fed Proc 45:1456–1460, 1986.

74. Illingworth CM: Trapped fingers and amputated finger tips in children. J Pediatr Surg 9:853–858, 1974.

75. Toole BP, Gross J: The extracellular matrix of the regenerating newt limb: Synthesis and removal of hyaluronate prior to differentiation. Dev Biol 25:57–77, 1971.

76. Smith GN, Toole BP, Gross J: Hyaluronidase activity and glycosaminoglycan synthesis in the amputated newt limb: Comparison of denervated, nonregenerating limbs with regenerates. Dev Biol 43:221–232, 1975.

77. Mescher AL, Munain SI: Changes in the extracellular matrix and glycosaminoglycan synthesis during the institution of regeneration in adult newt forelimbs. Anat Rec 214:424–431, 1986.

78. Kulyk WM, Zalik SE, Demitriov E: Hyaluronic acid activity in the newt iris during lens regeneration. Exp Cell Res 172:180–191, 1987.

79. Toole BP, Trelstad RL: Hyaluronate production and removal during corneal development in the chick. Dev Biol 26:28–35, 1971.

80. Feinberg RN, Beebe DC: Hyaluronate in vasculogenesis. Science 220:455–459, 1982.

81. Auspruck DH: Distribution of hyaluronic acid and sulfated glycosaminoglycans during blood vessel development of the chick chorioallantoic membrane. Am J Anat 177:313–331, 1986.

82. West DC, Hampson IN, Arnold F, et al: Angiogenesis induced by degradation products of hyaluronic acid. Science 228:1324–1326, 1985.

83. Heingard D, Paulsson M: Structure and metabolism of proteoglycans. In Piez KA, Reddi AH (eds): Extracellular Matrix Biochemistry. New York, Elsevier, 1984, pp 277–280.

84. Abatangelo G, Martelli M, Vecchia P: Healing of hyaluronic acid-enriched wounds: Histologic observations. J Surg Res 35:410–416, 1983.

IV
REPAIR OF SPECIFIC TISSUES

22

THE SKIN

Bruce A. Mast, M.D.

The importance to survival of adequate wound healing is perhaps best exemplified by the fact that the ancient Greeks ascribed mystical powers to proper wound healing. Those inflicted with wounds would retreat to the temple of the god Aesculapius where it was thought that his serpent would lick their wounds while they slept and thereby cause them to heal.[1] Certainly our understanding of wound healing is much greater now, although some of the mysticism remains. This elegant, integrated process involves a variety of cell groups acting in concert to establish the integrity of injured tissue. Although most of our knowledge of wound healing has evolved from the study of tissue repair of skin, it is thought that many of the same principles apply to repair mechanisms in other tissues and structures.

This chapter presents an overview of dermal wound healing, many aspects of which are discussed in greater detail elsewhere in this text. Since this is a process of the integument, the anatomy of skin will be considered first, followed by a discussion of the normal healing process, factors that affect healing, the effects of aging, and finally, models that are used in the study of healing.

ANATOMY OF SKIN

The skin, also known as the cutis or integument, has a surface area of 1.5 to 2.0 m^2, making it the largest organ of the body.[2] Normal skin is essential for the survival of the animal because it provides thermal regulation, prevents dehydration through evaporative water loss, and acts as a barrier against chemical and infectious insults. The importance of this protective barrier is evidenced by the high mortality associated with toxic epidermal necrolysis, a condition in which total epidermal sloughing can occur. The skin is not a uniform organ, its appearance and thickness varying according to anatomical site. For instance, the skin of the soles of the feet is thickest (8 mm), whereas, the skin of the eyelids is the thinnest (1 mm).[2]

This skin is anatomically divided into two layers: the epidermis, or cuticle, and the dermis, or corium (Fig. 22–1). The epidermis is the superficial, protective layer, and the dermis provides the firmness and elasticity of healthy skin. These two layers make up the true skin; the subcutaneous tissue, or subcutis, is deep to the dermis, apposed to the fascia, and is sometimes included as part of the anatomy of the skin.[2]

Each layer of the skin consists of various cell types or structures. The epidermis is completely cellular, typically made up of a keratinized, stratified, squamous epithelium that contains five histologically distinct cell types. These cells are organized into layers that are arranged superficial to deep: horny layer (stratum corneum), clear layer (stratum lucidum), granular layer (stratum granulosum), prickle-cell layer (stratum spinosum), and basal layer (stratum basale). The two deepest layers are sometimes grouped together as the stratum germinativum since these cells are responsible for the normal physiological regeneration of the more superficial cells.[2]

The dermis is subdivided into two layers: the papillary dermis and the reticular dermis. The dermal papillae and epidermal rete pegs provide a close, undulating layer juxtaposition between epidermis and dermis. The more superficial papillary dermis contains a rich supply of blood vessels that penetrate from the deeper layers. Also contained within this layer are numerous nerve endings, thermoreceptors, and

344

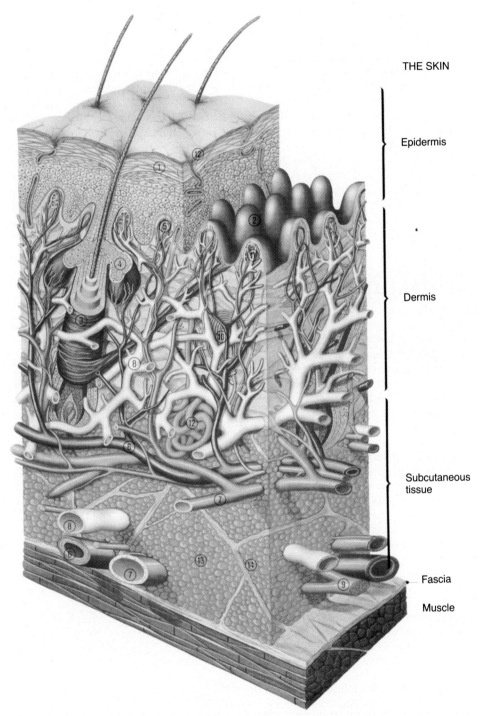

THE SKIN

Epidermis

Dermis

Subcutaneous
tissue

Fascia

Muscle

Figure 22–1. Anatomical features of the skin. (1) Horny layer (stratum corneum); (2) papillae of the dermis; (3) hair follicle; (4) sebaceous gland; (5) capillary loop with initial lymphatic vessel; (6) artery or arteriole respectively; (7) vein or venule respectively; (8) lymphatic vessel; (9) nerve; (10) Pacini's corpuscles; (11) Meissner's corpuscles; (12) sweat gland with excretory duct; (13) subcutaneous fatty tissue pads accumulated between the fibrous bands; (14) fibrous bands (retinacula cutis). (From Asmussen PD: Compendium Medical. Vol. 1, Einführung und Grundlagen: Rohstoffe, die Haut, Klebetechnologie. Hamburg, Beiersdorf AG, 1986, p. 43.)

cryoreceptors. The deeper, reticular dermis is mainly a layer of connective tissue in which fibroblasts are surrounded by a matrix of collagen, elastin, and proteoglycans that provide the structural support for the skin.[2] The reticular dermis also contains the dermal appendages: hair follicles and sweat glands. The hair and sweat ducts extend upward through the epidermis. The crypts of the hair follicles are important in that they are in continuity with the epidermis and therefore can be a source of epidermal regeneration.

The subcutaneous tissue is deep to the dermis and contains a variety of cells: adipocytes, fibroblasts, histiocytes, plasma cells, lymphocytes, and mast cells.[2] Many of these cells are involved in the processing of foreign antigens that may be traumatically introduced into skin. Dendritic cells of the dermis have a similar function.

THE NORMAL HEALING RESPONSE

The overall healing response can be classified into several different types in which there are differing contributions of connective tissue deposition, epithelialization, and contraction. The actual contribution of each of these processes varies depending on the type of wound or the corresponding tissue defect that is to be repaired. Furthermore, the type of therapeutic intervention can affect the type of healing that occurs. Wounds that have been closed shortly after injury by apposition of the cut edges as a result of suturing or stapling heal by *primary intention*. Connective tissue deposition is the primary means by which these wounds heal. Wounds whose edges remain open heal by *secondary intention*; the main mechanism of healing is contraction, with additional contributions made by epithelialization and connective tissue deposition. Wounds that are left open for 1 to 2 days and then surgically closed heal by *delayed primary intention*. Bacterially contaminated wounds are often treated this way to permit early wound care for the prevention

of infection. These wounds heal by a combination of all three processes, although collagen deposition is the principal process. Partial thickness wounds such as abrasions or superficial burns do not penetrate the dermis and therefore, connective tissue deposition does not play a role in healing. These wounds heal mainly as a result of epithelialization (see Table 22–1).

The actual biology of wound healing has been studied extensively. The process of healing is an intricate, organized response to tissue injury that involves cellular and extracellular matrix components (Fig. 22–2). The complexity of this process has been simplified for descriptive purposes by Schilling, who divided the healing response into four broad categories that approximately coincide with the temporal sequence of normal healing: hemostasis, inflammation, proliferation, and remodeling.[3]

Hemostasis

The events responsible for normal wound healing are initiated at the precise moment tissue trauma occurs. Upon injury, the epidermal and dermal elements are disrupted and the cutaneous vasculature is severed, causing peripheral blood cells to spill into the wound site. As the platelets come into contact with damaged collagen and other tissue debris, they aggregate and degranulate. The released alpha granules contain factors that affect clotting as well as potent polypeptide growth factors.[4] The deposition and polymerization of fibrin occurs, as well as continued aggregation of platelets, thus forming a thrombus. The formation of a thrombus within the wound in conjunction with reactive vasoconstriction of the traumatized vessels leads to hemostasis. This thrombus is thought to act as a scaffold, providing a substrate to which inflammatory cells attach and migrate into the wound site.[3, 5]

Platelets are the first cellular elements to enter the wound site. In addition to their hemostatic role, they influence the subsequent cellular response within the wound. Platelets

Table 22–1. RELATIVE CONTRIBUTION OF THE THREE PRINCIPAL MECHANISMS OF WOUND HEALING IN DIFFERENT TYPES OF WOUNDS

Healing Mechanism	Type of Wound		
	Sutured (Primary Intention)	Open (Secondary Intention)	Partial-Thickness
Contraction	0	+ + +	0
Epithelialization	+	+	+ + +
Connective tissue deposition	+ + +	+ +	0

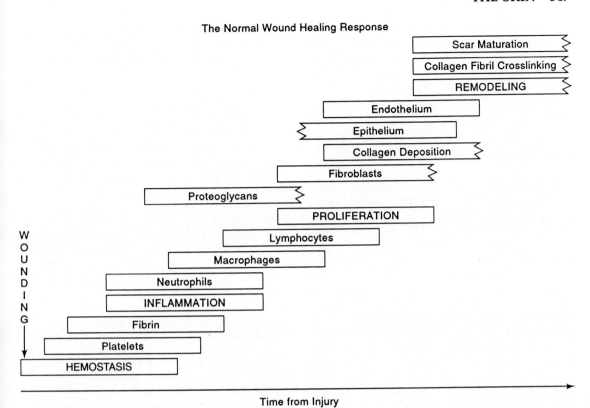

Figure 22–2. Temporal relationship between the multiple processes occurring in dermal wound healing.

release platelet-derived growth factor (PDGF), which is a chemoattractant for smooth muscle cells[6] and fibroblasts.[7] Transforming growth factor-β (TGF-β) is also released by platelets[8] and has a similar chemoattractive effect for inflammatory cells and fibroblasts.

Inflammation

Following thrombus formation, secondary vasodilatation and increased capillary permeability ensue, resulting in the initiation of acute inflammation as neutrophils enter the wound site. The neutrophils primarily have an immunological function, controlling local bacterial contamination and aiding in the debridement of devitalized tissue.[3] Neutrophil infiltration peaks at about 24 hours postwounding, and slowly recedes as monocytes enter the wound. These circulating monocytes are converted into macrophages as they continue to destroy bacteria and debride the wound. Similar to platelets, macrophages also have an integral function related to subsequent healing events.[9] For instance, when guinea pigs were made monocytopenic with hydrocortisone and antimonocyte serum, fibroblast recruitment and collagen deposition were significantly delayed at wound

sites.[10] The importance of macrophages lies in their secretion of growth factors, such as TGF-β, which stimulate the proliferation of fibroblasts as well as positively affecting collagen synthesis.[8] Additionally, other cytokines, such as interleukin-1 (IL-1) and tumor necrosis factor (TNF) are released from macrophages. (The role of growth hormones in the healing response is discussed in detail in Chapter 14.)

Other inflammatory cells implicated in normal wound healing are lymphocytes, plasma cells, and mast cells. The role of lymphocytes is not fully understood. Barbul and associates[11] found that wounds of adult rats thymectomized at 4 to 8 weeks of age had increased breaking strength. Suppressor T lymphocytes were postulated as being negative regulators in healing. However, the observation that treatment of rats with cyclosporine A, which suppresses T-cell–dependent immunity, results in decreased wound strength suggests that lymphocytes may have a positive role in the completion of normal healing.[4] (The relationship of lymphocytes and the healing response is reviewed in greater detail in Chapter 17.)

The composition of the wound matrix changes during the inflammatory phase. Fibrin is the initial component of the matrix, largely as a result of hemostasis. As vascular permeability increases during the onset of acute inflammation, transudation of plasma components ensues, resulting in the entry of complement, antibodies, and other plasma components into the wound. During this transudation, fibrin is replaced by glycosaminoglycans and proteoglycan.[3, 5]

Proliferative Phase

In full-thickness wounds, connective tissue deposition, especially collagen crosslinking, is the major process responsible for the repair of the violated dermis, and the key cell is the fibroblast. Beginning approximately 3 to 4 days postwounding, fibroblast infiltration and proliferation are prominent. This is largely in response to the previous events in the wound that have resulted in the secretion of growth factors that affect the migration and activity of these cells. Proliferation of endothelial cells also occurs as neovascularization proceeds. Epithelialization is prominent at this time, especially in partial-thickness wounds or wounds healing by secondary intention. The cellular migration that occurs is guided by the provisional matrix that exists within the wound, anatomical tissue planes, and planes aligned according to the tension across the wound.[3]

The entry of fibroblasts into the wound is crucial to the healing process since these cells synthesize collagen, the primary structural component of the repaired tissue. The production of collagen is an elaborate process involving several intracellular and extracellular events.[12] (Phillips and Wenstrup present an in-depth discussion of the biosynthesis of this highly conserved protein in Chapter 9.)

The deposition of collagen into the wound is coincident with the degradation of proteoglycans. Collagen is the final and permanent component of the wound matrix. The rate of collagen deposition in rat wounds, as indicated by total hydroxyproline content, was measured by Madden and Peacock.[13] A rapid and linear accumulation of radiolabeled hydroxyproline was observed in these wounds starting at 2 days and peaking at 14 days after wounding, the time period corresponding with the influx of fibroblasts. The deposition of radiolabeled collagen within the wounds was always significantly greater than in uninjured skin. During the following 10 weeks, a gradual reduction in the hydroxyproline content of the wounds occurred, although it continuously remained greater than the content within normal skin. The progressive deposition of collagen in the early healing period was later corroborated by the measurement of collagenase digestible radiolabeled protein, which is a specific determinant of collagen synthesis.[14]

In addition to fibroblasts, collagen is produced by smooth muscle cells, epithelial cells, and endothelial cells.[15] There are numerous collagen types that differ by their component chains. Type III collagen is synthesized and deposited as the initial form of collagen in healing wounds, but it is quickly replaced by type I, the predominant collagen of skin.[12] Since collagen is the main structural protein of connective tissue it provides the tensile strength for organs such as skin and bone and likewise, for healed wounds. Indeed, an increase in tensile strength has been correlated with an increase in the hydroxyproline content of rat and rabbit wounds.[16]

Remodeling

Remodeling is the last and longest phase of healing. During this period the exuberant neovascularization of early granulation tissue recedes as repair continues.[3] The principal processes occurring during this phase are the dynamic remodeling of collagen and the formation of the mature scar. The net deposition of collagen in virtually all tissues, including wounds, is a balance between collagenolytic activity and collagen synthesis,[17] such that production and degradation are ongoing, opposing processes. Elevated collagenolytic activity has been detected in wounds as long as 20 years after wounding.[17]

During remodeling, the tensile strength of the wound continues to increase despite a reduction in the rate of collagen synthesis.[13] This gain in strength is a result of structural modification of the newly deposited collagen. Levenson and co-workers observed marked changes in the histological appearance of the collagen deposited within rat wounds.[18] The collagen present in wounds after 5 days of healing consisted of fine, unorganized fibrils. Over the ensuing weeks and months, fibril diameter increased, fascicles formed, and the fibers became more compact. However, the wound collagen never achieved the bundled, organized pattern of normal dermal collagen (Fig. 22–3). Doillon and associates studied the structure of wound collagen in greater detail by means of scanning electron microscopy.[19] They found that there was a progressive increase in the diameter of collagen fibers, as well as a positive correlation between wound tensile strength and fiber di-

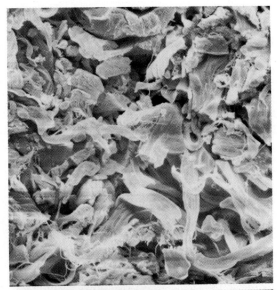

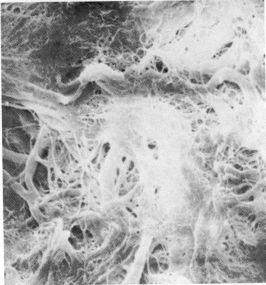

Figure 22–3. Scanning electron micrograph of normal dermis *(top panel)* and normal scar *(lower panel).* ×17,000. (Reprinted with permission from Diegelmann RF, et al: Fibrogenic processes during tissue repair. In Nimni ME (ed): Collagen: Biochemistry and Biomechanics, vol 2. Boca Raton, FL, CRC Press, 1988, p 122. Copyright CRC Press, Boca Raton, FL.)

ameter. Therefore, it appears that much of the gain in strength in repaired tissue is a result of structural modification of collagen, rather than continued deposition. Crosslinking of collagen fibrils is largely responsible for these modifications. The formation of these covalent bonds between collagen molecules is mediated by the enzyme lysyl oxidase[12, 15] and provides increasing strength to the wound.

Remodeling is a dynamic process in which scar maturation occurs for months to years after the initial synthesis of collagen by fibroblasts. However, this is an imperfect process since the wound collagen never achieves the normal structure of dermal collagen. This is reflected in the fact that the strength of healed tissue never equals that of uninjured skin. The increase in tensile strength of rat wounds plateaus approximately 3 months following injury, reaching an apparent maximum strength measured at 1 year postwounding that is only 80 percent of the tensile strength of normal skin.[18] The ongoing process of remodeling can be observed clinically. Oftentimes scars are erythematous and raised soon after healing, but with time the redness and prominence diminish.

Open Wound Contraction

Contraction is the process by which the area of tissue loss in an open wound decreases by a concentric reduction in the size of the wound. This process should not be confused with contracture, which is excessive scar formation across joints or opposing areas of skin resulting in a cosmetic and/or functional deficit and which is the consequence of contraction.

As the term "contraction" denotes, this process is thought to be secondary to actual movement of the wound edges. Myofibroblasts are the cells thought to be responsible for this phenomenon. These specialized fibroblasts contain the contractile protein actin[20] and other specialized features that may indicate that these cells participate in unified movement.[21] An alternative theory suggests a dynamic interaction between individual fibroblasts and the collagenous matrix of the injured tissue. This hypothesis suggests that myofibroblasts are merely quiescent fibroblasts rather than contractile cells.[22]

Contraction is a vital aspect of open wound healing. The size of the tissue defect is reduced so that a lesser degree of connective tissue deposition and epithelialization is required. Contraction predominates in traumatic open wounds as well as contaminated surgical wounds that are packed open and then subjected to dressing changes. In either case, the contribution of contraction to the healing of these wounds is great.

FACTORS THAT AFFECT HEALING

A consequence of the complexity of wound healing as a multiple integrated process is the variety of conditions that can impair it. This section first reviews several systemic conditions and therapeutic interventions that adversely affect the healing response and then considers ways in which tissue repair might be improved.

Bacterial Infection

Gross bacterial infection of a wound certainly delays or even reverses the healing response. Local destruction of tissue by bacterial growth and enzymatic action as well as prolongation of the inflammatory phase of healing are responsible. However, the abundance of normal bacterial flora of the skin suggests that virtually all wounds are contaminated to some degree. Yet contamination does not always lead to infection or deficient healing. Perhaps this is best exemplified by burn wounds, in which a bacterial count of as much as 100,000 is acceptable prior to skin grafting. Furthermore, it is interesting to note that controlled bacterial infection may actually accelerate healing. Tenorio and coworkers found that rat wounds experimentally infected with gram-negative bacteria demonstrated a more vigorous inflammatory response and greater tensile strength over that of controls.[23] However, there is a fine line between eliciting a more favorable inflammatory response and overwhelming it, with resultant gross infection and impaired healing.

Malnutrition

Patients with malnutrition have long been observed to have wound healing problems. Animal studies have confirmed a healing impairment following massive loss of body weight. Irvin found that the strength of skin and abdominal wounds, as well as colonic anastomoses, was significantly less in rats that were protein starved for 8 weeks.[24] Similarly, Daly and coworkers found that the bursting strength of colonic anastomoses was positively correlated with the serum albumin level of the rats; i.e., the higher the albumin level or less severe the protein malnutrition, the higher the bursting strength.[25] Severe protein malnutrition affects body protein metabolism and thus may exert effects on collagen synthesis and connective tissue deposition. Moreover, the severely malnourished patient is immunosuppressed, thus affecting the inflammatory phase of healing. Local control of bacterial contamination may not be as efficient, leading to an increased likelihood of wound infection. This suppression

can also blunt the proliferative phase of healing as macrophage infiltration and the cytokines they elicit are reduced.

The malnourished patient may also have deficiencies in vitamins and trace elements. Depletion of vitamin C, or ascorbic acid, causes an altered healing response that manifests as the disease scurvy. The absence of this cofactor needed for proline and lysine hydroxylation results in an abnormal amino acid sequence in procollagen such that the molecules are rapidly degraded within the cell. Abnormal collagen synthesis in this condition results in impaired wound healing and the disruption of old wounds as collagenolytic activity continues unabated despite improper collagen synthesis.[26] Several other vitamins, including riboflavin, pyridoxine, and thiamine, are involved in healing, probably as cofactors in crosslinking of collagen.[26] Zinc is required for the activities of RNA and DNA polymerases, and a deficiency of this element may retard epithelialization and fibroblast proliferation. Ferrous iron is a cofactor in the hydroxylation step of collagen synthesis, and copper is needed for the oxidative deamination of lysine, which is requisite to crosslinking.[12] Deficiencies of these substances may affect matrix synthesis. (A complete discussion of the effects of malnourishment on wound healing is presented in Chapter 15.)

Tissue Oxygenation

The healing response is a metabolically active process. Oxygen is required for the efficient supply of energy necessary for the various steps of healing. Furthermore, oxygen is directly involved as a substrate in oxidative destruction of bacteria by neutrophils and macrophages and in the hydroxylation of proline and lysine. Therefore, conditions that result in reduced tissue oxygenation may impair healing. In this way, hypovolemia resulting in reflex vasoconstriction and the shunting of blood away from skin,[27, 28] uncorrected anemia,[29] hypoxemia,[30] and poor extremity perfusion secondary to peripheral vascular disease[31] may cause impaired healing.

Medication: Corticosteroids, Cytotoxic Agents, and Immunosuppressives

Systemic corticosteroid therapy has multiple effects on wound healing. The inflammatory response necessary for healing may be blunted. This anti-inflammatory effect is thought to be mediated via stabilization of lysosomal enzymes, thereby preventing the secretion of acid hydrolases.[32] The blunted inflammatory response may, in turn, result in the observed impairment in capillary budding, inhibition of fibroblast proliferation, decreased protein synthesis, and diminished epithelialization.[15] Systemic therapy with vitamin A has been shown to reverse steroid-induced healing deficiencies in linear and open wounds.[32, 33] Vitamin A is thought to counteract the effect of steroids by labilization of lysosomes within inflammatory cells, thus restoring the efficiency of the early healing response.[32] Therefore, the administration of steroids following the manifestation of inflammation should have a minimal effect on healing and indeed, this has been demonstrated in rats by Sandberg.[34] Cortisone therapy instituted 2 or more days following wounding had no significant effect on tensile strength or hydroxyproline content of wounds, whereas these healing parameters were significantly reduced when therapy was begun prior to that time.

The effect of anticancer drugs on healing is of particular interest to clinicians since effective cancer therapy often involves a combination of surgery and chemotherapy. A variety of antineoplastic drugs have been shown to reduce the breaking strength of cutaneous wounds in experimental animals when administered at therapeutic levels.[35] These cytotoxic agents render their therapeutic effect by interfering with DNA or RNA synthesis, cell division, or protein synthesis.[27] Consequently, their effect on healing occurs primarily during the proliferative phase.[15] Additionally, many patients receiving chemotherapy are systemically neutropenic and more prone to wound infection, which further impairs healing.[27]

Immunosuppressives such as steroids, azathioprine, and cyclosporine A are used in the treatment of a variety of conditions, most often for the prevention of rejection following organ transplantation. The therapeutic effect of these drugs is due to a blunting of the normal immune response, and cells involved in the inflammatory response of healing are likewise affected, causing a potential deficiency in tissue repair.

Surgery is often undertaken in patients receiving one or more of these medications. It is vital to be cognizant of the potential adverse impact upon healing of these agents, so that patient care can be modified appropriately. Thus, administration of these drugs may be delayed immediately following surgery if possible, or skin sutures or staples should remain in place for a longer period. If such safeguards are taken, clinically significant healing problems should be kept to a minimum.

Diabetes

Diabetes is a systemic disease that results from an insufficient level of insulin or a relative insensitivity to this hormone's actions, such that serum glucose levels are elevated. The effects of diabetes on the body are multiple, as are the effects on healing.[36]

Animal experiments on diabetic rats have demonstrated diminished wound strength correlated with a deficient production of connective tissue. Goodson and Hunt[37] demonstrated that wounds of diabetic rats had significantly reduced tensile strength and hydroxyproline content compared to those of controls. Insulin treatment for the first 11 days following wounding resulted in wound hydroxyproline content similar to that in nondiabetic rats.

Diabetes is also known to alter the function of leukocytes in such a way that chemotaxis, phagocytosis, and intracellular bacterial killing are all diminished.[27] These effects would be expected to lead to impaired healing due to a less efficient inflammatory response, and the altered functions of neutrophils, macrophages, and lymphocytes can cause diminished fibroblast proliferation and collagen deposition. Moreover, altered leukocyte function is implicated in the prospective observation that the incidence of surgical wound infections is five times higher in diabetics.[38] These findings suggest that diminished collagen synthesis in diabetic animals is probably secondary to an impaired inflammatory response leading to an attenuated proliferative phase rather than due to direct interference with collagen synthesis.[27]

Occlusive peripheral vascular and microvascular disease are more common in diabetics. These conditions result in reduced cutaneous blood flow and can potentially impair healing. Clinically relevant poor perfusion was demonstrated by Barnes and colleagues[31] who evaluated peripheral vasculature using digital photoplethysmography. Diabetics required a higher distal perfusion pressure compared to nondiabetics to heal lower extremity amputation sites. Diabetes also causes peripheral neuropathy, and the resultant impaired sensation leading to repeated trauma to tissue and wounds combined with poor perfusion may cause a further delay in healing.

Improvement of Healing

Attempts to improve the healing process center on systemic treatment of the patient or manipulation of the local wound environment to make conditions more favorable for normal healing. The most obvious systemic treatment is the correction of an identified deficiency that causes impaired healing. Examples are vitamin C administration for scurvy and correction of malnutrition with hyperalimentation. Insulin therapy and/or careful serum glucose control in diabetics can ameliorate several healing defects including altered leukocyte function, fibroblast proliferation, and collagen synthesis.[36] In addition to these obvious deficiencies, nutritional substances have been identified that may positively affect wound healing, yet they may not be suspected of being deficient in patients. Barbul and associates[39, 40] have demonstrated a positive healing effect of arginine that may be mediated through lymphocyte stimulation. They postulate that arginine may be an "essential" amino acid in traumatized animals.

Growth factors are integral components in the regulation of the healing response. Since their discovery, their potential for augmentation of the repair process has stirred much interest. Grotendorst and co-workers studied the effect of PDGF administration on healing in rats using Hunt-Schilling wound chambers. Compared to normals, the treated rats demonstrated an apparent improvement in the early repair response as indicated by an earlier infiltration of fibroblasts, elevated DNA synthesis, and greater hydroxyproline content during the first 2 weeks. Moreover, treatment with PDGF restored a normal healing response in diabetic animals with a healing impairment.[41] In corroboration of these findings, Pierce and others showed that incisional rat wounds treated with PDGF had a significantly greater breaking strength than normals.[61] Similar findings have resulted from animal studies in which wounds were treated with TGF-β.[8, 42, 43] Human studies with various growth factors are currently underway.

THE EFFECT OF AGING

It is well known to even a casual observer that the repair of injured tissue is altered as aging occurs. Adults who have sustained a laceration or sprained an ankle realize that such injuries healed more rapidly when they were children. A multitude of studies reveals that aging affects almost all aspects of the healing response.[44]

Open Wounds

One of the earliest attempts to scientifically delineate the effect of aging on wound healing was the work of Carrell and DuNouy during World War I.[45] These investigators found that increasing age was correlated with a slower rate of contraction and closure of open traumatic wounds: 20 year old patients closed their wounds in 40 days, compared to 56 days for 30 year olds and 76 days for 40 year olds. These observations were corroborated by laboratory experiments in which uniform open wounds were created on the backs of young and old rats.[44]

Closed Wounds

The effect of aging on closed, linear wounds was first studied by Howes and Harvey, who evaluated the healing of incisions in the stomachs of young and old rats.[46] Every 2 days following wounding the bursting strength of the wounds were measured. Compared to the young rats, older animals showed a delayed increase in breaking strength and an earlier plateau in strength gain. Furthermore, the final bursting strength of the younger wounds was greater than that of the older wounds. A more recent study by Gottrup found that there was no significant difference in the breaking strength or breaking energy of stomach or duodenal wounds in young and old rats.[47] Perhaps this discrepancy can be explained by the fact that measurements in the more recent study were performed only at postwounding days 7 and 20, times that are later than the reported healing delay from the earlier study.

Sussman evaluated cutaneous, linear wounds and observed that younger rats had wounds that were thicker and had a greater breaking strength.[48] These findings suggest that connective tissue deposition was diminished in the wounds of older animals. In agreement with this conclusion is Vilijanto's observation that the amount of hydroxyproline incorporated into cellulose sponges within human wound sites had a negative correlation with increasing age.[49]

The cellularity of wounds as related to age has also been studied. The DNA and RNA ribose content of young rat wounds was higher than in older wounds.[50] Additionally, monocyte and macrophage infiltration occurred earlier in the wounds of younger versus older children,[51] and significantly more fibroblasts were observed in wounds of young mice and rats compared to old animals 3 days after wounding.[44] Fibroblast activity has also been observed to be diminished in older patients. Fibroblasts from punch biopsies of older people had a reduced outgrowth rate in culture.[52] It has also been observed that collagen production from human skin biopsies decreases with increasing age.[53] Therefore, it appears that older animals have delayed proliferation or recruitment of cells in response to tissue injury and that collagen production may be reduced.

The dynamics of collagen deposition have been studied using experimentally induced granuloma wounds.[54–56] While young rat wounds contained less connective tissue 7 days after injury, at 14 days the older animals had less. Additionally, at all times, the breaking strength of wounds of younger animals was greater.[55] In another experiment, the total hydroxyproline content of wounds of young and old rats was essentially the same, but the young animals exhibited a greater rate of collagen synthesis as indicated by proline hydroxylation.[50] It appears, therefore, that while no clear-cut quantitative difference in connective tissue formation in wounds of young and old animals has been demonstrated, qualitative differences exist in that collagen formation is more rapid and efficient in young animals.

Epithelialization

The above studies indicate that wound contraction and connective tissue deposition are delayed as aging proceeds, and evidence exists that the same is true of epithelialization. Epidermal blisters created with ammonium hydroxide on the arms of human volunteers had a significantly shorter healing time in subjects under 35 years of age compared to those older than 65 years.[52] Another wound that heals mostly by epithelialization is the donor site of split-thickness skin grafts. Fatah and Ward found that 95 percent of these injuries were healed by 21 days in patients less than 60 years old, whereas only 80 percent of the donor sites were healed by 20 days postwounding in older patients.[57]

Clinical Relevance

It is obvious that aging has an adverse effect on wound healing. The defects appear to be related to cellular proliferation and/or recruitment, altered collagen deposition and remodeling, diminished contraction of open wounds, and delayed epithelialization. The clinical relevance of these deficits is exemplified by the fact that the incidence of dehiscence of surgical abdominal incisions increases linearly with increasing age.[58] However, major surgical procedures are being performed upon an increasingly elderly population and most of these patients do not experience problems in wound healing. For instance, no significant increase in the wound complication rate following major head and neck surgery was observed in elderly patients.[59] Although the healing response is "deficient" in older patients, it is clinically adequate in most cases. The elderly have a greater incidence of systemic medical conditions[59] that adversely effect healing, and it is the combination of the effects of these conditions and the effects of aging that sets the stage for inadequate healing.

ANIMAL MODELS FOR WOUND HEALING RESEARCH

The investigation of the biology of wound healing has long depended on the use of various models.[60] Many in vitro techniques are available, but their limitations are obvious. It is for these reasons that animal models are crucial in wound healing research.

Rodents, especially rats, are used most often in healing studies. The rodent healing response is similar to that in humans, with excessive collagen deposition leading to scar formation. However, the fact that keloids, hypertrophic scars, and intra-abdominal adhesions do not occur and that there is no requirement for dietary ascorbic acid indicates that healing in this animal is not identical to human wound healing. Some investigators think the guinea pig is a better model of human healing because ascorbic acid is not synthesized by the animal but must be supplied in the diet. Still, other studies have used rabbits because of their larger size. Although primates are phylogenetically closest to humans, they are not good models since exuberant scar formation is not characteristic of their healing response.

As long as the selected animal used in studies heals by scarring, the particular mammalian species used will probably not affect the results. Rats will most likely continue to be the most often used model because of their low cost, relative ease of handling, and nondemanding care.

CONCLUSION

Wound healing is a complex process in which a variety of cellular and matrix components act in concert to establish the integrity of injured tissue. The response can be broadly divided into four phases in which specific processes occur. Many medical conditions or treatments exist that impair or improve the processes occurring during these phases. Anything that affects these individual processes has the potential to affect the successful completion of healing, thus illustrating the interdependency of the individual components of the repair response.

References

1. Reed BR, Clark RAF: Cutaneous tissue repair: Practical implications of current knowledge. II. J Am Acad Dermatol 13:919–941, 1985.
2. Asmussen PD: The Skin. In Compendium Medical, vol 1, Einfürung und Grundlagen: Rohstoffe, die Haut, Klebetechnologie. Hamburg, AG Biersdorf, 1986, p 6.
3. Schilling JA: Wound healing. Surg Clin North Am 56:859–874, 1976.
4. Pessa ME, Kirby KI, Copeland EM: Growth factors and determinants of wound repair. J Surg Res 42:207–217, 1987.
5. Weigel PH, Fuller GM, LeBoeuf RD: A model for the role of hyaluronic acid and fibrin in the early events during the inflammatory response and wound healing. J Theor Biol 119:219–234, 1986.
6. Grotendorst GR, Chang T, Seppa HEJ, et al: Platelet-derived growth factor is a chemoattractant for vascular smooth muscle cells. J Cell Physiol 113:261–266, 1983.
7. Seppa HEJ, Grotendorst GR, Seppa SI, et al: The platelet-derived growth factor is a chemoattractant for fibroblasts. J Cell Biol 92:584–588, 1982.
8. Roberts AB, Sporn MR, Assoian RK, et al: Transforming growth factor type β: Rapid induction of fibrosis and angiogenesis in vivo and stimulation of collagen formation in vitro. Proc Natl Acad Sci USA 83:4167–4171, 1986.
9. Diegelmann RF, Cohen IK, Kaplan AM: The role of macrophages in wound repair: A review. Plast Reconstr Surg 68:107–113, 1981.
10. Leibovich SJ, Ross R: The role of the macrophage in wound repair. A study with hydrocortisone and anti-macrophage serum. Am J Pathol 78:71–100, 1975.
11. Barbul A, Sisto D, Rettura G, et al: Thymic inhibition of wound healing: Abrogation by adult thymectomy. J Surg Res 32:338–342, 1982.
12. Jackson DS: Development of fibrosis. Cell proliferation and collagen biosynthesis. Ann Rheum Dis (Suppl) 36:2–4, 1977.
13. Madden JW, Peacock EE: Studies on the biology of collagen during wound healing. I. Rate of collagen synthesis and deposition in cutaneous wounds of the rat. Surgery 64:288–294, 1968.
14. Diegelmann RF, Rothkopf LC, Cohen IK: Measurement of collagen biosynthesis during wound healing. J Surg Res 19:239–243, 1975.
15. Stevenson TR, Mathes SJ: Wound healing. In Miller TA, Rowlands BJ, (eds): Physiologic Basis of Modern Surgical Care. St. Louis, CV Mosby, 1988, pp 1010–1013.
16. Sandberg N, Zederfeldt B: The tensile strength of healing wounds and collagen formation in rats and rabbits. Acta Chir Scand 126:187–196, 1963.
17. Peacock EE Jr: Collagenolysis: The other side of the equation. World J Surg 4:297–302, 1980.
18. Levenson SM, Geever EF, Crowley LV, et al: The healing of rat skin wounds. Ann Surg 161:293–308, 1965.
19. Doillon CJ, Dunn MG, Bender E, et al: Collagen fiber formation in repair tissue: Development of strength and toughness. Coll Rel Res 5:481–492, 1985.
20. Gabbiani G, Hirschel BJ, Ryan B, et al: Granulation tissue as a contractile organ. J Exp Med 135:719–734, 1972.
21. Gabbiani G, Runngger-Brandle E: The fibroblast. In Glynn LE (ed): Tissue Repair and Regeneration. Amsterdam, Elsevier/North-Holland, 1981, pp 22–29.
22. Ehrlich HP: Wound closure: Evidence of cooperation between fibroblasts and collagen matrix. Eye 2:149–157, 1988.
23. Tenorio A, Jindrak K, Weiner M, et al: Accelerated healing in infected wounds. Surg Gynecol Obstet 142:537–543, 1976.
24. Irvin TT: Effects of malnutrition and hyperalimentation on wound healing. Surg Gynecol Obstet 146:33–37, 1978.
25. Daly JM, Vars HM, Dudrick SJ: Effects of protein depletion of colonic anastomoses. Surg Gynecol Obstet 134:15–21, 1972.
26. Ruberg RL: Role of nutrition in wound healing. Surg Clin North Am 64:705–714, 1984.
27. Carrico TJ, Mehrhof AI, Cohen IK: Biology of wound healing. Surg Clin North Am 64:721–733, 1984.
28. Sandberg N, Zederfelt B: Influence of acute hemorrhage on wound healing in the rabbit. Acta Chir Scand 118:367–371, 1959/1960.
29. Sandblom P: The tensile strength of healing wounds. Systemic factors, anemia and dehydration. Acta Chir Scand (Suppl)89, 1944.
30. Uitto J, Prockop DJ: Synthesis and secretion of under-hydroxylated procollagen at various temperatures by cells subject to temporary anoxia. Biochem Biophys Res Commun 60:414–423, 1974.
31. Barnes RW, Thornhill B, Nix L, et al: Prediction of amputation wound healing: Roles of Doppler untrasound and digit plethysmography. Arch Surg 116:80–83, 1981.
32. Ehrlich HP, Hunt TK: Effects of cortisone and vitamin A on wound healing. Ann Surg 167:324–328, 1968.
33. Hunt TK, Ehrlich HP, Garcia JA, et al: Effects of vitamin A on reversing the inhibitory effect of cortisone on healing of open wounds in animals and man. Ann Surg 170:633–641, 1969.
34. Sandberg N: Time relationship between administration of cortisone and wound healing in rats. Acta Chir Scand 127:446–455, 1964.
35. Cohen SC, Gabelnick HL, Johnson RK, et al: Effects of antineoplastic agents on wound healing in mice. Surgery 78:238–244, 1975.
36. McMurry JF: Wound healing with diabetes mellitus. Better glucose control for better wound healing in diabetics. Surg Clin North Am 64:769–778, 1984.
37. Goodson WH, Hunt TK: Studies of wound healing in experimental diabetes mellitus. J Surg Res 22:221–227, 1977.

38. Cruse PJE, Foord R: A prospective study of 23,649 surgical wounds. Arch Surg 107:206–210, 1973.
39. Barbul A, Wasserdrug BA, Seifter E, et al: Immunostimulatory effects of arginine in normal and injured rats. J Surg Res 29:228–235, 1980.
40. Barbul A, Rettura G, Levenson S, et al: Wound healing and thymotropic effects of arginine: A pituitary mechanism of action. Am J Clin Nutr 37:786–794, 1983.
41. Grotendorst GR, Martin GR, Pencev D, et al: Stimulation of granulation tissue formation by platelet-derived growth factor in normal and diabetic rats. J Clin Invest 76:2323–2329, 1985.
42. Mustoe TA, Pierce GF, Thomason A, et al: Accelerated healing of incisional wounds in rats induced by transforming growth factor-β. Science 237:1333–1336, 1987.
43. Brown GL, Curtsinger LJ, White M, et al: Acceleration of tensile strength of incisions treated with EGF and TGF-β. Ann Surg 208:788–794, 1988.
44. Goodson WH, Hunt TK: Wound healing and aging. J Invest Dermatol 73:88–91, 1979.
45. Carrell A, DuNouy P: Cicatrization of wounds. J Exp Med 34:339–348, 1921.
46. Howes EL, Harvey SC: The age factor in the velocity of the growth of fibroblasts in the healing wound. J Exp Med 55:577–590, 1932.
47. Gottrup F: Healing of incisional wounds in stomach and duodenum: The influence of aging. Acta Chir Scand 147:363–369, 1981.
48. Sussman MD: Aging of connective tissue: Physical properties of healing wounds in young and old rats. Am J Physiol 224:1167–1171, 1973.
49. Vilijanto JA: A sponge implant method for testing connective tissue regeneration in surgical patients. Acta Chir Scand 135:297–300, 1969.
50. Heikkinen E, Aalto M, Vihersaari T, et al: Age factor in the formation and metabolism of experimental granulation tissue. J Gerontol 26:294–298, 1971.
51. Vilijanto JA, Raekallio J: Wound healing in children as assessed by the CELLSTIC method. J Pediatr Surg 11:43–49, 1976.
52. Kligman AM: Perspectives and problems in cutaneous gerontology. J Invest Dermatol 73:39–46, 1979.
53. Uitto J: A method for studying collagen biosynthesis in human skin biopsies in vitro. Biochim Biophys Acta 201:438–445, 1970.
54. Forscher BK, Cecil HC: Some effects of age on the biochemistry of acute inflammation. Gerontologia 2:174–182, 1958.
55. Holm-Pedersen P, Zederfeldt B: Granulation tissue formation in subcutaneously implanted cellulose sponges in young and old rats. Scand J Plast Reconstr Surg 5:13–16, 1971.
56. Houck JC, Jacob RA: The effect of age on the chemistry of inflammation. J Invest Dermatol 42:377–381, 1964.
57. Fatah MF, Ward CM: The morbidity of spit-skin graft donor sites in the elderly: The case for mesh grafting the donor site. Br J Plast Surg 37:184–190, 1984.
58. Mendoza CB, Postlethwait RW, Johnson WD: Incidence of wound disruption following operation. Arch Surg 101:396–398, 1970.
59. McGuirt WF, Loevy S, McCabe BF, et al: The risks of major head and neck surgery in the aged population. Laryngoscope 87:1378–1382, 1977.
60. Cohen IK, Mast BA: Models of wound healing. J Trauma (Suppl) 30:S149–S155, 1990.
61. Pierce GF, Mustoe TA, Senior RM, et al: In vivo incisional wound healing augmented by platelet-derived growth factor and recombinant c-sis gene homodimeric proteins. J Exp Med 167:974–987, 1988.

23

BONE AND CARTILAGINOUS TISSUE

Isaac L. Wornom, III, M.D., and Steven R. Buchman, M.D.

Fracture repair is a complex and dynamic process that incorporates physical, biochemical, and biomechanical forces into a network of coordinated interactions. These repair processes culminate in a fracture site that when healed may be virtually indistinguishable from the preinjured state. At the moment of fracture, the healing process is initiated by an array of mechanisms triggered by the injury. These are regulated by detailed feedback phenomena influenced by the unique injuries associated with each fracture. Perturbations in the environment of the injured bone may disrupt this delicately balanced regulation and lead to nonunion. Much of the early response to injury in bone parallels those in wound healing in soft tissues but the later aspects of fracture healing are largely a recapitulation of early bone formation, translating into a healthy, functional, and structurally sound bone.

Perhaps one of the most extraordinary properties of bone is the ability to heal with practically no scar. Indeed some authors take issue with the term "bone healing" and claim a more appropriate description would be "bone regeneration."[1] Suffice it to say that bone has the ability to regain normal physical characteristics and structural anatomy in response to injury.

Many texts attempt to explain fracture repair in terms of stages of bone healing.[2, 3] Although this may be an easy way to compartmentalize the healing process, it clouds the underlying tenets of bone repair. Bone healing results from a continuum of interactions and overlapping phases that make up the healing process. Due to the lack of uniform and specific gradations in fracture repair, references to stages or sharp demarcations are avoided and a more descrip-

tive approach is used to explain the macroscopic, histological, cellular, and biochemical processes that lead to healed bone.

MACROSCOPIC ASPECTS OF FRACTURE REPAIR

When a bone sustains impact, energy is transferred and the resultant force is dissipated through it. The magnitude and direction of force, the rate of loading, and the duration of stress determine whether the affected bone will fail. Fracture happens when the maximum limit of strain or force is surpassed.

Upon breaking a bone, multiple events occur at the fracture site aside from the loss of structural integrity. The soft tissue envelope around the fracture is disrupted, often with associated damage to adjacent muscles, tendons, and ligaments. The marrow is often injured and the blood supply is compromised as blood vessels rupture. Bleeding ensues with resultant hematoma formation at the site of injury (Fig. 23–1).

The clinical signs vary with each fracture and may consist of pain and tenderness, deformity, and decreased range of motion. Occasionally, a functional deficit can be elicited as well as a possible neurovascular injury.

The fracture site just after injury is a milieu of devitalized soft tissues, clot, dead bone, and necrotic marrow. As the healing process commences the nonviable elements are degraded and digested and the hematoma liquefies and resorbs. The region of bone bordering the af-

356

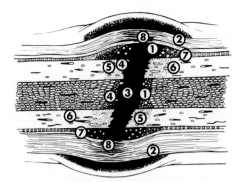

Figure 23–1. Initial injury. 1. The continuity of the periosteum, cortical bone, and medullary trabeculae is broken. 2. Injured muscle and surrounding soft tissue. 3. Hematoma must be infiltrated or eliminated to allow bridging of the gap. 4. Dead osteocytes. 5. Empty haversian canals. *Note:* Osteocytes and osteogenic cells in the vicinity of the fracture die. 6. Undamaged haversian canals from which vascular osteogenesis begins. 7. Cambium layer of periosteum, which forms primary intramembranous bone as well as fibrocartilage callus. 8. Fibrous layer of periosteum seals off callus from external soft tissues. *Note:* This fracture may be treated with or without internal fixation. (From Connolly JF: DePalma's The Management of Fractures and Dislocations. Philadelphia, WB Saunders, 1981, p 14.)

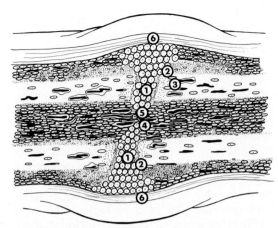

Figure 23–2. Four to six weeks after injury. 1. The fracture gap is still open but has been filled with cartilage. 2. Some bone has been formed on the cortical fragments by oppositional ossification. 3. The haversian canals are slowly being revascularized. 4. Medullary revascularization is occurring rapidly. 5. Bone spicules promote oppositional new bone formation. 6. The fibrous layer of periosteum has sealed off the callus. (From Connolly JF: DePalma's The Management of Fractures and Dislocations. Philadelphia, WB Saunders, 1981, p 15.)

fected area undergoes revascularization, which can be seen grossly as the formation of granulation tissue. This tissue bridges the fracture site and incorporates the interfragmentary gaps. The clinical signs associated with revascularization are inflammation with evidence of swelling and erythema.

After three to four days a collar of soft tissue begins to form around the bone in the region of the fracture, which is referred to as the *soft callus*. The soft callus may take up to a month to form and binds the fracture fragments (Fig. 23–2). It provides an internal splint for the injured bone and helps to achieve fibrocartilaginous union of the fracture site. The callus forms externally along the bone shaft as well as internally along the marrow cavity and works to limit motion at the injured area. This natural form of internal fixation helps to prevent possible reinjury by immobilizing the fracture and protecting against disruption of newly formed blood vessels and granulation tissue. Clinically, the end of pain and inflammation corresponds to the formation of soft callus.

Hard callus is formed by mineralization of the soft callus and conversion to bone. The formation of hard callus may take up to 2 months and upon completion represents bony union (Fig. 23–3). Stability at the fracture site increases with the formation of hard callus since the bone fragments are no longer mobile. The bond is considered substantial enough to allow weightbearing. Once the hard callus is formed and union is achieved the fracture site will appear healed radiographically. However, there is often excess bone, which may be visible externally and may fill the marrow cavity internally.

A process of modeling and remodeling begins to replace the cortical callus with dense compact

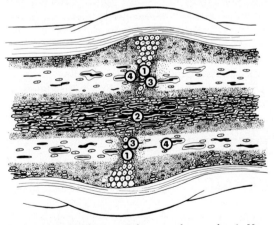

Figure 23–3. Healing at eight to twelve weeks. 1. Vascular bridging of the external cartilage has produced endochondral ossification and an external callus. This callus is oriented perpendicular to the fractured cortices. 2. The longitudinal bridging of the fracture occurs in the medullary canal. 3. Some bridging through the fracture cortices is occurring as a result of haversian remodeling. 4. Remodeling will continue to form longitudinal osteons and increase the bone strength. (From Connolly JF: DePalma's The Management of Fractures and Dislocations. Philadelphia, WB Saunders, 1981, p 15.)

bone. These changes may take years and serve to reshape the bone to more normal contours and restore the integrity of the marrow cavity. Gradually the orientation of the bone begins to reflect the strains and loads of use. Modeling ensures that the forces transmitted through the bone are supported by its architecture. Slowly old bone is resorbed and new bone is deposited to return the fracture site to its original form. In the case of a displaced fracture, these forces work to elicit the best possible conjunction of form and biomechanical function. At the completion of the healing process, some residual thickening may be seen radiographically but fractures often heal so well that the fracture site is indistinguishable from normal bone.

In some instances, bone may undergo *primary healing* after a fracture without a cartilage intermediate. In this case there is minimal evidence of either soft or hard callus formation and bone is formed directly. The new bone bridges the fracture site and modeling and remodeling begin immediately. Lack of motion, close apposition, and compression of bone at the fracture site foster this process. This is the method of bone healing most commonly seen with open reduction and internal fixation with compression plates (Fig. 23–4).

Many different local conditions can influence fracture healing. Severe trauma with associated extensive injury to adjacent soft tissues may retard bone healing, and an inadequate reduction or undue distraction at the fracture site can also compromise fracture repair. Inadequate immobilization or tissue interposition between fractured bones may lead to delayed or even nonunion. Concurrent malignancy or infection or a previous history of irradiation at the fracture site may also impede the healing process. (Delayed union and nonunion are discussed in more detail later in the chapter.)

HISTOLOGICAL ASPECTS OF FRACTURE REPAIR

The disruption of the blood supply to a bone when a fracture takes place leads to ischemia and cell death.[4] The amount of necrotic bone correlates with the number of ischemic areas created by the interruption of the intracortical blood supply and the destruction of the medullary and periosteal capillary systems. Soft tissue and marrow elements are disrupted and the periosteum is split along with fragmentation of bone and shearing of blood vessels. Local

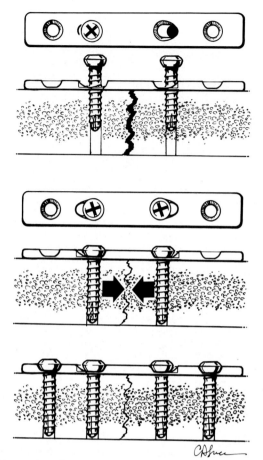

Figure 23–4. Diagram showing the use of a compression plate. A four-hole plate is shown with the inner holes being eccentrically shaped so that as the screws are tightened the heads fall into the wider portion and compress the edges of the fracture. Bone repair after this treatment occurs without a cartilage intermediate. (From Cutting C: Repair and grafting of bone. In McCarthy J (ed): Plastic Surgery, vol 1. Philadelphia, WB Saunders, 1990, p 591.)

osteocyte death leads to release of lysosomal enzymes with subsequent destruction of collagenous and noncollagenous organic matrix. Hematoma floods the wound and the inflammatory response ensues. Local tissue reaction results in widespread vasodilatation and edema (Fig. 23–5).[5]

As in healing in other tissues, many blood-borne elements are contained in the hematoma and provide the first population of cells at the fracture site.[6] As the clot forms, platelet deposition occurs and a fibrin scaffold develops, which allows migration of new cells to the site of injury from the marrow, the endosteum, and the cambium layer of the periosteum.[7] The early inflammatory cells include macrophages, polymorphonuclear leukocytes, and mast cells.[6, 8] In addition, osteoclasts derived from a

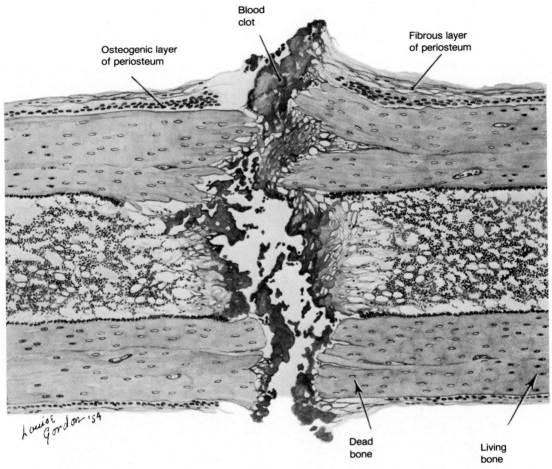

Figure 23–5. Diagrammatic representation of a longitudinal section of a 2-day-old rib fracture (rabbit). (From Ham AW, Harris WR: Repair and transplantation of bone. In Bourne GH (ed): The Biochemistry and Physiology of Bone, vol 3, 2nd ed. New York, Academic Press, 1971, p 338.)

syncytial consolidation of monocytes of osteogenic and hematological origin can be seen early on.[9, 10] Macrophages and giant cells begin to remove necrotic debris and resorb hematoma, as osteoclasts resorb and remove dead bone while digesting and eroding fracture surfaces.[11]

Too few cells are present at the initial time of fracture for successful repair to be achieved during the prolonged healing process. To remedy this, precursor mesenchymal cells and osteoprogenitor cells proliferate and migrate into the wound from adjacent muscle and marrow as well as from local layers of endosteum and the cambium layer of the periosteum.[1, 12] These cells contribute to the earliest formation of bone at the fracture site.[13] The blood supply to the fracture is initially periosteal in origin, with some contribution from the endosteum, but as the clot continues to organize, endothelial cells and smooth muscle cells migrate along the fibrin scaffold with ingrowth of capillary buds and granulation tissue.[14, 15]

The development of a new capillary system provides the pool needed for ongoing replacement of cells during fracture repair. There is an influx of mononuclear cells from the blood and local differentiation of cells of the cambium layer of the periosteum. These local precursor cells differentiate into osteoblasts, fibroblasts, and chondroblasts and produce osteoid, collagen, and cartilage.[16, 17] Initially type I, II, and III collagen is deposited, but as the soft callus matures, type I collagen predominates, forming the framework on which mineralization occurs.[18] With the onset of hard callus formation, there is intensive regeneration of new haversian systems, and as the fracture site remodels, these systems realign to accommodate the stresses placed on the injured bone.

As osteoclastic degradation of devitalized fracture fragments continues there is an increase of cellularity and protein synthesis at the fracture site. The periosteum thickens and a collar of tissue grows around the fragmented bone that consists of inflammatory cells, the differentiating pluripotential cells, and their products. These cells, which differentiate into fibroblasts, chondroblasts, and osteoblasts, soon produce fibrous tissue, cartilage, and immature woven bone, which is called the soft callus. Found at the external portion of the bone and within the medullary cavity, the soft callus binds the fracture site (Fig. 23–6). This cellular and tissue interaction culminates with a state of fibrous union, bridging and stabilizing the broken bone.[11] The larger the diameter of the callus the more mechanical advantage it possesses.[19] The main constituent of the soft callus is unmineralized cartilage, especially at the more peripheral areas. The balance of cartilage, fibrous tissue, and bone in the soft callus is poorly understood but seems to be controlled by differences in local factors such as degree of bone displacement, vascularity, soft tissue injury, and fracture contamination. How these local effects modulate soft callus formation is currently the subject of active research.

The cartilage of the soft callus gradually converts to bone by a process of endochondral ossification. The cartilage intermediate, made up of primarily type II collagen, undergoes degradation, and the cells of the soft callus begin to synthesize and secrete new matrix composed chiefly of type I collagen.[3, 20] Calcium hydroxyapatite is deposited in the matrix, and the resultant calcified collagen structure forms a slender perforated labyrinth of interconnecting spaces that are invaded by developing blood vessels (Fig. 23–7).[1] Osteoprogenitor cells migrate along the new vascular channels and form a layer on the calcified remnants of cartilage matrix. These osteogenic cells differentiate into osteoblasts, which lay down new immature woven bone with random organization of collagen elements.[21] The woven bone forms a network of fine trabeculae in the interstices of the

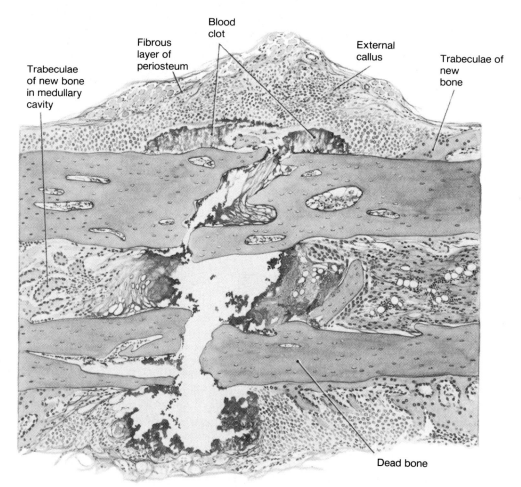

Blood clot

Fibrous layer of periosteum

External callus

Trabeculae of new bone

Trabeculae of new bone in medullary cavity

Dead bone

Figure 23–6. Diagrammatic representation of a longitudinal section of a 1-week-old rib fracture (rabbit). (From Ham AW, Harris WR: Repair and transplantation of bone. In Bourne GH (ed): The Biochemistry and Physiology of Bone, vol 3, 2nd ed. New York, Academic Press, 1971, p 338.)

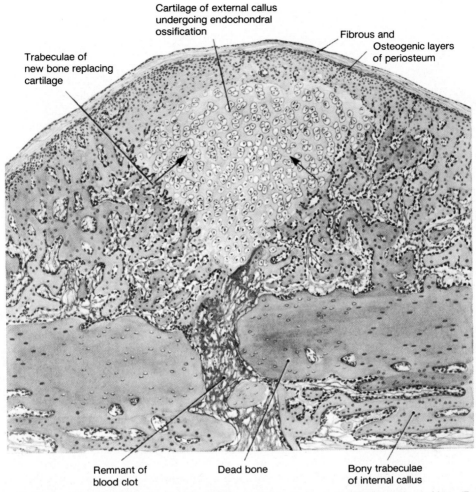

Cartilage of external callus
undergoing endochondral
ossification

Fibrous and
Osteogenic layers
of periosteum

Trabeculae of
new bone replacing
cartilage

Remnant of
blood clot

Dead bone

Bony trabeculae
of internal callus

Figure 23–7. Diagrammatic representation of a longitudinal section of a 2-week-old rib fracture (rabbit). (From Ham AW, Harris WR: Repair and transplantation of bone. In Bourne GH (ed): The Biochemistry and Physiology of Bone, vol 3, 2nd ed. New York, Academic Press, 1971, p 338.)

capillary channels. This immature woven bone results in bony union of the fracture site; weight stress can be placed on the fracture when this stage is complete.

Once bony union is achieved, the fracture site still does not resemble the architecture of the original bone, nor does it have normal strength and stability. To restore the original form and function, the bone undergoes modeling and remodeling. Modeling refers to a group of cellular interactions that result in a normalization of bony macrostructure. Remodeling refers to the cell-mediated breakdown and formation of bone leading to a stable orientation of bony infrastructure in response to applied forces. These processes work concurrently to complete the sequence of events of bone healing.[22] Histologically, the hard callus is made up of woven bone, which haphazardly follows the patterns of capillary ingrowth rather than the lines of force. A highly organized set of succes-

sive layers of mature bone, called lamellar bone, replaces woven bone under the influence of functional stresses (Fig. 23–8).

Cellular modules or units of osteoclasts and osteoblasts are activated in sequences of both bone resorption and formation to convert the bulbous contours of the hard callus to the original bony architecture.[23] First, the osteoclasts resorb the inefficient surplus of irregular woven bone not subjected to strains or loads. Osteoblasts then deposit a new organic matrix of lamellar bone that later mineralizes, resulting in new struts of mature bone laid down along the lines of stress. These sequences repeat themselves, re-establishing the marrow cavity as well as restoring the structure of the normal haversian systems (Fig. 23–8).[22] Once the bone is healed, the processes of modeling and remodeling continue on a smaller scale as a normal homeostatic mechanism to deal with the changing demands on the bony skeleton.

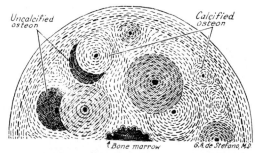

Figure 23–8. Cross section of compact bone as seen by microradiography. Note that the osteons are oriented in the longitudinal axis of the long bone. The dark masses represent recent decalcified osteons, and the light masses represent older calcified osteons. (From Cutting C: Repair and grafting of bone. In McCarthy J (ed): Plastic Surgery, vol. 1. Philadelphia, WB Saunders, 1990, p 584.)

Primary bone healing, referred to previously, represents another form of fracture repair, which histologically does not follow the sequence of events just described. In this case, mechanical factors such as lack of motion and close apposition of the fracture site, as occurs in the proper application of rigid compression plates, allows direct internal remodeling and intracortical healing to take place (Fig. 23–9).

There is no inflammatory phase, cartilaginous intermediate, or callus formation.[24] Existent osteoprogenitor cells differentiate into osteoblasts, and locally derived osteoclasts of osteogenic or hematological origin direct bone healing. Cones of cutting osteoclasts move across the fracture line, resorbing dead bone.

Another cone of osteoblasts trails behind, depositing woven bone parallel to the axis of the long bone.[25] The process is similar to the intramembranous ossification that takes place in the embryological development of flat bones. Primary bone healing incorporates and connects haversian systems, remodeling the bone at the fracture site. New osteons traverse the fragments of the broken bone, culminating in direct osteonal union.

Primary bone healing occurs in fractures treated with open reduction and rigid internal fixation when the fractured bone ends are closely apposed and immobilized. Also of importance in this situation is the stripping of the periosteum, which is done around the fracture site to expose the fracture and apply the rigid fixation. Some authors feel that this can actually delay union.[26]

BIOCHEMICAL ASPECTS OF BONE HEALING

The theory of regional acceleratory phenomenon (RAP) was developed to explain the complex network of regulatory controls initiating and maintaining fracture repair (Fig. 23–10).[27] This theory states that the ultimate healing of a fracture occurs via a series of interrelated cellular events controlled by local and blood-borne proteins. RAP starts with local changes resulting from an injury to bone and relates these changes to perturbations of local cells. Autocrine, para-

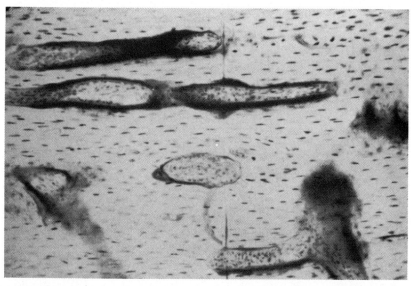

Figure 23–9. Histological characteristics of primary bone healing 12 weeks after internal fixation with a compression plate. There is direct haversian system remodeling and no resorption of the compressed surfaces. (From Hayes WC: Biomechanics of fracture treatment. In Heppenstall RB (ed): Fracture Treatment and Healing. Philadelphia, WB Saunders, 1980, p 140.)

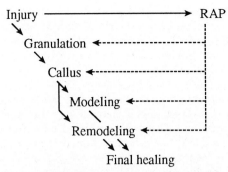

Figure 23–10. Diagrammatic representation of the relationship of the regional acceleratory phenomenon (RAP) with bone healing processes. (From Frost HM: The biology of fracture healing. Clin Orthop Rel Res 248:288, 1989.)

crine, and endocrine factors produced by these cells initiate biochemical changes leading to a well-coordinated cascade of reactions between cells and their products, resulting in fracture repair.

These processes remain unclear. Close examination of the fracture healing process coupled with review of results of extensive research in bone healing provides clues to this network of interactions leading to bone healing. These interactions may contribute to the communication, timing, and influence of specific elements responsible for bone repair and could potentially lead to pharmacological intervention to enhance bone repair.

Bone repair is initiated by the activation or induction of local and blood-borne cells and their subsequent proliferation and interaction. Examples include the processes of osteoinduction and osteoconduction as outlined by Urist.[28] Osteoinduction involves the transformation of mesenchymal pluripotential cells into bone-forming cells by means of chemical, humoral, and/or physical signals. Osteoconduction refers to the ingrowth of capillaries and osteoprogenitor cells into the fracture from the surrounding bone and soft tissues, interconnecting the fragments and leading to gradual formation of new bone. It has also been referred to as "creeping substitution" in the case of bone graft healing.[29] These processes, both of which are active and important in fracture repair, appear to be controlled by local proteins produced by cells at the fracture site and influenced by endocrine proteins as well.

Inductive Factors

There is experimental evidence for a group of inductive factors called osteogenins, which are protein or protein complexes isolated from demineralized bone.[30] One such osteogenin, called bone morphogenetic protein (BMP), has been studied extensively. BMP is thought to cause local cells at the site of injury to become active in the healing process. An intramuscular implant of BMP-rich matrix has been shown experimentally to cause de novo bone synthesis in soft tissue apart from bone.[31]

Urist has characterized and isolated this collagenase-resistant glycoprotein. The identification of this substance is based on its ability to induce mesenchymal perivascular connective tissue cells into bone-forming osteoprogenitor cells.[32] This bioassay is accomplished by placing a sample of tissue or periosteal BMP in a muscle pouch, subcutaneous space, or diffusion chamber and noting induction of cartilage and woven bone within 10 days, lamellar bone within 20 days, and ossicle-containing bone marrow within 30 days.

Active work is underway to purify BMP (the least abundant of the approximately 25 classified bone matrix proteins). It has been extracted and partially purified from the demineralized bones of rabbits, cows, and humans. The molecular structure of BMP has been cleaved to produce the smallest protein with osteoinductive activity. This protein has a molecular weight of between 15 and 35,000 Da and has been termed primary osteogenic factor. When placed in porous block hydroxyapatite, it increases the amount of bone deposition over that in implant blocks without the factor.[33] The amino acid sequence of this protein has been determined, and investigation of its effects on bone healing is ongoing.

The effects of BMP in animal models of bone repair have been extensively studied. Skull defects in adult rhesus monkeys treated with BMP show more complete bone regeneration than defects implanted with bovine serum albumin. The BMP-induced osteogenesis in monkeys follows a histological sequence of mesenchymal cell proliferation, cartilage differentiation, woven bone formation, and lamellar bone formation with near complete healing at 16 weeks of a 14 to 20 mm defect.[34] Similar findings in sheep and dogs have also been reported.[35, 36]

Bone morphogenetic protein has also been shown to induce bone repair in an ulnar defect in dogs that heals with a nonunion with no treatment. In this study, autologous bone graft also lead to bone union with a similar sequence of cellular events as the skull defects in the rhesus monkeys: 4 weeks, fibrocartilage, cartilage, and woven bone; 8 weeks, resorption of cartilage and replacement with woven bone; 12 weeks, woven bone remodeled to lamellar bone.[37]

Urist has suggested that BMP acts in both of these situations by causing differentiation of perivascular connective tissue cells into chondroblasts and osteoprogenitor cells, thus stimulating the regenerative power of the osteoprogenitor cells already present in the periosteum and the endosteum. The evidence for the perivascular connective tissue cell as the target for BMP comes from experimental work on bone induced by BMP in muscle pouches.[38]

Cell culture studies have shown that BMP stimulates DNA synthesis and cell replication in fetal rat calvaria and rat kidney fibroblast cell lines. Not surprisingly, this effect was seen only in the periosteum and not in periosteum-free bone, as the periosteum is where the nondifferentiated cells reside. In these same studies, BMP enhanced ^{3}H-proline incorporation into collagenase-digestible and noncollagen protein but did not alter fetal rat calvarial cell alkaline phosphatase activity. As the BMP used in this study was only partially purified, it is unknown whether the mitogenic effect was due to BMP alone or to a different bone matrix protein that was copurified with the BMP.[39]

Growth Factors

Many growth factors and regulatory protein complexes have been isolated that experimentally influence various portions of the bone healing cascade.[40] These substances are thought to be temporally released to both fit into the schema of fracture repair and to drive the coordinated cellular interaction needed for an ordered progression toward bone regeneration.

These factors, be they systemic or local, have been shown in cell culture studies and animal studies to have many different mitogenic, chemotactic, and secretory effects on cells that are present at the fracture site. These effects seem to control the progression of morphological and physiological events during bone repair.

The cells involved in the early stages of bone repair are essentially those present in any early traumatic wound. Bleeding at the fracture site leads to platelet aggregation and clot formation. Some polymorphonuclear leukocytes (PMNs), macrophages, and fibroblasts are attracted to the area of the injured bone in the first several hours and days after injury, when multiple chemoattractant factors and mitogens are probably present, but the actual mediators have not been precisely identified.[17] Many growth factors have been shown to affect various cells and processes important in the different stages of bone repair. Their names and the experimental evidence linking them to bone repair are listed in Table 23–1.[41]

As soon as a fracture occurs, a local network of interactions is initiated. In fact, the occasional failure of bone repair may in part be due to perturbations in the activation of local factors. As blood and blood-borne elements accumulate at the fracture site, platelets are deposited and platelet-derived growth factor (PDGF) is released. PDGF has been shown to elicit an endothelial response and to promote fibroblast proliferation. In addition, PDGF enhances cartilage synthesis and production of type II collagen.[83, 84] Concurrent prostaglandin release recruits monocyte precursors that can then differentiate into osteoclasts. Prostaglandins have been shown to increase the size and number of osteoclasts that can cause profound effects on bone resorption.[85] Lymphokines and monokines derived from blood-borne elements in the hematoma can act as mitogens, recruiting and directing cells to move into the wound and begin to divide.[86, 87] Local fibroblasts release fibroblast growth factor (FGF), which is angiogenic and may serve to foster neovascularization of the fracture site and early formation of granulation tissue.[88] Kallikreins also stimulate the release of vasoactive and angiogenic factors that can affect the local blood supply. Local lymphocytes and monocytes release osteoclast activating factor (OAF), which stimulates osteoclasts to resorb bone.[89] Transforming growth factor-β (TGF-β) has been implicated as a local mitogen spurring proliferation of cells and stimulating bone collagen synthesis and the expansion of osteoblastic cells.[90] Cartilage growth factor (CGF) is active in the production of type II collagen, and plasma fibronectin has been shown to anchor cells to ground substance and to participate in collagen production.[91] A myriad of other mediators such as epidermal growth factor, angiogenic growth factor, and tumor necrosis factor have been found at the fracture site.

As can be seen from the previous discussion, protein-to-cell interactions in bone repair are extremely complex and not yet completely understood. Once these interactions are characterized and the proteins sequenced and produced by recombinant DNA techniques, their therapeutic potential will likely become realized. Possible clinical areas of application include treatment of acute fractures prone to nonunion, management of nonunions, and improved craniofacial onlay bone grafting.

Table 23–1. POTENTIAL ROLE OF PROTEINS AND GROWTH FACTORS IN BONE REPAIR*

Vascular Ingrowth

Plasma fibronectin
  anchors cells in the ground substance (42)†
  required for collagen formation (43)

Endothelial cell–derived growth factor mitogenic (44, 45)

Macrophage–derived growth factor C
  mitogenic for (rat) osteoblastlike cells and chondrocytes (46)

Callus Formation

Platelet-derived growth factor
  mitogenic for fibroblasts (47), bone cells (48)
  activates monocytes and promotes bone resorption (49)

Epidermal cell growth factor (transforming growth factor-1)
  mitogenic (50, 51) for cartilage (52), bone (53–55)
  inhibits type I bone collagen synthesis (56–59)

Fibroblast growth factor
  mitogenic for cartilage (60), fibroblasts (61)

Insulin-like growth factor (somatomedin C)
  chondrocyte proliferation (52, 62)
  chondrocyte proteoglycan synthesis (63)

Nerve growth factor
  mitogenic (64)

Transforming growth factor-β
  mitogenic for bone cells (48)

Cartilage growth factor 1
  mitogenic for cartilage cells in callus (65–67)

Cartilage growth factor-2
  morphogen required for production of type II collagen (68)

Bone growth factors-1, 2, 3
  stimulate type I (bone) collagen production (69, 70)

Osteoclast activating factor
  stimulates development of resorptive ultrastructure in osteoclast (71–73)

Bone Formation/Remodeling Phase

Epidermal growth factor
  promotes bone resorption (74–76)

Fibroblast growth factor
  promotes (high dose) bone resorption (76)

Insulin
  synergistic effect with bone growth protein (77)

Interleukins (monocyte products)

IL-1 fibroblast proliferation (78, 79)
  collagenase production (80)
  prostaglandin production (80)

IL-2 T-cell growth factor aids resorption via osteoclast-activating factor production (81, 82)

*Modified from Simmons DJ: Fracture healing perspectives. Clin Orthop Rel Res 200:105–106, 1985.
†Numbers in parentheses refer to references.

BIOPHYSICAL CHARACTERISTICS OF BONE HEALING

The biophysical elements of oxygen tension and bioelectric potentials are important factors in fracture healing. Oxygen gradients and electric charges generated by a fracture have an important influence on bone regeneration.[1] They work in concert with the local biochemical phenomena to influence the bone healing process.

Oxygen Tension

Changes in oxygen tension influence the formation of bone and cartilage at the fracture site. Relatively hypoxic cells in settings of low oxygen tension are more likely to form cartilage intermediates during bone formation.[92] Histologically, nests of persistent cartilage are formed in areas of the fracture callus most distant from the capillary buds. Conversely, higher oxygen tensions are related to the promotion of direct bone healing. In fact, the requisite immobilization needed for primary bone healing is thought to be due to the need to maintain higher oxygen tensions at the fracture site. Rigid fixation may accomplish this by preventing reinjury to blood vessels and preserving oxygen delivery to the wound.[11, 93]

Although higher oxygen tensions may generate bone without a cartilage intermediate, it should be noted that this level of oxygen tension is only high relative to other areas of healing bone. In fact, the overall partial pressure of oxygen found in tissue during bone repair is low when compared to systemic values. In general, low oxygen tension favors bone healing.[94] Experimental evidence of in vitro bone growth shows optimal results in a setting of a low partial pressure of oxygen.[95]

Bone and cartilage cells follow a mostly anaerobic metabolic pathway. The fracture hematoma has a lower pH than serum, and lactate production increases and peaks during the metabolically active period of soft callus formation. This increase in acid production is in keeping with biochemical evidence of glycolytic enzyme patterns during the proliferation of bone and cartilage cells.[1] Brighton's studies support the theory that tissue hypoxia may well play a role in endochondral ossification at the fracture callus. Hypertrophic chondrocytes which have sequestered calcium in their mitochondria release their stores when all of the glycogen available for anaerobic metabolism is consumed. The released calcium aids in the nucleation and mineralization of surrounding matrix.[1, 95, 96]

There is increased vascularity and blood flow in a fresh fracture site (Fig. 23–11). Blood flow peaks at 10 days and may take up to 2 months to normalize.[97] Despite the increase in perfusion, the oxygen tension in the fracture hematoma is low (Fig. 23–12). In fact, research using microelectrodes indicates that oxygen tension is also low in freshly formed fracture cartilage and bone.[94] Furthermore, other experiments confirm that partial pressure of oxygen is low

in fresh fracture callus and that oxygen consumption during active bone formation is not increased.[98]

The coincidence of increased blood flow, steady state oxygen consumption, and low oxygen tensions at the fracture site seems contradictory. However, if hypoxia and oxygen utilization are thought of as being measured at the cellular level, a more cogent explanation becomes apparent. If the cellular proliferation at the growing fracture callus outstrips the augmented blood supply, then each cell will show low oxygen tension and a lower than expected

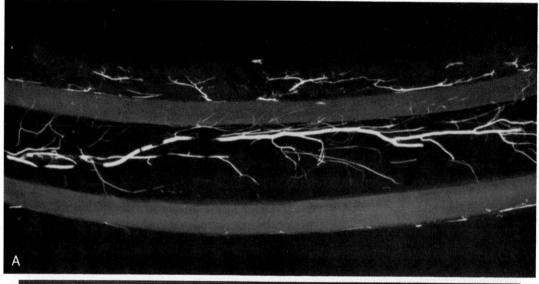

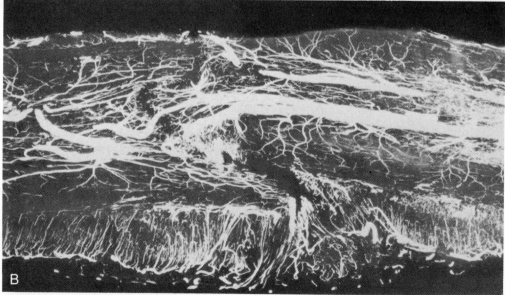

Figure 23–11. *A,* Microgram of the midshaft of a normal dog radius with the circulation in a resting state. Note the prominence of the medullary vessels. *B,* Microangiogram of 3-week-old displaced radial fracture with re-establishment of the medullary circulation. The extensive periosteal callus shows the characteristic arrangement of blood vessels perpendicular to the cortical surface (×6). (From Heppenstall RB: Fracture healing. In Heppenstall RB (ed): Fracture Treatment and Healing. Philadelphia, WB Saunders, 1980, p 48.)

Figure 23–12. The tissue oxygen, carbon dioxide, and oxygen consumption values obtained in healing dog rib defects as a function of time. Of interest was the fact that at 3 to 4 weeks, when bone was actively being formed, the oxygen tension remained low and was associated with slightly elevated carbon dioxide tension and no evidence of an increase in oxygen consumption above that of normal bone. (From Heppenstall RB: Fracture healing. In Heppenstall RB (ed): Fracture Healing and Treatment. Philadelphia, WB Saunders, 1980, p 53.)

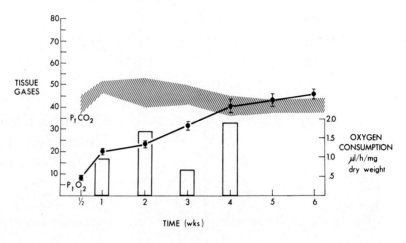

oxygen consumption. So despite increased perfusion to a fracture site, an increase in cell number greater than the concomitant rise in blood supply would lead to a relative state of hypoxia at the cellular level (Fig. 23–13).[1] Perhaps it is this oxygen gradient across the fracture callus that drives the formidable stimulus of induction of bone repair. Although not fully substantiated, this theory remains an active area of continued research.

Bioelectrical Effects

Wolff's law, published at the end of the 19th century, states that a bone develops the structure most suited to resist the forces acting upon it, or more plainly put, "form follows func-

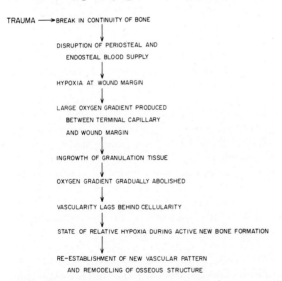

Figure 23–13. A hypothetical sequence of events in relation to oxygen and fracture healing. (From Heppenstall RB: Fracture healing. In Heppenstall RB (ed): Fracture Healing and Treatment. Philadelphia, WB Saunders, 1980, p 55.)

tion."[99] Basset proposed that mechanical changes to bone modify the behavior of the bone cells.[100] Cellular processes and external mechanical forces require a common level of communication in order to exert influence on one another. The phenomenon of piezoelectricity provides that level of communication and may be the medium by which the physical manifestations of Wolff's law are realized. Piezoelectricity is the generation of electric polarity by pressure in a crystalline substance such as mineralized bone. Alterations in bioelectrical potentials in bone can experimentally influence osteogenesis, and these signals may have a role in controlling bone cell activity and bone structure.

Stress-generated potentials act on bone with distinct polarity so that compressive forces show electronegativity while tensile forces produce electropositivity (Fig. 23–14). Additionally, concave surfaces tend to be electronegative and convex surfaces electropositive.[101, 102] Clinically, bone develops a more significant callus on an electronegative concave surface following fracture reduction.[3] Studies have also shown that regions of electropositivity are osteoclastic and regions of electronegativity osteoblastic.[103] Such evidence suggests a role for bioelectrical potentials in bone repair.

Bioelectrical potentials recorded from a fresh fracture callus are strongly negative at the beginning of the healing process and slowly revert to normal as healing progresses.[104] This supports the concept that active bone growth and repair are electronegative. The process has also been reproduced experimentally to show that when electricity is applied to bone at specific currents and voltages, the result is osteoblastic new bone formation. These findings have been exploited clinically in the treatment of fracture nonunion.[105] Bioelectricity may also play a role in the

PIEZOELECTRIC EFFECT

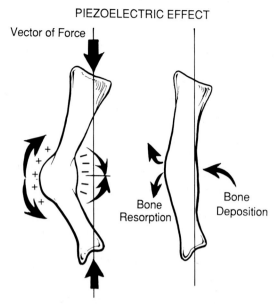

Figure 23–14. Electrical signals arise when bone is stressed. Note that the area under compression is electronegative and the area under tension is electropositive. A long bone that has healed with an angulation will remodel through the piezoelectric effect. Electronegativity causes bone deposition and electropositivity causes bone resorption, the net result of which is gradual straightening of the bone. (From Cutting C: Repair and grafting of bone. In McCarthy J (ed): Plastic Surgery, vol 1. Philadelphia, WB Saunders, 1990, p 598.)

sequence of bone mineralization and calcium deposition during the formation of crystalline lattice of bone. Piezoelectrical effects may fine tune or direct local bioelectrical phenomena vital to ordered bone healing.

BIOMECHANICAL ASPECTS OF BONE HEALING

The biomechanical influences on fracture healing consist of the application of mechanical forces and their effects on healing bone. These forces—tension, bending, and torsion—represent the spectrum of mechanical properties that normal bone must accommodate.

In general, as a fracture heals it becomes stiffer and stronger, with bending stiffness returning more rapidly than bending strength.[106] In addition, the ability to elongate the healing bone gradually diminishes.[107] Initially, the bone fails through the area of the healing fracture but as the repair process continues the bone gains strength and resists alteration. Ultimately, a completely healed bone should have an equal probability of failure at or outside the site of

previous injury.[108] The temporal relationship between fracture repair and full restoration of structural integrity is related to the site of injury and a myriad of other variables affecting fracture healing.

Delayed Union and Nonunion: Failure of Bone Repair

Each fracture has a unique temporal sequence of bone healing. The particular type of fracture incurred in conjunction with the special characteristics of the injured bone combine to determine the time frame of healing. Delayed union is said to occur when a fracture requires a longer than expected time to heal with no clinical or radiographically apparent reason that it cannot do so. In the case of nonunion, there is a termination of the bone healing process, with cessation of bone repair and bone regeneration.

The incidence of nonunion in long bone fractures is about 5 percent and is rare in children. Bones of the axial skeleton show a lower incidence of nonunion compared to long bones, while certain other bones such as the distal tibia, radius, ulna, and the carponavicular bones show a higher incidence.[109] Histological examination of the fracture site reveals normal elements of bone healing to be present. However, cartilage and fibrous tissue persist that normally would have been replaced by bone (Fig. 23–15).

Many delayed unions and nonunions are considered idiopathic in origin. One of the difficulties in discovering the causes of nonunion is the lack of a good animal model. A vast array of systemic factors have been implicated in both the promotion and the impairment of fracture healing (Table 23–2).[2] Unfortunately, their influence on bone repair remains controversial: many of these factors have been shown to slow the repair process in one group of experiments while accelerating the repair process in others. However, a judicious review of the literature will often reveal that these investigations focused on different aspects of the healing process or reported a variance in the dose/response relationship and in fact do not represent opposing or competing points of view. Further experimental inquiry into the intricate mechanisms of the factors that influence bone healing will help to rectify these discrepancies and provide a unified view of the systemic influences on local fracture repair.

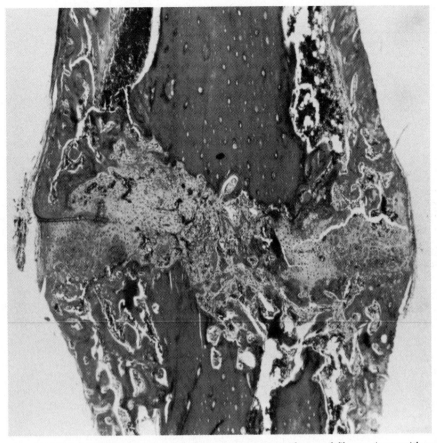

Figure 23–15. Longitudinal section of a nonunion. Note the persistent cartilage and fibrous tissue with no progression toward new bone formation at the fracture site. (From Heppenstall RB: Fracture healing. In Heppenstall RB (ed): Fracture Healing and Treatment. Philadelphia, WB Saunders, 1980, p 45.)

Etiology of Impaired Union

As stated earlier, union of fractures with associated clinical conditions such as malignancy and infection or those with tissue interposition or distraction at the fracture site can be delayed or absent. In extensive traumatic injury to bone, there is often massive destruction of adjacent soft tissues, and the wound healing process in such injuries may be affected by prioritization at the cellular level. Competing metabolic needs and inflammatory stimuli may cause an imbalance of fibroblastic and osteoblastic differentiation and an impaired union. If the injury results in a significant depletion of blood supply to the fracture site, all cellular activity could be suppressed, leading to a failure of callus formation. Full-blown pseudarthrosis can occur. Histologically, a pseudarthritic nonunion consists of a cellular mass of collagen and ground substance making up a fibrinoid complex that is hydroscopic and exudes a pseudosynovial

fluid. The result is a large fluid-filled cavity with a synovial-type lining.

Inadequate fixation with repeated manipulation of the fracture site may also lead to a failure to form proper callus. In this scenario, a cleft forms at the end of the fracture and a false joint can develop. However, it is important that the fracture site be subjected to some mechanical force since exercise increases the rate of repair.[110] Clinicians have developed varied weightbearing techniques to exploit these findings.[111] Promotion of bone healing through early use of a fractured extremity can probably be best explained by the bioelectrical phenomena discussed earlier.

Age can also contribute to delayed or nonunion. Animal studies and clinical observations support the notion that fracture healing slows with age.[13] In the case of massive bone loss, the size of the gap may exceed the capacity of the healing process to span it, resulting in a nonunion. If avascular necrosis of bone occurs as a result of fracture, the affected bone is entirely dependent on exogenous sources for blood sup-

Table 23–2. SYSTEMIC FACTORS
INFLUENCING BONE HEALING

Factors Claimed to Promote Bone Healing	Factors Claimed to Retard Bone Healing
Growth hormone	Corticosteroids
Triiodothyronine	Alloxan diabetes
Thyroxine	Castration
Thyrotropin	Vitamin A, high dose
Calcitonin	Vitamin D, high dose
Insulin	Rachitis
Vitamin A	Anemia
Vitamin D	Aminoacetonitrile
Anabolic steroids	β-Aminopropionitrile
Chondroitin sulphate	Bone wax
Hyaluronidase	Delayed manipulation
Anticoagulants	Denervation
(dicumarol)	Hyperbaric oxygen
Ultrasonics	(6 hr, 2 atm daily)
Electric currents	Anticoagulants
Hyperbaric oxygen	(dicumarol)
(2 hr, 3 atm daily)	
Physical exercise	

From Cruess RL: Healing of bone tendon and ligament. In Rockwood CA, Green DP: Fractures. Philadelphia, JB Lippincott, 1984, p 153.

ply and ingrowth of capillaries, a situation predisposing to impaired union. Disease states affecting bone such as Paget's disease can also lead to delayed or nonunion.

The diagnosis of delayed union has clinical relevance, as the method of fracture treatment can be altered to enhance bone repair and prevent nonunion. Factors that can cause delayed union and increase the incidence of nonunion can be classified as local or systemic. Local factors include the mechanism of injury, degree of trauma, and method of treatment, while the systemic factors influence the entire patient and his or her ability to heal. The systemic factors are listed in Table 23–2 and the local factors in Table 23–3. Although systemic factors can be important clinically, it is the local factors that play the predominant role in influencing the development of delayed or nonunion.

Extensive soft tissue disruption at the fracture site seems to delay bone healing. This is thought by most investigators to be caused by a decrease in the blood supply to the fracture through disruption of the surrounding cortical blood supply directly through the periosteum. Although most of the blood supply to the fracture site comes through the endosteum, some blood is supplied from the periphery and with massive soft tissue injury, this outer cortical blood supply can be lost. In addition, it is thought that soft tissue injury around the fracture can lead to an alteration in the electrical potentials and compressive forces at the fracture site thereby retarding the healing process.[109] These alterations in active electrical potentials and compressive forces can delay bone repair by mechanisms not yet well understood.

Loss of bone at the fracture site clearly will delay healing; however, in certain open fractures, such as in the distal tibia, with severe comminution and contamination, debridement of devitalized bone fragments is required to prevent osteomyelitis. When defects are created, by either the injury or the treatment, delayed union and nonunion are likely to occur if bone grafting is not employed. Grafting is usually done on a delayed basis after coverage of the wound with a vascularized muscle flap.[112]

Inadequate reduction contributes to delayed union and nonunion as a larger amount of callus is required to bridge the fracture gap. In addition, pedicled vascularized muscle can interpose itself between the bone ends and inhibit callus formation,[109] although it has been shown that most large devitalized soft tissue fragments will scar and ossify.[113]

There has been a reevaluation of the effects of immobilization on fracture treatment over the past several years. Twenty years ago almost all authors recommended rigid immobilization for all long bone fractures. Now, however, it is felt that rigid compression of the bone ends with active contraction of the surrounding muscles has no detrimental effect on, and may even stimulate, bone repair.[109] As mentioned, this beneficial effect may result from alteration in the electrical potentials around the healing bone. There is no question that rigidly immobilized long bone fractures treated with compression plates heal differently than those undergoing closed treatment.

Certain anatomical fracture sites have a high incidence of delayed union or nonunion due primarily to the convergence of several local factors. Particularly troublesome are fractures of the navicular bone at the wrist, subcapital fractures of the hip, and fractures of the lower third of the tibia.

Table 23–3. LOCAL FACTORS THAT CAN
LEAD TO DELAYED UNION AND
NONUNION

Site of fracture
Soft tissue injury
Bone loss
Inadequate reduction
Inadequate immobilization
Infection
Radiation
Malignancy at fracture site
Poor arterial flow to fracture site

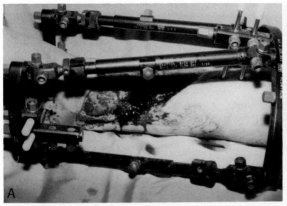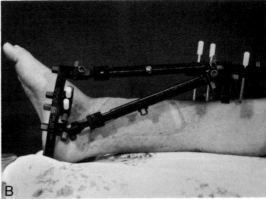

Figure 23–16. A patient with massive soft tissue loss associated with an open tibial fracture treated with a muscle flap. *A,* Appearance of open tibial fracture after debridement. *B,* Progression of healing 6 weeks after closure with free latissimus dorsi muscle flap covered by split-thickness skin graft.

Fractures of the navicular bone are the most frequently missed fractures in adults as a radiological abnormality may not be apparent at the time of injury. A high percentage of patients develop avascular necrosis of the proximal part of the navicular bone with transverse fractures because the bone has no muscle attachments and is surrounded almost entirely by articular cartilage. The primary blood supply enters the bone distally and the lack of periosteum makes healing dependent on the endosteal blood supply, which is disrupted by a transverse fracture.[109]

Vascular supply is also one of the problems in subcapital fractures at the hip joint. The blood supply to the femoral head is tenuous, and displaced fractures through the neck frequently interrupt it. The periosteum over the neck is thin and easily disrupted, and as in the navicular bone, fracture healing is heavily dependent on the endosteal blood supply. In addition, these fractures are usually very unstable. All of these factors lead to a high incidence of avascular necrosis of the femoral head, nonunion, and subsequent degenerative joint disease of the hip.[109]

Distal fractures of the tibia are prone to delayed union and nonunion because of the presence of open fracture and the degree of associated soft tissue disruption. These fractures frequently are open and contaminated, setting the stage for osteomyelitis and delayed union or nonunion. Current treatment protocols of serial debridement, delayed closure with muscle flaps, and delayed bone grafting appear to be decreasing the incidence of these complications.[112]

Infection can cause delayed union or nonunion in open fractures or after open reduction and internal fixation. Open fractures are thus treated with immediate surgical irrigation and debridement in an effort to prevent the development of infection. Cultures are done immediately and antibiotics are given.

Massive soft tissue injury can accompany open fractures of the tibia and fibula. These injuries frequently require muscle flaps from local tissues or from distant sites (i.e., free tissue transfer) (Fig. 23–16). Experimental work suggests that these muscle flaps can decrease the incidence of chronic osteomyelitis by bringing new vascularized tissue into the wound. These flaps also appear to enhance polymorphonuclear leukocyte function at the fracture site and improve the clearance of dead bone.[114, 115] Others have shown muscle flaps to be superior to skin flaps in initiating the repair of devascularized cortical bone and callus formation of the fracture site.[116]

Treatment of Nonunion

In a nonunion, the fracture site retains the ability to form bone, as evidenced by the successful re-initiation of healing with other treatment. In order to treat a nonunion, the environment at the fracture site must be altered in favor of union. Bone healing can be restarted by bone grafting (see next section) or electrical stimulation.

Surgical intervention can remove the cartilage and scar of a pseudoarthritic nonunion and revitalize the sclerotic ends of a fracture. Autogenous bone grafting can dramatically influence the constituents of a fracture site, and this treatment has resulted in a significant rate of nonunion healing.

In the 1950s, Fukada and Yasuda showed that direct current applied to bone fosters osteogenesis in the region of the cathode.[102] The further discovery of piezoelectrical effects in the crystalline lattice of mineralized bone matrix led to the application of exogenous electrical current to fracture sites to stimulate bone healing. By the 1970s, these bioelectrical phenomena were being applied to the treatment of nonunited fractures in humans.[101, 105] Continued experimentation and refinement of electrical stimulation techniques have resulted in acceleration of fracture healing in delayed unions and a significant rate of nonunion healing both in the laboratory and in clinical practice. The various methods of providing electrical stimulation to bone can be described in terms of voltage gradients, total current, and current density at the target fracture site. In the case of nonunion, electrical stimulation is now a viable alternative to bone grafting and is apparently equally efficacious in re-initiating the healing process.[117] Case reports employing a range of different stimulation methods demonstrate a 75 to 90 percent rate of nonunion healing. In addition, electrical stimulation has been used to treat avascular necrosis and pseudarthroses and even to augment fresh fracture healing.[118]

Healing of Bone Grafts

Bone grafts are used to improve healing of fractures in which bone has been lost, to replace missing pieces of bone after trauma or surgical removal, as interposition grafts after movement of major bone segments, particularly in the craniofacial skeleton, as onlay grafts to alter facial contour, and to stimulate bone repair in delayed or nonunions. The healing of these grafts involves many of the principles and processes already discussed. However, bone graft healing differs from the healing of fractures, in certain ways. In addition, there is substantial interest at present in mechanisms to improve survival of onlay grafts to the face and in the use of bone graft substitutes such as hydroxyapatite and cadaver bone allografts.

Osteogenesis and osteoconduction are the primary mechanisms by which bone grafts "take" (Fig. 23–17), however, osteoinduction, or the transformation of local undifferentiated cells into bone-forming cells, may also be involved. Osteogenesis is the formation of new bone by surviving cells within the graft. This mechanism is a major factor in vascularized bone transfers in which the blood supply to the graft is either maintained by a vascular pedicle or reconstituted with a microvascular anastomosis. It is less important when free grafts of

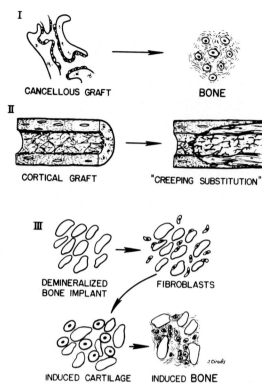

Figure 23–17. Mechanisms of bone regeneration after bone grafting. I, Osteogenesis. Cancellous bone grafts transfer preosteoblasts and osteoblasts that form new bone. II, Osteoconduction. Cortical bone grafts function as a scaffold for the ingrowth of bone from the recipient bed. III, Osteoinduction. Demineralized bone implants induce transformation of local mesenchymal cells into bone-forming cells. (From Motoki DS, Mulliken JB: The healing of bone and cartilage. Clin Plast Surg 817:529, 1990.)

cancellous bone are used because these grafts rapidly revascularize from surrounding bone and soft tissue.[119] Most nonvascularized free bone grafts heal through osteoconduction, which is the process by which blood vessels and cells from the surrounding tissues grow into the graft and use it as a scaffold for the deposition of new bone as the old dead bone is resorbed (Fig. 23–18).[120] This slow and incompletely understood process has been termed "creeping substitution."[121]

The healing process differs in cortical grafts and cancellous bone grafts, since they possess different structural and healing properties. During the first week after grafting, all bone grafts are subjected to an intense inflammatory response. During the second week, this inflammation is gradually replaced by proliferating fibroblasts and osteoclasts around the periphery of the graft. While this is occurring outside the graft, osteocytic autolysis with necrosis of tissue within the haversian canals and marrow spaces is taking place within the bone.[120, 122, 123]

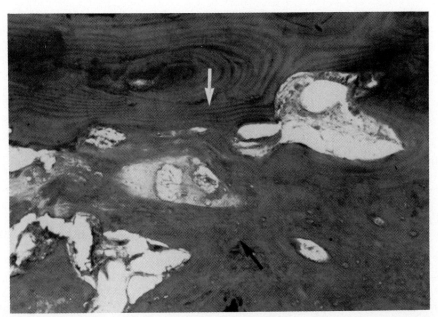

Figure 23–18. Photomicrograph of bone graft healing by osteoconduction. The ingrowth of blood vessels and osteoprogenitor cells from adjacent recipient site bone results in resorption of the graft (*white arrow;* note empty lacunae) and deposition of new bone (*black arrow*). (From Motoki DS, Mulliken JB: The healing of bone and cartilage. Clin Plast Surg 817:529, 1990.)

Invading blood vessels revascularize cancellous grafts within 2 weeks. Cells lining the trabeculae either brought there from the blood or differentiated from premature mesenchymal cells in the vicinity of the graft appear to differentiate into osteoblasts and deposit a seam of osteoid around the old bone. This necrotic old bone, which has undergone osteocytic autolysis, is then gradually resorbed by osteoclasts and the graft is replaced by new bone.[120]

In contrast, cortical grafts vascularize much more slowly than cancellous grafts; the process can require 1 to 2 months more.[124] The new blood vessels growing into the graft must follow the Volkmann and haversian canals.[124, 125] While vascular ingrowth is occurring, osteoclasts begin to resorb peripheral haversian systems.[123] Osteoblasts then arrive and manufacture osteoid where resorption has taken place. Resorption and osteoid production occur simultaneously with revascularization. The revascularized areas are resorbed and replaced with viable new bone. In cortical grafts, there are areas of nonvascularized bone that seem to become isolated from osteoclastic activity, remaining as islands of necrotic bone within the viable bone graft.[125]

These differences in healing of cancellous and cortical bone grafts are reflected in marked variations in porosity, strength, and the amount of new bone formed over time (Fig. 23–19).[125]

If bone grafts are used to replace missing parts of the skeleton and if infection is con-trolled and soft tissue cover is adequate, healing is generally predictable with a good chance of graft take and uncomplicated bone repair. When they are used as onlay grafts, most commonly to alter facial contour either for recon-

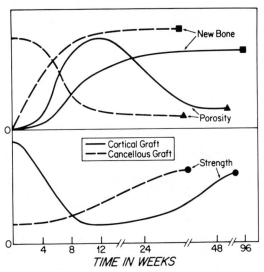

Figure 23–19. Differences between rate of new bone formation, porosity, and mechanical strength in cancellous versus cortical grafts. Cancellous grafts initially strengthen because repair begins with new bone formation. Cortical grafts weaken initially because repair starts with osteoclastic resorption that increases the internal porosity of the graft. (From Motoki DS, Mulliken JB: The healing of bone and cartilage. Clin Plast Surg 817:529, 1990.)

structive or aesthetic reasons, their survival is less predictable. While numerous animal studies have investigated this phenomenon, the exact mechanisms contributing to this unpredictable repair are only beginning to be understood.

Experimentally a greater volume of onlay bone graft survives when there is periosteum on the graft surface[126, 127] and graft orientation is such that the cortical surface is in contact with soft tissue and cancellous surface is in contact with the underlying bone.[126–128] Bone of embryological origin such as membranous bone appears to maintain a higher volume than endochondral grafts,[129, 130] and rigid fixation of the grafts seems to improve the volume of bone graft surviving, particularly with endochondral grafts in areas of high motion.[131, 132] In addition, systemic factors such as age and nutritional status are important, as are local factors such as excessive scar in the host bed, inadequate soft tissue coverage, and radiation.

Whitaker has proposed the biologic boundary theory of onlay bone survival, which states that the body has a known "boundary" or structure.[133] Clearly, onlay bone grafts are used to change this structure, and their resorption may be influenced by how far from the individuals "biologic boundary" the graft extends. For example, an onlay bone graft to the nose after a nasoethmoid complex fracture that aims to restore the preinjured appearance would presumably resorb less than an onlay graft to the zygoma in a patient with Treacher-Collins syndrome, which would exceed the biologic boundary. There are certainly other reasons why these changes occur, but perhaps this theory can provide a unified explanation for the many observations that have been made regarding onlay bone grafts.

Bone Graft Substitutes

Due to donor site morbidity, limited availability of autogenous bone, and the unpredictable behavior of autogenous bone grafts, several bone graft substitutes are currently in clinical use. The most notable of these are hydroxyapatite and cadaver bone allografts.

Calcium hydroxyapatite $(Ca_{10}[PO_4]_6[OH]_2)$ crystals are the major inorganic constituent of bone and teeth. This material can be manmade as either a dense ceramic or a porous material, the latter having a definite propensity for bone ingrowth.[134] The most common pore size is 200 μ, depending on how it is prepared. It is available either as granules, commonly used for

augmentation of the atrophied alveolar ridge,[135] or as blocks used as interposition and onlay grafts to the facial skeleton.[136]

This material has osteoconductive properties as manifested by bone ingrowth documented in both experimental and clinical studies.[134, 137–146] Backscatter electron microscopy techniques show mean values of 18 percent bone and 33.5 percent fibrovascular tissue in hydroxyapatite implants removed several months after implantation into human maxillofacial bones.[146] There appears to be minimal resorption of the inorganic matrix over time as documented by the absence of osteoclastic activity and the fact that implant blocks remain distinguishable from surrounding bone both grossly and radiologically over time.[136] This implant material is not replaced by bone, but rather seems to supply a scaffold into which bone that is in contact with the material can grow (Fig. 23–20).

Cadaver allografts, in contrast, do not remain indistinguishable from surrounding tissues. They virtually all resorb and are replaced to varying degrees by new bone via the process of

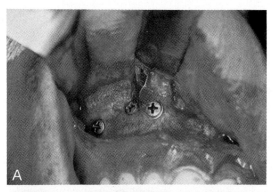
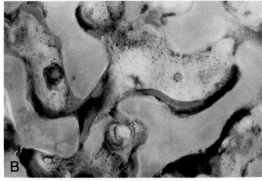

Figure 23–20. Gross (*A*) and histologic (*B*) appearance of porous block hydroxyapatite 14 months (gross) and 4 months (histologic) after implantation. Note that grossly the bone-implant interface remains well delineated. Histologically, the implant matrix remains intact with bone deposition against the walls (Villanueva-Goldner stain $\times 10$). (From Rosen HM, McFarland MM: The biologic behavior of hydroxyapatite implanted into the maxillofacial skeleton. Plast Reconstr Surg 85:718–723, 1990.)

creeping substitution. Their survival is unpredictable and for that reason they are rarely used alone for alveolar ridge augmentation or inlay or onlay grafts to the facial skeleton. Excellent results have been reported in mandibular reconstruction using a combination of a tray of decalcified cadaver mandible surrounded by cancellous bone graft. The cadaver bone gradually resorbs as the cancellous bone graft is replaced by new bone. This technique has been used in combination with hyperbaric oxygen therapy in the radiated mandible and results appear comparable to those with vascularized free bone transfers.[147]

CARTILAGE HEALING AND REPAIR

From Hippocrates to the present age it is universally allowed that ulcerated cartilage is a troublesome thing and that, once destroyed, it is not repaired.[148]

Cartilage as a tissue consists of cells, the chondrocytes, surrounded by an extracellular matrix, fibers, and water. The extracellular matrix is made up of several proteoglycans that are synthesized by the chondrocytes. The chief glycosaminoglycans that are bound to the protein core of the proteoglycans of cartilage are hyaluronic acid, chondroitin-4-sulfate, and keratan sulfate (Fig. 23–21). These are polymerized with type II collagen and various mixtures of elastic fibers. This relationship gives cartilage its structure.

Unlike bone, cartilage has no blood or lymphatic vessels so nutrition is primarily by diffusion of nutrients through the proteoglycan-collagen-water matrix. The perichondrium is an extremely vascular tissue with a rich capillary network that is felt to contribute substantially to the nutrition of the surrounding cartilage.

Cartilage is classified according to the predominant fiber type. Hyaline cartilage covers the articular surface of joints, forms the cartilage of the rib cage, and is the skeletal support of the tracheobronchial tree and nose. Elastic cartilage, in which elastin predominates in the extracellular matrix, is found in the external ear and areas of the larynx. Fibrocartilage gives strong support to the intervertebral discs and tendon attachments to bone.

Superficial Injury and Repair of Joint Cartilage

Upon superficial laceration or fracture of cartilage there is a disruption of the proteoglycan-

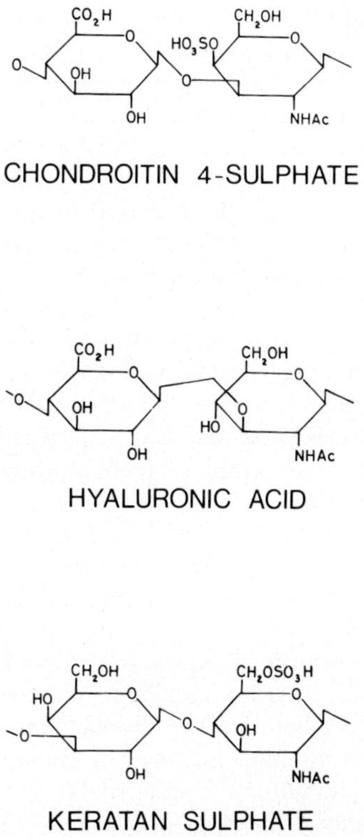

CHONDROITIN 4-SULPHATE

HYALURONIC ACID

KERATAN SULPHATE

Figure 23–21. The repeating units of the glycosaminoglycans found in bone tissue and cartilage tissue. (From Triffitt JT: The organic matrix of bone tissue. In Urist MR (ed): Fundamental and Clinical Bone Physiology. Philadelphia, JB Lippincott, 1980, p 73.)

collagen matrix and injury to cellular constituents. Due to the absence of blood vessels, there is no inflammatory response; rather, there is some loss of matrix and an increase in proteoglycan and collagen synthesis by the chondrocytes. There may or may not be an increase in mitotic activity among the chondrocytes as reflected in increased tritiated thymidine uptake. When a functioning joint is subjected to the constant impact of outside forces, the long-term response of the cartilage depends on whether or not the injury leads to progressive degeneration of the remainder of the joint cartilage.[149]

Due to the avascular nature of cartilage, a superficial injury is totally dependent on the chondrocyte for repair. The chondrocytes must proliferate, synthesize the necessary proteoglycans and collagen, and then incorporate the building blocks into a matrix with a semblance to the preinjured state. Unfortunately the chondrocyte's attempt to reconstitute its environment often falls short, and the overall regenerative power of cartilage is usually inadequate.[150] Cartilage repair is limited and slow and frequently leaves persistent structural defects in response to superficial injury.

As opposed to the relatively dormant state of the chondrocyte in normal adult cartilage, superficial injury is associated with an increase in cellular proliferation at the injury site. In partial-thickness lacerations of cartilage, a distinct zone of necrosis can be seen adjacent to the injury, ghost cells can be found in the lacunae of chondrocytes, and there is evidence of damage to the surrounding matrix.[151, 152]

Just behind the zone of necrosis is a zone of proliferation, which consists of replicating chondrocytes. This is demonstrated experimentally as an increased uptake of radiolabeled thymidine.[153] There is an associated increase in glycosoaminoglycan and collagen synthesis with electron microscopic evidence of increased intracellular activity.[151] The majority of synthesized collagen is type II, although type I collagen has been isolated in the pericellular region of chondrocytes.[154, 155]

Since a superficial injury is localized only to cartilage, there is no associated damage to the blood vessels beneath the cartilage in the subchondral bone and in turn no inflammatory reaction. The injury is essentially isolated by the avascular properties of cartilage. There is no evidence of a cascade of multicellular response nor is there formation of a fibrin clot to act as a scaffold for repair. Nearby perichondrium can assist in the proliferation of chondrocytes, but overall the increase in synthesis and number of local cells evoked by a superficial laceration is short lived. Insufficient cell population and inadequate production of matrix usually culminates in failure to achieve complete healing of a defect. A study by Ghadially and others followed the repair of superficial injuries to cartilage by electron microscopy over a 2-year period.[156] They found no difference in appearance of the wounds at 2 years when compared to the same wounds immediately after injury.

Deep Injury of Joint Cartilage

In contrast to superficial injury, deep lacerations that breach the subchondral bone produce an exuberant inflammatory response. Full-thickness injury encroaches on local blood vessels, causing hemorrhage and allowing for an inflammatory response with subsequent mediation of cellular activity toward repair. Extension of an injury to subchondral bone provides an extrinsic means of cartilage healing. The bone and synovial tissue may be used as a source of reparative cells. Although the cartilage itself does not change its normal response to injury, the exposure to vascular channels of surrounding tissue allows ingrowth of granulation tissue. Blood vessels carry blood-borne elements that migrate to the wound and stimulate local cells, inducing an inflammatory reaction. Inflamed articular cartilage associated with deep injury contains a variety of factors that act as catalysts for the healing process. Interleukin-1 has chemotactic activity and may induce the production of chondrocyte proteases. In addition mononuclear cell factor (MCF), catabolin, and lymphocyte activating factor (LAF) may serve as messengers that stimulate the production of enzymes from chondrocytes.[157-159] In pathologically healing joint cartilage, PGE_2 has been implicated in the release of calcium and may foster the deposition of calcium crystals in the joint.[157] As the inflammatory response subsides, the granulation tissue continues to fill the defect and bonds to the cartilage surface. Fibroblasts migrate along with the vascular ingrowth and begin to synthesize fibrous tissue, which undergoes chondrification. Fibrocartilage intermediates are found spanning the gap of the injury. Gradually, hyaline cartilage is formed, which heals the wound and helps to restore the structural and functional integrity of the original cartilage. The durability and quality of repair depend on the clinical parameters surrounding the deep cartilage injury and the institution of a successful sequence of extrinsic healing. Whether or not normal function is restored or chronic arthritis and joint dysfunction develop is determined by the degree of trauma and the adequacy of the healing response.

Articular and growth plate cartilage display bioelectrical properties. Electronegative charges are associated with areas of growth and may have many similarities to the reparative and regenerative processes of bone.[160] Perhaps the piezoelectrical phenomenon found in bone has a correlate in cartilage healing. Evidence supports the use of continuous passive motion to foster cartilage repair in full-thickness articular defects (Fig. 23–22).[161] The mechanisms and regulation of cartilage repair await further clarification and may provide a fertile area for research on the progression of joint disease such as osteoarthritis and the proper treatment of joint injuries.

Healing of Cartilage Grafts

Grafts of autogenous cartilage are used extensively to alter nasal form in rhinoplasty and to

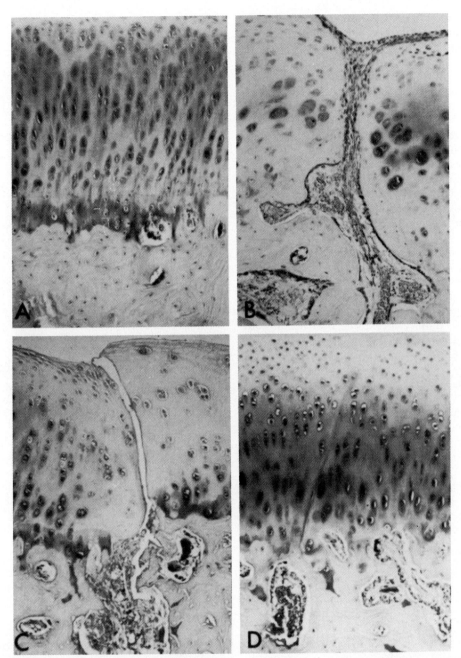

Figure 23–22. Photomicrograph of the experimental fracture site in articular cartilage (safranin O stain). *A,* Normal intact articular cartilage of the femoral condyle of a rabbit. *B,* After 4 weeks of cast immobilization the fracture in the cartilage has healed by fibrous scar tissue. *C,* After 4 weeks of cage activity the fracture has failed to heal. *D,* After 4 weeks of continuous passive motion the fracture in the cartilage has healed well by cartilage. (From Salter RB: Textbook of Disorders and Injuries of the Musculoskeletal System, p 365. © 1983, The Williams & Wilkins Co., Baltimore.)

reconstruct the external ear and the eyelid. These grafts appear to maintain structure and volume over time with minimal resorption. Growth of these grafts has been experimentally demonstrated.[162] It is felt that because cartilage has no blood vessels and is nourished by diffusion, the chondrocytes are able to continue to live by diffusion and maintain the surrounding matrix in their new site. This allows rib cartilage to remain structurally sound when carved into an ear and ear cartilage to remain elastic and pliable when transferred to the nasal tip.[163]

Carving and contouring of cartilage can alter the balance in tension between the outer and inner layers and produce warping of the cartilage over time. This has been particularly important clinically in rib cartilage grafts to the dorsum of the nose and seems to be reduced by carving in balanced cross section (Figs. 23–23 and 24).[163] The propensity of cartilage to warp over time when manipulated or injured also undoubtedly is important in the deviation of a fractured nasal septum some time after injury.

Cartilage can also be grafted with skin as a composite graft to restore structural integrity and skin cover. The most common transfer is from the ear to the nasal rim. The maximum size graft that can be transferred varies with the character of the bed but is approximately 1.0 to 1.5 cm in diameter. Healing of these grafts is similar to that of skin grafts, with the take of the skin maintaining the underlying cartilage. Cartilage allografts have been used as implants as well, but they resorb to varying degrees over time and do not maintain their volume as well as autografts.[164, 165] This is presumably due to antigenic stimulation of the host leading to inflammation and resorption.

CONCLUSION

In bone, the inflammatory phase and particularly the release of growth factors are of critical

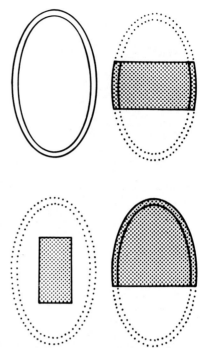

Figure 23–24. Four basic, balanced cross sections of rib cartilage (assuming a symmetric distribution of stresses). While these assumptions do not always hold true over time, carving in this manner can produce nonbending grafts. (From Gibson T, Davis WB: The distortion of autogenous grafts: Its cause and prevention. Br J Plast Surg 10:257, 1958.)

importance to the repair of damaged tissue. One can see that growth factors are central biological regulators that orchestrate the repair of tissue, in this case the formation and remodeling of callus. Therefore, this aspect of tissue repair is common to both soft and hard tissue repair.

Because of its biomechanical properties, piezoelectrical potentials generated in bone appear to significantly affect the healing process. Whereas this effect has been well-documented in bone both in research and in clinical settings, the importance of electrical fields in soft tissue healing remains speculative. Future research may determine if this bioelectrical effect is restricted to hard tissue. Of particular importance is the possibility that biophysical properties such as piezoelectrical potentials can be manipulated to foster functional cartilage repair. The repair of damaged joint cartilage without the formation of a type I collagenous scar awaits significant experimental and clinical advances before consistent clinical results are possible.

The study of bone and cartilage healing continues to be a challenging field of study, with many of the fundamental regulatory mechanisms controlling these yet to be elucidated.

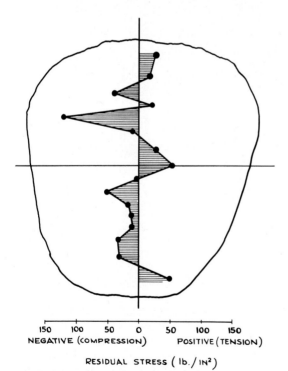

RESIDUAL STRESS (lb. / IN²)

150	100	50	0	50	100	150
NEGATIVE (COMPRESSION)				POSITIVE (TENSION)		

Figure 23–23. Alternating compression and tension stresses in a cartilaginous rib from a 50-year-old male. (From Gibson T: Cartilage grafts. Br Med Bull 21:153, 1965.)

The next decade should see major advances, particularly in the area of growth factors, with application to the clinical setting not far beyond.

REFERENCES

1. Brighton CT: Principles of fracture healing. In Murry JA (ed): Instructional Course Lectures. St. Louis, CV Mosby, 1984, pp 60–82.
2. Cruess RL: Healing of bone, tendon, and ligament. In Rockwood CA, Green DP (eds): Fractures in Adults. Philadelphia, JB Lippincott, 1984, pp 147–169.
3. Simmons DJ: Fracture healing. In Urist MR (ed): Fundamental and Clinical Bone Physiology. Philadelphia, JB Lippincott, 1980, pp 283–330.
4. Uam AW: A histologic study of the early phases of bone repair. J Bone Joint Surg 12:827–844, 1930.
5. Wray JB: Acute changes in femoral arterial blood flow after closed tibial fractures in dogs. J Bone Joint Surg 6A:1261–1268, 1964.
6. Beufu C, Xuemmy T: Ultra structure investigation of experimental fracture healing. I. Electromicroscopic observation of cellular activity. Chin Med J 92:530–535, 1979.
7. Potts WJ: The role of the hematoma in fracture healing. Surg Gynecol Obstet 57:318–324, 1933.
8. Duthie RB, Barker AN: The histochemistry of the pre-osseous stage of bone repair studied by autoradiography. J Bone Joint Surg 37B:691–710, 1955.
9. Gothlin G, Ericsson JLE: The osteoclast: review of ultrastructure, origin, and structure-function relationship. Clin Orthop 120:201–231, 1976.
10. Simmons DJ, Kahn AJ: Cell lineage in fracture healing in chimeric bone grafts. Calcif Tiss Res 27:247–253, 1974.
11. Ashhurst DE: The influence of mechanical conditions on the healing of experimental fractures in the rabbit: A microscopic study. Trans R Soc Lond B313:271–302, 1986.
12. Ashton BA, Allen TD, Howlett CR, et al: Formation of bone and cartilage by marrow stromal cells in diffusion chambers in vivo. Clin Orthop 151:294–307, 1980.
13. Tonna EA, Cronkite EP: The periosteum: Autoradiographic studies on cellular proliferation and transformation utilizing tritiated thymidine. Clin Orthop 30:218–233, 1963.
14. Trueta J: The role of the vessels in osteogenesis. J Bone Joint Surg 45B:402–418, 1963.
15. Rhinelorder FW, Baragri RA: Microangiography in bone healing. I. Undisplaced closed fractures. J Bone Joint Surg 44A:1273–1298, 1962.
16. Sandberg M, Aro H, Multimaki P, et al: In situ localization of collagen production by chondrocytes and osteoblasts in fracture callus. J Bone Joint Surg 71A:69–77, 1989.
17. Nemeth, GG, Bolander ME, Martin GR, et al: Growth factors and their role in wound and fracture healing. In Hunt TK, Pines E, Barbul A, et al (eds): Growth Factors and Other Aspects of Wound Healing. Biological and Clinical Implications. New York, Alan R. Liss, 1989, pp 1–17.
18. Lane JM, Boskey AL, Li WKP, et al: A temporal study of collagen, proteoglycans, lipids and mineral constituents in a model of endochondral osseus repair. Metab Bone Dis Rel Dis 1:319–324, 1979.
19. Davy DT, Connolly JF: The biomechanical behavior of healing canine radii and ribs. J Biomech 15:235–247, 1982.
20. Lane J, Suda M, Von der Mark K, et al: Immunofluorescent localization of structural collagen types in endochondral fracture repair. J Orthop Res 4:318–329, 1986.
21. Wheater PR, Burkill UG, Daniels VG: Functional Histology. London, Churchill Livingstone, 1980.
22. Frost HM: Skeletal physiology and bone remodeling. In Urist MR (ed): Fundamental and Clinical Bone Physiology. Philadelphia, JB Lippincott, 1980, pp 208–241.
23. Frost HM: Bone Remodeling and Its Relation to Metabolic Bone Disease. Springfield, IL, Charles C Thomas, 1973.
24. Rahn BA, Gallinaro P, Baltensperger A, et al: Primary bone healing. An experimental study in the rabbit. J Bone Joint Surg 53A:783–786, 1971.
25. Perren SM: Physical and biological aspects of fracture healing with special reference to internal fixation. Clin Orthop 138:175–196, 1979.
26. McKibbon B: The biology of fracture healing in long bones. J Bone Joint Surg 60B:150–162, 1978.
27. Frost HM: The biology of fracture healing. I. An overview for clinicians. Clin Orthop 248:283–293, 1989.
28. Urist MR: Bone transplantation. In Urist MR (ed): Fundamental and Clinical Bone Physiology. Philadelphia, JB Lippincott, 1980, pp 331–368.
29. Phemister DB: The fate of transplanted bone and regenerative power in its various constituents. Surg Gynecol Obstet 19:303–333, 1914.
30. Sampath TK, Mothokumaran N, Reddi AH, et al: Isolation of osteogenin and extracellular matrix associated bone inductive protein by heparin affinity chromatography. Proc Natl Acad Sci USA 84:7109–7113, 1987.
31. Urist MR: Bone formation by autoinduction. Science 150:893–899, 1965.
32. Urist MR, Delange RJ, Finerman GAM: Bone cell differentiation and growth factors. Science 220:680–686, 1983.
33. Miller TA, Kobayashi M, Douglas W, et al: The induction of bone by an osteogenic factor and the conduction of bone by porous hydroxyapatite. A preliminary laboratory study. Abstr Am Assoc Plast Surg 61–62, 1989.
34. Ferguson D, Davis WL, Hurst MR, et al: Bovine bone morphogenetic protein (bBMP) fraction induced repair of craniotomy defects in the rhesus monkey (Macaca sepciosa). Clin Orthop Rel Res 219:251–258, 1987.
35. Lindholm TC, Lindholm TS, Alitalo I, et al: Bovine bone morphogenetic protein (bBMP) induced repair of skull trephine defects in sheep. Clin Orthop Rel Res 227:265–268, 1988.
36. Sato K, Urist MR: Induced regeneration of calvaria by bone morphogenetic protein (BMP) in dogs. Clin Orthop Rel Res 197:301–311, 1985.
37. Nilsson OS, Urist MR, Davson EG, et al: Bone repair induced by bone morphogenetic protein in ulnar defects in dogs. J Bone Joint Surg 68B:635–642, 1986.
38. Lindholm TS, Urist MR: A quantitative analysis of new bone formation by induction in composite grafts of bone marrow and bone matrix. Clin Orthop 150:288–300, 1980.
39. Canalis E, Centrella M, Urist MR: Effect of partially purified bone morphogenetic protein on DNA synthesis and cell replication in calvarial and fibro-

blast cultures. Clin Orthop Rel Res 198:289–296, 1985.

40. Reddi AH, Ma SS, Cunningham NS, et al: Induction and maintenance of new bone formation by growth and differentiation factors. Ann Chir Gynaecol 77:189–192, 1988.

41. Simmons DJ: Fracture healing perspectives. Clin Orthop Rel Res 200:100–113, 1985.

42. Purves LR, Purves M, Hickman R, et al: The role of plasma fibronectin. Suid-Afrikaanse Tydskrif vir Wetenskap, 80:469–474, 1984.

43. Weiss RE, Reddi AH: Synthesis and location of fibronectin during collagenous matrix-mesenchymal cell interaction and differentiation of cartilage and bone. Proc Natl Acad Sci USA 77:2074–2078, 1980.

44. DiCorleto PE, Gajdusek CM, Schwartz SM, et al: Biochemical properties of the endothelium derived growth factor: Comparison to other growth factors. J Cell Physiol 114:339–345, 1983.

45. Gajdusek CM: Release of endothelial cell-derived growth factor (ECDGF) by heparin. J Cell Physiol 121:13–21, 1984.

46. Rifas L, Shen V, Mitchell K, et al: Macrophage-derived growth factor for osteoblast-like cells and chondrocytes. Proc Natl Acad Sci USA 81:4558–4562, 1984.

47. Williams LT, Antoniades HN, Goetzl EJ: Platelet-derived growth factor stimulates mouse 3T3 cell mitogenesis and leukocyte chemotaxis through different structural determinants. J Clin Invest 72:1759–1763, 1983.

48. Canalis E: Effect of growth factors on bone cell replication and differentiation. Clin Orthop 193:246–263, 1985.

49. Key LL Jr, Carnes DL Jr, Weichselbaum P, et al: Platelet-derived growth factor stimulates bone resorption by monocyte monolayers. Endocrinology 112:761–762, 1983.

50. Feldman EJ, Aures D, Grossman MJ: Epidermal growth factor stimulates ornithine decarboxylase activity in the digestive tract of mouse. Proc Soc Exp Biol Med 159:400–408, 1978.

51. Franklin JD, Lynch JB: Effects of topical applications of epidermal growth factor on wound healing. Plast Reconstr Surg 64:766–770, 1979.

52. Hill DJ, Holder AT, Seid J, et al: Increased thymidine incorporation into fetal rat cartilage in vitro in the presence of human somatomedin, epidermal growth factor and other growth factors. Endocrinology 96:489–497, 1983.

53. Canalis E, Raisz LG: Effect of epidermal growth factor on bone formation in vitro. Endocrinology 104:862–869, 1979.

54. Graves DT, Owen AJ, Antoniades HN: Evidence that a human osteosarcoma cell line which secretes a mitogen similar to platelet-derived growth factor requires growth factors present in platelet-poor plasma. Cancer Res 43:83–87, 1983.

55. Ng KW, Patridge NC, Niall M, et al: Epidermal growth factor receptors in clonal lines of a rat osteogeneic sarcoma and in osteoblast-rich rat bone cells. Calcif Tissue Int 35:298–303, 1983.

56. Canalis E, Peck WA, Raisz LG: Stimulation of DNA and collagen synthesis by autologous growth factor in cultured fetal rat calvaria. Science 210:1021–1023, 1980.

57. Hata HH, Jori H, Nagai Y, et al: Selective inhibition of Type I collagen synthesis in osteoblastic cells by epidermal growth factor. Endocrinology 115:867–876, 1984.

58. Kumegawa M, Hiramatsu M, Hatakeyama K, et al:

Effects of epidermal growth factor on osteoblastic cells. Calcif Tissue Int 35:542–548, 1983.

59. Osaki Y, Tsunoi M, Hakeda Y, et al: Immunocytochemical study of collagen in epidermal growth factor (EGF)-treated osteoblastic cells. J Histochem Cytochem 32:1231–1233, 1984.

60. Adolphe M, Froger B, Ronot X, et al: Cell multiplication and Type II collagen production by rabbit articular chondrocytes cultivated in a defined medium. Exper Cell Res 155:527–536, 1984.

61. Wellmitz G, Petzold E, Jentzsch KD, et al: The effect of brain fraction with fibroblast growth factor activity on regeneration and differentiation of articular cartilage. Exper Pathol (Jena) 18:282–287, 1980.

62. Jennings J, Buchanan F, Freeman D, et al: Stimulation of chick embryo cartilage sulfate and thymidine uptake: Comparison of human serum, purified somatomedins, and other growth factors. J Clin Endocrinol Metab 51:1166–1170, 1980.

63. Nevo Z: Somatomedins as regulators of proteoglycan synthesis. Connect Tiss Res 10:109–113, 1982.

64. Huff KR, Guroff G: Nerve growth factor–induced reduction in epidermal growth factor responsiveness and epidermal growth factor receptors in PC12 cells: An aspect of cell differentiation. Biochem Biophys Res Commun 89:175–180, 1979.

65. Azizkhan JC, Klagsbrun M: Chondrocytes contain a growth factor that is localized in the nucleus and is associated with chromatin. Proc Natl Acad Sci USA 77:2762–2766, 1980.

66. Klagsbrun M, Langer R, Levenson R, et al: The stimulation of DNA synthesis and cell division in chondrocytes and 3T3 cells as a growth factor isolated from cartilage. Exper Cell Res 105:99–109, 1977.

67. Klagsbrun M, Smith S: Purification of a cartilage derived growth factor. J Biol Chem 25:10859–10866, 1980.

68. Shen V, Rifas L, Kohler G, et al: Fetal rat chondrocytes sequentially elaborate separate growth- and differentiation-promoting peptides during their development in vitro. Endocrinology 116:920–925, 1985.

69. Kuhlman RE: Functioning enzyme systems in skeletal tissue and their relationship to structure. In Urist MR (ed): Fundamental and Clinical Physiology. Philadelphia, JB Lippincott, 1980, pp 172–207.

70. Peck WA, Rifas L: Regulation of osteoblast activity and the osteoblast-osteocyte transformation. In Massry S, Letteri J, Ritz ER (eds): Regulation of Phosphate and Mineral Metabolism. New York, Plenum Press, 1982, pp 393–400.

71. Holtrop ME, Raisz LG, King GJ: The response of osteoclasts to prostaglandin and osteoclast activating factor as measured by ultrastructural morphometry. In Horton JE, Tarpley TM, Davis WF (eds): Mechanisms of Localized Bone Loss. Calcified Tissue Abstracts. Information Retrieval, 1977, p 13.

72. Horton JE, Raisz LG, Simmons HA, et al: Bone resorbing activity in supernatant fluid from cultured human peripheral blood leukocytes. Science 177:793–795, 1972.

73. Raisz LG, Luben RA, Mundy GR, et al: Effect of osteoclast activating factor from human leukocytes on bone metabolism. J Clin Invest 56:408–413, 1975.

74. Chikuma T, Kato T, Hiramatsu M, et al: Effect of epidermal growth factor on dipeptidyl-aminopeptidase and collagenase-like peptidase activities in cloned osteoblastic cells. J Biochem 95:283–286, 1984.

75. Lorenzo JA, Quinton J, Sousa S, et al: Effects of

DNA and prostaglandin inhibitors on the stimulation of resorption by epidermal growth factor in fetal rat long bone cultures. J Clin Invest 77:1897–1902, 1982.

76. Tashjian AH, Levine L: Epidermal growth factor stimulates prostaglandin production and bone resorption in cultured mouse calvaria. Biochem Biophys Res Commun 85:966–975, 1978.

77. Dieter A, Prins A, Lipman JM, et al: Effect of purified growth factors on rabbit articular chondrocytes in monolayer culture. I. DNA synthesis. Arthritis Rheum 25:1217–1227, 1982.

78. Beresford JN, Gallagher JA, Gowen M, et al: The effects of monocyte-conditioned medium and interleukin I on the synthesis of collagenous and non-collagenous proteins by mouse bone and human bone cells in vitro. Biochim Biophys Acta 801:58–65, 1984.

79. Schmidt JA, Mizel SB, Cohen D, et al: Interleukin I, a potential regulator of fibroblast proliferation. J Immunol 128:2177–2182, 1982.

80. Millis AJT, Hoyle M, Field B: Human fibroblast conditioned media contains growth-promoting activities for low density cells. J Cell Physiol 93:17–24, 1977.

81. Cheever MA, Thompson JA, Kern DE, et al: Interleukin-2 administered in vivo induces the growth and augments the function of cultured T cells in vivo. J Biol Response Mod 3:462–467, 1984.

82. Smith KA: T-cell growth factor. Immunol Rev 51:337–357, 1980.

83. Howes R, Bowness JM, Grotendorst GR, et al: Platelet derived growth factor enhances demineralized bone matrix induced cartilage and bone formation. Calcif Tissue Int 42:34–38, 1988.

84. Grotendorst GR, Grotendorst CA, Gilman T, et al: Production of growth factors (PDGF & TGFβ) at the site of tissue repair. In Hunt TK, Pines E, Barbul A (eds): Growth Factors and Other Aspects of Wound Healing: Biological and Clinical Implications. New York, Alan R. Liss, 1988, pp 47–54.

85. Dominquez J, Mundy GR: Monocytes mediate bone resorption by prostaglandin production. Calcif Tissue Int 31:29–34, 1980.

86. Schmidt JA, Mizel SB, Cohen D, et al: Interleukin I, a potential regulator of fibroblast proliferation. J Immunol, 128:2177–2182, 1982.

87. Barbul A: Role of T cell dependent immune system in wound healing. In Hunt TK, Pines E, Barbul A (eds): Growth Factors and Other Aspects of Wound Healing: Biological and Clinical Implications. New York, Alan R. Liss, 1989, pp 161–175.

88. McGrath MH: Peptide growth factors and wound healing. In Rudolph R, Miller SU (eds): Wound Healing. Philadelphia, WB Saunders, 1990, pp 421–432.

89. Luben RA, Mundy GR, Trummel CL: Partial purification of osteoclast activating factor from phytohemagglutinin stimulated human leukocytes. J Clin Invest 53:1473–1480, 1974.

90. Sporn MB, Roberts AB: Transforming growth factor-B: Multiple actions and potential clinical applications. JAMA 262:938–941, 1989.

91. Weiss RE, Reddi AH: Role of fibronectin in collagenous matrix-induced mesenchymal cell proliferation and differentiation in vivo. Exper Cell Res 133:247–254, 1981.

92. Bassett CAL: Current concepts of bone formation. J Bone Joint Surg 44A:1217–1244, 1962.

93. Jargiello DM, Caplan AJ: The establishment of vascular-derived microenvironments in the developing chicken wing. Dev Biol 97:364–374, 1983.

94. Brighton CT, Krebs AG: Oxygen tension of healing fractures in the rabbit. J Bone Joint Surg 54A:323–332, 1972.

95. Brighton CT, Hay RD, Sobel LW, et al: In vitro epiphyseal plate growth in various oxygen tensions. J Bone Joint Surg 51A:1383–1396, 1969.

96. Brighton CT, Wirt RM: Mitochondrial calcium and its role in calcification. Clin Orthop 100:406–416, 1974.

97. Brockes M: The Blood Supply of Bone. New York, Appleton-Century-Crofts, 1971.

98. Heppenstall RB, Grislig G: Tissue gas tensions and oxygen consumption and healing bone defects. Clin Orthop 106:357–365, 1975.

99. Wolff J: Das gaetz der Transformation. Transformation der Knocken. Berlin, Hirschwald, 1892.

100. Bassett CAL: Biophysical principles affect bone structure. In Bovine GU (ed): The Biochemistry and Physiology of Bone. New York, Academic Press, 1971.

101. Bassett CAL, Becker RO: Generation of electrical potentials by bone in response to mechanical stress. Science 137:1063–1064, 1962.

102. Fukada E, Yasuda I: On the piezoelectric effect of bone. J Physiol Soc Jpn 12:1158–1166, 1957.

103. Bassett CAL: Review: Biological significance of piezoelectricity. Calcif Tissue Res 1:252–272, 1968.

104. Friedenberg ZB, Brighton CT: Bioelectric potentials in bone. J Bone Joint Surg 48(A):915–923, 1966.

105. Brighton CT: The semi-invasive method of treating non-union with direct current. Orthop Clin N Am 15:33–45, 1984.

106. Davy DT, Connolly JF: The biomechanical behavior of healing canine radii and ribs. J Biomech 15:235–247, 1982.

107. Christel P, Cerf G, Pilla AA: Evolution des propriétés mecaniques du cal de fracture jusqua consolidation chèz le rat. J Biophys Med Nucl 5:21–33, 1981.

108. White AA, Panjabi MM, Southwick WO, et al: The four biomechanical stages of fracture repair. J Bone Joint Surg 59A:188–192, 1977.

109. Heppenstall RB: Delayed union, non-union, and pseudarthrosis. In Heppenstall RB (ed): Fracture Treatment and Healing. Philadelphia, WB Saunders, 1980, pp 80–96.

110. Frankel VU, Bystein AU: Orthopaedic Biomechanics. Philadelphia, Lea & Febiger, 1970.

111. Sarmiento A, Mullis DL, Latta LL, et al: A quantitative comparative analysis of fracture healing under the influence of compression plating vs. closed weight-bearing treatment. Clin Orthop 149:232–239, 1980.

112. Yaremchuk MJ, Brimback RJ, Menson PN, et al: Acute and definitive management of traumatic osteocutaneous defects of the lower extremity. Plast Reconstr Surg 80:1–12, 1987.

113. Urist MR, Matzet R Jr, McLean FC: The pathogenesis and treatment of delayed union and non-union. A survey of eighty-five ununited fractures of the shaft of the tibia and one hundred control cases with similar injuries. J Bone Joint Surg 34A:931–967, 1954.

114. Eshima I, Mathes SJ, Paty P: Comparison of the intracellular bacterial killing of leukocytes in musculocutaneous and random-pattern flaps. Plast Reconstr Surg 86:541–547, 1990.

115. Maseum M, Greenburg BM, Hoffman C, et al: Comparative bacterial clearances of muscle and skin/subcutaneous tissues with and without dead bone: A laboratory study. Plast Reconstr Surg 85:773–781, 1990.

116. Richards RR, Orsini EC, Maheavey JL, et al: The influence of muscle flap coverage on the repair of

devascularized tibial cortex: An experimental investigation in the dog. Plast Reconstr Surg 79:946–956, 1982.

117. Bassett CAL, Mitchell SN, Gaston SR, et al: Treatment of ununited tibial diaphyseal fractures with pulsing electromagnetic fields. J Bone Joint Surg 62A:511–523, 1981.

118. Lavine SL, Grodzinsky AJ: Electrical stimulation of repair of bone. J Bone Joint Surg 69A:626–630, 1987.

119. Goldberg VM, Shaffer JW, Field G, et al: Biology of vascularized bone grafts. Orthop Clin North Am 18:197–205, 1987.

120. Motoki DS, Mulliken JB: The healing of bone and cartilage. Clin Plast Surg 17:527–544, 1990.

121. Phemister DB: The state of transplanted bone and regenerative power of its various constituents. Surg Gynecol Obstet 19:303–333, 1914.

122. Burchardt H: The biology of bone graft repair. Clin Orthop 174:28–42, 1983.

123. Burchardt H: Biology of bone transplantation. Orthop Clin N Am 18:187–196, 1987.

124. Delea J, Trueta J: Vascularization of bone grafts in the anterior chamber of the eye. J Bone Joint Surg 47B:319–329, 1965.

125. Enneking WF, Burchardt H, Puhl JJ, et al: Physical and biological aspects of repair in dog cortical bone transplants. J Bone Joint Surg 57A:237–252, 1975.

126. Knize DM: The influence of periosteum and calcitonin on onlay graft survival. Plast Reconstr Surg 53:190–199, 1974.

127. Thompson N, Casson JA: Experimental onlay bone grafts to the jaws. A preliminary study in dogs. Plast Reconstr Surg 46:341–348, 1970.

128. Zins JE, Kusiak JF, Whitaker LA, et al: The influence of recipient site on bone grafts to the face. Plast Reconstr Surg 73:371–379, 1984.

129. Smith JD, Abramson M: Membranes vs. endochondral bone autografts. Arch Otolaryngol 99:203–205, 1974.

130. Zins JE, Whitaker CA: Membranes versus endochondral bone: Implications for craniofacial reconstruction. Plast Reconstr Surg 72:778–785, 1983.

131. Phillips JH, Rahn BA: Fixation effects on membranous and endochondral onlay bone-graft resorption. Plast Reconstr Surg 92:872–877, 1988.

132. Lin KY, Bartlett SP, Yaremchuk MJ, et al: The effect of rigid fixation on the survival of onlay bone grafts: An experimental study. Plast Reconstr Surg 86:449–456, 1990.

133. Whitaker LA: Biological boundaries: A concept in facial skeletal restructuring. Clin Plast Surg 16:1–10, 1989.

134. Holmes RE: Bone regeneration within a coralline hydroxyapatite implant. Plast Reconstr Surg 63:626–633, 1979.

135. Deeb ME, Waite DE, Mainous EG: Correction of the deficient alveolar ridge. Clin Plast Surg 16:733–748, 1989.

136. Rosen HM, McFarland MM: The biologic behavior of hydroxyapatite implanted into the maxillofacial skeleton. Plast Reconstr Surg 85:718–723, 1990.

137. Chiroff RT, White EW, Weber KN, et al: Tissue ingrowth of replamineform implant. J Biomed Mater Res 9:29–45, 1975.

138. Finn RA, Bell WH, Brammer JA: Interpositional "grafting" with autogenous bone and coralline hydroxyapatite. Maxillofac Surg 8:217–227, 1980.

139. Piecuch JF, Topazian RG, Skoly S, et al: Experimental ridge augmentation with porous hydroxyapatite implants. J Dent Res 62:148–154, 1983.

140. Wolford LM, Wardrop RW, Hartog JM: Coralline porous hydroxyapatite as a bone graft substitute in orthognathic surgery. J Oral Maxillofac Surg 45:1034–1042, 1987.

141. Kenney EB, Lekovic V, Han T, et al: The use of porous hydroxyapatite implants in periodontal defects. I. Clinical results after six months. J Periodontol 56:82–88, 1985.

142. Kenney EB, Lekovic V, SaFerreira JC, et al: Bone formation within porous hydroxyapatite implants in human periodontal defects. J Periodontol 57:76–83, 1986.

143. Bucholz RW, Holmes RE, Mooney V: Synthetic hydroxyapatite as a bone-graft substitute in traumatic defects of long bones. Transactions of the 53rd Annual Meeting of the American Academy of Orthopaedic Surgeons. New Orleans, 1986, p 149.

144. Piecuch JF: Augmentation of the atrophic edentulous ridge with porous replamineform hydroxyapatite. Dent Clin North Am 30:291–305, 1986.

145. Salyer KE, Hall CD: Porous hydroxyapatite as an onlay graft in maxillofacial surgery. Plast Reconstr Surg 84:236–244, 1989.

146. Holmes RE, Wardrop RW, Wolford LM: Hydroxyapatite as a bone graft substitute in orthognathic surgery: Histologic and histometric findings. J Oral Maxillofac Surg 46:661–671, 1988.

147. Marx RE, Ames JR: The use of hyperbaric oxygen therapy in bony reconstruction of the irradiated or tissue-deficient patient. J Oral Maxillofac Surg 40:4120–4200, 1982.

148. Hunter W: Study of the structure and diseases of articulating cartilage. Philos Trans R Soc 42:514–521, 1743.

149. Albright JA, Musra RP: Mechanisms of resorption and remodeling of cartilage. In Hall BK (ed): Cartilage: Biomedical Aspects. Vol. 3. New York, Academic Press, 1983, pp 49–86.

150. Campbell CJ: The healing of cartilage defects. Clin Orthop 64:45–63, 1964.

151. Fuller JA, Ghadially FN: Ultrastructural observations on surgically produced partial thickness defects in articular cartilage. Clin Orthop 86:193–205, 1972.

152. Mankin HJ: Localization of tritiated thymidine in articular cartilage of rabbits. II. Repair in immature cartilage. J Bone Joint Surg 44A:688–698, 1962.

153. Mankin HJ, Boyle CJ: The acute effects of lacerative injury on DNA and protein synthesis in articular cartilage. In Baset CAL (ed): Cartilage Degradation and Repair, Washington, DC, National Academy of Science, N.R.L., 1967, pp 185–199.

154. Kosher RA: The chondrocyte and chondroblast. In Hall BK (ed): Cartilage: Structure, Function and Biochemistry. New York, Academic Press, 1983, pp 59–85.

155. Gay S, Müller PK, Lemmen C, et al: Immunohistological study on collagen in cartilage-bone metamorphosis and degenerative osteoarthrosis. Klin Wschr 54:969–976, 1976.

156. Ghadially JA, Thomas I, Oryschak AF, et al: Long-term results of deep defects in articular cartilages: A scanning electron microscopic study. Virchow Arch Cell Pathol 25:125–136, 1977.

157. Dayer JM, Krane SM, Goldring SR, et al: Cellular and humoral factors modulate connective tissue destruction and repair in arthritic diseases. Semin Arthritis Rheum 11:77–81, 1981.

158. Mizel SB: Characterization of lymphocyte activating factor obtained from the murine macrophage cell line P388b. In DeWeck AL, et al (eds): Biochemical Char-

acterization of Lymphokines. New York, Academic Press, 1980, pp 401–418.

159. Dee R, Goral A, Blyznak N: Articular cartilage. In Dee R, Mango E, Hurst LC, et al (eds): Principles of Orthopaedic Practice. Vol. 1. New York, McGraw-Hill, 1988, pp 24–32.

160. Hall BK: Bioelectricity and cartilage. In Hall BK (ed): Cartilage: Biomedical Aspects. New York, Academic Press, 1983, pp 309–338.

161. Salter RB, Simmonds DF, Malcolm BW, et al: The biological effect of continuous passive motion on the healing of full thickness defects in articular cartilage. J Bone Joint Surg 62A:1232–1251, 1980.

162. Stoll DA, Furnus DW: The growth of cartilage trans-

plants in baby rabbits. Plast Reconstr Surg 45:356–359, 1970.

163. Gibson T, Davis WB: The distortion of autogenous cartilage grafts: Its cause and prevention. Br J Plast Surg 10:257–274, 1958.

164. Converse JM: The resorption and shrinkage of maternal ear cartilage used as living homografts: Follow-up report of 21 Gillie's patients. In Converse JM (ed): Reconstructive and Plastic Surgery. Philadelphia, WB Saunders, 1977, p 308.

165. Krutchinskij GV, Schvedi A: Attempt to reconstruct the auricle using ear cartilage from a living donor. Acta Chir Plast (Prague) 26:100–106, 1984.

24
TENDON AND LIGAMENT

Peter C. Amadio, M.D.

Tendon and ligament are specialized connective tissues that link muscle to bone and bone to bone, respectively. These tissues are generally similar in their composition, consisting of parallel bundles of collagen fibers interspersed with spindle-shaped cells.[1] The fibers are oriented in the direction of and generally serve to resist tensile stress. Despite the general similarity of tendon and ligament, specialized modifications of these tissues do occur in response to local mechanical and nutritional environments, and these localized differences may affect the response of tendon or ligament tissue to injury. This chapter discusses the general structure of tendon and ligament tissue; specialized structures that may occur in response to mechanical and nutritional factors; the general response to injury; the response of specialized structures to injury; and research efforts to improve the rate or quality of healing of these tissues.

GENERAL STRUCTURE OF TENDON AND LIGAMENT

The spindle-shaped fibrocytes typical of tendon and ligament secrete a matrix that consists predominantly of type I collagen but also has a significant component of dermatan sulfate–containing, low molecular weight, nonaggregating proteoglycan.[2, 3] The type and amount of proteoglycan serves to regulate the size and packing of the collagen fibrils and thus tissue strength, which is proportional to the collagen fibril diameter.[4, 5] The type and amount of proteoglycan synthesis appears also to be affected by the mechanical environment to which

the tendon or ligament is exposed,[6, 7] although how this is mediated is unknown. Stress-induced electrical potentials[8] or a direct mechanical effect on pericellular proteoglycans[3] and specialized collagens[9] may serve as signals recognizable by the cell and may result in change in proteoglycan synthesis. Regardless of the details of the regulatory process, in adult tissue the typical tendon or ligament has a bimodal distribution of collagen fibril diameters, with clustering at 100 nm and 200 nm.[5, 10] However, this distribution appears to vary with tissue loading, with a greater shift towards higher fibril diameters with increasing tensile loads and unimodal distribution in tendons that experience compressive loading (see below).

At the molecular level, as discussed in chapter 8, the collagen fibrils consist of helically arranged bundles of tropocollagen molecules in 64 nm quarter-stagger arrangement and the tropocollagen molecules themselves are in a helical arrangement of two α1 (I) and one α2 (I) collagen chain, each molecule itself helical.[11]

In a hierarchy[12] reminiscent of the fractal scaling seen in other biological tissues,[13] the collagen fibrils are themselves wound into fascicles that in turn can often be seen to spiral, particularly in tendons (Fig. 24–1). A characteristic crimp structure is also seen in tendons and ligaments at rest.[14, 15] This waviness histologically and even grossly seems to represent some inherent structural slackness, which is removed by application of a small amount of tensile stress. This initial stress results in a fairly large strain, or change in length, that is nonlinear in nature; after the crimp is removed, the stress-strain relationship in tendon and ligament remains linear until close to the failure point (Fig. 24–2).[16, 17]

Developmentally, both tendon and ligament begin as undifferentiated mesenchymal tissue

HIERARCHY OF TENDON STRUCTURE

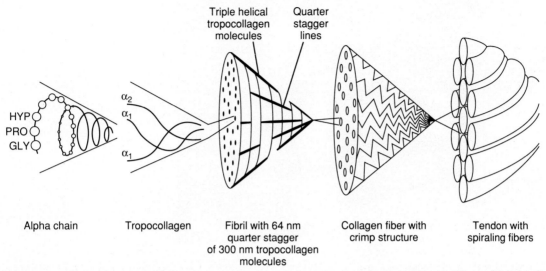

Figure 24–1. Hierarchy of tendon structure. (Modified from Kastelic J, Galeski A, Baer E: The multicomposite structure of tendon. Conn Tiss Res 6:11–23, 1978.)

that differentiates in response to muscular tension and joint movement, respectively.[18, 19] In embryos experimentally treated to prevent muscular and joint development, differentiation of tendon and ligament is aborted.[20] In normal development, these structures are well-differentiated in the fetus but the collagen fibrils have a unimodal size distribution. The typical tendon and ligament are vascularized via small vessels that enter at multiple levels from the surrounding areolar tissue. Blood flow is low, averaging less than 10 ml per 100 grams per minute.[21]

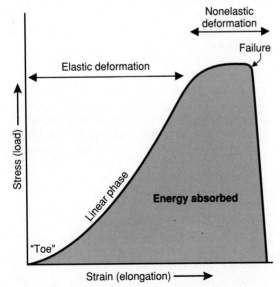

Figure 24–2. Stress-strain curve for typical tendon or ligament.

SPECIALIZED STRUCTURES

Although the preceding general description reflects the organization of tendons and ligaments, there are specialized locations where different structures and arrangements exist. One such specialized arrangement occurs where tendon crosses a joint. Where the tendon crosses the concavity of a joint, as on either side of the wrist or the flexor surface of the fingers, the loose areolar connective tissues surrounding the tendon are replaced by dense fibrous condensations of collagen fibers running at right angles to the tendon and serving to hold the tendon close to the axis of joint motion.[22, 23] Although such a mechanical arrangement decreases the moment arm and thus the net effect of the given tendon force on joint motion, by keeping the tendon close to the joint, it does maximize the joint movement arc provided by a given amount of tendon excursion. This is a point of particular importance in muscle-tendon units that cross more than one joint and for which conservation of excursion is critical.[24, 25] The fibrous condensations are commonly known as pulleys and in humans are most prominent in the hand as the annular and cruciate pulleys of the digits and at the wrist as the flexor and extensor retinacula.

Within the close tolerance of the pulley systems, flexor tendons are covered by a single cell layer epitenon.[26] In the fingers, the pulley system is perforated at the midproximal phalanx

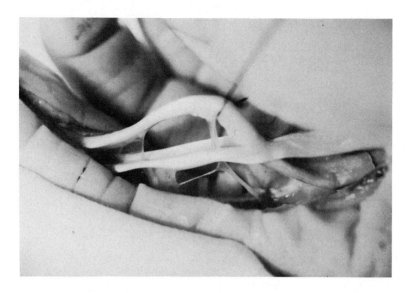

Figure 24–3. The vincula of a human flexor tendon. Notice the broad short vincula to the profundus and superficialis distally and the longer, thinner long vincula to the profundus and superficialis proximally.

and proximal interphalangeal joint levels by vessels that reach the dorsal surface of the tendons by synovial-lined vincula (Fig. 24–3). The epitenon, vincular synovium, and synoviocytes lining the pulleys form a topologically continuous layer that normally secretes synovial fluid to lubricate tendon motion.[26]

Especially in the finger, this specialized arrangement is important for two effects on tendon biology. In addition to the tensional forces transmitted along the tendon, a compression force is added when the tendon comes in contact with the pulley system.[27] The tendon matrix adapts to the compression forces by specific changes in composition and organization seen most obviously in quadrupeds, where the changes are abetted by weightbearing, although to a lesser extent in primates.

The archetypical tissue designed to resist compressive forces is cartilage. In cartilage, the collagen fibers are thin, randomly arranged or arranged in loose arcades, and mixed with a high molecular weight aggregating chondroitin sulfate– and keratan sulfate–containing proteoglycan in a highly hydrated gel. The cells in cartilage are rounded in shape and located within lacunae, specialized pericellular environments that appear matrix free on routine histology but actually contain specialized collagens and proteoglycans.[28] This "compressive pattern" of soft tissue structure mechanically serves as a hydraulic unit able to deform by displacement of water out of the highly electrostatic matrix under compression, then re-imbibing water and resuming its shape when the compression is relieved.[28] In cartilage, which is avascular, this fluid pumping system also serves to promote the flow of nutrients in from, and metabolites out to, the synovial fluid. Tendon under compression is very similar in appearance and composition to fibrocartilage (Fig. 24–4). In the organization of its matrix, it lies midway between uncompressed tendon or ligament on the one hand and hyaline cartilage on the other (Table 24–1).[27]

The response of noncalcified connective tissue to stress by modification of matrix structure is reminiscent of that seen in bone, where this phenomenon is commonly referred to as Wolff's law (Fig. 24–5).[29] In noncalcified tissues, the form-function relationship must take into consideration both tensional and compressive forces and may also be depicted schematically (Fig. 24–6).

As mentioned previously, areas of tendon compression have a different blood supply than noncompressed tendon or ligament. In noncompressed areas, circumferential vascular areolar tissue provides similar vascular nutrition to each point along the length of the tendon or ligament. In compressed areas, nutrition comes from segmental vessels called vincula.[30] Between these segmental vessels and especially in areas of high compressive forces, the tendon may be completely avascular, presumably relying on synovial fluid pumping for nutrition. Such pumping has been observed experimentally, and small canaliculi seem to be present to carry nutrients into the depths of the tendon.[31]

RESPONSE TO INJURY

Tendon and ligaments may be subjected to a variety of injuries, but these can be generally grouped into three categories: laceration, rupture, and cumulative stress. Tendon and liga-

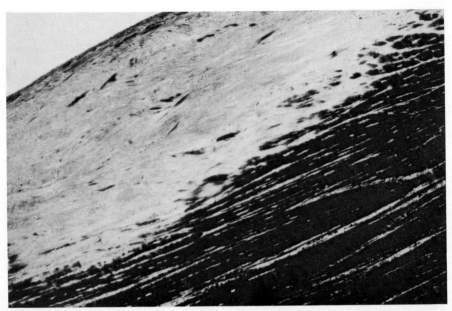

Figure 24–4. Histology of canine flexor tendon in an area exposed to compression (*top left*) and tension (*bottom right*). Note in the compressive area the dispersed nature of the collagen fibers, decreased collagen staining, and rounded appearance of cells. Histologically, this area stains positively for proteoglycan. In the tensile area, note the heavily stained parallel collagen fibers with spindle-shaped cells interspersed. This area stains negatively for proteoglycan.

Table 24–1. COMPARISON OF TENDON UNDER COMPRESSIVE OR TENSIONAL
FORCES AND CARTILAGE

	Tendon Under Tension	Tendon Under Compression	Articular Cartilage
Cells	Along collagen fibers	In lacunae	In lacunae
Blood supply	Vascular	Avascular	Avascular
Glycosaminoglycan	DS*	C-6-S*	C-6-S
Proteoglycan	90% LMW*	50% HMW*	95% HMW
Collagen	Type I	Type I	Type II
Fibril size	Large	Small	Small
Fibril orientation	Parallel to tension	Random	Random

*DS = dermatan sulfate; LMW = low molecular weight; HMW = high molecular weight; C-6-S = chondroitin-6-sulfate.

Figure 24–5. Wolff's law of bone.

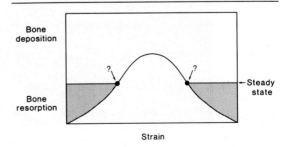

MECHANICAL "WINDOW" OF WOLFF'S LAW

Bone deposition

Bone resorption

Steady state

Strain

WOLFF'S LAW OF SOFT TISSUE

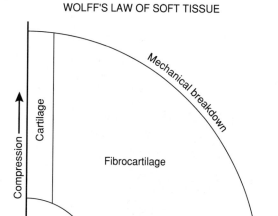

Figure 24–6. Proposed scheme for Wolff's law of soft tissue.

ment respond to laceration as would any incised tissue. Depending upon the degree of bacterial contamination and crush, there is some necrosis at the incised surface. Due either to joint motion or to muscular action, there is often a separation of the incised surfaces. The resulting defect heals, as would any wound, with hema-

toma organization, cellular migration, and scar formation (Fig. 24–7). All the typical elements associated with scar, including random collagen fibril orientation, mixtures of type I and type III collagen and increased water content, DNA content, and total glycosaminoglycan content, are present.[32–34] As the parallel collagen fibers of the two cut ends of the tendon or ligament merge with the disorganized mesh work of collagen fibers in the scar, they tend to transmit at least a portion of the normal physiological stress through the scar, which may serve to organize the scar collagen network in a direction parallel to that of the tendon or ligament as the scar remodels. Although this remodeling process is substantially complete after 3 to 4 months, biochemical differences in collagen type and arrangement, water content, DNA content, and glycosaminoglycan content persist indefinitely and the material properties of these scars never equal those of intact tendon or ligament.[35] If the incised tissue is sutured to reduce gap formation, the extent of mechanical derangement is reduced but not eliminated.[35]

Rupture of tendon or ligament affects the tissue variably, depending in part upon the rate of elongation, or strain rate of the injury. Although tendon or ligament material properties are not strain rate–sensitive, those of bone are, so that a relatively slow strain rate will usually

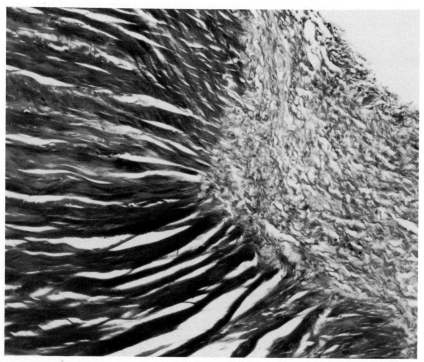

Figure 24–7. Photomicrograph showing healing of a partially lacerated canine flexor tendon by in-migration of cells from the epitenon ($\times 100$).

cause avulsion of the tendon or ligament insertion from bone whereas a more rapid rate will be associated with a midsubstance tear.[36] A tendon or ligament avulsed from its insertion is unlikely to heal unless surgically reattached. Even when reattached, the specialized fixation structure described earlier probably does not re-form, although careful studies in this area are lacking.

Midsubstance tendon or ligament ruptures occur either through aberrant tissue or as the result of high strain rates, as mentioned previously. Either case represents a major disruption of tissue structure, with a typical "rag mop" appearance of the ruptured ends. Structurally, microscopic failure occurs in the collagen fibrils before gross separation occurs,[37] so that just before failure, the tissue lengthens considerably with minimal additional force input creating a second nonlinear part of the tendon stress-strain relationship, similar to that seen when initial stress is applied and the crimp structure is eliminated.[35, 38] This additional degree of injury away from the actual visible site of failure results in larger areas of necrotic tendon or ligament, which must be removed in the course of healing, and consequently a larger scar than would occur with a clean laceration, even if surgical repair is undertaken. Ultimate material properties and functional capabilities after tendon or ligament midsubstance rupture are therefore usually poorer than one would expect with an incised wound.[39, 40]

Cumulative stress on cadaver tendon or ligament will result eventually in tissue failure, given sufficient force and repetitions. Even at lower levels of stress and repetition, microscopic failure and deformation will occur.[41] In living tissue, the possibility for repair and synthesis of a newer, stronger matrix exists and indeed will occur after exercise, although the magnitude of the increase is limited, with work hypertrophy usually not exceeding 50 percent.[42] Hypovascular tendons, such as the sheathed digital tendons, may have a decreased capacity for work hypertrophy.[43] Much of this work hypertrophy actually represents increased crosslinking of existing collagen fibers, creating fibers of greater cross-sectional area and therefore tensile strength.[5, 42] Thus the body efficiently reorganizes existing interstitial proteins and reduces the need for new synthesis. Collagen turnover in tendon and ligament tissue is quite slow, with half-lives estimated at 300 to 500 days, and the time frame for work hypertrophy is consequently long, measured in months to years.[44]

In vivo cumulative stress that exceeds the

Wolff's law capacity for work hypertrophy will result in tendon or ligament breakdown, usually preceded by focal cellular necrosis and matrix calcification.[45] Areas of particular risk for cumulative stress degeneration appear to be those with reduced or absent blood supply, as in the supraspinatus tendon of the shoulder, which commonly ruptures, and in the finger flexors, which may become edematous and trigger through the flexor sheath.[45]

HEALING OF TENDON LACERATIONS WITHIN THE DIGITAL SHEATH

Tendon healing in the digital sheath has been the subject of intense research interest for many years. The finger flexors must glide approximately 3 cm to provide full finger motion, and an additional 3 cm of glide is taken up at the wrist.[22] Adhesions that bind a tendon to its fibrous sheath, which is less than 1 mm away, prevent gliding and result in gross impairment of hand function. Surgeons attempting to repair tendons within the digital sheath are thus faced with the imposing challenge of achieving healing of two structures, tendon and sheath, less than a millimeter apart while preventing them from participating in the same wound response and healing to each other. Clinical attempts at tendon repair in the digital sheath in the past were met so often with failure that the sheath became known as "no man's land."[46]

By trial and error, gentle surgical technique and early mobilization of the repair site were found to improve the results of tendon repair in the digital sheath. These and other aspects of tendon healing within the digital sheath are discussed herein, grouped by variables relating to the injury and those under control of the surgeon.

Among the injury variables, tendon vascularity has been shown to have a clear effect on the quality of tendon healing.[47] Clinically, the results of tendon repair in digits with vincular injury are worse than those without such damage. Repairs with excision of the superficialis tendon, through which the long vinculum to the profundus courses, also produce worse results than repairs in which the superficialis is left intact or repaired.[48] In both instances, the hypovascular tendons heal with significantly less motion and presumably more in the way of scar adhesions than tendons with more normal circulatory patterns. Experimentally, several studies have investigated the effect of avascularity or hypovascularity in chicken tendon injuries and all have shown a significant detriment from hypovascularity, reflected in decreased matrix synthesis within the tendon, decreased ultimate strength and motion of the injured tendon, and more severe adhesion formation.[49-52]

On a more basic level, gross studies of vascularity do not address the question of whether the injured tendon can muster sufficient metabolic response to heal without obligatory "help" from surrounding tissues, which would come via vascular neogenesis and adhesion formation. Fortunately, considerable experimental evidence now exists to show that tenocytes are not effete, but instead are rather robust metabolically. They retain the potential to vary their synthetic ability in response to the stress of injury,[53] and they retain the ability to dedifferentiate, divide, and migrate.[54] Such activities can be shown to occur even in the complete absence of vascularity in tissue culture and various heterotopic implantation experiments (Fig. 24–8).[55-57]

Histologically, it appears that the cells with the greatest potential for metabolic change in flexor tendons within the digital sheath are those on the tendon surface.[58, 59] These epitendinous cells are topologically identical to the tendon sheath cells, which of course are the cells that, when they migrate across the synovial space to participate in tendon healing, form the adhesions that are the enemy of tendon gliding.

It is ironic that in the case of tendon healing within the digital sheath, the same cell layer is at once hero and villain; proof of the possibility of adhesion-free "intrinsic healing" and the inevitability of adhesion formation and "extrinsic healing." Viewed in such a light, the question of ideal healing of tendon within the digital sheath takes on a new form, in which one might consider the possibility of variable stimulation of cells based upon their attachment to structures that differ in mechanical function.

The effect of mechanical stimulation on tendon healing has been the focus of much recent research. The concept of Wolff's law as it pertains to soft tissue has already been introduced. Tensile stress has been shown in a number of experimental systems to increase the rate and organization of collagen synthesis.[60-62] In the case of an injured tendon, the possibility of gap formation at the injury site as a result of tensile stress must be borne in mind, however; such a stimulus could become a two-edged sword, increasing synthetic rate but simultaneously drawing the injured tendon ends further apart, destroying the normal anatomical length-tension relationship as well as increasing the size of the space to be filled with scar. Indeed, such gapping after early mobilization of flexor tendon injuries has been implicated as the source of the 10 to 20 percent weakness of grip noted in digits with repaired tendons.[63] Of course, such weakness could also be the result of tendon

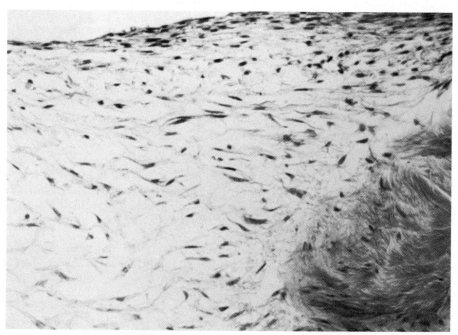

Figure 24–8. Photomicrograph of the edge of a tendon explant in a plasma clot showing cells migrating away from the explant after 5 days in culture (×64). (From Graham MF, Becker H, Cohen IK, et al: Intrinsic tendon fibroplasia: Documentation *in vitro*. J Orthop Res 1:251–256, 1984.)

adhesions' dissipating the power of muscular contraction proximal to the point of force application. To overcome the tendency for gap formation, a variety of suture techniques have been advised. Those with a locking or grasping component function best at reducing gap, although of course the tensile strength of any tendon suture remains much less than that of an intact tendon, which may resist forces measured in the hundreds of kilograms.[64] Even the strongest tendon suture is capable of resisting only 1 to 2 kg without gapping.[64]

In addition to tension, motion has a salutary effect on tendon healing, as it facilitates pumping of synovial nutrients. Such motion may also serve to disrupt vascular buds crossing the synovial space and therefore to disrupt or lengthen adhesions.[65–67]

Surgical technique and tissue handling are also critical to the quality of the result after tendon repair. In a series of detailed studies, Potenza investigated the effect of tissue handling and superficialis excision in a dog model and demonstrated conclusively the importance of preservation of all anatomical structures and delicate handling of injured tendon ends.[68, 69]

Combining all the above data, tendon healing within the digital sheath can be seen as a complex process involving some modifiable and some nonmodifiable factors. Currently modifiable factors include the amount of stress placed on the repair, surgical technique, and the type of suture used. Nonmodifiable factors include the beginning vascularity of the injured tendon ends and the extent of initial tissue injury. One would imagine that a partial injury could bear more stress than a completely lacerated and sutured tendon, and that one possessing intact vascularity would function best, and this is indeed so. Such tendons can heal without apparent adhesions and with restoration of normal strength and motion both experimentally and clinically due to a continued ability to move.[70] In contrast, repair of completely divided tendons usually produces restoration of 75 to 90 percent of normal motion, with reduced strength.

The question of sheath closure versus sheath excision frequently arises in regard to tendon healing within the digital sheath. Those who favor closure argue for the normal biomechanics of tendon movement and the beneficial effects of restoring a closed synovial space on nutrition and lubrication.[57, 71] Those who opt for excision argue a reduction in the potential for adhesions to a rigid sheath, by physical elimination of the sheath.[72] Current data suggest that excision of the membraneous sheath has no apparent effect on tendon healing.[47] This may be due to the fact that this layer recellularizes rapidly and can effectively recreate a closed sheath system in a few days similarly to the recellularization of peritoneum or like surfaces. The fibrous sheath is a different matter. When fibrous pulleys are excised, the flexor tendon is permitted to bowstring away from the finger joints. As the tendon bowstrings, its moment arm and mechanical advantage for flexion increase.[22, 23] As the mechanical advantage and moment arm of the extensor are fixed, a relative imbalance develops, predisposing to flexion contracture. This is all the more so in a situation of acute injury and healing, since hematoma between tendon and joint is likely to cellularize and form a dense contracting scar, further limiting joint motion. For this mechanical reason, the fibrous sheath should not be excised. With increasing pulley excision, tendon excursion produces a decreasing amount of joint angular motion per unit of excursion, so that total flexion capacity decreases.[22] Clinical results of tendon repair and sheath excision are, in fact, significantly worse than similar repairs done with preservation of the fibrous sheath.

HEALING OF TENDON GRAFTS WITHIN THE DIGITAL SHEATH

When primary tendon healing does not occur, it may on occasion be necessary to excise the injured tendon and replace it with a tendon graft. If the graft is thin, fresh, and autogenous, it may retain significant viability from diffusion, particularly if it is passed through an intact or reconstructed sheath.[73] If the graft is thick or heterologous, it must be recellularized from surrounding tissue.[74] Such a recellularization process usually, if not always, involves the ingrowth of adhesions, and thus the potential results of tendon grafting are generally inferior to those that can be expected from repair of viable tendon.[75] Nonetheless, the results are often functional, with roughly two thirds of total digital motion restored on average.[76] Somewhat poorer results can be expected from tendon allografts, where additional fibrosis induced by immunological incompatibility must also be taken into consideration.[77]

TENDON AND LIGAMENT SUBSTITUTES

Tendon and ligament substitutes can be divided into two groups: true prosthetic replacements and synthetic devices designed to augment a tissue repair. Among these devices, three main areas require discussion: biocompatibility; material properties of the implant; and fixation of the implant.

Biocompatibility of synthetic fibers must take into consideration not only any toxic effect from the substance to be used on a molecular basis or compatibility of the implant in the form in which it is originally inserted but also compatibility of the implant in the form it may take in vivo after considerable use. Some synthetic materials undergo changes in structure after extended periods in vivo, particularly in response to repetitive movement, compression, and abrasion. Particulate debris may develop with dimensions small enough to become cellular irritants, even though the intact implant shows no evidence of irritability. Two classic examples in which biocompatibility of the intact implant is generally good but fragmentation of the implant occurs, are carbon filament implants[78] and implants containing silicone elastomers.[79] In both cases, after repeated use, microfragmentation may occur resulting in local inflammation and failure of the implanted device. Inflammation secondary to debris from metal wear or microfragmentation of methylmethacrylate are other common examples, more often related to reconstruction of bone or joints.

Material properties of a tendon or ligament replacement are clearly important and should, where possible, mimic the material properties of normal tendon or ligamentous tissue.[80] With true prosthetic replacements, the device must be strong enough to withstand repeated stress under physiological loads without failure. As an augmenting device, the device should provide for load sharing with host tissue. As host tissue may not adhere well to the implant, perception of tension transmitted through the implant may be poor, and the host response thereby enfeebled.[80]

Fixation of artificial tendon and ligament devices is another major issue. There are two aspects to this question, one of which is fixation at an appropriate length and tension that mimics the physiological situation; the other is fixation that is strong enough to withstand repetitive loading without loosening. In regard to the former, detailed information about joint biomechanics and the role of ligament joint stability is crucial and often lags behind clinical use of ligament replacement. With the latter, fixation by biological ingrowth to form a composite structure appears to be the most promising, but remains under investigation.[81] Among the materials that appear most promising as tendon or ligament prostheses are polyester textiles[82] and Gore-tex[83] (expanded polyterafluoroethylene fiber) (Table 24–2). At present, however, tendon and ligament prostheses and implants remain predominately investigational devices without demonstrable superiority or even parity to primary repair or autograft reconstruction.[84, 85] Their current use is generally limited to salvage situations where no autogenous reconstruction is possible or practical, preferably in a research setting.

STIMULATION OF TENDON AND LIGAMENT HEALING

Given the relative hypocellularity of tendon and ligament, methods to further stimulate cel-

Table 24–2. TENDON AND LIGAMENT SUBSTITUES

Material	Advantages	Disadvantages	References
Xenograft	Biological geometry Initial strength	Ingrowth fixation strength Reactivity (glutaraldehyde leaching) Immunogenicity	96, 98, 99
Dacron	Versatile—many weaves, shapes Low reactivity Initial strength May be coated where ingrowth not desired	Limited ingrowth fixation	81, 82
PTFE*	Versatility of shape, structure Low reactivity Initial strength	Limited ingrowth fixation	83, 97
Carbon fiber	Ingrowth potential Initial strength	Limited ingrowth fixation strength Reactivity of fibers	78, 84
Woven nylon	Biocompatibility Initial strength Low reactivity	Limited ingrowth fixation	97

*Expanded polytetrafluoroethylene (Gore-tex).

lular synthesis and replication could provide for more rapid and stronger tendon healing. Two areas have been investigated in this regard. Electrical stimulation of tendon healing, the focus of several recent reports,[86, 87] is known to improve the quality of bone healing, and in a short-term in vitro study, some effect on proline synthesis was also noted in rabbit tendon explants subjected to pulsed electromagnetic fields.[87] Direct electrical stimulation has also been shown to have a positive effect on tendon healing in an experimental model.[86] Polypeptide growth factors stimulate wound healing and would appear to be another focus for future research (see Chapter 14).[88] Nonsteroidal anti-inflammatory drugs may also have a direct effect on the quality of tendon healing.[89]

REDUCTION OF TENDON ADHESIONS IN EXPERIMENTAL MODELS

Clinically, tendon adhesions can be minimized by gentle tissue handling and early mobilization. Other interventions have also been investigated. Probably the substance studied most has been hyaluronic acid.[90–92] Hyaluronic acid–enriched wounds may heal faster, due to facilitation of cellular migration.[92] (The importance of glycosaminoglycans in wound healing is discussed in Chapter 11.) It also appears to reduce tendon adhesions in experimental models.[90] The mechanism for adhesion reduction by hyaluronic acid is not clear but may involve an inhibition of vascular neogenesis.[91]

Other chemical compounds may also serve to reduce tendon adhesion formation. Proline analogues may reduce collagen synthesis in general and thereby have an indirect effect on tendon adhesion but also on tendon strength, and unless locally delivered, on collagen throughout the body.[93] The same can be said for anti-crosslinking agents such as β-aminopropionitrile.[94] However, such drugs seem currently too toxic for clinical use.

Mechanical devices that may serve to disrupt adhesions have also been studied. Ultrasonic vibrations appear to have some effect on adhesions both in the laboratory and clinically.[95]

TENDON AND LIGAMENT HEALING IN THE FUTURE

Progress in the quality and predictability of tendon and ligament healing in the future will probably take several forms. Better understanding of the biology and regulation of wound healing on a cellular level will probably result in the development of factors that will stimulate the ability of local tissues to heal. By combining these with specific mechanical stimulation, it may be possible to augment healing of only one portion of a wound, which would be of particular applicability in tendon healing in the digit. Hyaluronic acid or some other substance may prove useful as a blocking agent to inhibit adhesion formation. Finally, tendon and ligament substitutes may take the form of porous textiles coated with biological adhesion factors to facilitate ingrowth both for augmentation and for fixation. Devices coated with fibronectin may permit cells to adhere directly to the implant fibers and thus better perceive forces transmitted along the implant fibers, stimulating organized matrix synthesis.

REFERENCES

1. Amiel D, Frank C, Harwood F, et al: Tendons and ligaments: A morphological and biochemical comparison. J Orthop Res 1:257–265, 1984.
2. Scott JE, Haigh M: Proteoglycan-type I collagen fibril interactions in bone and non-calcifying connective tissues. Biochem Rep 5:71–81, 1985.
3. Poole AR: Proteoglycans in health and disease: Structures and functions. Biochem J 236:1–14, 1986.
4. Vogel KG, Paulsson M, Heinegård D: Specific inhibition of type I and type II collagen fibrillogenesis by the small proteoglycan of tendon. Biochem J 223:587–597, 1984.
5. Parry DAD, Barnes GRG, Craig AS: A comparison of the size distribution of collagen fibrils in connective tissues as a function of age and a possible relation between fibril size distribution and mechanical properties. Proc R Soc Lond 203:305–321, 1978.
6. Gillard GC, Merrilees MJ, Bell-Booth PG, et al: The proteoglycan content and the axial periodicity of collagen in tendon. Biochem J 163:145–151, 1977.
7. Gillard GC, Reilly HC, Bell-Booth PG, et al: The influence of mechanical forces on the glycosaminoglycan content of the rabbit flexor digitorum profundus tendon. Conn Tiss Res 7:37–46, 1979.
8. Grodzinsky AJ, Shoenfeld NA: Tensile forces induced in collagen by means of electromechanochemical transductive coupling. Presented at the First Cleveland Symposium on Macromolecules, Structure and Properties of Biopolymers, Case Western Reserve University, Cleveland, October, 1976.
9. Piez KA: Collagen types: A review. In Development and Diseases of Cartilage and Bone Matrix. New York, Alan R. Liss, 1987, pp 1–19.
10. Okuda Y, Gorski JP, Amadio PC: Effect of postnatal age on the ultrastructure of six anatomical areas of canine flexor digitorum profundus tendon. J Orth Res 5:231–241, 1987.
11. Kastelic J, Galeski A, Baer E: The multicomposite structure of tendon. Conn Tiss Res 6:11–23, 1978.
12. Baer E, Hiltner A, Keith HD: Hierarchical structure in polymeric materials. Science 235:1015–1022, 1987.

13. West BJ, Goldberger AL: Physiology in fractal dimensions. Am Sci 75:354–365, 1987.
14. Evans HJ, Barbenel JC, Steel TR, et al: Structure and mechanics of tendon. Symp Soc Exp Biol 34:465–469, 1980.
15. Betsch DF, Baer E: Structure and mechanical properties of rat tail tendon. Biorheology 17:83–94, 1980.
16. Schwerdt A, Constantinesco A, Chambron J: Dynamic viscoelastic behaviour of the human tendon in vitro. J Biomech 13:913–922, 1980.
17. Lanir Y: Structure-strength relations in mammalian tendon. Biophys J 24:541–554, 1978.
18. Chaplin DM, Greenlee TK Jr: The development of human digital tendons. J Anat 120(2):253–274, 1975.
19. Greenlee TK Jr, Beckham C, Pike D: A fine structured study of the development of the chick flexor digital tendon: A model for synovial sheathed tendon healing. Am J Anat 143:303–314, 1976.
20. Amadio PC, Jaeger SH, Hunter JM: Nutritional aspects of tendon healing. In Hunter JM, Schneider LH, Mackin EJ, et al (eds): Rehabilitation of the Hand, 2nd ed. St. Louis, CV Mosby, 1984, pp 255–260.
21. Tothill P, Hooper G: Measurement of tendon blood flow in rabbits by microsphere uptake and ^{133}Xe washout. J Hand Surg 10B:17–20, 1985.
22. Idler RS: Anatomy and biomechanics of the digital flexor tendons. Symposium on Flexor Tendon Surgery. Hand Clin 1:3–11, 1985.
23. Delattre JF, Ducasse A, Flament JB, et al: The mechanical role of the digital fibrous sheath: Application to reconstructive surgery of the flexor tendons. Anat Clin 5:187–197, 1983.
24. Solonen KA, Hoyer P: Positioning of the pulley mechanism when reconstructing deep flexor tendons of fingers. Acta Orthop Scand 38:321–328, 1967.
25. Peterson WW, Manske PR, Bollinger BA, et al: Effect of pulley excision on flexor tendon biomechanics. J Orthop Res 4:96–101, 1986.
26. Inoue H, Takasugi H, Akahori O: Surface study of tenosynovium in hens and humans by electron microscopy. Hand 8:222–227, 1976.
27. Okuda Y, Gorski JP, An K-N, et al: Biochemical, histological, and biomechanical analyses of canine tendon. J Orthop Res 5:60–68, 1987.
28. Broom ND, Poole CA: Articular cartilage collagen and proteoglycans: Their functional interdependency. Arthritis Rheum 26:1111–1119, 1983.
29. Arem AJ, Madden JW: Is there a Wolff's law for connective tissue? Surg Forum 25:512–514, 1974.
30. Lundborg G, Myrhage R, Rydevik B: The vascularization of human flexor tendons within the digital synovial sheath region—structural and functional aspects. J Hand Surg 2:417–427, 1977.
31. Weber ER: Nutritional pathways for flexor tendons in the digital theca. In Hunter JM, Schneider LH, Mackin EJ (eds): Tendon Surgery in the Hand. St. Louis, CV Mosby, 1987, pp 91–99.
32. Gelberman RH, Manske PR, Akeson WH, et al: Flexor tendon repair. J Orthop Res 4:119–128, 1986.
33. Reiderer-Henderson MA, Nachemson A, Hendrix MJC, et al: Sheathed tendon repair: Type III collagen synthesis in the wound area and by tendon synovial cells in culture. Trans Orthop Res Soc 8:26, 1983 (abstract).
34. Reid T, Flint MH: Changes in glycosaminoglycan content of healing rabbit tendon. J Embryol Exp Morphol 31:489–495, 1974.
35. Frank C, Amiel D, Woo SL-Y, et al: Normal ligament properties and ligament healing. Clin Orthop Rel Res 196:15–25, 1985.
36. Woo SL-Y, Gomez MA, Seguchi Y, et al: Measurement

of mechanical properties of ligament substance from a bone-ligament-bone preparation. J Orthop Res 1:22–29, 1983 (abstract).
37. Minns RJ, Steven FS: Local denaturation of collagen fibers during the mechanical rupture of collagenous fibrous tissue. Ann Rheum Dis 39:164–167, 1980.
38. Woo SL-Y: Mechanical properties of tendons and ligaments. Biorheology 19:385–396, 1982.
39. Frank C, Amiel D, Akeson WH: Healing of the medial collateral ligament of the knee. Acta Orthop Scand 54:917–923, 1983.
40. Steiner M: Biomechanics of tendon healing. J Biomech 15:951–958, 1982.
41. Goldstein SA, Armstrong TJ, Chaffin DB, et al: Analysis of cumulative strain in tendons and tendon sheaths. J Biomech 20:1–6, 1987.
42. Woo SL-Y, Ritter MA, Amiel D, et al: The biochemical and biomechanical properties of swine tendons: Long term effects of exercise. Conn Tiss Res 7:177–183, 1980.
43. Woo SL-Y, Gomez MA, Woo Y-K, et al: Mechanical properties of tendons and ligaments. The relationships of immobilization and exercise on tissue remodelling. Biorheology 19:397–408, 1982.
44. Neuberger A, Perrone JC, Slack HGB: The relative metabolic inertia of tendon collagen in the rat. Biochem J 49:199–204, 1951.
45. Józsa L, Bálint BJ, Réffy A: Calcifying tendinopathy. Arch Orthop Traum Surg 97:305–307, 1980.
46. Bunnell S: Surgery of the Hand, 3rd ed. Philadelphia, JB Lippincott, 1956.
47. Amadio PC, Hunter JM, Jaeger SH, et al: The effects of vincular injury on the results of flexor tendon surgery in zone 2. J Hand Surg 10A:626–632, 1985.
48. Lister GD, Kleinert HE, Kutz HE, et al: Primary flexor tendon repair followed by immediate controlled mobilization. J Hand Surg 2:441–451, 1977.
49. Pennington DG: The influence of tendon sheath integrity and vincular blood supply on adhesion formation following tendon repair in hens. Br J Plast Surg 32:302–306, 1979.
50. Matthews JP: Vascular changes in flexor tendons after injury and repair: An experimental study. Injury 8:227–233, 1977.
51. Banes AJ, Enterline D, Bevin AG, et al: Effects of trauma and partial devascularization on protein synthesis in the avian flexor profundus tendon. J Trauma 21:505–512, 1981.
52. Kain CC, Russell JE, Manske PR, et al: The effect of sheath integrity and proximity to laceration in the healing flexor tendon: A biomechanical study. Trans Orthop Res Soc 12:163, 1987 (abstract).
53. Landi AP, Altman FP, Pringle DJ, et al: Oxidative enzyme activity in rabbit intrasynovial flexor tendons. J Surg Res 29:287–292, 1980.
54. Graham MF, Becker H, Cohen IK, et al: Intrinsic tendon fibroplasia: Documentation by in vitro studies. J Orthop Res 1:251–256, 1984.
55. Gelberman RH, Manske PR, Vande Berg JS, et al: Flexor tendon repair in vitro: A comparative histologic study of the rabbit, chicken, dog, and monkey. J Orthop Res 2:39–48, 1984.
56. Becker H, Graham MF, Cohen IK, et al: Intrinsic tendon cell proliferation in tissue culture. J Hand Surg 6:616–619, 1981.
57. Lundborg G, Rank F: Experimental intrinsic healing of flexor tendons based upon synovial fluid nutrition. J Hand Surg 3:21–31, 1978.
58. Manske PR, Lesker PA, Gelberman RH, et al: Intrinsic restoration of the flexor tendon surface in the nonhuman primate. J Hand Surg 10A:632–637, 1985.

59. Manske PR, Lesker PA: Histologic evidence of intrinsic flexor tendon repair in various experimental animals. Clin Orthop Rel Res 182:297–304, 1984.
60. Slack C, Flint MH, Thompson BM: The effect of tensional load on isolated embryonic chick tendons in organ culture. Conn Tiss Res 12:229–247, 1984.
61. Videman T, Eronen I, Candolin T: Effects of motion load changes on tendon tissues and articular cartilage. Scand J Work Environ Health 5:56–67, 1979.
62. Leung DYM, Glagov S, Mathews MB: A new *in vitro* system for studying cell response to mechanical stimulation. Exp Cell Res 109:285–298, 1977.
63. Ejeskär A: Finger flexion force and hand grip strength after tendon repair. J Hand Surg 7:61–65, 1982.
64. Urbaniak JR, Cahill JD Jr, Mortenson RA: Tendon suturing methods: Analysis of tensile strengths. In Hunter JM, Schneider LH (eds): AAOS Symposium on Tendon Surgery in the Hand. St. Louis, CV Mosby, 1975, pp 70–80.
65. Strickland JW, Glogovac SV: Digital function following flexor tendon repair in Zone II: A comparison of immobilization and controlled passive motion techniques. J Hand Surg 5:537–542, 1980.
66. Hitchcock TF, Light TR, Bunch WH, et al: The effect of immediate constrained digital motion on the strength of flexor tendon repairs in chickens. J Hand Surg 12A:590–595, 1987.
67. Woo SL-Y, Gelberman RH, Cobb NG, et al: The importance of controlled passive mobilization on flexor tendon healing. Acta Orthop Scand 52:615–622, 1981.
68. Potenza AD: Prevention of adhesions to healing digital flexor tendons. JAMA 187:187–191, 1964.
69. Potenza AD: Effect of associated trauma on healing of divided tendons. J Trauma 2:175–184, 1962.
70. Bishop AT, Cooney WP III, Wood MB: Treatment of partial flexor tendon lacerations: The effect of tenorrhaphy and early protected mobilization. J Trauma 26:301–312, 1986.
71. Lister GD: Incision and closure of the flexor sheath during primary tendon repair. Hand 15:123–135, 1983.
72. Verdan CE: Primary repair of flexor tendons. J Bone Joint Surg 42A:647–657, 1960.
73. Manske PR, Lesker PA, Bridwell K: Experimental studies in chickens on the initial nutrition of tendon grafts. J Hand Surg 4:565–575, 1979.
74. Potenza AD: The healing of autogenous tendon grafts within the flexor digital sheath in dogs. J Bone Joint Surg 46A:1462–1484, 1964.
75. Verdan CE: Half a century of flexor-tendon surgery. J Bone Joint Surg 54A:472–491, 1972.
76. Boyes JH, Stark HH: Flexor-tendon grafts in the fingers and thumb. J Bone Joint Surg 53A:1332–1342, 1971.
77. Hirasawa Y, Shikata Y, Nakamura T, et al: Experimental study on tendon transplantation using allograft. Arch Jpn Chir 53:273–286, 1984.
78. King JB, Bulstrode C: Polylactate-coated carbon fiber in extra-articular reconstruction of the unstable knee. Clin Orthop Rel Res 196:139–142, 1985.
79. Worsing RA Jr, Engber WD, Lange TA: Reactive synovitis from particulate silastic. J Bone Joint Surg 64A:581–585, 1982.
80. Goodship AE, Wilcock SA, Shah JS: The development of tissue around various prosthetic implants used as replacements for ligaments and tendons. Clin Orthop Rel Res 196:61–68, 1985.
81. Jaeger SH, Hunter JM, Schneider PJ, et al: Development of a long term tendon prosthesis. In Hunter JM, Schneider LH, Mackin EJ (eds): Tendon Surgery in the Hand. St. Louis, CV Mosby, 1987, pp 293–302.
82. Park JP, Grana WA, Chitwood JS: A high-strength Dacron augmentation for cruciate ligament reconstruction: A two-year canine study. Clin Orthop Rel Res 196:175–185, 1985.
83. Bolton CW, Bruchman WC: The GORE-TEX™ expanded polytetrafluoroethylene prosthetic ligament: An *in vitro* and *in vivo* evaluation. Clin Orthop Rel Res 196:202–213, 1985.
84. Strum GM, Larson RL: Clinical experience and early results of carbon fiber augmentation of anterior cruciate reconstruction of the knee. Clin Orthop Rel Res 196:124–138, 1985.
85. McPherson GK, Mendenhall HV, Gibbons DF, et al: Experimental mechanical and histologic evaluation of the Kennedy ligament augmentation device. Clin Orthop Rel Res 196:186–195, 1985.
86. Nelson AJ, Owoeye I, Spielholz N, et al: Uses of pulsed electrical stimulation for tendon healing. In Hunter JM, Schneider LH, Mackin EJ (eds): Tendon Surgery in the Hand. St. Louis, CV Mosby, 1987, pp 109–111.
87. Nessler JP, Mass DP: Direct-current electrical stimulation of tendon healing *in vitro*. Clin Orthop Rel Res 217:303–311, 1987.
88. Kaplan J: Polypeptide-binding membrane receptors: Analysis and classification. Science 212:14–20, 1981.
89. Kulick MI, Smith S, Hadler K: Oral ibuprofen: Evaluation of its effect on peritendinous adhesions and the breaking strength of a tenorrhaphy. J Hand Surg 11A:110–120, 1986.
90. Thomas SC, Jones LC, Hungerford DS: Hyaluronic acid and its effect on postoperative adhesions in the rabbit flexor tendon: A preliminary look. Clin Orthop Rel Res 206:281–289, 1986.
91. Feinberg RN, Beebe DC: Hyaluronate in vasculogenesis. Science 220:1177–1179, 1983.
92. Abatangelo G, Martelli M, Vecchia P: Healing of hyaluronic acid–enriched wounds: Histological observations. J Surg Res 35:410–416, 1983.
93. Bora FW Jr, Lane JM, Prockop DJ: Inhibitors of collagen biosynthesis as a means of controlling scar formation in tendon injury. J Bone Joint Surg 54A:1501–1508, 1972.
94. Porat S, Rousso M, Shoshan S: Improvement of gliding function of flexor tendons by topically applied enriched collagen solution. J Bone Joint Surg 62B:208–213, 1980.
95. Stevenson JH, Pang CY, Lindsay WK, et al: Functional, mechanical, and biochemical assessment of ultrasound therapy on tendon healing in the chicken toe. Plast Reconstr Surg 77:965–970, 1986.
96. Allen PR, Amis AA, Jones MM, et al: Bovine glutaraldehyde treated tendon as a graft. J Bone Joint Surg 67B:159, 1985 (abstract).
97. Dunlap J, McCarthy JA, Joyce ME, et al: Biomechanical and histologic evaluations of pulley reconstructions in nonhuman primates. J Hand Surg 16A:57–63, 1990.
98. Ellingsworth LR, DeLustro F, Brennan JE, et al: The human immune response to reconstituted bovine collagen. J Immunol 136:877–882, 1986.
99. Smith DJ, Jones CS, Hull M, et al: Bioprosthesis in hand surgery. J Surg Res 41:378–387, 1986.

25

ACUTE LUNG INJURY

Marshall I. Hertz, M.D., Linda S. Snyder, M.D.,
Keith R. Harmon, M.D., and Peter B. Bitterman, M.D.

Although dramatic improvements have been made in sophisticated critical care and ventilatory support for patients suffering from acute lung injury, the most severe form of this injury still carries a mortality in excess of 50 per cent.[1-3] Careful epidemiological studies of patient deaths following severe acute lung injury reveal two important features that may provide a clue as to why patients die: (1) in nearly all cases successful supportive care is provided during the first week after the disease becomes manifest with most deaths occurring between one and three weeks after the onset of respiratory insufficiency; and (2) respiratory failure, either directly or as a result of complications attributable to prolonged mechanical ventilation, constitutes a major reason for mortality.[3] These observations support the conclusion that one fundamental determinant of survival in patients following acute lung injury is the ability of alveolar repair to occur in a timely and orderly fashion. Implicit in this concept is that the pathology underlying the initial alveolar injury, for example, sepsis or pancreatitis, must be promptly controlled.

To understand the process of alveolar repair, it is necessary to define the cellular and biochemical nature of the structural derangements that occur after lung injury and to consider the molecular mechanisms leading to reconstitution of the alveolus. To accomplish this, research directed at elucidating mechanisms of lung injury and repair are reviewed. In those instances in which knowledge of the cellular repair processes in the alveolus is incomplete, analogous repair and cell replication in other tissues are examined.

DEFINITION OF ACUTE LUNG INJURY

Acute lung injury can be defined as a rapid alteration of alveolar structures leading to impairment of the gas exchange apparatus following exposure to noxious environmental or endogenous agents. Clinicians from nearly all disciplines, including surgery, internal medicine, pediatrics, and anesthesiology, regularly confront this problem. Acute lung injury can range in severity from the modest and reversible biochemical and functional impairment following exposure to 100 per cent oxygen for relatively brief intervals (less than 24 hours)[4] to the devastating respiratory failure of the adult respiratory distress syndrome (ARDS), the most severe form of acute lung injury with an attendant mortality risk of up to 70 per cent.[2] As an indication of the magnitude of the problem, the National Heart, Lung, and Blood Institute Task Force on respiratory diseases estimated that in 1976 at least 150,000 cases of ARDS were treated nationwide.[5]

In clinically significant lung injury, the disease process begins with structural and functional alterations of alveolar parenchymal cells resulting from direct interaction of the noxious agent with critical cellular macromolecules (Fig. 25–1).[6-12] In addition to this direct cytotoxicity, an inflammatory response involving predominantly neutrophils, mononuclear phagocytes (macrophages), and platelets ensues.[13-18] By releasing toxic mediators such as oxidant species and proteolytic enzymes, these inflammatory cells cause additional parenchymal cytotoxicity.[19-21] It is the resultant parenchymal cell

396

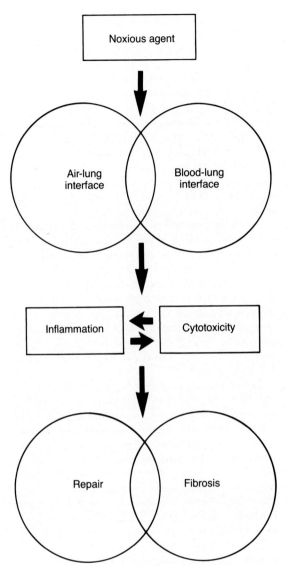

Figure 25–1. Pathogenesis of acute lung injury. The process begins when a noxious agent injures the air-lung interface (e.g., aspiration) or the blood-lung interface (e.g., sepsis). In either instance there is a transmural inflammatory response inflicting further alveolar injury and leading to cell death. Repair begins promptly and can result in nearly complete restoration of normal structure and function. However, to a variable extent, acute and subacute fibrosis can subvert the repair process. (From Cerra FB (ed): Critical Care: State of the Art. Fullerton, Society of Critical Care Medicine, 1987, p 353.)

dysfunction and death that manifest in the patient as respiratory insufficiency.

Clinically, the earliest sign of lung injury is tachypnea, which may precede the onset of dyspnea by hours or even days. At this stage, the patient has an increased alveolar to arterial oxygen gradient and the chest film usually shows increased interstitial markings, reflecting interstitial pulmonary edema. As the injury

progresses, alveolar flooding leads to frank hypoxemia and diffuse alveolar opacities on radiography. The hypoxemia in these patients is difficult to overcome with increased inspired oxygen tensions due to the microanatomical shunting of blood resulting from alveolar flooding and collapse. In addition, gas exchange is also adversely affected by increased dead space ventilation. In mechanically ventilated patients, the compliance of the respiratory system progressively decreases.[22] Signs of systemic illness may also be present, including fever, increased oxygen consumption, decreased systemic vascular resistance, and increased cardiac index. This constellation of findings, referred to as "sepsis syndrome," may or may not be associated with an identified source of infection.

Acute lung injury may occur as an isolated organ failure or as a component of multiple organ failure syndrome (MOFS), a systemic disorder characterized by concurrent or sequential failure of the coagulation system, liver, kidneys, and brain (Fig. 25–2). When acute lung injury occurs as isolated organ failure, a wide spectrum of clinical outcomes is possible, ranging from complete recovery to death.

Clinical management of acute lung injury requires a sophisticated level of supportive care that includes control of inspired gas concentration, mechanical ventilation, and manipulations to optimize hemodynamic status and oxygen delivery. Elimination of the noxious agent when possible (for example, treatment of sepsis) is of paramount importance. These management strategies are based on an improved understanding of the pathophysiology of respiratory

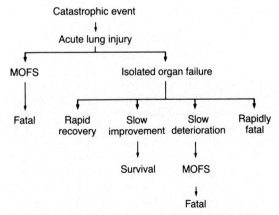

Figure 25–2. Clinical course of acute lung injury. Following a catastrophic event, acute lung injury may occur as isolated organ failure or as a component of the systemic disorder involving the coagulation system, kidneys, liver, and brain; referred to as multiple organ failure syndrome (MOFS). When lung injury occurs as an isolated organ failure a wide spectrum of clinical courses and outcomes may ensue.

insufficiency following acute lung injury.[23-25] However, in spite of our ability to provide excellent supportive care, patient outcomes vary from functionally complete repair of the alveolar structures to acute and subacute massive alveolar fibrosis leading to death or severe disability.[3, 26-30] Therefore, those factors that determine whether repair or fibrosis occurs form the foundation for designing therapeutic approaches during the interval of lung repair.

ANATOMY OF ACUTE LUNG INJURY

Our current state of knowledge regarding the response of the lung to acute injury has its basis in a detailed understanding of alveolar anatomy. The normal gas exchange apparatus can be conceptualized as consisting of three anatomical compartments: the capillary endothelium, comprising the blood-lung interface; the epithelium, constituting the air-lung interface; and the interstitium, which separates the endothelium from the epithelium (Fig. 25–3).

The pulmonary microvessels enter the acinus as muscularized arterioles (external diameter approximately 150 μm).[31] They gradually arborize, appearing as typical capillaries (external diameter 15 μm) once within the alveolar wall. As vessel diameter decreases, two morphological changes occur. First, mesenchymal cell subtype and distribution change. Pulmonary interstitial mesenchymal cells, ontogenically derived from embryonic mesenchyme, include five subtypes of cells: fibroblasts, interstitial cells, myofibroblasts, pericytes, and smooth muscle cells. Each is distinguished by its location and ultrastructural features.[32-45] Smooth muscle cells and pericytes (in addition to vascular endothelial cells, which are also derived from embryonic mesenchyme) are the primary mesenchymal cell constituents of the vascular wall.[34, 46, 47] The continuous envelope of smooth muscle cells within the largest intra-acinar microvessels becomes discontinuous, spiraling within the vessel wall in a helical orientation along an axis parallel to the direction of blood flow (Fig. 25–4).[32] Smooth muscle cell density gradually decreases as the microvessels approach the alveolar wall, and no smooth muscle cells are present within the alveolar capillary wall. The alveolar capillaries are typical microvascular structures with a single endothelial cell layer connected by tight junctions resting on a basement membrane.[31, 48, 49] Pericytes are intimately associated with the

capillary endothelium, internal to the basal lamina.[31, 49] These cells replicate under hypoxic stress[50] and provide signals to the capillary endothelial cells. They may have a significant role in vascular remodeling.[51]

Second, the internal and external elastic laminae gradually thin as the microvessels approach the alveolus. Within the gas exchange apparatus, the internal elastic lamina terminates and only the external elastic lamina remains.[31] The alveolar epithelium, also connected by tight junctions, consists almost exclusively of type 1 and type 2 cells (Fig. 25–5). Type 1 epithelial cells are flat with attenuated cytoplasm and few subcellular organelles, while type 2 epithelial cells are cuboidal and possess microvilli on their apical surface. Although type 2 cells outnumber type 1 cells by a ratio of 2:1, type 1 cells cover over 95 per cent of the air-lung interface. Type 2 cells contain cytoplasmic lamellar bodies and are responsible for the production of pulmonary surfactant. In addition, type 2 cells are the progenitor cell of the alveolar epithelium, capable of replication to replace cells that are lost following injury.[52]

The interstitium is that region of the alveolar wall bounded by and including the epithelial and endothelial basement membranes. It consists of cells and stroma as well as the two basement membranes. The major cellular constituents of the interstitium are mesenchymal cells;[47] also present are immune and inflammatory cells, predominantly macrophages with a few lymphocytes. Neutrophils are rarely found in the normal lung.[46, 48, 52] The stroma comprises several classes of connective tissue macromolecules including collagens type I and III, elastin, fibronectin, and proteoglycans.[47] The connective tissue elements of the basement membranes include collagen type IV, laminin, and fibronectin.[53] Over a large portion of the gas exchange surface, the endothelial and epithelial basement membranes are a single fused structure virtually excluding additional elements of the interstitial space from this portion of the alveolar wall.[49] The interstitium serves as a scaffolding for the remaining parenchymal elements, defining the general outline of the alveolar structures.

Current concepts of the sequelae of acute lung injury are derived from two sources: (1) morphological studies of patients from whom postmortem or biopsy material was available; and (2) systematic morphological and cytokinetic studies in animal models. Within a few hours following lung injury, the alveolar interstitium is expanded in those regions where two distinct basement membranes are observed

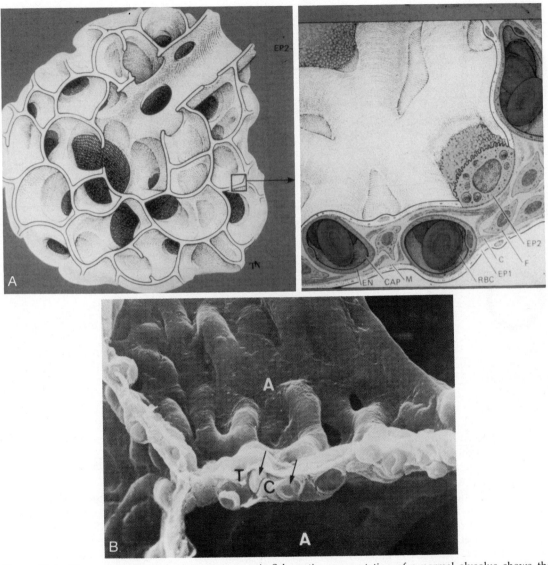

Figure 25–3. The normal gas exchange apparatus. *A,* Schematic representation of a normal alveolus shows the capillary endothelium (EN) and endothelial basement membrane (M), comprising the blood-lung interface; the epithelium, made up of type 1 (EP1) and type 2 (EP2) epithelial cells, comprising the air-lung interface; and the interstitium, containing collagen (C), which separates the endothelium from the epithelium. Red blood cells (RBC) may be seen within the alveolar capillaries (CAP), and interstitial mesenchymal cells are shown (F). *B,* Scanning electron micrograph of the alveolar structures shows capillaries (C), containing red blood cells, between alveoli (A), containing air, with the blood separated from the air by a thin tissue barrier (T). (From Weibel ER: Is the lung built reasonably? Am Rev Resp Dis 128:752–760, 1983.)

(Fig. 25–6).[13, 28, 54, 55] The interstitium contains an increased volume of fluid with higher concentration of plasma proteins characterized by a shift toward higher molecular weight species.[56, 57] Aggregates of leukocytes and platelets are present within the pulmonary microvasculature (Fig. 25–6).[18, 58] Although the capillary endothelial cells appear morphologically intact, the altered fluid and macromolecular transport properties of the blood-lung interface indicate functional impairment.[13, 54, 55, 58] In addition, there is damage to the air-lung interface with ultrastructural evidence of type 1 cell injury.[13, 54, 55, 58] As early as one day after injury, there is accumulation of inflammatory cells, particularly neutrophils, mononuclear phagocytes, and platelets within the alveolar interstitium as well as evidence of fibrin deposition.[13, 54, 55, 58] Within the first couple of days, type 1 cells are lost. The epithelial basement membrane develops gaps leaving the interstitium in direct communication with the alveolar airspace (Fig. 25–7). The air-lung interface becomes a denuded basement membrane except for scattered type 2

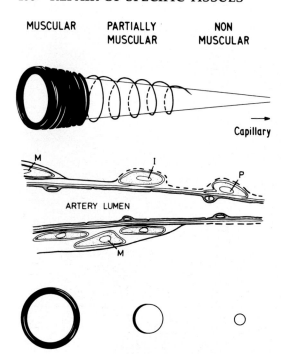

Figure 25–4. Microvascular muscle spiral. The continuous envelope of smooth muscle cells (M) within the largest intra-acinar microvessels is replaced by a discontinuous spiral before disappearing in precapillary microvessels. I = intermediate cell; P = pericyte. (From Reid L, Fried R, Geggel R, et al: Anatomy of pulmonary hypertensive states. In Bergofsky EH (ed): Abnormal Pulmonary Circulation. New York, Churchill Livingstone, 1986, pp 221–264.)

cells.[13, 24, 58] As the epithelial cells of the air-lung interface die, the primary barrier to the flux of water and solutes from the capillary into the alveolar air space is lost.[59] This results in alveolar flooding and the severe impairment in gas exchange characteristic of these patients. By the second or third day of injury, intravascular coagulation in association with platelet and leukocyte aggregation leads to endothelial cell dysfunction and death.[54, 55] Endothelial cell death is a particularly prominent feature of capillary injury where basement membrane within the alveolar wall is observed in the absence of identifiable endothelial cells (Fig. 25–8). The interstitium begins to manifest stromal disorganization, with structural changes in collagen and elastin.[13, 55, 58] Therefore, this explosive process injures each of the three major anatomical compartments of the alveolus,

leaving an essentially dead epithelial air-lung interface, a disordered interstitium, and a functionally impaired endothelial blood-lung interface.

MECHANISMS OF ALVEOLAR REPAIR

When alveolar repair is effective, all three anatomical compartments are coordinately restored (Table 25–1). There is prompt replication of type 2 epithelial cells, re-establishing the air-lung interface, followed by their proportional differentiation into type 1 cells. Rapid but controlled replication of mesenchymal cells occurs in association with orderly synthesis of stromal connective tissue elements. Metabolic reconsti-

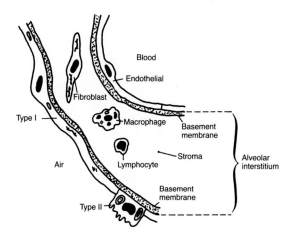

Figure 25–5. Schematic of the alveolar structures. The alveolar capillaries possess a single endothelial cell layer resting on a basement membrane. The epithelium is composed almost exclusively of type 1 and type 2 cells. The interstitium is composed of cells (predominantly mesenchymal), stroma, and the two basement membranes (epithelial and endothelial), which are fused to form a single structure over much of the gas exchange apparatus.

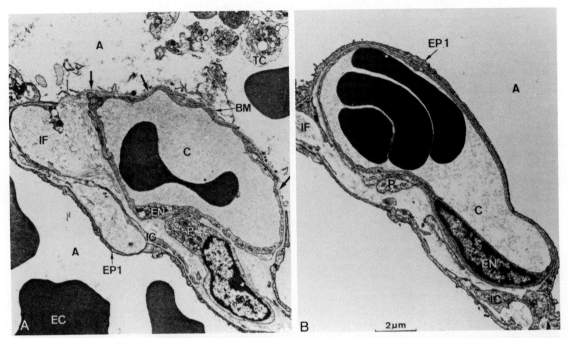

Figure 25–6. The alveolus immediately following acute lung injury. *A,* Alveoli of a 16-year-old male suffering the effects of severe trauma, 7 hours after a motor vehicle accident. There is an increased amount of interstitial fluid (IF). The alveolar air spaces (A) contain aggregates of leukocytes and platelets (TC). The type 1 epithelial cells (EP1) are damaged (*arrows*), exposing a denuded basement membrane (BM). C = capillary; EN = endothelial cell; IC = interstitial cell; P = pericyte. *B,* Normal alveolus for comparison. (From Bachofen M, Weibel ER: Structural alterations of lung parenchyma in the adult respiratory distress syndrome. Clin Chest Med 3:35–56, 1982.)

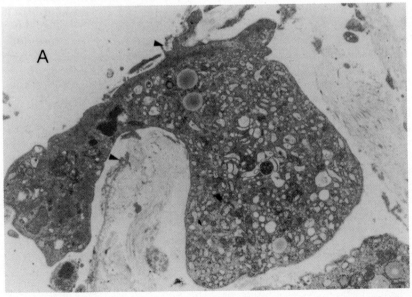

Figure 25–7. Within a few days following acute lung injury the epithelial basement membrane develops gaps (*arrows*), leaving the interstitium in direct communication with the alveolar airspace (A). An interstitial mesenchymal cell is entering the airspace through the gap. (From Fukuda Y, Ishizaki M, Masuda Y, et al: The role of intraalveolar fibrosis in the process of pulmonary structural remodeling in patients with diffuse alveolar damage. Am J Pathol 126:171–182, 1987.)

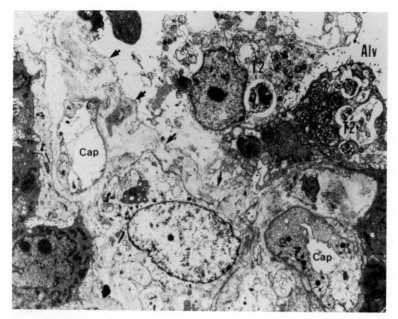

Figure 25–8. Endothelial cell death following acute lung injury. The capillaries (Cap) are lined by endothelial cells containing ballooning cytoplasm. Also shown is a necrotic type 2 epithelial cell (T2). Arrows indicate partial denudation of epithelial basement membrane. Alv = alveolar airspace. (From Katzenstein AA, Myers JL, Mazur MU: Acute interstitial pneumonia: A clinicopathologic, ultrastructural, and cell kinetic study. Am J Surg Pathol 10:256–267, 1986.)

tution of the endothelial cells, coupled with cell migration, replication, and re-establishment of vascular lumenal patency, completes the process of effective alveolar repair.

Interstitium

The interstitium consists of two basic elements, cells and stroma. Mesenchymal cells, accounting for 90 per cent of all cells within the interstitium, have a central role as the effector cells of the interstitial repair process. Two features of mesenchymal cell biology form the foundation for understanding the complex events occurring in the interstitium following lung injury: (1) mesenchymal cell replication and migration; and (2) mesenchymal cell connective tissue metabolism.

During the days to weeks following acute lung injury within the inflammatory alveolar microenvironment, mesenchymal cell replication ensues, leading to an expansion of the mesenchymal cell population within the alveolar wall.[13, 54, 55] In addition, mesenchymal cell migration through gaps in the epithelial basement membrane from the interstitium into the alveolar airspace is followed by cellular replication resulting in intra-alveolar fibrosis and ablation of gas exchange (Figs. 25–7 and 25–9).[60] In those instances when relatively normal lung architecture is to be restored, mesenchymal cell migration and replication and thus the evolution of the fibrotic process appear to be self-limited, occurring concurrently with the restoration of a nearly normal alveolar epithelium. However, in many patients normal alveolar architecture is not restored, as continued mesenchymal cell migration and replication lead to further increases in the number of mesenchymal cells and increased quantities of their connective tissue matrix within the alveolar wall and airspace.[54, 55, 61] This results in a fibrotic, noncompliant lung that is incapable of effective gas exchange. Thus, the clinical outcome following acute lung injury is critically dependent on the mesenchymal cell response, which currently can be neither predicted nor controlled. Therefore, in order to understand the process of interstitial repair following acute

Table 25–1. EVENTS OF ALVEOLAR REPAIR FOLLOWING ACUTE LUNG INJURY

Interstitium	Air-Lung Interface	Blood-Lung Interface
Replication of mesenchymal cells	Replication of type 2 cells	Metabolic reconstitution
Reconstitution of stroma	Differentiation into type 1 cells	Replication of endothelial cells and mesenchymal cells
Control of mesenchymal cell replication		Control of mesenchymal cell replication and reestablishment of vascular luminal patency

From Cerra FB (ed): Critical Care: State of the Art. Fullerton, Society of Critical Care Medicine, 1987, p 355.

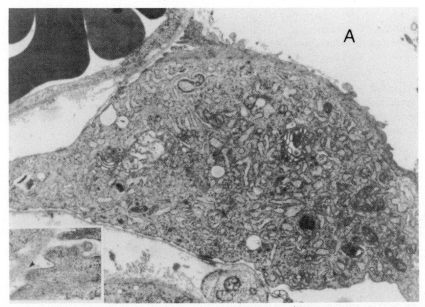

Figure 25–9. Intra-alveolar fibrosis. Mesenchymal cell migration through gaps in the epithelial basement membrane into the alveolar airspace (A), followed by cellular replication, has resulted in intra-alveolar fibrosis. Insert: visualization of extracellular filaments between mesenchymal cell and basement membrane (*arrow*). (From Fukuda Y, Ishizaki M, Masuda Y, et al: The role of intra-alveolar fibrosis in the process of pulmonary structural remodeling in patients with diffuse alveolar damage. Am J Pathol 126:171–182, 1987.)

lung injury, it is necessary to identify those signals within the alveolus that function to enhance as well as inhibit mesenchymal cell replication. These signals have been most extensively studied in the context of the chronic fibrotic lung disorders.

Lessons from the Chronic Fibrotic Lung Disorders

The chronic fibrotic lung diseases are a heterogeneous group of disorders characterized by proliferation and accumulation of mesenchymal cells within the pulmonary interstitium, resulting in structural derangements in alveolar architecture and loss of functioning alveolar capillary units.[62] Although more than 100 agents are known to cause chronic pulmonary fibrosis, in two thirds of cases no cause can be identified.

In cases of pulmonary fibrosis induced by known agents, subacute or chronic exposure to the injurious agent results in persistent alveolar inflammation.[63] In addition, in the interstitial lung diseases of unknown cause, alveolar inflammation is a prominent feature, although the putative inflammatory stimuli remain largely undefined. Significantly, in nearly all instances of environmental or idiopathic lung fibrosis, activated alveolar macrophages play a central role in the inflammatory response.[62–65]

One of the best-studied chronic fibrotic lung diseases of unknown cause is idiopathic pulmonary fibrosis (IPF). Morphologically, IPF is characterized by persistent alveolar inflammation with alveolar macrophages predominating and other inflammatory cells also present. There is an accompanying expansion of the alveolar interstitium by large numbers of mesenchymal cells and stromal elements.[62, 65] With progressive interstitial fibrosis and distortion of the alveolar architecture, the lung is rendered noncompliant and inefficient in its gas-exchange function, manifesting in the patient as slowly progressive respiratory insufficiency with low arterial oxygen tension. IPF typically has an aggressive clinical course and is usually fatal an average of 3 to 6 years after the onset of symptoms.[66–68]

The generally accepted pathogenetic hypothesis for the evolution of the fibrotic process is as follows: Chronic alveolar inflammation, induced by a known or unknown stimulus, leads to replication of interstitial mesenchymal cells and pulmonary fibrosis. In clinically established IPF and the other chronic fibrotic lung disorders, alveolar inflammation and interstitial fibrosis appear to coexist throughout the evolution of the disease process.[62–65] The most convincing evidence currently available to support a causative relationship between alveolar inflammation and pulmonary fibrosis derives from families affected by an inherited form of idiopathic pulmonary fibrosis in which alveolar inflammation has been detected prior to clinical evidence of pulmonary dysfunction.[69] Whether these individuals will develop clinically evident pulmonary fibrosis is unknown and will be of critical importance in the assessment of the influence of alveolar inflammation on mesenchymal cell replication in the chronic fibrotic lung disorders.

Identifying the signals that regulate mesenchymal cell replication as well as the sources of these signals is central to understanding the evolution of the fibrotic process. Current concepts suggest that regulation of mesenchymal cell replication occurs primarily in the G_0/G_1 phase of the cell cycle. (See Chapter 4 for detailed information on regulatory mechanisms of the cell cycle.) These events are controlled by growth factors, peptides of molecular mass generally between 5000 and 35,000 daltons, that interact with specific cell surface receptors in the nanomolar to picomolar range, providing defined signals for cellular replication.[70]

Several characterized growth factors released by alveolar macrophages are likely to be involved in chronic interstitial fibrosis. For example, alveolar macrophages obtained from patients with idiopathic pulmonary fibrosis spontaneously release increased amounts of platelet-derived growth factor (PDGF).[71] This 30,000 dalton cationic glycoprotein provides a specific signal in G_0, causing lung mesenchymal cells to enter the G_1 phase of the cell cycle.[72] In addition, PDGF is a potent chemoattractant for a variety of mesenchymal cells,[73] including those from the lung, thereby providing a means of recruiting lung mesenchymal cells to regions of active inflammation. A second molecule released spontaneously in markedly excess amounts by macrophages from patients with fibrotic lung disorders is fibronectin.[74] This 440,000 dalton glycoprotein also provides a signal early in G_0/G_1.[75] Like PDGF, fibronectin is a potent chemoattractant for mesenchymal cells.[74] The alveolar macrophage-derived growth factor (AMDGF) is a 20,000 dalton peptide closely related to insulin-like growth factor-1 (IGF-1), whose release by lung macrophages from normal individuals is undetectable. However, it is invariably released by lung macrophages from patients with progressive fibrotic lung disorders.[76] It acts somewhat later in G_1 in a coordinate fashion with either fibronectin or PDGF to signal lung mesenchymal cells to enter the S phase of the cell cycle and thus undergo DNA synthesis and cell division.[75] A final molecule released by alveolar macrophages in some of the chronic granulomatous lung disorders is the 15,000 dalton peptide interleu-

kin-1.[77] While not providing a primary signal for cell replication, interleukin-1 is capable of inducing autocrine PDGF production by cultured fibroblasts, thereby providing an indirect mitogenic signal.[78, 79] Perhaps by a similar mechanism, interleukin-1 has been found to enhance the mesenchymal cell response to submaximal concentrations of primary growth-promoting signals.[79]

Mesenchymal Cell Replication and Migration Following Acute Lung Injury

The growth factors within the alveolar structures that serve to modulate mesenchymal cell replication following acute lung injury remain undefined. However, based on an extensive body of knowledge concerning the control of mesenchymal cell replication in vitro, coupled with current understanding of the modulation of mesenchymal cell replication in the chronic fibrotic lung disorders and during wound healing, some of the growth modulators that may be important following acute lung injury can be surmised (Table 25–2).

There are a number of potential sources of growth factors for mesenchymal cells following acute lung injury. Conceptually, they can be considered in three groups within the alveolar structures: (1) resident cells that are induced to release growth factors by the altered milieu; (2) cells recruited to the alveolar structures that are induced to release growth factors; and (3) soluble mediators transported from the plasma in increased concentration.

Resident Cells. Among the resident cells, alveolar macrophages, the representative of the mononuclear phagocyte family of cells present in the lung, are a rich source of growth factors for lung mesenchymal cells.[74, 75, 80–88] Mononuclear phagocytes from both blood and lung can be induced to release PDGF by a variety of inflammatory signals (e.g., endotoxin).[82, 88] In addition, PDGF is a potent chemoattractant for a variety of mesenchymal cells,[73] including those from the lung, thereby providing a means of recruiting lung mesenchymal cells to regions of active inflammation. As noted before, alveolar macrophages of patients with chronic fibrotic lung disorders produce increased amounts of several other known growth factors for mesenchymal cells including fibronectin, AMDGF, and interleukin-1. At present there is no clear evidence that they play a role in the fibrosis

Table 25–2. GROWTH FACTORS FOR MESENCHYMAL CELLS

Source	Growth Factor*	Role in Chronic Interstitial Lung Disorders
Resident cells		
Alveolar macrophages	PDGF	Yes
	Fibronectin	Yes
	AMDGF	Yes
	IL-1	Yes†
Mesenchymal cells	IGF	?
	PDGF	?
Endothelial cells	PDGF	?
Recruited cells		
Platelets	PDGF	?
	TGF-β	?
	TGF-α	?
Circulation	Fibronectin	?
	IGF	?
	EGF	?

*PDGF = platelet-derived growth factor; AMDGF = alveolar macrophage–derived growth factors; IL-1 = interleukin-1; IGF = insulin-like growth factors; TGF = transforming growth factor; EGF = epidermal growth factor.
†Documented only in the granulomatous lung disorders.
From Cerra FB (ed): Critical Care: State of the Art. Fullerton, Society of Critical Care Medicine, 1987, p 356.

observed following acute lung injury. Nonetheless, as lung injury and repair evolve, increased numbers of mononuclear phagocytes are found within the alveolar wall.[13, 89] Moreover, a variety of the signals known to be capable of stimulating macrophage growth factor release, for example, endotoxin, are present in most circumstances associated with acute lung injury. Thus, it is reasonable to suspect an important role for growth factors released by macrophages in the physiological reconstitution of the alveolar interstitium and in the pathogenesis of acute alveolar fibrosis.

A second type of resident cell that may be an important source of growth factors for lung mesenchymal cells are the mesenchymal cells themselves. Lung mesenchymal cells can be stimulated to produce certain growth factors, including IGF.[90] In this regard, one important signal for autocrine IGF production is known to be PDGF,[91] and another is likely to be AMDGF.[92] As a group, the IGFs range in molecular mass from 5000 to 20,000 daltons and interact at the target cell surface with one of two distinct receptors.[92] Lung mesenchymal cells have receptors for both IGF-1 and IGF-2.[93] The specific type of IGF produced by mesenchymal cells appears to depend on their differentiated state, with fetal mesenchymal cells producing more IGF-2 and adult cells more IGF-1,[93] although this has not been firmly established with freshly isolated mesenchymal cells from the human lung. The IGFs deliver a specific signal late in the G_1 phase of the cell cycle a few hours prior to entry into S phase.[94, 95] Recent evidence suggests that vas-

cular mesenchymal cells may also be capable of the autocrine production of a PDGF-like molecule.[96] Whether lung mesenchymal cells following acute lung injury behave similarly remains unexplored.

A final resident cell known to be capable of producing a growth factor for mesenchymal cells is the endothelial cell. Specifically relevant to acute lung injury, components of the coagulation cascade such as thrombin[97] and factor Xa[98] are capable of stimulating endothelial cell production of a PDGF-like molecule. Whether the microvascular cells following acute lung injury locally release PDGF remains undefined.

Recruited Cells. The predominant cells recruited to the alveolar structures during the first several days after acute lung injury are neutrophils, platelets, and additional macrophages. Neutrophils do not appear to play a major role in stimulating lung mesenchymal cell replication. However, platelets are a well-known source of growth factors for mesenchymal cells. Among the factors produced by platelets are PDGF and an epidermal growth factor (EGF)-like molecule capable of stimulating mesenchymal cell replication that may be identical to transforming growth factor-α (TGF-α).[99] Similarly, recent evidence also suggests that activated macrophages are capable of releasing EGF/TGF-α.[100] While the biochemical evidence that these molecules are present remains incomplete, the morphological evidence of degranulated platelets and activated macrophages within the alveolar interstitium strongly supports a potential role for these factors.[13] After the first couple of weeks there is less morphological information regarding the recruited cell populations that are present within the alveolar structures.

Circulation. The circulation may also be an important source of growth factors for lung mesenchymal cells following lung injury. The circulation contains platelet release products as well as inflammatory cell mediators. In addition, the circulation ordinarily contains high concentrations of fibronectin,[101] IGF,[102] and very likely EGF as well.[103] With the abolition of normal barrier function, macromolecules present in plasma are over-represented in the alveolar interstitium.[57] Thus, products not normally present in the circulation and increased concentrations of growth-promoting agents normally present in the circulation may both play a role in signaling lung mesenchymal cell replication during lung repair. In view of this plethora of regulatory signals for lung mesenchymal cells, it is important to recognize that there is limited information regarding which of these factors are present following acute lung injury or during lung repair. It remains a task for future investigators to identify and purify the major growth-promoting signals directing the process of mesenchymal cell replication during lung repair.

Equally important to a thorough understanding of the process of interstitial repair following acute lung injury is the identification of signals that inhibit the process of mesenchymal cell replication and therefore serve to control and limit the fibrotic process. The principal class of mediators known to inhibit mesenchymal cell replication are the E series prostaglandins (PGE),[78, 104–106] although other agents such as TGF-β may be important. (Chapter 18 presents a detailed discussion of the eicosanoids involved in the wound healing process.) Molecules inhibiting mesenchymal cell replication derive from resident cells, recruited cells, and plasma. Both PGE and TGF-β are known to be produced by alveolar macrophages,[107] and in addition, alveolar macrophages can be stimulated to release an as yet uncharacterized macromolecule that stimulates autocrine PGE production by mesenchymal cells.[104–106] Among the recruited cells, both neutrophils and platelets are potential sources of arachidonic acid metabolites as well as other modulators of mesenchymal cell replication.[108, 109] Plasma may also serve as a source of E series prostaglandins as well as proteins that may directly, or by serving as binding moieties for growth factors, actually inhibit mesenchymal cell replication.[110, 111] Given the importance of controlling mesenchymal cell replication following acute lung injury, it is notable that neither PGE, TGF-β, nor other putative inhibitors have been measured or clearly identified within the gas exchange apparatus in this clinical setting. Correctly applying the lessons learned from basic studies of mesenchymal cell biology as well as from studies of the chronic fibrotic lung disorders and wound healing may permit identification of the basic molecular and cellular events associated with mesenchymal cell replication following acute lung injury.

Mesenchymal Cell Connective Tissue Metabolism

Stromal reconstitution as well as restoration of the cellular populations within the interstitium constitutes a critical step in the repair of the gas exchange apparatus. Our knowledge of the sequelae of damage to the interstitium following lung injury is derived from detailed immunohistochemical, ultrastructural, and molecular studies of acute lung injury in patients as well as animal models. In some patients, reconstitution of stromal elements permits a return to near normal interstitial anatomy, but in many patients, acute fibrosis occurs. The interstitium is expanded with collagen, elastin, fibronectin, and other extracellular matrix proteins that extend from the interstitium into the alveolar air space, obliterating the air-lung interface.

Some insight into the pathogenesis of acute alveolar fibrosis is provided by bleomycin-induced lung injury in the hamster.[112] In this model of lung injury, current evidence suggests that the transcriptional activity of genes coding for type I procollagen, elastin, and fibronectin is selectively increased, resulting in elevated levels of the respective mRNAs coding for these three extracellular matrix proteins.[113–115] The result is an expanded interstitium with increased deposition of collagen, elastin, and proteoglycans as well as intra-alveolar fibrosis.

While transcriptional activity of connective tissue genes has not been assessed in patients following acute lung injury, biochemical analysis indicates there is an accumulation of type I and III collagen in the expanded interstitium.[116] Type III collagen predominates during early repair, and type I collagen in the later stages.[116] The basement membrane is disrupted early in the course of lung injury with invasion of the alveolar air space by collagens similar in type to those present in the adjacent interstitium.[116] Detailed ultrastructural studies of lung tissue from patients with acute lung injury reveal gaps in the epithelial basement membrane through which myofibroblasts migrate, replicate, and release connective tissue macromolecules, leading to intra-alveolar fibrosis (Fig. 25–7).[60]

Based on the diametric outcomes possible following acute lung injury (i.e., repair or acute fibrosis), it is apparent that identification of the signals that regulate the synthesis and degradation as well as the distribution of newly formed stromal elements is essential to a thorough knowledge of alveolar repair. This active area of investigation has resulted in the identification of several molecules that may play a role. One of these is transforming growth factor-β (TGF-β), a 25 kDa peptide found in platelets and produced by mononuclear phagocytes and endothelial cells.[117–120] This molecule is capable of enhancing the formation of extracellular matrix as well as inhibiting its degradation. TGF-β stimulates mesenchymal cell collagen and fibronectin synthesis.[121] In addition, TGF-β inhibits the proteolytic degradation of newly formed matrix proteins by (1) an increase in the formation and secretion of a plasminogen activator inhibitor,[122] and (2) a decrease in the secretion of three different types of proteinases, including a plasminogen activator.[123]

AIR-LUNG INTERFACE

Since the alveolar epithelium constitutes the primary barrier to the flux of salt and water from the capillary into the alveolar air space, restoration of epithelial integrity is a central event in the termination of alveolar flooding and the resumption of gas exchange.[59] There are two distinct phases leading to repair of the air-lung interface: (1) replication of type 2 epithelial cells, and (2) their differentiation into type 1 epithelial cells. Although an active area of investigation, essentially no information is available regarding the molecular signaling of the differentiation of type 2 cells into type 1 cells. Therefore, the remainder of this discussion will focus on type 2 cell replication.

Cytokinetic information in a murine model of acute lung injury suggests that reconstitution of the air-lung interface by replication of type 2 epithelial cells begins within 2 or 3 days following acute lung injury.[124] These observations have been corroborated by systematic morphological studies in a primate model of ARDS[89] as well as in patients,[125] suggesting that a similar sequence of events occurs in clinically significant lung injuries (Fig. 25–10). Despite the recognized importance of timely and orderly type 2 cell replication in lung repair, there is no information regarding which signals within the altered alveolar microenvironment direct the process of epithelial replication. Despite the paucity of direct information, recent studies examining the replication of freshly isolated type 2 cells in culture have provided some insights.

Consistent with the behavior of other epithelial cells, both a suitable substratum and the presence of specific growth regulatory molecules are important in controlling the replication of type 2 epithelial cells. For example, type 2 cells attach to the connective tissue matrix by interacting with a specific attachment factor. In contrast to other epithelial cells examined, however, fibronectin rather than laminin appears to serve this function.[126] Once appropriately attached, type 2 cells are capable of responding to specific growth-promoting signals provided by resident cells, recruited cells, and macromolecules in plasma.

Among the resident cells, alveolar macrophages are capable of releasing an as yet uncharacterized factor capable of augmenting DNA synthesis in rat type 2 cells.[127] In addition, mononuclear phagocytes are capable of releasing EGF/TGF-α.[100] In this regard, alveolar type 2 cells express EGF receptors on their surface[128] and increase their rate of DNA synthesis in response to this ligand.[129] Although it has not been formally demonstrated, type 2 cells would likely also respond to TGF-α, which shares with EGF a nanomolar affinity for the EGF receptor.[130] Additional investigations will undoubtedly help to elucidate the possible significance of EGF and TGF-α in lung repair.

Another potential source of growth factors for epithelial cells in addition to the alveolar macrophage is the lung mesenchymal cell. Rat fetal lung mesenchymal cells produce pneumocyte-stimulating factor, an approximately 10,000 dalton protein that stimulates fetal rat type 2 cells to synthesize surfactant.[131] Its activity as a possible growth factor for type 2 cells has not been defined, but since mesenchymal cells following lung injury divide and appear morphologically less differentiated, it is possible that pneumocyte-stimulating factor is released; however, this concept remains unexplored. In addition, mesenchymal cells can be induced to release IGFs, which not only are important for mesenchymal cell replication but also appear to be required for the replication of nearly all normal diploid cells studied to date.[132]

Among the recruited cells, macrophages and platelets are potential sources of growth factors for epithelial cells. As discussed previously,

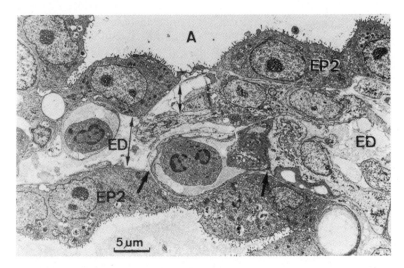

Figure 25–10. Electron micrograph of alveolar structures 5 days following acute lung injury. Replication of type 2 epithelial cells (EP2) has resulted in an epithelium made up almost exclusively of type 2 cells. Interstitial edema (ED) is still present. A = alveolar airspace. (From Bachofen M, Weibel ER: Structural alterations of lung parenchyma in the adult respiratory distress syndrome. Clin Chest Med 3:35–56, 1982.)

macrophages are capable of modulating type 2 cell DNA synthesis.[127] Platelets as well as macrophages release an EGF-like molecule that may share with EGF the ability to stimulate type 2 cell DNA synthesis.[133, 134]

Plasma contains IGF[102] and EGF,[103] and may contain other molecules capable of stimulating type 2 cell replication. Direct demonstration that plasma, serum, or its individual components besides IGF and EGF can modulate type 2 cell replication is lacking. In some epithelial cell systems (e.g., bronchial epithelial cells) serum inhibits replication, rather than stimulating it.[135] The recent purification from serum of a molecule that terminates replication and signals differentiation of epithelial cells may be highly relevant to the process of alveolar repair.[136] The relative stimulatory and/or inhibitory activity of plasma components for type 2 cells remains an area of active investigation.

BLOOD-LUNG INTERFACE

The anatomical events of acute lung injury and repair, detailed in patients as well as animal models, provide the basis for evaluating the molecular mechanisms that determine the effectiveness of the repair process. At the blood-lung interface the injurious agent induces an integral alteration in the normally nonthrombogenic pulmonary endothelium[137, 138] so that intravascular coagulation ensues. The resultant platelet and leukocyte aggregation, in conjunction with biomolecules that mediate inflammation and cellular injury, results in microvascular endothelial cell dysfunction and death.[139, 140] Ultrastructurally, endothelial cells are swollen with rarefied cytoplasm, dilated endoplasmic

reticulum, and swollen mitochondria (Fig. 25–8). Morphologically, cells become separated from their basement membrane.[139, 140] Eventually the number of capillaries decreases while their basement membranes appear frayed and reduplicated.[141] When an effective pulmonary circulation is to be re-established, endothelial cell replication along the structural framework provided by the denuded basement membranes apparently takes place.[140, 141] Though the exact microanatomy in the reconstituted lung of patients surviving acute lung injury remains to be detailed and direct hemodynamic measurements are lacking, the recovery of nearly normal lung function in some of these patients suggests that effective reconstitution of the blood-lung interface has occurred.[142]

In marked contrast, in many patients failure of effective repair occurs, contributing to development of an abnormal gas exchange apparatus and progressive respiratory failure. In this circumstance, the most significant changes result from dramatic alterations in vascular mesenchymal cell number and distribution.[31, 140, 143, 144] Intra-acinar smooth muscle cells and pericytes replicate and migrate peripherally along the vessel wall toward the alveolus.[49, 145, 146] The media and intima of the largest precapillary microvessels are markedly expanded by replicating mesenchymal cells, resulting in a significant decrease in luminal diameter. Partially muscular and nonmuscular precapillary microvessels as well as capillaries undergo a rapid process of muscularization as mesenchymal cell replication and migration occur. This substantially decreases luminal diameter in vessels that normally contribute little to total pulmonary vascular resistance. In some regions, re-endothelialization is incomplete; in others, it follows irregular patterns conferred by reduplicated basement membranes. Based on these detailed morphological events, an initial pathogenetic paradigm would account for the apparently opposing influences of microvascular repair that result in reconstitution of the microvascular bed and muscularization in which mesenchymal cell replication and migration lead to a marked increase in vascular resistance.

Microvascular Repair

Endothelial cell migration and replication are controlled by exogenous growth regulatory signals termed angiogenesis factors,[147, 148] and a number of these factors have been defined. Two major classes of heparin-binding angiogenesis factors have been identified.[147, 149, 150] The first class includes acidic fibroblast growth factor (FGF), or endothelial cell growth factor. Acidic FGF is a 140 amino acid polypeptide with a molecular mass of 15,000 to 18,000 daltons.[147, 151, 152] The second class includes basic FGF, which is a 146 amino acid polypeptide with a molecular mass of 16,000 to 18,500 daltons.[147, 153] Basic FGF has been found in various tissues and cells, including tissue macrophages.[148, 154, 155] Both classes of heparin-binding growth factors stimulate endothelial cell chemotaxis and replication and induce in vivo angiogenesis.[147]

Several non–heparin-binding angiogenic factors have also been described. Transforming growth factor-α (TGF-α), a <10,000 dalton polypeptide, is a direct-acting angiogenesis factor that is expressed by wound macrophages and that has mitogenic activity for endothelial cells in vitro and promotes angiogenesis in vivo.[156] Unlike TGF-α, transforming growth factor-β (TGF-β) appears to induce angiogenesis indirectly. A recent study has shown that TGF-β is chemotactic for monocytes and induces their expression of angiogenic activity.[157] Tumor necrosis factor-α (TNF-α) is a 17,000-dalton polypeptide that is an inflammatory mediator produced by macrophages.[158, 159] TNF-α has been reported to cause angiogenesis in vivo, but recent evidence suggests that, as with TGF-β, this effect may be secondary to the induction of inflammation.[121, 160–162]

Angiogenesis factors that induce endothelial cell migration but not proliferation in vitro yet cause in vivo angiogenesis have been isolated from wound fluids.[121, 160, 161] Purification is incomplete, but the wound fluid factor(s) appears to be a low molecular weight peptide. While unproved, the cellular source of wound fluid angiogenesis factor(s) is thought to be macrophages because wounds deficient in macrophages generally lack vascular ingrowth. A number of other molecules relevant to endothelial cell motility and replication have been described, including angiogenin and prostaglandins.[147, 148, 162–164]

While the signals within the pulmonary microenvironment that serve to modulate endothelial cell migration and replication following acute lung injury remain undefined, available data support the concept that angiogenesis factors, in part derived from alveolar macrophages, have a role in the vascular repair that follows lung injury. First, although the factor that regulates wound-associated angiogenesis is incompletely characterized, wounds rich in macrophages elaborate angiogenesis factor(s) and stimulate vascular ingrowth, while those deficient in macrophages do not. Second, macrophages are known to produce other factors capable of modulating angiogenesis including basic FGF, TGF-α, and TNFα.[148, 156, 162, 165] Therefore, the importance of angiogenesis factors as primary signals for endothelial cell migration and replication, coupled with the fact that macrophages, a source of characterized angiogenesis factors, are present in increased numbers in proximity to pulmonary microvessels following diffuse acute lung injury, supports the hypothesis that reconstitution of the blood-lung interface may be mediated by macrophage-derived angiogenesis factors.

Muscularization

Extensive evidence indicates that growth factors have an important role in controlling mesenchymal cell replication and migration, two primary processes leading to muscularization (see "Interstitium," above). Among the growth factors acting on mesenchymal cells, both PDGF and fibronectin are potent mesenchymal cell chemoattractants.[73, 74] While the role of fibronectin remains unexplored, the potential role of PDGF in the process of muscularization of the pulmonary microcirculation is strengthened by two observations: (1) platelets adhere to areas of denuded or damaged endothelium and likely degranulate, providing one plausible cellular source of PDGF;[13] and (2) intravascular coagulation with thrombin generation is an ongoing process at the endothelial surface, and thrombin is known to induce endothelial cell production of PDGF.[97] These observations implicate PDGF in the process of vascular muscularization.

In addition to the direct mechanical and hemodynamic disturbances associated with excessive mesenchymal cell replication and migration within the vessel wall, muscularization may also influence re-establishment of an intact blood-lung interface. Both smooth muscle cells and pericytes, cells in intimate contact with pulmonary microvascular endothelial cells, increase markedly during the muscularization process. In vitro, both of these mesenchymal cell types inhibit endothelial cell replication, and this inhibition depends on physical contact with the endothelial cells and varies directly with the ratio of mesenchymal cells to endothelial cells.[51] Thus, ineffective microvascular repair may result from the contact-dependent inhibitory effect of vascular mesenchymal cells on endothelial cell replication.

FUTURE DIRECTIONS

Significant progress has been made in achieving a better understanding of the pathogenetic mechanisms of acute lung injury. Unfortunately, this knowledge has not yet been translated into improved patient survival.[1-3, 166-169] To be effective, therapy intended to limit the extent of the initial injury must be administered soon after the injury. In current practice, this is rarely possible due to three factors: (1) the 6 to 24 hour lag between the onset of injury and the first appearance of clinical signs and symptoms; (2) the frightening rapidity with which patients develop fulminant respiratory failure following these earliest clinical findings; and (3) the inability to predict which at-risk patients will develop ARDS. For these reasons, improving the prognosis following acute lung injury will likely be achieved by developing therapies designed to enhance the lung repair process, and this will require a better understanding of the cellular and molecular events of lung repair.

Clinical investigation of the repair phase of acute lung injury has begun in several centers with an expansion of the data base of patients with lung injury. Although patients can be stratified into good and poor prognosis groups on the basis of multiple physiological parameters at the onset of illness,[1, 2, 166] these classification schemes remain imperfect. Information correlating the physiological parameters of illness with cellular and biochemical abnormalities at the site of injury are of critical importance. In such studies, comprehensive physiological and metabolic testing in concert with repeated bronchoalveolar lavage following the onset of illness will be carried out. Physiological and metabolic indicators of pulmonary performance and systemic sepsis syndrome can

then be correlated with inflammatory mediators and growth regulatory substances present in the alveolar microenvironment. It is conceivable that a profile of bronchoalveolar lavage fluid and cellular constituents will emerge as containing the proper balance of growth factors and growth inhibiting activities to promote normal alveolar repair, portending a good prognosis. Likewise, patients who do poorly may have a recognizable biochemical and cellular profile that differs from that of the survivors.

In addition to clinical and analytical studies of lavage fluid recovered from patients with acute lung injury, research examining the basic mechanisms of mesenchymal, epithelial, and endothelial cell growth regulation is of central importance. Particularly important are studies of how growth factor–receptor interactions direct growth regulatory gene expression. Elucidating the basic mechanisms of cell replication and the fundamental scientific principles of organ repair will likely lead to improved treatment strategies following acute lung injury.

Current therapy for acute lung injury is limited to sophisticated ventilatory and circulatory support measures. As increasing knowledge permits more precise prediction of which patients will develop acute lung injury and our understanding of the pathogenesis of lung injury improves, specific therapies to limit injury will emerge. For example, since an excess of proteolytic enzymes and toxic oxygen metabolites contributes to the alveolar injury,[6-12, 19-21] delivery of antiproteases and antioxidant substances to the alveolar surface warrants consideration. In addition, trials of surfactant replacement to limit the adverse effects of positive pressure ventilation are under way.

Therapeutic advances based on an improved understanding of the alveolar repair process are also on the horizon. To promote alveolar repair, molecules will be identified and developed that accelerate epithelial cell replication, limit mesenchymal cell replication, and promote endothelial cell replication and reconstitution. Ideally, these substances will be delivered to the alveoli by the inhalational route to maximize their therapeutic efficacy while minimizing their systemic activity.

Additional comprehensive epidemiological studies based on biochemical and cellular as well as physiological parameters will permit better assignment of patients to prognostic categories at diagnosis. This will enable clinicians to identify patients in whom recovery is likely without therapy, those who require therapy to improve outcome, and those who are unlikely to recover even if given maximal support and therapy. Young patients in the latter category, if identified early in the course of their illness, could be considered for lung transplantation.

The prognosis following severe acute lung injury has not improved over the past 20 years despite advances in supportive care.[1-3, 166-169] Improving survival will depend upon a coordinated multidisciplinary approach by medical scientists and clinicians.

References

1. Fowler AA, Hamman RF, Zerbe GO, et al: Adult respiratory distress syndrome: Prognosis after onset. Am Rev Resp Dis 132:472–478, 1985.
2. Kaplan RL, Sahn SA, Petty TL: Incidence and outcome of the respiratory distress syndrome in gram-negative sepsis. Arch Intern Med 139:867–869, 1979.
3. Montgomery AB, Stager MA, Carrico CJ, et al: Causes of mortality in patients with the adult respiratory distress syndrome. Am Rev Resp Dis 132:485–489, 1985.
4. Davis WB, Rennard SI, Bitterman PB, et al: Pulmonary oxygen toxicity: Early reversible changes in human alveolar structures induced by hyperoxia. N Engl J Med 309:878–883, 1983.
5. Pontoppidan H, Huttemeier PC, Quinn DA: Etiology, demography, and outcome in acute respiratory failure. In Zapol WM, Falke KJ (eds): Acute Respiratory Failure. New York, Marcel Dekker, 1985, pp 1–21.
6. McGuire WW, Spragg RG, Cohen AB, et al: Studies on the pathogenesis of the adult respiratory distress syndrome. J Clin Invest 69:543–553, 1982.
7. Schraufstatter IU, Revak SD, Cochrane CG: Proteases and oxidants in experimental pulmonary inflammatory injury. J Clin Invest 73:1175–1184, 1984.
8. Lee CT, Fein AM, Lippman M, et al: Elastolytic activity in pulmonary lavage fluid from patients with adult respiratory distress syndrome. N Engl J Med 304:192–196, 1981.
9. Fantone JC, Ward PA: Role of oxygen-derived free radicals and metabolites in leukocyte dependent inflammatory reactions. Am J Pathol 107:397–418, 1982.
10. Klebonoff SJ: The iron-H_2O_2-iodide cytotoxic system. J Exp Med 156:1262–1267, 1982.
11. Fridovich I: Superoxide radical: An endogenous toxicant. Annu Rev Pharmacol Toxicol 23:235–257, 1983.
12. McCord JM: Oxygen-derived free radicals in post-ischemic tissue injury. N Engl J Med 312:159–163, 1985.
13. Bachofen M, Weibel ER: Structural alterations of lung parenchyma in the adult respiratory distress syndrome. Clin Chest Med 3:35–56, 1982.
14. Henson PM, Larson GL, Webster RO, et al: Pulmonary microvascular alterations and lung injury produced by complement fragments: Synergistic effect of complement activation, neutrophil sequestration, and prostaglandins. Ann NY Acad Sci 384:287–299, 1982.
15. Till GO, Johnson NJ, Kunkel R, et al: Intravascular activation of complement and acute lung injury. Dependency on neutrophils and toxic oxygen metabolites. J Clin Invest 69:1126–1135, 1982.
16. Weiland JE, Davis WB, Holter JF, et al: Lung neutrophils in the adult respiratory distress syndrome: Clinical and pathophysiological significance. Am Rev Resp Dis 133:216–225, 1986.
17. Schoenberger CI, Rennard SI, Bitterman PB, et al: Paraquat induced pulmonary fibrosis. Role of the alveolitis in modulating the development of fibrosis. Am Rev Resp Dis 129:168–173, 1984.
18. Hammerschmidt DE: Activation of the complement system and of granulocytes in lung injury: The adult respiratory distress syndrome. Adv Inflamm Res 5:147–171, 1983.
19. Tate RM, Van Benthuysen KM, Shasby DM, et al: Oxygen radical–mediated permeability edema and vasoconstriction in isolated perfused rabbit lungs. Am Rev Resp Dis 126:802–806, 1982.
20. White CW, Repine JE: Pulmonary antioxidant defense mechanisms. Exp Lung Res 8:81–96, 1985.
21. Martin WJ, Gadek JE, Hunninghake GW, et al: Oxidant injury of lung parenchymal cells. J Clin Invest 68:1277–1288, 1981.
22. Bell RC, Coalson JJ, Smith JD, et al: Multiple system organ failure and infection in adult respiratory distress syndrome. Ann Int Med 99:293–298, 1983.
23. Bone RC: Treatment of severe hypoxemia due to the adult respiratory distress syndrome. Arch Intern Med 140:85–89, 1980.
24. Prewitt RM, McCarthy J, Wood LDH: Treatment of acute low pressure pulmonary edema in dogs. Relative effects of hydrostatic and oncotic pressure, nitroprusside, and positive end-expiratory pressure. J Clin Invest 67:409–418, 1981.
25. Petty TL, Fowler AA: Another look at ARDS. Chest 82:98–103, 1982.
26. Alberts WM, Priest GR, Moser KM: The outlook for survivors of ARDS. Chest 84:272–274, 1983.
27. Lakshminarayan S, Stanford RE, Petty TL: Prognosis after recovery from adult respiratory distress syndrome. Am Rev Resp Dis 113:7–15, 1976.
28. Lamy M, Fallat RJ, Koeniger E, et al: Pathologic features and mechanisms of hypoxemia in adult respiratory distress syndrome. Am Rev Resp Dis 114:267–284, 1976.
29. Douglas ME, Downs JB: Pulmonary function following severe acute respiratory failure and high levels of positive end-expiratory pressure. Chest 71:18–23, 1977.
30. Elliott CG, Morris AH, Cengiz M: Pulmonary function and gas exchange in survivors of adult respiratory distress syndrome. Am Rev Resp Dis 123:492–495, 1981.
31. Meyrick B: The structure and ultrastructure of the pulmonary microvasculature. In Will JA, Dawson CA, Weir EK, et al (eds): The Pulmonary Circulation in Health and Disease. Orlando, Academic Press, 27–39, 1987.
32. Reid L: The 1978 J. Burns Amberson lecture. The pulmonary circulation: Remodeling in growth and disease. Am Rev Resp Dis 119:531–546, 1979.
33. Meyrick B, Reid L: Ultrastructural features of the distended pulmonary arteries of the normal rat. Anat Rec 193:71–98, 1979.
34. Bradley KH, Kawanami O, Ferrans VJ, et al: The fibroblast of human alveolar structure: A differentiated cell with a major role in lung structures and function. In Harris CC, Trump BF, Stoner GD (eds): Methods in Cell Biology, vol. 21. New York, Academic Press, 1980, pp 37–64.
35. Ross R: The connective tissue fiber forming cell. In Ramachandran GN (ed): Treatise on Collagen. New York, Academic Press, 1968, pp 2–82.
36. Ross R: The fibroblast and wound repair. Biol Rev Cambridge Philos Soc 43:51–96, 1968.
37. Brandes D, Murphy DG, Anton EB, et al: Ultrastructural and cytochemical changes in cultured human lung cells. J Ultrastruct Res 39:465–483, 1972.

38. Kuhn C: The cells of the lung and their organelles. In Crystal RG (ed): The Biochemical Basis of Pulmonary Function. New York, Marcel Dekker, 1976, pp 3–48.

39. Vaccarro C, Brody JS: Ultrastructure of developing alveoli. I. The role of the interstitial fibroblast. Anat Rec 192:467–480, 1978.

40. Brody JS, Vaccaro C: Postnatal formation of alveoli: Interstitial events and physiologic consequences. Fed Proc 38:215–223, 1979.

41. O'Hare KH, Reiss OK, Vatter AE: Esterases in developing and adult rat lung I. Biochemical and electron microscopic observations. J Histochem Cytochem 19:97–115, 1971.

42. Askin FB, Kuhn C: The cellular origin of pulmonary surfactant. Lab Invest 25:260–268, 1971.

43. Kapanci Y, Assimacopoulos A, Irle C, et al: "Contractile interstitial cells" in pulmonary alveolar septa: A possible regulator of ventilation/perfusion ratio? Ultrastructural, immunofluorescence and in vitro studies. J Cell Biol 60:375–392, 1974.

44. Ryan GB, Cliff WJ, Gabbiani G, et al: Myofibroblasts in an avascular fibrous tissue. Lab Invest 29:197–206, 1973.

45. Rhodin JA: Ultrastructure of mammalian venous capillaries, venules, and small collecting veins. J Ultrastruct Res 25:452–500, 1968.

46. Weibel ER: Morphologic basis of alveolar-capillary gas exchange. Physiol Rev 53:419–495, 1975.

47. Bitterman PB, Rennard SI, Crystal RG: Environmental lung disease and the interstitium. Clin Chest Med 2:393–412, 1981.

48. Burri PH: Morphology and respiratory function of the alveolar unit. Int Arch Allergy Appl Immunol (Suppl) 1:2–12, 1985.

49. Meyrick B, Reid L: The alveolar wall. Br J Dis Chest 64:121–140, 1970.

50. Meyrick B, Reid L: Hypoxia and incorporation of ^{3}H-thymidine by cells of the rat pulmonary arteries and alveolar wall. Am J Pathol 96:51–70, 1979.

51. Orlidge A, D'Amore PA: Inhibition of capillary endothelial cell growth by pericytes and smooth muscle cells. J Cell Biol 105:1455–1462, 1987.

52. Crapo JD, Barry BE, Gehr P, et al: Cell numbers and characteristics of the normal human lung. Am Rev Resp Dis 126:332–337, 1982.

53. Furthmayr H, Roll FJ, Madri JA: Composition of basement membrane as viewed with the electron microscope. In Kuehn K, Schoene HH, Timpel R (eds): New Trends in Basement Membrane Research. New York, Raven Press, 1982, pp 31–48.

54. Pietra GG, Ruttner JR, Wust W, et al: The lung after trauma and shock—fine structure of the alveolar capillary barrier in 23 autopsies. J Trauma 21:454–462, 1981.

55. Bachofen M, Weibel ER: Alteration of the gas exchange apparatus in adult respiratory insufficiency associated with septicemia. Am Rev Resp Dis 116:589–615, 1977.

56. Brigham KL, Bowers RE, Haynes J: Increased sheep lung vascular permeability caused by E. coli endotoxin. Circ Res 45:292–297, 1976.

57. Holter JF, Weiland JE, Pacht ER, et al: Protein permeability in the adult respiratory distress syndrome. Loss of size selectivity of the alveolar epithelium. J Clin Invest 78:1513–1522, 1986.

58. Schnells G, Voigt WH, Redl H, et al: Electron-microscopic investigation of lung biopsies in patients with post-traumatic respiratory insufficiency. Acta Chir Scand (Suppl) 499:9–20, 1980.

59. Wangensteen OD, Witmers LE Jr, Johnson JA: Permeability of the mammalian blood gas barrier and its components. Am J Physiol 216:719–727, 1969.

60. Fukuda Y, Ishizaki M, Masuda Y, et al: The role of intraalveolar fibrosis in the process of pulmonary structural remodeling in patients with diffuse alveolar damage. Am J Pathol 126:171–182, 1987.

61. Zapol WM, Trelstad RL, Coffey JW, et al: Pulmonary fibrosis in severe acute respiratory insufficiency. Am Rev Resp Dis 119:542–554, 1979.

62. Crystal RG, Bitterman PB, Rennard SI, et al: Interstitial lung diseases of unknown cause: Disorders characterized by chronic inflammation of the lower respiratory tract. N Engl J Med 310:154–165, 235–244, 1984.

63. Bitterman PB, Rennard SI, Crystal RG: Environmental lung disease and the interstitium. Clin Chest Med 2:393–412, 1981.

64. Crystal RG, Gadek JE, Ferrans VJ, et al: Interstitial lung disease: Current concepts of pathogenesis, staging and therapy. Am J Med 70:542–568, 1981.

65. Crystal RG, Fulmer JD, Roberts WC, et al: Idiopathic pulmonary fibrosis: Clinical, histologic, radiographic, physiologic, scintigraphic, cytologic, and biochemical aspects. Ann Intern Med 85:769–788, 1976.

66. Stack HR, Choo-Kang YFJ, Heard BE: The prognosis of cryptogenic fibrosing alveolitis. Thorax 27:535–542, 1972.

67. Carrington CB, Gaensler EA, Coutu RE, et al: Natural history and treated course of usual and desquamative interstitial pneumonia. N Engl J Med 298:801–809, 1978.

68. Turner-Warwick M, Burrows B, Johnson A: Cryptogenic fibrosing alveolitis: Clinical features and their influence on survival. Thorax 35:171–180, 1980.

69. Bitterman PB, Rennard SI, Keogh BA, et al: Familial idiopathic pulmonary fibrosis: Evidence of lung inflammation in unaffected family members. N Engl J Med 314:1343–1347, 1986.

70. Underwood LE, VanWyk JJ: Normal and aberrant growth. In Wilson JD, Foster DW (eds): Textbook of Endocrinology. Philadelphia, WB Saunders, 1985, 155–205.

71. Martinet Y, Rom WN, Grotendorst GR, et al: Exaggerated spontaneous release of platelet-derived growth factor by alveolar macrophages from patients with idiopathic pulmonary fibrosis. N Engl J Med 317:202–209, 1987.

72. Pledger WJ, Stiles CD, Antoniades N, et al: An ordered sequence of events is required before BALB/C-3T3 cells become committed to DNA synthesis. Proc Natl Acad Sci USA 75:2839–2843, 1978.

73. Grotendorst GR: Alteration of the chemotactic response of NIH/3T3 cells to PDGF by growth factors, transformation, and tumor promoters. Cell 36:279–285, 1984.

74. Rennard SI, Hunninghake GW, Bitterman PB, et al: Production of fibronectin by the human alveolar macrophage: Mechanism for the recruitment of fibroblasts to sites of tissue injury in interstitial lung disease. Proc Natl Acad Sci USA 78:7147–7151, 1981.

75. Bitterman PB, Rennard S, Adelberg S, et al: Role of fibronectin as a growth factor for fibroblasts. J Cell Biol 97:1925–1932, 1983.

76. Bitterman PB, Adelberg S, Crystal RG: Mechanisms of pulmonary fibrosis: spontaneous release of the alveolar macrophage derived growth factor in the interstitial lung disorders. J Clin Invest 72:1801–1813, 1983.

77. Hunninghake GW: Release of interleukin-1 by alveolar macrophages of patients with active pulmonary sarcoidosis. Am Rev Resp Dis 129:569–572, 1984.

78. Bitterman PB, Wewers MD, Rennard SI, et al: Modulation of alveolar macrophage-driven fibroblast proliferation by alternative macrophage mediators. J Clin Invest 77:700–708, 1986.

79. Raines EW, Dower SK, Ross R: Interleukin-1 mitogenic activity for fibroblasts and smooth muscle cells is due to PDGF-AA. Science 243:393–396, 1989.

80. Bitterman PB, Adelberg S, Crystal RG: Mechanisms of pulmonary fibrosis: Spontaneous release of the alveolar macrophage derived growth factor in the interstitial lung disorders. J Clin Invest 72:1801–1813, 1983.

81. Bitterman PB, Rennard SI, Hunninghake GW, et al: Human alveolar macrophage growth factor for fibroblasts. Regulation and partial characterization. J Clin Invest 70:806–822, 1982.

82. DeLustro F, Sherer GK, LeRoy EC: Human monocyte stimulation of fibroblast growth by a soluble mediator(s). Res J Reticuloendothel Soc 28:519–532, 1981.

83. Glenn KC, Ross R: Human monocyte-derived growth factor(s) for mesenchymal cells: Activation of secretion by endotoxin and concanavalin A. Cell 25:603–615, 1981.

84. Mornex JF, Martinet Y, Yamauchi K, et al: Spontaneous expression of the c-sis gene and release of a platelet-derived growth factor-like molecule by human alveolar macrophages. J Clin Invest 78:61–66, 1986.

85. Leibovich SJ, Ross R: A macrophage-dependent factor that stimulates the proliferation of fibroblasts in vitro. Am J Pathol 84:501–513, 1976.

86. Schmidt JA, Oliver CN, Lepe Zuniga L, et al: Interleukin-1, a potential regulator of fibroblast proliferation. J Immunol 128:2177–2182, 1982.

87. Schmidt JA, Oliver CN, Lepe Zuniga L, et al: Silica-stimulated monocytes release fibroblast proliferation factors identical to interleukin-1. A potential role for interleukin-1 in the pathogenesis of silicosis. J Clin Invest 73:1462–1472, 1984.

88. Martinet Y, Bitterman PB, Mornex JF, et al: Activated human monocytes express the c-sis proto-oncogene and release a mediator with platelet-derived growth factor-like activity. Nature 319:158–160, 1986.

89. Kapanci Y, Weibel ER, Kaplan HP, et al: Pathogenesis and reversibility of the pulmonary lesions of oxygen toxicity in monkeys. Lab Invest 20:101–118, 1969.

90. Bitterman PB, Rennard SI, Nissley SP, et al: Insulin-like growth factor production by fibroblasts: Stimulation by alveolar macrophage derived growth factor. Clin Res 30:385A, 1982.

91. Clemmons DR, Underwood LE, Van Wyk JJ: Hormonal control of immunoreactive somatomedin production by cultured human fibroblasts. J Clin Invest 67:10–19, 1981.

92. King GL, Kahn RC, Rechler MM, et al: Direct demonstration of separate receptors for growth and metabolic activities of insulin and multiplication stimulating activity (an insulin-like growth factor) using antibodies to the insulin receptor. J Clin Invest 66:130–140, 1980.

93. Rechler MM, Nissley SP: The nature and regulation of the receptors for insulin-like growth factors. Ann Rev Physiol 47:425–442, 1985.

94. Stiles CD, Capone GT, Scher HN, et al: Dual control of cell growth by somatomedins and platelet-derived growth factor. Proc Natl Acad Sci USA 76:1279–1283, 1979.

95. Wharton W: Hormonal regulation of discrete portions of the cell cycle: Commitment to DNA synthesis is commitment to cellular division. J Cell Physiol 117:423–429, 1983.

96. Nilsson J, Sjolund M, Palmberg L, et al: Arterial smooth muscle cells in primary culture produce a platelet derived growth factor-like protein. Proc Natl Acad Sci USA 82:4418–4422, 1985.

97. Harlan JM, Thompson PJ, Ross RR, et al: Alpha-thrombin induces release of platelet-derived growth factor-like molecule(s) by cultured human endothelial cells. J Cell Biol 103:1129–1133, 1986.

98. Gajdusek C, Carbon S, Ross R, et al: Activation of coagulation releases endothelial cell mitogens. J Cell Biol 103:419–428, 1986.

99. Lee DC, Rose TM, Webb NR, et al: Cloning and sequence analysis of a cDNA for rat transforming growth factor-alpha. Nature 313:489–491, 1985.

100. Sporn MB, Roberts AB: Peptide growth factors in inflammation, tissue repair, and cancer. J Clin Invest 78:329–332, 1986.

101. Rennard SI, Crystal RG: Fibronectin in human bronchopulmonary lavage fluid. Elevation in patients with interstitial lung disease. J Clin Invest 69:113–122, 1981.

102. Merimee TJ, Zapf J, Frosech ER: Dwarfism in the pygmy: An isolated deficiency of insulin-like growth factor 1. N Engl J Med 305:965–968, 1981.

103. Carpenter G: Epidermal growth factor: Biology and receptor metabolism. J Cell Sci (Suppl) 3:1–9, 1985.

104. Elias JA, Zusier RB, Rossman MD, et al: Inhibition of lung fibroblast growth by lung mononuclear cells. Am Rev Respir Dis 130:810–816, 1984.

105. Clark JG, Kostal KM, Marino BA: Modulation of collagen production following bleomycin-induced pulmonary fibrosis in hamsters. J Biol Chem 257:8098–8105, 1982.

106. Korn JH, Halushka PV, Leroy EC: Mononuclear cell modulation of connective tissue function. Suppression of fibroblast growth by stimulation of endogenous prostaglandin production. J Clin Invest 65:543–554, 1980.

107. Morley J, Bray MA, Jones RW, et al: Prostaglandin and thromboxane production by human and guinea pig macrophages and leukocytes. Prostaglandins 17:729–746, 1979.

108. Borgeat P, Samuelsson B: Transformation of arachidonic acid by polymorphonuclear leukocytes. J Biol Chem 254:2643–2649, 1979.

109. Smith JB, Ingerman C, Kocsis JJ, et al: Formation of prostaglandins during the aggregation of human blood platelets. J Clin Invest 52:965–969, 1973.

110. Allerga J, Tautlein J, Demers L, et al: Peripheral plasma determinations of prostaglandin E in asthmatics. J Allerg Clin Immunol 58:546–550, 1976.

111. Huang JS, Huang SS, Deuel TF: Specific covalent binding of platelet-derived growth factor to human plasma alpha-macroglobulin. Proc Natl Acad Sci USA 81:342–346, 1984.

112. Clark JG, Overton BA, Marino BA, et al: Collagen biosynthesis in bleomycin-induced pulmonary fibrosis in hamsters. J Lab Clin Med 96:943–953, 1980.

113. Raghow R, Lurie S, Seyer JM, et al: Profiles of steady state levels of messenger RNAs coding for type I procollagen, elastin, and fibronectin in hamster lungs undergoing bleomycin-induced interstitial pulmonary fibrosis. J Clin Invest 76:1733–1739, 1985.

114. Kelly J, Chrin L, Shull S, et al: Bleomycin selectively elevates mRNA levels for procollagen and fibronectin following acute lung injury. Biochem Biophys Res Comm 131:836–843, 1985.

115. Raghow R, Kang AH, Pidikiti D: Phenotypic plasticity of extracellular matrix gene expression in cultured hamster lung fibroblasts. J Biol Chem 262:8409–8415, 1987.

116. Raghu G, Striker LJ, Hudson LD, et al: Extracellular matrix in normal and fibrotic human lungs. Am Rev Resp Dis 131:281–289, 1985.

117. Sporn MB, Roberts AB, Wakefield LM, et al: Some recent advances in the chemistry and biology of transforming growth factor. J Cell Biol 105:1039–1045, 1987.

118. Sporn MB, Roberts AB, Wakefield LM, et al: Transforming growth factor-beta: Biological function and chemical structure. Science 233:532–534, 1986.

119. Hannan R, Kowrembanas, Flanders K, et al: Human endothelial cells synthesize fibroblast growth factor and transforming growth factor-beta. J Cell Biol 105:22(abstract), 1987.

120. Assoian RK, Fleurdelys BE, Stevenson HC, et al: Expression and secretion of type β transforming growth factor by activated human macrophages. Proc Natl Acad Sci USA 84:6020–6024, 1987.

121. Roberts AB, Sporn MB, Assoian RK, et al: Transforming growth factor type β: rapid induction of fibrosis and angiogenesis *in vivo* and stimulation of collagen formation *in vitro*. Proc Natl Acad Sci USA 83:4167–4171, 1986.

122. Laiho M, Sahesela O, Andreasen PA, et al: Enhanced production and extracellular deposition of the endothelial-type plasminogen activator inhibitor in cultured human lung fibroblasts by transforming growth factor beta. J Cell Biol 103:2403–2410, 1986.

123. Chiang CP, Nielsen-Hamilton M: Opposite and selective effects of epidermal growth factor and human platelet transforming growth factor-beta on the production of secreted proteins by murine 3T3 cells and human fibroblasts. J Biol Chem 261:10478–10481, 1986.

124. Adamson IYR, Bowden DH, Cote MQ, et al: Lung injury induced by butylated hydroxytoluene. Cytodynamic and biochemical studies in mice. Lab Invest 36:26–32, 1977.

125. Schlag G, Redl HR: Morphology of the human lung after traumatic injury. In Zapol UM, Falke KJ (eds): Acute Respiratory Failure. New York, Marcel Dekker, 1985, pp 161–183.

126. Clark AF, Mason RJ, Folkvord JM, et al: Fibronectin mediates adherence of rat alveolar type II epithelial cells via the fibroblastic cell-attachment domain. J Clin Invest 77:1831–1840, 1986.

127. Leslie CC, McCormick-Shannon K, Cook JL, et al: Macrophages stimulate DNA synthesis in rat alveolar type II cells. Am Rev Resp Dis 132:1246–1252, 1985.

128. Blundell TL, Humbel RE: Hormone families: Pancreatic hormones and homologous growth factors. Nature 287:781–787, 1980.

129. Leslie CC, McCormick-Shannon K, Robinson PC, et al: Stimulation of DNA synthesis in cultured rat alveolar type II cells. Exp Lung Res 8:53–66, 1985.

130. Marquardt H, Hunkapiller MW, Hood LE, et al: Rat transforming growth factor type I: Structure and relation to epidermal growth factor. Science 223:1079–1082, 1984.

131. Post M, Barsoumian A, Smith BT: The cellular mechanism of glucocorticoid acceleration of fetal lung maturation. Fibroblast pneumonocyte factor stimulates choline-phosphate cytidylyl transferase activity. J Biol Chem 261:2179–2184, 1986.

132. Keller GH, Ladda RL: Correlation between phosphatidylcholine labeling and hormone receptor levels in alveolar type II epithelial cells: Effects of dexamethasone and epidermal growth factor. Arch Biochem Biophys 211:321–326, 1981.

133. Assoian RK, Grotendorst GR, Miller DM, et al: Cellular transformation by coordinated action of three peptide growth factors from human platelets. Nature 309:804–806, 1984.

134. Oka Y, Orth DN: Human plasma epidermal growth factor/beta-urogastrone is associated with blood platelets. J Clin Invest 72:249–259, 1983.

135. Lechner JF, Haugen A, McClendon IA, et al: Clonal growth of normal adult human bronchial epithelial cells in a serum-free medium. In Vitro 18:633–642, 1982.

136. Wier ML, Scott RE: Aproliferin. A human plasma protein that induces the irreversible loss of proliferative potential associated with terminal differentiation. Am J Pathol 125:546–554, 1986.

137. Ryan US: Endothelial cell activation response. In Ryan US (ed): Pulmonary Endothelium in Health and Disease, vol 32. New York, Marcel Dekker, 1987, pp 1–33.

138. Hill NS, Fanberg BC: Clinical correlates of endothelial dysfunction. In Ryan US (ed): Pulmonary Endothelium in Health and Disease, vol 32. New York, Marcel Dekker, 1987, pp 351–371.

139. Jones R, Zapol WM, Tomashefski JF, et al: Pulmonary vascular pathology: Human and experimental studies. In Zapol WM, Falke KJ (eds): Acute Respiratory Failure. New York, Marcel Dekker, 1985, pp 23–160.

140. Tomashefski JF Jr, Davies P, Boegs C: The pulmonary vascular lesions of the adult respiratory distress syndrome. Am J Pathol 112:112–126, 1983.

141. Katzenstein AA, Myers JL, Mazur MU: Acute interstitial pneumonia: A clinicopathologic, ultrastructural, and cell kinetic study. Am J Surg Pathol 10:256–267, 1986.

142. Ingbar DH, Matthay RA: Pulmonary sequelae and lung repair in survivors of the adult respiratory distress syndrome. Crit Care Clin 2:629–665, 1986.

143. Zapol WM, Snider MT, Rie MA, et al: Pulmonary circulation during acute respiratory distress syndrome. In Zapol WM, Falke KJ (eds): Acute Respiratory Failure. New York, Marcel Dekker, 1985, pp 242–274.

144. Zapol WM, Jones R: Vascular components of ARDS: Clinical pulmonary hemodynamics and morphology. Am Rev Resp Dis 136(2):471–474, 1987.

145. Meyrick B, Fujiwara K, Reid L: Smooth muscle myosin in precursor and mature smooth muscle cells in normal pulmonary arteries and the effect of hypoxia. Exper Lung Res 2:303–313, 1981.

146. Hislop A, Reid L: New findings in pulmonary arteries of rats with hypoxia-induced pulmonary hypertension. Br J Exp Pathol 57:542–554, 1976.

147. Folkman J, Klagsbrun M: Angiogenic factors. Science 235:442–447, 1987.

148. Zetter BR: Angiogenesis: State of the art. Chest (Suppl) 93:159–166, 1988.

149. Lobb RR, Fett JW: Purification of two distinct growth factors from bovine neural tissue by heparin affinity chromatography. Biochemistry 23:6295–6299, 1984.

150. Esch F, Baird, Ling N, et al: Primary structure of bovine pituitary basic fibroblast growth factor (FGF) and comparison with the amino-terminal sequence of bovine brain acidic FGF. Proc Natl Acad Sci USA 82:6507–6511, 1985.

151. Gimenez-Gallego G, Rodkey J, Bennett C, et al: Brain-derived acidic fibroblast growth factor: Complete amino acid sequence and homologies. Science 230:1385–1388, 1985.

152. Jaye M, Howk R, Burgess W, et al: Human endothelial cell growth factor: Cloning, nucleotide sequence, and chromosome localization. Science 233:541–545, 1986.

153. Abraham JA, Mergia A, Whang JL, et al: Nucleotide

sequence of a bovine clone encoding the angiogenic protein, basic fibroblast growth factor. Science 233:545–548, 1986.

154. Folkman J, Klagsbrun M, Sasse J, et al: A heparin-binding angiogenic protein-basic fibroblast growth factor is stored within basement membrane. Am J Pathol 130:393–400, 1988.

155. Baird A, Moumede P, Bohlen P: Immunoreactive fibroblast growth factor in cells of peritoneal exudate suggests its identity with macrophage-derived growth factor. Biochem Biophys Res Commun 126:258–363, 1985.

156. Leibovich SJ, Polverini PJ, Shepard HM, et al: Macrophage-induced angiogenesis is mediated by tumor necrosis factor-α. Nature 329:630–632, 1987.

157. Polverini PJ, Cotron RS, Gimbrone MA, et al: Activated macrophages induce vascular proliferation. Nature 269:804–806, 1977.

158. Beutler B, Greenwald D, Hulmes JD, et al: Identity of tumour necrosis factor and the macrophage-secreted factor cachectin. Nature 316:552–554, 1985.

159. Bachwich PR, Lynch JP, Larrick J, et al: Tumor necrosis factor production by human sarcoid alveolar macrophages. Am J Pathol 125:421–425, 1986.

160. Banda MJ, Knighton DR, Hunt TK, et al: Isolation of a nonmitogenic angiogenesis factor from wound fluid. Cell Biol 79:7773–7777, 1982.

161. Knighton DR, Hunt TK, Scheuenstuhl H, et al: Oxygen tension regulates the expression of angiogenesis factor by macrophages. Science 221:1283–1285, 1983.

162. Schreiber AB, Winkler ME, Derynck R: Transforming growth factor-α: A more potent angiogenic mediator than epiderminal growth factor. Science 232:1250–1253, 1986.

163. Fett JW, Strydom DJ, Lobb RR, et al: Isolation and characterization of angiogenin, an angiogenic protein from human carcinoma cells. Biochemistry 24:5480–5486, 1985.

164. Weiner HL, Weiner LH, Swain JL: Tissue distribution and developmental expression of the messenger RNA encoding angiogenin. Science 237:280–282, 1987.

165. Baird A, Mormede P, Bohlen P: Immunoreactive fibroblast growth factor in cells of peritoneal exudate suggests its identity with macrophage-derived growth factor. Biochem Biophys Res Comm 126:358–364, 1985.

166. Fein AM, Lippmann M, Holteman H, et al: The risk factors, incidence, and prognosis of acute respiratory distress syndrome following septicemia. Chest 83:40–43, 1983.

167. Fowler AA, Hamman RF, Good JT, et al: Adult respiratory distress syndrome: Risk with common predispositions. Ann Intern Med 593–597, 1983.

168. Pepe PE, Potkin RT, Reus DH, et al: Clinical predictors of the adult respiratory distress syndrome. Am J Surg 144:124–129, 1982.

169. Ashbaugh DG, Bigelow DB, Petty TL: Acute respiratory distress in adults. Lancet 2:319–323, 1967.

26

HEPATIC FIBROSIS

Jerome M. Seyer, Ph.D., and Rajendra Raghow, Ph.D.

HEPATIC LOBULE

The human liver is a massive organ representing nearly 2 percent of the total body weight. The organization of its cellular and extracellular components has evolved to optimally carry out its major functions. The hepatic lobule (Fig. 26–1), the basic anatomical unit of the liver, is made up of an epithelial parenchyma and a complex array of anastomosing vascular sinusoids.[1] The microvasculature of the lobule is an anatomical and functional unit referred to as the portal triad, which comprises three vessels; the hepatic arteriole, the portal venule, and the bile duct. This area is separated from the surrounding liver parenchyma by a connective tissue matrix. The peripheral meeting place of several lobules occurs at a portal triad with the liver cell plates converging toward the central hepatic veins. The lobule is divided into three functional zones.[2] Zone 1 represents the most direct route of blood flow from the portal triad to the central vein, and zone 3 is the farthest away from the predicted passage of blood. Conceivably, cells in zone 3 would be more susceptible to anoxia.

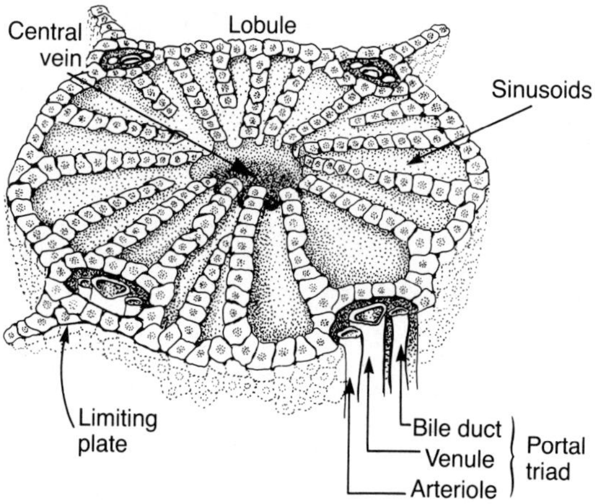

SINUSOIDAL SYSTEM

The sinusoids, which receive a mixture of portal and arterial blood, are specialized hepatic sinuses containing a one cell thick, porous lining of endothelial and Kupffer cells with a segmented basement membrane (Fig. 26–2). This primitive basement membrane–like structure contains type IV collagen but not laminin and can hardly be expected to retain plasma proteins. Adjacent to and surrounding the sinusoid is a perisinusoidal space (space of Disse) separating endothelial cells and the sinusoidal lumen from the liver cells. Fine fibers of type I and III collagen (reticulin) are sparsely distributed in this region together with a few lipocytes, or Ito cells. A rapid and alternating exchange of fluid and solutes takes place between the sinusoidal lumen and the liver cells. Sinusoidal fluid freely enters the central vein in the absence of any limiting plate. A system of elaborate sphincters, both outlet and inlet, regulates blood flow and drainage from the hepatic parenchyma.[3]

BILIARY SYSTEM

The biliary passages begin with fine bile canaliculi between individual hepatic cells (Fig. 26–2). This network of bile canaliculi is drained by the cholangioles, or ductiles, and enters a definable bile duct or tubule in or near the portal triad.[4] These ductile cells form a tubular arrangement with a surrounding basement membrane and, at a further distance, a typical

Figure 26–1. Architecture of the hepatic lobules.

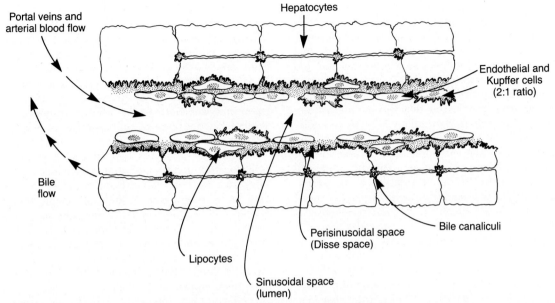

Figure 26–2. Liver cell plate with microvasculature.

connective tissue structure containing interstitial collagen types I and III.

CELLULAR COMPONENTS

The cellular organization of the liver is dominated by its major cell component, the hepatocyte, which occupies nearly 80 percent of the cellular space[5] and accounts for 60-70 percent of the total cells.[6] The other cellular components are represented primarily by sinusoidal cells, including Kupffer cells, epithelial cells, and lipocytes (Ito cells) in an approximate ratio of 4:2:1.[7]

Hepatocytes

The hepatocyte is a large multifunctional cell actively engaged in the processes of resorption and secretion. Tissue spaces between these cells are not sealed by gap junctions and this allows the cells to be exposed to sinusoidal fluid over a greater surface area. The portal tracts are surrounded by hepatocytes that are extremely vulnerable to cellular injury in chronic liver diseases. The concentration of xenobiotics or their metabolites declines toward the central vein, thereby exposing the hepatocytes of the limiting plate to a higher concentration of these substances compared with centrolobular hepatocytes.[4] For instance, xenobiotics such as allyl alcohol and bromobenzene have been shown to induce selective zonal damage and dramatically affect the function of the remaining cells in this region. In contrast, hepatocytes in the centrolobular area are more likely to suffer hypoxic injury since they reside further away from the fresh arterial blood.[2]

Efforts to cultivate hepatocytes that proliferate and maintain their phenotype in culture have been only marginally successful. In addition to very strict requirements for soluble factors, which include autologous serum from partially hepatectomized animals, investigators have used a variety of matrix components as substrates coated on the culture dishes. Bissel and colleagues reported that of the matrix components tested, type I collagen substrates were inadequate in maintaining cell proliferation.[8] However, the biomatrix extracted from normal or regenerating liver was conducive to cell proliferation.[9] In addition to the influence on cell proliferation, the dramatic loss of liver-specific gene expression was substantially lessened by plating cells onto collagenous or biomatrix substrate. Therefore, it was hypothesized that hepatocellular proliferation as well as regulation of hepatocyte-specific gene expression was dependent both on a specific hormonal milieu and on contact between hepatocytes and their surrounding extracellular matrix components.

Receptors that recognize and respond to various matrix components on cell surfaces have received much attention. Receptors for fibronectin, vitronectin, and laminin have been isolated and purified by immunological techniques such as affinity chromatography with matrix components as ligands. A common sequence recognized by a number of such cell receptors is the tripeptide Arg-Gly-Asp (RGD).[10] A widespread occurrence of receptor proteins that recognize RGD-containing sequences has led to the suggestion that these proteins (named integrins) are critical to cellular metabolism.[11] It has been postulated that the common function of integrins is to mediate cell-cell and cell–extracellular matrix interactions. Although the precise identity and molecular interactions of different forms of integrins on different cell types remain to be elucidated, it has been established that such interactions play a crucial role in physiologically important processes. It has been suggested that the transduction of a signal after the binding of the ligand to its receptor occurs through its interaction with the cytoskeletal elements, the interactive components of which could include vinculin, talin, actin, and tropomyosin.[12] Thus, integrins may be envisaged as transmembrane links between the extracellular matrix ligands and the cytoskeleton. How such binding of matrix ligands to integrins might signal nuclear events (e.g., changes in the rates of liver-specific gene expressions) in either an intact organ or in cultured hepatocytes is an intriguing question that will undoubtedly warrant more intense investigations.

Nonparenchymal Cells

Kupffer cells are the major phagocytic cells of the liver and are considered akin to resident macrophages.[13] In the normal liver they are distributed in larger numbers near the periportal zone, but they become more numerous near the central vein after tissue injury.[14] They have a number of phagosomes resembling lysosomes that contain hydrolytic enzymes such as acid phosphatase, esterases α- and β-glucuronidase. Collagenase, gelatinases, and type IV and type V collagenases are also produced by Kupffer cells; these enzymes are not stored but rather are secreted immediately.[15] In a damaged liver, Kupffer cells enlarge and appear more active with a greater number of lysosomes and an increased quantity of rough endoplasmic reticulum. Biochemically, they react to phorbol esters and lipopolysaccharide in the same manner as alveolar macrophages.[16, 17]

Normal liver contains approximately twice as many sinusoidal endothelial cells as Kupffer cells.[7] The endothelial cells normally function only to provide a semipermeable barrier; however, in damaged liver they are believed to

produce a "true" basement membrane, thereby transforming the sinusoid into a capillary (see below). Evidence has been presented that sinusoidal endothelial cells differ significantly from large vessel or capillary endothelial cells. In vivo, they take up acetoacetylated low-density lipoproteins.[18] They produce type IV collagen and lack both factor VIII-R antigen and Weibel-Palade bodies, the absence of which distinguishes them from other endothelial cells.

Ito cells, or lipocytes, are vitamin A storage cells located in the perisinusoidal spaces.[19, 20] They can be readily localized after feeding a diet high in vitamin A and observing their fluorescence. Their hepatic function has not been positively defined, but studies have demonstrated an ability in culture to produce extracellular matrix components including type I and type III interstitial collagen.[21] In vivo, they have been shown to produce laminin and type IV collagen, key elements of basement membranes.[22, 23] Clearly, their collagen phenotype is not stable, and more studies are needed to define their physiological function. Numerically, they represent approximately one fourth of the sinusoidal lining endothelial cells, not an insignificant number. The location of these cells in the space of Disse is critical, since excess extracellular matrix formation in this region severely restricts passage of fluids to and from the hepatocyte.

Fibroblasts and myofibroblasts are also present in normal liver, especially in portal tracts and central canals.[24–26] Except during liver injury, these cells are present at very low levels. Fibroblasts, and particularly myofibroblasts, readily grow out of liver tissue explants. In culture, fibroblasts synthesize mainly type I and type III collagens (90 percent type I), fibronectin, glycosaminoglycans, and under certain circumstances, collagenase and gelatinase.[27] Myofibroblasts in culture produce type III and type V collagens and elastin.[28] Again, the role of these two cells in normal adult liver remains obscure. Other cells identified in the liver include smooth muscle cells, a liver connective tissue cell (different from smooth muscle cell), ductile cells, Schwann cells, and histiocytes, all having a special role pertaining to the parent tissue.

HEPATIC EXTRACELLULAR MATRIX

Liver tissue contains a relatively small amount of extracellular matrix compared to other organs. The collagen content of human liver is approximately 2 percent, but livers of other animals have much less (rats have 0.55 percent collagen).[26, 29] Not surprisingly, the interstitial collagens, type I and type III, represent 70 to 80 percent of the total hepatic collagens (Table 26–1). As expected, type IV (basement membrane–associated), type V (pericellular), and type VI (microfibrillar) collagens are present in lesser amounts[30] and collagen types VII, VIII, XII, and XIV are in extremely small amounts.

A number of well-described noncollagenous glycoproteins are also found in the extracellular matrix of the liver. The most abundant is fibronectin, which directs cell adhesion to the extracellular matrix. Laminin is limited to typical basement membrane structures and is not present in areas containing interstitial collagens of the liver.[31] Other intrinsic components of basement membrane include entactin and heparan sulfate proteoglycan.[32, 33] Entactin is an adhesion glycoprotein found in hepatic and other parenchymal tissues that has not yet been chemically characterized. The heparan sulfate proteoglycan is chemically distinct from the typical extracellular matrix heparan sulfate proteoglycan.

Glycosaminoglycans are also present in hepatic tissue. As noted, heparan sulfate is located in basement membrane structures, but this represents only a small fraction of the total hepatic extracellular matrix. Ninomiya and coworkers[34] reported that the glycosaminoglycans consist of 10 percent hyaluronic acid, 7 percent dermatan sulfate, 7 percent chondroitin sulfate, and 75 percent heparan sulfate. Their functional role appears to be restricted to water binding and lubrication as predicted for other tissues. Rapid turnover rates measured in damaged liver give evidence of their role in regenerating hepatic tissue.

The hepatic lobule (Fig. 26–3) contains a sparse extracellular matrix composed primarily of thin delicate fibrils of type I and type III collagens and fibronectin both in the perisinusoidal space of Disse and around the hepatocyte microvilli. At times, the hepatocyte appears to be in direct contact with interstitial collagen.[22] This relationship is clearly unique, since other cells of ectodermal or endodermal origin are normally separated from the interstitium by a basement membrane. Reticular fibers previously described in hepatic tissue, although present, are not considered as a separate entity here since they consist not only of type III collagen but also of a less defined mixture of type I collagen and various glycoproteins.[35] Dense fibers of type I and type III collagens are located at inflection or turning points of the sinusoids, leaving the impression that these collagen bundles may provide a structural scaffold upon which the hepatocyte cell plates rest and that they form a continuous honeycombed collagenous structure within the lobule. Some thin fibrils are infrequently found in spaces between the hepatocytes.

Fibronectin, on the other hand, is normally found only in the space of Disse and its location does not always correlate with the position of interstitial collagen fibrils.[23] Fibronectin is more closely aligned to the microvilli of the hepatocyte, suggesting that (1) the hepatocytes are primarily responsible for its secretion as opposed to endothelial sinusoidal lining cells, and (2) the fibronectin may form a "primitive" matrix alone, without any type I collagen. Structures such as this occur in developmental conditions but, in those cases, the fibronectin is eventually replaced by a true basement membrane.[36] This, of course, does not occur in the liver and the fibronectin matrix may be retained to provide a partial barrier between hepatocytes and sinusoids. In addition, it may act as a bridge between hepatocytes and sinusoidal cells.

Type IV collagen is located along the sinusoids as revealed by conventional light microscopy.[32] Studies using thick sections for light microscopy demonstrated a continuous struc-

Table 26–1. COLLAGEN TYPES FOUND IN HEPATIC AND RELATED TISSUE

Collagen*	Site	Structure
Type I	Interstitial matrix	$[\alpha1(I)]_2\alpha2(I)$
Type III	Interstitial matrix	$[\alpha1(III)]_3$
Type IV	Basement membrane	$[\alpha1(IV)]_2\alpha2(IV)$
Type V	Pericellular, interstitial	$[\alpha1(V)]_2\alpha2(V)$ or
		$[\alpha1(V)\alpha2(V)\alpha3(V)]$
Type VI	Microfibrillar structures	Unknown
Type VII†	Anchoring fibrils	$[\alpha1(VII)]_2$
Type VIII†	Endothelial cell product	Unknown
Type XII†	Product of fibroblast	Unknown

*This list does not include type II, IX, X, and XI collagens, which are restricted to cartilaginous tissue.
†Type VII, VIII, and XII collagens have not been specifically isolated from hepatic tissue but they almost certainly are present in trace amounts.

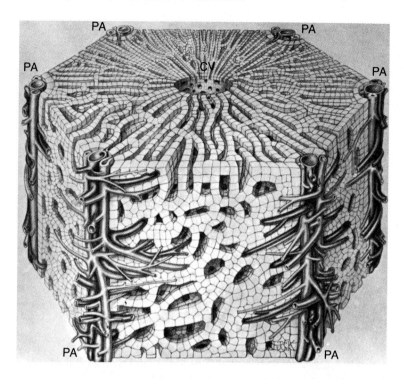

Figure 26–3. Liver lobule; schematic view. The central vein (CV) lies in the center of the figure, surrounded by anastomosing cords of blocklike hepatocytes. About the periphery of the schema are six portal areas (PA) consisting of branches of the portal vein, the hepatic artery, and the bile duct. (From Jones CM, Spring-Mills H: Histology, 4th ed. New York, McGraw-Hill, 1977, p. 701.)

ture. However, when ultrathin sections and immunohistochemistry were used for immuno-electron microscopy, type IV collagen was seen as "discontinuous bundles" rather than as sheets.[22] The location of these segmented bundles rules out any role in the selective filtration generally ascribed to type IV collagen and basement membrane in other tissues. Therefore, its functional role remains undetermined, but two theories have been proposed: (1) a continuous layer of laminin and type IV collagen were initially formed but destroyed by proteases that more rapidly removed laminin leaving only remnants of type IV collagen; or (2) the type IV collagen may play an adhesive role, binding hepatocytes and sinusoidal cells. As alluded to previously, laminin is conspicuously missing in these areas. Absence of laminin and heparan sulfate in the perisinusoidal spaces rules out the possibility of any permanent basement membrane structure in this region of the lobule.

The portal triads contain a significant concentration of extracellular matrix.[26] True basement membrane structures containing type IV collagen, laminin, and heparan sulfate glycosaminoglycan are abundant. The type IV collagen is localized around smooth muscle cells of blood vessels, bile duct and ductules, nerve axons, hepatic arteries, and lymphatic vessels. Anti–type IV antibodies localize the type IV collagen equally in the lamina rara and the lamina densa.[36a] Laminin is equally abundant in the same basement membrane structures of the

portal triads. Although not identified, heparan sulfate would be expected to have distribution similar to that of type IV collagen and laminin. Type I and type III collagens appear as dense fibers in the stroma of all blood vessels and ducts of the portal triads. Fibronectin in this area is closely associated with the interstitial collagens of the vessel stroma in the portal triads.

The extracellular matrix of the central veins contains a structure similar to that found in the portal triads. Both type IV collagen and laminin form a continuous endothelial basement membranous sheath around the vessel, and types I and III collagen and fibronectin form the supporting perivasculature in the stroma of the central vein. The largest bundles of type I collagen, however, are located, together with fibronectin, in the liver capsule. The dense fibrous connective tissues follow and form thin perivascular sheets around entering veins, arterioles, and bile ducts until they meet their terminal ramification where they merge with the adventia of the portal vein and hepatic artery in the portal triads.[1]

HEPATIC FIBROSIS

When human hepatic tissue sustains an acute injury such as a weekend alcoholic binge by an individual or when a single injection of carbon tetrachloride (CCl_4) is administered to rats, fatty metamorphosis develops with elevated synthesis of fibronectin, laminin, type I collagen, and type IV collagen in the liver. If no further hepatoxins are administered, the liver will completely regenerate to a state indistinguishable from the original hepatic architecture. It is thought that under conditions of repeated injury, as in chronic alcohol consumption or CCl_4 administration, the regenerative process becomes overwhelmed and fibrotic scar tissue accumulates in the parenchyma. In hepatic tissue, the collagen content increases five to seven fold in alcoholic liver cirrhosis.[26] The factors that distinguish normal reparative processes from detrimental scar formation remain largely unknown and a challenge to investigators of liver diseases. Chronicity of liver damage is certainly an important aspect of liver fibrosis. The general method of CCl_4 administration in rats requires biweekly administration of the hepatotoxin. Animals receiving similar injections spaced 10 days apart never develop cirrhosis;[37, 38] presumably, sufficient regeneration occurs during this 10-day period to prevent chronic liver damage. Perhaps the determining factors may reside in the extracellular matrix and its relation to specific liver cells. Hepatic cirrhosis has multiple etiologies and forms, yet all types have common features such as excess interconnecting fibrous scars, disorganized parenchymal architecture, regenerating nodules, and loss of normal vascular relationships.

Cirrhotogenic Agents

Most studies on hepatic fibrosis have centered on animal models because of the difficulty in obtaining adequate amounts of viable human liver tissue by biopsy and in obtaining follow-up specimens. Baboons have been used by Zern and associates to study alcoholic liver disease.[39] After chronic ethanol administration, these primates develop fatty metamorphosis, chronic active hepatitis, and cirrhosis in a manner similar to humans. Unfortunately, the expense of maintaining such a primate center is beyond the resources of most investigators. Studies of alcoholic liver disease in other animals, including rodents and miniature pigs, have been useful for studying psychological dependence and withdrawal but the damaging effect of ethanol on their liver tissue has not been convincing. Therefore, other hepatotoxins have been used extensively for measuring hepatic fibrosis.

Cameron and Karunartne[37] reported in 1936 that repeated administration of CCl_4 to rats induced cirrhosis of the liver. Since then, many other animal species as well as different routes of administration have been used to carefully follow the disease progression. These studies have been based on the premise that CCl_4-induced cirrhosis of the liver is an adequate model of alcoholic cirrhosis in humans, and histological and biochemical changes that develop in the chronically treated animal do indeed mimic those seen in human cirrhoses of several etiological types.[40] The response of individual animals to CCl_4, like that of humans to alcohol, is highly variable. Morphologically, the major features of liver disease (Fig. 26–4) in both cases are basically similar: (1) the normal liver architecture is replaced by nodules of regenerating cells with segmentation of the liver by connective tissue septa, (2) bile ducts proliferate, and (3) portal to central vein anastomosis develops within the connective tissue septa. The major differences, however, are due to the role of hepatocyte necrosis in the animal model that results in increased collagen accumulation. In the baboon model and in certain types of human cirrhosis, necrosis may not be the stimulus for fibrosis.[39] Additionally, the initial lesion in CCl_4-induced cirrhosis is centrilobular, but in alcoholic cirrhosis such lesions rarely lead to cirrhosis. Hepatocellular carcinoma is associated with different types of human liver cirrhosis including alcoholic but except for the mouse, hepatic carcinoma does not occur in CCl_4-induced cirrhosis unless additional carcinogenic substances are administered. Despite these differences, sufficient similarities have made CCl_4-induced hepatic injury the model of choice for studies of hepatic fibrosis. The experimental cirrhosis is completely reversible for up to 5 weeks despite the formation of thin septa and small nodules of liver cell regeneration. But after 10 weeks, thick connective tissue septa and regenerative nodules are abundant and these remain for months after discontinuation of the hepatotoxin.[26]

A number of other hepatotoxins or inciting agents have been used to induce cirrhosis. Repeated injection of heterologous serum, specifically albumin, causes an inflammatory reaction in the portal triads, edema, and eventually destruction of the limiting plate.[41] Inflammatory cells are recruited into the area and septa are formed that radiate from the portal tract into the parenchyma. They progress to the central vein with development of small blood vessels connecting portal veins and central veins. Surprisingly, fatty metamorphosis, extensive hepatocellular necrosis, and regeneration are minimal in contrast to Laennec's cirrhosis, which is

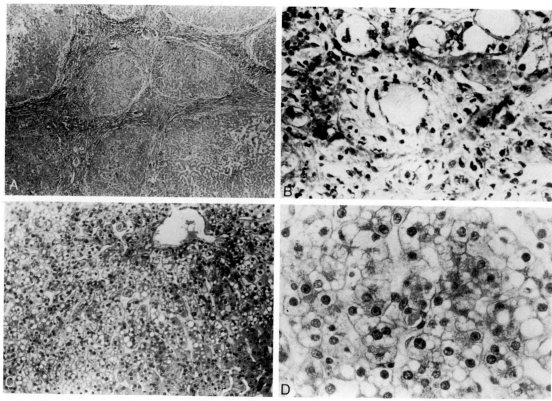

Figure 26–4. Photomicrographs demonstrating the difference in CCl$_4$ injury from alcoholic liver injury. *A,* Nodules of regenerating liver are outlined by bands of fibrous septae. This represents a late regenerating stage of alcoholic cirrhosis in a patient who discontinued alcohol use many years prior to this biopsy. (Masson's trichrome stain, ×5.) *B,* A central vein (terminal hepatic venule) with intimal fibrosis and ballooning of the pericentral hepatocyte. This lesion, called central hyalin sclerosis, is typical of early stages of alcoholic cirrhosis. (Masson's trichrome stain, ×40.) *C,* Microvesicular steatosis around a central vein in a patient with acute carbon tetrachloride toxicity. The periportal hepatocytes (*lower right corner*) are spared. (Masson's trichrome stain, ×10.) *D,* The pericentral hepatocytes demonstrate small vacuoles of fat. The hepatocytes themselves are not ballooned although there is disarray and an acidophylic (apoptotic) body seen in the center of this field. (Masson's trichrome stain, ×40.) (Courtesy of Caroline A. Reily, M.D., Gastroenterology Division, Department of Medicine, University of Tennessee, Memphis, TN.)

recognized by the regular formation of small nodules and thin septa.[1] Fibroblasts accumulate in the portal tract as part of the inflammatory reaction.

Ligation of the bile duct produces cirrhosis as expected, much akin to primary or secondary biliary cirrhosis.[42] An inflammatory reaction develops with extensive bile duct proliferation and periductile fibrosis. Eventually connective tissue septa bridge the portal tracts, and after 30 days most of the normal lobular architecture is destroyed and replaced by regenerative nodules; decompensated cirrhosis with development of ascites is one of the characteristic features of biliary cirrhosis.

Thioacetamide, like CCl$_4$, induces centrilobular necrosis and degeneration by 13 weeks.[43] A reversed lobular pattern occurs with the portal triad appearing to have become the center of the lobule. Parenchymal regeneration is stimulated in the periportal areas. Nodules ap-

pear within 28 weeks in the periportal area along with thin septa. The nodules became very large, cholangiofibrosis occurs, and a mild inflammatory response with neutrophils, lymphoctyes, and macrophages can be seen.

Choline deficiency induced as a result of a high-fat, low-protein diet produces fatty metamorphosis, degeneration, and frequent inflammatory cell infiltration. Nodular regeneration does not occur until 47 weeks and is combined with diffuse fibrosis and ductile proliferation.[44]

Hepatic Necrosis

Central necrosis results many times from low oxygen tension due to exposure to chemical toxins (O$_2$ is used to metabolize these agents), infection, shock, and cardiac failure causing passive congestion or any other affliction resulting in oxygen depletion. Periportal necrosis generally results from an inflammation in the portal triads that extends into the limiting plate and peripheral zone; examples include chronic viral hepatitis and chronic biliary obstruction.

Steatosis of long standing also leads to necrosis, primarily in the central zone. During the process of liver cell degeneration, isolated, viable hepatocytes multiply with the formation of regenerative nodules.

Biliary obstruction results in connective tissue formation around the bile ducts, but this does not extend into the parenchyma or disrupt the lobular architecture. Later, irritation due to excess bile and other inflammatory reactions around the portal tract initiate formation of septa leading to cirrhosis as described previously.

In summary, hepatic necrosis represents a common pathway to liver cirrhosis. The end result is a consistent pattern of extensive septa formation, portal vein–hepatic vein shunts through these septa, and many regenerating nodules. The parenchymal network of the new liver nodules lacks the organized orientation present in the normal liver lobule.

Collagen Production

The biochemical events that occur in hepatic fibrosis and cirrhosis have been extensively studied in regard to collagen production. As stated previously, most hepatic cell types are capable of producing different collagen types but primarily the interstitial collagens. The cells designated as the most likely collagen sources include hepatocytes, lipocytes, fibroblasts, and myofibroblasts; however, the evidence is primarily indirect (Table 26–2). It is of note that the cellular composition of the cirrhotic liver has not been accurately determined, but fibroblasts and myofibroblasts can be readily grown from explants of cirrhotic liver.

A change in amino acid pools and certain transfer RNA (tRNA) isoacceptor species has been identified in diseased liver tissue. For instance, granulation tissue contains more prolyl-tRNA than normal liver.[45] After administration of CCl_4 to rats, there is a tenfold increase in all tRNA and all three isoacceptor species of prolyl-tRNA are elevated.[46] Proline metabolism appears to have a special role in damaged liver tissue since in fibrotic and cirrhotic rat or human liver tissue, free proline levels are increased two to four fold. This could be accounted for partly by decreased prolyl oxidase activity in, for example, CCl_4-fibrotic rat liver, thereby reducing its catabolism. In fact, using liver slices in vitro, Ehrinpreiss and associates[47] demonstrated that collagen production is rate dependent on levels of proline in the culture media up to 0.2 mM. Arginine rather than glutamic acid is the major precursor of proline in both normal and fibrotic rat liver.[48]

The activity of prolyl 4-hydroxylase, the enzyme required for the hydroxylation of procollagen prolyl residues, was found to be elevated in both human fibrotic liver samples and in samples of chemically induced rat liver fibrosis.[49] The amount of enzyme activity correlates well with elevated collagen production in fibrosis. However, the levels of hepatic prolyl hydroxylase(s) are generally not considered to be rate limiting despite the large increase in collagen synthesis in fibrotic liver. In chemically induced fibrosis, studies have indicated that elevated enzymatic activity may precede the increase in the rate of collagen deposition.

Lysyl oxidase enzyme converts lysine residues of both collagen and elastin to allysine or hydroxyallysine. Lysyl oxidase activity of CCl_4 and human cirrhotic liver (needle biopsy) correlates well with anticipated increases in collagen synthesis.[50] This enzyme has been found to be a better indicator of liver collagen deposition than the other post-translational enzymes discussed previously: a 30-fold increase in enzymatic activity was found in the CCl_4-damaged rat liver. Additionally, lysyl oxidase levels in the serum were increased in parallel with changes in the liver.

CELLULAR SOURCE OF HEPATIC COLLAGEN IN FIBROSIS

Fibroblasts or fibroblast-like cells have long been considered the major source of all extracellular matrix, in particular that of interstitial collagen. For this reason, fibroblasts have generally been implicated as the causative cell in fibrotic tissue of liver, lung, and dermal scars. Fibroblasts are normally not present in large numbers in the liver but may be recruited from surrounding tissues if necessary. However, it has been demonstrated that most cells, endothelial and epithelial cells in particular, have the potential to produce not only type IV collagen for their basement membrane structures but also varying amounts of interstitial types I, III, and V collagen. Given the correct signal, it appears that most, if not all, cells of the liver may contribute to its characteristic extracellular

Table 26–2. RATIO OF DIFFERENT COLLAGEN TYPES SYNTHESIZED BY
RAT LIVER CELLS IN CULTURE

Liver Cells	Percentage of Cells	Collagen Types			
		I	III	IV	V
Fibroblasts	Transient	95	5	0	Trace
Hepatocytes	70	6	38	19	36
Lipocytes	10	70	30		0
Endothelial cells	20			Immuno-	
Kupffer cells	10			fluorescence	
				positive	

matrix during normal growth, regeneration, and fibrosis.

Hepatocytes in primary culture produce collagen, as mentioned previously. The amount of collagen produced by these cells can be modulated by obtaining hepatocytes from regenerating rat liver or from hepatocytes of CCl_4-injured livers, which produce approximately three times more collagen than cells from sham-operated animals. Transformed hepatocytes or cells from hepatoma cell lines produced 20-fold more collagen even though some continued to produce albumin. These studies confirm that the hepatocytes, given the correct stimulus, can produce interstitial collagen. This was further illustrated by the use of cDNA probes encoding for type I collagen chains; in situ hybridization of the corresponding mRNA in tissue sections identified a low level of mRNA–specific type I collagen.[51] Martinez-Hernandez[22] was able to localize type I collagen antigen inside the hepatocyte organelles by electron immunohistochemical methods.

Ito cells, or lipocytes, have also been proposed as a major source of fibrotic liver collagen. Early studies have shown a correlation in their location and the position of new collagens produced by rat hepatic tissue after CCl_4 injury. Tissue sections stained positive for type III collagen in and around these vitamin A–containing lipocytes.[21] In cell culture, lipocytes synthesized substantial amounts of collagen, estimated to be about 5 percent of their total protein, whereas, collagen production by sinusoidal endothelial cells and hepatocytes was quantitated to be 1.72 and 0.23 percent, respectively. Therefore, on the basis of the ratio of collagen to noncollagen protein synthesis, lipocytes produce 20- to 30-fold more collagen than do hepatocytes and threefold more than the endothelial cells. Thus, lipocytes resemble fibroblasts in respect to collagen production, but clearly they are not fibroblasts since desmin, a unique intermediate filament protein, and some type IV collagen are typically synthesized by lipocytes.[52] Regardless, the lipocytes have been implicated in increased local collagen

accumulation at both the periphery of the hepatic lobule and within the space of Disse.

The endothelial cells that line the sinusoid are also potential collagen-producers; in vivo they synthesize types III, IV, and V collagen. However, endothelial cells often alter their collagen phenotype in vitro to primarily produce interstitial types I and III collagen, making them likely hepatic collagen producers in cirrhosis.

The remaining two cell types are fibroblasts and myofibroblasts. Both are transient cells present in insufficient number to cause fibrosis in the normal liver but capable of being recruited by chemotactic stimuli. Although myofibroblasts are found in the baboon liver in sufficient numbers to cause fibrosis after alcoholic liver injury, fibroblasts have long been primarily implicated. The fibroblasts play a major role in dermal scar formation, pulmonary fibrosis, and other wound-healing conditions. Fibroblasts produce primarily type I collagen, with less than 10 percent type III collagen found in culture.

Sufficient information on the role of fibroblasts has accumulated to allow some generalizations. Fibroblasts may be recruited into an area by a number of well-defined chemotactic agents, including collagen alpha chains, fibronectin, and peptides derived from collagen, elastin, and fibronectin.[53] Therefore, autolytic digestion of these extracellular matrix molecules in the liver during injury and necrosis will attract fibroblast into the area. Other chemotactic agents present during inflammation such as platelet-derived growth factor and a chemotactic substance released from T lymphocytes,[54, 55] as well as enzymes released from neutrophils, macrophages and Kupffer cells that degrade liver extracellular matrix, could assist in recruiting fibroblasts into the damaged area. Fibroblasts can then be stimulated to or inhibited from proliferating by an additional set of proteins released from inflammatory cells at the site of injury. Those now recognized include a host of cytokines including interleukin-1, transforming growth factor-β, tumor necrosis factor-α and -β and platelet-derived growth factor. In this manner, the number of fibroblasts present in injured liver can increase rapidly via chemical mediators released from a variety of inflammatory or resident liver cells.

We have isolated a "fibrogenic factor" from thioacetamide- or CCl_4-damaged rat liver and human cirrhotic liver.[56, 57] The fibrogenic component has been demonstrated to specifically stimulate collagen (types I and III) but not noncollagen protein synthesis by fibroblasts. This factor stimulates type V collagen production in a rhabdomyosarcoma cell line (A204) as well as types I and IV collagen production by mesangial cells.[57, 58] These results point toward a global effect of the fibrogenic factor and suggest that collagen protein synthesis is specifically affected in a variety of target cells. This in situ collagen production–stimulating factor is not mitogenic and exemplifies how local components developed through tissue injury can lead to elevated collagen production in a very specific area.

Based on data from runoff transcripts of nascent procollagen mRNA, it was concluded that the fibrogenic factor affects transcription of type I collagen genes. Attempts are currently being made to identify the chemical composition of this factor but are hampered by the instability of the factor itself. Previous studies had determined it to be resistant to proteolytic digestion (pronase and trypsin) but destroyed by phospholipase C, an enzyme that cleaves between glycerol and phosphate in phospholipids. This information, combined with its chemical content (6.8% hexose, 13% protein, and 3% phosphorus), led to the suggestion that it may be a proteophospholipid.[56] The factor becomes opalescent with time in aqueous solution, a physical change that can be inhibited by storage under nitrogen atmosphere. It is believed that the opalescence may be a result of oxidation and may also occur in vivo; hence the factor may be generated in injured hepatic tissue and activated by in situ oxidation. It is present in liver 4 days after an initial CCl_4 injection, but maximum activity occurs at the time of maximum collagen synthesis, i.e., after 21 to 60 days of chronic hepatotoxin administration.

Other mediators of fibroblast collagen synthesis have been isolated from injured tissues. McGee and colleagues found a small molecular weight component (less that 5,000 daltons) in CCl_4-injured rat liver[59] that was different from our own. Igarashi identified 22,000 and 5,000 dalton components from CCl_4-injured rat liver that also stimulated collagen biosynthesis by dermal fibroblasts.[60]

In summary, many cells of the liver have the potential to synthesize collagen. It is now recognized that the individual hepatic cells (i.e., hepatocytes, endothelial cells, and ductile cells) contain their own collagen synthetic capability and probably do produce their extracellular matrix during normal growth and regeneration. This most likely includes types I, III, and V collagen by hepatocytes and types III and IV by endothelial and ductile cells. During tissue injury and fibrosis, collagen production becomes more complicated. Added to this confusion is the instability of the collagen phenotype of these cells after isolation and growth in the artificial system of cell culture. Until proven otherwise, it must be assumed that phenotypic instability must also occur in situ, allowing hepatocytes to produce collagens for the extracellular matrix of the liver cell plates. In effect, the hepatocyte may attempt to protect itself by producing a new collagen matrix. The source of the additional collagen deposited in the Disse space between the sinusoid and the hepatocyte remains uncertain but is extremely important. Cells in this region include lipocytes and hepatocytes. Lipocytes are the major candidates, since they are more active and have a fibroblast-like phenotype (synthesizing primarily types I and III collagen).

Fibrosis in the portal tract and in the periductal region most likely results from the action of fibroblasts. An inflammatory response is generally associated with fibrosis in these areas, a reaction similar to that found in dermal scar formation. Fibroblasts can be identified in the area, and collagen deposits are much larger than would be anticipated from hepatocytes, ductile cells, or capillary endothelium. Myofibroblasts may also be present in these regions, but insufficient information is available to make this assertion.

COLLAGEN DEGRADATION

The accumulation of collagen fibers in hepatic fibrosis and cirrhosis represents a composite of both collagen synthesis and degradation. Collagen degradation itself is a rigidly controlled process; secretion of collagen-degrading enzymes is restricted to specific cell types.[61] Kupffer cells in liver tissue are the major source of these hepatic enzymes (i.e., collagenase, gelatinase, and proteoglycanase). During inflammation, resident neutrophils, monocytes, and fibroblasts are recruited, providing additional sources of degradative enzymes and thereby contributing to extracellular tissue degradation. Collagenase and gelatinase enzymes are produced and secreted in latent forms and are activated in vivo by such proteases as thrombin and plasminogen activator. Lipocytes have been shown to produce a 72 kDa gelatinase (type IV collagenase).[62]

In addition to the latent and active forms of collagenase, significant levels of tissue inhibitor of metalloproteinase (TIMP) have been detected in normal and cirrhotic human livers.[63] This 35,000 dalton protein inhibits the previously mentioned metalloproteinases noncompetitively by irreversibly binding to the enzyme stoichiometrically. TIMP is widespread in tissues and plasma. Using immunohistochemical methods, our laboratory was able to identify elevated levels of TIMP in human cirrhotic liver, but the precise source of hepatic TIMP remains uncertain. Fibroblasts are capable of producing it and serum contains significant levels of the circulating inhibitor.[63]

Collagenolysis in hepatic tissue has been difficult to estimate. Much of the early work erroneously measured lysosomal enzyme activity or collagenolytic cathepsins at an acid pH. These enzymes are capable of removing only the nonhelical telopeptides of collagen molecules and hence are not considered effective during in vivo collagen destruction. Whether active hepatic collagenase is present in normal rat or human liver remains unresolved. The same was true for culture supernates of purified Kupffer cells; activation of culture supernates by trypsin, KSCN, or aminophenylmercuric acetate (APMA) was found to be necessary before enzyme activity could be demonstrated.[64] Liver explants on an in vitro collagen gel showed evidence of increased collagen lysis in experimental CCl_4-induced rat livers during the early reversible phase of disease: the activity decreased with advanced or irreversible CCl_4-induced cirrhosis. Collagenase was also located immunohistochemically on newly formed collagen septa but was absent on the more advanced, thickened septa of irreversible cirrhosis.[65]

Collagenase activity against type I and type IV collagens in humans has been measured in extracts of needle biopsies of alcoholic livers.[64] Most samples showed an increase in interstitial type I collagenase activity, although consistent but variable decreases in type IV collagenase activity were noted. When samples were correlated with and without lobular distortion, those containing distortion showed the lowest type IV collagenase activity. Lack of adequate

type IV degrading activity by lipocytes may account for an accumulation of new basement membrane collagen during lobular disorganization and may explain capillarization of hepatic sinusoids.

The role of inhibitors in liver cirrhosis has not been investigated satisfactorily. Perez-Tamayo and Montfort[66] reported that the addition of hepatic tissue extracts to a collagenase assay system did not inhibit enzymatic activity and hence no inhibitors were apparently present. This may not be a valid assumption, since TIMP binds irreversibly to the enzymes and, unless excess amounts are present, it would not be available to inhibit enzymatic activity under conditions of enzyme excess. Our laboratory used immunohistochemical methods with monospecific antibodies to localize TIMP in primary biliary cirrhosis. A diffuse area was observed along the sinusoids, but higher levels were present along the septa, suggesting that it may indeed be bound irreversibly to the enzyme at these locations.

In summary, collagenase activity plays a major role in remodeling during the acute or the early reversible phase of CCl_4-induced cirrhosis, but its activity is decreased later, suggesting that irreversibility of hepatic fibrosis may be in part due to a lack of enzyme activity rather than elevated collagen synthesis. Discontinuation of the hepatotoxin at an early, reversible stage results in a rapid return to baseline enzyme levels within 2 weeks. An understanding of the role of TIMP during CCl_4-induced rat liver cirrhosis may help explain the lower collagenolytic activity at later stages of cirrhosis. This has been suggested by the observation of high levels of TIMP outlining the septa; these are resistant to collagenase digestion.

EXTRACELLULAR MATRIX ALTERATIONS DURING FIBROSIS IDENTIFIED IMMUNOLOGICALLY

The chronological order of events occurring in liver cirrhosis has been extensively studied histologically in both humans and animal models. Recently Martinez-Hernandez[23] reported a time course study of cirrhosis in the rat CCl_4 model (see Fig. 26–4).

The first 5 weeks of CCl_4 administration were primarily a period of steatosis. Although evidence of cirrhosis was present, the deposition of fibronectin occurred within the lobule in a pattern outlining anticipated septa formation. This, together with an increase in fibronectin in the space of Disse, is consistent with the hypothesis that fibronectin deposition may precede connective tissue formation,[67] a proposition developed from studies of scar formation. This may indeed be the scaffold upon which other matrix components become deposited and directed. After 5 to 10 weeks, thin, delicate strands of type I collagen were deposited in the same location as fibronectin. During this period of fatty metamorphosis and septal formation, type I collagen radiated from the central veins with the formation of clearly evident septa dissecting the lobule. Only the hepatocytes in the portal periphery appeared normal, the others showed extensive necrosis, especially in the central lobular area. During the later septal stage, dense collagen fibers were located in the space of Disse. Ito cells (lipocytes) lost some of their lipid droplets and appeared to be producing collagen. A few fibroblast-like cells were located in the area of increased septa formation. Inflammatory cells were also present. The final stage, referred to as the period of true cirrhosis, saw extensive regenerating nodule formation, bile duct proliferation, and formation of arterioles and venules within the newly formed septa. Fibronectin and type I collagen deposition continued with more extensive deposits.

The alterations in the extracellular matrix were also followed by the appearance of monospecific antibodies directed against the basement membrane components laminin and type IV collagen. Type IV collagen deposition appeared very early, after only 2 weeks of CCl_4 administration. Surprisingly, the type IV collagen deposition paralleled that of fibronectin. Type IV collagen deposits lined some sinusoids. Laminin deposition, on the other hand, lagged behind type IV collagen production by 2 weeks in the same manner as type I collagen lagged behind fibronectin.

During the final cirrhosis stage, deposition of basement membrane components continued. Sinusoidal endothelial cells and Ito cells both contained high levels of both laminin and type IV collagen. True basement membrane structures became continuous around some of the sinusoids, converting them from the leaky exchange system separating hepatocytes from the sinusoidal lumen to a true capillary.

LIVER REGENERATION AND GROWTH

The liver has been an excellent system for the study of growth regulation. Normally an adult hepatocyte undergoes only one or two divisions in its lifetime. However, regeneration, or more precisely compensatory growth after loss of liver tissue, can readily be induced by partial hepatectomy. As much as 70 percent of the rat liver can be excised and the remaining lobes can still regenerate to an equivalent size and cell number within 2 weeks.[68]

The sequence of events following partial hepatectomy has been divided into two phases: an initial hypertrophic stage (10 to 12 hours in the rat), and a phase of hyperplasia with DNA replication and cell division. During hypertrophy, cells are considered to be preparing for DNA replication by going from the G_0 to the G_1 phase of the cell cycle. At the peak of DNA synthesis in regenerating liver, approximately 40 percent of the cells incorporate labeled thymidine into DNA after short labeling exposure and are considered to be in the S phase.[69] By 70 hours 90 to 95 percent of young adult and 70 to 75 percent of old adult rat hepatocytes have divided at least once. Hepatocyte ploidy increases after regeneration (10 and 50 percent increase in tetra- and octaploid nuclei, respectively), while the proportion of binucleate hepatocytes decreases from 25 to 30 percent to 10 percent. Ductal, endothelial, and Kupffer cells also divide after partial hepatectomy, but peak DNA synthesis occurs 24 to 36 hours later than in hepatocytes.[70]

Immediately (2 hours) after partial hepatectomy, a number of biochemical events occur, many being physiological adaptations necessary for the survival of an animal with only 30 percent of its liver capacity.[69] For example, changes occur in the urea cycle almost immediately, thereby avoiding toxicity due to high blood ammonia levels. During this period, the amino acid and nucleotide precursor pools increase rapidly to accommodate anticipated cell proliferation. The amount of poly (A)$^+$ RNA in the cytoplasm increases more rapidly than total cytoplasmic RNA, indicating a possible increase in synthesis of ribosomal proteins and/or DNA synthesizing enzymes.[71] The abundance of specific individual RNA sequences changes after partial hepatectomy, although their role remains to be established. When polysomal poly (A)$^+$ RNA both before and after partial hepatectomy was compared, no qualitative changes were found, but both increases and decreases in the abundance of some transcripts were seen in regenerating liver. Transcripts of cellular oncogenes, for example, were among the mRNAs that increased during DNA synthesis and liver regeneration.[70] The ras and myc oncogenes were elevated three- to fourfold above normal and this corresponded exactly with the major wave of DNA synthesis; in fact, the *ras* gene expression slightly preceded the peak of DNA synthesis.[72]

In summary, hepatocytes in adult animals are stimulated to enlarge and divide in response to a reduction in liver mass. They respond by changing the amount of existing mRNAs without significantly altering the type of transcripts produced in the cell. The alterations in mRNA transcripts differ from those associated with fetal liver development or in adult liver as the result of hormonal changes. The ratio of albumin to α-fetoprotein remains nearly constant in adult and regenerating liver but is dramatically different in the fetal liver. It therefore appears that regeneration has little resemblance to fetal development. Rather, changes in specific mRNA species, either up or down, permit the transition of a hepatocyte from a resting to a dividing state. Messenger RNA coding for oncodevelopmental proteins is only slightly elevated, followed by a period of maximum DNA synthesis. Obviously, more extensive studies will reveal the identity and role of many new transcripts that are elevated in the regenerating liver.

DIAGNOSTIC MARKERS OF HEPATIC FIBROSIS

Excess collagen synthesis and deposition characterize hepatic fibrosis. Therefore, it appears quite likely that certain aspects of collagen metabolism can act as markers for liver fibrosis. Hydroxyproline is an abundant amino acid found in collagen, and serum levels of hydroxyproline and hydroxyproline-containing peptides were measured to predict aberrant hepatic collagen metabolism.[73] However, the urinary hydroxyproline values showed no consistent relationship to the histological aspects of liver disease. Additionally, other disorders of connective tissue metabolism and normal bone metabolism completely obliterated the minimal effects of liver disease on urinary hydroxyproline.

Elevated collagen production in hepatic fibrosis has been quantitated by measuring prolyl and lysyl hydroxylases, and uridine diphosphoryl glucosyl and galactosyl transferases, enzymes involved in post-translational modification of procollagen chains.[74, 75] Although elevated levels of these enzymes paralleled increased rates of collagen production, these measurements required the use of liver biopsy samples and were therefore of limited use as routine screening tests. The best correlation was obtained from the measurement of lysyl oxidase: a 30-fold increase in enzyme activity was found in biopsy tissue.[76] Additionally, sufficient amounts of this extracellular enzyme were released into the serum to allow its quantitation.

The major development in diagnostic tests for elevated collagen production in hepatic fibrosis in the past 10 years has been a radioimmunoassay for type III procollagen peptide in serum in human liver diseases.[77] As stated previously, the major interstitial collagens of human liver are type I and type III, which are found in nearly equal amounts. During procollagen synthesis, polypeptide chains are produced that have both NH_2 and COOH terminal procollagen peptides. The terminal procollagen peptides are excised by procollagen peptidases, rendering the collagen molecule insoluble in physiological fluids. These propeptide fragments are released into serum. The NH_2 terminal propeptide of type III collagen and the COOH terminal propeptide of type I collagen contain interchain disulfide crosslinks that help to maintain their globular structure and resist somewhat the proteolytic degradation that occurs during passage into serum.[78] In contrast, the NH_2 terminal propeptide of type I collagen does not contain interchain crosslinks and is presumably rapidly degraded by tissue-neutral proteases.

Early studies with serum from patients with alcoholic liver disease showed significant (2- to 20-fold) elevation of the NH_2 terminal propeptide.[77] Normal levels of peptide are estimated at 7 ng per milliliter; peptide content of up to 160 ng per milliliter was present in some patients with alcoholic liver disease. Surprisingly, the highest level was found in serum of patients with chronic active hepatitis and lower levels occurred during the later stages of alcoholic liver cirrhosis. Peptide levels are also slightly elevated in 20 percent of patients with rheumatoid arthritis and other diseases such as systemic sclerosis and lung fibrosis. Procollagen peptide levels in alcoholic patients correlated well with portal inflammation and periportal necrosis. Serum parameters such as bilirubin, SGOT, and IgG showed a significant but weaker correlation.[79] Serum propeptide levels are also elevated in primary biliary cirrhosis, and they promptly regress to normal after liver transplantation.

A commercial radioimmunoassay diagnostic kit is now available for rapid, noninvasive testing for ongoing fibrosis and the development of cirrhosis. Elevated serum type III propeptides appear to be dependent on the rapid rate of ongoing fibrosis. Several studies using these protocols have been completed and a number of conclusions can be drawn. It is believed that the *rate* of ongoing fibrosis is an important determinant in elevated peptide levels. Moreover, in primary biliary cirrhosis, elevated peptide levels may be a better indicator of progression than histological stage, and in alcoholic hepatitis, the serum propeptide values are very high and decline when the disease subsides. Finally, in acute viral hepatitis they are high but normalize within 1 to 6 months. If the serum propeptide levels remain high, chronic active hepatitis was diagnosed in a retrospective study; thus the assay was capable of distinguishing between chronic active hepatitis (high) and chronic persistent hepatitis (low).[78]

A major problem with the earlier radioimmunoassay (RIA) for propeptide III levels in serum was its apparent lack of reliability due to the variable degrees of degradation of the propeptide, yielding different fragments with unequal affinity for the antibody. This has been circumvented by the use of FAB fragments of the antibody, and the currently available FAB-RIA assay yields linear results with both large and small fragments of the type III procollagen propeptide. The FAB-RIA assay showed a positive correlation in liver biopsies with a morphometric measurement of portal tract area and the number of fibroblasts present.[80] Patients undergoing treatment with penacillamine, azathioprine, or prednisone had normal serum propeptide levels.

From these studies, it is apparent that levels of serum procollagen type III peptides can be useful for distinguishing between fibrotic and nonfibrotic liver disease. However, long-term follow-up studies of patients with elevated serum peptide levels have yet to be conducted. Will they develop cirrhosis faster? Will peptide levels be valuable for assessing a decline in fibrosis as the result of therapy? In any event, the measurement of serum levels of type III propeptide will remain a valuable tool for differentiating subgroups of liver diseases. It remains to be determined whether the propeptide level occurs as the result of type III collagen synthesis, degradation, clearance of the propeptide, or remodeling as opposed to net degradation of the fibrotic matrix. It should be remembered that peptide levels are elevated in infants, growing children, and pregnant mothers in whom both synthesis and remodeling are occurring at a rapid pace. It may also be beneficial to measure degradation products of type IV collagen and laminin, since these are directly related to net degradation of the fibrotic matrix.

CONCLUSION

The liver is a complex, multifunctional organ that acts as the collection point for most toxic chemicals that enter the bloodstream. It is not surprising that an elaborate set of detoxification mechanisms exists, and in certain situations these mechanisms become overwhelmed and hepatic injury is inevitable. Fortunately, a large reserve of hepatic tissue is present and hepatic shutdown occurs only in extreme cases. This is evident by the fact that 70 percent of the hepatic tissue in rats can be removed without the liver being compromised to any degree.

How hepatic tissue regenerates so rapidly after partial hepatectomy, and presumably after acute liver injury, has long been a mystery. Future studies involving the role of oncogenes, including *ras* and *myc*, and growth factors such as platelet-derived growth factor, epidermal growth factor, and transforming growth factor-α and -β (TGF-α and -β) to name only a few, will help to explain how individual cells of the liver communicate with each other through soluble, chemical mediators to maintain normal or abnormal function. In addition, inflammatory cells produce a variety of lymphokines, monokines, and cytokines that can be expected to modulate all hepatic cells in acute or chronic injury, thereby explaining how excess collagen may be deposited. Two major factors are TGF-β, which stimulates collagen production in scar tissue, and tumor necrosis factor-α and -β, (TNF-α and -β) which have lytic effects such as stimulation of collagenase production in tissue damage and remodeling. It is recognized that hepatic fibrosis may result from an overproduction of such factors as TGF-β and/or a decrease in TNF-α or some other kinin. Investigations of liver disease therefore require quantitation of these mediators as well as collagen and collagenase production. At the same time, the use of molecular biology techniques enables the investigator to examine hepatic tissue in a more global manner through the use of cDNA probes that encode individual proteins. Steady-state levels of a number of mRNAs can be quantitated simultaneously, giving the investigator a much clearer picture of the complex hepatic tissue metabolism. It has already been seen how in situ hybridization can pinpoint the exact cell type currently producing an excess of a specific mRNA and presumably a specific protein. These techniques will allow us to move beyond the isolated cell cultures into in vivo tissue where various cells and cell types communicate extensively through contact and chemical mediators.

References

1. Netter FH: Digestive system. III; liver, biliary tract, and pancreas. In Oppenheimer E (ed): The CIBA Collection of Medical Illustrations, vol 3. New York, RR Donnelley, 1976, pp 1–31, 60–120.
2. Rappaport AM, Hiraki GY: The anatomical pattern of lesions in the liver. Acta Anat 32:126–140, 1958.
3. Popper H: Correlation of hepatic function and structure based on liver biopsy studies. In Liver Injury. Transactions of the 9th Conference. New York, Macy Foundation, 1951.
4. Popper H, Elias H: Histogenesis of hepatic cirrhosis studied by the three dimensional approach. Am J Pathol 31:405–432, 1955.
5. Hutterer F, Rubin E, Singer EJ, et al: Quantitative relation of cell proliferation and fibrogenesis in the liver. Cancer Res 21:206–215, 1961.
6. Rubin E, Hutterer F, Popper H: Cell proliferation and fiber formation in chronic carbon tetrachloride intoxication. A morphologic and chemical study. Am J Pathol 42:715–728, 1963.
7. Irving MG, Roll FJ, Bissell DM: Sinusoidal endothelial cells from normal rat liver: Isolation, culture and collagen phenotype. Hepatology 1:520–529, 1981.
8. Bissell DM, Hammaker LE, Meyer DA: Parenchymal cells from adult rat liver non-proliferating monolayer culture. I. Functional studies. J Cell Biol 59:722–734, 1973.
9. Rojkind M, Gatmaitan Z, Mackensen S, et al: Connective tissue biomatrix: Its isolation and utilization for long-term cultures of normal rat hepatocytes. J Cell Biol 87:255–263, 1980.
10. Yamada KM: Fibronectin and other structural proteins. In Hay ED (ed): Cell Biology of Extracellular Matrix. New York, Plenum Press, 1981, p 95–114.
11. Hynes RO: Integrins: A family of cell surface receptors. Cell 48:549–554, 1987.
12. Suzuki S, Argraves WS, Pytela R, et al: cDNA and amino acid sequences of the cell adhesion protein receptor recognizing vitronectin reveal a transmembrane domain and homologies with other adhesion protein receptors. Proc Natl Acad Sci USA 83:8614–8618, 1986.
13. Fujiwara K, Sakai T, Oda T, et al: The presence of collagenase in Kupffer cells of rat liver. Biochem Biophys Res Commun 54:531–537, 1973.
14. Maruyama K, Feinman L, Fainsilver Z, et al: Mammalian collagenase increases in early alcoholic liver disease and decreases with cirrhosis. Gastroenterology 80:1341, 1981 (abstract).
15. Kashiwazaki K, Hibbs MS, Seyer JM, et al: Stimulation of interstitial collagenase in co-cultures of rat hepatocyte and sinusoidal cells. Gastroenterology 90:829–836, 1986.
16. Maruyama K, Okazaki I, Kobayashi T, et al: Collagenase production by rabbit liver cells in monolayer culture. J Lab Clin Med 102:543–550, 1983.
17. Irving MG, Roll FJ, Huang S, et al: Characterization and culture of sinusoidal endothelium from normal rat liver: Lipoprotein uptake and collagen phenotype. Gastroenterology 87:1233–1247, 1984.
18. Wagner DD, Olmsted JB, Marder VJ: Immunolocalization of von Willebrand protein in Weibel-Palade bodies of human endothelial cells. J Cell Biol 95:355–360, 1982.
19. Friedman SL, Roll FJ: Isolation and culture of hepatic lipocytes, Kupffer cells, and sinusoidal endothelial cells by density gradient centrifugation with Stractan. Anal Biochem 161:207–218, 1987.
20. Wake K: Perisinusoidal stellate cells (fat-storing cells, interstitial cells, lipocytes), their related structure in and around the liver sinusoids, and vitamin A–storing cells in extrahepatic organs. Int Rev Cytol 66:303–353, 1980.
21. Kent G, Gay S, Inouye T, et al: Vitamin A–containing lipocytes and formation of type III collagen in liver injury. Proc Natl Acad Sci USA 73:3719–3722, 1976.
22. Martinez-Hernandez A: The hepatic extracellular matrix. I. Electron immunohistochemical studies in normal rat liver. Lab Invest 51:57–74, 1984.
23. Martinez-Hernandez A: The hepatic extracellular matrix. II. Electron immunohistochemical studies in rats with CCl₄-induced cirrhosis. Lab Invest 53:166–186, 1985.
24. Gabbiani G, Lelouis M, Bailey AJ, et al: Collagen and myofibroblasts of granulation tissue. Virchows Arch (Cell Pathol) 21:133–145, 1976.
25. Bhathal PS: Presence of modified fibroblasts in cirrhotic livers in man. Pathology 4:139–144, 1972.
26. Popper H, Udenfriend S: Hepatic fibrosis. Correlation of biochemical and morphologic investigations. Am J Med 49:707–721, 1970.
27. Ross R: The connective tissue fiber forming cell. In Ramachandran GN (ed): Treatise on Collagen, vol 2. New York, Academic Press, 1968, pp 1–82.
28. Leo MA, Mak KM, Savolainen ER, et al: Isolation and culture of myofibroblasts from rat liver. Proc Soc Exp Biol Med 180:382–391, 1985.
29. Seyer JM: Interstitial collagen polymorphism in rat liver with CCl₄-induced cirrhosis. Biochim Biophys Acta 629:490–498, 1980.
30. Timpl R, Engle J: Type VI collagen. In Burgeson R, Mayne R (eds): Structure and Function of Collagen Types. New York, Academic Press, 1987, pp 105–144.
31. Rohde H, Wick G, Timpl R: Immunochemical characterization of the basement membrane glycoprotein laminin. Eur J Biochem 102:195–201, 1979.
32. Hahn E, Wick G, Pencev D, et al: Distribution of basement membrane proteins in normal and fibrotic human liver: collagen IV, laminin, and fibronectin. Gut 21:63–71, 1980.
33. Carlin BE, Durkin ME, Bender B, et al: Synthesis of laminin and entactin by F9 cells induced with retinoic acid and dibutyryl cyclic AMP. J Biol Chem 258:7729–7737, 1983.
34. Ninomiya Y, Hata RI, Nagai Y: Active synthesis of glycosaminoglycans by liver parenchymal cells in primary culture. Biochim Biophys Acta 675:248–255, 1981.
35. Kjellen L, Oldberg A, Hook M: Cell-surface heparan sulfate. Mechanisms of proteoglycan-cell association. J Biol Chem 255:10407–10413, 1980.
36. Hahn EG, Gauss-Muller V, Hormann H, et al: Enhanced production of fibronectin, a transformation-sensitive glycoprotein, by malignant human hepatocytes. Liver 1:159–160, 1981.

36a. Laurie GW, Leblond CP, Martin GR: Localization of type IV collagen, laminin, heparan sulfate proteoglycan, and fibronectin to basal lamina of basement membranes. J Cell Biol 95:340–349, 1982.

37. Cameron GR, Karunaratne WAE: Carbon tetrachloride cirrhosis in relation to liver regeneration. J Pathol Bacteriol 42:1–26, 1936.

38. Morrione TG: Factors influencing collagen content in experimental cirrhosis. Am J Pathol 25:273–280, 1949.

39. Zern MA, Leo MA, Giambrone MA, et al: Increased type I procollagen mRNA levels and in vitro protein synthesis in the baboon model of chronic alcoholic liver disease. Gastroenterology 89:1123–1131, 1985.

40. Perez-Tomayo P: Is cirrhosis of the liver experimentally produced by CCl₄ an adequate model of human cirrhosis? Gastroenterology 3:112–120, 1983.

41. Paronetto F, Popper H: Chronic liver injury induced by immunologic reactions. Am J Pathol 49:1087–1095, 1966.

42. Kunntouras J, Billing BH, Scheuer PJ: Prolonged bile duct obstruction: A new experimental model for cirrhosis in the rat. Br J Exp Pathol 65:305–311, 1984.

43. Gupta DN: Nodular cirrhosis and metastasizing tumours produced in the liver of rats by prolonged feeding with thioacetamide. J Pathol Bacteriol 72:415–426, 1956.

44. Hartroft WS: Hepatic cancer. Nutritional factors and the production by dietary choline deficiency of cancer *de novo* in mice. Gastroenterology 37:669–688, 1959.

45. Lanks KW, Weinstein IB: Quantitative differences in proline tRNA content of rat liver and granulation tissue. Biochem Biophys Res Commun 40:708–715, 1970.

46 Rojkind M, Dunn MA: Hepatic fibrosis. Gastroenterology 76:849–863, 1979.

47. Ehrinpreiss MN, Giambrone MA, Rojkind M: Liver proline oxidase activity and collagen synthesis in rats with cirrhosis induced by carbon tetrachloride. Biochim Biophys Acta 629:184–193, 1980.

48. Dunn MA, Rojkind M, Hait PK, et al: Conversion of arginine to proline in murine schistosomiasis. Gastroenterology 75:1010–1015, 1978.

49. Risteli J, Kivirikko KI: Activities of prolyl hydroxylase, lysyl hydroxylase, collagen galactosyltransferase and collagen glucosyltransferase in the liver of rats with hepatic injury. Biochem J 144:115–122, 1974.

50. Hahn EG, Hochweiss S, Berk PD: Diagnostic parameters of altered collagen turnover. In Berk, PD, Castro-Malaspina H, Wasserman LR (eds): New York, Alan R. Liss, 1984, pp 335–342.

51. Saber MA, Zern MA, Shafritz DA: Use of *in situ* hybridization to identify collagen and albumin mRNAs in isolated rat hepatocytes. Proc Natl Acad Sci USA 80:4017–4020, 1983.

52. Friedman SL, Roll FJ, Boyles J: Hepatic lipocytes: The principal collagen–producing cells of normal rat liver. Proc Natl Acad Sci USA 82:8681–8685, 1985.

53. Postlethwaite AE, Seyer JM, Kang AH: Chemotactic attraction of human fibroblasts to type I, II, and III collagens and collagen-derived peptides. Proc Natl Acad Sci USA 75:871–875, 1978.

54. Seppa H, Grotendorst GR, Seppa G, et al: Platelet-derived growth factor is chemotactic for fibroblasts. J Cell Biol 92:584–591, 1982.

55. Postlethwaite AE, Snyderman R, Kang AH: The chemotactic attraction of human fibroblasts to a lymphocyte-derived factor. J Exp Med 114:1188–1196, 1976.

56. Hatahara T, Seyer JM: Isolation of a fibrogenic factor from CCl₄-damaged rat liver. Biochim Biophys Acta 716:377–382, 1982.

57. Raghow R, Gossage D, Seyer JM, et al: Transcriptional regulation of type I collagen genes in cultured fibroblasts by a factor isolated from thioacetamide-induced fibrotic rat liver. J Biol Chem 259:12718–12723, 1984.

58. Choe I, Aycock RS, Raghow R, et al: A hepatic fibrogenic factor stimulates the synthesis of types I, III and V procollagens in cultured cells. J Biol Chem 262:5408–5413, 1987.

59. McGee JO'D, O'Hare RP, Patrick RS: Stimulation of the collagen biosynthetic pathway by factors isolated from experimentally injured liver. Nature [New Biol] 243:121–123, 1973.

60. Igarashi S: Identification of a fibrogenic component from fibrotic rat liver. Hepat Jpn 18:10–14, 1977.

61. Harris ED, Krane SM: Collagenases. N Engl J Med 291:557–563, 1974.

62. Arthur MJP, Friedman SL, Roll FJ, et al: Lipocytes from normal rat liver release a neutral metalloproteinase that degrades basement membrane (type IV) collagen. J Clin Invest 84:1076–1085, 1990.

63. Welgus HG, Stricklin GP: Human skin fibroblast collagenase inhibitor. J Biol Chem 258:12259–12264, 1983.

64. Maruyama K, Feinman L, Okazaki I, et al: Direct measurement of neutral collagenase activity in homogenates from baboon and human liver. Biochim Biophys Acta 658:124–141, 1981.

65. Hutterer F, Eisenstadt M, Rubin E: Turnover of hepatic collagen in reversible and irreversible fibrosis. Experientia 26:244–245, 1970.

66. Perez-Tamayo R, Montfort I: The susceptibility of hepatic collagen to homologous collagenase in human and experimental cirrhosis of the liver. Am J Pathol 100:427–440, 1980.

67. Raghow R, Lurie S, Seyer JM, et al: Profiles of steady-state levels of messenger RNAs coding for type I procollagen, elastin and fibronectin in hamster lungs undergoing bleomycin-induced interstitial pulmonary fibrosis. J Clin Invest 76:1733–1739, 1985.

68. Harkness RD: The spatial distribution of dividing cells in the liver of the rat after partial hepatectomy. J Physiol 116:373–379, 1952.

69. Fausto N: Messenger RNA in regeneration liver; implication for the understanding of regulated growth. Mol Cell Biochem 59:131–147, 1984.

70. Fausto N, Shank PR: Oncogene expression in liver regeneration and hepatocarcinogenesis. Hepatology 3:1016–1023, 1983.

71. Church R, McCarthy BJ: Changes in nuclear and cytoplasmic RNA in regenerating mouse liver. Proc Natl Acad Sci USA 58:1548–1555, 1967.

72. Goyette M, Petropoulos DJ, Shank PR, et al: Expression of an oncogene during liver regeneration. Science 219:510–512, 1983.

73. Kershenobich D, Garcia-Tsao G, Saldana SA, et al: Relationship between blood lactic acid and serum proline in alcoholic liver cirrhosis. Gastroenterology 80:1012–1015, 1981.

74. Kuutti-Savolainen ER, Risteli J, Miettinen TA, et al: Collagen biosynthesis enzymes in serum and hepatic tissue in liver disease. I. Prolyl hydroxylase. Eur J Clin Invest 9:89–95, 1979.

75. Kuuti-Savolainen ER, Anttinen H, Miettinen TA, et al: Collagen biosynthesis enzymes in serum and hepatic

tissue in liver disease. II. Galactosylhydroxylysyl glucosyltransferase. Eur J Clin Invest 9:97–101, 1979.

76. Siegel RC: Lysyl oxidase. Int Rev Conn Tissue Res 8:73–118, 1980.

77. Rohde H, Vargas L, Hahn E, et al: Radioimmunoassay for type III procollagen peptide and its application to human liver disease. Eur J Clin Invest 9:451–459, 1979.

78. Hahn E: Blood analysis of liver fibrosis. Hepatology 1:67–73, 1984.

79. Frei H, Zimmerman A, Weigand K: The N-terminal propeptide of collagen type III in serum reflects activity and degree of fibrosis in patients with chronic liver disease. Hepatology 4:830–834, 1984.

80. Rohde H, Langer J, Krieg T, et al: Serum and urine analysis of the aminoterminal procollagen peptide type III by radioimmunoassay with antibody FAB fragments. Coll Rel Res 3:371–379, 1983.

27

THE ALIMENTARY CANAL

Martin F. Graham, M.D.; and Peter Blomquist, M.D., Ph.D., and Bengt Zederfeldt, M.D., Ph.D.

This topic will be approached from two standpoints. The first examines the healing response that follows injury and inflammation, and the second examines the healing of surgical incisions and anastomoses

FUNCTIONAL MORPHOLOGY

When approaching the pathophysiology of healing in the gastrointestinal tract it must be remembered that this is a hollow muscular organ lined by epithelium, with a number of discrete connective-tissue and mesenchymal cell layers (Fig. 27–1). The intestine is divided physically into two major elements: the mucosa, a layer consisting of epithelium, lamina propria, and muscularis mucosae; and the deep muscle layer or muscularis propria. These two major layers are connected by a third layer, the submucosa, which is a discrete band of connective tissue containing blood vessels and lymphatics. The outside of the intestine is coated by a layer of connective tissue known as the serosa, which is an extension of the peritoneum. This arrangement of layers is found along the entire length of the gastrointestinal tract with the exception of the proximal third of the esophagus. Additionally, most of the duodenum and the rectum have no serosa because they are extraperitoneal.

Mucosa

The luminal surface of the mucosa consists of a layer of *epithelial cells* that form glands, pits, villi, or crypts depending on the region of the gut. This layer is columnar and one cell thick throughout the entire gastrointestinal tract with the exception of the esophagus, where it is stratified and squamous. The epithelial cell layer is in a continuously dynamic state known as "epithelial renewal," [1] whereby undifferentiated cells from a proliferative zone within the layer divide, differentiate, and migrate to the luminal surface where they are sloughed. This process takes from 3 to 8 days.

The structure of *basement membrane* appears to be similar in different tissues[2] and has been well conserved through evolution.[3] Although the ultrastructure of human intestinal epithelial basement membrane has not been studied, it is generally assumed that it is similar to that of epithelia from other tissues.[4] The structural core of basement membrane is a sheet of type IV collagen molecules arranged in a reticular structure.[5] This constitutes the lamina densa of

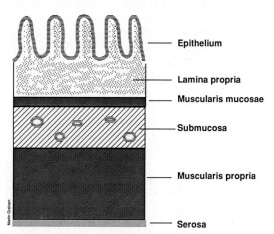

Figure 27–1. Schematic representation of the multiple cell layers in the gastrointestinal tract wall.

- Epithelium
- Lamina propria
- Muscularis mucosae
- Submucosa
- Muscularis propria
- Serosa

433

the basement membrane. The sheet of type IV collagen is coated by heparan sulfate proteoglycan, which is thought to provide a cationic shield against the passage of anionic macromolecules.[6] Laminin is the constituent of the lamina lucida and anchors the epithelial cell to the lamina densa.[4] It is widely accepted that the basement membrane is produced and deposited by the epithelial cells.

The *lamina propria* is a loose connective tissue that supports the epithelium and consists of collagen types I, III, and V[7] and elastin.[8] A network of capillaries and lymphatics in the lamina propria facilitates absorption and secretion. An array of mesenchymal cells including smooth muscle cells, subepithelial myofibroblasts, and fibroblasts in the lamina propria of the villi have recently been described and characterized.[9, 10] Inflammatory cells such as plasma cells, lymphocytes, macrophages, mast cells, and eosinophils are a significant feature of the normal lamina propria and play an important role in the immune function of the intestine.[11]

The *muscularis mucosa* is a thin layer of smooth muscle cells 2 to 5 cells thick that separates the lamina propria from the submucosa. The precise function of this layer of cells has not been delineated, but it is assumed to contribute to effective intestinal motility.

Submucosa

The submucosa is a loose meshwork, predominantly of collagen with some elastin and numerous vessels. The majority of the collagen in the intestinal wall is in the submucosa, and biochemical analysis shows it to consist of 68 percent type I, 20 percent type III, and 12 percent type V collagen.[12] Interestingly, a similar collagen composition has been found in human aorta,[13] another hollow muscular organ. It appears that in hollow muscular organs, smooth muscle cells play a significant role in the production and maintenance of the extracellular matrix of the organ, and the intestine is no exception. Recent in vitro studies have demonstrated that human intestinal smooth muscle cells produce large amounts of collagen types I, III, and V[14] compared to human dermal fibroblasts.[14] It should be assumed, therefore, that as the submucosal collagen connects two smooth muscle cell layers, it is produced and maintained by the smooth muscle cells of those layers.

The submucosal collagen is relatively rich in type V collagen compared to other tissues such as skin (~ 2% type V[15]), and gingiva (~ 1%[16]) when extracted by similar methods. The relative abundance of this collagen type in the bowel wall raises the question of its physiological function. The role of type V collagen in the structure and function of other human tissue has not, as yet, been clearly delineated; however, recent studies of type V collagen in human amnion and placenta suggest that it is a network of anchoring fibrils connecting cells with interstitial collagens.[17, 18] In addition, it has been demonstrated that smooth muscle cells bind preferentially to, and have glycoprotein receptors for, type V collagen.[19, 20] Although the precise function of the submucosal connective tissue network has not been defined, it appears to attach, in a compliant fashion, the mucosa to the deeper muscular layers (Fig. 27–2). It therefore seems plausible that type V collagen in the submucosa serves to connect the two smooth muscle cell layers and the interstitial collagens of the submucosal matrix.

Muscularis Propria

This layer consists of densely packed smooth muscle cells surrounded by thin collagen fibrils 30 to 35 nm in diameter. These fibrils coalesce to form collagen fibers, which constitute the intramuscular septae. Analysis of the collagen types in human intestinal muscle reveals a predominance of types I and III with smaller amounts of V.[21] The collagenous network in visceral smooth muscle, which is three times more abundant than in skeletal muscle, is thought to act as an intramuscular tendon for the transmission of longitudinal forces between groups of smooth muscle cells.[22] Hypertrophy of intestinal muscle secondary to experimentally induced obstruction is associated with an increase in the collagen content of the bowel wall,[23, 24] particularly in the muscle layer.[24]

Ultrastructurally, the collagen fibrils emanate from the smooth muscle cells.[24, 25] As alluded to previously, the collagenous network in the normal muscularis propria is produced and maintained by the smooth muscle cells themselves. Within the muscle bundles there are larger spaces occupied by nerves, capillaries, and interstitial cells. The identity of these interstitial cells is controversial, but they are thought to be either modified sympathetic neurons, immature smooth muscle cells, or modified fibroblasts.[22]

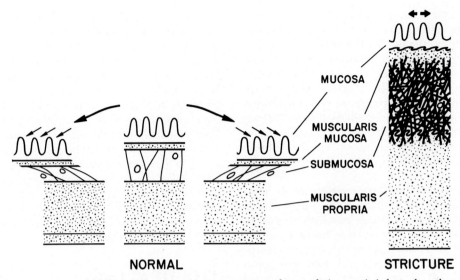

Figure 27–2. The normal compliant relationship between mucosa and muscularis propria is lost when the submucosa becomes fibrotic. (From Graham MF, Diegelmann RF, Elson CD, et al: Collagen content and types in the intestinal strictures of Crohn's disease. Gastroenterology 94:257–265, 1988.)

INJURY PATTERNS AND RESPONSE IN THE INTESTINE

Little is known about the pathophysiology of repair in the gastrointestinal tract. A large body of work has been performed on the repair processes of the gastric epithelium in response to acute injury, but these studies have not ventured beyond the epithelial basal lamina. Clinical, pathological, and laboratory-derived data on the reparative response in acid-peptic disease of the stomach—a pervasive and ubiquitous inflammatory disease in humans—can provide a conceptual framework within which to develop an understanding of some principles of repair in the bowel.

The human stomach is continuously subjected, under physiological conditions, to the injurious combination of hydrochloric acid and pepsin. This digestive mixture can overcome the gastric epithelium's innate defenses against autodigestion and can cause injury under a number of circumstances: if gastric acid is produced in excessive amounts; if those defenses are compromised by drugs such as corticosteroids or chemotherapeutic agents or if the mucosa is exposed to toxins such as aspirin or alcohol. Injury will also result if there is excessive contact between this peptic mixture and epithelia that are not designed to withstand it such as those in the esophagus and duodenum. Minor degrees of epithelial disruption are undoubtedly occurring continuously in these mucosae and would result in severe inflammation

if a mechanism were not available for rapid, efficient reconstitution of the epithelium. Studies performed both in vivo and in vitro have demonstrated that such a mechanism exists. Short-term exposure (10 min to 1 hour) of gastric or duodenal mucosa to a variety of injurious agents results in necrosis and detachment of the epithelium. In areas where the basal lamina remains intact, surrounding epithelial cells begin migrating into the defect within minutes and seal the epithelium within 1 to 2 hours following injury.[26, 27] Neither cell proliferation nor inflammation is involved in this remarkably rapid process. Recent studies suggest that contraction of the villae by myofibroblasts in the lamina propria plays a role in this epithelial reconstitution.[28]

It should be emphasized that this process of reconstitution will occur only if the basal lamina remains intact. If the injury penetrates through the basal lamina into the lamina propria, vessels will be disrupted and inflammation will ensue. In this latter setting, the epithelium will heal more slowly by a process of mitosis and proliferation. When the epithelium is disrupted and inflammation is present but confined to the mucosa, the lesion is classified as an erosion. When the injury penetrates through the muscularis mucosae and into the submucosa, an ulcer results. This distinction is important because it has a bearing on the quality of the subsequent healing response.

With the advent of the flexible gastroscope, gastroenterologists have had the opportunity to correlate the gross appearance of these lesions with their histopathology and with their patterns of both clinical and histological healing. The major determinant of the pattern of healing appears to be the depth of the lesion. Erosions, (lesions confined to the mucosa) will heal completely without either clinical or histological evidence of scar.[29] The mucosa therefore appears to heal itself by processes of reconstitution and regeneration rather than by repair. Deeper lesions that have penetrated into the submucosa and muscularis propria (ulcers) will always demonstrate some degree of fibrotic repair in the deeper layers.[30]

The degree of this fibrosis and its reversibility depend on the chronicity of the insult. Acute ulcers are defined as those in which a minimal fibrotic response is seen but because of the relatively short duration of the injury, resorption of the scar will occur and there will be no longstanding morphological or functional changes. In chronic ulcers, fibrosis in the deeper layers is significant and results in major, irreversible changes in morphology. Grossly, there is often distortion of the tissue, producing stenosis in the esophagus and duodenum or an "hour-glass" constriction in the stomach. If the lesion is circumferential, a tight, obstructive stricture results. Microscopically, chronic peptic ulcers have a characteristic appearance.[30] In the earlier stages there is extensive fibrosis of the submucosa and hypertrophy of the muscularis propria. Later, the muscularis propria is replaced entirely by fibrous scar, which then constitutes the base of the ulcer.

Utilizing these observations, a model for the reparative response of the bowel to injury can be proposed: the quality of the reparative response of the bowel to injury is determined by both the depth and the chronicity of the injury. Injury confined to the mucosa heals with a complete return to normal morphology by processes of reconstitution and regeneration rather than by healing with scar deposition. Injury involving the deeper layers of the bowel wall elicits a fibrotic response that, depending on chronicity, is often irreversible and can result in functional impairment (Fig. 27–3). This conceptual framework will be utilized in the examination of the healing response to other forms of injury to the gastrointestinal tract.

THE HEALING RESPONSE IN SPECIFIC CLINICO-PATHOLOGICAL STATES

Schistosomiasis

Schistosomiasis, a disease affecting 200 million people worldwide, provides a fascinating example of the healing response of the intestine. This is because the connective tissue response of the intestinal wall to the *Schistosoma* egg plays an indispensible role in the life cycle of the invading parasite. One can extrapolate from

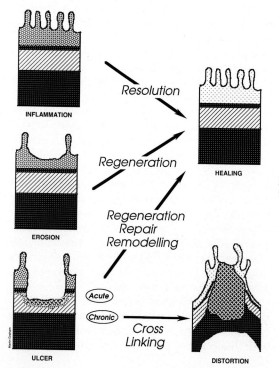

Figure 27–3. Pattern of gastrointestinal repair depends on the depth of mucosal inflammation.

studies of the pathophysiology of the schistosomal granuloma in the intestinal wall to formulate a general concept of the intestinal response to injury. These studies, which in the main have focused on the immunology of the disease, have been greatly facilitated by the development of a murine model.

Schistosoma mansoni, hematobium, and japonicum are ubiquitous parasites in Egypt, Africa, the Caribbean basin, Brazil, and the Far East. Humans are infected by wading or swimming in infested water. The cercaria, or larvae, penetrate the skin, enter the circulation, and lodge in the liver where they mature into adult worms, which then migrate upstream into the terminal mesenteric venules in the case of S. *mansoni* and S. *japonicum* and deposit their eggs in the intestinal submucosa. To complete the life cycle, the eggs must migrate from the submucosa through the mucosa and into the intestinal lumen to be excreted in the feces. Approximately 50 percent of the deposited eggs manage to accomplish this task. The balance, however, either remain trapped in the intestinal wall or are swept up in the mesenteric circulation to lodge in the intrahepatic portal radicles. These entrapped eggs elicit a granulomatous response from the host tissue and the resultant fibrosis in liver and bowel is responsible for the significant morbidity of the disease.

The schistosome egg facilitates its passage through the mucosa by secreting lytic enzymes through its shell.[31] These enzymes are thought to evoke the cell-mediated immune response that produces the granulomas.[32] When the intestine of the mouse is examined from 6 to 20 weeks postinfection, eggs are present in the mucosa and the muscularis in an equal distribution.[33] However, while granuloma formation with fibrosis is pronounced around the eggs in the muscularis, minimal or no reaction is seen around the eggs in the mucosa.[33, 34] In fact, the majority of the eggs in the mucosa remain morphologically intact with no collagen and only eosinophils and degenerating epithelial cells surrounding them.[34] Similar findings have been noted in human specimens.[35] The granulomata in the muscularis evolve as follows: At 6 to 8 weeks after infection the eggs are surrounded mainly by eosinophils and some neutrophils, plasma cells, lymphocytes, and epithelioid cells. At this stage there is minimal fibrosis. Twenty weeks following infection, the granuloma is predominantly collagenous with few surrounding eosinophils, although the disrupted egg shell contains macrophages.[34] The connective tissue composition of these intestinal granulomata has recently been characterized using immunofluorescent techniques and they appear to be made up of collagen types I and III in equal proportions and by fibronectin. Type V collagen was not examined.[36] Interestingly, significant differences in the genesis of ileal, colonic, and hepatic granulomata have been described. Those in the ileum are smaller, do not modulate with time, and contain far fewer lymphocytes.[37, 38] The reason for these differences is not known but a clear distinction between mucosal and muscularis granulomata was not made in those studies. Unfortunately, the mesenchymal cell response in these granulomata has not been well characterized to date but could be easily studied.

An interesting facet of the pathology in this model is the lack of a granulomatous/fibrotic response to injury in the ileal mucosa when compared to the muscularis. It is fascinating that this phenomenon plays an important role in the life cycle of the parasite, which utilizes the peculiar healing response of the different layers of the intestinal wall to facilitate its life cycle. However, more importantly, this observation does agree with the concept that the mucosa does not respond to injury by producing scar whereas the deeper layers of the intestine do.

Crohn's Disease

In the Western world, a striking and ubiquitous intestinal fibrotic healing response is seen in the strictures that complicate Crohn's disease, a chronic, idiopathic inflammatory bowel disease that affects the terminal ileum and cecum most frequently but can involve any part of the gastrointestinal tract from the mouth to the anus. Stricture formation is seen so frequently in Crohn's disease that it is considered a characteristic feature and not a complication of this disease. The hallmark of this inflammatory process that distinguishes it from most other chronic inflammatory bowel diseases is inflammation seated in the submucosa rather than the mucosa. This is similar to the inflammatory process seen in intestinal tuberculosis, with which it is often confused. The inflammatory process extends both luminally through the mucosa and serosally through the muscularis propria and it is classically termed "transmural." Dense submucosal fibrosis and thickening of the muscular layers ensue. The mucosa loses its compliant attachment to the muscularis propria to which it becomes firmly adherent (see Fig. 27–2).[12] The thickening of the deeper layers leads to stenosis and the loss of mucosal compliance and impairs physiological propulsion of the luminal contents. Both of these phenomena contribute to the subtle obstructive symptoms (nausea, anorexia, and abdominal pain) that characterize this disease in its earlier stages and are largely responsible for the indolent morbidity that manifests in weight loss and cachexia. Progression of the fibrotic lesions to stricture and then to frank obstruction necessitates surgical resection, but recurrences of the strictures are frequent at the anastomotic site.

Despite the frequent occurrence of these strictures and the significant morbidity associated with them, their pathogenesis had not, until recently, been studied systematically. Of help in understanding this process would be the identification of the mesenchymal cell or cells involved in the response, the character of the extracellular matrix involved, and the relationship between the chronic inflammation and the connective tissue response.

Gross histological reports have merely described thickening and fibrosis of the intestinal wall. More recently, a proliferation of smooth muscle cells of the muscularis mucosa extending into the submucosa has been described.[12] An ultrastructural study of inflamed bowel without stricture demonstrated similar findings in the muscularis mucosae and submucosa.[39] There was an increase in the size and number of smooth muscle cells of the muscularis mucosae, often extending into the submucosa and through to the muscularis propria. In addition, these smooth muscle cells were intimately related to new collagen fibrils and to elastin. The abnormal submucosa contained fragmented, disorganized collagen fibers. A prominent fibroblast response was seen only in a case that had presented acutely with a perforation.

Biochemical quantitation of intestinal connective tissue in Crohn's disease has yielded conflicting results. In one study, analysis of strictures compared to uninvolved areas demonstrated an increase in glycosaminoglycan hexosamine but not an increase in collagen as measured by hydroxyproline quantitation.[40] In another study, quantitation of prolyl hydroxylase activity in rectal biopsy specimens revealed a threefold increase in patients with Crohn's disease compared to controls and to patients with ulcerative colitis.[41] In a more recent study,[12] quantitation by high-performance liquid chromatography of hydroxyproline in full-thickness specimens of intestinal wall demonstrated a significant increase in collagen content in strictured bowel compared to grossly normal bowel. The collagen content of bowel that was inflamed but not strictured was not significantly increased. Interestingly, the collagen content of colon resected from patients with ulcerative colitis was significantly less than that of control colon. The bowel in ulcerative colitis has a tendency to dilate and perforate rather than to stricture. The inflammation in ulcerative colitis therefore appears to result in an increased turnover and a depletion of extracellular matrix rather than in an accumulation of matrix as seen in Crohn's disease.

Biochemical analysis of the collagen types accumulating in these strictures has revealed a 50 percent increase in the relative amount of type V.[12] An accumulation of type V collagen in strictured bowel was also demonstrated by immunohistology.

The relative abundance of types III and V collagen in both normal (20%, 12%) and strictured (24%, 17%) bowel,[12] in combination with the histological data cited previously, substantiates the role of smooth muscle cells in the production of the collagenous extracellular matrix in both the normal and the diseased intestine. To further evaluate this concept, human intestinal smooth muscle (HISM) cells have been isolated from normal human jejunum, grown in culture,[42] and studied with regard to collagen production.[14] When proliferating in the presence of 10 percent fetal calf serum, HISM cells increased collagen production at the expense of noncollagen protein production. This response to serum appears to be peculiar to intestinal smooth muscle cells as a similar response was not seen in either human uterine or aortic smooth muscle cells.[43] When confluent, HISM cells produced twice as much collagen relative to noncollagen protein as human dermal fibroblasts cultured under identical conditions. These data demonstrate that collagen synthesis is a significant function of HISM cells and that this function is augmented by serum. Serum can be conceptualized as an inflammatory milieu containing relatively large amounts of inflammatory mediators such as platelet-derived growth factor and transforming growth factor-β (TGF-β). Recently published studies have demonstrated that TGF-β selectively augments collagen synthesis by HISM cells.[44] Therefore, it is likely that the intestinal smooth muscle cell is an important target of inflammation in the intestinal wall and has, in addition to its contractile function, the responsibility of producing a healing matrix in response to injury.

In terms of down-regulation of HISM cell function, the effects of heparin, protamine, corticosteroids, and cyclic nucleotides have been studied. Heparan sulfate significantly inhibited proliferation,[45] altered the profile of secreted proteins,[46] and inhibited the contraction of collagen lattices by HISM cells but did not selectively inhibit collagen synthesis.[45] Protamine sulfate, on the other hand, selectively inhibited collagen production without effects on noncollagen synthesis or DNA synthesis.[47] This effect was in part related to both the lysine moiety in protamine and to the molecule's positive charge. Corticosteroids had no effect on collagen production by HISM cells in contradistinction to a 90 percent inhibition of this function in a control line of human dermal fibroblasts.[48] Elevation of cAMP levels by exposure to cholera toxin, isobutylmethylxanthine, or forskolin resulted in a selective inhibition of collagen synthesis[49] as has been reported for fibroblasts.

Another characteristic feature of Crohn's disease is the development of intestinal fistulae, tracts from the bowel lumen through the bowel wall and out into the peritoneal cavity. The tract can be walled off in the peritoneum as an abscess or can communicate with adjacent loops of bowel or adjacent viscera such as the bladder or vagina. The morbidity associated with these lesions is severe and management is extremely difficult. These lesions can be conceptualized as a failure of the healing response in the bowel wall. Characteristically in Crohn's disease, the tissue necrosis in the submucosa that results from the severe chronic inflammation there is met by a vigorous connective tissue response. A healing matrix is deposited in an effort to seal off the liquefying tissue. Stenosis and stricture may result, but the bowel nevertheless remains intact. In certain locations the liquefaction process overwhelms the scarring response and a fissure breaks through to both the luminal and the serosal surfaces forming a fistula.

Ascorbate deficiency has been investigated as a possible factor in the pathogenesis of these fistulae. Ascorbate is an essential cofactor in collagen synthesis, particularly in human intestinal smooth muscle cells,[14] and a deficiency thereof could well impair the capacity of the smooth muscle cells to produce adequate scar. One study demonstrated a decrease in ascorbate levels in plasma, normal bowel, and diseased bowel of Crohn's patients with intestinal fistulae compared to Crohn's patients without fistulae.[50] However, a similar but more recent study did not reveal any differences in ascorbate levels.[51] The discrepancy between the two studies may simply reflect the improved nutritional management, often parenteral, that is currently afforded patients with severe bowel disease. Interestingly, both of these studies showed an increased concentration of ascorbate in diseased bowel compared to normal bowel in both the fistula and nonfistula groups.

Ulcerative colitis is another chronic, idiopathic bowel disease probably of similar etiology but differing from Crohn's disease in that the inflammation is confined to the mucosa and does not extend into the submucosa. In ulcerative colitis, the intestinal inflammation is not accompanied by a mesenchymal cell or connective tissue healing response and strictures are rare. Those strictures that do occur are thought to be due to hypertrophy and contracture of the muscularis mucosae and not to fibrosis.[52]

Collagenous Colitis

Collagenous colitis refers to the histopathological finding of a thick collagen layer beneath the intercryptal colonic epithelium in patients, mostly elderly and female, with watery diarrhea.[53] Acute and chronic inflammation in the lamina propria and epithelial cell damage are invariably present and often precede the connective tissue changes, which can be progressive.[54] Ultrastructural studies have demonstrated alterations in the epithelial basement membrane, including a complete absence of the basal lamina. In certain cases, an increase in thickness of the basement membrane was noted, whereas in other cases decreased thickness was apparent, which was contiguous with an abnormal accumulation of fibrillar collagen.[55]

The etiology of this disease is currently unknown, but it is thought to be a primarily inflammatory phenomenon of varied etiologies with the connective tissue changes following secondarily.[56] The conventional wisdom regarding the pathogenesis of the collagen band is that because epithelial cell turnover is reduced, pericryptal fibroblasts spend longer in the mature phase and therefore produce more collagen.[57] The authors suspect that this theory is way off the mark because epithelial cell turnover should be increased in the presence of inflammation, and there is no evidence that pericryptal fibroblasts are producing the abnormal collagen. Our hypothesis regarding pathogenesis, particularly in light of the ultrastructural findings, is that the inflammation triggers the epithelial cells to produce fibrillar collagen rather than the normal basement membrane; this could readily be tested in an in vitro system.

Celiac Disease

Celiac disease, or gluten-sensitive enteropathy, is another chronic inflammatory disease involving the small intestine. The chronic lymphocytic infiltrate in the lamina propria results in the destruction of the mucosal villi, leaving a characteristic "flat lesion." Despite the severe nature of this inflammatory process in and confined to the mucosa, a healing response is not seen and removal of the offending antigen, gluten, from the diet results in complete resolution of the inflammation, and a return to normal mucosal morphology presumably by regeneration. This disease entity provides another example of how inflammation confined to the mucosa, even though severe and chronic, will repair without fibrosis.

Intestinal Ischemia

Ischemia is a frequent cause of intestinal injury and has been extensively studied in animal models. Common etiologies in humans include vascular thrombosis, hypovolemic shock, neonatal necrotizing enterocolitis, volvulus, and a variety of vasculitides. The pathological response to ischemia in the bowel is a coagulative necrosis, which is initially seen in the mucosa because it is the layer most sensitive to anoxia. Three clinicopathological patterns of inflammation and subsequent healing have been described,[58] depending on the depth of the injury, which in turn is determined by the degree to which blood flow has been compromised. In the least severe form, the coagulative necrosis extends into the submucosa and may involve the muscularis propria to a small degree. This depth of injury is invariably followed by fibrosis and stricture formation. In these strictures, the submucosa is expanded by a dense accumulation of scar, which sometimes extends into a necrotic muscularis propria.[59] The mesenchymal cells involved in this particular healing response have not been studied or defined. In the third and most severe pattern of injury, coagulative necrosis penetrates through to the serosa and results in transmural infarction of the bowel. In this situation healing cannot proceed and intestinal gangrene ensues.

Radiation Injury

Radiation therapy to the abdomen and pelvis is another frequent cause of intestinal injury. Mucosal biopsies in the immediate postirradiation phase reveal mucosal necrosis.[60] If the injury is severe enough, focal necrosis of the whole thickness of the bowel can occur at this early stage, with perforation and fistula formation. The epithelium regenerates through a dysplastic process with abnormal mitoses,[61] producing convoluted folds and ridges. There is vascular congestion, edema, and a proliferation of fibroblasts in the lamina propria.[62] Later, extensive and progressive submucosal, muscular, and serosal fibrosis occurs with a striking hyalinization of the accumulated collagen.[63] Arteriolar endarteritis and proliferation are characteristically seen. Strictures are the end result of this fibrotic healing response and may occur many years after the radiation injury.

Tuberculosis

Tuberculosis is the classic infectious bowel disease that results in intestinal fibrosis. A fibrotic healing response would be expected in this disease, according to the model proposed, because the inflammation in tuberculosis is transmural and resembles that in Crohn's disease. The majority of infectious enterocolitides are confined to the mucosa and do not result in fibrosis. In its earlier stages, intestinal tuberculosis presents as large annular or circular ulcers overlying transmural caseating granulomas.[64] With time, the lesions in the bowel wall become progressively fibrotic, leading to either the hypertrophic[65] or the ulceroconstrictive[66] forms of the disease. In these strictures, large amounts of scar tissue accumulate in the submucosa and the muscularis propria, making them difficult to differentiate from the strictures of Crohn's disease or intestinal ischemia.[67]

Lye Ingestion

The ingestion of lye is a common cause of severe esophageal injury, particularly in the pediatric population.[68] The source of the lye is usually household drain cleaner that has either been carelessly left within the reach of a toddler or deliberately ingested. Dilute solutions of lye induce only erythema of the mucosa, a superficial lesion that heals spontaneously without any sequelae. When the ingested lye is in either a concentrated liquid or a crystalline form, the inflammation is severe and results in ulceration of the mucosa with penetration into the deeper layers. Strictures are a frequent and tragic consequence of this insult. Parenteral corticosteroid therapy prevented stricture formation in a feline model of lye esophagitis,[69] and steroids are therefore given whenever endoscopy demonstrates an injury of moderate severity. However, controlled trials to demonstrate the efficacy of this therapy in humans have yet to be performed.

Epidermolysis Bullosa

Epidermolysis bullosa (EB) is a chronic hereditary blistering disease thought to be due to excessive production of collagenase by fibroblasts.[70] This abnormality results in the separation of the squamous epithelium of skin and mucous membranes from the underlying dermis. In the milder forms of the disease, EB simplex and junctional EB, the collagenolysis occurs superficially within the epithelium or between the epithelium and the dermis. In the severe and frequently fatal form, EB dystrophica, lysis occurs within the dermis, and because the epithelium cannot regenerate adequately, chronic inflammation and scarring ensue. In this form of the disease, esophageal strictures often complicate the clinical course, requiring dilatation, resection, or esophageal replacement.[71] It is assumed in these cases that chronic inflammation has been ongoing in the deeper layers of the esophagus and that the strictures result from the depth of the chronic injury.

These examples of clinical intestinal pathology all appear to fit the model that has been proposed for healing in the bowel. They will, of course, have to be examined in greater detail in order to document their pathophysiology more precisely. However, it is probable that general rules will be applicable to mechanisms of healing in the gastrointestinal tract whether the injury is in esophagus, ileum, or bile duct and irrespective of the nature of the injury.

From a teleological standpoint, the variation in the healing response of the intestine based on the depth of the injury makes sense. Injury confined to the mucosa would not be life threatening and therefore would not require a robust connective tissue response. In addition, healing of the mucosa with accumulation of scar would not be desirable, as this would impair absorptive function. The reconstitutive and regenerative processes that have evolved for mucosal repair are therefore certainly advantageous. In contrast, injury penetrating through to, or arising in, the deeper layers of the bowel wall presents a more significant problem for the organism. This latter pathological situation could threaten life because perforation would ensue if repair was not adequate, and vigorous healing response with the production of dense scar would be desirable if not mandatory. The mesenchymal cells of the deeper layers of the bowel wall therefore respond to injury by producing and laying down a resilient matrix. This healing process in the deeper layers of the bowel wall, although efficacious and advantageous from the point of view of survival of the organism, has the disadvantage of potential functional impairment because stenosis and stricturing are its frequent end products.

HEALING OF SURGICAL INCISIONS IN THE GASTROINTESTINAL TRACT

In addition to the multiple disease states discussed in the preceding sections that require gastrointestinal healing, surgical resection of the alimentary canal represents another common insult requiring repair. Based on the extensive surgical studies of tissue repair following surgery, the next section examines specific types of surgical injury and their subsequent healing.

The major complications of intestinal anastomoses, especially those of the colon, rectum, and esophagus, are anastomotic leakage and dehiscence, which are associated with a high morbidity and mortality rate.[72-74] In clinical investigations, there are large variations in the reported incidence of anastomotic failure. The rate of clinically apparent anastomotic complications in the large bowel varies between 2 and 18 percent.[72-80] In two prospective studies, when early contrast enemas and radiological examination of the anastomosis were obtained routinely after colonic surgery, the incidence of leakage was 51 and 40 percent, respectively.[75, 81] In the esophagus, a leakage rate between 5 and 21 percent is reported, which is associated with even higher morbidity and mortality than in the large intestine.[82-88] Anastomoses of the small intestine have a lower complication rate than those of the colon and esophagus. After small intestinal operations for morbid obesity, leakage rates of between 1 and 4 percent have been reported;[89-93] however, these studies reported only the most serious leaks. In an earlier clinical study of both large and small intestinal anastomoses, a similar incidence of anastomotic leaks was reported in different parts of the intestine located within the peritoneal cavity.[94]

Due to variations in experimental protocols, it is difficult to give exact figures for complication rates within various regions of the alimentary canal. However, the frequency is high overall and the consequences often serious. The greatest morbidity is found in dehiscences occurring in extraperitoneal locations, e.g., esophagus and rectum. The absence of a serosal outer layer and omentum to wrap around the anastomosis and seal it off might be one explanation; another might be that there are differences in healing capacity as such in different areas of the alimentary tract.

The subject of healing of gastrointestinal anastomoses has received much attention from investigators. Theoretically, wound complications in the alimentary canal such as dehiscence, leakage, and even late stricture formation may be due to defects in sutures, insufficient wound margin tissue strength, or abnormalities in the healing sequence.

Wound Margin Strength and Anastomotic Healing

As mentioned before, the sequence of events in the healing of intestinal anastomoses is similar to that elsewhere in the body.[95] The mechanical strength of the intact intestinal wall is provided mainly by the fibrous connective tissue in the submucosa.[96] This tissue is rather uniformly distributed in the alimentary canal and is the only layer strong enough to support sutures.[96] Its main constituent is collagen.[97, 98]

Anastomotic healing means that new fibrous tissue bridges the wall defect, and with time this tissue, and its collagen content, becomes the determining factor in anastomotic strength.[97, 99] Thus, studies of both pre-existing and newly formed collagen in the bowel wall should be of major interest for understanding the intestinal healing process and thus the underlying mechanisms for complications.

During the first 3 to 4 postoperative days (i.e., the inflammatory phase) the integrity of a gastrointestinal anastomosis is dependent on fibrin sealing the wound gap and making it leak proof. The tensile strength at this point is completely dependent on the suture strength and the suture holding capacity of the intestinal wall (i.e., the amount and structure of collagen supporting the sutures in the wound margin) and on the number of sutures and direction of pull upon them.[100–102] Defective sutures should be a rare cause of dehiscence of intestinal anastomoses. Choosing an adequate suture material that retains its strength and tying the knots securely will eliminate this problem.

When mechanical tests of intestinal anastomoses are performed, the initial strength can be almost as strong as that of intact tissue.[103]

Initial breaking strengths of anastomoses are similar in the esophagus, the duodenum, and the colon, but are less in the ileum.[104] This may imply certain differences in the quality of the connective tissue in different regions.

When healing is compared in the ileum and colon, there are some differences in time sequence and magnitude of biochemical changes in the anastomotic region.[105] These differences do not, however, indicate impaired healing in the colon. Instead, the collagen content in the anastomotic area increases more and earlier in the colon than in the small intestine. Earlier studies have shown conflicting results in comparisons of healing in the small and large intestine.[106, 107]

The most critical time for anastomotic integrity is during the first postoperative days, when the wound margin strength is markedly reduced.[102–104, 106–109] It has been suggested that this loss of anastomotic strength is due to collagen degradation in the wound margin. Hawley and associates found increased collagenolytic activity in the mucosa, most apparent adjacent to the anastomosis but also present to some extent in the whole gastrointestinal tract.[110] Other authors have reported an early increase of collagen synthesis in the intestine after anastomosis, which is interpreted as a response to increased collagenolytic activity.[105, 111]

Adamson and co-workers demonstrated that incisional skin wounds are surrounded by what they called a "biochemically active" zone where collagen breakdown is prominent in the first postoperative week.[112] A reduction of collagen that extends rather far from the transection line has also been found in the colon and stomach.[102, 110, 113, 114] In all these studies the amount of collagen was determined as hydroxyproline concentration. However, the concentration of hydroxyproline does not necessarily represent the actual amount of collagen in this situation, which is influenced by changes in proteins other than collagen, predominantly plasma proteins accumulating as part of the inflammatory reaction.[99, 105, 115] Irvin and Hunt[99] found an actual decrease in collagen content in the anastomotic area on the order of 25 percent on the third postoperative day, while other, more recent studies have not found any evidence of collagen breakdown with net reduction of collagen content or change in collagen solubility in the early postoperative period.[105, 115, 116] Therefore, the early loss of mechanical integrity does not correlate with the amount of collagen nor with changes in collagen solubility. Instead, the collagen fibers may have undergone some structural changes not revealed by current methods.

The decrease in tissue strength seems to be related to neutrophils, which accumulate early in the wound margin.[117] By giving rats antineutrophil serum, the decrease in anastomotic strength can be avoided.[118] It is suggested that the decrease in tissue strength is partly due to collagen degradation mediated by the generation of oxygen free radicals or by the release of neutral proteinases.[119] Certain proteinase inhibitors and oxygen free radical scavengers have been demonstrated to have a beneficial effect on early wound strength in the intestine.[118, 120–122] Therefore, there might be a future role in intestinal surgery for inhibitors of neutrophil proteinases and oxygen radicals.

One can speculate that when anastomotic complications such as dehiscence and leakage occur they are caused by local infection or trauma, with an increased accumulation of neutrophils mediating an excessive degradation of collagen in or around the anastomotic line. To counteract the enhanced breakdown of collagen, its synthesis may increase as a protective response.

Thus, the early decrease in anastomotic margin strength, which is a general reaction to surgical trauma, is probably of major importance for the development of anastomotic complications. After these first 3 to 4 critical postoperative days, collagen synthesis predominates in and around the anastomosis. The rapid net gain in anastomotic strength that follows is due to an increasing amount of tissue bridging the anastomosis and increased suture-holding capacity of the adjacent intestinal wall.[99, 103, 109, 115, 123, 124] In experimental studies, anastomotic strength, with and without sutures, was already the same after 1 week in the colon[125] and after 14 days in the ileum.[103] These observations indicate that anastomotic suture support is of minor or no importance 1 to 2 weeks after the procedure. Thus, modern synthetic, resorbable suture materials can be used safely for this type of anastomosis. In long-term studies of breaking strengths of incisional wounds in the colon of dogs, anastomotic strength 14 days after operation was 45 percent of the intact bowel wall and still only about 70 percent of normal after 4 months.[126]

Mucosal Healing Following Incision

As mentioned, the mucosal wounds at all levels of the alimentary tract are repaired by migration and hyperplasia of the epithelial cells to cover the defect.[26, 27] In incisional wounds, the epithelial cells cover the granulation tissue to form a barrier to the intestinal contents, and this mucosal layer probably inhibits excessive inflammation and connective tissue formation that might lead to stricture.[127] However, it remains an open question whether these events are of major importance in the development of anastomotic strength.

Anastomotic Healing in the Alimentary Canal

Although certain controversies exist, it is useful to consider anastomotic integrity as a fine balance between synthesis and lysis of collagen. This equilibrium is influenced by numerous factors that can contribute to anastomotic complications. In the literature these are often divided into *systemic* and *local* factors, and attempts have been made to determine their significance when isolated. Experimental studies are usually necessary, since the effects of major procedures and coexisting disease make it almost impossible to assess the significance of findings in relation to wound healing in the clinical setting.

Systemic Determinants

Among the systemic factors the *age* of the patient is probably the most important variable affecting morbidity and mortality rates after intestinal procedures.[72, 73, 80, 94] The incidence of dehiscence after colonic resection and anastomosis is greater in elderly patients.[73, 94] Many factors may be involved, including malnutrition, atherosclerosis, circulatory impairment, and coexisting malignancy.

In clinical studies, *protein malnutrition* seems to be associated with an increased incidence of anastomotic dehiscence after colon surgery,[94] and experimental studies have shown that rats deprived of protein have reduced bursting strength of colonic anastomoses.[128] Irvin and Hunt showed the healing of colonic anastomoses to be affected, as evidenced by decreased tensile strength and collagen synthesis, only in animals fed low levels of protein for 7 weeks.[129] The clinical implication of this study is that a minor degree of protein depletion for a short time has no significant effect.

Vitamin deficiency may be of some relevance to intestinal healing, since ascorbic acid, is one of the cofactors in conversion of proline to hydroxyproline.[95] Supplemental vitamin A has been shown to have a beneficial effect on healing of colonic anastomoses,[130] and it seems to counteract the impaired healing seen after irradiation.[131, 132]

Experimental studies indicate that *corticosteroids* impair wound healing, mainly by modifying the initial inflammatory response.[133] The healing process in the rat stomach is adversely affected by long-term cortisol treatment.[134] In clinical studies, however, therapeutic doses of corticosteroids have not been demonstrated to be harmful to intestinal anastomoses.[73]

The healing of intestinal anastomoses was not affected by *septicemia*[135] or *distant trauma*[136] in experimental studies. In contrast, *hypoxia* was detrimental to colonic anastomoses,[137] but *hyperoxygenation* had no apparent effect on the healing of uncomplicated or ischemic colonic anastomoses in rats.[138]

Local Determinants

Many local factors have been associated with anastomotic failure. The *blood supply* to the anastomotic area should be carefully preserved by adequate surgical technique. *Tension* over the anastomosis should be avoided since this might adversely affect the local blood supply. Reduction in blood volume of 10 percent decreases the colonic blood flow by almost 30 percent,[139] meaning that even a small amount of bleeding could be deleterious to anastomoses at risk. Esophageal and colorectal anastomoses carry an especially high incidence of failure, which might to a certain extent depend on poor blood supply. Clinical studies have shown that excessive blood loss is associated with an increased incidence of anastomotic failure in colorectal surgery.[73, 140]

In clinical as well as experimental studies, local *peritoneal sepsis* has an adverse effect on the healing of intestinal anastomoses.[76, 141-143] Hawley and co-workers showed that anastomotic leakage and abscess formation are accompanied by increased collagenolytic activity, which might contribute to the anastomotic breakdown.[110] However, many times in clinical practice it is impossible to establish whether infection is the cause or effect of anastomotic leakage.

There is strong evidence from both clinical and experimental studies that *fecal loading* is an important factor in the breakdown of intestinal anastomoses, although the exact mechanisms are not fully known. One possibility is that the fecal bulk distends the anastomosis and causes the sutures to cut through the weakened wound margin tissue in the early phase of repair. Irvin and Goligher showed a 24 percent incidence of anastomotic dehiscence when the colon was badly prepared compared to 7 percent when it was well prepared.[94] Furthermore, experimental studies have shown that fecal loading was accompanied by a high frequency of anastomotic complications following surgery on the left colon.[111, 113, 144, 145] Jiborn and colleagues found that the synthesis of collagen was markedly increased in the bowel wall of animals with colonic dilatation and fecal stagnation after left colon resection compared to animals with uncomplicated healing.[111] They concluded that a high collagen synthesis rate was a good marker for complications. Fecal stagnation proximal to an experimental colonic stenosis is also accompanied by enhanced collagen turnover and increased collagen deposition.[146] These changes in collagen metabolism imply that the healing capacity per se is not adversely affected if surgery is performed in an obstructed and loaded bowel, even though a high complication rate is found.

In acute colonic obstruction and to prevent complications in high-risk colorectal anastomoses, diversion of the fecal contents by a proximal *colostomy* is often done. However, several authors have reported a considerable incidence of anastomotic dehiscence despite this procedure.[72, 73, 75, 147, 148] Clinical studies have demonstrated that a proximal diverting colostomy does not prevent anastomotic failure as such, but may spare the patient its septic complications.[94, 149-152] Experimentally, a diverting colostomy leads to a confined and markedly reduced collagen response in the anastomotic area, paralleled by retarded anastomotic strength development[125, 153] compared to the ordinary healing pattern of left colon anastomosis. The passage of stool through the anastomosis thus seems to be of importance for development of anastomotic strength. In these studies anastomotic healing was macroscopically uncomplicated, and there was some indication that the colostomy prevents complications such as abscesses and adhesions.

Radiotherapy is increasingly used in the preoperative and postoperative management of different gynecological and gastrointestinal cancers. However, it is well known that there is a significantly increased risk of anastomotic failure and of spontaneous perforation of the intestine after radiotherapy.[154-157] Schrock and associates found a threefold increase in anastomotic dehiscence following radiotherapy in clinical practice,[73] and Murphy and co-workers showed that preoperative irradiation markedly decreased the bursting strength of colon anastomoses in rats irradiated 24 hours previously.[158] Long-term changes after radiotherapy include fibrosis, stricture, and ischemia resulting from hyalinization of blood vessels[159, 160] and these often complicate wound repair.[161]

The value of *drains* in the peritoneal cavity to prevent the accumulation of potentially infected fluids close to the anastomosis is not settled. In fact many studies have shown that drains are detrimental to anastomotic healing by potentiating infections.[162-167]

Suture Technique

Another important local factor is the suture technique used for performing the anastomosis. In recent years the benefits of *everting* versus *inverting* techniques have been much debated. In principle, serosa-to-serosa inversion of gastrointestinal anastomoses is considered preferable[168-170] to the everting, mucosa-to-mucosa technique.[171] Some controversy exists whether one or two layers of sutures should be used. Single-layer technique is preferred by some authors,[77, 78, 170-172] while others have the opposite opinion.[74, 173-175] In experimental studies *interrupted sutures* have been demonstrated to be superior to *continuous sutures*,[111, 113] although the advantage is yet to be proved clinically.

CONCLUSION

The gut has unique requirements for repair, and mammals have developed specific healing mechanisms that maximize the closure of the wound to ensure that the intestinal contents do not escape. Unfortunately, tissue repair in this setting is influenced by multiple systemic and local factors that can impair healing or lead to stenosis of the organ. Consequently, research should be directed toward understanding the tissue repair mechanisms in depth so that healing can be optimized without producing functional impairment.

References

1. Eastwood GL: Gastrointestinal epithelial renewal. Gastroenterology 72:962–975, 1977.
2. Mayne R, Wiedemann H, Dessau W, et al: Structural and immunological characterisation of type IV collagen isolated from chicken tissues. Eur J Biochem 126:417–423, 1982.
3. Noelken ME, Wisdom BJ, Dean DC, et al: Intestinal basement membrane of *Ascaris suum*. J Biol Chem 261:4706–4714, 1986.
4. Stanley JR, Woodley DT, Katz SI, et al: Structure and function of basement membrane. J Invest Dermatol (Suppl) 79:69–72, 1982.
5. Timpl R, Wiedemann H, van Delden V, et al: A network model for the organisation of type IV collagen molecules in basement membranes. Eur J Biochem 120:203–224, 1981.
6. Kanwar YS, Farquar MG: Isolation of glycosaminoglycans (heparan sulfate) from glomerular basement membranes. Proc Natl Acad Sci USA 76:4493–4497, 1979.
7. Gay S, Miller EJ: Collagen in the physiology and pathology of connective tissue. New York, Gustav Fischer Verlag, 1978, p 32.
8. Ito S: Functional gastric morphology. In Johnson LR (ed): Physiology of the Gastrointestinal Tract, 2nd ed. New York, Raven Press, 1987, p 845.
9. Fulcheri E, Cantino D, Bussolati G: Presence of intramucosal smooth muscle cells in normal human and rat colon. Basic Appl Histochem 29:337–344, 1985.
10. Joyce NC, Haire MF, Palade GE: Morphologic and biochemical evidence for a contractile cell network within the rat intestinal mucosa. Gastroenterology 92:68–81, 1987.
11. Elson CO, Kagnoff MF, Fiocchi C, et al: Intestinal immunity and inflammation: Recent progress. Gastroenterology 91:746–768, 1986.
12. Graham MF, Diegelmann RF, Elson CO, et al: Collagen content and types in the intestinal strictures of Crohn's disease. Gastroenterology 94:257–265, 1988.
13. Morton LF, Barnes MJ: Collagen polymorphism in the normal and diseased blood vessel wall. Investigation of collagens type I, III and V. Atherosclerosis 42:41–51, 1982.
14. Graham MF, Drucker DEM, Diegelmann RF, et al: Collagen synthesis by human intestinal smooth muscle cells in culture. Gastroenterology 92:400–405, 1987.
15. Elstow SF, Weiss JB: Extraction, isolation and characterization of neutral salt soluble type V collagen from fetal calf skin. Coll Rel Res 3:181–194, 1983.
16. Narayanan AS, Engel LD, Page RC: The effect of chronic inflammation on the composition of collagen types in human connective tissue. Coll Rel Res 3:323–334, 1983.
17. Modesti A, Kalebic T, Scarpa S, et al: Type V collagen in human amnion is a 12 nm fibrillar component of the pericellular interstitium. Eur J Cell Biol 35:246–255, 1984.
18. Adachi E, Hayashi T: In vitro formation of fine fibrils with a D-periodic banding pattern from type V collagen. Coll Rel Res 5:225–232, 1985.
19. Grotendorst GR, Seppa HEJ, Kleinman HK, et al: Attachment of smooth muscle cells to collagen and their migration toward platelet derived growth factor. Proc Natl Acad Sci USA 78:3669–3672, 1981.
20. Leushner JRA, Haust MD: Glycoproteins on the surface of smooth muscle cells involved in their interaction with type V collagen. Can J Biochem Cell Biol 63:1176–1182, 1985.
21. Epstein EH Jr, Munderloh NH: Isolation and characterization of human [α1(III)]₃ collagen and tissue distribution of [α1(I)]₂α2 and [α1(III)]₃ collagens. J Biol Chem 250:9304–9312, 1975.
22. Gabella G: Structure of muscles and nerves in the gastrointestinal tract. In Johnson LR (ed): Physiology of the Gastrointestinal Tract, 2nd ed. New York, Raven Press, 1987, pp 335–381.
23. Stromberg BV, Klein L: Collagen dynamics of partial small bowel obstruction. Am J Surg 148:257–261, 1984.
24. Gabella G, Yamey A: Synthesis of collagen by smooth

muscle in the hypertrophic intestine. Q J Exp Physiol 62:227–264, 1977.

25. Gabella G: Hypertrophic smooth muscle. V. Collagen and other extracellular materials. Vascularization. Cell Tissue Res 235:275–283, 1984.

26. Ito S, Lacy ER: Morphology of rat gastric mucosal damage, and restitution in the presence of luminal ethanol. Gastroenterology 88:250–260, 1985.

27. Feil W, Wenzl E, Vattay P, et al: Repair of rabbit duodenal mucosa after acid injury in vivo and in vitro. Gastroenterology 92:1973–1986, 1987.

28. Moore R, Madara J: Ileal epithelial repair following injury: A rapid process aided by villus contraction. Gastroenterology 94:309 (abstr), 1988.

29. Morgan AG, MacAdam WAF, Pyrah RD, et al: Multiple recurring gastric erosions (aphthous ulcers). Gut 17:633–639, 1976.

30. Morson BC, Dawson IMP: Gastrointestinal Pathology, 2nd ed. Oxford, Blackwell Scientific, 1979, pp 125–129.

31. Warren KS: The immunopathogenesis of schistosomiasis: A multidisciplinary approach. Trans R Soc Trop Med Hyg 66:417–432, 1972.

32. Pelley RP, Warren KS: Immunoregulation in chronic infectious disease: Schistosomiasis as a model. J Clin Invest Dermatol 71:49–55, 1978.

33. Domingo EO, Warren KS: Pathology and pathophysiology of the small intestine in murine Schistosomiasis mansoni, including a review of the literature. Gastroenterology 56:231–240, 1969.

34. Bogitsh BJ, Wikel SK: Schistosoma mansoni: Ultrastructural observations on the small intestine of the murine host. Exp Parasitol 35:68–79, 1974.

35. Morson BC, Dawson IMP: Gastrointestinal Pathology, 2nd ed. Oxford, Blackwell Scientific, 1979, p 522.

36. Grimaud JA, Boros DL, Takiya C, et al: Collagen isotypes, laminin and fibronectin in granulomas of the liver and intestines of Schistosoma mansoni–infected mice. Am J Trop Med Hyg 37:335–344, 1987.

37. Weinstock JV, Boros DL: Heterogeneity of the granulomatous response in the liver, colon, ileum, and ileal Peyer's patches to schistosome eggs in murine Schistosomiasis mansoni. J Immunol 127:1906–1909, 1981.

38. Weinstock JV, Boros DL: Organ-dependent differences in composition and function observed in hepatic and intestinal granulomas isolated from mice with Schistosomiasis mansoni. J Immunol 130:418–422, 1983.

39. Dvorak AM, Osage JE, Monahan RA, et al: Crohn's disease: Transmission electron microscopic studies. III. Target tissues. Proliferation of and injury to smooth muscle and the autonomic nervous system. Hum Pathol 11:620–634, 1980.

40. Seppala PO, Viljanto J, Lehtonen A: Biochemical analysis of the intestinal wall in a case of regional enteritis (Crohn's disease). Acta Chir Scand 139:79–83, 1973.

41. Farthing MJG, Dick AP, Heslop G, et al: Prolyl hydroxylase activity in serum and rectal mucosa in inflammatory bowel disease. Gut 19:743–747, 1978.

42. Graham MF, Diegelmann RF, Elson CO, et al: Isolation and culture of human intestinal smooth muscle cells. Proc Soc Exp Biol Med 176:503–507, 1984.

43. Perr HA, Graham MF, Diegelmann RF, et al: Influence of tissue of origin on the response of human smooth muscle cells to serum. J Cell Biol 105:212A (abstr), 1987.

44. Graham MF, Bryson GR, Diegelmann RF: Transforming growth factor β_1 selectively augments collagen production by human intestinal smooth muscle cells. Gastroenterology 99:447–453, 1990.

45. Graham MF, Drucker DEM, Perr HA, et al: Heparin modulates human intestinal smooth muscle cell proliferation, protein synthesis and lattice contraction. Gastroenterology 93:801–809, 1987.

46. Cochran DL, Perr HA, Graham MF, et al: Heparin induces specific protein release from human intestinal smooth muscle cells. Biochem Biophys Res Commun 142:542–551, 1987.

47. Perr HA, Drucker DEM, Cochran, DL, et al: Protamine selectively inhibits collagen synthesis by human intestinal smooth muscle and other mesenchymal cells. J Cell Physiol 140:463–470, 1989.

48. Graham MF, Drucker DEM, Diegelmann RF, et al: Collagen synthesis by human intestinal smooth muscle cells in vitro is resistant to inhibition by corticosteroids. J Cell Biol 101:95A, 1985 (abstract).

49. Perr HA, Graham MF, Diegelmann RF, et al: Cyclic nucleotides regulate collagen production by human intestinal smooth muscle cells. Gastroenterology 96:1521–1528, 1989.

50. Gerson CD, Fabry EM: Ascorbic acid deficiency and fistula formation in regional enteritis. Gastroenterology 67:952–956, 1974.

51. Pettit SH, Irving MH: Does local intestinal ascorbate deficiency predispose to fistula formation in Crohn's disease? Dis Colon Rectum 30:552–557, 1987.

52. Goulston SJM, McGovern VJ: The nature of benign strictures in ulcerative colitis. N Engl J Med 2:281–295, 1969.

53. Lindstrom CG: "Collagenous colitis" with watery diarrhea. A new entity. Pathol Eur 11:87–89, 1976.

54. Kingham JGC, Levison DA, Morson BC, et al: Collagenous colitis. Gut 27:578–580, 1986.

55. Fausa O, Foerster A, Hovig T: Collagenous colitis. A clinical, histological and ultrastructural study. Scand J Gastroenterol (Suppl) 107:8–23, 1985.

56. Jessurun J, Yardley JH, Lee EL, et al: Microscopic and collagenous colitis: Different names for the same condition? Gastroenterology 91:1583–1584, 1986 (letter to the editor).

57. Pascal RR, Kaye GI, Lane N: Colonic pericryptal fibroblast sheath: Replication, migration and cytodifferentiation of a mesenchymal cell system in adult tissue. Gastroenterology 54:835–851, 1968.

58. Norris HT: Reexamination of the spectrum of ischemic bowel disease. In Norris HT (ed): Pathology of the Colon, Small Intestine and Anus. New York, Churchill Livingstone, 1983.

59. Morson BC, Dawson IMP: Gastrointestinal Pathology, 2nd ed. Oxford, Blackwell Scientific, 1979, pp 389–391.

60. Wiernick G: Radiation damage and repair in the human jejunal mucosa. J Pathol Bacteriol 91:389–394, 1966.

61. Cuthbertson AM: The surgical implication of irradiation damage to the bowel. Aust NZ J Surg 36:33–39, 1966.

62. Graham JB, Villalba RJ: Damage to the small intestine by radiotherapy. Surg Gynecol Obstet 116:665–668, 1963.

63. Morson BC, Dawson IMP: Gastrointestinal Pathology, 2nd ed. Oxford, Blackwell Scientific, 1979, p 564.

64. Tandon HD, Prakash A: Pathology of intestinal tuberculosis and its distinction from Crohn's disease. Gut 13:260–269, 1972.

65. Anand SS: Hypertrophic ileocecal tuberculosis in India with a record of fifty hemicolectomies. Ann R Coll Surg 19:205–210, 1956.

66. Tandon HD, Prakash A, Rao VB, et al: Ulceroconstrictive disorders of the intestine in Northern India: A pathologic study. Indian J Med Res 54:129–141, 1966.

67. Morson BC, Dawson IMP: Gastrointestinal Pathology, 2nd ed. Oxford, Blackwell Scientific, 1979, pp 275–278.
68. Leape LL, Ashcraft KW, Scarpelli DG, et al: Hazard to health—liquid lye. N Engl J Med 284:578–588, 1971.
69. Haller JA, Bachman K: The comparative effect of current therapy on experimental caustic burns of the esophagus. Pediatrics 34:236–245, 1964.
70. Bauer EA, Gedde-Dahl T, Eisen AZ: The role of human skin collagenase in epidermolysis bullosa. J Invest Dermatol 68:119–124, 1977.
71. Fonkalsrud EW, Ament ME: Surgical management of esophageal stricture due to recessive dystrophic epidermolysis bullosa. J Pediatr Surg 12:221–226, 1977.
72. Debas HT, Thomson FB: A critical review of colectomy with anastomosis. Surg Gynecol Obstet 135:747–752, 1972.
73. Schrock TR, Deveney CW, Dunphy JE: Factors contributing to leakage of colonic anastomoses. Ann Surg 177:513–518, 1973.
74. Fielding LP, Stewart-Brown S, Blesovsky L, et al: Anastomotic integrity after operations for large bowel cancer: A multicentre study. Br Med J 281:411–414, 1980.
75. Goligher JC, Graham WG, de Dombal FT: Anastomotic dehiscence after anterior resection of rectum and sigmoid. Br J Surg 57:109–118, 1970.
76. Morgenstern L, Yamakawa T, Ben-Shosan M, et al: Anastomotic leakage after low colonic anastomosis. Am J Surg 123:104–109, 1972.
77. Matheson NA, Irving AD: Single layer anastomosis after recto-sigmoid resection. Br J Surg 62:239–242, 1975.
78. Everett WG: A comparison of one layer and two layer techniques for colorectal anastomosis. Br J Surg 62:135–140, 1975.
79. Wilson SM, Beahrs OH: The curative treatment of carcinoma of the sigmoid, rectosigmoid and rectum. Ann Surg 183:556–563, 1976.
80. Tagart REB: Colorectal anastomosis: Factors influencing success. J R Soc Med 74:111–118, 1981.
81. Young HL, Wheeler MH: Results of a prospective randomized double-blind trial of aprotinin in colonic surgery. World J Surg 8:367–373, 1984.
82. Gunnlaugsson GH, Wychulis AR, Roland C, et al: Analysis of the records of 1657 patients with carcinoma of the esophagus and cardia of the stomach. Surg Gynecol Obstet 130:997–1005, 1970.
83. Inberg MV, Linna MI, Scheinin TM, et al: Anastomotic leakage after excision of esophageal and high gastric carcinoma. Am J Surg 122:540–544, 1971.
84. Hermreck AS, Crawford DG: The esophageal anastomotic leak. Am J Surg 132:794–798, 1976.
85. Alfonso A, Rosen P, Guerra O, et al: Adenocarcinoma of the proximal third of the stomach. Am J Surg 134:326–330, 1977.
86. Papachristou DN, Fortner JC: Anastomotic failure complicating total gastrectomy and esophagogastrectomy for cancer of the stomach. Am J Surg 138:399–402, 1979.
87. Wilson SE, Stone R, Scully M, et al: Modern management of anastomotic leak after esophago-gastrectomy. Am J Surg 144:95–99, 1982.
88. Kirkpatrick JR, Siegel T: Gastrojejunal disruptions. Arch Surg 119:659–663, 1984.
89. Alden JF: Gastric and jejunal bypass. Arch Surg 112:799–804, 1977.
90. Bray GA: Current status of intestinal bypass surgery in the treatment of obesity. Diabetes 26:1072–1079, 1977.
91. Griffen WO Jr, Young VL, Stevenson CC: A prospective comparison of gastric and jejunal bypass procedures for morbid obesity. Ann Surg 186:500–507, 1977.
92. Butler CM, Pilkington TRE, Gazet J-C: Complications of jejuno-ileal bypass surgery. In Maxwell JP, Pilkington TRE, Gazet J-C (eds): Surgical Management of Obesity. London, London Academic Press, 1980, pp 209–219.
93. McFarland RJ, Gazet J-C, Pilkington TRE: A 13-year review of jejunal bypass. Br J Surg 72:82–87, 1985.
94. Irvin TT, Goligher JC: Aetiology of disruption of intestinal anastomoses. Br J Surg 60:461–464, 1973.
95. Irvin TT: Wound Healing. Principle and Practice. London, Chapman and Hall, 1981.
96. Halstead WS: Circular suture of the intestine—an experimental study. Am J Med Sci 94:436–461, 1887.
97. Peacock EE Jr, van Winkle W Jr: The biochemistry and the environment of wounds and their relation to wound strength. In Peacock EE Jr, van Winkle W Jr (eds): Wound Repair. Philadelphia, WB Saunders, 1976, pp 145–202.
98. Lord MG, Valies P, Broughton AC: A morphologic study of the submucosa of the large intestine. Surg Gynecol Obstet 145:55–60, 1977.
99. Irvin TT, Hunt TK: Reappraisal of the healing process of anastomoses of the colon. Surg Gynecol Obstet 138:741–746, 1974.
100. Howes EL, Harvey SC: The strength of the healing wound in relation to the holding strength of the catgut suture. N Engl J Med 200:1285–1290, 1929.
101. Howes EL: The immediate strength of the sutured wound. Surgery 7:24–31, 1940.
102. Cronin K, Jackson DS, Dunphy JE: Changing bursting strength and collagen content of the healing colon. Surg Gynecol Obstet 26:747–753, 1968.
103. Jönsson K, Jiborn H, Zederfeldt B: Breaking strength of small intestinal anastomoses. Am J Surg 145:800–803, 1983.
104. Högström H, Haglund U: Postoperative decrease in suture holding capacity in laparotomy wounds and anastomoses. Acta Chir Scand 151:533–535, 1985.
105. Jönsson K, Jiborn H, Zederfeldt B: Comparison of healing in the left colon and ileum. Changes in collagen content and collagen synthesis in the intestinal wall after ileal and colonic anastomoses in the rat. Acta Chir Scand 151:537–541, 1985.
106. Wise L, McAlister W, Stein T, et al: Studies on healing of anastomoses of small and large intestines. Surg Gynecol Obstet 141:190–194, 1975.
107. Hesp FLEM, Hendiks T, Lubbers EJC, et al: Wound healing in the intestinal wall. A comparison between experimental ileal and colonic anastomoses. Dis Colon Rectum 27:99–104, 1984.
108. Chlumsky V: Experimentelle Untersuchungen über die verschiedenen Methoden der Darmvereinigung. Bruns Beitr Klin Chir 25:539–600, 1899.
109. Blomquist P, Jiborn H, Zederfeldt B: The effect of relative bowel rest on healing of colonic anastomosis. Breaking strength and collagen in the colonic wall following left colon resection and anastomosis in the rat. Acta Chir Scand 150:681–685, 1984.
110. Hawley PR, Faulk WP, Hunt TK, et al: Collagenase activity in the gastrointestinal tract. Br J Surg 57:896–899, 1970.
111. Jiborn H, Ahonen J, Zederfeldt B: Healing of experimental colonic anastomoses. Effects of suture technique on collagen metabolism in the colonic wall. Am J Surg 139:406–413, 1980.
112. Adamson RJ, Musco F, Enquist IF: The chemical dimensions of healing incision. Surg Gynecol Obstet 123:515–521, 1966.

113. Jiborn H, Ahonen J, Zederfeldt B: Healing of experimental colonic anastomoses. The effect of suture technique on collagen concentration in the colonic wall. Am J Surg 135:334–340, 1978.

114. Gottrup F: Healing of incisional wounds in stomach and duodenum: Collagen distribution and relation to mechanical strength. Am J Surg 141:222–227, 1981.

115. Blomquist P, Ahonen J, Jiborn H, et al: The effect of relative bowel rest on healing of colonic anastomoses. Collagen synthesis and content in the colonic wall after left colon resection and anastomosis in the rat. Acta Chir Scand 150:677–681, 1984.

116. Högström H, Bondeson L, Haglund U: Neutrophil-induced decrease in wound margin strength after intestinal anastomosis—influence on collagen and mechanisms of granulocyte action. Eur Surg Res 20:260–266, 1988.

117. Ryan GB, Majno G: Acute inflammation. Am J Pathol 86:183–276, 1977.

118. Högström H, Haglund U: Neutropenia prevents decrease in strength of rat intestinal anastomosis: Partial effect of oxygen free radical scavengers and allopurinol. Surgery 99:716–720, 1986.

119. Murphy P: The Neutrophil. New York, Plenum Press, 1976.

120. Young HL, Wheeler MH: Collagenase inhibition in the healing colon. J R Soc Med 76:32–36, 1983.

121. Högström H, Haglund U, Zederfeldt B: Beneficial effect of proteinase inhibitors on early breaking strength of intestinal anastomosis. Acta Chir Scand 151:529–532, 1985.

122. Shandall AA, Williams GT, Hallett MB, et al: Colonic healing: A role for polymorphonuclear leukocytes and oxygen radical production. Br J Surg 73:225–228, 1986.

123. Herrmann JB, Woodward SC, Pulaski EJ: Healing of colonic anastomoses in the rat. Surg Gynecol Obstet 119:269–275, 1964.

124. Jiborn H, Ahonen J, Zederfeldt B: Healing of experimental colonic anastomoses. Breaking strength of the colon after left colon resection and anastomosis. Am J Surg 136:595–599, 1978.

125. Blomquist P, Jiborn H, Zederfeldt B: Effect of diverting colostomy on breaking strength of anastomoses after resection of the left side of the colon. Am J Surg 149:712–715, 1985.

126. Van Winkle W Jr, Hastings JC, Barker E, et al: Role of the fibroblast in controlling rate and extent of repair in wounds of various tissues. In Kulonen E, Pikkarainen J (eds): Biology of Fibroblast. New York, Academic Press, 1973, pp 559–570.

127. Deveney CW, Dunphy JE: Wound healing in the gastrointestinal tract. In Hunt TK, Dunphy JE (eds): Fundamentals of Wound Management. New York, Appleton-Century-Crofts, 1979, pp 569–593.

128. Daly JM, Vars HM, Dudrick SJ: Effects of protein depletion on strength of colonic anastomoses. Surg Gynecol Obstet 134:15–21, 1972.

129. Irvin TT, Hunt TK: Effect of malnutrition on colonic healing. Ann Surg 180:765–771, 1974.

130. Bark S, Rettura G, Goldman D, et al: Effects of supplemental vitamin A on the healing of colon anastomoses. J Surg Res 36:470–474, 1984.

131. Levenson SM, Gruber CA, Rettura G, et al: Supplemental vitamin A prevents the acute radiation-induced defect in wound healing. Ann Surg 200:106–124, 1984.

132. Winsey K, Simon RJ, Levenson SM, et al: Effect of supplemental vitamin A on colon anastomotic healing in rats given preoperative irradiation. Am J Surg 153:153–156, 1987.

133. Ehrlich P, Hunt TK: Effects of cortisone and vitamin A on wound healing. Ann Surg 167:324–328, 1968.

134. Gottrup F, Oxlund H: Healing of incisional wounds in stomach and duodenum.: The effect of long-term cortisol treatment. J Surg Res 31:165–71, 1981.

135. Högström H, Jiborn H, Zederfeldt B, et al: Influence of intraperitoneal *Escherichia coli* with septicemia on the healing of colonic anastomoses and skin wounds. An experimental study in the rat. Eur Surg Res 17:128–132, 1985.

136. Irvin TT, Hunt TK: Pathogenesis and prevention of disruption of colonic anastomoses in traumatized rats. Br J Surg 61:437–439, 1974.

137. Shandall A, Lowndes R, Young HL: Colonic anastomotic healing and oxygen tension. Br J Surg 72:606–609, 1985.

138. Kirk D, Irvin TT: The role of O_2 therapy in the healing of experimental skin wounds and colonic anastomoses. Br J Surg 64:100–103, 1977.

139. Gilmour DG, Aitkenhead AR, Hothersall AP, et al: The effect of hypovolaemia on colonic blood flow in the dog. Br J Surg 67:82–84, 1980.

140. Whitaker BL, Dixon RA, Greatorex G: Anastomotic failure in relation to blood transfusion and blood loss. J R Soc Med 63:751, 1970.

141. Rothenbeg H, Chassin J, Scher S, et al: Bowel anastomosis in the presence of peritonitis. Surg Forum 10:201–203, 1959.

142. Yamakawa T, Patin CS, Sobel S, et al: Healing of colonic anastomoses following resection for experimental "Diverticulitis". Arch Surg 103:17–20, 1971.

143. Irvin TT: Collagen metabolism in infected colonic anastomoses. Surg Gynecol Obstet 143:220–224, 1976.

144. Smith SRG, Connolly JC, Gilmore OJA: The effect of faecal loading on colonic anastomotic healing. Br J Surg 70:49–50, 1983.

145. Törnqvist A, Blomquist P, Jiborn H, et al: Anastomotic healing after resection of left colon stenosis: Effect on collagen metabolism and anastomotic strength. An experimental study in the rat. Dis Colon Rectum 33:217–221, 1990.

146. Törnqvist A, Blomquist P, Jiborn H, et al: The effect of stenosis on collagen metabolism in the colonic wall. Studies in the rat. Acta Chir Scand 154:389–393, 1988.

147. Hoier-Madsen K, Bech Hansen J, Lindenberg J: Anastomotic leakage following resection for cancer of the colon and rectum. Acta Chir Scand 141:304–309, 1975.

148. Wara P, Sörensen K, Berg V: Proximal fecal diversion: Review of ten years' experience. Dis Colon Rectum 24:114–119, 1981.

149. Smithwick RH: Surgical treatment of diverticulitis of the sigmoid. Am J Surg 99:192–205, 1960.

150. Colcock BP: Surgical treatment of diverticulitis. Twenty years experience. Am J Surg 115:264–270, 1968.

151. Botsford TW, Zollinger RM Jr: Diverticulitis of the colon. Surg Gynecol Obstet 128:1209–1214, 1969.

152. Garnjobst W, Hardwick C: Further criteria for anastomosis in diverticulitis of the sigmoid colon. Am J Surg 120:264–289, 1970.

153. Udén P, Blomquist P, Jiborn H, et al: Influence of proximal colostomy on the healing of a left colon anastomosis: An experimental study in the rat. Br J Surg 75:325–329, 1988.

154. Calame RJ, Wallach RC: An analysis of the complication of the radiologic treatment of carcinoma of the cervix. Surg Gynecol Obstet 125:39–44, 1967.

155. Smith AN, Douglas M, McClean N, et al: Intestinal complications of pelvic irradiation for gynecologic cancer. Surg Gynecol Obstet 127:721–728, 1968.

156. Wellwood JM, Jackson BT: The intestinal complications of radiotherapy. Br J Surg 60:814–818, 1973.

157. Osborne JW, Prasad KN, Zimmerman GR: Changes in the rat intestine after X-irradiation of exteriorized short segments of ileum. Radiat Res 43:131–142, 1979.

158. Murphy K, Frith C, Lang N, et al: Effects of radiotherapy on healing of colonic anastomoses. Surg Forum 31:222–223, 1980.

159. Warren S, Friedman NB: Pathology and pathologic diagnosis of radiation lesions in the gastrointestinal tract. Am J Pathol 18:499–514, 1942.

160. Berthrong M, Fajardo LF: Radiation injury in surgical pathology. II. Alimentary tract. Am J Surg Pathol 4:153–178, 1981.

161. Ormiston M: A study of rat intestinal wound healing in the presence of radiation injury. Br J Surg 72:56–58, 1985.

162. Berliner SD, Burson LC, Lear PE: Intraperitoneal drains in surgery of the colon. Am J Surg 113:646–647, 1967.

163. Manz CW, LaTendresse C, Sako Y: The detrimental effects of drains on colonic anastomoses: An experimental study. Dis Colon Rectum 13:17–25, 1970.

164. Duthie HL: Drainage of the abdomen. N Engl J Med 287:1081–1083, 1972.

165. Crowson WN, Wilson CS: An experimental study of the effects of drains on colon and anastomosis. Am J Surg 39:597–601, 1973.

166. Ravitch MM, Brolin R, Kolter J, et al: Studies in the healing of intestinal anastomoses. World J Surg 65:627–637, 1981.

167. Smith SRG, Connolly JC, Crane PW, et al: The effect of surgical drainage materials on colonic healing. Br J Surg 69:153–155, 1982.

168. Hargreaves AW, Keddie NC: Colonic anastomosis. A clinical and experimental study. Br J Surg 55:774–777, 1968.

169. Trueblood HW, Nelsen TS, Kohatsu S, et al: Wound healing in the colon: Comparison of inverted and everted closures. Surgery 65:919–930, 1969.

170. Irvin TT, Edwards JP: Comparison of single-layer inverting, two-layer inverting, and everting anastomoses in the rabbit colon. Br J Surg 60:453–457, 1973.

171. Getzen LC, Holloway CK: Comparative study of intestinal anastomotic healing in inverted and everted closures. Surg Gynecol Obstet 123:1219–1277, 1966.

172. Gambee LP, Garnjobst W, Hardwick CE: Ten years experience with a single layer anastomosis in colon surgery. Am J Surg 92:222–227, 1956.

173. McAdams AJ, Meikle G, Medina R: An experimental comparison of inversion and eversion colonic anastomoses. Dis Colon Rectum 12:1–6, 1969.

174. Irvin TT, Goligher JC, Johnston D: A randomized prospective clinical trial of single-layer and two-layer inverting intestinal anastomoses. Br J Surg 60:457–460, 1973.

175. Goligher JC, Lee PWG, Simpkins KC, et al: A controlled comparison of one- and two-layer techniques of suture for high and low colorectal anastomoses. Br J Surg 64:609–614, 1977.

28

PERIPHERAL NERVE INJURY

Roger D. Madison, Ph.D., Simon J. Archibald, Ph.D., and Christian Krarup, M.D., Ph.D.

This chapter addresses several aspects of wound healing related to peripheral nerves and gives an overview of the normal anatomy and physiology of peripheral nerves, as well as a detailed description of peripheral nerve injuries and repair. Nerve injury and subsequent repair are major problems confronting modern medicine. It has been estimated that more than 200,000 nerve repair procedures are performed yearly in the United States.[1] Much of the impetus for more reliable nerve repair procedures came about due to the large number of traumatic nerve injuries experienced during World War II and subsequent conflicts. Peripheral nerve degeneration also complicates many metabolic, immunological, and hereditary disorders. A more detailed understanding of the various processes that control regeneration in traumatic lesions may also contribute to more rational treatment of related peripheral nerve disorders.

Following axonal transection in the peripheral nervous system (PNS), a series of remarkably consistent changes take place. Phagocytic cells remove degenerating axons and myelin within the distal stump; this is termed wallerian degeneration. Regenerating axonal sprouts extend from the proximal stump and their growth cones actively probe and interact with their immediate surroundings.[2, 3] Schwann cells ensheathe and remyelinate the regrowing axons. Some of the regenerating axons elongate to successfully reinnervate their original targets and form functional connections. Unfortunately, this axonal regeneration usually does not result in normal nerve function or morphology. The poor functional outcome of clinical nerve repair has motivated research on the basic mechanisms of peripheral nerve regeneration.

A peripheral nerve is a complex arrangement of axons, nonneuronal cells, and extracellular elements. These different components each contribute to the regenerative process, but it remains necessary to clarify their respective contributions.

Functional nerve regeneration requires the successful completion of three major tasks. First, the parent cell bodies must survive axonal transection. Second, these neurons must regenerate axons that grow across the site of initial transection and enter the distal nerve stump. Third, regenerating axons must seek out and reconnect to their correct end-organ targets. This chapter discusses aspects of all three of these key areas.

The first two sections review the basic anatomy and physiology of peripheral nerves. These two sections will especially be useful for the reader with little previous exposure to the subject. More experienced readers may wish to proceed directly to the third section of the chapter, which reviews the current status of the field of peripheral nerve repair, both clinically and experimentally.

The preparation of this chapter, as well as some of the work reported herein, was made possible in part by NIH grant NS22404 (RM) and the Merit Review Program of the Veterans Administration (RM).

NORMAL ANATOMY OF PERIPHERAL NERVES

A peripheral nerve trunk is made up of six major components: nerve fibers, fasciculi, connective tissues, blood vessels, lymphatics and tissue spaces, and nervi nervorum.[2]

Nerve Fibers. Nerve fibers from several segments of the spinal cord are grouped together in plexus formations, from which emerge the major peripheral nerves (Fig. 28–1). In these plexuses, motor and sensory nerves from different segments of the spinal cord and sympathetic fibers are intermingled and rearranged. As a result, each peripheral nerve contains motor and sensory fibers from a number of cord segments in addition to postganglionic sympathetic fibers.

The interior aspect of the axons, termed axoplasm, is a viscous fluid enclosed by a membrane, the axolemma, which is 65 to 80 Å thick (Fig. 28–2A). The axoplasm contains microtubules and neurofilaments, which are its main constituents; mitochondria, endoplasmic reticulum, and granular vesicula structures are also present. Running in unbroken courses down the length of the axon, neurotubules and neurofilaments help to impart rigidity to an otherwise viscous fluid and are also involved in axoplasmic transport. In nonmyelinated fibers, neurotubules outnumber neurofilaments; the reverse is true for myelinated fibers.[4]

In nonmyelinated fibers, several axons may be surrounded by a single Schwann cell with its basement membrane (Fig. 28–2C). This complex in turn is surrounded by the connective tissue covering of the endoneurium.[5] In myeli-

nated fibers, each Schwann cell is associated with only one axon (Fig. 28–2A and B). The axonal sheath consists of a Schwann cell-myelin complex. The axon is surrounded by a layer of myelin, formed by the Schwann cell, which is divided into segments along the length of the nerve fiber. Each segment, or internodal region, contains one Schwann cell with its nucleus situated midway along the node. In the paranodal region the cross-sectional outline of the axon becomes crenated (Fig. 28–2B). The myelin sheath follows the form of the axon and becomes indented, and the grooves formed in the outer surfaces of the myelin sheath are filled with Schwann cell cytoplasm. Where the myelin terminates, the columns of cytoplasm fuse to form a collar around the axon, termed the node of Ranvier. The myelin thickness gradually decreases as the node is approached.[6] The nodes of Ranvier are devoid of myelin sheath and are surrounded by the cytoplasm of the two adjacent Schwann cells whose boundaries are found at the node. The basement membrane and the outer endoneurial sheath are continuous across the region of the node.

Connective Tissues. The *epineurium* consists of areolar connective tissue that separates the fasciculi and holds them loosely together (Fig. 28–2D). This tissue becomes condensed on the surface of the nerve trunk to form a defined sheath surrounding the enclosed fasciculi. The collagen fibrils of the tissue are mostly longitudinal, although some are arranged in a random, open criss-cross fashion.[5, 7] The fibrils are generally thicker (60 to 100 nm) than those in the perineurium or the endoneurium; some scattered elastin fibers are also found. Adipose tissue is rarely seen within the fasciculi, but it can form conspicuous interfascicular elements in the epineurium of larger nerve trunks. The epineurium protects the fasciculi from excessive extension, and provides a loose matrix that cushions them against deforming forces.[2] The epineurium and perineurium are the common placement sites for sutures during direct surgical repair of a transected peripheral nerve.

The *perineurium,* a dense and distinctive sheath of connective tissue that surrounds the nerve fibers and the endoneurium of the fasciculus, consists of three concentric layers. The internal and middle layers are composed of flattened cells with long processes and a basement membrane. The boundaries of the perineurial cells form tight junctions and their basement membranes fuse to form a single intervening membrane. This arrangement of cells forms a diffusion barrier that prevents free passage of proteins and other molecules and

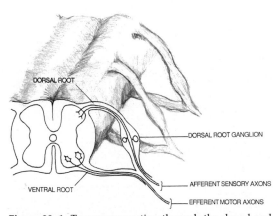

Figure 28–1. Transverse section through the dorsal and ventral roots of the spinal cord showing location of the motor and sensory neurons whose myelinated and unmyelinated axonal processes form the major part of the peripheral nervous system.

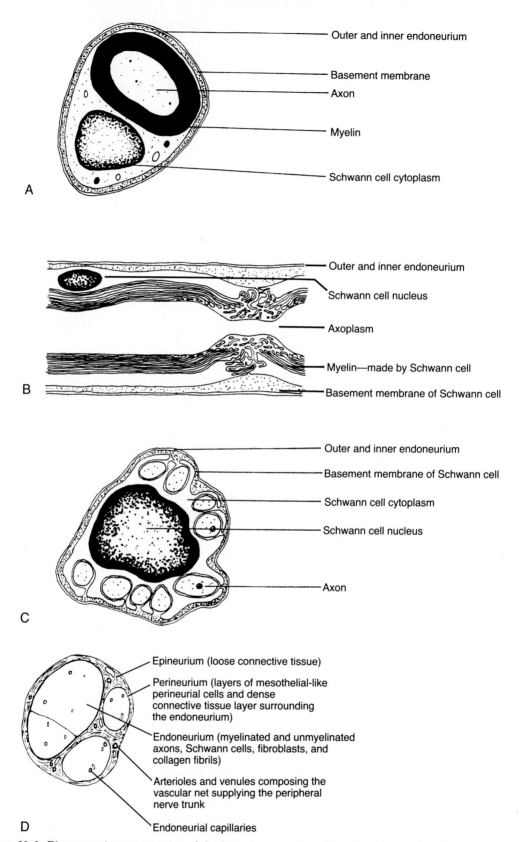

Figure 28–2. Diagrammatic representation of the basic features of myelinated and unmyelinated axons, based on light and transmission electron micrographs. *A,* Transverse section through a myelinated axon. *B,* Longitudinal section of a myelinated axon showing a node of Ranvier. *C,* transverse section of a group of unmyelinated axons and their supporting Schwann cell. *D,* Transverse section showing the funicular arrangement and the major tissues of the peripheral nerve trunk.

452

helps prevent the spread of infection and inflammation into the fasciculus.[8, 9] Nerve trunks passing through areas of infection remain unaffected while the perineurium is intact, but if it is breached the infection enters the fasciculi and rapidly spreads proximally and distally. Infections within the fasciculi (e.g., leprosy) are confined within the nerve bundle by the perineurium. The perineurium also helps to give physical strength to the nerve during extension.[10] The external layer is a zone of gradual transitions from the perineurium to the epineurium where the collagen fibers become progressively thicker and lose their orderly arrangement. The lamellar pattern is replaced by a more open arrangement and the perineurial cells are replaced by fibroblasts of the epineurium.

The *endoneurium* is the supporting connective tissue that fills the fasciculus and provides packing between nerve fibers. Fine intrafascicular septa partly subdivide the nerve fibers into smaller groupings. There are also spaces in the endoneurium that are filled with extracellular fluid. The endoneurium is composed of fibroblasts and collagen fibrils and forms a tube of loosely packed fibrils around each nerve fiber; the endoneurial tube is occupied by the Schwann cell and the axon.[5]

Fasciculi. The peripheral nerve trunk is made up of one or more fasciculi. The fasciculus is a bundle of nerve fibers surrounded by a thin but strong laminated cellular layer, the perineurium. The pattern of fasciculi in the cross-section of the nerve trunk is not constant down its length (Fig. 28–3). The fasciculi branch, reform, and branch repeatedly down the length of the nerve. The fascicular pattern of nerve trunks removed from the same level in different subjects, or from the same level of the contra-

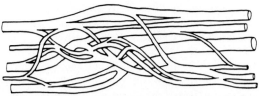

Figure 28–3. Funicular plexus formation over a distance of 3 cm. The funiculi are continually diverging and reanastomosing as they course down the nerve trunk, causing dramatic changes in the funicular pattern over very short distances. (Adapted from Sunderland S: Nerves and Nerve Injuries. New York, Churchill Livingstone, 1978.)

lateral limb in the same subject, can differ considerably. The diameter of peripheral nerve fasciculi in humans ranges from 0.04 mm to 2.0 mm with an occasional fasciculus of 4.0 mm in diameter. The accepted nomenclature for fascicular patterns is mono-, oligo-, and polyfascicular. The plexus formation between fascicles decreases in the distal portions of the extremities.[2]

Blood Vessels. Peripheral nerves are abundantly vascularized throughout their length (Fig. 28–4). The "arteriae nervorum" are blood vessels that enter and terminate within the nerve trunk. They are derived from the main vessel of the limb or its main branches and they supply the nerve exclusively. Other vessels come from muscular and cutaneous branches that are destined to supply extraneural tissues predominantly. Macroscopic arterioles are usually visible on the surface of large peripheral nerves, and their longitudinal arrangement can aid in the alignment of proximal and distal nerve stumps during direct surgical repair. The intraneural pattern of the venous network generally corresponds to the arterial pattern; however, the number of intrafascicular venules appears

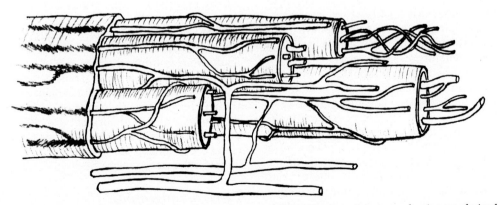

Figure 28–4. Arrangement of the blood vessels supplying a peripheral nerve. Arteries and veins are derived from the major vessels accompanying the nerve and descend into the epineurium. These in turn give rise to arterioles and venules, which supply the intrafascicular capillary network of the endoneurium.

to exceed the number of arterioles. They drain into the principal vein, veins or venus plexus associated with the neighboring artery.

The endothelial cells of the endoneurial capillaries have tight junctions, and they are normally impermeable to a wide range of substances and form the blood-nerve barrier, the peripheral nerve equivalent of the blood-brain barrier of the central nervous system. The junctions of endothelial cells in the epineurial and perineurial capillaries are not as tight, and thus some leakage occurs into the surrounding tissues.[11]

Lymphatics. The lymphatic capillary network in the epineurium is drained by lymphatic channels accompanying the arteries that supply the nerve trunk. There are no true lymphatic capillaries within the fasciculi, but there are fluid-filled endoneurial spaces between the nerve fibers. Fluid exchange between the extrafascicular lymphatics and these spaces is prevented by the perineurium, which provides an effective barrier between the two systems.[11]

Nervi Nervorum. Nerve trunks are supplied by special nerves, the nervi nervorum, which originate from fibers within the nerve and the perivascular plexuses. They are distributed to all three levels of connective tissue as diffuse plexuses. Both sympathetic and sensory fibers are represented in the nervi nervorum.

PERIPHERAL NERVE INJURIES

Peripheral nerve injuries can be divided into several broad categories or classes.[2, 12, 13] Perhaps the most useful divisions are neurapraxia, axonotmesis, and neurotmesis (Table 28–1). Although some authors and practitioners prefer to further subdivide peripheral nerve injuries,[14] these three categories of peripheral nerve lesions are widely used and are of importance from both a prognostic and a therapeutic point of view. Damage to peripheral nerves usually includes elements of both nerve conduction (neurapraxia) and loss of axonal continuity in compression/contusion/division (axonotmesis and neurotmesis). Lesions causing paralysis of nerve function without loss of axonal continuity are usually due to compression of the nerve and are associated with demyelination. The clinical signs of weakness and sensory loss in neurapraxia may be as severe as those due to complete loss of axonal continuity, but it is important to recognize these injuries as distinct from loss of axonal continuity because the prognosis is markedly different. Electrophysiological stud-

ies are of prime importance in this regard to show the presence of viable fibers on the distal side of the lesion, thus demonstrating axonal continuity. It must, however, be recognized that this distinction may not be possible in the *acute* situation, as wallerian degeneration occurs over several days after nerve injury, during which time conduction is possible along the distal nerve stump. Studies performed in this intermediate period may give the impression of conduction block due to loss of continuity rather than to focal abnormalities of conduction properties.

To arrive at a correct diagnosis, multiple assessments are often necessary to document whether the nerve response distal to the lesion diminishes, suggesting the presence of wallerian degeneration. Even though prominent signs of denervation may be evident in the electromyogram (EMG) of a muscle innervated by a damaged nerve, the presence of a large amplitude muscle response when stimulating distal to the lesion is usually associated with complete recovery over weeks to months. Demonstration of continued conduction from even just a few axons indicates that the nerve is in continuity and suggests that functional recovery may occur without surgical intervention.

Functional Assessment of Nerve Injuries

Electromyography and nerve conduction studies are used to assess the structure and function of the peripheral nervous system, and to document the presence of nerve damage and determine the nature and anatomical extent of the lesion. Correct classification is important, as recovery is dependent on the nature of the underlying lesion, and may aid in evaluating whether surgical exploration and repair are needed.

With respect to pathology, electrophysiological studies are limited in that inferences are made from findings that are rarely specific for particular types of lesions. Hence, it is important to assess the signs of abnormality in quantitative terms and to consider a number of different criteria of abnormality, including evidence of denervation and reinnervation of muscle and conduction along different segments of motor and sensory nerve fibers.

Electromyography

EMG is performed to evaluate the presence of denervation and reinnervation of muscle fi-

Table 28–1. CLASSIFICATION OF PERIPHERAL NERVE INJURIES

Classification	Characteristics
I (Neurapraxia)	Focal conduction block either transient due to ischemia or compression, etc., or more delayed but still reversible, e.g., focal demyelination
II (Axonotmesis)	Interruption of axonal continuity but preservation of Schwann cell basal lamina tubes
III (Neurotmesis)	Interruption of axonal and Schwann cell basal lamina tubes

bers and loss of motor units. Electrical signals are recorded during rest, weak effort, and maximal effort, using a concentric or a monopolar needle inserted into the muscle. The electrical activity of normal muscle at rest is almost completely absent. When the muscle is voluntarily activated, discrete motor unit action potentials are produced at weak effort. The frequency of the motor unit action potentials increases with the strength of contraction until they merge and individual motor unit action potentials can no longer be discerned on the EMG.

At various times after denervation, spontaneous activity in the form of fibrillation potentials and positive sharp waves is generated by individual muscle fibers. Denervated muscle begins to show fibrillation potentials several days after the nerve injury. The period between the injury and the appearance of fibrillation potentials is related to the distance of the nerve lesion from the muscle. The absence of fibrillation activity does not rule out denervation of muscle fibers; cyclic spontaneous activity has been demonstrated in noninnervated muscle fibers in culture.

During weak effort, summated potentials generated by individual motor units are recorded and evaluated according to their duration, amplitude, and shape. The duration of the motor unit potential is dependent on the number of muscle fibers in the motor unit, their density, and the territory covered. Due to the arrangement of the motor unit, the motor unit potentials often become complex and polyphasic with prolonged duration and increased amplitude. Because of the wide variability of the duration and amplitude of motor unit potentials recorded from individual muscles, it is necessary to record multiple potentials from different sites and to treat these parameters in a statistical manner. In addition, the characteristics of motor unit potentials vary in different muscles and with age, which should be taken into consideration when comparing findings in patients and normal subjects.

During maximal effort, the potentials from individual motor units are recorded simultaneously, giving rise to the so-called interference pattern. In neurogenic disorders, the motor units supplied by affected motor fibers do not contribute to the activity and if a sufficient number are lost, the pattern is reduced; if the condition is severe, the pattern becomes discrete, with each individual motor unit potential standing out against the background.[15, 16]

Nerve Conduction Studies

Conduction along peripheral nerves is studied by electrically stimulating the nerve and recording evoked muscle and nerve action potentials. The technique produces a synchronous triggering of all the motor units within the muscle. The action potential recorded by this method is a summation of action potentials from motor units or nerve fibers and is therefore termed the compound muscle or nerve action potential (Fig. 28–5).

Stimulation of a peripheral nerve supplying a totally denervated muscle does not produce a muscle response. The first signs of reinnervation are small amplitude action potentials. With progressive reinnervation of the muscle and maturation of regenerated fibers the amplitude of the action potentials increases and the shape becomes less polyphasic.[17]

Electrical activity from muscle activated voluntarily or by electrical stimulation of the parent nerve provides early evidence of reinnervation. In animal experiments where it is not possible to measure the electromyogram of voluntary contractions, recording of electrically evoked motor response is the only method by which neuromuscular function can be directly assessed.

Examination of the conduction of motor and sensory fibers helps to determine whether abnormalities are widespread or focal and whether the clinical symptoms are due to loss of axons or abnormalities in conduction. Measurements

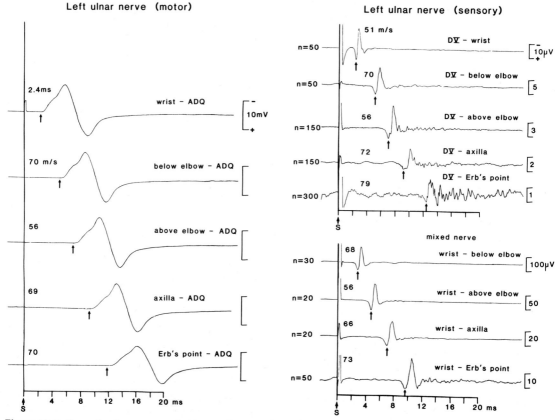

Figure 28–5. Example of a nerve conduction study carried out on the normal ulnar nerve of a human. *Left,* Compound action potentials from the abductor digiti V evoked by stimulation of the ulnar nerve at the wrist, below the elbow, above the elbow, at the axilla, and at Erb's point. The distal motor latency is indicated above the top trace and the conduction velocity along the different segments between the traces. *Right top,* Compound sensory nerve action potentials evoked from digit V. The responses were recorded from the ulnar nerve via needle electrodes placed close to the nerve. The conduction velocities are indicated above the traces. The number of responses averaged is indicated to the left of the traces (n). *Right bottom,* Mixed nerve compound action potentials evoked at the wrist and recorded from the ulnar nerve. The conduction velocities are indicated above the traces. The number of responses averaged is indicated to the left of the traces (n).

are made of the amplitude, shape, and conduction velocity of the evoked action potential. Motor fibers are studied by stimulating the nerve at different sites along its course, and the evoked muscle action potential is recorded from an appropriate muscle (Fig. 28–6). The muscle response is recorded via an electrode with a large surface area to allow pick-up from the whole muscle. The amplitude is measured peak-to-peak or from baseline to the negative peak; the latency of the response from the stimulus artefact to the take-off from baseline (Fig. 28–7A). The conduction velocity is calculated between different stimulation points by the difference in the latency. The conduction velocity is an expression of the fastest conducting fiber(s) in the nerve and may be normal even in severe lesions if the spared fiber(s) are of large caliber. However, if the largest fibers degenerate, the conduction velocity is reduced due to fiber loss.

The motor nerve conduction velocity in a regenerating nerve is a function of the axon diameter, the internodal length, and the extent of remyelination of the axon. Increase in the axon diameter and the myelin thickness produces a corresponding increase in the conduction velocity.[15, 16] The accuracy of measurements of motor conduction velocity is affected by a number of variables, including temperature, age of subject, the accuracy of the length measurement between the stimulating electrodes, and the course of the peripheral nerve within the limb being studied. These factors are potential sources of measurement error.

Sensory fibers are studied by stimulating a sensory branch and recording the orthodromic response from the nerve (Figs. 28–6 and 7B). The stimulating electrodes used may be placed on the skin, or, if greater resolution is required, needle electrodes are placed close to the nerve.

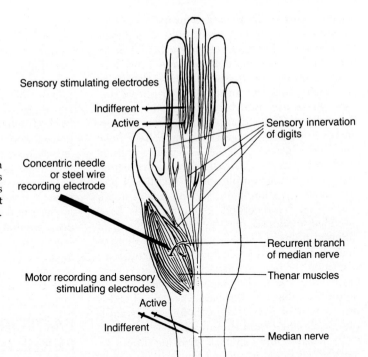

Figure 28–6. Median nerve innervation of the monkey hand, with the positions of recording and stimulating electrodes used in electrophysiological assessment of motor and sensory function indicated.

The amplitude of the compound sensory nerve action potential is measured peak-to-peak, and the conduction velocity is calculated from the latency to the first positive peak (Fig. 28–7B). This method provides information only about a restricted part of the fibers in the nerve; thus the conduction velocity provides information about only the very large fibers. The main component of the sensory action potential is derived from fibers more than 7 μ in diameter and the peak-to-peak amplitude is determined by fibers of at least 9 μ. In order to obtain accurate information about smaller caliber nerve fibers, it is necessary to average the

responses to 256 to 1024 stimuli. In normal nerve, the condition velocity of smaller fibers is about 15 m per second, i.e., the components of the response originate from fibers 4 to 5 μ in diameter. A substantially lower minimum conduction velocity indicates the presence of abnormal fibers in the nerve, and regenerating fibers may have velocities as low as 2 to 5 m per second.[15, 16]

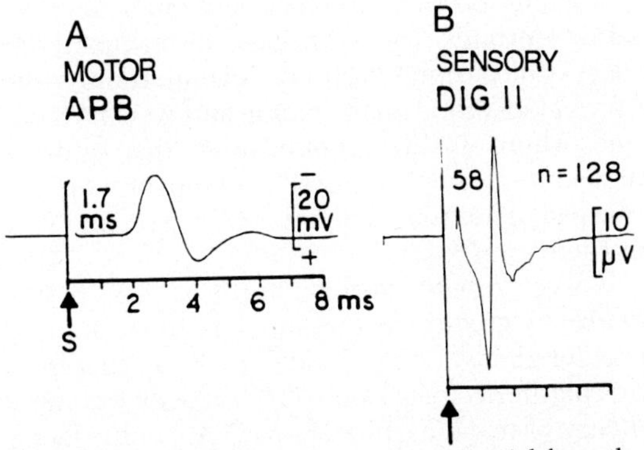

In partial nerve lesions, the surviving fibers have normal conduction velocities, and any reduction of the nerve conduction velocity is due to loss of fast conducting fibers. This indicates that the evaluation of the nerve conduction velocity cannot be performed without analysis of the amplitude and shape of the potential. Substantial reductions in conduction velocity, out of proportion to the apparent loss of fibers, usually indicate that additional abnormalities are present, such as compression-induced demyelination of surviving fibers. In complete nerve lesions, the conduction velocity of newly regenerated fibers may be as low as 1 to 3 m per second in promyelinated nerve fibers.

Experimental Electrophysiological Methods

The two major methodological approaches for the physiological study of regenerating peripheral nerve are in vitro recordings of responses from regenerated nerve and reinnervated target

A
MOTOR
APB

1.7 ms
20 mV
+
2 4 6 8 ms
↑
S

B
SENSORY
DIG II

58 n = 128
10 μV
↑

Figure 28–7. A, Normal motor action potential from the abductor pollicis brevis muscle following stimulation of the median nerve at the wrist. B, Normal sensory action potential recorded from the median nerve at the wrist following stimulation at the base of digit II.

organs (muscle fibers and sensory receptors) and longitudinal in vivo recordings to delineate the recovery of conduction properties of nerve fibers after wallerian degeneration caused by physical injury.[18-20] In such studies, the action potentials evoked in muscles or peripheral sensory nerves are used to gauge regeneration of nerve fibers. The action potentials from sensory nerves in humans[17, 20] and monkeys[21] have been recorded through needle electrodes placed close to the nerve. Using electronic averaging, responses with an amplitude of 0.05 to 0.1 μV, generated by stimulation of just a few nerve fibers, can be recorded. Such methods have provided evidence for the varying effects of different types of nerve lesions, such as demyelination with conduction block, acrylamide intoxication, or nerve constriction, on the regenerative processes. The major limitation of these methods is that no information is gained about the growth of nerve fibers before a response can be obtained from the muscle.

To localize the front of growing fibers, a method has been developed that utilizes highly sensitive and stable electrodes chronically implanted around a cat peripheral nerve (Fig. 28–8).[15, 16] The multicontact configuration is used first to determine elongation of the growing fibers and subsequently to observe the rate and level of maturation. By applying high-intensity stimuli through the different leads in the nerve cuff electrode distal to the site of the lesion, the most distal site at which nerve fibers could be excited was determined in serial studies (Fig. 28–9). By relating this site to the time after the nerve lesion, the rate of progression of excitability could be calculated to be 3.2 mm per day (Fig. 28–10). This corresponds well with the rate of regenerating axons in cat nerve of 3 to 4 mm per day as determined by other methods. In contrast, when nerve fibers had to grow through a constriction, the rate of elongation was about 30 percent slower (2.2 mm per day). The delay in regeneration after a simple crush lesion was 8 days, and this was not prolonged by a constriction. Thus, the delay in reinnervation of muscle fibers when a nerve had to regenerate through a constriction[19] was due to reduced rate of growth of nerve fibers distal to the constriction rather than to a local delay at the site of the lesion. With this model, responses are evoked from a constant site, and the amplitude and conduction velocity of the action potentials from regenerated fibers can be followed to ascertain the degree of maturation. The conduction velocity in newly regenerated fibers was found to be 1 to 2 m per second as

opposed to the 90 to 100 m per second in normal cat tibial nerve. This method allows determination of conduction along promyelinated fibers. Gradually this conduction velocity increases to a maximum of about 80 to 90 percent of normal (Fig. 28–11). In parallel with the increase in velocity, the amplitude of the evoked action potential increased to the low normal range after simple crush injury, whereas it remained markedly depressed after constriction distal to the crush.

In summary, with longitudinal in vivo recordings, it is possible to follow axon regeneration in the same animal and compare the temporal development of the regenerative phenomena during their different phases. It is also possible to quantify the effects of different lesions and treatment procedures, such as the implantation of nerve guide conduits.

FACTORS AFFECTING PERIPHERAL NERVE REPAIR

Factors Affecting Neuronal Survival and Axonal Elongation

Rapid advances in basic neurobiology are leading to new insights into the molecular mechanisms involved in axonal regeneration in the peripheral nervous system. Recent studies have shown that specific cell adhesion molecules, growth factors, and receptors are intimately involved in the process of axonal elongation and regeneration. These advances in the basic understanding of axonal growth are considered before the difficult area of clinical repair of damaged peripheral nerve is explored.

Role of Growth Factors and Specific Proteins. Certainly the most basic prerequisite for successful peripheral nerve regeneration is the survival of the primary motor and sensory neuron. There is little doubt now that specific molecules (growth factors) can help support the survival of neurons that have sustained an injury to their axon.[22-25]

Nerve growth factor (NGF) is the model neuronal growth factor and has been studied now for almost four decades.[26, 27] Emerging from this plethora of work on NGF has been a general theory of trophic connections.[28] A trophic factor is produced by the end-organ target tissue where innervating nerve terminals take up the factor and retrogradely transport it to their cell

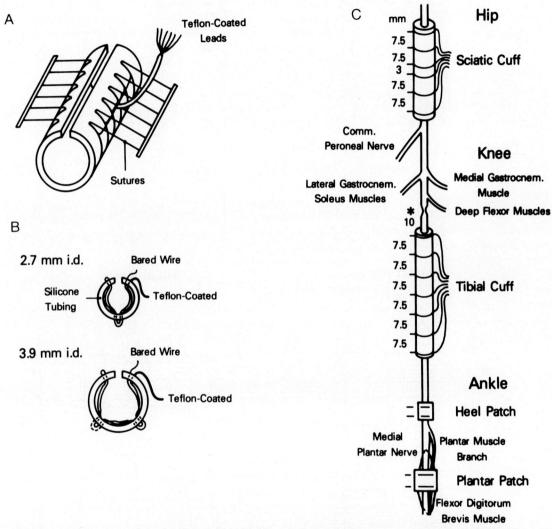

Figure 28–8. Schematic representation of cuff and patch electrodes implanted in the hindlimb of cat. *A,* Silicone cuff electrode with external closing sutures and Teflon-coated cables connecting the leads to the back pack socket. *B,* Placement of leads along the internal circumference of the cuff electrode. The internal diameter (i.d.) of the tibial cuff was 2.7 mm and that of the sciatic cuff 3.9 mm. *C,* Full complement of cuff and patch electrodes at hindlimb nerves and muscle. The distances between contacts are indicated. Patch-electrodes had interlead distances of 5 to 7 mm. The bare leads were placed on Dacron-reinforced silicone sheeting. The heel patch was placed facing the plantar nerve just distal to the calcaneus and the plantar patch facing the flexor digitorum brevis muscle and the medial branch of the plantar nerve. The * indicates the position of the nerve lesion distal to the leg branches of the tibial nerve (From Krarup C, Loeb GE: Conduction studies in peripheral cat nerve using implanted electrodes. I. Methods and findings in controls. Muscle Nerve 11:922–932, 1988.)

N10 Regeneration After a Crush Lesion

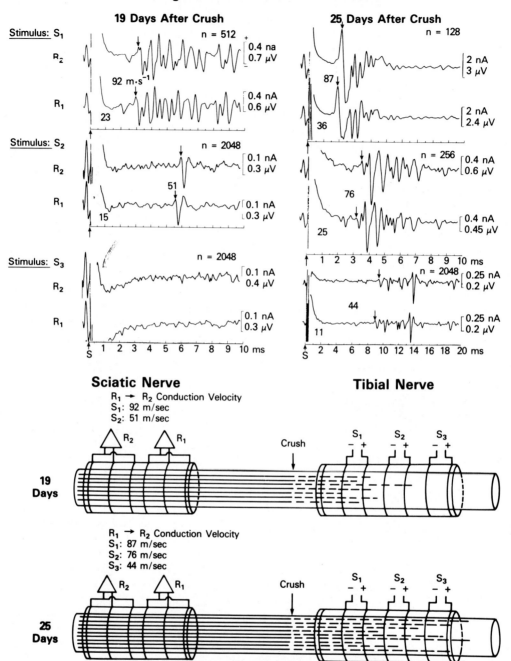

Figure 28–9. Progression of excitability along the denervated portion of the nerve and characterization of fastest regenerating fibers. *Above,* The tibial nerve distal to crush was stimulated at three different sites (S_1, S_2, S_3) and the evoked ascending nerve action potential recorded at two sites (R_1, R_2) along the sciatic nerve proximal to crush. The stimulus site S_1 was 19 mm *(upper pair of traces)*, S_2 was 34 mm *(middle pair)*, and S_3 was 49 mm *(lower pair)* distal to the lesion. The conduction velocity from the site of stimulation to R_1 is indicated below the traces and between R_1 and R_2 *(arrows)* between the traces. The number of averaged responses (n) is indicated. Nineteen days after crush an action potential was evoked from S_1 and S_2 but not from S_3. When the study was repeated 6 days later (25 days after crush), a potential was also present from S_3, but more distal stimulation did not evoke a response. *Below,* Schematic interpretation of the findings in the traces above. Nineteen days after crush a number of nerve fibers responded to the most proximal stimulus site (S_1) giving rise to the polyspike potential but only a single fiber responded at S_2. After further regeneration, a number of fibers responded at all three sites of stimulation. The conduction velocity proximal to the site of crush suggests that the response from the most distal excitable site was slower than that from more proximal sites of stimulation. (From Krarup C, Loeb GE, Pezeshkpour GH: Conduction studies in peripheral cat nerve using implanted electrodes. II. The effects of prolonged constriction on regeneration of crushed nerve fibers. Muscle Nerve 11:933–944, 1988.)

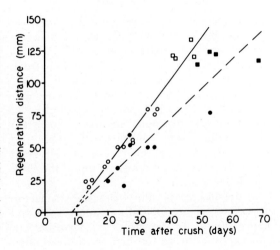

Figure 28–10. Relationship between the distance of excitability (mm, ordinate) and the time (days, abscissa) after crush alone *(open symbols)* and crush plus constriction *(solid symbols)*. The distance was determined by the most distal excitable site along the nerve from the site of crush. Linear regression lines (P <0.001) were fitted by least squares after crush alone *(solid line,* r=0.98, n=16) with a slope of 3.24 mm/day, and after crush plus constriction *(dashed line,* r=0.90, n=12) with a slope of 2.23 mm/day. After crush alone, the slope was 45 percent steeper (P <0.02) than after crush plus constriction. The regression lines were extrapolated to zero distance to show the delay (8 days) in start of regeneration. In crush plus constriction, the constricting cuff was place 5 mm along the distance of regeneration axis. (From Krarup C, Loeb GE, Pezeshkpour GH: Conduction studies in peripheral cat nerve using implanted electrodes. II. The effects of prolonged constriction on regeneration of crushed nerve fibers. Muscle Nerve 11:933–944, 1988.)

bodies. Once in the cell soma the factor may have many effects, especially in terms of gene regulation. NGF exhibits all of these effects for sympathetic and dorsal root ganglia (sensory) neurons.

Since NGF was discovered, many other neuronal growth factors have been discovered and the list is still growing. In the PNS, several growth factors have now been shown to promote survival of primary motor or sensory (or auto-

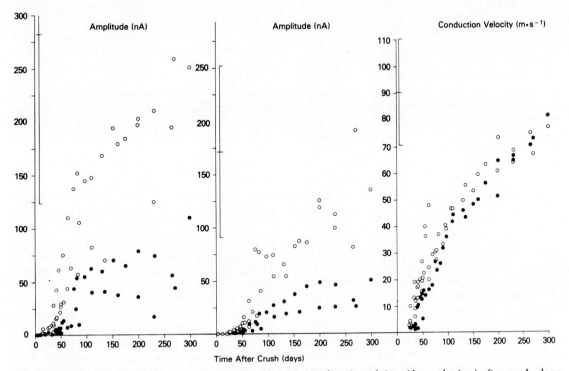

Figure 28–11. Composite of recovery of conduction properties as function of time (days, abscissa) after crush alone (○, five nerves) and crush plus constriction (●, four nerves). *Left,* Amplitude (nA, ordinate) of the ascending action potential in the sciatic nerve evoked at the tibial nerve 18 to 25 mm distal to crush. The mean and lower 95 percent confidence limit in control nerves is shown to the right of the ordinate. *Middle,* as in the left panel, values were obtained by stimulating the tibial nerve 48 to 55 mm distal to the lesion. Mean ± 95 percent confidence limits from control indicated to the right of the ordinate. *Right,* Conduction velocity (m · s^{-1}) between the two sites of stimulation. Mean ± 95 percent confidence limits from control indicated to the right of the ordinate. (From Krarup C, Loeb GE, Pezeshkpour GH: Conduction studies in peripheral cat nerve using implanted electrodes. II. The effects of prolonged constriction on regeneration of crushed nerve fibers. Muscle Nerve 11:933–944, 1988.)

nomic nervous system) neurons. Brain-derived neurotrophic factor (BDNF) was originally isolated from brain extracts as a 12 kDa basic protein.[29] BDNF has been shown in vitro to stimulate survival of dorsal root ganglia (DRG) neurons, as well as other primary sensory neurons such as trigeminal, nodose, vestibular, and mesencephalic trigeminal neurons.[29] Recent in vivo studies have confirmed the ability of BDNF to decrease the extent of cell death normally seen during development of the DRG and nodose ganglia.[30]

Basic and acidic fibroblast growth factors (bFGF, aFGF) are potent mitogens that have a high affinity for heparin.[31, 32] Madison and colleagues[33, 34] were the first to show an effect for aFGF in vivo in terms of supporting neuronal survival following peripheral nerve transection and repair. Interestingly, this stimulatory effect was seen for sensory neurons much more than for motor neurons. This finding reinforces the idea that different growth factors in the PNS may well have specific effects on only sensory, motor, or autonomic neurons. Other studies have also shown that bFGF stimulates axonal regeneration in the PNS,[35, 36] although it is not clear whether there is a preferential effect on sensory versus motor neuron survival as has been shown for aFGF.[33, 34]

Neuroleukin (NLK), a 63 kDa protein isolated from skeletal muscle, stimulates outgrowth from spinal cord neurons.[37] More recent studies, based on known DNA sequence identities, have shown that NLK is phosphoglucose isomerase, a glycolytic enzyme.[38] NLK has been shown to increase survival of both spinal cord motoneurons and sensory neurons from chick DRG.[37]

Ciliary neuronotrophic factor (CNTF) is a growth factor originally isolated from conditioned medium that is present in many tissues, (e.g., heart, sciatic nerve, eye).[39, 40] CNTF has been shown in vitro to increase survival of ciliary, DRG, and sympathetic neurons. CNTF has recently been cloned and sequenced by Lin and colleagues[40] and is currently under intense investigation to determine if the survival effects of this molecule can be shown in vivo.

Even this short list of neuronal growth factors active in the PNS belies the complexity of the problem, since many of these same factors have been shown to influence neurons in the central nervous system as well. In this fashion, imbalances in these growth factors could exert indirect influences on primary sensory and motor neurons via a direct effect on CNS neurons, which then influence the PNS.

Cell Adhesion Molecules. The list of defined molecules involved in cell-cell and cell-sub-

strate interactions is growing even faster than that of neuronal growth factors. Although earlier classification schemes for such molecules concentrated on in vitro function, more recent systems have tried to separate such molecules based on their cellular or extracellular location.[41] Thus the nomenclature has progressed from CAMs (cell adhesion molecule), SAMs (substrate adhesion molecule), and neurite outgrowth-promoting factor, to one that emphasizes the location of the molecule as either a cell surface molecule (involved with cell-cell interactions) or an extracellular matrix molecule (mediates cell-substrate interactions).[41–43]

The cell surface adhesion molecules pertinent to the PNS that are best understood are NCAM (neural cell adhesion molecule); NgCAM (Neuron-glia), also known as L1; MAG (myelin-associated glycoprotein); and N-cadherin.[41–43] Both NCAM and L1 are expressed during development of the PNS, being found on Schwann cells prior to a 1:1 association typical of the myelinating Schwann cell. Once Schwann cells have begun to myelinate axons, the expression of L1 and NCAM is reduced.[44]

In terms of extracellular matrix molecules implicated in nerve regeneration, the most studied are laminin and fibronectin and molecular complexes containing these extracellular matrix molecules.[45–47] Laminin has been shown in vitro to influence many different cell types, including the morphology and elongation of Schwann cells.[48] A laminin-containing gel has been shown to increase the rate of peripheral nerve regeneration in vivo (discussed further on).[49]

The actual contributions of cell adhesion and extracellular matrix molecules to peripheral nerve regeneration in vivo are not well understood, although rapid advances are being made. It has been shown that after nerve transection L1 and NCAM reappear on many Schwann cells, with the same temporal expression as during normal development.[44, 50, 51] Interestingly, NGF has been shown to increase expression of L1 on Schwann cells in culture.[52] Thus, it is likely that there is a dynamic interplay between neuronal growth factor production and the expression of cell adhesion molecules.

Non-neuronal Cells and Receptors. Two non-neuronal cells that no doubt contribute significantly to nerve repair are the Schwann cell and the macrophage.[53] Macrophages have usually been thought of as serving only to remove degenerating myelin; however, it has also been known for some time that they can act as general effector cells for wound healing.[54] Macrophages may influence endothelial cell migration,[55] present a mitogen to Schwann cells that is derived from myelin,[56] and help to induce the secretion of NGF from denervated Schwann cells.[57]

Schwann cells have long been implicated in peripheral nerve regeneration,[58] and recently Johnson and colleagues have begun to uncover the possible molecular connections between Schwann cells and regenerating axons.[59, 60] These studies have shown that following nerve transection, both NGF production and expression of low-affinity NGF receptors on Schwann cells are dramatically increased. This increased expression in the distal stump is then reduced once axonal contact has been re-established.[60] From this has arisen the theory that loss of axonal contact leads to increased NGF receptor and protein production by Schwann cells in the distal stump, the low-affinity NGF receptor on the surface of the Schwann cell binds the NGF in an autocrine fashion, the bound NGF is then transferred to the high-affinity NGF receptor located on the regenerating axon, and the NGF is then transported back to the parent cell body.[60]

It is this complicated interplay among non-neuronal cells, growth factors, cell adhesion molecules, and axons that leads to peripheral nerve regeneration. Given the complexity of the problem, one may wonder how any functional recovery occurs following nerve damage and clinical repair, and as discussed in the following section, a satisfactory clinical outcome after peripheral nerve repair is still far from routine.

Axonal Regeneration Following Nerve Injury and Repair

This section reviews the current standard clinical approaches to repair injured peripheral nerves.[2, 14, 61, 62] As discussed previously, our understanding of the basic underlying mechanisms of peripheral nerve regeneration has been advancing rapidly. However, despite recent progress in basic neurobiology, the clinical value of this basic knowledge for the surgeon faced with the formidable task of nerve repair is still quite limited.

The type of surgical repair that is carried out is directly related to the type and extent of the nerve injury. As mentioned, peripheral nerve injuries can be divided into three broad categories, neurapraxia, axonotmesis, and neurotmesis (see Table 28–1).[2, 12, 13]

It is generally accepted that if there is still continuity of the axoplasm through the lesion site (class I injury, neurapraxia) it is best to simply wait and assess nerve regeneration or restoration of conduction properties, since no surgical procedure can improve upon the intact nerve fascicle. Likewise, there are legitimate reasons to simply wait and assess recovery following a class II injury (axonotmesis), the rationale being that as long as the original Schwann cell basal lamina tube remains intact the regenerating axon is more likely to successfully cross the lesion site and eventually reconnect to its appropriate end-organ target. The more difficult task for the surgeon is the class III injury (neurotmesis) in which there is complete severance of the nerve fascicle and associated Schwann cell tubes. This type of injury also usually involves disruption of soft tissue surrounding the nerve, which makes surgical management all the more difficult.

The major clinical objective in repair of class III injuries is to restore continuity between the proximal and distal nerve stumps, without which functional recovery is virtually impossible. In cases in which the distal and proximal nerve stumps can be identified and brought into continuity, it is generally accepted that a direct suture repair is the preferred treatment. There are several schools of thought concerning the preferred type of direct suture repair, and these are discussed later. However, in cases in which there is a nerve gap distance that must be bridged, it may be impossible to bring the cut nerve stumps into close enough proximity to achieve a direct suture repair, and some type of intervening material must be used. The most commonly used material is an autograft of a peripheral nerve harvested from the patient, e.g., a sural nerve autograft. However, there is renewed interest in the use of different types of biomaterials, both natural and synthetic, as nerve guide tubes or conduits; this is commonly referred to as "entubulation repair."

Direct Surgical Repair of Transected Peripheral Nerves

The main types of direct suture repair are epineurial and perineurial (Fig. 28–12), the difference being whether the suture material is drawn through the perineurium or the epineurium of the nerve fascicle. In a multifasciculated nerve, perineurial repair offers the advantage of direct alignment of individual fascicles in the

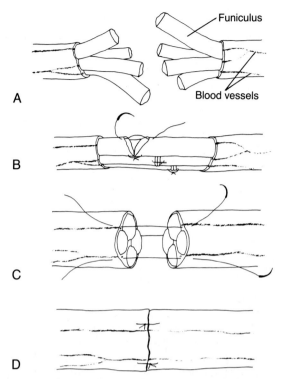

Figure 28–12. Methods of anastomosis of multifunicular peripheral nerve trunks. Comparison of perineurial repair and epineurial repair. *A*, In perineurial repair the funiculi are dissected free of the ensheathing layer of endoneurial connective tissue to allow their individual manipulation. The nerve stumps are positioned to provide the best alignment of the funiculi. *B*, Microsutures are placed within the perineurial sheath, care being taken not to penetrate the extremely delicate endoneurial tissue. The sutures are tied so that each anastomosis is tension free. *C*, Epineurial repair is easier and less time consuming to perform than perineurial suture. The loss in accuracy of the funicular ligament is compensated for by the reduced manipulation of the nerve stumps during the repair procedure. *D*, Using anatomical markers such as the epineurial blood vessels, the nerve stumps are positioned to provide the best alignment of the proximal and distal funicular patterns. Tensionless microsutures are placed within the epineurial sheath.

proximal stump with their corresponding fascicles in the distal stump. There is still no clear indication of which technique is superior for nerve repair despite many clinical and experimental studies comparing them. Some of the most convincing experimental comparison studies used retrograde transport of horseradish peroxidase to ascertain the degree to which motor neurons would correctly reinnervate their appropriate muscles following rat sciatic nerve repair.[63–65] These studies suggested a higher degree of accuracy of muscle reinnervation following group fascicular repair (perineurial) compared to epineurial repair. However, other studies have not found such a difference and the subject remains controversial.[66]

Tissue glues, most notably composed of fibrin, have also been used to join transected nerve stumps together. Recent studies have claimed superior,[67] inferior,[68] or equal[69] results for nerve repair with fibrin glues compared to nerve suturing. A major problem with these glues is the possibility of the two nerve stumps becoming disconnected when placed under stress due to joint and muscle movement.[68] Surgical tape has also been tested as a means of connecting transected nerve stumps.[70] Despite these investigations, direct suturing is still much more common than tissue adhesives or tape.

Nerve Autografting

It is generally accepted that better results are obtained by directly joining nerve stumps than by using an intervening material if the two stumps of a severed nerve can be brought into continuity without tension at the junction site. The distance at which stress at the junction site becomes a problem is debatable, but most surgeons agree that a nerve gap distance within the hand or forearm of greater than a few centimeters (e.g., 2 to 5 cm) should not be bridged by direct contact.[71–74] Some surgeons believe that tension will become a factor at the repair site if direct surgical repair cannot be carried out with the extremity in a neutral position.

The process and types of nerve autografting procedures are similar to those discussed for direct suture repair. The most common donor nerves used in autografting are the sural nerve and the lateral and medial antebrachial cutaneous nerve. These sensory nerves are used because the loss of sensation due to harvesting is usually well tolerated by the patient.

There has been debate over whether a nerve graft that is transferred with its vascular supply intact (vascularized graft) performs better than one that is not vascularized at the time of grafting. The theoretical advantages of using vascularized grafts include the ability of the graft to be well vascularized even if placed in a severely compromised host vascular bed and the presumption that even very long grafts (e.g., more than 10 cm) would still have access to a good blood supply.[75, 76] Since most nerve grafts become well-vascularized from the recipient vascular bed, it is not clear that grafting the vascular supply with the nerve actually leads to better vascularization of the graft in a normal host vascular bed. Results from experimental studies in animals do not clearly support or invalidate the use of these grafts.[77–82] Terzis and Breidenbach[82] have made an extensive series of cadaveric dissections to identify which nerves might be the most useful for vascularized nerve grafts. They considered the type and consistency of blood supply to the potential donor nerve, the accessibility of the donor nerve, and the length and neural tissue area of the donor nerve, and based on these criteria the following nerves were identified as the best potential donor nerves for vascularized nerve grafts: superficial radial, ulnar, sural, anterior tibial, superficial peroneal, and saphenous.

Whether or not one uses a vascularized or nonvascularized donor graft, there is still the decision of whether to carry out an epineurial or perineurial (e.g., group fascicular) repair (see Fig. 28–12). Several studies have noted that in all cases care must be taken to avoid tension at the suture lines of the nerve graft and recipient nerve. However, the terms "epineurial" and "perineurial" actually refer to the placement of sutures rather than the fascicular pattern of the nerve being repaired.[74] It is certainly generally agreed that on a gross modality level (e.g., motor vs. sensory), if individual fascicles can be identified as belonging to motor or sensory nerves, then corresponding fascicles should be connected.

Motor and sensory nerves can be identified by anatomical, physiological, and histochemical properties specific to the respective fascicles. Sunderland published a classical description of the interchanging patterns of fascicles of the median, ulnar, and radial nerves in 1945, and since then several anatomical mappings of major fascicular patterns of the major peripheral nerves have been published.[2, 83–86] The quickly interchanging fascicular patterns along the length of a peripheral nerve make identification of any single fasciculus difficult (see Figure 28–3). However, this plexus formation dramatically decreases in the distal extremity, which makes surgical manipulation and repair at this level more satisfactory.

Histochemical differences between motor and sensory fascicles have also been used for identification.[87, 88] The presence of acetylcholinesterase and choline acetyltransferase indicates motor fibers,[87] and the presence of carbonic anhydrase has been used to identify sensory fibers.[88] There is even evidence that the amount of carbonic anhydrase within sensory neurons and their axons may be dependent on whether the neuron innervates muscle (e.g., muscle spindles) or skin.[88]

Electrical stimulation has also been used to differentiate motor and sensory fascicles.[89] This technique is necessarily limited to the proximal nerve stump, since conduction in the distal nerve stump occurs only during the first few days after transection. The clinical use of electrical stimulation as an aid in peripheral nerve surgery has recently been reviewed.[90] This simple but very specific technique is probably underutilized in the surgical evaluation of the proximal stump.

The distinction of modality-specific fascicles is limited to the distal portions of nerve trunks, as individual nerves approach their end-organ targets. The segregation of motor and sensory fibers into distinct fascicles breaks down as one progresses more proximally toward the spinal cord and dorsal root ganglia, such that at proximal levels (e.g., brachial plexus) there may be a random mixing of sensory and motor fibers within fascicles. Thus, repair in the proximal portions of a nerve trunk is more likely to result in the mismatching of regenerating motor and sensory fibers and lead to aberrant regeneration.

Complications of Direct Nerve Suture and Grafts

Axonal escape at the suture line is a possibility in direct suture repair and nerve autografting. Obviously if axons escape at the suture line and do not enter the distal nerve stump they will have no chance of reaching the distal end-organ target to restore function. In addition, axonal escape at the suture line can lead to formation of a neuroma with potential painful consequences.[91, 92] Since a nerve autograft will have two suture lines as opposed to one in direct surgical repair, it stands to reason that there is an increased risk of axonal escape from an autograft repair. On the other hand, too much tension at the suture line has been shown to give poor results. Excellent surgical technique is required to bring the two cut nerve stumps together for a direct end-to-end repair while at the same time avoiding tension at the suture line. As mentioned, when it is felt that tension will result at the suture line, a nerve autograft is indicated.

Additional complications of nerve autografting have recently been reviewed by Millesi.[71, 93] They include failure of graft survival and vascularization, potential caliber difference between donor nerve and injured nerve, and unavailability of donor nerves. Because the nerve autograft is vascularized from its recipient bed by small vessels, the center of a thick donor graft will be revascularized more slowly than a thin one. This reasoning has led to the use of vascularized nerve grafts, but the clinical benefit of such grafts over nonvascularized nerve grafts has not been demonstrated. If there is a large difference between the caliber of the nerve to be repaired and the donor nerve, one must either group segments of the donor nerve together to approximate the size of the injured nerve (cable graft) or dissect out the individual fascicles of the injured nerve and repair them with single segments of the donor nerve. Finally, in cases of severe injury, enough donor nerve may not be available without sacrificing important sensory or motor function.

Results of Direct Suture Repair

Mackinnon and Dellon have given one of the most comprehensive reviews of functional recovery following nerve repair.[14] These authors used the rating scales shown in Tables 28–2 and 28–3 to assess sensory and motor recovery, respectively. These scales are a modification of Highet and Sanders' scheme for rating functional outcome.[95] They applied these rating scales to many of the published large clinical studies since World War II for which there was enough information to gauge the results. If one looks only at results for median nerve repair at the level of the wrist (Table 28–4), it can be seen that motor recovery is usually better than sensory recovery but that only a very few patients fully recover motor and sensory function. The results of median nerve repair with autografting are shown in Table 28–5. Approximately 2 percent of patients recovered to S4, 24 percent to S3, 20 percent to M5, and 13 percent to M4.

ENTUBULATION REPAIR OF TRANSECTED PERIPHERAL NERVES

As discussed before, current standard clinical practice for the repair of human peripheral nerve injuries favors the direct anastomosis of proximal and distal nerve stumps. Unfortunately, there are many clinical situations in which direct realignment of nerve fascicles is impossible, including severe laceration and injuries in which a segment of nerve has been damaged or removed and the proximal and distal nerve stumps are separated by too great a distance to permit direct suturing. In these cases, the necessary bridging is usually accomplished by a nerve autograft, e.g., a portion of sural nerve from the patients leg is grafted to

Table 28–2. CLASSIFICATION OF MOTOR RECOVERY

Grade	Motor Recovery
M0	No contraction
M1	Return of perceptible contraction in the proximal muscles
M2	Return of perceptible contraction in both proximal and distal muscles
M3	Return of function in both proximal and distal muscles to such a degree that all important muscles are sufficiently powerful to act against gravity
M4	All muscles act against strong resistance and some independent movements are possible
M5	Full recovery in all muscles

From Mackinnon SE, Dellon AL: Surgery of the Peripheral Nerve. New York, Thieme Medical Publishers, 1988.

bridge a damaged median nerve in the arm. Unfortunately, the results of such nerve grafting are not entirely satisfactory.

Bridging a nerve gap with a tubular prosthesis, entubulation repair is a promising alternative nerve repair strategy. The use of such "nerve guide conduits" is especially applicable when direct realignment of nerve fascicles is impossible.

Entubulation repair has gained renewed interest recently as a useful model to study basic mechanisms of peripheral nerve regeneration in vivo. The effects of gap length, distal stump components, and initial ingrowth were studied by both Longo and Lundborg and colleagues by bridging transected rat sciatic nerves with silicone tubes.[96, 97] They provoked rats to form subcutaneous mesothelial tubes, which were

Table 28–3. CLASSIFICATION OF SENSORY RECOVERY*

Grade	Recovery of Sensibility
S0	No recovery of sensibility in the autonomous zone of the nerve
S1	Recovery of deep cutaneous pain sensibility with the autonomous zone of the nerve
S1+	Recovery of superficial pain sensibility
S2	Recovery of superficial pain and some touch sensibility
S2+	As in S2, but with overresponse
S3	Recovery of pain and touch sensibility with disappearance of overresponse†
S3+	As in S3, but localization of the stimulus is good and there is imperfect recovery of two-point discrimination†
S4	Complete recovery†

*From Mackinnon SE, Dellon AL: Surgery of the Peripheral Nerve. New York, Thieme Medical Publishers, 1988.
†These classifications were modified to include classic two-point discrimination ranges as follows: S3 has two-point discrimination greater than 15 mm, S3+ includes 7 to 15 mm range, S4 includes 2 to 6 mm range.

Table 28–4. RESULTS OF MEDIAN NERVE REPAIR—LOW

Repair Timing	No. Cases	Age (yr)	% Children	Follow-up (yr)	Motor Recovery (%)				Sensory Recovery (%)				
					M2	M3	M4	M5	S2	S2+	S3	S3+	S4
All	235	Adults	0	2	67				27		73		
Secondary	290	Adults	0	5	31	14	18	0	47	15	30	9	0.2
Secondary	244	Adults	0	4	11	23	29	31	17	28	14	18	
Secondary	52		16	5	21	27	39	0	21	15	40	25	0
Primary	54		16	1–7	35	0	65	0					
Secondary	24		16	1–7	50	0	50	0	3	0	26	71	0
All	46			2–24									9
All	27	<14	100	Long	0	0	27	65	4	0	4	7	86
All	16	>14	0	Long	13	20	27	13	17	0	17	61	0
Primary	38	3–81	26	2–31	13	37	11	0	15	33	13	5	0
Secondary	20	3–81	26	2–31	25	35	25	0	20	29	32	4	0
Primary	40			1–12	25	38	15	7	50	0	7	10	3
Primary	15	<14	100	4–11	20	13	40	27	0	0	0	27	73
Primary	17	>14	0	4–11	30	23	18	29	22	18	18	41	0
All	10	5–58	33	1–3	30	70			30		70		
All	26		35	1					0		88	8	4
Secondary	110			5	5	47		44	4	5	47	44	0
Secondary	95	Adults	0	1	61		39	0	61		39		0
Primary	14		6	2–11	0	43	57	0	7	7	29	57	0

From Mackinnon SE, Dellon AL: Surgery of the Peripheral Nerve. New York, Thieme Medical Publishers, 1988.

reinforced with wire coils, and then used the tubes to repair several nerves. The same investigators went on to use silicone tubes and defined the early sequence of events within the chamber bounded by the tube that led to effective regeneration.[98, 99] They described the initial formation of a fibrin-rich extracellular matrix containing blood-derived cells, followed by invasion of endothelial, fibroblastic, and Schwann cells from both ends of the tube. Nerve fibers subsequently formed a cable enclosed within a connective tissue capsule, separated from the inner wall of the tube of a fluid-filled space. In effect, then, the tube lumen serves to house a "wound healing" environment that is the immediate milieu for the regenerative process. In this model, the lumen of the tube serves to separate degenerating material that may cause physical obstructions to the regenerating tissues and provides a controlled experimental chamber where individual PNS components can be studied under normal or experimentally modified conditions.

Entubulation has several theoretical advantages over other nerve repair methods. Tube repair appears to limit the ingrowth of fibroblasts into the repair site and thus avoids excessive collagen and scar formation. In addition, it provides directional guidance to the regenerating axons and prevents axonal escape into the area surrounding the repair site. Trophic factors from the injury site may become concentrated within the lumen of the tube and serve to facilitate axonal growth.[97]

Many biodegradable and nonbiodegradable materials have been used to assist regeneration of peripheral nerves, including polylactate/polyglycolate copolymers,[100, 101] acrylic copoly-

Table 28–5. RESULTS OF MEDIAN NERVE GRAFT

Gap Grafted (cm)	No. Cases	Age (yr)	% Children	Follow-up (yr)	Motor Recovery (%)				Sensory Recovery (%)				
					M2	M3	M4	M5	S2	S2+	S3	S3+	S4
3–15	32			1–15									3
5–15	11	Adult		2–3	0	36	18	0	10	18	45	18	0
>7	33			>5	0	69	0	0	21	0	69	0	0
2–20	38	8–62	3	5–11	7	21	14	46	3	0	60	34	3
5–10	8	17–38	0	1.5–2.5	12	0	50	0	13	0	12	63	12
4–15	6			1.5–2.5		33	16	33				33	
>2	8	15–57	0	1–5	0	0	0		0	37	38	25	0
4–6	5	5–71	2–6		average M2+			0	average S2			0	

From Mackinnon SE, Dellon AL: Surgery of the Peripheral Nerve. New York, Thieme Medical Publishers, 1988.

mers,[102, 103] polyvinylidene fluoride (PVDF),[104, 105] polyglactin mesh,[106] Millipore filter material,[107] silicone,[97–99] Gore-tex,[108] arterial cuffs,[109–111] preformed mesothelial tubes,[112] collagen,[113–118] polylactates,[49, 119] and various other synthetic polyester.[120, 121] Some major criteria for a useful nerve guide are control over the rate of resorption and the change in mechanical properties with time in vivo, the permeability properties of the conduit membrane, the surgical technique used to stabilize the nerve stumps within the conduits, and flexibility in terms of manufacturing various sizes of conduits. Although each of the materials listed has some advantages, none has been found to be entirely satisfactory. Disadvantages of such materials include elicitation of foreign body response, induction of scar tissue, difficulty in application, and for the nonbiodegradable materials, a secondary operation for removal of the implant.[122]

The ideal implantable nerve guide must meet the following requirements: (1) complete bioresorbability via the normal metabolic pathways of the host organism; (2) nontoxicity, nonantigenicity, and noncarcinogenicity; (3) resorption at controllable rates to be compatible with axon growth so that the guide maintains mechanical integrity until axons have successfully grown through it; (4) physical growth properties that allow suitable flexibility to avoid compression neuropathies and allow suturability; and (5) amenability to custom fabrication so that channel dimensions can be made appropriate for the particular nerve to be repaired.

Most recent studies of entubulation repair have continued to focus on events within the chamber itself. To quantify experimental variations to either the lumen of the tube or tubular composition, investigators have measured the number of axons found at midtube level.[98, 112] These studies suggest that low-intensity fields, multiple injections of biochemical agents, and permeability of the tubular prothesis all stimulate axonal regeneration.[104, 105, 123] However, axonal branching may be a confounding factor in studies that use only number of axons within the tube as a quantitative measure of successful regeneration.

Effects of Protein Additives on Nerve Guide Tubes

Neurite outgrowth is profoundly influenced by the adhesive properties of a substrate with which a neuron interacts. Several molecules of the extracellular matrix (ECM) can promote attachment and process outgrowth from a variety of neurons in culture, such as laminin, fibronectin, and collagen types I and IV.[47, 124, 125] Although there are differences in the neuronal responses to these and other adhesive glycoproteins in vitro, neurite outgrowth of several different central and peripheral neuronal cell types is stimulated by laminin as a substrate.

Earlier studies have clearly shown that bioresorbable tubes filled with a laminin containing gel (Matrigel)[49] or acidic fibroblast growth factor (aFGF)[33, 34] displayed an accelerated rate of regeneration. Matrigel is a solubilized tissue basement membrane containing laminin, collagen type IV, heparan sulfate proteoglycan, and entactin. Axons had completely crossed a 4 mm nerve gap in Matrigel-filled tubes by 2 weeks but not in initially empty tubes. In the studies with aFGF, the growth factor was added to a collagen-filled nerve guide that connected the two cut ends of the rat sciatic nerve. After 4 weeks, horseradish peroxidase was applied to the sciatic nerve distal to the nerve guide repair to retrogradely label primary motor and sensory neurons that had regenerated an axon through the nerve guide. It is interesting to note that the survival-promoting effects of aFGF were found to be specific for sensory rather than motor primary neurons (Fig. 28–13).

It has also been shown that the maximum nerve gap distance that can be successfully bridged is increased by adding either collagen or Matrigel to implanted tubes.[126] Enhanced regeneration also occurred in silicone tubes filled with collagen gels or saline compared to empty tubes.[127, 128] However, the influence of additives is dependent upon the composition of the tube itself. For instance, Valentini and coworkers[129] have shown that if one fills a permeable tube, as opposed to an impermeable silicone or Tygon tube, with Matrigel, the additive may actually impede axonal regeneration. There is thus a complex interplay between the composition of the tube and the gel additives. It is clear, however, that additives to a tubular repair site significantly influence the regeneration outcome.

Studies with empty silicone tubes have shown that within 7 days postimplantation, proximal and distal stumps are connected by a fibrin bridge. This fibrin matrix contains various blood-derived cells (erthyrocytes, leukocytes, and macrophages), fibroblasts, and ECM components.[98, 130] It has been suggested from light microscopic studies and transmission electron microscopic analysis[130] that this structure forms a primary scaffolding for orienting the migration of fibroblasts, Schwann cells, and eventually axonal processes. In empty tubes, fibroblasts

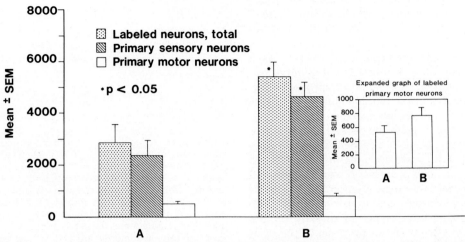

Figure 28–13. A comparison of total horseradish peroxidase–labeled primary neurons, primary labeled sensory neurons, and primary labeled motor neurons in nerve guides filled with collagen plus heparin (group A, n = 6) versus collagen plus heparin plus acidic fibroblast growth factor (aFGF) (group B, n = 6). (From Cordeiro PG, Seckel BR, Lipton SA, et al: Acidic fibroblast growth factor enhances peripheral nerve regeneration in vivo. Plast Reconstr Surg 83:1013–1019, 1989.)

proliferate and invade the fibrin matrix from both nerve stumps to form a concentric cellular layer around the fibrin matrix.[130] These layers of concentric cells eventually form a perineurium,[131] although not necessarily a normal one.[132] Similar results are found with tubes filled with protein additives.[133]

Glial cell surfaces themselves appear to have the ability to support neurite outgrowth.[134–137] For instance, Schwann cells can support extensive neurite outgrowth from embryonic retinal neurons. However, neurite outgrowth is affected equally well by Schwann cells that either express or do not express ECM.[137] Thus, Schwann cells themselves may also function as preferred substrates for axonal attachment and growth due to the presence of cell adhesion molecules on their surfaces. It is unlikely that only one or even several ECM molecules are responsible for the ability of certain tissues to promote axonal growth. Rather, there is a complicated interrelationship among ECM molecules, cell surface substrates such as adhesion molecules, and eventual axonal growth and guidance.

Comparison with Standard Nerve Autografting in Rodents and Non-human Primates

There is a growing body of evidence that an entubulation repair is as effective as conventional nerve grafting to repair transected nerves

as judged physiologically[138–141] and anatomically.[138, 142, 143] In cases in which alignment of fascicles cannot be obtained, the implantation of a nerve guide may be as effective as the implantation of a nerve autograft.

We have recently completed studies comparing entubulation repair of peripheral nerve with a collagen-based nerve guide to the more standard nerve graft procedure in rodents and nonhuman primates.[21, 115–117, 144] The collagen-based nerve guide conduits used for these studies were provided by Colla-Tec, Inc., Plainsboro, NJ, and have been described previously.[21, 115–117, 144] These collagen guides had an average pore size sufficiently large for macromolecules such as bovine serum albumin (MW = 68 kDa) to readily diffuse across the membrane of the nerve guide conduits.[144]

Rats were divided equally among three surgical protocols with additional animals placed into normal and negative control groups. Under deep anesthesia all animals except the normal control group received transection of the left sciatic nerve midway between the sciatic notch and the popliteal space. For the direct repair group the nerve was repaired using two perineurial 10-0 microsutures. For the nerve autograft group a 4 mm segment of the nerve was removed, reversed, rotated 180° along its axis, and sutured to the proximal and distal nerve stumps with two 10-0 microsutures at each junction. The nerve guide repair animals had a 4 mm segment of nerve removed, and the proximal and distal nerve stumps were sutured into the nerve guide by a single 10-0 suture connecting the conduit wall and perineurium of the nerve stump about 1 mm from the transected face of the nerve. This resulted in a 4 mm nerve gap distance (Fig. 28–14). As a negative control, a 4 mm segment of nerve was removed with no subsequent repair procedure. As a normal control, physiological assessments were carried out on five naive animals.

Figure 28–15 shows the evoked muscle action potentials recorded via a concentric needle electrode from the gastrocnemius muscle at 4 and 12 weeks following nerve repair. Compound muscle action potentials (MAPs) from each recording site were evoked by two platinum wire stimulating electrodes placed directly on the sciatic nerve trunk 5 mm proximal to the transection site, amplified, averaged (n = 64), and recorded with a computer-based data acquisition system.

The peak-to-peak amplitude of the MAP from the gastrocnemius was measured from averaged responses. At 4 weeks the amplitude of the MAP from the suture group was significantly greater than in the other three surgical groups (analysis of variance; p <0.01, Student-Newman-Keuls test). There were no statistically significant differences among any of the surgical groups at 12 weeks.

The maximum peak-to-peak amplitude of the MAP is a function of three factors: the population of motor nerve fibers responding to the stimulus, the synchronization of their response, and the size of the motor unit innervated by

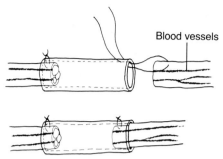

Figure 28–14. Entubulation repair of a peripheral nerve trunk using a collagen-based nerve guide conduit. The microsuture is passed through the wall, into the lumen of the nerve guide, and then through the endoneurial sheath 1 to 2 mm away from the cut face of the nerve stump. The suture is then passed back through the lumen and then the wall of the tube. Pulling on both ends of the suture draws the nerve stump into the nerve guide. Tensionless sutures are tied to hold the nerve stumps in position.

the axons. As axon regeneration and remyelination proceed, more muscle fibers are recruited and their response becomes increasingly more synchronized, thereby increasing the amplitude of the MAP.

The greater degree of recovery in the direct repair group at 4 weeks was not surprising, as there was no nerve gap to be bridged. A greater delay would have been expected in the two repair groups with a nerve gap while nerve fibers were elongating through the nerve guide or the autograft. However, no greater initial delay was observed in the nerve guide compared with the autograft group, and all four

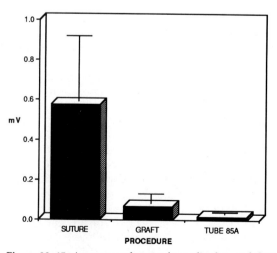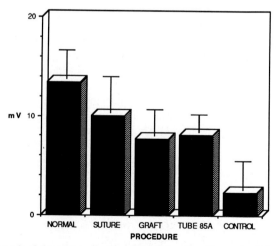

Figure 28–15. Average peak-to-peak amplitudes, and their standard deviations for the evoked muscle action potential from rat gastrocnemius muscle at 4 (*left*) and 12 (*right*) weeks following sciatic nerve transection and repair. (From Archibald SJ, Krarup C, Shefner J, et al: A collagen-based nerve guide conduit for peripheral nerve repair: An electrophysiological study of nerve regeneration in rodents and nonhuman primates. J Comp Neurol 306:685–696. Copyright © 1991 by Wiley-Liss. Reprinted by permission of Wiley-Liss, a division of John Wiley and Sons, Inc.)

surgical repair groups displayed similar levels of recovery of the MAP amplitudes at 12 weeks. This suggests that the delayed muscle reinnervation seen in the other groups, compared to the direct repair group, did not cause any irreversible denervation changes in the distal nerve stump or in the muscle. It is important to note that at 12 weeks following surgery all experimental surgical groups displayed significantly greater amplitudes than the negative control in which the nerve gap was left unbridged. At this same time point, the nerve guide group performed as well as the autograft group and the direct suture group.

Thus, based on the EMG assessment in the rat sciatic nerve model at 12 weeks, regeneration through the collagen-based nerve guide conduits was similar to that after direct repair of the transected sciatic nerve or a nerve autograft. At 12 weeks there was partial recovery of MAP amplitude activity in the negative control group. Thus some axons managed to successfully reinnervate the distal nerve stump even though a nerve repair procedure had not been performed. Previous studies have also noted that the rat peripheral nervous system has a great capacity for spontaneous regeneration.[145]

In contrast to this spontaneous regeneration in lower animals, a wealth of clinical and experimental data show that when a peripheral nerve is completely transected in humans and nonhuman primates, the vast majority of axons form a large endbulb neuroma, and only a very few axons successfully reach the distal nerve stump unaided.[2, 92] We were thus prompted to test the collagen-based nerve guides in the nonhuman primate, using the transected median nerve as a model.[115, 116]

The median nerves of adult male monkeys (*Macaca fascicularis*) were transected 2 cm above the wrist. Four animals had bilateral transections with an interval of 2 to 4 months between surgeries and two animals received unilateral transections. The nerve deficit was then repaired with the aid of an operating microscope by either (1) a nerve autograft, in which a 4 mm segment of the nerve was removed, reversed, rotated 180° along its axis, and sutured to the proximal and distal nerve stumps with two 10-0 microsutures at each junction, or (2) a nerve guide repair, in which a 4 mm segment of nerve was removed and the proximal and distal nerve stumps sutured into the nerve guide with a single 10/0 suture at each stump. Clinically, an autografting procedure usually involves harvesting the sural nerve and performing a cable-grafting procedure. We reasoned that using the portion of excised me-

dian nerve would be a more rigorous control because it would allow a more accurate anastomosis than the smaller diameter sural nerve and yet not be too large to become well vascularized from the host vascular bed.

Beginning 1 month following surgery, serial assessments of motor and sensory nerve function were performed under general anaesthesia. The recovery of the compound muscle action potential (MAP) of the abductor pollicis brevis (APB) muscle of the thumb, which is exclusively innervated by the median nerve (see Fig. 28–6), was followed by stimulating the median nerve at the wrist and recording the MAP at the APB muscle. To assess sensory nerve function, the digital nerves of digit II were stimulated through surface ring electrodes or steel pins placed close to the nerves. The evoked sensory nerve action potential (SAP) was recorded via the same needle placed close to the median nerve at the wrist that was previously used to evoke the MAP (see Fig. 28–6). To detect the small SAP during early regeneration, 512 to 1024 responses were averaged, allowing recording of responses with amplitudes of $0.1\mu V$.

All of the animals tolerated the initial surgery and subsequent physiological procedures well; none of the monkeys displayed complications such as self-mutilation, pressure ulcers, sensory neglect, infection, overt signs of discomfort, or inability to use the affected hand for grooming or eating.

The MAP amplitude gradually recovered to the normal average in all monkeys within a period of 162 to 760 days (Fig. 28–16). The amplitude of the MAP reached the low normal value of 11 mV at an average of 226 days (range 174 to 314 days) after nerve guide repair and 320 days (range 229 to 616 days) after graft repair. This difference suggested that recovery might be faster with a nerve guide tube than with a graft.

To compare the rate of recovery of the MAP response between the two repair techniques we fit an exponential curve of the following type to the data:

$$\text{MAP amplitude} = a * e^{b/\text{days after section}}$$

where a is the final value reached and b is the slope of recovery. When fitted to the MAP amplitude of the individual nerves as a function of time, S-shaped regression curves with high correlation coefficients ($r = 0.7199–0.9866$, $p < 0.01$) were obtained for each of the nerves (Fig. 28–16). A paired t-test ($p < 0.02$) of the slopes of the curves suggested that recovery in

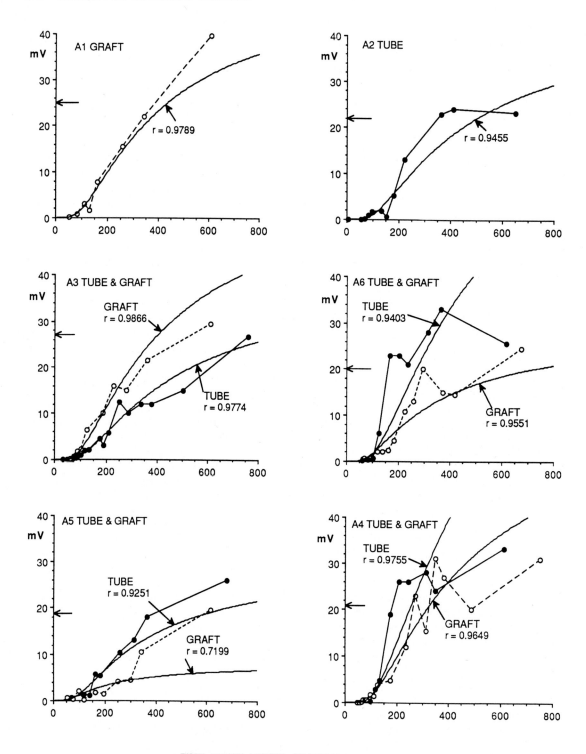

TIME AFTER NERVE SECTION (days)

Figure 28–16. Amplitude of the muscle action potential evoked at the wrist and recorded from the abductor pollicis brevis muscle as a function of time following nerve repair. The presurgery baseline levels for each animal are indicated by an arrow pointing to the ordinate. Curves, based on the least square method after logarithmic transformation, were fitted to values from nerves repaired with a collagen-based nerve guide tube *(solid line)* or by nerve autografting *(dashed line).* (From Archibald SJ, Krarup C, Shefner J, et al: A collagen-based nerve guide conduit for peripheral nerve repair. An electrophysiological study of nerve regeneration in rodents and nonhuman primates. J Comp Neurol 306:685–696. Copyright © 1991 by Wiley-Liss. Reprinted by permission of Wiley-Liss, a division of John Wiley and Sons, Inc.)

the nerve guide group was on average 28 percent faster than in the graft group (Fig. 28–17A). The final extrapolated value reached was not significantly different in the two groups. Similarly, the difference in amplitude of the final MAP recorded was not statistically different between the two groups (nerve guide: average 26.2 mV, range 19.4–33.2 mV; graft: 28.8 mV, range 19.6–39.7 mV). This final reading was performed on average 664 days (range 613 to 760) after nerve guide repair and 654 days (range 609 to 753) after graft repair.

In all cases the latency of the evoked MAP response from the APB returned to normal baseline levels (Fig. 28–17C). A comparison of the recovery rate of the MAP latency was made by using the same curve fit analysis as for the MAP amplitudes. The slopes and final values

of the recovery curves were similar in the nerves repaired by nerve guides and by grafts (p < 0.5).

The amplitudes of the evoked sensory response, obtained by stimulating digit II and recording the SAP at the level of the wrist in serial observations, are shown in Figure 28–17B. The same type of curve fit analysis as used for the MAP amplitudes revealed no statistically significant differences between the two groups in the recovery rate of SAP amplitude or conduction velocity or in the final level of recovery. The conduction velocity increased to 80 to 90 percent of normal mean conduction velocity (Fig. 28–17D).

Although the results from the monkey studies indicate a statistically significant increased rate of recovery of the MAP amplitude in nerves

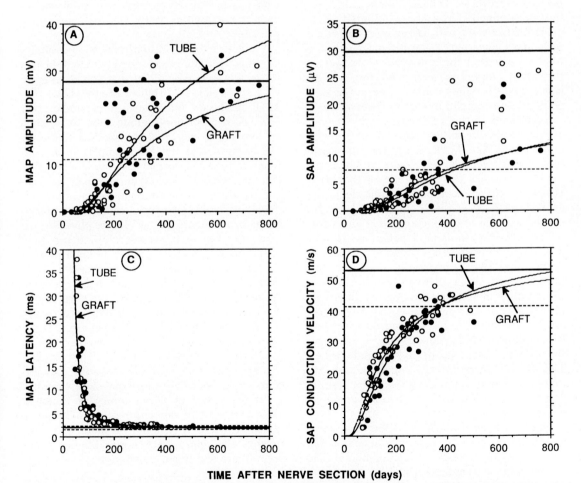

TIME AFTER NERVE SECTION (days)

Figure 28–17. Pooled assessments of motor and sensory function collapsed into graft *(open circle)* and tube *(solid circle)* treatment groups. The solid lines in each panel represent the mean normal value and the dotted lines represent the 95 percent confidence limits. The regression curves represent the mean from each of five nerves in the two treatment groups and are based on the least square method after logarithmic transformation. *A,* Amplitude of the evoked muscle action potential (MAP) abductor pollicis brevis. *B,* Amplitude of the evoked sensory nerve action potential (SAP). *C,* Latencies of the evoked MAP. *D,* Conduction velocities of the evoked SAP. (From Archibald SJ, Krarup C, Shefner J, et al: A collagen-based nerve guide conduit for peripheral nerve repair: An electrophysiological study of nerve regeneration in rodents and nonhuman primates. J Comp Neurol 306:685–696. Copyright © 1991 by Wiley-Liss. Reprinted by permission of Wiley-Liss, a division of John Wiley and Sons, Inc.)

repaired with conduits compared with nerve autografts, this difference must be interpreted with caution. The findings in this study are based on a small number of animals (N = 6), and the differences in rates of recovery varied markedly among animals. On inspection of the individual graphs of MAP amplitude recovery, it appears that three of the four bilaterally implanted animals (A4–6) showed an increased recovery rate of MAP amplitudes for the nerve repaired with a collagen nerve guide tube (Fig. 28–16). One of the four bilaterally implanted animals (A3) showed an increased recovery rate of MAP amplitudes for the nerves repaired with a nerve autograft, and the two animals that had unilateral short-gap repairs demonstrated equivalent rates of recovery. Perhaps the most accurate conclusion from these data is that nerve repair with a collagen nerve guide conduit is as effective as a nerve autograft. However, further work with larger numbers of animals and longer nerve gap distances will help to clarify whether the faster rate of recovery of the MAP amplitude seen with the collagen nerve guide conduits compared to nerve autografts is a meaningful biological observation.

Recordings of the SAP may provide a more accurate estimate of the degree of nerve regeneration than the MAP, since the amplifying effect of different muscle fibers in the motor units determines the amplitude of the MAP. However, the peak-to-peak amplitude of the evoked SAP is markedly influenced by the synchronization of conduction along fibers contributing to the compound potential. Thus in newly regenerated nerve compared to normal nerve, the SAP is markedly dispersed and therefore provides a relatively poor measure of the number of regenerated sensory fibers. In the monkey study, the SAP during late regeneration became better synchronized with similar amplitudes and recovery curves for nerve repair with autografts or nerve guide tubes. This finding suggests that the growth and maturation of nerve fibers into the distal sensory domain was similar with the two repair procedures.

The latency of the MAP and the conduction velocity of the SAP are measures of conduction velocity of the fastest conducting fibers. The latency and the conduction velocity are measures of the degree of maturation of the fastest conducting fibers and the recovery is influenced by both myelination and increases in the diameter of the regenerated fibers.[15, 16] The exponential recovery curves of both the MAP latency and the SAP conduction velocity were similar after nerve guide and autograft repair,

indicating that the conduction properties of the fastest conducting fibers and the degree of maturation were the same in the two groups.

We interpret the results from this study as very encouraging. One might expect that axonal regeneration in the nerve guide group would be somewhat delayed as well as suboptimal compared to that in the graft group, due to the 4 mm gap between nerve ends. Although the nerve autograft group also had a 4 mm distance to bridge, this gap was filled with the grafted nerve. Taken together, these data argue strongly that the nerve guide conduits promote rapid and functional nerve regeneration in nonhuman primates in vivo. This study demonstrates that in terms of recovery of the evoked compound muscle and sensory action potential, a bioresorbable collagen nerve guide was at least comparable in performance to an autologous nerve graft in both rats and nonhuman primates.

We have also begun to explore the possibility of using collagen-based nerve guide tubes to repair longer nerve defects that would be more clinically relevant. Figure 28–18 shows the MAP amplitude and latency in a monkey that received a 2 cm nerve guide tube to repair a 15 mm nerve defect of the median nerve. It can be seen that the MAP amplitude and latency returned to normal baseline levels within 600 to 700 days following nerve repair.

The results with nonhuman primates are valuable for several reasons. Most importantly, these experiments followed the physiological recovery over long periods of time (up to 2 years) rather than just making a single physiological assessment at the time of sacrifice. Such data allow comparison of not only the final degree of recovery but also the rate of recovery. As discussed previously, to avoid possible denervation atrophy of the end-organ target (e.g., muscle), one would like nerve regeneration to proceed as rapidly as possible. The monkey results are also important because the data are from a model of nerve injury that closely mimics a prevalent site of nerve injury in humans. However, even if rapid nerve regeneration is obtained, there is still the problem of reconnecting the appropriate nerve fibers to the appropriate end organ target.

Specificity of Functional Reinnervation

Perhaps the fundamental problem in peripheral nerve repair is the inability to direct the regenerating axons to reinnervate their original

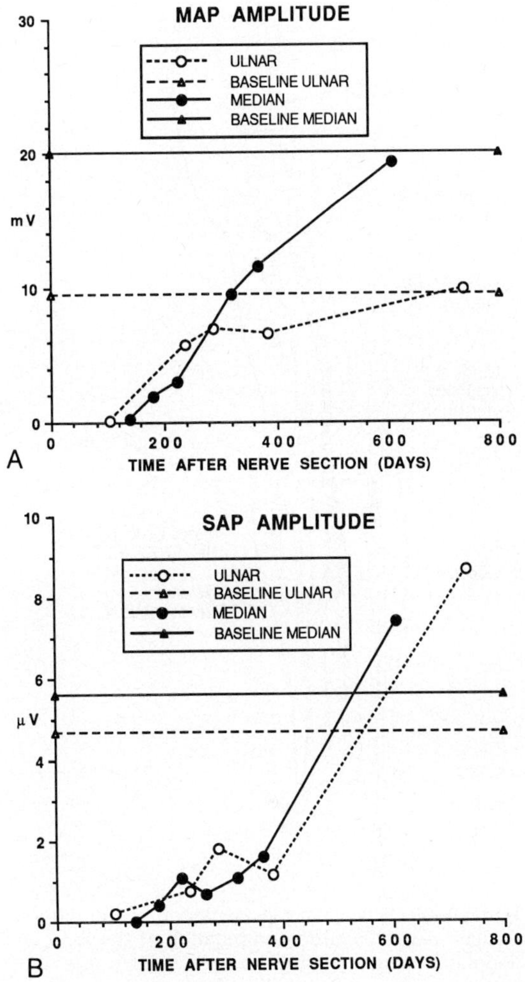

Figure 28–18. Evoked motor (MAP) and sensory (SAP) responses after repair of a 15 mm nerve gap with a long tube in the median and ulnar nerves. The nerves had previously been repaired with a polylactate nerve guide to bridge a 4 mm deficit. Note that these previous baseline levels were reached 600 to 750 days postimplantation of a 2 cm collagen nerve guide. B, Latency of the evoked MAP. (From Archibald SJ, Krarup C, Shefner J, et al: A collagen-based nerve guide conduit for peripheral nerve repair: An electrophysiological study of nerve regeneration in rodents and nonhuman primates. J Comp Neurol 306:685–696, 1991.)

targets. It is not enough for regenerating axons to simply successfully cross the injury site; if they do not reinnervate their original targets the result can be aberrant sensory and motor regeneration and recovery as illustrated by the following clinical case.[20]

Case History

M.M., a 22 year old male, had his left arm amputated at the distal third of the humerus in a combined section-avulsion injury in a motor vehicle accident. After a cold-ischemic time of 4 to 5 hours the arm was reattached at the humerus with a compression plate after shortening of the bone by 4 to 6 cm (Fig. 28–19). The brachial artery and communicating veins were anastomosed under the operating microscope.

Due to the combination of section and avulsion injuries of peripheral nerves, several different types of nerve repair were necessary over a period of 7 to 8 months for re-establishment of continuity of nerves, preparation of vascularized beds for nerve grafts, and repair of skin defects. The ulnar nerve was repaired by direct anastomosis, after minor resection of contused stumps, the day after the accident (Fig. 28–19). Seven months after the injury, after preparation of vascularized nerve beds, the median and radial nerves were reconstructed in stages. The median nerve had been avulsed high at the upper arm level and a large gap existed between proximal and distal stumps. Both vascularized and nonvascularized grafts were used to provide sufficient peripheral nerve graft material.

In spite of the severe injury, the extremity remained well vascularized and no necrosis of digits occurred. The first signs of motor recovery in the hand were seen approximately 9 months after the injury, and the first signs of sensation were present about 1 year after the injury. Over the next several years sensation to most modalities (e.g., pin prick, temperature,

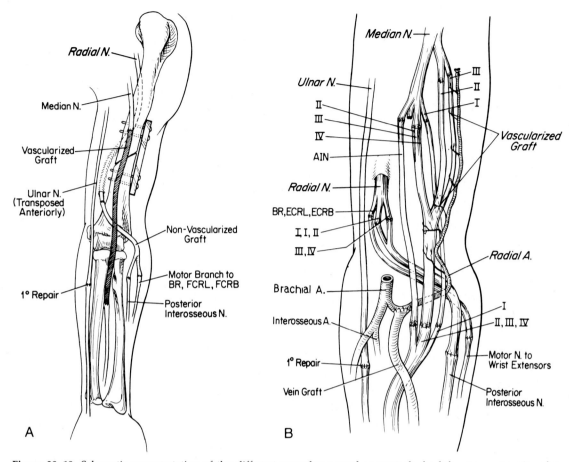

Figure 28–19. Schematic representation of the different procedures used to reattach the left upper extremity after traumatic section-avulsion amputation at the level of the humerus. *A,* The shaft of the humerus was fixed after shortening using a compression plate. The ulnar nerve was repaired by end-to-end suture (1° repair), the median nerve was repaired by combined vascularized and nonvascularized grafting, and the radial nerve was repaired by nonvascularized sural nerve grafting. *B,* The different fascicles of the median nerve were identified proximally by electrical stimulation and distally from Sunderland's fascicular anatomy. The vascularized graft was obtained from the denervated stump of the superficial radial nerve and the radial artery. The nerve was cut at the wrist, swung around with the artery, and the distal end was sutured to the proximal ends of the median nerve (fascicles supplying digits I, II, III, and motor fascicle to thenar muscles). Nonvascularized sural nerve grafts were used to connect the fascicle to the anterior interosseous nerve (AIN). The radial nerve to the wrist and finger extensors and sensory branches was anastomosed using sural nerve graft. The brachial artery was reconnected to the radial artery using a venous graft. (Br = brachioradialis; FCRL = flexor carpi radialis longus; FCRB = flexor carpi radialis brevis; ECRL = extensor carpi radialis longus; ELRB = extensor carpi radialis brevis; AIN = anterior interosseus nerve.) (From Krarup C, Upton J, Craeger MA: Nerve regeneration and reinnervation after limb amputation and replantation. Clinical and physiological findings. Muscle Nerve 13:291–304, 1990.)

light touch but not vibration) had returned to some extent. Although the sensation of touch had recovered, the localization of the touch stimulus was markedly deficient.

Extensive neurological and electrophysiological testing was carried out 3½ years after the injury. Touch stimuli were applied with a fine brush and the patient was asked to localize the stimulus on an observer's hand (Fig. 28–20). Localization was deficient within the median as well as the ulnar innervated areas. Some touch stimuli applied to the median innervated area of the digits and palm were localized to ulnar

innervated areas, suggesting aberrant reinnervation of median nerve–innervated areas by fibers from the ulnar nerve. There was no improvement of localization on follow-up tests up to 1 year after the first examination.

The clinical and physiological findings in this patient with extensive nerve injuries show that even in cases of severe injury, axonal regeneration in humans can occur over extremely long distances. However, the findings also indicate that the specificity of reinnervation is low, contributing to the poor prognosis for functional recovery following severe nerve injuries.

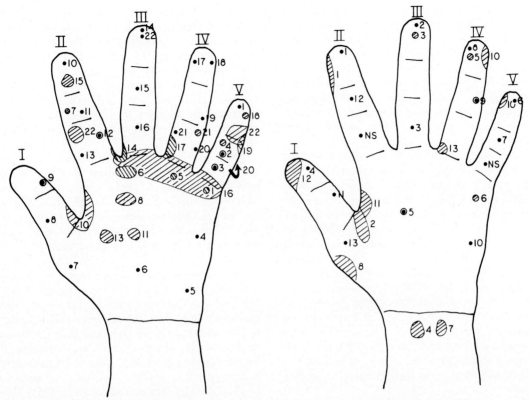

Figure 28–20. Localization of touch stimuli applied to the volar aspect of the reinnervated left hand on two occasions with a 7 month interval. The solid circles indicate the site of application using a fine brush and the correspondingly numbered hatched areas indicate the localization of the stimulus on an observer's hand. The size of the hatched area approximates the size of the area indicated by the patient. A solid circle within a large open circle indicates correct localization of the site of stimulation. NS denotes failure to appreciate the stimulus. As indicated, localization was deficient on both occasions. At some sites of stimulation, two areas were identified and there appeared to be overlap between median and ulnar innervated areas (e.g., #22 at digit III localized to both digit II and V). (From Krarup C, Upton J, and Craeger MA: Nerve regeneration and reinnervation after limb amputation and replantation: Clinical and physiological findings. Muscle Nerve 13:291–304, 1990.)

From the preceding section, it is clear that significant "mistakes" can be made by regenerating axons in terms of reinnervating appropriate end-organ targets. This mismatching of regenerating sensory and motor fibers results in impaired sensory and motor function. Two major unresolved questions within the field of peripheral nerve regeneration are how many axons selectively reinnervate their appropriate distal end-organ targets and what role these distal targets play in "neurotropic" guidance of regenerating axons. Recent animal studies have begun to address these questions experimentally.

Animal Experiments Regarding Specificity of Reinnervation

The hypothesis that distal targets can guide regenerating axons toward them was termed neurotropism, or chemotaxis, early in this century by Cajal.[58] In terms of appropriate reinnervation of targets during peripheral nerve regeneration, neurotropism would have to operate at three distinctly different levels of the peripheral nerve: (1) at the tissue level (generic neurotropism), whereby regenerating axons grow toward distal nerve stumps rather than nonnerve tissue such as surrounding connective tissue and skin; (2) at the level of the nerve trunk (specific neurotropism), as demonstrated by the growth of axons from motor neurons toward distal motor fascicles rather than sensory fascicles and vice versa; and (3) at the distal end-organ target, exemplified by the correct topographical reinnervation of muscle or the selective reinnervation of specific sensory receptors.

Brushart and Seiler[146, 147] have begun to study modality-specific regeneration (e.g., motor vs. sensory), utilizing the two terminal branches of the femoral nerve of the rat as a model. The femoral nerve of the rat divides into one purely sensory branch (continuing as the saphenous nerve and local cutaneous innervation) and a motor branch to the quadriceps muscle just distal to the inguinal ligament. Both branches are nearly equal in gross size and axoplasmic area, and the modality identity of the regenerated axons can be determined by retrograde transport of tracers from either branch to primary motor or sensory neurons.

Motor axons, when given equal access to the distal motor or sensory branches at the distal ends of a Y-shaped tube, will preferentially grow into the distal motor stump when the femoral nerve is inserted into the proximal stem of the tube.[147] This preferential reinnervation of the motor branch is also seen following simple transection and repair of the parent femoral nerve.[146] In these studies, sensory axons also displayed a greater affinity to reinnervate the sensory as opposed to the motor branch. As powerful as this model is, it was impossible to determine whether the motoneurons or sensory neurons that projected into the motor branch following transection and repair were from the original neuronal pools that projected into this branch.

Madison and colleagues[148–151] have refined the femoral nerve regeneration model to be able to determine on the individual motor and sensory neuron level how many neurons of the original neuron pool (both sensory and motor) have regenerated back into their original nerve stumps following transection and repair of the parent femoral nerve.

The neuronal pools to the quadriceps muscle in the rat can be permanently labeled by applying the fluorescent dye DiI (1,1′dioctadecyl-3,3,3′,3′ tetramethylindocarbocyanine perchlorate)[152] to the motor branch of the femoral nerve to the quadriceps muscle. The stump of the motor branch was inserted into a polyethylene tube and a 3% suspension of DiI was loaded into the tube via a custom syringe holder. Following a 1 hour exposure to the DiI, the polyethylene tube with the DiI was carefully removed, the proximal nerve stump carefully cleaned with saline to remove excess DiI, and the motor branch repaired with two 10-0 nylon sutures.[148–151]

For our qualitative pilot studies, three animals each were perfused following 1 or 2 week survival periods to check for the extent and quality of the DiI labeling. Animals were processed for qualitative examination by cryostat frozen section (24 μ thick) with dye-labeled motoneurons clearly visible in all animals. Although previous studies suggested that DiI was severely affected by frozen sectioning,[152] we had no difficulty with frozen sections. We suspect that this is because rather than picking the frozen section up on a microscope slide and allowing it to dry, we collected the frozen sections into buffer and examined them as wet-mounts. Although some label persists if the sections are allowed to air dry, the label is weaker than in wet-mounts and can become severely distorted.

Our qualitative analysis revealed (1) that there was a fairly consistent location of the motoneuron pool to the muscle, and (2) that although a survival time of 1 week was sufficient to label the motoneurons, a 2 week or greater survival time increased the intensity of the label such that localization and quantification would be easier.

For our quantitative experiments, we needed a second label which would be compatible with DiI and also display a similar efficacy of retrograde labeling. Ten animals received exposure to DiI as described, and 6 weeks later the motor branch of the femoral nerve was re-exposed, retransected immediately proximal to the original transection, and exposed to a 5% solution of Fluorogold.* Animals were perfused 5 days later and the spinal cords were processed for fluorescence histochemistry. Cryostat sections were cut at 24 μ and collected into buffer. Sections were then mounted onto glass slides, coverslipped with a glycerol solution with 0.04% p-phenylenediamine,[153] and examined with the fluorescence microscope. One animal died during the surgery, so only nine animals were available for quantitative analysis.

Fluorogold worked very well as the second tracer. The dye is quite stable in tissue from animals perfused with room-temperature solutions, it does not fade quickly during examination with the fluorescence microscope, and labeled neurons remain stable in tissue from animals perfused with room-temperature solutions. Labeled neurons remain stable for weeks to months in sections or tissue which are kept in the refrigerator. With this model, we have been able to demonstrate a greater than 98 percent overlap of the two tracers in the motoneuron pool to the quadriceps muscle. Results of the quantitative analysis of single and double labeled neurons are listed in Table 28–6.

These results can be analyzed in several different ways (Fig. 28–21). Most importantly, the very high degree of overlap of the two labels shows that both dyes not only labeled the same number of motoneurons but also la-

---

*Fluorochrome, Inc., Englewood, CO.

Table 28–6. SINGLE AND DOUBLE LABELED NEURONS 47 DAYS FOLLOWING DIL EXPOSURE AND 5 DAYS FOLLOWING FLUOROGOLD EXPOSURE TO THE MOTOR NERVE TO THE QUADRICEPS MUSCLE*

Animal (#)	Doubled Labeled	Dil Alone	Flurogold Alone	Total Motoneuron Pool
89-2-A1	354	1	22	355
89-2-A2	379	0	2	379
89-2-A3	321	2	0	323
89-2-A4	408	0	1	408
89-2-A5	431	2	13	433
89-2-A6	443	1	0	444
89-2-A7	424	1	0	425
89-2-A8	414	6	1	420
89-2-A9	393	4	2	397
Mean ± std. dev.	396±37	2±2	4.5±7.2	398±37

*All cell counts have been corrected for split cell counts using the formula by Konigsmark, 1970:[154] $t/(t+d)$ where t = thickness of section and d = mean nuclear diameter. We used 24-μ thick sections, and analysis of 100 labeled neurons yielded a mean nuclear diameter of 19 μ.

beled the exact same motoneurons when applied to the motor branch at widely spaced intervals. The number of double-labeled neurons represented neurons that originally projected an axon into the motor branch and that maintained that projection following transection and direct suture repair of the motor branch. By combining the double-labeled neurons and Dil-alone neurons, the average size of the original motoneuron pool (400 ± 40; mean ± std. dev.) could be estimated. The number of Dil-alone neurons represented original motoneurons that either did not survive the original transection, or withdrew their axons proximal to the site of Fluorogold application. The very small number of Fluorogold-alone neurons (4.5 ± 7.2; mean ± std. dev.) represented either motoneurons whose axons did not transport Dil or motoneurons that were labeled by leakage of the Fluorogold.

These data reveal several important aspects of this model system. (1) Applying Dil and Fluorogold to the motor branch at widely different times resulted in the vast majority of motoneurons becoming labeled with both dyes. (2) Following transection of the motor branch and direct suture repair, a very high percentage of motoneurons maintained their axonal projections into the motor branch (~98 to 99%). The number of motoneurons that either could not transport Dil or were spuriously labeled by Fluorogold was very small (<3%).

Taken as a whole, these data suggest that it is possible to reliably label the original motoneuron pool to the quadriceps muscle by a relatively short exposure to Dil. Motoneurons retain the Dil label for extended periods of time and thus for practical purposes, are permanently labeled according to their initial axonal projection. Also important is the fact that following the Dil procedure, virtually all of the original motoneuron pool still projects into the motor branch to the quadriceps. This is an extremely important point because if the process of labeling the original motoneuron pool to the muscle resulted in disruption of that pool, interpretation of the data would be impossible.

Because the femoral nerve is a mixed peripheral nerve that terminally divides into a purely motor branch (to the quadriceps muscle) and a purely sensory branch (saphenous nerve), it will be possible to directly test the hypothesis that neurotropism and/or neurotrophism exists at the level of a mixed nerve trunk following nerve transection and repair. Toward this end, we have begun to look at the degree of accuracy of regeneration in this model system following femoral nerve transection and repair.[148] In five rats that underwent the prelabeling protocol described previously and then received femoral nerve transection, all but 25 percent of the motor neurons had correctly regenerated into the motor branch by 4 weeks.

Using this technique, it will be possible to quantitatively compare various nerve repair strategies in terms of the degree of "correct" regeneration at the level of the individual neuron.

Factors Influencing Functional Clinical Outcome

Aspects of regeneration that influence recovery of function include elongation of neurites, maturation of regenerated axons, reinnervation

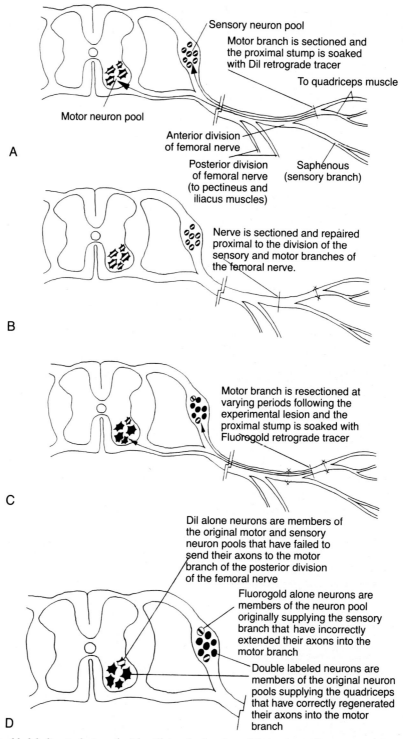

Figure 28–21. Double labeling technique for identifying the location of the motor and sensory neuron pools supplying axons in normal and regenerated peripheral nerve. *A,* The original neuron pools are labeled by applying a fluorescent retrograde tracer (DiI) to the motor branch of the femoral nerve to the quadriceps muscle. *B,* The experimental manipulation of the nerve trunk is performed proximal to the saphenous branch of the femoral nerve. *C,* Following varying periods of axonal regeneration, a second fluorescent retrograde tracer (Fluorogold) is applied distal to the experimental lesion and proximal to the primary labeling site. *D,* Thick sections of the dorsal root ganglions and the ventral motor columns of the spinal cord show populations of DiI alone, Fluorogold alone, and double labeled neurons.

of target organs, specificity of reinnervation, and possible associated plasticity of the central nervous system. It is likely that factors thought to influence functional recovery after lesions of the peripheral nervous system, including the age of the patient, the severity and site of the lesion, and the presence of underlying systemic disorders, can affect any or all of these regeneration variables.

Age. It is clinically accepted that recovery of function after nerve lesions is better in juveniles than in adults. For instance, children had greater recovery of two-point discrimination measured at least 5 years after nerve repair.[155] Buchthal and Kuhl[17] followed three patients with complete section and suture and one with partial section of the median nerve at the wrist. In these cases there was a relationship between the cumulative amplitude of the dispersed sensory action potential recorded with a near-nerve electrode and recovery of touch sensation. The recovery of both the electrophysiological parameters and the clinical deficit was three times faster in children than in adults. Tackmann and associates[156] also found a correlation between cumulative amplitude and two-point discrimination but not vibratory threshold. However, Ballantyne and Campbell[157] and Tallis and coworkers,[158] using surface electrodes to record the sensory nerve action potential, detected no relationship between recovery and age. Measurements of the rate of regeneration of sensory fibers in humans indicate a value of about 1 to 2 mm per day[17, 159] and of 1.0 to 2.5 mm per day in motor fibers.[160] Whether the rate is faster in children than in adults is uncertain.

In experimental animals there is little evidence regarding the specific influence of age on nerve regeneration. It has been suggested that recovery of physiological characteristics in rats is more complete in nerve crush performed before the age of 3 weeks compared with crush at 4 months.[161] However, it is well known that degeneration of the motoneuron and to some extent the sensory neuron takes place if the lesion occurs during the very early postnatal age.[162, 163] Such cell body degeneration would of course preclude regeneration, but it is unknown to what extent this phenomenon occurs in newborn humans.

Site and Type of Injury. There is little doubt that recovery following extensive injury is poorer than after less severe nerve lesions. This difference may be related to the fact that more extensive injury usually is localized more proximally along the limb than the less severe injury. Thomas and colleagues[164] showed that control of motor function after median or ulnar

nerve section and suture was better with distal rather than proximal lesions due to the greater degree of misdirection of regenerating axons. Although aberrant reinnervation is important when recovery is considered, growth of regenerating fibers may also be contributory, as indicated by the much better recovery of the ulnar than of the median nerve in the patient with a severe proximal lesion described in the case history presented earlier.[20] The ulnar nerve had been repaired by primary suture, whereas the extensive defect in the median nerve was repaired by nerve grafts. In Tackmann and associates' paper,[156] the values presented also suggested that recovery of the cumulative amplitude was more complete in nerves repaired with direct suture than when a nerve graft had been inserted. However, Ballantyne and Campbell[157] did not find such a difference.

Degeneration caused by acute crush of the nerve is relatively rare in humans[159] but has been extensively investigated in experimental animals.[19] Regeneration is usually rapid and complete due to the maintained connection of Schwann cell tubes across the lesion.[165] In monkeys, aberrant reinnervation of sensory receptors occurred to a much greater extent after nerve section and suture than after nerve crush, and recovery of receptor function was delayed and less complete.[166]

Reinnervation of receptors has been investigated in patients using microneurographic techniques.[167] Such studies indicate that, for example, pacinian corpuscles are not reinnervated following wallerian degeneration, confirming findings in the baboon.[166] Thus, even though sensory fibers can be demonstrated electrophysiologically and it can be shown that tactile receptors are reinnervated,[20] vibratory sensation is usually not recovered in patients with nerve lesions. This discrepancy emphasizes the fact that while physiological studies accurately indicate recovery of some functions, poor correlation exists between such studies and other sensory clinical aspects.

Aberrant reinnervation after section and suture of peripheral nerve is common. Such abnormalities in reinnervation are frequent early in the regeneration period but tend to decrease with time.[166] However, in humans, faulty localization of stimuli persists for many years after the nerve lesion;[168, 169] microneurographic studies done up to 12 years after the lesion indicate that receptor innervation remained abnormal.[170] Persistent disturbances in localization of touch stimuli occur in spite of attempts at re-education.[20, 167] In monkeys recovery of topographical organization of the cortex has been shown to occur after nerve crush, whereas disorganization remains after nerve section and suture.[171]

The persistent disturbances in sensory and motor function after nerve section and repair as opposed to nerve crush emphasize that functional recovery is a complex interaction among regeneration, reinnervation, maturation of morphological and physiological receptor and nerve fiber function, and alterations of central nervous system connections. All these factors have to be taken into consideration when the effects of the type and site of the nerve lesion and the age of the patient are evaluated.

Systemic Disorders. Regeneration of peripheral axons requires extensive changes in cell body metabolism and axonal transport. It is likely that underlying systemic or hereditary disorders in the individual patient have an effect on nerve regeneration. This relationship is poorly understood in humans, but it is of interest that regeneration in patients with alcoholic polyneuropathy is relatively rare,[172] suggesting that a possible toxic effect interferes with regeneration. On the other hand, regeneration of axons appeared to occur side-by-side with axon degeneration in cats intoxicated by acrylamide.[173] Even though disruption of axonal continuity is a strong stimulus for regeneration, nerve regeneration after crush injury in the rat intoxicated with acrylamide was markedly slowed and maturation was impaired,[174] suggesting that interference with neurofilament transport impaired the normal processes of nerve elongation, fiber caliber increase, and remyelination. In rats intoxicated with vincristine, which disrupts microtubules in the axon and causes a neuropathy in humans, regeneration after nerve crush was delayed as investigated electrophysiologically,[175] and the caliber and myelination of regenerated fibers were decreased.[176]

CONCLUSION

This chapter describes the basic anatomy and physiology of peripheral nerves as they relate to the repair of damaged peripheral nerves. Careful evaluation of the extent of peripheral nerve damage is crucial to the choice of treatment. This is especially important in determining whether the lesion results in loss of axonal continuity (axonotmesis) or the less severe simple loss of electrical conduction (neurapraxia).

Knowledge of the basic mechanisms of peripheral nerve regeneration is increasing rapidly, along with our understanding of neuronal growth factors and cell adhesion molecules that can influence primary neuronal survival and eventual axonal elongation. Specific non-neuronal cells and receptor expression and regulation are also important in peripheral nerve regeneration. There is a complicated interplay among non-neuronal cells, growth factors, cell adhesion molecules, and axons that leads to peripheral nerve regeneration. Perhaps the most basic problem in peripheral nerve regeneration is the ability (or lack thereof) of axons to correctly reinnervate their original targets.

The peripheral nerve surgeon faced with the daunting task of repairing human peripheral nerve injuries must choose from among the procedures available for repair of damaged peripheral nerves. However, it is still not clear which procedures are the most efficacious for a given nerve injury. It is not definitively known whether a vascularized graft performs better than a nonvascularized graft, or whether fascicular repair gives a better functional outcome than epineurial repair of a multifasciculated nerve.

Much more work needs to be done using quantitative models of peripheral nerve repair before the "best" nerve repair procedure is determined. It is encouraging, however, that rapid advances are being made in elucidating the basic mechanisms involved in axonal regeneration and pathway selection following peripheral nerve injury in animal models. The difficult task for the future will be to apply this experimental knowledge to the surgical and clinical treatment of human peripheral nerve injuries.

References

1. Medical Devices and Diagnostic Industry. Washington, DC, U.S. Government Printing Office, August 5, 1985, p. 3.
2. Sunderland S: Nerves and Nerve Injuries. New York, Churchill Livingstone, 1978.
3. Lubinska, L: Axoplasmic streaming in regeneration and in normal fibers. Prog Brain Res 13:1–17, 1964.
4. Friede RL, Samorajski T: Axon caliber related to neurofilaments and microtubules in sciatic nerve fibers of rats and mice. Anat Rec 167:379–387, 1970.
5. Thomas PK: The connective tissue of peripheral nerve: An electron microscope study. J Anat Lond 97:35–44, 1963.
6. Berthold C-H: Ultrastructure of the node-paranode of mature feline ventral and lumbar spinal-root fibres. Acta Soc Med Upsal (Suppl) 9:37–70, 1968.
7. Gamble HJ, Eames RA: An electrom microscope study of the connective tissues of human peripheral nerves. J Anat 99:655–663, 1965.
8. Thomas PK, Jones DG: The cellular response to nerve injury. II. Regeneration of the perineurium after nerve injury. J Anat 101:45–55, 1967.
9. Denny-Brown D: Importance of neural fibroblasts in the regeneration of nerve. Arch Neuro Psychiat Chicago 55:171–215, 1946.

10. Sunderland S, Bradley KC: The perineurium of peripheral nerves. Anat Rec 113:125–141, 1952.
11. Orsson Y: Studies on vascular permeability in peripheral nerves. IV. Distribution of intravenously injected protein tracers in the peripheral nervous system of various species. Acta Neuropathol (Berl) 17:114–126, 1971.
12. Seddon HJ: Surgical Disorders of the Peripheral Nerves. Baltimore, Williams & Wilkins, 1972.
13. Thomas PK: Clinical aspects of PNS regeneration. Adv Neurol 47:9–29, 1988.
14. Mackinnon SE, Dellon AL: Surgery of the Peripheral Nerve. New York, Thieme Medical Publishers, 1988.
15. Krarup C, Loeb GE: Conduction studies in peripheral cat nerve using implanted electrodes I. Methods and findings in controls. Muscle Nerve 11:922–932, 1988.
16. Krarup C, Loeb GE, Pezeshkpour GH: Conduction studies in peripheral cat nerve using implanted electrodes: II. The effects of prolonged constriction on regeneration of crushed nerve fibers. Muscle and Nerve 11:933–944, 1988.
17. Buchthal, F, Kuhl V: Nerve conduction, tactile sensibility, and the electromyogram after suture or compression of peripheral nerve: A longitudinal study in man. J Neurol Neurosurg Psychiatry 42:436–451, 1979.
18. Gilliatt RW, Fowler TJ, Redge P: Peripheral neuropathy in baboons. In Meldrum BS, Marsden CD (eds): Advances in Neurology, vol 10. New York, Raven Press, 1975, pp 253–272.
19. Krarup C, Gilliatt RW: Some effects of prolonged constriction on nerve regeneration in the rabbit. J Neurol Sci 68:1–14, 1985.
20. Krarup C, Upton J, Creager MA: Nerve regeneration and reinnervation after limb amputation and replantation: Clinical and physiological findings. Muscle Nerve 13:291–304, 1990.
21. Krarup C, Archibald S, Madison R, et al: Peripheral nerve regeneration supported by an implanted nerve guide tube: An electrophysiological study in the monkey. Muscle Nerve 11:977, 1988.
22. Berg DK: New neuronal growth factors. Ann Rev Neurosci 7:149–170, 1984.
23. Crutcher KA: The role of growth factors in neuronal development and plasticity. CRC Crit Rev Clin Neurobiol 2:297–333, 1986.
24. Walicke PA: Novel neurotrophic factors, receptors, and oncogenes. Ann Rev Neurosci 12:103–126, 1989.
25. Lipton SA: Growth factors for neuronal survival and process regeneration. Implications in the mammalian central nervous system. Arch Neurol 46:1241–1248, 1989.
26. Levi-Montalcini R, Hamburger V: Selective growth-stimulating effects of mouse sarcoma on the sensory and sympathetic nervous system of the chick embryo. J Exp Zool 116:321–361, 1951.
27. Levi-Montalcini R: The nerve growth factor 35 years later. Science 237:1154–1162, 1987.
28. Purves D: Body and Brain. A Trophic Theory of Neural Connections. Cambridge, Harvard University Press, 1988.
29. Lindsay RM, Thoenen H, Barde YA: Placode and neural crest–derived sensory neurons are responsive at early developmental stages to brain-derived neurotrophic factor. Dev Biol 112:319–328, 1985.
30. Hofer MM, Barde YA: Brain-derived neurotrophic factor prevents neuronal death in vivo. Nature 331:261–262, 1988.
31. D'Amore PA, Klagsbrun M: Endothelial cell mitogens derived from retina and hypothalamus: Biochemical

and biological similarities. Cell Biol 99:1545–1549, 1984.
32. Gospodarowicz D, Cheng J, Lui GM, et al: Isolation of brain fibroblast growth factor by heparin-sepharose affinity chromatography: Identity with pituitary fibroblast growth factor. Proc Natl Acad Sci USA 81:6963–6967, 1984.
33. Cordeiro PG, Madison R, Seckel BR: Acidic fibroblast growth factor (aFGF) enhances axon regeneration in a nerve guide model. Plast Reconstr Surg Mtg, 1988 (abstr).
34. Cordeiro, PG, Seckel BR, Lipton SA et al: Acidic growth factor enhances peripheral nerve regeneration in vivo. Plast Reconstr Surg 83:1013–1019, 1989.
35. Cuevas P, Baird A, Guillemin R: Stimulation of neovascularization and regeneration of the rat sciatic nerve by basic fibroblast growth factor. J Cell Biochem (Suppl) 11B:192, 1987 (abstr).
36. Danielsen N, Pettmann B, Vahlsing HL, et al: Fibroblast growth factor effects on peripheral nerve regeneration in a silicone chamber model. J Neurosci Res 20:320–330, 1988.
37. Gurney ME, Heinrich SP, Lee MR et al: Molecular cloning and expression of neuroleukin, a neurotrophic factor for spinal and sensory neurons. Science 234:566–574, 1986.
38. Gurney ME: Letter to the editor. Nature 332:456–457, 1988.
39. Varon S, Manthorpe M, Adler R: Cholinergic neuronotrophic factors. I. Survival, neurite outgrowth and choline acetyltransferase activity in monolayer cultures from chick embryo ciliary ganglia. Brain Res 173:29–45, 1979.
40. Lin L-FH, Mismer, D Lile, JD, et al: Purification, cloning, and expression of ciliary neurotrophic factor (CNTF). Science 246:1023–1025, 1989.
41. Lander AD: Understanding the molecules of neural cell contacts: Emerging patterns of structure and function. Trends in Neuroscience 12:189–195, 1989.
42. Edelman GM: Cell adhesion molecules in the regulation of animal form and tissue pattern. Annu Rev Cell Biol 2:81–116, 1986.
43. Jessell TM: Adhesion molecules and the hierarchy of neural development. Neuron 1:3–13, 1988.
44. Schachner M: Families of neural adhesion molecules. Ciba Foundation Symposium 145, pp 156–172.
45. Hay ED: Cell Biology of Extracellular Matrix. New York, Plenum Press, 1981.
46. Chiu AY, Matthew WD, Patterson PH: A monoclonal antibody that blocks the activity of a neurite regeneration-promoting factor: Studies on the binding site and its localization in vivo. Cell Biol 103:1383–1398, 1986.
47. Rogers SL, Letourneau PC, Palm SL, et al: Neurite extension by peripheral and central nervous system neurons in response to substratum-bound fibronectin and laminin. Dev Biol 98:212–220, 1983.
48. Kleinman HK, McGarvey ML, Hassel JR et al: Basement membrane complexes with biological activity. Biochemistry 25:312–318, 1986.
49. Madison R, Da Silva CF, Dikkes P, et al: Increased rate of peripheral nerve regeneration using bioresorbable nerve guides and a laminin containing gel. Exp Neurol 88:767–772, 1985.
50. Nieke J, Schachner M: Expression of the neural cell adhesion molecules L1 and N-CAM and their common carbohydrate epitope L2/HNK-1 during development and after transection of the mouse sciatic nerve. Differentiation 30:141–151, 1985.
51. Martini R, Schachner M: Immunoelectron-micro-

scopic localization of neural cell adhesion molecules (L1, N-CAM, MAG) and their shared carbohydrate epitope and myelin basic protein (MBP) in developing sciatic nerve. Cell Biol 103:2439–2448, 1988.

52. Seilheimer B, Schachner M: Regulation of neural cell adhesion molecule expression on cultured mouse Schwann cells by nerve growth factor. EMBO J 6:1611–1616, 1987.

53. Hall SM: Regeneration in the peripheral nervous system. Neuropathol Appl Neurobiol 15:513–529, 1989.

54. Leibovich SJ, Ross R: The role of the macrophage in wound repair. A study with hydrocortisone and anti-macrophage serum. Am J Path 78:71–99, 1975.

55. Hunt TK, Knighton DR, Thakral KK, et al: Studies on inflammation and wound healing: Angiogenesis and collagen synthesis stimulated in vivo by resident and activated wound macrophages. Surgery 96:48–54, 1984.

56. Baichwal RR, Bigbee JW, DeVries GH: Macrophage-mediated myelin-related mitogenic factor for cultured Schwann cells. Proc Natl Acad Sci USA 85:1701–1705, 1988.

57. Lindholm D, Heumann R, Meyer M, et al: Interleukin-1 regulates synthesis of nerve growth factor in non-neuronal cells of rat sciatic nerve. Nature (London) 330:658–659, 1987.

58. Cajal RS: Experiments dealing with the transplantation of nerves and their products designed to prove especially an attractive or neurotrophic action on nerve sprouts. Degeneration and Regeneration of the Nervous System. New York, Hafner Press, 1928, pp 329–361.

59. Taniuchi M, Clark HB, Johnson Jr EM: Induction of nerve growth factor receptor in Schwann cells after axotomy. Proc Natl Acad Sci USA 83:4094–4098, 1986.

60. Taniuchi M, Clark HB, Schweitzer JB, et al: Expression of nerve growth factor receptors by Schwann cells of axotomised peripheral nerves. Ultrastructural location, suppression by axonal contact. Neurosci 8:664–681, 1988.

61. Daniel RK, Terzis JK: Reconstructive Microsurgery. Boston, Little, Brown, 1977.

62. Terzis JK: Microreconstruction of Nerve Injuries. Philadelphia, WB Saunders, 1987.

63. Brushart TM, Mesulam MM: Alteration in connections between muscle and anterior horn motoneurons after peripheral nerve repair. Science 208:603–605, 1980.

64. Brushart TM, Tarlov E, Mesulam MM: A comparison of motor neuron pool organization after epineurial and perineurial repair of the rat sciatic nerve. Orthop Trans 4:19–20, 1980.

65. Brushart TM, Henry EW, Mesulam M: Reorganization of muscle afferent projections accompanies peripheral nerve regeneration. Neuroscience 6:2053–2061, 1981.

66. Orgel MG: Epineurial versus perineurial repair of peripheral nerves. In Terzis JK (ed): Microreconstruction of Nerve Injuries. Philadelphia, WB Saunders, 1987, pp 97–100.

67. Bento RF, Miniti A: Comparison between fibrin tissue adhesive, epineurial suture and natural union in infratemporal facial nerve of cats. Acta Otolaryngol (Suppl) 465:1–36, 1989.

68. Cruz NI, Debs N, Fiol RE: Evaluation of fibrin glue in rat sciatic nerve repairs. Plast Reconstr Surg 78:369–373, 1986.

69. Becker CM, Gueuning CO, Graff GL: Sutures or fibrin glue for divided rat nerves: Schwann cell and muscle metabolism. Microsurgery 6:1–10, 1985.

70. Freeman BS, Perry J, Brown D: Experimental study of surgical tape for nerve anastomosis. Plast Reconstr Surg 43:174–179, 1969.

71. Millesi H: Reappraisal of nerve repair. Surg Clin North Am 61:321–340, 1981.

72. Terzis JK, Faibisoff BA, Williams B: The nerve gap: Suture under tension versus graft. Plast Reconstr Surg 56:166–170, 1975.

73. Miyamoto Y, Tsuge K: Effects of tension on interneural microcirculation in end to end neurorrhaphy. In Gorio A, Millesi H, Mingrino S (eds): Post-traumatic Peripheral Nerve Regeneration. New York, Raven Press, 1981, pp 81–91.

74. Millesi H, Meissl G: Consequences of tension at the suture site. In Gorio A, Millesi H, Mingrino S (eds): Posttraumatic Peripheral Nerve Regeneration. New York, Raven Press, 1981, pp 277–279.

75. Taylor GI, Ham FJ: The free vascularized nerve graft. Plast Reconstr Surg 57:413–426, 1976.

76. Bonney G, Birch R, Jamieson AM, et al: Experience with vascularized nerve grafts. In Terzis JK (ed): Microreconstruction of Nerve Injuries. Philadelphia, WB Saunders, 1987, pp 403–414.

77. Settergren CR, Wood MB: Comparison of blood flow in free vascularized versus nonvascularized nerve grafts. J Reconstr Microsurg 1:95–101, 1984.

78. Lind R, Wood MB: Comparison of the patterns of early revascularization of conventional versus vascularized nerve grafts in the canine. J Reconstr Microsurg 2:229–234, 1986.

79. Seckel BR, Ryan SE, Simons JE, et al: Vascularized versus nonvascularized nerve grafts. An experimental structural comparison. Plast Reconstr Surg 78:211–220, 1986.

80. Gu YD, Wu MM, Zheng Y, et al: Arterialized venous free sural nerve grafting. J Plast Surg 15:332–339, 1985.

81. Gilbert A: Vascularized sural nerve graft. In Terzis JK (ed): Microreconstruction of Nerve Injuries. Philadelphia, WB Saunders, 1987, pp 117–126.

82. Terzis JK, Breidenbach WC: The anatomy of free vascularized nerve grafts. In Terzis JK (ed): Microreconstruction of Nerve Injuries. Philadelphia, WB Saunders, 1987, pp 101–116.

83. Chow JA, Van Beek AL, Meyer DC, et al: Surgical significance of the motor fascicular group of the ulnar nerve in the forearm. J Hand Surg 10:867–872, 1985.

84. Jabaley ME, Wallace WH, Heckler FR: Internal topography of major nerves in the forearm and hand: A current view. J Hand Surg 5:1–18, 1980.

85. Williams HB, Jabaley, ME: The importance of interneural anatomy of the peripheral nerves to nerve repair in the forearm and hand. Hand Clin 2:689–707, 1986.

86. Shizhen Z, Xiangluo T, Muzhil I: The microsurgical anatomy of peripheral nerves. In Shizhen Z, Youngjian H, Wencyun Y (eds): Microsurgical Anatomy. Lancaster, England, MTP Press, 1985, pp 299–350.

87. He YS, Zhong SZ: Acetylcholinesterase: Histochemical identification of motor and sensory fascicles in human peripheral nerve and its use during operation. Plast Reconstr Surg 82:125–132, 1988.

88. Peyronnard JM, Charron L, Lavoie J, et al: Carbonic anhydrase and horseradish peroxidase: Double labelling of rat dorsal root ganglion neurons innervating motor and sensory peripheral nerves. Anat Embryol 177:353–359, 1988.

89. Hakstian RW: Funicular orientation by direct stimulation: An aid to peripheral nerve repair. J Bone Joint Surg 50:1178–1186.

90. Gaul JS: Electrical fascicle identification as an adjunct to nerve repair. Hand Clin 2:709–722, 1986.

91. Williams HB: The painful stump neuroma and its treatment. In Terzis JK (ed): Microreconstruction of Nerve Injuries. Philadelphia, WB Saunders, 1987, pp 161–171.

92. Dellon AL, Mackinnon SE: Basic scientific and clinical applications of peripheral nerve regeneration. Surg Ann 20:59–100, 1988.

93. Millesi H: Nerve grafting. Chap. 18. In Terzis JK (ed): Microreconstruction of Nerve Injuries. Philadelphia, WB Saunders, 1987, pp 223–237.

94. Zachery RB, Homes W: Primary suture of nerves. Surg Gynecol Obstet 82:632–651, 1946.

95. Highet WB, Sanders FK: The effects of stretching nerves after suture. Br J Surg 30:355–363, 1943.

96. Lundborg G, Longo FM, Varon S: Nerve regeneration model and trophic factors in vivo. Brain Res 232:157–161, 1982.

97. Longo FM, Skaper SD, Manthorpe M, et al: Temporal changes of neuronotrophic activities accumulating in vivo within nerve regeneration chambers. Exp Neurol 81:756–769, 1983.

98. Lundborg G, Gelberman RH, Longo FM, et al: In vivo regeneration of cut nerves encased in silicone tubes. J Neuropathol Exp Neurol 41:412–422, 1982.

99. Lundborg G, Dahlin LB, Danielsen N, et al: Nerve regeneration in silicone chambers: Influence of gap length and of distal stump components. Exp Neurol 76:361–375, 1982.

100. Reid, RL, Cutright DE, Garrison JS: Biodegradable cuff an adjunct to peripheral nerve repair: A study in dogs. Hand 10:259–266, 1978.

101. Dellon AL, Mackinnon SE: Alternative to the classical nerve graft with a bioabsorbable polyglycolic acid tube. Plastic Reconstr Surg 82:849–856, 1988.

102. Uzman BG, Villegas GM: Mouse sciatic nerve regeneration through semipermeable tubes: A quantitative model. J Neurosci Res 9:325–338, 1983.

103. Hurtado H, Knoops B, DeAguilar P: Rat sciatic nerve regeneration in semipermeable artificial tubes. Exp Neurol 97:751–757, 1987.

104. Aebischer P, Valentini RF, Dario P, et al: Piezoelectric guidance channels enhance regeneration in the mouse sciatic nerve after axotomy. Brain Res 436:165–168, 1987.

105. Aebischer P, Guenard V, Winn SR, et al: Blind-ended semipermeable guidance channels support peripheral nerve regeneration in the absence of a distal nerve stump. Brain Res 454:179–187, 1988.

106. Molander H, Olsson Y, Engkvist O, et al: Regeneration of peripheral nerve through a polyglactin tube. Muscle Nerve 5:54–57, 1982.

107. Noback CR, Husby J, Giorado JM, et al: Neural regeneration across long gaps in mammalian peripheral nerves: Early morphological findings. Anat Rec 131:633–647, 1958.

108. Young BL, Begovac P, Stuart DG, et al: An effective sleeving technique in nerve repair. J Neurosci Meth 10:51–58, 1984.

109. Zachery RB, Holmes W: Primary suture of nerves. Surg Gynecol Obstet 82:632–651, 1946.

110. Weiss P, Davis H: Pressure block in nerves provided with arterial sleeves. J Neurophysiol 6:269–286, 1943.

111. Weiss P, Taylor AC: Guides for nerve regeneration across gaps. J Neurosurg 3:375–389, 1946.

112. Lungborg G, Dahlin LB, Danielsen NP, et al: Reorganization and orientation of regenerating nerve fibers, perineurium, and epineurium in preformed mesothelial tubes: an experimental study on the sciatic nerve of rats. J Neurosci Res 6:265–281, 1981.

113. Braun RM: Experimental peripheral nerve repair tubulation. Surg Forum 15:452–454, 1964.

114. Kline DG, Hayes GJ: The use of a resorbable wrapper for peripheral nerve repair. J Neurosurg 21:737–750, 1964.

115. Archibald SJ, Krarup C, Shefner J, et al: Semipermeable collagen-based nerve guide tubes are as effective as standard nerve grafts to repair transected peripheral nerves: An electrophysiological study in the non-human primate. Soc Neurosci Absts 15:125.18, 1989.

116. Archibald SJ, Krarup C, Shefner J, et al: A collagen-based nerve guide conduit for peripheral nerve repair: An electrophysiological study of nerve regeneration in rodents and non-human primates. J Comp Neurol 306:685–696, 1991.

117. Archibald SJ, Madison R: Functional recovery following rat sciatic nerve regeneration through collagen nerve guide tubes: Comparison of direct anastomosis, nerve graft and entubulation repair. Soc Neurosci Absts 14:204.7, 1988.

118. MacKinnon S, Dellon L, Hudson A, et al: Nerve regeneration through a pseudosynovial sheath in a primate model. Plast Reconstr Surg 75:833–839, 1984.

119. Madison R, Disman RL, Myilas E, et al: Non-toxic nerve guide tubes support neovascular growth in transected rat optic nerve. Exp Neurol 86:448–461, 1984.

120. Nyilas E, Chiu TH, Sidman et al: Peripheral nerve repair with bioresorbable prosthesis. Trans Am Soc Artif Intern Organs 29:307–313, 1983.

121. Henry EW, Chiu TH, Nyilas E, et al: Nerve regeneration through biodegradable polyester tubes. Exp Neurol 90:652–656, 1985.

122. Merle M, Dellon, AL, Campbell JN, et al: Complications from silicone-polymer intubulation of nerves. Microsurgery 10:130–133, 1989.

123. Aebischer P, Guenard V, Brace S: Peripheral nerve regeneration through blind-ended semipermeable guidance channels: Effect of the molecular weight cutoff. J Neurosci 9:3590–3595, 1989.

124. Akers RM, Mosher DF Lilien JE: Promotion of retinal neurite outgrowth by substrate bound fibronectin. Dev Biol 86:179–188, 1981.

125. Hall DE, Neugebauer KM, Richardt LF: Embryonic neural retinal cell response to extracellular matrix proteins: Developmental changes and effects of the cell substratum attachment antibody (CSAT). J Cell Biol 104:623–634, 1987.

126. Madison RD, Da Silva CF, Dikkes P: Entubulation repair with protein additives increases the maximum nerve gap distance successfully bridged with tubular prostheses. Brain Res 447:325–334, 1988.

127. Satou T, Nishida S, Hirama S, et al: A morphological study of the effects of collagen gel matrix on regeneration of severed rat sciatic nerve in silicone tubes. Acta Pathol Jpn 36:199–208, 1986.

128. Williams LR, Varon S: Modification of fibrin matrix formations in situ enhances nerve regeneration in silicone chamber. J Comp Neurol 231:209–220, 1985.

129. Valentini RF, Aebischer P, Winn SR, et al: Collagen and laminin-containing gels impeded peripheral nerve regeneration through semipermeable nerve guidance channels. Exp Neurol 98:350–356, 1987.

130. Williams LR, Longo FM Powell HC, et al: Spatial-temporal progress of peripheral nerve regeneration within a silicone chamber: Parameters for a bioassay. J Comp Neurol 218:460–470, 1983.

131. Scaravilli F: The influence of distal environment on peripheral nerve regeneration across a gap. J Neurocytol 13:1027–1041, 1984.

132. Jenq CB, Coggeshall RE: Numbers of regenerating axons in parent and tributary peripheral nerves in the rat. Brain Res 326:27–40, 1985.

133. Kljavin IJ, Madison RD: PNS axonal regeneration within tubular prostheses: effects of laminin and collagen matrices on cellular ingrowth. Scanning Microsc 1:17–29, 1991.

134. McCaffery CA, Raju TR, Bennett MR: Effects of cultured astroglia on the survival of neonatal rat retinal ganglion cells in vivo. Dev Biol 104:441–448, 1984.

135. Nobel M, Fok-Seang J, Cohen J: Glia are a unique substitute for the in vitro growth of central nervous system neurons. J. Neurosci 4:1892–1903, 1984.

136. Fallon JR: Preferential outgrowth of central nervous system neurites on astrocytes and Schwann cells as compared with nonglial cells in vitro. J Cell Biol 100:198–207, 1985.

137. Kleitman N, Simon DK, Schachner M, et al: Growth of embryonic retinal neurites elicited by contact with Schwann cell surfaces is blocked by antibodies to L1. Exp Neurol 102:298–306, 1988.

138. Rosen JM, Hentz VR, Kaplan EN: Fascicular tubulization: A cellular approach to peripheral nerve repair. Ann Plast Surg 11:397–411, 1983.

139. Molander H, Engkvist O, Haaglund J, et al: Nerve repair using a polyglactin tube and nerve graft: An experimental study in the rabbit. Biomaterials 4:276–280, 1983.

140. Restrepo Y, Merle M, Michon J, et al; Fascicular nerve graft using an empty perineurial tube: An experimental study in the rabbit. Microsurgery 4:105–112, 1983.

141. Fields RD, Ellisman MH: Axons regenerated through silicone tube splices: Conduction properties. Exp Neurol 92:48–60, 1986.

142. Ashur H, Vilner Y, Finsterbush A, et al: Extent of fiber regeneration after peripheral nerve repair: Silicone splint versus suture, gap repair versus graft. Exp Neurol 97:365–374, 1987.

143. Field RD, Ellisman MH: Axons regenerated through silicone tube splices: Functional morphology. Exp Neurol 92:61–74, 1986.

144. Li S-T, Archibald SJ, Krarup C, et al: The development of collagen nerve conduits that promote peripheral nerve regeneration. Adv Biopolymer Tech. In press.

145. MacKinnon SE, Hudson AR, Hunter DA: Histologic assessment of nerve regeneration in the rat. Plast Reconstr Surg 76:384–488, 1985.

146. Brushart TME, Preferential reinnervation of motor nerves by regenerating motor axons. J Neurosci 8:1026–1031, 1987.

147. Brushart TME, Seiler WA: Selective reinnervation of distal motor stumps by peripheral motor axons. Exp. Neurol 97:289–300, 1987.

148. Madison RD, Archibald SJ, Meadows S: Permanent labeling of motoneuron pools: Accuracy of regeneration analyzed at the single neuron level. Soc Neurosci Absts 16:336.2, 1990.

149. Madison RD, Archibald SJ: Single neuron level analysis of the accuracy of regeneration of a motor neuron pool to appropriate target muscle. Proc 3rd Vienna Muscle Symposium. In press.

150. Harsh C, Archibald SA, Madison RD: Double labelling of saphenous nerve neuron pools: A model for determining the accuracy of regeneration at the single neuron level. J Neurosci Meth (In Press).

151. Harsh C., Archibald SJ, Madison RD: Double labeling of saphenous nerve neuron pool allows determination of accuracy of axon regeneration at the single neuron

152. level, 1991 Meeting Joint Section on Disorders of the Spine and Peripheral Nerves. Am Assoc Neurol Surg Congress of Neurol Surg, New Orleans, 1991.

152. Godement P, Vanselow J, Thanos S, et al: A study in developing visual systems with a new method of staining neurones and processes in fixed tissue. Development 101:697–713, 1987.

153. Dodd J, Solter D, Jessel TM: Monoclonal antibodies against carbohydrate differentiation antigens identify subsets of primary sensory neurons. Nature 311:469–472, 1984.

154. Konigsmark BE: Methods for the counting of neurons. In Nauta WJH, Ebbesson SOE (eds): Contemporary Research Methods in Neuroanatomy. New York, Springer-Verlag, 1970, pp 315–340.

155. Almquist E, Eeg-Olofsson O: Sensory-nerve conduction velocity and two-point discrimination in sutured nerves. J Bone Joint Surg 32A:791–796, 1979.

156. Tackmann W, Brennwald J, Nigst H: Sensory electroneurographic parameters and clinical recovery of sensibility in sutured human nerves. J Neurol 229:195–206, 1983.

157. Ballantyne JP, Campbell MJ: Electrophysiological study after surgical repair of sectioned human peripheral nerves. J Neurol Neurosurg Psychiatry 36:797–805, 1973.

158. Tallis R, Staniforth P, Fisher TR: Neurophysiological studies of autogenous sural nerve grafts. J Neurol Neurosurg Psychiatry 41:677–683, 1978.

159. Trojaborg W: Rate of recovery in motor and sensory fibres of the radial nerve: Clinical and electrophysiological aspects. J Neurol Neurosurg Psychiatry 33:625–638, 1970.

160. Hodes R, Larrabe MG, German W: The human electromyogram in response to nerve stimulation and the conduction velocity of motor axons. Arch Neurol Psychiatry 60:340–365, 1948.

161. Bowe CM, Kocsis JD, Waxman SG, et al: Physiological properties of regenerated rat sciatic nerve following lesions at different postnatal ages. Dev Brain Res 34:123–131, 1987.

162. Schmalbruch H: Motoneuron death after sciatic nerve section in newborn rats. J Comp Neurol 224:252–258, 1984.

163. Schmalbruch H: Loss of sensory neurons after sciatic nerve section in the rat. Anat Rec 219:323–329, 1987.

164. Thomas CK, Stein RB, Gordon T, et al: Patterns of reinnervation and motor unit recruitment in human hand muscles after complete ulnar and median nerve section and resuture. J Neurol Neurosurg Psychiatry 50:259–268, 1987.

165. Thomas PK: Invited review: Focal nerve injury: Guidance factors during axonal regeneration. Muscle Nerve 2:796–802, 1989.

166. Terzis JK, Dykes RW: Reinnervation of glabrous skin in baboons: Proportion of cutaneous mechanoreceptors subsequent to nerve transection. J Neurophysiol 44:1214–1225, 1980.

167. Mackel R: Human cutaneous mechanoreceptors during regeneration: Physiology and interpretation. Ann Neurol 18:165–172, 1985.

168. Ford FR, Woodhall B: Phenomena due to misdirection of regenerating fibers of cranial, spinal, and autonomic nerves. Arch Surg 36:480–496, 1938.

169. Hawkins GL: Faulty sensory localization in nerve regeneration: An index of functional recovery following suture. J Neurosurg 5:11–18, 1948.

170. Hallin RG, Wiesenfeld Z, Lindblom U: Neurophysiological studies on patients with sutured median nerves: Faulty sensory localization in nerve regener-

ation and its physiological correlates. Exp Neurol 73:90–106, 1981.

171. Wall JT, Felleman DJ, Kaas JH: Recovery of normal topography in the somatosensory cortex of monkeys after nerve crush and regeneration. Science 221:771–773, 1983.

172. Behse F, Buchthal F: Alcoholic neuropathy: clinical, electrophysiological, and biopsy findings. Ann Neurol 2:95–110, 1977.

173. Schaumburg HH, Wisniewski HM, Spencer PS: Ultrastructural studies of the dying-back process. I. Peripheral nerve terminal and axon degeneration in systemic acrylamide intoxication. J Neuropathol Exp Neurol 33:260–284, 1974.

174. Morgan-Hughes JA, Sinclair S, Durston JHJ: The pattern of peripheral nerve regeneration induced by crush in rats with severe acrylamide neuropathy. Brain 97:235–250, 1974.

175. Shiraishi S, Le Quesne PM, Gajree T: The effect of vincristine on nerve regeneration in the rat. An electrophysiological study. J Neurol Sci 71:9–17, 1985.

176. Shiraishi S, Le Quesne PM, Gajree T, et al: Morphometric effects of vincristine on nerve regeneration in the rat. J Neurol Sci 71:165–181, 1985.

V

CLINICAL MANAGEMENT OF HEALING TISSUES

29

FACTITIOUS PROBLEMS IN WOUND HEALING

Scott Brenman, M.D., and Donald Serafin, M.D.

Factitious, or self-induced, disorders were known to Hippocrates,[1] and physicians since have had the challenge of diagnosing and treating patients who either initiated their condition or interfered with their recovery. Such patients both fascinate and torment the treating physician who has been trained to believe that every patient would like to get well. The physician accepts with difficulty, and frequently anger, a patient found to be contributing to his or her own problem. Factitious disorders are often diagnosed only after exhaustive, expensive, and often invasive studies have failed to produce another cause. Not only misled in the diagnosis, the physician may in fact have been an unknowing accomplice in the patient's scheme to remain in the sick role. By being aware of the nature of factitious disorders, recognizing the personality types prone to these conditions, and understanding the psychopathology involved, physicians can diagnose and more effectively treat these most complex problems.

PSYCHIATRIC PROFILES

The skin is highly vulnerable to self-inflicted lesions because it is so accessible and because it serves as an important medium of communication between the individual and the social environment.[2] As a barrier, the skin may yield to pressures from both inside and out. Disorders of wound healing may be manifestations of psychoneuroses. Sufferers of factitious skin lesions can range from the sane but dishonest (typical malingerers) to the severely disturbed, as in Munchausen's syndrome.[3] The increase in

third party payers and disability insurance has led to a proliferation of these cases in physicians' offices, clinics, and hospitals.[4] The true incidence of factitious wounds remains unknown, though it is probably much higher than appreciated because of the lack of awareness of this problem and the difficulty in establishing the diagnosis.

Although various personality disorders are associated with factitious skin disorders, the best known, because of its bizarre manifestations, is Munchausen's syndrome, first defined by Ascher in 1951.[5] Named in memory of Baron Karl Freidrich Hieronymous von Munchausen, an 18th century cavalry officer who enjoyed a reputation for telling wildly exaggerated tales of his life, this syndrome denotes an impostor who typically wanders from one emergency room to the next seeking attention for fraudulent medical claims. The Munchausen patient typically feigns severe illness or injury, presents a dramatic but plausible history, and is willing to undergo extensive and often invasive diagnostic and therapeutic procedures for the self-inflicted problem. These patients usually have a history of frequent hospitalizations and show evidence of many previous operations. When confronted about a possible factitious etiology for their problem, they typically become aggressive and unruly and depart the hospital against medical advice. Oftentimes, no ulterior motive is evident for their behavior, though many satisfy a need to be the center of interest and attention by submitting to the patient role. Others may truly hold a grudge against doctors and hospitals and find satisfaction in deceiving them. The desire for drugs, free lodging, and escape from the police are more obvious motives for their behavior, although these are frequently well hidden behind elaborately contrived clinical presentations. It is likely that various personality disorders such as masochism, hysteria, schizophrenia, or other neuroses and psychoses underlie this disorder. Munchausen's syndrome (discussed further under Personality Disorders) is only part of the spectrum of factitious wound healing problems which will be further described.

By inflicting various injuries or exacerbating pre-existing lesions, patients may seek secondary gain such as attention, sympathy, financial reward, drugs, relief from career or family responsibilities, or protracted dependency from the sick role they maintain. Usually such patients display some abnormal psychological features that are apparent except to the patient and the family.[6] According to the DSMIII classification of the American Psychiatric Association, the characteristics of patients with factitious wounds fall along the spectrum of borderline personalities, from malingerers to neurotics to psychotics. Each of these psychopathologies will be discussed individually, although there does tend to be considerable overlap between the categories.

Malingerers

Malingerers (the term originally was applied to soldiers seeking to evade duty) deliberately and consciously attempt to simulate symptoms or injury to deceive the physician and achieve their own selfish ends. Malingerers may employ chemical, mechanical, or bacterial agents to induce their desired effect, and the resulting signs and symptoms may be completely baffling to the unsuspecting physician.[7] This type of self-mutilator feigns severe pain and disability, although he inflicts wounds upon himself without regard for the pain.[8] The patient, usually male, generally denies any knowledge of the cause of the lesions and radiates a nonchalance and objectivity out of context with the supposed degree of injury. Similarly, there is usually a marked discrepancy between the disability claimed by the patient and the actual physical findings.[9] The malingerer frequently reacts unfavorably to suggested diagnostic studies and is poorly compliant with treatment regimens.

Menninger isolated the essential elements in malingering as wishes for suffering, concealment, self-injury, and provocation of distress in others.[10] Malingerers also tend to be masochistic and exhibitionistic.[11] In their efforts to deceive, these patients indicate a displacement of aggression from the original source onto the unsuspecting physician. They initiate a competitive contest with the physician and when the deceit is uncovered, they receive their "punishment."[8] Because of this deeper motivation plus the need to derive secondary gain from their disorders, they likely will discharge themselves from the care of the physician whose efforts are primarily directed towards their recovery.

When confronted with a patient harboring both a suspicious lesion and features of antisocial behavior, the physician must ask what the patient has to gain from his disability. It is suggested that the physician sufficiently suspicious of a factitious etiology should confront the patient with the possibility, though it will likely be denied. The physician should recommend psychiatric evaluation as part of the treatment plan.

Personality Disorders

The highly complex factors in the make-up of patients who cannot adequately control the release of psychic energy may cause acts of self-mutilation. Unlike malingering, in which the material objective is fairly obvious, the most notable feature of psychiatric disturbances associated with factitious wounding is the apparent senselessness of it. However, the intrapsychic gains from suffering and prolonged disability are a result of poorly adapted response to stress in an unbalanced personality. There is no better example of this maladaptation than in the Munchausen patient previously described. The underlying psychopathology is varied and the psychodynamics have yet to be clearly defined, though pathological lying and deceit are at the center of the syndrome.[12] The very term "Munchausen" connotes pleasure in lying and these patients need to deceive and experience the feeling of superiority over those who have been "duped."[13] Frequently, Munchausen patients have had some relationship with a physician who was an important figure in their childhood, either as a parent or authority figure.[6] The physician became an object of love and hate, and by assuming the patient role the Munchausen patient is able to remain close to doctors while finding satisfaction in frustrating them. These patients frequently work in allied health fields and may gain a credible medical knowledge which enables them to present with a very elaborate and convincing history. However, once their deception is revealed, they typically become belligerent and leave the hospital against medical advice in pursuit of another unwitting physician who will accept their story and comply with their subconscious need for suffering. Crippling deformities and incapacitating operative procedures have been borne with fortitude in pursuit of their objectives.[11] This masochistic behavior may connote a pathological way of living and their wandering from one hospital to the next may be a search for intimacy.[14]

Neuroses

Neurotic excoriators tend to inflict or perpetuate their lesions because of poor coping with immediate situational crises, usually involving family or work. Typically female, with a peak age of onset between 30 and 45, the neurotic excoriator freely admits her morbid preoccupation with the skin.[8] To some degree she recognizes the compulsive nature of her behavior, but she does not understand why she does it, nor is she necessarily concerned about the scarring she is causing. These patients tend to be underaggressive, passive, and dependent. They may have repressed hostility toward authority and seek self-punishment out of guilt for the hostility. Described by Menninger as "focal suicide,"[10] the behavior of the neurotic excoriator arises from primary aggressive tendencies directed toward herself. While able to function marginally most of the time, a new source of stress may lead to a misguided response. For example, an elderly parent living with the patient may lead her to feel resentment for her burden, and out of guilt for such feelings she may turn the hostility towards herself.

Most neurotic excoriators are unaware of the cause and effect relationship between their neurotic behavior and their disease, although they will admit to scratching or treating their wounds.[3] Psychiatric therapy is sought to help provide some insight into the patient's self-directed aggression. No attempt to stop the excoriating by admonishing the patient will work. On occasion antianxiety or antidepressant medications such as benzodiazapam, amitriptyline, or pimozide may be effective.[2]

The habitual or compulsive manipulator tends to aggravate pre-existing lesions and differs from the neurotic excoriator only in degree. Unable to tolerate imperfection in the skin, these patients are overly concerned with cleanliness and order. They manipulate the lesions under the pretense of treating them dutifully, but only succeed in prolonging the recovery or producing new lesions. This, however, gives them the satisfaction of a self-perpetuating job.

These patients deny, either consciously or unconsciously, all responsibility for the damage they have brought upon themselves. There may be a long history of psychogenic illness, with the skin lesions a new manifestation of a deeper problem. Of note is that approximately 5% of these patients in one study had anorexia nervosa.[15]

Whereas the compulsive patient needs to take care of everything herself, the hysteric with a self-inflicted wound needs to be cared for by someone else. This dependency is a secondary gain, the primary gain being the conversion of anxiety into a physical form such as a cutaneous deformity. Because a manner of homeostasis is achieved, the patient appears calm, exhibiting "la belle indifference" toward her wound. The hysteric patient tends to have an immature style of relating and a poor self image and to lead an impulsive life marked by repetitive self-destructive behavior.[12] The main purpose for perpetuating the skin lesions is to elicit sympathy, attention, and pity through these morbid acts. The hysteric substitutes normal relationships for clinical situations where she can remain dependent in the passive patient role.

Depressed patients may manipulate their wounds in order to require surgery, which provides a "legitimate" excuse for avoiding a life crisis.[7] There is generally a better prognosis for depressed patients, with recovery often occurring after improvement in the difficult life situation.[15] In summary, the psychological characteristic of any patient with a nonhealing wound should be considered as a possible contributing cause. Carney examined a series of 42 patients with artifactual illness, and found that 61 percent were emotionally deprived in childhood and 90 percent in adulthood, 54 percent were psychopathic, and 50 percent were in the health professions.[11] Because of this complex interplay between mind and body, early psychiatric consultation should be obtained when a factitious source for poor wound healing is suspected. An empathetic supportive approach from the primary treating physician will be significantly more effective than direct confrontation, anger, or censure.

CHARACTERISTICS OF FACTITIOUS LESIONS

Factitious lesions frequently present with a bizarre appearance bearing little resemblance to any known disease process. They do not appear "natural," that is, they may have regular borders, geometric designs, or be arranged in patterns.[16] Lesions that appear to be at right angles to the normal distribution of the neurovascular bundles are also suspicious, as most cutaneous disorders follow the direction of underlying vessels, nerves, or lymphatics. Generally, self-inflicted lesions occur on sites accessible to the handedness of the patient and are seldom symmetrically distributed.[17] Thus, a right-handed person will usually spare the right hand and arm and unilaterally mutilate the left side of the body. Though generally placed on the exposed surfaces of the face, neck, hands, chest, abdomen, or legs, these self-inflicted lesions may appear in such "unreachable" areas as the interscapular region through ingenuity or the hand of an accomplice.[16]

Factitious lesions tend to appear suddenly in previously normal skin, often overnight. They are surrounded by normal skin and are fully "evolved", unlike genuine skin diseases.[6] Because even self-inflicted wounds have a tendency to heal, the patient may have a variety of lesions of different ages with areas of new and old scarring. When nonhealing wounds arising out of natural causes such as insect bites, burns, stasis ulcers, or pressure sores become progressively worse with the usual therapeutic methods, one should suspect factitious interference. These lesions may appear chronically infected, present as progressive necrosis, or be manipulated by the patient to produce a model of the original lesions, a form of pathomimicry.[18] Left exposed, these wounds remain unhealed, but when protected from the patient in an occlusive dressing or cast, they tend to heal in the absence of diabetes or vascular impairment.

Many methods used to cause self-inflicted lesions or interfere with their normal healing have been described. Excoriation with fingernails, teeth, or other sharp objects leaves ulcers with various degrees of infection present. Inoculation with feces, urine, saliva, milk, bacteria, drugs, or other contaminants tends to produce abscesses. Cigarette burns leave small blisters, whereas burns with caustics such as phenol, alkali, or acids may cause extensive full-thickness skin loss. These lesions may leave a characteristic "tail," or guttate, where the fluid has run down the skin.[4] The necrosis tends to be superficial in factitious lesions as compared to the deeper gangrene of vascular insufficiency. A limb that is mysteriously swollen with no history of previous tumor surgery, radiation therapy, or possibility of filariasis is also highly suspect for factitious etiology.[19] The presence of a circumferential band around the extremity

with edema noted only distal to this line is a strong indication that a tourniquet has been recently employed.

ESTABLISHING THE DIAGNOSIS

In diagnosing a factitious wound-healing problem one must take into consideration the nature of the skin lesion and the personality of the patient. It is unwise to entertain the diagnosis in an emotionally mature, stable individual, although intelligence and social status should not exclude a factitious etiology if the lesion looks suspicious.[20] Various other causes must be included in the differential diagnosis even if the patient fits the personality profile of a factitious excoriator. Excluded by a thorough history and physical examination and appropriate laboratory and pathology studies are all forms of vasculitis, including erythema nodosum, drug eruptions, tertiary syphilis, polyarteritis nodosum, rheumatoid arthritis, giant cell arteritis, and lupus.[20] Diabetes, vascular insufficiency, malignancy, sensory nerve lesions, defects of the immune system, synergistic infections, and pyoderma granulosa associated with ulcerative colitis must also be ruled out. Infestations with scabies, pediculosis, eczema, or other dermatoses must be considered. Drugs can cause cholestasis with pruritus. Primary disorders of the kidneys, liver, pancreas, and lymphatic system can have cutaneous manifestations. Deficiencies of vitamin B_{12}, vitamin C, iron, and folate need to be excluded.

The patient with a factitious wound will be unwilling to offer much information regarding the onset of the lesions, providing a "hollow history."[17] With enough questioning, the physician may be able to detect inconsistencies in the patient's description of the lesion's evolution. Patients with genuine cutaneous disorders tend to complain of a greater area of irritation and excoriate less fiercely than factitious excoriators who present with localized heavily ulcerated lesions but deny scratching or itching.[20]

It is characteristic of factitious wounds that an extensive series of special studies is negative or produces equivocal results. Once the diagnosis of a self-inflicted lesion is entertained, it is difficult to confirm unless the patient is observed traumatizing the wound or acknowledges involvement. The purpose of confirming the diagnosis is to proceed with appropriate psychiatric care for the underlying disorders.

Litmus paper or Clinitest strips may reveal

chemically produced lesions. Tetracycline or fluorescein when applied topically to a wound will fluoresce on the patient's fingers under a Wood's lamp if the patient has been tampering with the wound.[21] The wound should be protected in a cast or bulky dressing to cover but not totally prevent the patient so motivated from manipulating the wound. After an adequate period of privacy, ultraviolet examination showing fluorescence under the nails or in the nail folds provides confirmation.

Treatment of the wounds involves adequate debridement and skin grafts where necessary followed by protection in a well-padded plaster cast. Dressing changes are performed as necessary, although the patient is not left alone while the wound is exposed.

Once the diagnosis is made, the approach to the patient is one of empathy, not accusation. The physician must try to retain the patient's confidence, although this is difficult because of feelings of isolation, guilt, and fear of disclosure. The physician should stress the need for the cooperative efforts of a psychiatrist to help resolve the underlying problem. The implication should be that successful therapy requires the involvement of not only the patient and the physician, but of the patient's family as well.[22]

Despite these efforts, the overall prognosis is not good because the personality defect is likely to persist. Although the lesion may heal, another is likely to take its place unless the patient's motivation and response to psychotherapy is strong. Periodic recurrences during periods of stress are common and may occur even during sleep.[16] Mallot reported six patients whose lesions healed in plaster, with all but one developing new or recurrent lesions after the casts were removed.[23]

Case Reports

Case 1*

MM, a 54 year old white female, reported being bitten by a brown recluse spider on the left thumb and dorsum of the right hand in December, 1983 (Fig. 29–1 A). She underwent debridement and split thickness skin grafting, though necrosis on the right hand progressed

_____

* Courtesy of Dr. Joseph E. Kutz.

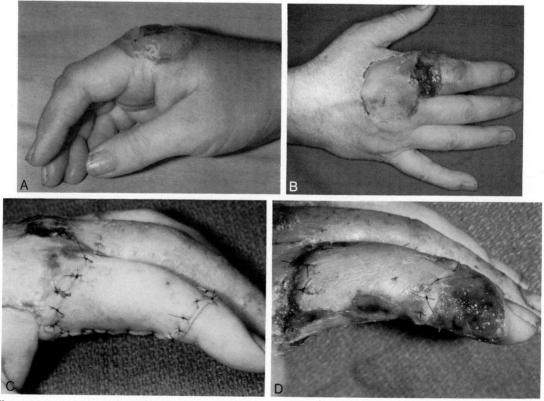

Figure 29–1. A, Right hand at presentation. B, Same hand following skin grafting. C, Left hand 6 months later. D, Development of ulceration in grafted digit.

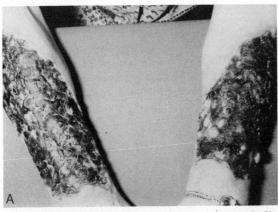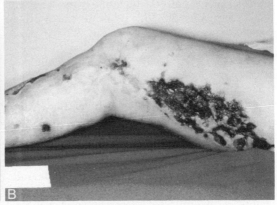

Figure 29–2. *A*, Forearms at presentation. *B*, Skin breakdown on left lateral thigh 1½ years later.

to the right index finger, requiring debridement and full-thickness skin grafting (Fig. 29–1*B*).

In June 1984 she presented with a grossly infected left hand wound from an alleged minor injury 2 weeks previously. This required debridement and split-thickness skin grafting to the dorsum of the left hand. Pathological examination revealed pseudoepitheliomatous hyperplasia. Later in the same month she developed necrosis of her left index finder from the metacarpal phalangeal to the proximal interphalangeal joint, which was debrided and skin grafted (Fig. 29–1*C*). Ulceration subsequently developed distally (Fig. 29–1*D*).

Psychiatric evaluation for possible factitious origin of these wounds was obtained. Although the patient did not appear particularly concerned about the condition of her hands she vehemently denied the possibility of self infliction. She showed marked dependency and strong use of denial, although the psychiatrist found no evidence of major psychopathology. The patient was unwilling to look for a potential source of unconscious contribution to the nonhealing of the ulcers and was lost to follow-up.

Case 2*

JM, a 52 year old divorced licensed practical nurse, presented in February, 1985 with infected "dog bites" she sustained several weeks previously (Fig. 29–2 *A*). She required multiple debridement and skin grafts for full-thickness skin loss with eventual healing over several months. Periodic outpatient follow-up revealed intermittent episodes of marked bilateral hand edema and superficial breakdown at the grafted sites, which healed in bilateral forearm casts. After removal of the casts, she developed sig-

nificant *Pseudomonas* infections of both arms that required further debridement and skin grafting.

In October, 1986, she presented with a 10 × 40 cm area of full-thickness skin loss on her lateral thigh in the area of a previous split-thickness skin graft donor site (Fig. 29–2*B*). According to the patient, this started as a superficial abrasion. While undergoing debridement and grafting to her leg, a full medical work-up failed to detect any organic cause for her nonhealing ulcers. A psychiatric evaluation found the patient to be angry and tense but without signs of depression or psychosis. There was evidence of Talwin abuse, which the patient was taking for chronic pain. When it was suggested that the lesions could be self-inflicted, she refused further evaluation and left against medical advice. She returned several months later requiring skin grafting of a "burn" to her left middle finger and later required coverage of her index finger and right antecubital fossa for full-thickness skin loss.

Case 3†

DC, a 32 year old white female Jehovah's Witness, had a history of a right dorsal hand burn at age 11 that required seven different skin grafts to obtain healing. She also had radiation therapy to her hand for treatment of hypertrophic scarring. She now presented with persistent ulceration on the dorsum of her right hand felt initially to be radiation necrosis or neoplasia (Fig. 29–3 *A*). Biopsy showed no signs of squamous cell carcinoma. A free lateral arm flap was applied to the area after adequate debridement. Three weeks after free tissue transfer the distal margin of the flap ulcerated

---

* Courtesy of Dr. Harold E. Kleinert.

†Courtesy of Dr. Thomas Wolff.

with periods of episodic bleeding from the edge of the flap (Fig. 29–3B). While in the waiting room during an office visit, the patient massively bled from the flap with a drop in hemoglobin to 5.5 g per deciliter. Because of religious prohibitions against blood transfusion, the vascular pedicle of the flap was ligated to control the bleeding. The patient left the hospital immediately after surgery against medical advice. Subsequently, the distal margin of the flap healed but a new area of ulceration near the center of the flap later developed (Fig. 29–3C).

The arm was placed in a cast with the wound covered with tetracycline powder "to promote healing." Several weeks later the cast was removed and the wound found to be further excoriated. Examination with a Wood's lamp revealed fluorescent material (tetracycline) tracking throughout the cast, indicating use of a long, sharp instrument, probably a coat hanger. The patient denied interfering with her wound, refused psychiatric consultation, and was lost to follow-up.

Case 4*

JH, a 34 year old bricklayer, sustained a third-degree burn of the right forearm with hydrochloric acid that required multiple debridements and skin grafts. Despite this treatment, persistent ulceration in the region of the burn required a rotation flap to the dorsum of the right hand, which also failed to adequately heal. Five months after the original injury a free lateral arm flap was placed in the area. The flap was the site of recurrent fistula and abscess formation despite repeated debridements and antibiotic therapy. During one debridement cotton cloth material was detected under the flap, which the patient admitted placing there when confronted with the possibility of factitious interference. After further debridement and skin grafting the wound healed and the patient returned to work 1 year after the initial injury.

*Courtesy of Dr. Thomas Wolff.

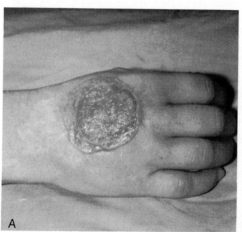
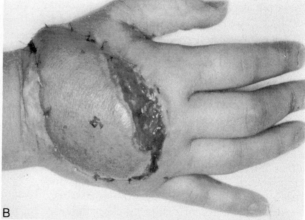
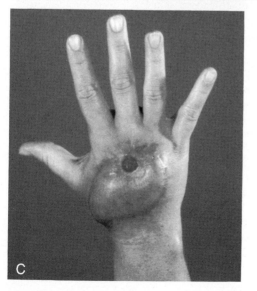

Figure 29–3. A, Ulcerated right dorsal hand. B, Distal marginal ulceration following free lateral arm flap. C, Subsequent ulceration in center of the flap.

Case 5*

A 35 year old chronically depressed house-wife presented with a chronic suprapubic ulceration of 2½ years' duration (Fig. 29–4 A). Soon after admission to the hospital a vesicocutaneous fistula was noted. The patient had a past history of problems with wound healing with a breakdown of an episiotomy wound immediately following the birth of her last child. Clinical and laboratory findings were within normal limits, including fibroblast cultures, humoral immunity studies, quantitative studies of cutaneous hypersensitivity, and extensive gastrointestinal and genitourinary studies.

The patient underwent wound debridement, urinary bladder fistula closure, and a gracilis musculocutaneous flap rotated into the pelvis to cover the vesical suture line. On the fifth postoperative day a recurrent vesicocutaneous fistula was noted, which was temporally associated with conversations regarding imminent discharge from the hospital. A psychiatric consultation was obtained and a depressive reaction

*Courtesy of Dr. Donald Serafin.

secondary to prolonged hospitalization and disability was diagnosed.

As factitious disease became increasingly more suspect, tetracycline tincture of benzoin mixture was applied topically to the wound. The results were equivocal. A progressive worsening of the wound was noted early one morning when a member of the operating team surprised the patient. Her fingers were noted to be beneath the dressing of the wound with gross blood on the fingertips. The patient was confronted by her primary physician.

An island tensor fascia lata flap was subsequently transferred to the suprapubic defect following closure of the vesicocutaneous fistula. Postoperatively the wound was protected with a plaster shield. The patient did well for 2 weeks, and the plaster shield was discontinued. Early in the third postoperative week a small area of ulceration was noted both in the suprapubic area and in the donor site of the lateral thigh of the tensor fascia lata flap. These wounds were secondarily closed. The patient began complaining of pain in the right lateral thigh. The entire staff supported this symptom complex and reinforced the patient's perception that

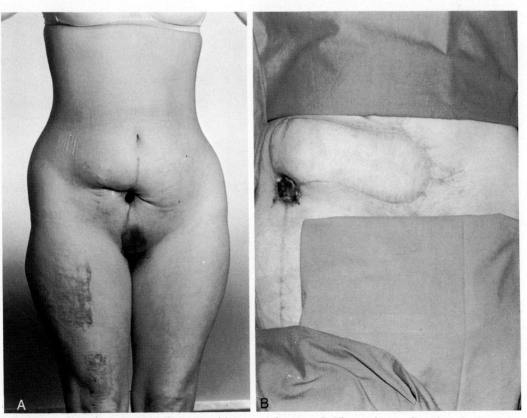

Figure 29–4. *A,* Chronic suprapubic ulceration of 2½ years' duration. *B,* Ulcerated wound on the superior aspect of the donor site.

the donor site would cause future difficulties. The patient was finally discharged following 70 days of hospitalization. One month following discharge a chronic ulcerated wound was noted in the superior aspect of the donor site (Fig. 29–4B). The suprapubic wound remained closed, however.

DISCUSSION

A review of these case reports points up not only the difficulty in establishing a diagnosis of factitious ulceration but also the chronicity of the disorder as well. Cutaneous manifestations often reflect intermittent exacerbations of the underlying psychiatric disorder. Cures are rare, but disease-free intervals can occur. Of the five patients reported, one returned to his previous employment, and three showed little or no improvement in spite of extensive treatment and hospitalization. One patient with a life-threatening vesicocutaneous fistula responded to surgical treatment and intense in-hospital psychotherapy. However, factitious ulceration recurred at another anatomical site.

Adequate treatment depends first on the establishment of the diagnosis, which is often difficult, time consuming, and costly. Depressed patients and truly psychotic patients can be helped with medication. Confrontation of the patient by the primary physician is useful in the treatment of hospitalized patients with sufficient personality assets to enable them to make a mature adaptation. Patients with limited coping skills, however, are more difficult to treat. Therapy is directed at encouraging the patient to give up the illness-feigning behavior, but these patients frequently reject further attempts at psychiatric treatment.

Malingering can often be treated, provided the secondary goals and benefits are identified and no longer made available. The threat of loss of hospitalization, workmen's compensation, or employment may be sufficient to permit healing of factitious wounds. This sequence of discovery of malingering, confrontation, and treatment is described in Case 4.

CONCLUSIONS

Various personality profiles and psychiatric disorders are associated with factitious ulceration. The difficulty in diagnosis, the chronicity of the disease, and its unlikelihood of perma-

nent cure are discouraging to physicians who attempt to treat these patients.

In establishing the diagnosis, the history of repeated unsuccessful treatment attempts by multiple physicians should be noted. Inconsistencies in the development or description of the lesions evolution are often noted. Patients with localized heavy ulcerated lesions often complain of pruritus but deny excoriation. Factitious lesions have some distinguishing characteristics. They may have regular borders, geometric designs, or may be arranged in patterns; they may be at right angles to the normal distribution of the neurovascular bundles rather than following them as do most cutaneous disorders. Self-inflicted lesions also occur in areas accessible to the dominant hand of the patient and are seldom distributed symmetrically. Most cutaneous lesions are located on the exposed surfaces of the face, neck, hands, or legs. Treatment must be directed concurrently at the wound and at the underlying psychiatric disorder.

References

1. Fras I: Factitial disease: An update. Psychosomatics 19:119–122, 1978.
2. Gupta MA, Gupta AK, Haberman HF: The self-inflicted dermatoses: A critical review. Gen Hosp Psychiatry 9:45–52, 1987.
3. Krupp NE: Self-caused skin ulcers. Psychosomatics 18:15–19, 1977.
4. Shafer N, Shafer R: Factitious diseases including Munchausen's syndrome. NY State J Med 80:594–603, 1980.
5. Asher R: Munchausen's syndrome. Lancet 1:339–341, 1951.
6. Eckert WG: The pathology of self-mutilation and destructive acts: A forensic study and review. J Forensic Sci 242–250, 1976.
7. Drinker H, Knorr NJ, Edgerton MT: Factitious wounds. Plast Reconstr Surg 50:458–461, 1972.
8. Waisman M: Pickers, pluckers and impostors: A panorama of cutaneous self mutilation. Postgrad Med 38:620–630, 1965.
9. Serafin D, Dimond M, France R: Factitious vesicocutaneous fistula: An enigma in diagnosis and treatment. Plast Reconstr Surg 72:81–87, 1983.
10. Menninger K: Man Against Himself. New York, Harcourt, Brace, and World, 1938.
11. Carney MWP, Brown JP: Clinical features and motives among 42 artifactual illness patients. Br J Med Psycho 56:57–66, 1983.
12. Aduan RP, Fauci AS, Dale DS, et al: Factitious fever and self-induced cases. Ann Intern Med 90:230–242, 1979.
13. Stone MH: Factitious illness. Bull Menninger Clin 41:239–254, 1977.
14. Scully RE, Mark EJ, McNeely BU: Case records of The Massachusetts General Hospital. N Engl J Med 311:108–115, 1984.

15. Sneddon I, Sneddon J: Self-inflicted injury: A followup study of 43 patients. Br Med J 3:527–530, 1975.
16. Agris J, Simmons CW: Factitious self-inflicted skin wounds. Plast Reconstr Surg 62:686–691, 1978.
17. Lyell A: Dermatitis artifacta and self-inflicted disease. Scott Med J 17:187–196, 1972
18. Millard LG: Dermatological pathomimicry: A form of patient maladjustment. Lancet 2:969–971, 1984.
19. Louis DS, Lamp MK, Greene TC: The upper extremity and psychiatric illness. J Hand Surg 10:687–693, 1985.
20. Lyell A: Cutaneous artifactual disease. J Acad Dermatol 1:391–407, 1979.
21. Phelps DB, Buchler V, Boswick JA: The diagnosis of factitious ulcer of the hand: A case report. Hand Surg 2:105–108, 1977.
22. Rees TD, Daniller A: Self-mutilation: Some problems in reconstruction. Plast Reconstr Surg 46:300–303, 1969.
23. Mallot IF, Farley LW, White WL: Psychic disturbances and wound healing. Plast Reconstr Surg 21:272–278, 1958.

30

KELOIDS AND EXCESSIVE DERMAL SCARRING

John C. Murray, M.D., and Sheldon R. Pinnell, M.D.

Keloids are fibrous growths that result from an abnormal connective tissue response to trauma, inflammation, surgery, or burns and occasionally seem to occur spontaneously. Keloids may be differentiated from hypertrophic scars even though both are characterized by an overabundant deposition of collagen in healed skin wounds. Keloids have been defined as abnormal scars extending beyond the confines of the original wound that rarely regress, whereas hypertrophic scars, while raised, frequently regress spontaneously and remain within the confines of the original wound (Fig. 30–1).[1] These uncontrolled growths frequently cause significant cosmetic and symptomatic problems. Often our efforts to treat keloids are disappointing despite a wide range of therapeutic options.

EPIDEMIOLOGY

Although the incidence of keloids remains unknown, random samplings of African populations suggest an incidence of approximately 6 to 16 percent.[2-4] The incidence is higher in blacks and in individuals with darker pigmentation.[5, 6] Keloids have been reported in nearly all races but not in albinos, again suggesting a relationship to skin pigmentation. In general, keloids occur between the ages of 10 and 30.[5, 7] Patients of any age may develop keloids, but keloid formation in prepubescent children[8] and older adults[6] is said to be rare, although the editors have observed numerous keloids in both groups. The incidence and median age of onset are equal for both sexes.[5, 6, 9]

ETIOLOGY

Various etiological factors such as trauma, tension, and hormones have been implicated in keloid formation. In most postpubescent and adult individuals, keloids occur within 1 year of local trauma.[7] Trauma may include surgery, lacerations, tattoos, burns, injections, bites, vaccinations, and unspecified or blunt trauma. Skin tension may also be a critical factor in keloid formation, since areas of highest tension, such as the upper back, shoulders, anterior

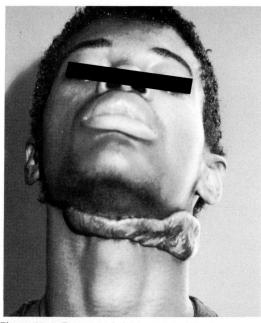

Figure 30–1. Recurrent keloid on the neck of a 17-year-old man that had been revised several times. (Patient photograph courtesy of I. K. Cohen, M.D.)

chest, and upper arms, are the most frequent sites of keloid formation. Local factors seem significant in that some individuals with keloids frequently have normal scars in other locations. Various aspects of wound healing such as orientation of the lines of relaxed skin tension, presence of infection, and dynamics of healing have been suggested as initiating or promoting factors in keloid formation, but the role of each remains speculative.[5, 10]

Certain observations have associated keloid formation with endocrinological factors. Estrogens have been implicated, since keloids frequently appear with puberty, resolve after menopause, and appear or enlarge during pregnancy.[7, 11] Fibroblast cultures of keloidal tissue have demonstrated increased androgen binding as compared to normal controls.[12]

Keloids have a familial predisposition. Although the exact inheritance pattern remains unknown, both autosomal recessive and autosomal dominant patterns have been reported.[3, 13] A positive family history is more likely in individuals with multiple severe keloids.[7] No association with HLA-A or HLA-B has been found.[14]

Keloid formation has been reported with other dermatological diseases, especially those characterized by inflammatory lesions in anatomical sites of high keloid predilection. Such diseases include dissecting cellulitis of the scalp, acne vulgaris, acne conglobata, hidradenitis suppurativa, pilonidal cyst, foreign body reaction, and local infections with herpes, smallpox, or vaccinia. Such associations are not surprising, given the inflammatory component. Keloid formation has also been described in Ehlers-Danlos syndrome,[15] Rubinstein-Taybi syndrome,[16] pachydermoperiostosis,[17] and scleroderma.[18] This association between connective tissue diseases and keloid formation is interesting, but its etiological significance remains speculative.

CLINICAL MANIFESTATIONS

The clinical manifestations of keloids are highly variable. Usually patients present for cosmetic reasons but keloids may be very symptomatic, and those that appear following sternotomy or thoracotomy seem particularly painful. Some patients note marked pruritus, and many associate more intense itching with periods of increased keloidal growth. Some even note changes with variations in barometric pressure.

Keloids commonly occur near a site of inflammation or injury, although many times patients have no memory of antecedent trauma. The extent of preceding trauma is often reflected in the size and configuration of the keloid. Earlobe keloids vary greatly: some may be 2 to 4 mm papules, while others are intralobular masses or pendulous nodular tumors.[19] Often the same earlobe may have normal epithelialized earring tracts next to tracts that have developed keloids. The configuration of keloids varies from evenly contoured extensions with regular borders to highly irregular clawlike projections. Such projections are commonly seen over the shoulders and chest, resulting from acne lesions, ruptured epidermal cysts, or local trauma.

As noted, keloids most commonly occur over the shoulders, anterior chest, upper arms, and mandibular angle. Other less frequently involved areas include the face, neck, and lower extremities.[2, 20] Keloids may occur anywhere, and more unusual sites have been reported such as the eyelids, genitalia, palms, soles,[6] cornea,[21] and mucous membranes.[7]

The clinical course of keloid formation is highly variable. Generally, they appear weeks or months following initial trauma or inflammation. Some will stabilize for a considerable period of time. Some lesions remain, while others enlarge and even undergo spontaneous suppurative necrosis and drainage.[22] It is speculated that such suppurative necrosis results from vascular compromise from keloid overgrowth or occlusion of a pilosebaceous unit and subsequent infection. Such suppuration is exquisitely painful and frequently recurs. In rare cases, keloids may regress spontaneously. Such involution is common in later years, as elderly patients commonly display flattened, resolved keloids that were prominent in years past. Keloid regression associated with cancer has been noted but never reported in the literature.

Malignant transformation of keloids has been observed, but such cases are rare and poorly documented.[7, 23] Lesions such as leiomyosarcoma and dermatofibrosarcoma protuberans may clinically resemble keloids,[24] and histopathological examination is critical in such cases to exclude malignancy.

PATHOLOGY

It has been assumed, but not demonstrated, that the early stages of both normal wound healing and keloid formation share similar histopathological changes. Both processes initially demonstrate an inflammatory stage that is followed by fibroplasia. Lesions demonstrate increased vascularity and a moderate perivascular mononuclear infiltrate along with early production of proteoglycan as well as collagen fibers and bundles.[25] The mononuclear cell infiltrate has moderate numbers of mast cells, plasma cells, and lymphocytes.[26] By the third week of wound healing, keloids demonstrate progressive fibroplasia, which continues without resolution. Keloids characteristically develop nodular vascular proliferations that are surrounded by fibroblasts. This nodular mass enlarges and transforms into a relatively avascular collection of collagen and proteoglycan. The persistent transformation of the swirl-like fibroblast clusters into collagen bundles or nodules is characteristic of keloid growth.[27] The number of fibroblasts increases as collagen bundles persist and remain disorganized. This increased collagen growth can compress and displace other skin appendages as well as flatten an otherwise normal epidermis.[28]

Persistence of the collagen nodules is not found in normal wound healing but is seen in hypertrophic scars.[29] Collagen nodules contain numerous fibroblasts and collagen fibrils, which are aligned in swirl-like clusters. These nodules contain few microvessels, as most blood vessels are located near the periphery, and many vessels are occluded or partially occluded by endothelial cells. A morphologically unique pericapillary cell, the myofibroblast, is present in keloids[30] that has characteristics of both fibroblasts and smooth muscle cells. The function of the myofibroblast remains speculative, but this cell has been described as more prevalent in actively growing keloids. Mature, stable keloids apparently have fewer myofibroblasts.

The morphology of collagen fibers has been studied by scanning electron microscopy.[31] In keloids, the collagen bundles are randomly aligned and discrete bundles are absent, and the keloid collagen fibers are loosely connected, with no orientation to the epithelial surface. In normal skin and mature scars, the collagen bundles lie parallel to the epithelial surface in discrete groups; fibers are closely packed and lie parallel to the surface.

PATHOGENESIS

Keloids demonstrate increased cellularity and enhanced metabolic activity. The increased cellularity is reflected by various parameters such as concentration of deoxyribonucleic acid (DNA) (normal 1.6 ± 0.3 ng/mg dry weight; keloid, 3.4 ± 0.3 ng/mg dry weight)[32]. Increased metabolic activity is demonstrated by elevated glycolytic enzyme activity and glycoprotein synthesis[33]. In spite of the increased cellularity and metabolic activity, keloid fibroblasts are similar to those of normal dermal fibroblasts: no differences could be detected in mean population doubling time, confluent density, cellular volume, or karyotype.[34] The only animal model system for keloids is the athymic nude mouse with transplanted human keloid tissue, making studies of the pathogenesis of keloids difficult.[35]

The abundant extracellular matrix accounts for most of the keloid bulk. Both glycoproteins[33, 36] and water[36, 37] are increased. Chondroitin-4-sulfate is the most prevalent glycoprotein in keloids and hypertrophic scars,[38] constituting 4.7 ± 0.7 percent of glycoprotein in normal skin and 26.4 ± 2.9 percent in hypertrophic scars. Most chondroitin-4-sulfate is preferentially located in active nodular areas in these scars.[39]

Hypertrophic scars contain minimal amounts of elastin.[40] Although hypertrophic scars and keloids are fibrous tumors, the collagen concentration is not significantly increased.[40] Collagen synthesis is increased in newly formed keloids[41] as measured by increased prolyl hydroxylase activity in keloid tissue.[42, 43] Studies of fibroblast cultures explanted from keloids reveal increased collagen synthesis relative to total protein synthesis (normal skin, $5.54 \pm 0.51\%$; keloid, $7.93 \pm 0.42\%$).[44] In other studies of fibroblast cultures from keloid explants, five of nine demonstrated increased procollagen production, while the other four cell lines were within normal control ranges.[45] In four of the keloid fibroblast lines with increased collagen production, type I procollagen mRNS levels were significantly increased. Such a correlation suggests that the increased collagen production is controlled at a transcriptional level. Other studies of fibroblast cultures from keloid explants revealed normal levels of types I and III procollagen mRNA levels, suggesting synthesis of normal amounts of collagen.[46] These variations in the amount of collagen synthesis may reflect only the clinical heterogeneity of sampled keloids.

Collagen synthesized in keloid tissue differs from that in normal dermis. Relative amounts of type III collagen appear increased, although this change may be minimal.[40, 47] Other studies report that the ratio of type I to type III collagen was significantly increased as compared to normal skin.[48] Again, these differences may be related to the sampling area or to keloid growth. The profile of reducible intermolecular crosslinks in keloid collagen is similar to that in young skin collagen.[40] Keloid collagen is more soluble than dermal collagen.[36, 40] Since collagen crosslinking depends upon lysyl oxidase, a copper-dependent enzyme, reduced copper levels in keloids may be important in abnormal crosslinking.[49] Type-specific collagen synthesis and collagen crosslinking are similar to those found in new granulation tissue or in embryonic skin.[50–53]

The overabundant deposition of collagen in keloids may result from decreased collagen degradation. In earlier studies, collagenase activity in keloids was reported to be normal,[54, 55] or increased,[37] but not diminished. Collagen degradation has been reported to be normal in tissue explants[54] and in keloid fibroblast cultures.[44] A more recent study reports that three of nine keloid cell lines had diminished degradation of newly synthesized collagen polypeptides. It is possible that the effectiveness of collagenase activity may be diminished even though collagenase levels are not decreased, and this may account for the altered collagen degradation. Collagenase is inhibited by α-macroglobulin and α_1-antitrypsin, both of which accumulate in keloids as demonstrated by immunofluorescent studies,[56] although the serum levels of these collagenase inhibitors are no different in patients with or without keloids. It is possible that glycoproteins such as the abundant chondroitin-4-sulfate found in hypertrophic scars may protect keloidal tissue by interfering with collagen degradation.[57]

The effect of corticosteroid on collagen synthesis and degradation is not completely understood, but studies in human skin fibroblast culture reveal that corticosteroids specifically inhibit collagen synthesis in addition to protein synthesis.[58, 59] Corticosteroid had less of an inhibitory effect on keloid fibroblast growth than on normal skin fibroblast growth.[59] Corticosteroids may also promote collagen degradation, since the deposition of serum proteins that inhibit collagenase may be reduced by corticosteroid therapy.[56, 60]

In summary, keloids are fibrous lesions with accumulation of extracellular matrix proteins, collagen, and proteoglycan. These lesions contain an abnormally high number of cells that synthesize collagen and glycoprotein. The glycoprotein and serum protease inhibitors coat the extracellular matrix and potentially limit remodeling and degradation by collagenase.

TREATMENT

The treatment of keloids remains a challenging problem. Numerous therapies have been described, and such diversity reflects the clinical heterogeneity of keloids as well as the variable therapeutic response. It is imperative to select the appropriate therapy for characteristic keloids.

Oral antihistamine administration is a helpful adjuvant therapy for certain keloid patients.[61] Antihistamines have been reported to inhibit in vitro proliferation of keloid fibroblast cultures.[62] Histologically, keloids often have an increased number of mast cells and, as mentioned, patients often suffer from intense pruritus.[61] Many of these patients describe reduced pruritus and subsequent reduction in local trauma with use of oral antihistamines. Control of pruritus is important because rubbing and scratching may release mast cell mediators that serve as growth factors.

Intralesional corticosteroid therapy is commonly used either alone[63] or following surgery.[4, 64, 65] Variations in response and recurrence rates with this regimen have been reported[66, 67] that are probably related to patient selection, clinical criteria for keloids, and duration of observation. Kiil reported that most keloids recurred within the first year after trauma and that some lesions may recur up to 5 years after therapy.[68] The recurrence rate in that study was 50 percent over 5 years. Additional intralesional triamcinolone therapy proved effective in some recurrent lesions. Griffith and co-workers reported that 5 of 56 keloids recurred within 4 years following intralesional triamcinolone therapy.[65]

Guidelines and recommendations for intralesional triamcinolone therapy vary considerably in the literature. Currently, several preparations of intralesional corticosteroids are available, but no advantage for one particular type has been clearly demonstrated. The dosage and administration have been arbitrary. Individual lesions or patients demonstrate variable clinical response to steroid injection, and this clinical variation can be addressed by varying the initial concentrations of triamcinolone acetonide from 10 to 40 mg per milliliter. Different lesions or different areas of the same lesion may be injected with 10 to 40 mg per milliliter so that the minimal effective dosage may be determined for each lesion[69] and subsequent injections may utilize the most appropriate dosage, thereby minimizing adverse effects.

Various delivery systems are available for injecting corticosteroids into keloids. The needle and syringe technique is efficient in delivering known quantities to a specific area. Use of the Luer-Lok needle and syringe is essential to avoid equipment separation. In general, a small-gauge (20 or 30) needle is used.

Injections can be spaced 0.5 to 1.0 cm apart over the entire lesion. The corticosteroid is injected into the mass to avoid superficial infiltration beneath the epidermis or deep deposition within adipose tissue. Superficial deposition may result in atrophy or depigmentation. In certain keloids (e.g., sternal keloids) preliminary lidocaine anesthesia may minimize patient discomfort. With repeated injections, the keloids are more easily infiltrated. Although injections are generally administered at monthly intervals or whenever the therapeutic benefit has waned, the treatment interval must be individualized according to patient response and may vary from 1 to 4 months.

Other delivery systems include mechanical injectors, such as spring or CO_2-powered devices.[70, 71] These mechanical injectors cause less discomfort for some patients, especially adolescents, and they are particularly useful in treating acne keloidalis and nuchal keloids. Care must be taken to direct mechanical injectors to avoid inadvertent infiltration into normal skin. Luer-Lok needle injection is often more efficient, as a significant amount of steroid solution may be wasted with mechanical injectors. Other mechanical devices include dental syringes such as the Ligmajet, which requires less effort to inject into these firm fibrous masses. Some clinicians prefer using 1 cc glass syringes, which may be fitted with metal finger handles to facilitate injection. Other mechanical injectors use a Luer-Lok needle and syringe attached to a repetitive pipette instrument[72] to deliver calibrated dosages by preset dispensing increments. Patient discomfort and ease of injection vary with each of these devices.

Intralesional corticosteroid may have adverse effects. Local complications include atrophy, depigmentation, telangiectasia, necrosis, ulceration, and Cushing's habitus. The risk of complications is greater if the corticosteroid is inadvertently injected into the surrounding dermis or subcutaneous tissue. One report described a patient who received intralesional corticosteroid injection for keloids and subsequently developed severe tuberculosis.[73] Fortunately such incidents are rare, but repeated injections of high-potency steroids can have widespread effects. After repeated injections, insoluble material from the corticosteroid preparations may be deposited beneath the epidermis, appearing white or faintly yellow and remaining for weeks to months. This complication can be minimized by placing the corticosteroid preparation in an ultrasound and/or sonication device before injection. Keloids injected with intralesional corticosteroids have revealed focal accumulations of mucinosis on histopathological examination.[74] Other findings include focal collections of foreign body type giant cells along with histiocytic reaction. The significance of these findings remains unclear, but this tissue reaction is presumed to be due to the corticosteroid injections.

Corticosteroid injections may be combined with other modalities.[64, 75] Ceilley and Babin describe using cryotherapy before intralesional injection of corticosteroids in order to induce edema and cellular disruption.[75] Following liquid nitrogen application, the fibrous tissue is less dense, and injections can penetrate tissue more easily and effectively. Cryotherapy with liquid nitrogen has been used alone, although the responses have been quite variable.[76] Zacarian has had good results with cryotherapy, especially with young keloids.[77] Unfortunately, some patients may note persistent depigmentation following cryotherapy.

Intralesional corticosteroid injections are frequently combined with surgery. Immediately following keloid excision, the wound edges may be injected with triamcinolone acetonide, and sutures may be left in place for an extra 5 days to minimize the potential for wound dehiscence. Intralesional treatment is then repeated at 3 to 4 week intervals. Such treatment intervals are arbitrary, and should be individualized according to the patient's response. Nevertheless, repeated adjuvant steroid injections appear necessary to minimize the chance of recurrence following excision. Often patients will report diminished pruritus and pain, and reduced size by the third or fourth week after steroid injection.

Keloids generally recur following simple excision, and the recurrence is often larger.[78] To avoid this, excision must be combined with adjuvant therapy, such as corticosteroid injection, radiation, pressure treatments, or oral medication, e.g., methotrexate, colchicine, penicillamine. When surgical excision is followed only by skin grafting, the recurrence rate has been reported to be 59 percent, and approximately half of the patients develop keloids in the donor site. Apfelberg and associates grafted the overlying epithelium after excision of the keloidal mass to avoid other donor sites,[79] and Pollack described removing flat pancakelike keloids and shelling out the keloidal bulk so that the superficial remnant could be grafted to the site.[80]

Surgical excision is most effective when inciting factors such as trapped hair follicles or epithelial cysts or tracts that may provide the initial stimulus for keloid growth are removed.

Surgical excision of earlobe keloids should involve removal of epithelial tract or cysts, since they tend to increase the recurrence rate. Pilosebaceous units should be removed with nuchal keloids, since they may provide the promoting stimulus for further fibrous growth. Often such nuchal lesions may respond well following surgical excision and repeated corticosteroid injection. Similarly, keloids in the mons pubis may be surgically excised if both the keloidal bulk and all pilosebaceous units are removed.

During keloid excision, tissue trauma should be minimized, and it is essential to avoid dead space, foreign material, hematoma, infection, and wound tension, since these factors may increase the possibility of recurrence. Surgical excisions must be carefully planned so that skin edges can be joined with minimal tension. Skin edges should parallel the relaxed skin tension lines if at all possible. Other surgical techniques that reduce skin edge tension such as Z-plasty and flap repair are commonly employed.[81] Residual keloid tissue may be purposefully left within the wound to minimize wound tension, and Cosman and Wolfe have reported that keloid remnants do not cause recurrence.[82] The reconstruction of earlobes following keloid excision often requires leaving some keloid remnant to maintain an acceptable cosmetic result.

Surgical excision of keloids has been performed using various types of lasers. Initial reports describe carbon dioxide laser surgery for nuchal[83] and earlobe keloids.[84] Although no controlled studies are available demonstrating the advantages of laser surgery over conventional scalpel surgery, these early reports do suggest a lower recurrence rate and a tendency for hypertrophic scar formation with recurrence. Argon lasers have been used with a multiple borehole technique, but this has not been effective.[85] The neodymium-yttrium-aluminum-garnet (Nd:YAG) laser has been reported to suppress collagen production specifically, both in fibroblast cultures and in normal skin.[86] Clinical trials using the Nd:YAG laser in a small number of patients have had encouraging results following low energy density irradiation.[87] The Nd:YAG laser was not used to totally remove excessive keloid tissue, but it has been shown to flatten and soften existing lesions. The role of laser surgery in keloid treatment requires further investigation. Lasers appear to modify wound healing by suppression of collagen synthesis in fibroblast cultures, and clinically this effect is demonstrated by the delayed healing times. Whether this scar alteration will prove to be beneficial when compared to conventional electrosurgery or simple scalpel excision remains to be seen. At the present time, laser therapy for keloid must be considered an experimental modality.

Surgical excision followed by pressure therapy has been recommended for earlobe keloids.[88] The keloid is debulked and the earlobe is rebuilt following removal of epithelial tracts, cysts, or foreign bodies. Pressure therapy must be continued for at least 4 to 6 months following surgery.[78] A spring pressure earring device (Napier Model #6238 or 6112) has provided excellent results.[89] Other pressure devices include elastic garments tightly fitted to involved bodily areas, including the face, neck, and upper trunk. Patient compliance remains a problem, since these devices must be worn continuously for long periods.

Other pressure devices have been designed for surgical wounds. Fujimori and associates described a synthetic polybutadine acrylate sponge with double-sided adhesive that was applied to the surgical scar 6 to 10 days postoperatively.[90] This device applied constant pressure to the surgical wound, and the incidence of recurrence was reportedly diminished. Pearce described an acrylic splint that can be fastened by acrylic screws following earlobe keloid excision.[91] He recommended that it be used for 18 to 24 months with only brief removal for hygienic purposes.

Steroid-impregnated tape was used in a series of 57 patients with recurrent earlobe keloids.[89] Patients used a large clip-on earring, and flurandrenolide tape was applied daily to cover the earlobe incision. Four recurrences among 57 patients were noted at 4-year follow-up. A variety of other techniques for treating earlobe keloids have been reported, but effective therapy seems to require surgical removal of cyst tracts or foreign body along with adjuvant therapy such as pressure devices or local steroid therapy.

Some investigators have reported low keloid recurrence (21% after 1 year) following combined surgery and radiation therapy.[92-94] In a series of 68 patients, 1500 rads were delivered in three equal doses. The first dose was delivered within hours after surgery and the other two doses were administered at 2 or 3 day intervals. In a series of 35 patients treated with immediate postoperative radiation, 1500 to 1800 rads of superficial x-rays were administered in five or six fractions over 12 to 14 days.[95] Keloids recurred in 5 of 35 patients who were followed from 6 to 24 months. Pigmentary change in the irradiated site was the only adverse effect.

Inalsingh reported good results in a series of

501 patients given superficial radiation with and without surgery.[96] Patients received 400 rads monthly in five or fewer treatments. Normal surrounding skin was shielded with lead cutouts. Good cosmetic results and relief of symptoms were noted in 76.5 percent of patients, while 15.1 percent had symptomatic relief only and 8.4 percent failed to respond. No adverse effects from radiation were observed during a 2-year follow-up.

Despite these impressive results, many investigators concerned about the carcinogenic effects of radiation therapy remain opposed to radiation therapy.[97] The medical literature holds many examples of postirradiation neoplasms as well as adverse effects from inadvertent radiation of other body structures.[98] Appropriate dosimetry and shielding can limit these adverse effects, and radiation therapy appears to be an effective adjuvant therapy.

Ionizing radiation may be delivered in other treatment regimens. In a series of 89 patients, electron beam therapy was given immediately postoperatively to 32 patients and to 57 nonsurgical patients.[99] The total dosage range was 1000 to 3000 rads. Electron beam therapy completely resolved lesions in 26.3 percent of the nonsurgical patients and improved symptoms without keloid resolution in 52.6 percent. The best results were seen in patients who received postoperative electron beam therapy: 74.1 percent were successfully treated.

Malaker and co-workers described postoperative radiation by interstitial radiotherapy administered to the base of the sutured wound edges.[100] During surgical excision, a plastic tube is placed in the wound between the cuticular and the subcutaneous sutures. The ends of the plastic tube emerge either at the end of or slightly beyond the excision. Radioactive iridium-192 wire is inserted into the plastic tubing so that a dose of 2000 rads is delivered at a point 2.5 mm from the axis of the wire opposite its midpoint. In a series of 31 keloids treated with this technique a 20 percent recurrence rate was noted. These lesions were followed for 2 years and no complications were noted.

Surgical excision has also been combined with oral medications. Peacock reported a series of 15 patients with severe keloids treated by surgical excision followed by induced lathyrism with β-aminopropionitrile fumarate (BAPN) or penicillamine and administration of colchicine.[101, 102] BAPN and penicillamine are lysyl oxidase inhibitors that interfere with formation of collagen crosslinking, while colchicine increases tissue collagenase activity and accelerates collagen degradation. When these patients

were followed for 18 months to 5 years no keloids were noted. Instead, patients developed hypertrophic scars at the surgical sites. No adverse effects were noted with this adjuvant medication.

Topical retinoids have been shown to soften and to reduce keloid growth. DeLimpens reported that daily applications of a 0.05% solution of retinoic acid reduced pruritus and keloid bulk in a group of 28 patients.[103] These patients were followed from 3 to 22 months and 77 percent noted improvement. Daly and associates reported a series of 41 patients treated with tretinoin cream (0.05%) in a double-blind controlled study.[104] A significant number of patients noted softening and shrinkage of the keloid as well as symptomatic improvement. When added to fibroblast cultures, tretinoin decreased fibroblast proliferation and reduced collagen synthesis.[105] Retinoids apparently can modify keloid growth, although the change may be minimal, as less than a 20 percent reduction in total volume of treated keloid was noted.

Nuchal keloids occur on the neck and occipital scalp of black men. Initially lesions are perifollicular papules and pustules that may present as a transepithelial elimination disorder.[106] Lesions may enlarge and clinically resemble keloids found elsewhere on the body. These lesions are treated by removing involved hairs and pilosebaceous glands, and administering intralesional corticosteroids. Patients are instructed to avoid grease and to use clear gel or glycerin solutions for hair care. Inflammatory lesions may be treated with topical tretinoin along with topical or oral antibiotics. Larger lesions respond to surgical excision. It is essential to remove pilosebaceous units along with keloidal bulk to minimize the risk of recurrence. Generally these patients do not have keloids elsewhere and the recurrence rate following total excision is low.

References

1. Peacock EE Jr, Madden JW, Trier WC: Biologic basis of treatment of keloid and hypertrophic scars. South Med J 63:755–760, 1970.
2. Oluwasanmi JO: Keloids in the African. Clin Plast Surg 1:179–195, 1974.
3. Omo-Dare P: Genetic studies on keloids. J Natl Med Assoc 67:428–432, 1975.
4. Barrett JL: Keloid. In Bergsma D (ed): Birth Defects: Atlas and Compendium. Baltimore, Williams & Wilkins, 1973, p 553.
5. Ketchum LD, Cohen IK, Masters FW: Hypertrophic scars and keloids: A collective review. Plast Reconstr Surg 53:140–454, 1974.
6. Kamin AJ: The etiology of keloids: A review of the

literature and a new hypothesis. S Afr Med J 38:913–916, 1964.

7. Cosman B, Crikelair GF, Gaulin JC, et al: The surgical treatment of keloids. Plast Reconstr Surg 27:335–358, 1961.

8. Monstala MFH, Abdel-Fattah AMA: Keloids of the earlobes in Egypt: Their rarity in childhood and their treatment. Br J Plast Surg 29:59–60, 1976.

9. Pamakrishnan KM, Thomas KP, Sundararajan CR: Study of 1000 patients with keloids in South India. Plast Reconstr Surg 53:276–280, 1977.

10. Ketchum LD: Hypertrophic scars and keloids. Clin Plast Surg 4:301–310, 1977.

11. Monstafa MFH, Abdel-Fallah AF: Presumptive evidence of the effect of pregnancy estrogens on keloid growth: Case report. Plast Reconstr Surg. 56:450–453, 1975.

12. Ford LC, King DF, Lagasse LD, et al: Increased binding in keloids: A preliminary communication. J Dermatol Surg Oncol 9:545–547, 1983.

13. Bloom D: Heredity keloids: A review of the literature and report of a family with multiple keloids in five generations. NY State J Med 56:511–519, 1956.

14. Cohen IK, McCoy BJ, Mohanakumar T et al: Immunoglobulin, complement and histocompatibility antigen studies in keloid patients. Plast Reconstr Surg 63:689–695, 1979.

15. Char F: Ehlers-Danlos syndrome. Birth Defects 8:300–301, 1972.

16. Kurwa AR: Rubinstein-Taybi syndrome and spontaneous keloids. Clin Exp Dermatol 4:251–254, 1978.

17. Hambrick GW, Carter DM: Pachydermoperiostosis. Touraine-Solente-Golie syndrome. Arch Dermatol 94:594–607, 1966.

18. Akintewe TA, Alabi GO: Scleroderma presenting with multiple keloids. Br Med J 291:448–499, 1985.

19. Abdel-Fattah AMA: Three distinct varieties of earlobe keloids in Egypt. Br J Plast Surg 31:261–262, 1978.

20. Crockett DJ: Regional keloid susceptibility. Br J Plast Surg 17:245–253, 1964.

21. O'Grady RB, Kirk HO: Corneal keloids. Am J Ophthalmol 73:206–213, 1972.

22. Onwukwe MF. The suppurative keloid. J Dermatol Surg Oncol 4:333–335, 1978.

23. Hayrati E, Hoomand A: The keloidal diathesis: A resistant state to malignancies. Plast Reconstr Surg 59:555–559, 1977.

24. Manalan SS, Cohen IK, Theograf SD: Dermatofibrosarcoma protuberans or keloid—a warning. Plast Reconstr Surg 54:96–98, 1974.

25. Mancini RF, Quaife JV: Histogenesis of experimentally produced keloids. J Invest Dermatol 38:143–150, 1962.

26. Kischer CW, Bailey JF: The mast cell in hypertrophic scars. Tex Rep Biol Med 30:327–338, 1972.

27. Linares HA, Larson DL: Early differential diagnosis between hypertrophic and nonhypertrophic healing. J Invest Dermatol 62:512–516, 1974.

28. Nikolowski W: Pathogenesis, Klinik and therapie des keloids. Arch Klin Exp Dermatol 212:550–569, 1961.

29. Linares HA, Kischer CW, Dobrkovsky M, et al: The histiotrophic organization of the hypertrophic scar in humans. J Invest Dermatol 59:323–331, 1972.

30. James WD, Besancenez DC, Odom RB: The ultrastructure of a keloid. J Am Acad Dermatol 3:50–57, 1980.

31. Knapp TR, Daniels JR, Kaplan EN: Pathological scar formation. Am J Pathol 56:47–63, 1977.

32. Hoopes JE, Su C-T, Im MJ: Enzyme activities in hypertrophic scars. Plast Reconstr Surg 47:132–137, 1971.

33. Shetlar MR, Dobrkovsky M, Linares H, et al: The hypertrophic scar. Glycoprotein and collagen components of burn scars. Proc Soc Exp Biol Med 138:298–300, 1971.

34. Russell JD, Witt WS: Cell size and growth characteristics of cultured fibroblasts isolated from normal and keloid tissue. Plast Reconstr Surg 57:207–212, 1976.

35. Shetlar MR, Shetlar CL, Hendricks L, et al: The use of athymic nude mice for the study of human keloids. Proc Soc Exp Biol Med 179:549–552, 1985.

36. Bazin S, Nicoletis C, Delaunay A: Intercellular matrix of hypertrophic scars and keloids. In Kulonen E, Pikkaranine J (eds): Biology of Fibroblast. London, Academic Press, 1973, pp 571–578.

37. Cohen IK, Diegelmann RF, Keiser HR: Collagen metabolism in keloid and hypertrophic scar. In Longacre JJ (ed): The ultrastructure of collagen. Springfield, IL, Charles C Thomas, 1973, pp 199–212.

38. Kischer CW, Shetlar MR: Collagen and mucopolysaccharides in the hypertrophic scar. Conn Tissue Res 2:205–213, 1974.

39. Shetlar MR, Shetlar CL, Linares HA: The hypertrophic scar: Location of glycosaminoglycans within scars. Burns 4:14–19, 1977.

40. Bailey AJ, Bazin S, Sims TJ, et al: Characterization of the collagen of human hypertrophic and normal scars. Biochim Biophys Acta 405:412–421, 1975.

41. Craig DP, Schofield JD, Jackson DS: Collagen biosynthesis in normal and hypertrophic scars and keloid as a function of the duration of the scar. Br J Surg 62:741–744, 1975.

42. Cohen IK, Keiser HR: Collagen synthesis in keloid and hypertrophic scar following intralesional use of triamcinolone. Surg Forum 24:521–523, 1973.

43. Fleckman PH, Jeffrey JJ, Eisen AZ: A sensitive microassay for prolyl hydroxylase: Activity in normal and psoriatic skin. J Invest Dermatol 60:46–52, 1973.

44. Diegelmann RF, Cohen IK, McCoy BJ: Growth kinetics and collagen synthesis of normal skin, normal scar, and keloid fibroblasts in vitro. J Cell Physiol 98:341–346, 1979.

45. Abergel RP, Pizzurro D, Meeker CA, et al: Biochemical composition of the connective tissue in keloids and analysis of collagen metabolism in keloid fibroblast cultures. J Invest Dermatol 84:384–390, 1985.

46. Ala-Kokko L, Rintala A, Savolainen ER: Collagen gene expression in keloids: analysis of collagen metabolism and type I, III, IV and V procollagen mRNAs in keloid tissue and keloid fibroblast cultures. J Invest Dermatol 89:238–244, 1987.

47. Weber L, Meigel WN, Spier W: Collagen polymorphism in pathologic human scars. Arch Dermatol Res 261:63–71, 1978.

48. Uitto J, Perejda AJ, Abergel RP, et al: Altered steady-state ratio of type I/III procollagen mRNAs correlates with selectively increased type I procollagen biosynthesis in cultured keloid fibroblasts. Proc Natl Acad Sci USA 82:5935–5939, 1985.

49. Psillakis JM, DeJorge FB, Sucena RC, et al: Water and electrolyte content of normal skin, scars and keloid. Plast Reconstr Surg 47:272–274, 1971.

50. Bailey AJ, Robins SP: Embryonic skin collagen. Replacement of the type of aldimine crosslinks during the early growth period. FEBS Lett 21:330–334, 1972.

51. Bailey AJ, Bazin S, Delaunay A: Changes in the nature of the collagen during development and resorption of granulation tissue. Biochem Biophys Acta 328:383–390, 1973.

52. Bailey AJ, Sims TJ, LeLous M, et al: Collagen polymorphism in experimental granulation tissue. Biochem Biophys Res Commun 66:1160–1165, 1975.

53. Gay S, Viljanto J, Rackallio J, et al: Collagen types in early phases of wound healing in children. Acta Chir Scand 144:205–211, 1978.
54. Milsom JP, Craig RDP: Collagen degradation in cultured keloid and hypertrophic scar tissue. Br J Dermatol 89:635–643, 1973.
55. McCoy BJ, Cohen IK: Collagenase in keloid biopsies and fibroblasts. Connect Tissue Res 9:181–185, 1982.
56. Diegelmann RF, Bryant CP, Cohen IK: Tissue alpha-globulins in keloid formation. Plast Reconstr Surg 59:418–423, 1977.
57. Linares HA, Larson DL: Proteoglycans and collagenase in hypertrophic scar formation. Plast Reconstr Surg 62:589–593, 1978.
58. Ponec M, Kempenaar JA, Van Der Meulen-Van Harskamp GA, et al: Effects of glucocorticosteroids on cultured human skin fibroblasts. IV. Specific decrease in the synthesis of collagen but no effect on its hydroxylation. Biochem Pharmacol 28:2777–2778, 1979.
59. McCoy BJ, Diegelmann RF, Cohen IK: *In vitro* inhibition of cell growth, collagen synthesis, and prolyl hydroxylase activity by triamcinolone acetonide. Proc Soc Exp Biol Med 163:216–222, 1980.
60. Ketchum LD, Robinson DW, Masters FW: The degeneration of mature collagen: A laboratory study. Plast Reconstr Surg 40:89–91, 1967.
61. Cohen IK, Beaven MA, Horakova S., et al: Histamine and collagen synthesis in keloid and hypertrophic scar. Surg Forum 23:509–511, 1972.
62. Topol BM, Lewis VL Jr, Benveniste K: The use of antihistamine to retard the growth of fibroblasts derived from human skin, scar, and keloid. Plast Reconstr Surg 68:227–232, 1981.
63. Maguire HC: Treatment of keloids with triamcinolone acetonide injected intralesionally. JAMA 192:325–327, 1965.
64. Minkowitz F: Regression of massive keloid following partial excision and post-operative intralesional administration of traimcinolone. Br J Plast Surg 20:432–435, 1967.
65. Griffith BH, Monroe CW, McKinney P: A follow-up study on the treatment of keloids with triamcinolone acetonide. Plast Reconstr Surg 46:145–150, 1970.
66. Ketchum LD, Smith J, Robinson DW, et al: Treatment of hypertrophic scars, keloids, and scar contracture by triamcinolone acetonide. Plast Reconstr Surg 38:209–218, 1966.
67. Griffith BH: Treatment of keloids with triamcinolone acetonide. Plast Reconstr Surg 38:202–208, 1966.
68. Kiil J: Keloids treated with topical injections of triamcinolone acetonide (Kenalog). Immediate and long term results. Scand J Plast Reconstr Surg 11:169–172, 1977.
69. Murray JC, Pollack SV, Pinnell SR: Keloids: A review. J Am Acad Dermatol 4:461–470, 1981.
70. Vallis CP: Intralesional injection of keloids and hypertrophic scars with the Dermojet. Plast Reconstr Surg 40:255–262, 1967.
71. Berry RB: A comparison of spring and CO_2 powered needleless injectors in the treatment of keloids with triamcinolone. Br J Plast Surg 34:458–461, 1981.
72. Tsur H, Blankstein A, Kon M, et al: New technique for intralesional steroid injections. Ann Plast Surg 18:83–84, 1987.
73. Amene P: Activation of pulmonary tuberculosis following intralesional corticosteroids. Arch Dermatol 119:361–362, 1983.
74. Santa Cruz DJ, Ulbright TM: Mucin-like changes in keloids. Am J Clin Pathol 75:18–22, 1981.
75. Ceilley RI, Babin RW: The combined use of cryosur-

76. Shepard JP, Dawber RPR: The response of keloid scars to cryotherapy. Plast Reconstr Surg 70:677–682, 1982.
77. Zacarian SA: Discussion of the response of keloid scars to cryosurgery. Plast Reconstr Surg 70:683, 1982.
78. DaCosta JC: Modern Surgery. Philadelphia; WB Saunders, 1931.
79. Apfelberg DB, Master MR, Lash H: The use of epidermis over a keloid as an autograft after resection of the keloid. J Dermatol Surg Oncol 2:409–411, 1976.
80. Pollack SV, Goslen JB: The surgical treatment of keloids. J Dermatol Surg Oncol 8:1045–1049, 1982.
81. Borges AF, Alexander JE: Relaxed skin tension lines, Z-plasty on scars and fusiform excision of lesions. Br J Plast surg 15:242–254, 1962.
82. Cosman B, Wolfe M: Correlation of keloid recurrence with completeness of local excision. A negative report. Plast Reconstr Surg 50:163–166, 1972.
83. Kantor GR, Ratz JL, Wheeland RG: Treatment of acne keloidalis nuchae with carbon dioxide laser. J Am Acad Dermatol 14:263–267, 1986.
84. Kantor GR, Wheeland RG, Barlen PL, et al: Treatment of earlobe keloids with carbon dioxide laser excision: A report of 16 cases. J Dermatol Surg Oncol 11:1063–1067, 1985.
85. Apfelberg DB, Maser MR, Lash H, et al: Preliminary results of argon and carbon dioxide laser treatment of keloid scars. Lasers Surg Med 4:283–290, 1984.
86. Abergel RP, Dwyer RM, Meeker CA, et al: Laser treatment of keloids: A clinical trial and *in vitro* study with Nd:YAG laser. Lasers Surg Med 4:291–295, 1984.
87. Abergel RP, Meeker CA, Lain TS, et al: Control of connective tissue metabolism by lasers: Recent developments and future prospects. J Am Acad Dermatol 11:1142–1150, 1984.
88. Brent B: The role of pressure therapy in management of earlobe keloids: Preliminary report of a controlled study. Ann Plast Reconstr Surg 1:579–581, 1978.
89. Rauscher GE, Kolmer WL: Treatment of recurrent earlobe keloids. Cutis 38:67–68, 1986.
90. Fujimori R, Hiramoto M, Ofuji S: Sponge fixation method for treatment of early scars. Plast Reconstr Surg 42:322–327, 1968.
91. Pearce HE: Postsurgical acrylic ear splints for keloids. J Dermatol Surg Oncol 12:583–585, 1986.
92. Cosman B, Crikelair GF, Ju DMC, et al: The surgical treatment of keloids. Plast Reconstr Surg 27:335–358, 1961.
93. Craig RDP, Pearson D: Early postoperative irradiation of keloid scars. Br J Plast Surg 18:369–376, 1965.
94. Ollstein RN, Siegel HW, Cillooley JF, et al: Treatment of keloids by combined surgical excision and immediate postoperative x-ray therapy. Ann Plast Surg 7:281–285, 1981.
95. Levy DS, Salter MM, Roth RE: Postoperative irradiation in the prevention of keloids. Am J Roentgenol 127:509–510, 1976.
96. Inalsingh CHA: An experience in treating five hundred and one patients with keloids. Johns Hopkins Med J 134:284–290, 1974.
97. Keloids and x-rays. Br Med J 3:592, 1974.
98. Hoffman S: Radiotherapy for keloids. Ann Plast Surg 9:265, 1982.
99. King GD, Salzman FA: Keloid scars: Analysis of 89 patients. Surg Clin North Am 50:595–598, 1970.
100. Malaker K, Ellis F, Paine CH: Keloid scars: A new

method of treatment combining surgery with interstitial radiotherapy. Clin Radiol 27:179–183, 1976.

101. Peacock EE: Pharmacologic control of surface scarring in human beings. Ann Surg 193:592–597, 1981.

102. Peacock EE: Control of wound healing and scar formation in surgical patients. Arch Surg 116:1325–1329, 1981.

103. DeLimpens J: The local treatment of hypertrophic scars and keloids with topical retinoic acid. Br J Dermatol 103:319–323, 1980.

104. Daly TJ, Golitz LE, Weston WL: A double-blind placebo-controlled efficacy study of tretinoin cream 0.05% in the treatment of keloids and hypertrophic scars. J Invest Dermatol 86:470, 1986 (abstract).

105. Daly TJ, Weston WL: Retinoid effects on fibroblast proliferation and collagen synthesis in vitro and on fibrotic disease in vivo. J Am Acad Dermatol 15:900–902, 1986.

106. Goette DK, Berger TG: Acne keloidalis nuchae. A transepithelial elimination disorder. Int J Dermatol 26:442–444, 1987.

31

SCLERODERMA (SYSTEMIC SCLEROSIS): COMPARISON WITH WOUND HEALING

E. Carwile LeRoy, M.D.

Why include a chapter on the diffuse connective tissue diseases, emphasizing scleroderma, in a text on wound healing? Because understanding of both scleroderma and wound healing may be advanced by a detailed comparison of the two processes. Wound healing represents a localized, tightly regulated fibrotic response in which inflammation, angiogenesis, and extracellular matrix formation and organization follow predictable patterns and move in stages toward a functionally efficient outcome. In contrast, the same processes of inflammation, altered angiogenesis, and extracellular matrix deposition occur in scleroderma, leading to hidebound skin, microvascular obliteration, vascular scarring, and circulatory insufficiency in vital organs. A complete understanding of both connective tissue disease pathobiology and wound healing biology will require more precise knowledge of connective tissue structure, cell-matrix interactions, angiogenesis, inflammation, responses to growth factors and cytokines, and the orderly termination of these activating and selecting processes.

DEFINITIONS AND CLINICAL COMMENTS

Connective tissue diseases are widespread afflictions of the diffuse interstitial connective tissues that can, and often do, affect contiguous organs and structures as well. Whether skin, muscle, joints, bone, or internal viscera (gut,

lungs, heart, kidneys, brain, pancreas, bone marrow) are affected usually determines the clinical label applied to the individual patient, as well as the prognosis and outcome. Approximately 10 percent of patients have features of more than one connective tissue disorder; here the term "overlap syndrome" (of two connective tissue diseases) is used. These disorders vary widely in extent of involvement and in the stages of inflammation, immune injury, proliferation, fibrosis and atrophy present at any point in time.[1] The major connective tissue diseases are presented in Table 31–1.

The connective tissue diseases (excluding inherited forms) are believed to have an autoimmune mechanism; i.e., the body's molecular

Table 31–1. MAJOR CONNECTIVE TISSUE DISORDERS

Rheumatoid arthritis

Osteoarthritis

Systemic lupus erythematosus

Scleroderma (systemic sclerosis, SSc)
  Dermatomyositis/polymyositis
  Sjögren's syndrome

Inherited connective tissue disorders
  Ehlers-Danlos syndrome
  Osteogenesis imperfecta
  Marfan's syndrome
  Pseudoxanthoma elasticum

Systemic vasculitis syndromes
  Polyarteritis
  Wegener's granulomatosis
  Behçet's disease

constituents, to which the individual's immune system had previously developed tolerance (nonrecognition), are now recognized as foreign antigens that trigger the immune response. Whether altered antigens or an altered immune system is primary in the autoimmune process is unknown; it remains probable that autoimmune phenomena may be secondary epiphenomena masking more specific, truly foreign activation of the immune system, such as by a virus.

Rheumatoid arthritis is a generalized multisystem disorder of immune regulation whose manifestations are consistent with widespread immune activation. Precise etiological agents, such as the Epstein-Barr virus, have failed the tests of specificity and of Koch's postulates[2] and the etiology remains unknown.

Systemic lupus erythematosus (SLE) is a multisystem disorder of immune regulation in which B-lymphocyte activation and autoantibodies to nuclear antigens seem to predominate. Target organs for immune injury are the skin, the hematopoietic stem cells, the kidneys, brain, and the lining tissue of the joints and serosal cavities. Immune complexes are uniformly present. Overlap between lupus and other connective tissue disorders, especially scleroderma, is common.[3]

Sjögren's syndrome is characterized by dry eyes and dry mouth secondary to diminished secretions due to autoimmune injury to the lacrimal and/or salivary apparatus. Alone, these findings are called the sicca complex; about half the time this complex is associated with rheumatoid arthritis, lupus, or scleroderma. The course is usually indolent with lymphadenopathy evolving into autonomous lymphoma after one to three decades.[4]

Dermatomyositis/polymyositis involves an immune injury to muscle. Patients with myositis have heterogeneous manifestations, creating confusion in classification and nomenclature. Since rheumatoid arthritis, lupus erythematosus, and scleroderma may be intrinsically associated with myositis, it is superfluous to attach other labels (mixed, overlap) to these disorders when myositis is present. One must be careful in interpreting the literature, because different authors classify connective tissue diseases differently, depending on the presence of myositis.[5]

The *inherited connective tissue disorders* include Marfan's syndrome, Ehlers-Danlos syndrome, osteogenesis imperfecta, pseudoxanthoma elasticum, homocysteinuria, and occasional disorders with overlapping features that are more difficult to classify. (Abnormalities of connective tissue are discussed in Chapter 9.)

The *systemic vasculitides* are too broad and ill-defined a category to be considered here. They are characterized by an intense inflammatory infiltration of all layers (intima, media, adventitia) of the arterial and arteriolar wall with destruction, organ insufficiency, and aneurysmal formation. Clinically, peripheral and visceral neuropathy and peripheral vascular insufficiency are the hallmarks.[6]

Osteoarthritis is a degenerative condition of the articular cartilage and subchondral bone that can be caused by trauma, infection, crystal-induced inflammation, autoimmune-mediated inflammation, metabolic deposition, and many other factors. Whether there are intrinsic or primary causes of articular (hyaline) cartilage failure remains to be fully answered.[7]

Since scleroderma is the main topic of this chapter, the reader is referred to standard texts on rheumatic disease for further discussion of other connective tissue disorders.

SCLERODERMA

Scleroderma is a spectrum of disorders characterized by subtle inflammatory changes, vascular obliteration, and fibrosis in association with autoimmune phenomena. Localized scleroderma consists of morphea (firm patches of scarring that may or may not show pigmentary changes), linear scleroderma (long strips of scarring, often with epidermal atrophy, usually in neurodermatome distribution that may be associated with growth retardation and bone atrophy [coup de sabre]), and generalized morphea (major portions of the body covered with isolated and/or confluent firm patches.[8]

Generalized scleroderma (systemic sclerosis, SSc) is a variably expressed disorder characterized by inflammation, vascular lesions, and fibrosis that affects the skin, gastrointestinal tract, lungs, joints, tendons, heart, and kidneys. Patients with systemic sclerosis seem to show two separate patterns of skin and internal organ involvement. The most prevalent pattern is called limited cutaneous systemic sclerosis (lSSc). These patients have a long history of Raynaud's phenomenon (episodic vasospasm of the digits, nose, and ears), skin thickening limited to the fingers, extremities, or face, and internal organ involvement limited to the second, third, and fourth decades of disease (with the exception of the esophagus which is affected early). This form can often be detected early, when the only clinical feature is Raynaud's phenomenon, by nailfold capillaroscopy and anticentromere antibody determinations.[9]

Fortunately affecting only a minority of SSc patients is diffuse cutaneous systemic sclerosis (dSSC), the more serious form of generalized scleroderma (Fig. 31–1). These patients may present with the abrupt onset of Raynaud's phenomenon, puffy hands, arms, face, and feet, rapid development of hidebound skin covering both extremities and trunk, and the appearance of hypertension with renal failure, progressive pulmonary alveolitis with interstitial fibrosis, severe gastrointestinal dysfunction, myocarditis with myocardial fibrosis, peripheral joint contractures, and ischemic ulcerations with necrosis of tissue. These manifestations, alone or in combination, may be fatal. With the exception of renal SSc, which has shown remarkable responsiveness to the newer antihypertensive medications including captopril and enalapril, the systemic manifestations are sufficiently resistant to therapy to make dSSc one of the most frequent causes of death among the diffuse connective tissue diseases.[10]

The major sign (taut skin proximal to the metacarpophalangeal joints) and several of the minor symptoms (interstitial lung disease, wide-mouthed colonic sacculations, digital infarcts, and esophageal hypomotility) of SSc are not infrequently associated with other connective tissue disorders; the most appropriate diagnostic term for this clinical situation is overlap syndrome of scleroderma and the other disorder (for example, SLE). Convention and usage exclude myositis and Sjögren's syndrome from this rule; i.e., SSc with myositis is SSc, not overlap, and SSc with sicca complex is both SSc and Sjögren's syndrome, not overlap. Most investigators agree with this use of the term "overlap."

There is much less agreement about a group of patients with features suggestive of one or more connective tissue disorders but insuffi-cient to confirm any one definitively. Most of these patients have Raynaud's phenomenon, some have esophageal hypomotility, and many have a variety of autoimmune phenomena. These patients are best diagnosed as having undifferentiated connective tissue syndromes (UCTS), because most of them will eventually develop a definite connective tissue disease.[11] Some investigators refer to this as mixed (MCTD) or early (ECTD) connective tissue disorder or use such hybrid terms as "sclerolu-pus." The nomenclature is confusing and one must determine which features patients reported in the literature actually have. The use of the term "scleroderma spectrum of disorders" serves to emphasize the broad and overlapping manifestations of these connective tissue disorders.

PATHOGENESIS

Fibrosis has been the clinical hallmark of SSc since Curzio described the first case in 1753. After Klemperer declared it, among others, a connective tissue ("collagen") disease in 1942, detailed characterization of the connective tissue ensued. In parallel investigations over the last 50 years, many investigators have emphasized the vascular and microvascular features of SSc. Interactions among connective tissue, anchorage-dependent cells, and angiogenesis give SSc and wound healing much in common (similar substrates, structures, and the skin as the primary arena), as well as much in contrast (usually, wound healing is tightly regulated and efficiently executed, returning ultimately to a virtually healthy state while the pathological fibrosis of SSc persists). Primary incisions in proximal sites of scleroderma patients heal on time and with appropriate configuration. This

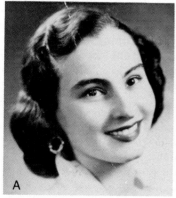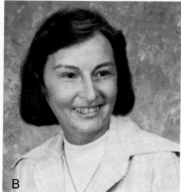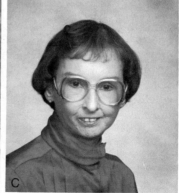

Figure 31–1. Photographs of a patient with scleroderma over a 34-year time span. *A,* Patient at age 20. *B,* Two years after diagnosis at age 42. *C,* Twelve years following diagnosis.

is in contrast to the indolent, poorly healing ulcers that occur over distal pressure sites. For the purposes of this discussion, tissue matrix, cellular, molecular, and regulatory factors are discussed separately, with immune, vascular, and connective tissue considerations intercalated.[12]

Tissue/Matrix

Connective tissue has many components, including, in the skin alone, collagens I, III, V, fibronectin, proteoglycans, and structural glycoproteins. The vasculature of connective tissue also contains collagens IV, V, VI, laminin, heparan sulfates, and structural glycoproteins.[13] Since both the connective tissue and the vasculature are affected in SSc, it should come as no surprise that most of the components of both that have been analyzed have been found to be abnormal. In a real sense, the histopathology that dominated study in the first half of this century has been confirmed in macromolecular or extracellular matrix terms in the present half century.

It has been difficult to quantify collagens in skin for several reasons: (1) healthy dermis is 85 percent collagen (largely type I); (2) collagens are insoluble; (3) histochemical, even immunohistochemical, techniques are at best semiquantitative; (4) the disease stage at which lesional samples are taken is important but often uncontrolled; and (5) the skin of different anatomical regions differs substantially in content and thickness of matrix.[14] It is thus understandable that early studies of total skin collagen in SSc showed little to no difference from controls. However, it came to be realized that the sclerotic process was replacing subcutaneous fat with connective tissue, which was indistinguishable from contiguous healthy dermis. Immunohistological examination of types I, III, and V collagen suggested increases.[15] In vitro biosynthetic studies involving lesional fibroblasts have been helpful in more precisely defining the collagens involved in quantitative terms.[16, 17]

Skin from SSc patients was analyzed for mucopolysaccharides (uronic acid and sulfated sugars) and usually found to contain elevated levels.[18] The precise proteoglycan involved was never clearly identified owing to the variable separation of chondroitin and heparan and keratan sulfates on ion-exchange columns after cetylpyridinium precipitation. Increased proteoglycan production is one of the earliest and most consistent matrix abnormalities observed

in the in vitro study of the SSc fibroblast. The major mucopolysaccharide found to be increased is hyaluronate.[19] (A complete discussion of proteoglycans is presented in Chapter 11.)

Fibronectin, an attachment protein of ubiquitous distribution produced by virtually every cell type studied, is present in the lesions of SSc, and its production by lesional fibroblasts in vitro is increased.[20] (The significance of fibronectin in normal wound healing is also discussed in Chapter 12.)

Cell culture studies have been the key to understanding the fibrotic, vascular, and immune features of SSc.

Fibroblast Studies

The first study indicating that the SSc fibroblast was unusual in its synthesis of matrix was published in 1972.[16] This report was the first in vitro demonstration of a propagable abnormality of anchorage-dependent lesional cells from a connective tissue disease. The initial observation was that SSc fibroblasts synthesize and secrete increased quantities of total collagen on a per-cell basis and that this increased collagen synthesis can be demonstrated in culture for up to 10 to 12 subpassages (propagable). Several laboratories have expanded and sharpened the focus of the initial report.[17, 21–23] First, the collagen synthesized is similar in type to that produced by healthy fibroblasts: about 80 percent type I and 20 percent type III. Second, SSc fibroblasts produce the usual amounts of collagenase with the usual activity. Third, in addition to collagens, SSc fibroblasts synthesize and secrete increased quantities of proteoglycan and fibronectin, raising a number of testable questions: (1) Do all lesional cells from fibrotic reactions show increased synthesis and secretion of such diverse molecules (collagens, proteoglycans, fibronectin) as does the SSc fibroblast? (2) Is the regulation of synthesis and secretion of these diverse components of the extracellular matrix coordinately controlled? (3) Is such a general increase in secretion and synthesis of collagens, proteoglycans, and attachment proteins (fibronectin) a general phenomenon of fibroblast activation? Answers to these questions could bring us closer to the ability to control the undesirable effects of fibrosis in humans.

Fibroblast activation is not the only hypothesis offered to explain the behavior of SSc fibroblasts. An alternative explanation involves amplification of a subset of fibroblasts already programmed to secrete and synthesize high levels of extracellular matrix. Consistent with this selection hypothesis is the fact that, despite their monotonous morphological homogeneity, fibroblasts are distinctly heterogenous with regard to proliferation and matrix synthesis.[24] Page and colleagues developed a probe to select and isolate the high matrix-synthesizing fibroblast. The first component of complement, C1q, binds selectively to these fibroblasts and induces mitogenesis; thus, both the selection and the amplification of the high matrix-synthesizing cell can be achieved in this instance by the same receptor-ligand interaction.[25] The data of Page and co-workers predicted that C1q would show increased binding to SSc fibroblasts.[26] We tested this hypothesis and found substantially greater amounts of C1q bound to SSc fibroblasts than to healthy fibroblasts (Fig. 31–2). Binding affinity of C1q to SSc fibroblasts has not yet been determined. Despite these technical limitations, C1q looks promising as a probe to identify and isolate the high matrix-producing fibroblast in all human fibrotic lesions to determine the basis of its preprogrammed high matrix-synthesizing state. C1q seems to bind via its collagenous portion. As yet, there is no evidence that fibronectin is the receptor, since neither trypsin treatment of cells nor the presence of antibodies to fibronectin affects C1q binding. Thus, the fibroblast membrane receptor for C1q remains unidentified.

Of perhaps equal significance to the high matrix-synthesizing phenotype of SSc fibroblasts is the realization, based on more recent evidence, that these cells exhibit unusual growth characteristics suggestive of abnormal growth regulation. Even in the early work, with collagen synthesis as an end point, it was observed that SSc fibroblasts were insensitive to serum deprivation compared with healthy fibroblasts.[27] Since the major serum mitogen for anchorage-dependent cells is platelet-derived growth factor (PDGF), studies with purified PDGF showed SSc fibroblasts to be insensitive to the isolated growth factor as well.[28] Present studies with multiple growth factors suggest that the insensitivity to PDGF observed with SSc fibroblasts in two different study formats is not associated with general growth factor insensitivity; to the contrary, when exposed to several combinations of growth factors, SSc fibroblasts show increased sensitivity over a prolonged period in vitro (Fig. 31–3). Whereas healthy cells show modest proliferative responses to combinations of PDGF, transforming growth factor-β (TGF-β), and epidermal growth factor (EGF), and whereas these responses decline substantially by the sixth to eighth subpassage, SSc fibroblasts show heightened responses, especially in the presence of EGF, that persist beyond the sixth to eighth subpassage. It remains to be determined whether these in vitro studies of fibroblast responses to growth factor combinations will have in vivo significance for the understanding of SSc.[27–29]

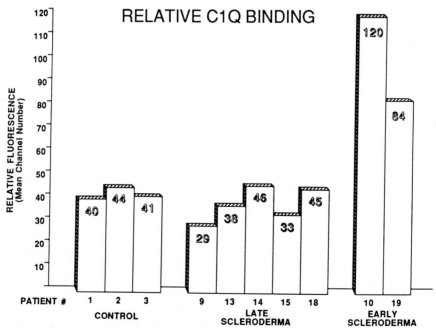

Figure 31–2. Relative fluorescence of cultured human dermal fibroblasts stained with fluorescein conjugated anti-C1q antibodies. (From Maxwell DB, Grotendorst CA, Grotendorst GR, et al: Fibroblast heterogeneity in scleroderma: C1q studies. J Rheumatol 14:756–759, 1987.)

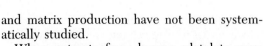

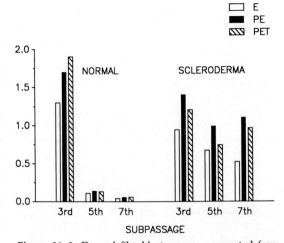

Figure 31–3. Dermal fibroblasts were propagated from punch biopsies of involved dorsal forearm skin of a patient with scleroderma and from a matched healthy volunteer by standard explant techniques. Monolayers were grown to confluence and exposed to previously determined optimal concentrations of epidermal growth factor (E), platelet-derived growth factor (P), or transforming growth factor-β (T) in all combinations (PE, PET) in 1 percent serum for 18 hours. Cultures were incubated with tritiated thymidine for 2 hours and harvested and the amount of incorporated label determined. Results are expressed as the ratio of cpm/cell with and without growth factor.

(Chapter 4 provides an in-depth discussion on the effect of growth factors on cell division.)

For nearly a decade it has been known that the sera of some patients with SSc inhibited the growth of endothelial cells while stimulating the growth of fibroblasts.[30] Since that time we and others have sought combinations of sera, conditioned media, and isolated growth factors that mimic as closely as possible this dual effect of scleroderma serum. Crude supernatants ("crude soups") of peripheral blood mononuclear cells from healthy and SSc subjects were found to be stimulatory both to fibroblast growth and to collagen production.[31] These crude soups also inhibited endothelial cell growth. Panning for adherent monocytes enriched this activity, whereas removal of adherent monocytes reduced activity. Postlethwaite and colleagues[32] and, independently, Agelli and Wahl[33] found both fibroblast stimulatory and fibroblast inhibitory activities in the crude soups of lymphocytes prepared and treated by a variety of techniques. Some, but not all, of these activities were reproduced by combinations of serum and interleukin-1 (IL-1), which is very likely present in the crude soups of all activated monocytes. IL-1, however, does not seem to be a sufficient explanation for all the activities observed in SSc serum. The effects of other interleukins (IL-2,3,4,5) on fibroblast growth

and matrix production have not been systematically studied.

When extracts from human platelets were studied for effects on fibroblasts, no distinctive patterns could be found. This may be due to the obvious fact that all in vitro cell studies are dependent on serum and that serum is essentially a platelet extract or to the fact that platelets contain multiple factors (e.g., PDGF, TGF-β, beta thromboglobulin, connective tissue activating peptide III) that blunt the full expression of one another.

The effects of PDGF on fibroblast behavior were well described by Ross and colleagues years ago.[33a] More recently, Varga and Jimenez along with others, including ourselves, have focused on the effects of TGF-β on fibroblast behavior.[34] In combination with serum, TGF-β is stimulatory to both fibroblast growth and collagen synthesis, perhaps via the autocrine stimulation of PDGF synthesis. Recalling the dual and dichotomous effects of SSc serum on fibroblasts and endothelial cells, we found that endothelial cells were exquisitely sensitive to picomolar concentrations of TGF-β and that the irreversible inhibition of endothelial cell growth was associated with a down-regulation of EGF receptors. In contrast, TGF-β up-regulates fibroblast EGF receptors, perhaps explaining the dichotomous behavior of this pleiotrophic growth factor. At the moment, TGF-β is a candidate for the SSc serum factor that injures endothelial cells and stimulates fibroblasts.[35]

It is possible that fibroblast selection/activation in SSc represents the absence of an inhibitory factor rather than the presence of a stimulatory factor. Interferon-γ, a cytokine capable of inhibiting fibroblast collagen synthesis, has been proposed as a potential therapeutic agent in SSc.[36] Diminished interferon-γ production by SSc cells or patients has not been reported as yet.

Endothelial Cells

Prominent intimal proliferation of arteries and obliterative proliferation of arterioles and capillaries have been observed histologically for over 50 years in tissues affected by scleroderma. These lesions bear remarkable similarity to those of chronic homograft rejection. In 1979, Kahaleh and associates propagated endothelial cells in vitro by the technique of Jaffé and showed that some scleroderma sera prevented endothelial cell proliferation and, in high concentrations, were directly cytotoxic.[30] These same sera demonstrated diminished capacity to neutralize the serum protease trypsin, which showed a strong negative correlation with cytotoxicity.[37] Protease inhibitors such as soybean trypsin inhibitor (Kunitz) inhibited cytotoxicity; it was concluded that a protease was present in scleroderma sera in concentrations sufficient to overcome the multiple serum protease inhibitors and that this protease was cytotoxic to endothelial cells. Direct isolation of this putative protease has not been achieved, but using selective substrates and inhibitors, it does not appear to be kallikrein, angiotensin-converting enzyme inhibitor, or plasminogen activator. T cells, monocytes, and mast cells all produce a variety of proteases.

On the basis of the autoimmune hypothesis, one might expect antibodies, selective or nonspecific, to be directed against endothelial cells and to have access to at least the surface of these cells. Occasional reports of antibodies to endothelial cells have not shown them to be selective either for endothelial cells or for SSc. The most selective of the autoantibodies for SSc are antibodies to centromere,[38] to topoisomerase I,[39] to ribonucleoprotein (RNP), to several nucleolar proteins presently being defined,[40] and to the matrix proteins type IV collagen and laminin.[41, 42] Several testable questions arise: (1) Could circulating antibodies to subcellular components injure endothelial cells in vivo? The present consensus seems to be that antibodies do not penetrate cell plasma membranes unless they recognize a peripheral cell membrane component and activate complement-dependent cell lysis or at least induce altered permeability to macromolecules. (2) Could antibodies to endothelial basement membrane components, the anchorage-dependent foundation for endothelial cell function composed largely of type IV collagen, laminin, and heparan sulfate, prevent the full phenotypic maturation of these cells and their orderly proliferation to resurface areas of vascular denudation and ultimately to impair the critical functions of nonthrombogenicity, prevention of platelet adhesiveness, and capillary permeability? (3) Could the autoimmunity and endothelial injury of SSc be better understood by asking whether specialized functions of endothelial cells (transport, shape change) expose either subcellular (e.g., topoisomerase I) components or matrix (laminin) to the immune system (e.g., it is known that endothelial cells can be induced to become antigen-presenting cells by expressing Ia antigens)? It would be of interest to see whether topoisomerase I is expressed on the surface of dividing or migrating endothelial cells. An activated endothelial cell expressing class II MHC (major histocompatibility complex) determi-

nants and containing topoisomerase I (topo I) on its surface could present this enzyme to appropriate T lymphocytes, and this could initiate an anti-topo I immune response, which would perpetuate the antioimmune attack on endothelial cells, including microvascular endothelial cells.

Autoantibodies, of course, are not the only effector of the immune response that could initiate endothelial cell injury. Cytolytic effector cells can also directly attack the vascular lining in vitro and in vivo. Recent interest in IL-2 for tumor chemotherapy has highlighted the serious side effects of the in vivo production of the lymphokine-activated killer, or LAK, cell, a T-lymphocyte, IL-2–independent cytolytic cell.[43] Similar cells (natural killer or large granular lymphocytes) could play a role in the endothelial cell damage in SSc, but as yet no proof of this exists.

There are conflicting data concerning the presence of endothelial cell cytotoxic activities in scleroderma sera.[44–46] Patients with other diagnoses (e.g., mixed connective tissue disease), which to our minds are part of the pathobiological spectrum of scleroderma-related disorders, have been shown to have endothelial cell–cytotoxic activity in their serum. Also, some investigators have observed low levels of cytotoxicity to fibroblast preparations (which could be explained by contamination of fibroblast cell cultures with microvascular endothelial cells). Despite these largely semantic and technical differences between the original and later reports, interesting new information has emerged from the pursuit of an endothelial cytotoxic factor in SSc. Deicher and colleagues recently observed two distinct endothelial cytotoxic factors in the sera of scleroderma patients: a large factor with activity similar to the original and a dialyzable, small molecular weight (<1000 daltons) factor, which has been isolated and identified by mass spectrometery/ gas liquid chromatography to be the arachidonate-derived, 5-lipoxygenase–dependent leukotriene LTB_4, one of the most potent leukocyte chemotactic factors but not previously shown to be cytotoxic to endothelial cells.[47] It seems likely that more than one type of leukocyte produces leukotriene and that there is more than one type of endothelial cytotoxic activity in scleroderma. More detailed studies are needed to evaluate the potential for proteases, cytokines, antibodies, and immediate inflammatory mediators (leukotrienes, serotonin, histamine) to be either primary or intermediary factors in the vascular disease of SSc through the mechanism of endothelial injury.

Most students of capillary permeability focus

on the gap junctions between endothelial cells and the heparan sulfate–rich glycocalyx surrounding endothelial cells as critical factors in maintaining the selectively permeable state that exists across the healthy endothelium. The disrupted morphology of endothelial cells in SSc makes it likely that permeability is deranged throughout the microvasculature in these patients. Direct in vivo studies of capillary permeability have not been carried out in SSc.

Platelets

In vivo evidence exists that platelet behavior is abnormal in SSc, presumably secondary to the loss of endothelial integrity. The proportion of platelets circulating in aggregates is distinctly increased,[48] and Fishman and co-workers have shown this to be characteristic of experimental endothelial injury.[49] In addition, plasma levels of the platelet alpha granule protein β-thromboglubulin (BTG) are elevated in SSc patients.[50] This offers an obvious and relatively safe way to attempt to intervene in the SSc process (with antiplatelet therapy); in the clinic, however, attempts to use dipyridamole and aspirin combinations in SSc patients have not demonstrated unequivocal therapeutic efficacy.[51] In fact, even large doses of these agents have not reduced elevated BTG levels to the normal range.

Monocytes/Lymphoctyes

In the early histological lesions of patients with scleroderma of all types, mononuclear leukocytes are plentiful. Surface markers identify these cells as about 80 percent T cells and 20 percent mixed B cells and monocytes.[52] A predominance of T cells is not specific for SSc since many inflammatory tissues contain large numbers of T cells. Certain models of fibrosis, such as the streptococcal cell wall injection model of Schwab and Cromartie, more recently studied by Agelli and Wahl, have been shown to be T-cell–dependent by virtue of resistance to induction in the T-cell–deficient nude (nu/nu) mouse.[33] To this point, no consistent evidence of a T-cell abnormality affecting fibroblast behavior has been observed in SSc patients,[53] although a variety of partially characterized activities from T cells have been identified that both stimulate and inhibit fibroblast proliferation and stimulate and inhibit fibroblast collagen and proteoglycan production. The potential for a T-cell role in the fibrosis of SSc remains; studies of tumor necrosis factor, α-lymphotoxins, and IL-2 are under way. In addition, monocytes, activated lymphocytes, and natural killer (NK) cells are potent sources of proteases, which have been implicated in the vasculotoxic reactions of SSc serum.

Mast Cells

Mast cells have been identified in vascular and epithelial tissues since Ehrlich synthesized the dyes to stain their prominent granules.[54] Moreover, the development of granulation and fibrotic responses to a variety of stimuli is associated with increased numbers of mast cells. Experimental fibrosis and mast cells have been linked since the turn of the century. Recently, a predominance of mast cells has been noted in involved SSc tissues,[55] in the immune model for SSc induced by a chronic graft-vs-host reaction,[56] and in the genetic mouse model for scleroderma, the tightskin (Tsk/+) mouse.[57] More than 20 years ago, Boucek and Alvarez observed a fibroblast-stimulating activity of the mast cell factor histamine.[58] Heparan sulfate, a major component of mast cell granules, exerts significant effects on cell proliferation in its own right and also acts to concentrate and provide a template for cationic growth factors to activate cells.[59] In addition, mast cells are reservoirs of the potent proteases tryptase and chymase, which are also used as markers to distinguish mucosal from interstitial mast cells.[60] Therefore, potentially at least, the mast cell contains a number of molecules that are capable of interacting with the microvasculature and with the interstitial fibroblast to induce responses similar to those seen in SSc. The prominence of mast cells in SSc provides a compelling basis to continue the pursuit of an immune pathogenesis because IL-3 and IL-4 are the most potent mast cell growth factors known.[61] The possibility that therapies for SSc can be developed around the inhibition of release of mast cell granules is greatly strengthened by the observation that disodium cromoglycate administration to Tsk/+ mice prevents the subsequent development of skin fibrosis.[57]

Cellular and Molecular Regulation (the Pathogenetic Hypothesis)

A major advance in molecular biology has been the development of methods for studying the regulation of gene expression. These tools can now be applied to the scleroderma fibroblast, a cell that exhibits in vitro, and presumably in vivo, a combined failure to regulate both extracellular matrix production and cell growth.

Over a 20-year span, the SSc fibroblast has been documented to express increased levels of production of collagen (types I and III and possibly type V), proteoglycans (types incompletely characterized, possibly hyaluronate, heparan sulfate, and keratan sulfate), and fibronectin. In metabolic terms of substrates, enzymes, and cofactors, few common pathways exist that explain so widespread and so autonomous a stimulation of such divergent connective tissue pathways unless these widely differing matrix species are under common promotor/enhancer regulation of gene expression. During the period of study of the SSc fibroblast, very little has been learned of the precise regulation of synthesis of any of these matrix species. Questions can now be asked regarding the

common regulation of multiple matrix molecules without complete understanding of the individual control of each molecular pathway separately. This would seem to be a valid approach to the study of the failure of regulation of matrix synthesis by the SSc fibroblast.

In addition to matrix synthesis, the SSc fibroblast also exhibits unusual growth characteristics. It remains insensitive to changes in its in vitro environment (serum, PDGF concentration) whether one measures collagen synthesis or cell proliferation. Ongoing studies are attempting to define the pattern of responses of healthy and SSc fibroblasts to multiple growth factors both by receptor expression and by competence gene expression (Fig. 31–4). It may be possible to expand the experimental parameters (within which matrix synthesis is studied separately from growth regulation) and ask

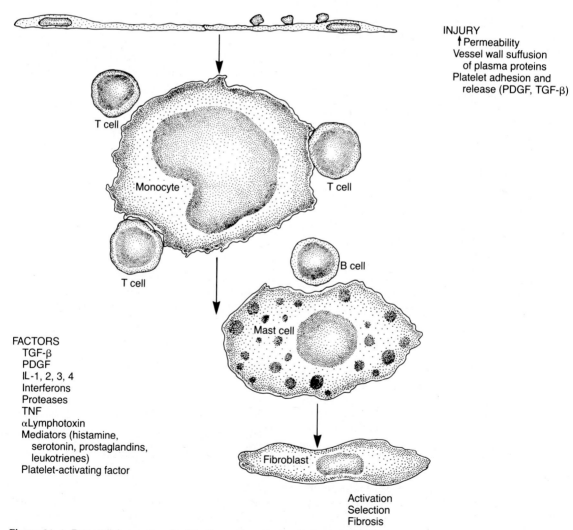

INJURY
↑Permeability
Vessel wall suffusion
  of plasma proteins
Platelet adhesion and
  release (PDGF, TGF-β)

T cell

Monocyte

T cell

T cell

B cell

FACTORS
  TGF-β
  PDGF
  IL-1, 2, 3, 4
  Interferons
  Proteases
  TNF
  αLymphotoxin
  Mediators (histamine,
    serotonin, prostaglandins,
    leukotrienes)
  Platelet-activating factor

Mast cell

Fibroblast

Activation
Selection
Fibrosis

Figure 31–4. Potential factors involved in the pathogenesis of scleroderma. PDGF = platelet-derived growth factor; TGF-β = tumor growth factor-β; IL = interleukin; TNF = tumor necrosis factor.

whether regulatory molecules can be identified that control both matrix production and growth. The SSc fibroblast represents a disease-derived cell in which the coordinate control of matrix production and cell growth regulation can be studied simultaneously.

Therapy

Agents or procedures that change the course of SSc have been few and far between. Almost everything has been tried at one time or another. Dissolving a scar seems natural enough in normal wound healing but has defied pharmacological intervention. This approach has been tested with antifibrotic agents such as potassium aminobenzoate, colchicine, and d-penicillamine (d-pen). Each of these agents has its proponents, but an effect on fibrosis has been difficult to demonstrate.

Clearly, the major success story in SSc has been the management and prevention of renal insufficiency, which is largely attributable to the family of inhibitors of angiotensin-converting enzymes, primarily captopril and later enalapril.[62] These agents, and the aggressive management of accelerated hypertension by dialysis and renal transplants, have improved the life expectancy and the quality of life for SSc patients with renal involvement. Patients are currently alive and fully functioning 8 to 10 years following the onset of the previously fatal scleroderma renal crisis. With these therapeutic advances, renal involvement is no longer the major cause of death in SSc, having been replaced by the pulmonary complications.

Colchicine has long been known to be a relatively safe drug both to treat and to prevent attacks of gouty arthritis. In cell biology studies, colchicine is known to disrupt microtubules and to prevent processing and secretion of macromolecules destined for export, such as matrix components. It was natural that colchicine would be tried for fibrotic states in the hope that it would prevent collagen deposition and possibly alter chemotaxis and proliferation as well. Investigators in Mexico City have used it to treat liver cirrhosis[63] and SSc.[64] SSc requires prolonged treatment to show skin effects, which makes the results difficult to evaluate because the taut skin of SSc patients is known to soften with time alone. Nonetheless, colchicine is safe, and the Mexico City group remains enthusiastic, despite short-term studies by other investigators that show no effect.

Enthusiasm has also developed for the treatment of pulmonary scleroderma (interstitial lung disease, fibrosing alveolitis, pulmonary fibrosis) by the long-term (18 to 36 months) administration of moderately large doses of d-pen.[65] This agent was originally introduced as a chelator of copper in patients with Wilson's disease; subsequently it was realized that d-pen interrupted the formation of collagen crosslinks in newly synthesized collagen (it has not been demonstrated to solubilize already crosslinked collagen), and on this basis it was introduced as a therapeutic agent in SSc. Subsequently, d-pen, with its free S-H group, has been demonstrated to have general immunosuppressive properties and has also been used in the treatment of rheumatoid arthritis. Its substantial toxicity led to gradual reduction in the recommended maximal dose; some of its side effects (e.g., myasthenia) mimic the autoimmune signs and symptoms for which it is prescribed. That d-pen is effective in SSc has not been documented by a controlled, prospective study. The recent studies of pulmonary involvement address the most prevalent life-threatening complication in SSc, severe interstitial lung disease with concomitant pulmonary hypertension and right heart failure. Bronchoalveolar lavage and gallium scan are being used to detect alveolitis and to elucidate its mechanisms in the hope of achieving early and more precise therapeutic intervention. It seems clear that glucocorticoids are not suitable for long-term therapy because of the side effects of osteopenia, cataracts, and skin thinning; short-term glucocorticoids are used for active alveolitis just as they are for the inflammatory and edematous features of SSc wherever they occur. Other proposed antifibrotic therapies, such as potassium aminobenzoate (Potaba), EDTA, methysergide, and tocopherol, have not stood the test of time.

Vasoactive Therapy

Vasoactive agents have been the standard therapy for the Raynaud's and peripheral vasospasms of SSc since the advent of tolazoline. Many different agents have been used, from drugs that dilate the smooth muscle directly to those that block sympathetic vasoconstriction by pharmacological sympathectomy to inhibitors of angiotensin generation. It seems inappropriate to review these agents here simply because they have all been replaced in the last 5 years by the calcium channel blockers nifedipine and diltiazem, which are more effective and have substantially fewer side effects. When these agents are coupled with captopril for hypertension and dipyridamole for microangiopathic hemolytic anemia,[66] they provide effective management for the vascular features of SSc. Local application of topical nitroglycerin over the digital arteries of fingers affected by severe pain, necrosis, or ischemic ulcers can be effective as well. In acute situations, stellate ganglion blockade can improve perfusion, and its efficacy can be monitored by skin temperature measurements. It must be kept in mind that the relentless reactive intimal proliferation of arterioles and the obliterative destruction of capillaries proceed despite vasoactive therapy and are presently unresponsive to all attempts to intervene.

CONCLUSION

One key to understanding SSc lies in explaining the intense and relentless fibrosis in the vascular intima and the diffuse interstitium in molecular terms. At the cellular level, this fibrosis is generated by direct injury to endothelium, activation/selection of fibroblasts, and subsequent autoimmune phenomena. Concerted studies of growth factors, cytokines, and inflammatory mediators are needed in order to provide a sound basis to prevent the intractable fibrosis of SSc.

Future clinical management will continue to focus on early detection of susceptible subjects, protection from environmental triggers, and intervention at the most basic pathophysiological level possible to interrupt the cycle of events that results in fibrosis. Innovative experimental therapies include mast cell blockade with ketotifin, collagen inhibition with interferon-γ, and active T-cell demolition with psoralen and photophoresis. These are imaginative therapeutic interventions yet to be proven in the clinical setting. Successful therapy will develop hand in hand with cellular and molecular understanding of the fibrosis and vascular injury of systemic sclerosis.

References

1. Christian CL: Connective tissue disease: overlap syndromes. In Cohen AS (ed): The Science and Practice of Clinical Medicine Rheumatology and Immunology, vol 4. New York, Grune & Stratton, 1979, pp 154–158.
2. Williams RC Jr, McCarty DJ: Clinical picture of rheumatoid arthritis. In McCarty DJ (ed): Arthritis and Allied Conditions, 10th ed. Philadelphia, Lea & Febiger, 1985, pp 605–619.
3. Reeves WH, Lahita RG: Clinical presentation of systemic lupus erythematosus in the adult. In Lahita RG (ed): Systemic Lupus Erythematosus. New York, John Wiley & Sons, 1987, pp 355–382.
4. Fischbach M, Talal N: Overlap syndromes: Mixed connective tissue disease and Sjögren's syndrome. In Lahita RG (ed): Systemic Lupus Erythematosus. New York, John Wiley & Sons, 1987, pp 413–420.
5. Bradley WG: Inflammatory diseases of muscle. In Kelley WN, Harris ED Jr, Ruddy S, et al (eds): Textbook of Rheumatology, 2nd ed. Philadelphia, WB Saunders, 1985, pp 1225–1245.
6. Cupps TR, Fauci AS: The Vasculitides: Major Problems in Internal Medicine. Philadelphia, WB Saunders, 1981.
7. Moskowitz RW: Clinical and laboratory findings in osteoarthritis. In McCarty DJ (ed): Arthritis and Allied Conditions. Philadelphia, Lea & Febiger, 1985, pp 1408–1432.
8. Braverman I: Morphea. In Demis DJ (ed): Clinical Dermatology, vol I, 14th ed. New York, Harper & Row, 1987.
9. LeRoy EC: Systemic sclerosis. In Kelley WN, Harris ED Jr, Ruddy S, et al (eds): Textbook of Rheumatology. Philadelphia, WB Saunders, 1981, pp 1211–1230.
10. LeRoy EC, Black C, Fleishmajer R, et al: Scleroderma (systemic sclerosis): classification, subsets, and pathogenesis. J Rheumatol 15:202–205, 1988.
11. LeRoy EC, Maricq HR, Kahaleh MB: Undifferentiated connective tissue syndromes. Arthritis Rheum 23:341–343, 1980.
12. LeRoy EC: The vascular defect in scleroderma (systemic sclerosis). Acta Med Scand (Suppl) 715:165–167, 1987.
13. Bachinger HP, LeRoy EC: Connective tissue in scleroderma (systemic sclerosis). Vascular emphasis. In Kuehn K, Krieg T (eds): Rheumatology. An Annual Review. Connective Tissue: Biological and Clinical Aspects. Basel, S. Karger, 1986, pp 430–450.
14. Cheung HS, Nicoloff JT, Kamiel MB, et al: Stimulation of fibroblast biosynthetic activity by serum of patients with pretibial myxedema. J Invest Dermatol 71:12–17, 1978.
15. Gay RE, Buckingham RB, Prince RK, et al: Collagen types synthesized in dermal fibroblast cultures from patients with early progressive systemic sclerosis. Arthritis Rheum 23:190–196, 1980.
16. LeRoy EC: Connective tissue synthesis by scleroderma skin fibroblasts in cell culture. J Exp Med 135:1351–1362, 1972.
17. Uitto J, Bauer EA, Eisen AZ: Scleroderma: Increased biosynthesis of triple helical type I and type III procollagens associated with unaltered expression of collagenase by skin fibroblasts in culture. J Clin Invest 64:921–930, 1979.
18. Uitto J, Helin G, Helin P, et al: Connective tissue in scleroderma. A biochemical study on the correlation of fractionated glycosaminoglycans and collagen in human skin. Acta Dermatovener (Stockholm) 51:401–406, 1971.
19. Buckingham RB, Prince RK, Rodnan GP: Progressive systemic sclerosis (PSS, scleroderma) dermal fibroblasts synthesize increased amounts of glycosaminoglycan. J Lab Clin Med 101:659–669, 1983.
20. Fleischmajer R, Perlish JS, Krieg T, et al: Variability in collagen and fibronectin synthesis by scleroderma fibroblasts in primary culture. J Invest Dermatol 76:400–403, 1981.
21. LeRoy EC: Increased collagen synthesis by scleroderma skin fibroblasts in vitro. J Clin Invest 54:880–889, 1974.
22. Buckingham RB, Prince RK, Rodnan GP, et al: Increased collagen accumulation in dermal fibroblast cultures from patients with progressive systemic

sclerosis (scleroderma). J Lab Clin Med 92:5–21, 1978.

23. Jimenez SA, McArthur W, Rosenbloom J: Inhibition of collagen synthesis by mononuclear cell supernates. J Exp Med 150:1421–1431, 1979.

24. Botstein GR, Sherer GK, LeRoy EC: Fibroblast selection in scleroderma. Arthritis Rheum 25:189–195, 1982.

25. Bordin S, Page RC, Narayanan AS: Heterogeneity of normal human diploid fibroblasts: Isolation and characterization of one phenotype. Science 223:171–173, 1984.

26. Maxwell DB, Grotendorst CA, Grotendorst GR, et al: Fibroblast heterogeneity in scleroderma: C1q studies. J Rheumatol 14:756–759, 1987.

27. LeRoy EC, Mercurio S, Shere GK: Replication and phenotypic expression of control and scleroderma human fibroblasts: Responses to growth factors. Proc Natl Acad Sci USA 79:1286–1290, 1982.

28. Ishikawa O, LeRoy EC, Trojanowska M: The mitogenic effect of TGF-β on human fibroblasts involves the induction of PDGF-α receptors. J Cell Physiol 145:181–186, 1990.

29. LeRoy EC, Kahaleh MB, Mercurio S: A fibroblast mitogen present in scleroderma but not control sera: Inhibition by proteinase inhibitors. Rheumatol Int 3:35–38, 1983.

30. Kahaleh MB, Shere GK, LeRoy EC: Endothelial injury in scleroderma. J Exp Med 149:1326–1335, 1979.

31. DeLustro F, LeRoy EC: Characterization of the release of human monocyte regulators of fibroblast proliferation. J Reticuloendothel Soc 31:295–305, 1982.

32. Postlethwaite AE, Smith GN, Mainardi CL, et al: Lymphocyte modulation of fibroblast function in vitro: Stimulation and inhibition of collagen production by different effector molecules. J Immunol 132:2470–2477, 1984.

33. Agelli M, Wahl SM: Cytokines and fibrosis. Clin Exp Rheumatol 4:379–388, 1986.

33a. Ross R, Vogel A: The platelet-derived growth factor. Cell 14:203–210, 1978.

34. Varga J, Jimenez SA: Stimulation of normal human fibroblast collagen production and processing by transforming growth factor-β. Biochem Biophys Res Commun 138:974–980, 1986.

35. Takehara K, LeRoy EC, Grotendorst GR: TGF-β inhibition of endothelial cell proliferation: alteration of EGF binding and EGF-induced growth regulatory (competence) gene expression. Cell 49:415–422, 1987.

36. Jimenez SA, Freundlich B, Rosenbloom J: Selective inhibition of excessive progressive systemic sclerosis (PSS) fibroblast collagen synthesis by recombinant gamma interferon. Arthritis Rheum (Suppl) 28:35, 1985.

37. Kahaleh MB, LeRoy EC: Endothelial injury in scleroderma. A protease mechanism. J Lab Clin Med 101:553–560, 1983.

38. Moroi Y, Peebles C, Fritzler MJ, et al: Autoantibody to centromere (kinetochore) in scleroderma sera. Proc Natl Acad Sci USA 77:1627–1631, 1980.

39. Bordwell B, Rothfield NF, Earnshaw WC: High titers of autoantibodies to topoisomerase I (Scl-70) in sera from scleroderma patients. Science 4739:737–740, 1986.

40. Reimer G, Rose KM, Scheer V, et al: Autoantibody to RNA polymerase I in scleroderma sera. J Clin Invest 79:65–72, 1987.

41. Mackel AM, DeLustro F, Harper FE, et al: Antibod-

ies to collagen in scleroderma. Arthritis Rheum 25:522–531, 1982.

42. Huffstutter JE, DeLustro FA, LeRoy EC: Cellular immunity to collagen and laminin in scleroderma. Arthritis Rheum 28:775–780, 1985.

43. Skibber JM, Lotze MT, Uppenkamp I, et al: Identification and expansion of human lymphokine-activated killer cells: Implications for the immunotherapy of cancer. J Surg Res 42:613–621, 1987.

44. Cohen S, Johnson AR, Hurd E: Cytoxicity of sera from patients with scleroderma. Arthritis Rheum 26:170–178, 1983.

45. Meyer O, Haim T, Dryll A, et al: Vascular endothelial cell injury in progressive systemic sclerosis and other connective tissue disease. Clin Exp Rheumatol 1:29–34, 1983.

46. Shanahan WR Jr, Korn JH: Cytotoxic activity of sera from scleroderma and other connective tissue diseases. Arthritis Rheum 25:1391–1395, 1982.

47. Drenk F, Mensing H, Serbin A, et al: Studies on endothelial cell cytotoxic activity in sera of patients with progressive systemic sclerosis, Raynaud syndrome, rheumatoid arthritis, and systemic lupus erythematosus. Rheumatol Int 5:259–263, 1985.

48. Kahaleh MB, Scharstein KK, LeRoy EC: Enhanced platelet adhesion to collagen in scleroderma. Effect of scleroderma plasma and scleroderma platelets. J Rheumatol 12:468–471, 1985.

49. Fishman JA, Ryan GB, Karnovsky MJ: Endothelial regeneration in the rat carotid artery and the significance of endothelial denudation in the pathogenesis of myointimal thickening. Lab Invest 32:339–351, 1975.

50. Kahaleh MB, Osborn I, LeRoy EC: Elevated levels of circulating platelet aggregates and beta-thromboglobulin in scleroderma. Ann Intern Med 96:610–613, 1982.

51. Takehara K, Grotendorst G, Silver R, et al: Dipyridamole decreases platelet-derived growth factor levels in human serum. Arteriosclerosis 7:152–158, 1987.

52. Roumm AD, Whiteside TL, Medsger TA Jr, et al: Lymphocytes in the skin of patients with progressive systemic sclerosis. Arthritis Rheum 27:645–653, 1984.

53. Freundlich B, Jimenez SA: Phenotype of peripheral blood lymphocytes in patients with progressive systemic sclerosis: Activated T lymphocytes and the effect of D-penicillamine therapy. Clin Exp Immunol 69:375–384, 1987.

54. Wasserman SI: The mast cell and the inflammatory response. In Pepys J, Edwards AM (eds): The Mast Cell. Its Role in Health and Disease. London, Pitman, 1979, pp 9–20.

55. Hawkins RA, Claman HN, Clark RAF, et al: Increased dermal mast cell populations in progressive systemic sclerosis: A link in chronic fibrosis? Ann Intern Med 102:182–186, 1985.

56. Claman HN: Mast cell depletion in murine chronic graft-verus-host disease. J Invest Dermatol 84:246–248, 1985.

57. Walker MA, Harley RA, LeRoy EC: Inhibition of fibrosis in TSK mice by blocking mast cell degranulation. J Rheumatol 14:299–301, 1987.

58. Boucek RJ, Alvarez TR: 5-Hydroxytryptamine: A cytospecific growth stimulator of cultured fibroblasts. Science 167:898–899, 1970.

59. Sporn MB, Roberts AB: Peptide growth factors and inflammation, tissue repair, and cancer. J Clin Invest 78:329–332, 1986.

60. Irani AM, Craig SS, DeBlois G, et al: Deficiency of the tryptase-positive, chymase-negative mast cell type

in gastrointestinal mucosa of patients with defective T lymphocyte function. J Immunol 138:4381–4386, 1987.

61. Crawford RM, Finbloom DS, Ohara J, et al: B cell stimulatory factor-1 (interleukin-4) activates macrophages for increased tumoricidal activity and expression of Ia antigens. J Immunol 139:135–141, 1987.

62. Whitman HH III, Case DB, Laragh JH, et al: Variable response to oral angiotensin-coverting enzyme blockade in hypertensive scleroderma patients. Arthritis Rheum 25:241–248, 1982.

63. Kershenobich D, Vargas F, Garcia-Tsao G, et al: Colchicine in the treatment of cirrhosis of the liver. N Engl J Med 318:1709–1713, 1988.

64. Alarcon-Segovia D, Ramos-Niembro R, DeKasap GI, et al: Long-term evaluation of colchicine in the treatment of scleroclerma. J Rheumatol 6:705–712, 1979.

65. Steen VD, Medsger TA Jr, Rodnan GP: d-Penicillamine therapy in progressive systemic sclerosis (scleroderma): A retrospective analysis. Ann Intern Med 97:652–659, 1982.

66. FitzGerald GA: Dipyridamole. N Engl J Med 316:1247–1257, 1987.

32

BURN SCAR AND SKIN EQUIVALENTS

Joseph V. Boykin, Jr., M.D., and Joseph A. Molnar, M.D., Ph.D.

The pathophysiological derangements that follow severe thermal injury are generally unequaled by other types of trauma. With injuries covering more than 30 percent of total body surface area (TBSA), significant hypovolemia and burn shock are observed, although inhalation injury remains the most frequent cause of early mortality. The presence of an inhalation injury will also significantly affect the overall mortality and morbidity of the burn patient. In addition to these acute problems, severe burns cause substantial depression of immune function, which places the patient at risk for life-threatening sepsis and related infectious complications. Recent advancements in our understanding of critical care, the nutritional requirements of the burn patient, and the increasing acceptance of early excision and grafting of selected burns have greatly improved the chances of survival for victims of severe thermal injury.

Crucial to the implementation of any clinical treatment plan is the promotion of burn wound healing and the timely coverage of the burn wound. Indeed, in the burn patient, the wound is the fundamental pathology to be treated. For the survivors of serious burn injuries, the burn scar serves as a visual reminder of their experience and, all too often, of our ineptitude at optimally controlling or modifying the environment of the burn wound (Fig. 32–1). While the factors that stimulate burn wound healing are no different from those encountered in other types of trauma, unchecked "healing" may often be accomplished at the expense of functional movement and cosmetic appearance.

In planning the treatment of severe burn injuries, one must anticipate the complications

of the wound before they have become established, and this requires a basic understanding of the phases of wound healing and the unique aspects of burn healing. Beyond this, the physician must develop an appreciation for the dedicated and resourceful team of nurses, therapists, counselors, and other specialists whose combined skills are needed to implement the treatment plan. It is through this team approach that the burn physician can optimize the healing environment of the burn wound, as well as the

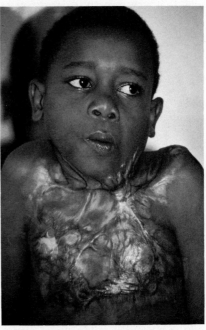

Figure 32–1. "Healed" deep partial-thickness burn injury displaying significant functional impairment and disfigurement.

motivation and enthusiasm of the patient. With these measures it is hoped that we not only can promote optimal wound healing and preserve function but also provide the patient with the skills needed to be self-sufficient and to maintain a reasonable quality of life.

BIOLOGICAL EFFECTS OF HEAT, COLD, AND CAUSTIC CHEMICALS

Humans exist within a narrow temperature continuum at the extremes of which they may experience irreversible thermal injury to skin and the supporting soft tissues. At temperatures above 120°F, scalding liquids in contact with intact skin for more than 5 minutes may cause partial-thickness injuries. This time interval for injury may be reduced to 1 second if the temperature of the liquid is increased to 155°F.[1] This time and temperature relationship also holds true for dry heat (Fig. 32–2). Conversely, prolonged exposure to extreme cold may induce frostbite. In the case of cold injury, ice crystal formation in the extracellular fluid leads to dehydration, electrolyte imbalance, and metabolic disruption secondary to the creation of an osmotic gradient that injures the cell directly.[2] Endothelial injury from cold exposure results in increased vascular permeability, thrombus formation, and microcirculatory impairment that may greatly extend the area of

tissue loss, but not to the degree of equivalent heat injury.[3–5]

Following a cutaneous burn, three zones of injury have been classically identified: coagulation, stasis, and hyperemia.[6] In the zone of coagulation, the incident heat causes an almost instantaneous destruction of protein.[7] Microcirculatory observations in a moderate scald burn have documented similar zones of abnormal capillary flow. These were identified as (1) a zone of complete capillary occlusion, where no capillary flow was observed; (2) a zone of partial capillary occlusion, where occluded capillaries were intermixed with normally perfused capillaries; and (3) a zone of hyperemia, with no capillary occlusion and an increased capillary flow.[8] Arteriovenous shunt pathways were observed to open following thermal injury and to supply the remaining capillaries in the zone of partial occlusion.

Arteriolar constriction and dilatation and venular dilatation were also observed in the intact scald-injured skin in this model.[8] Near-complete constriction of cutaneous arterioles was observed within the first 30 seconds of injury, with rebound arteriolar dilatation to 150 percent of preburn diameter at 60 seconds after burn. Venular dilatation was somewhat delayed after injury but plateaued by 30 seconds after injury when vessel diameter was likewise 150 percent of preburn diameter. Both arteriolar and venular diameters had returned to their preburn dimensions by 0.5 and 4 hours after injury, respectively. These observations suggest that

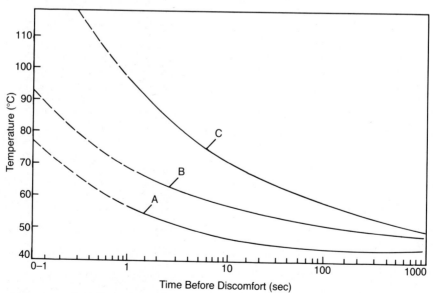

Figure 32–2. The relationship of dry heat and time in causing discomfort (*A*), partial-thickness (*B*), or full-thickness (*C*) cutaneous burns. Values less than 1 sec are extrapolations. (Reprinted by permission of the Council of the Institute of Mechanical Engineers from Lawrence JC, Bull JP: Thermal conditions which cause skin burns. J Inst Mech Eng 5:61–63, 1976.)

the microvascular reactivity of burned tissues is rather transient after moderate scald injury. These studies further documented platelet thromboembolism as the cause of complete and permanent microvascular occlusion, which led to dermal ischemia and an increased area of tissue loss after injury. Red cell aggregation and white cell adhesion to venular walls and diapedesis were also observed with this model within the first several hours after injury. Robson and associates demonstrated that specific inhibitors of thromboxane A_2 formation significantly increase the dermal perfusion in the zone of stasis (partially occluded capillary flow).[9] Supporting these findings is evidence that inhibition of thromboxane A_2 formation (or release) results in decreased platelet adherence and leukocyte and red blood cell adhesion to vessel walls.[10] It is possible that thromboxane may be responsible for the conversion of partial-thickness burn injuries to full-thickness burn injuries seen in postresuscitation dermal ischemia through similar mechanisms.

Several potent endogenous vasoactive mediators (e.g., prostaglandins, thromboxane, kinins, histamine, oxygen radicals, and various lipid peroxides) are released in increased amounts after burn injury and appear to promote permeability changes and platelet aggregation, which lead to burn edema formation and microvascular thromboembolism.[11–14] Following a severe thermal injury these vasoactive mediators play an important role in the development of burn hypovolemia and burn shock, which are discussed in a later section. An active area of research pertinent to the study of these mediators has been the efficacy of pharmacological antagonism in modifying the inflammatory and microvascular pathophysiology that follows thermal injury.

Interestingly, histamine release from heat-stimulated mast cells may be inhibited by cooling or immediate cold water treatment of burned skin.[15] Besides providing a prompt means of transferring heat away from thermally injured skin, cooling also substantially attenuates the microvascular response to a moderate scald injury and inhibits burn wound and remote edema formation.[16] Further studies of the effects of cooling in severe experimental burns have demonstrated a significant reduction in serum lactate levels and an enhancement of cardiovascular performance (mean arterial pressure and cardiac output) in cold water–treated animals.[17] While these observations have helped in understanding how cooling can modify some aspects of the pathophysiology of burn injury, the clinical application of cooling therapy remains limited to small (10% or less TBSA), uncomplicated burns.

Chemicals that contact the skin can destroy tissues by coagulation necrosis, protein precipitation (colliquation of tissue), cytoplasmic poisoning, or vascular thrombosis.[18] Acids promote collagen denaturation and subsequent degradation. Cellular dehydration and intercellular edema are observed with separation of the dermis and epidermis. Strong alkalis cause colliquation, a process in which water is extracted from tissue and protein precipitated. The treatment of acid and alkaline burns has been experimentally assessed using pH determinations after water lavage. In this study, skin burned with 50% NaOH required over 12 hours of water lavage before the pH returned to normal, while skin subjected to 30% acid required only 2 hours.[19] Beyond 1 hour, washing had little effect on lye burns because of the formation of soluble soaps and protein complexes with the proteins and fats of the skin, which facilitates passage of injurious hydroxyl ions to deeper layers of tissues. Hydrogen ions from acids are not similarly complexed.[16] Phosphorus is the only chemical whose mode of injury is that of a thermal burn as this compound burns in air at room temperature.

DEPTH OF BURN INJURY

While the cause and extent of burn injury are important considerations in the acute treatment and resuscitation of the burn victim, the depth of the burn injury is critical to ultimate patient morbidity and mortality and to the cosmetic result. Unfortunately, acute diagnosis of the depth of injury is extremely difficult even for the most experienced burn surgeons. Fluorescein,[19] laser Doppler flow,[20] and pulse-echo ultrasound[21] show promise as assessment methodologies.

Clinically, a burn is referred to as either a partial- or full-thickness injury. These terms refer to the relative thickness of the injured skin (epidermis and dermis) containing the epithelial appendages (sweat gland and sebaceous glands) that carry the regenerative potential for re-epithelialization. Partial-thickness injuries (previously termed first and second degree burns) are further categorized as superficial or deep partial-thickness injuries according to the length of time required for the wound to heal. Wounds that require less than 3 weeks to heal are considered to be superficial; those requiring more time are considered deep. The clinical significance of this classification relates to the presence of burn scar hypertrophy in the healed wound, which may have functional as well as aesthetic complications.

In a clinical study of the correlation of burn wound healing to the presence of burn scar hypertrophy, Deitch and co-workers[22] observed that when partial-thickness wounds healed in less than 3 weeks, 33 percent resulted in hypertrophic scars as opposed to 78 percent of those requiring more than 21 days to heal. This suggests that the extent of dermal destruction is directly related to hypertrophic scar formation. This information should also allow the burn surgeon to substantiate the need for excision and grafting in areas of burn injury where complete healing has not been achieved early and where the aesthetic or functional results might be significantly compromised by burn scar hypertrophy.

The full-thickness burn injury, or third degree burn, presents an environment in which spontaneous re-epithelialization is not possible because of the complete destruction of the dermal appendages. The entire thickness of the skin is involved, sometimes including the underlying fat, fascia, muscle, and bone. Following removal of the burn wound eschar, full-thickness injury requires coverage by autografting or flap techniques or with preparatory allografting or artificial skin dermal matrix. Because of the increased complications associated with burn wound sepsis in untreated, full-thickness wounds, early surgical excision and grafting are usually the preferred methods of treatment. Deep partial-thickness or full-thickness burns that remain unhealed over several years not only pose a threat of recurrent chronic infection but are also at risk of malignant degeneration into burn scar carcinoma (Marjolin's ulcer).[23]

METABOLIC, CARDIOVASCULAR, AND IMMUNE RESPONSE FOLLOWING THERMAL INJURY

Large body surface area thermal injury results in severe metabolic alterations due to both the loss of the normal physiological function of skin and the systemic response to trauma. The increase in metabolic rate that is seen in the postresuscitation period is much greater after thermal injury than in any other form of trauma or severe sepsis. A doubling of the basal metabolic rate (approximately 40 kcal per m^2 of surface area per hour) is documented when burn size exceeds 50 percent TBSA.[24, 25] While there is increased evaporative water loss from damaged skin, this does not entirely account for the magnitude of hypermetabolism.[25–27] Significant hypovolemia and burn shock are also observed. Clinical and experimental studies of the cardiovascular response to major burns have been the basis for the development of various formulas for burn shock resuscitation. Beyond the period of acute burn resuscitation, the severely burned patient is at risk for the development of burn wound sepsis or infectious complications that are related to a multifactorial depression in immune functions. The significant alterations in the metabolic, cardiovascular, and immune status of the burn victim are representative of the many interrelationships among caloric homeostasis, inflammation, and cellular and humoral defense mechanisms following severe burn injury.

Metabolic Response

The metabolic response to thermal injury has been the focus of intense investigation. This is the result of the need to support the burn patient, but it is also due to the fact that the burn patient represents a model of trauma. Modes of response in the burn patient are usually quantitatively greater but qualitatively similar to those in other trauma patients. Unfortunately, we are still developing methodology to accurately assess the metabolic and nutritional requirements of the burn patient. For example, only recently have we been able to determine that the caloric requirements of the burn patient are not nearly so large as previously thought, and this has led to the recognition of the deleterious effects of overnutrition, especially with carbohydrate.[28, 29]

Following thermal injury, an increase in release of high-energy substrates and in thermogenesis has been documented.[30] In addition, severe burns may increase oxygen consumption by as much as 100 percent due to septic complications and significant evaporative losses secondary to loss of epidermis requiring enormous expenditures of energy. Investigations have indicated that this increased thermogenesis and energy expenditure are associated with substrate cycling (triglyceride-fatty acid) due to β-adrenergic stimulation.[31] These findings appear to substantiate earlier studies that implicated catecholamines as mediators of the overall increase in metabolic rate in patients with burns.

Increased glucose production, as by gluconeogenic-glycolytic cycling, however, is not affected by adrenergic mechanisms.[30] Glucagon appears to be the primary stimulator of glucose production after burn injuries[32] and therefore functions as the second important mediator of the metabolic response after thermal injury.

Other hormonal imbalances may be initiated and maintained by afferent signals from the burn wound.[33] Increased circulating inflammatory mediators such as prostaglandin-E_2 and interleukin-1 are also involved in the promotion of the afferent signal by the central nervous system.[33] Early wound closure has been demonstrated to decrease the metabolic response after injury, but the mechanisms by which this is achieved are not understood.[34] Nevertheless, it is certain that the systemic effects of the burn wound on metabolic alterations are profound. Until the wound is closed, the inflammatory response continues and body metabolism remains altered. Further investigations of the role of inflammatory mediators in the modifications of hormonal and afferent mechanisms responsible for thermoregulation and caloric expenditure may allow us to better understand how burn wound closure may affect metabolism.

As documented by Hunt and colleagues,[35] the oxygen tension of the healing wound appears to correlate directly to the rate of healing, and wound healing may be accelerated as more oxygen is made available. Oxygen appears to increase the rate of fibroblast reproduction and collagen synthesis, and epithelial cell reproduction. Because of these relationships and the significantly increased metabolic demands for oxygen due to altered substrate metabolism, it is important that careful documentation of oxygen requirements be performed during the postresuscitation period. For these reasons some have advocated the use of hyperbaric oxygen in the treatment of burn wounds[36]; however, results of experimental studies have been contradictory.[37] Further experimental studies utilizing well-planned models of burn wound healing will hopefully allow clarification of these mixed observations.

In spite of these and other known oxygen requirements of the burn wound, studies to determine the metabolic characteristics of granulation tissue have demonstrated that anaerobic glycolysis (increased glucose consumption and accelerated lactate production) is its major source of energy.[38] The importance of the effects of lactate and oxygen on collagen synthesis by the fibroblast has only recently been documented.[39] The relative hypoxia of the ischemic wound causes macrophages to produce angiogenesis factor, which stimulates the growth of new blood vessels in wounds. This central hypoxia also causes fibroblasts to activate the enzymes for collagen synthesis.[40] A duplication of the hypoxic synthetic drive and increased collagen formation are observed in the presence of increased lactate concentration. Lactate also causes macrophages to produce an angiogenic factor even in the presence of oxygen.[41] Lactate is therefore an important mediator of collagen synthesis and neovascularization in the healing wound.

Alterations in micronutrient metabolism may lead to deficient healing of the burn wound. For example, early investigations of this problem have clearly established acute, significant depressions in plasma ascorbic acid, thiamine, and nicotinamide concentrations after severe burn injury.[42] Ascorbic acid and oxygen are required for hydroxylation of proline during collagen synthesis, which in turn is required for the maintenance of the triple-helical conformation.[43] Abnormal burn wound healing in this setting could relate to the imbalance of the "dynamic" mechanisms responsible for collagen remodeling. Because synthesis of new collagen is blocked during ascorbic acid deficiency, and because collagenolytic activity probably proceeds normally, abnormal or deficient scar formation may result from the accelerated degradation of the surrounding collagen matrix responsible for the transmission of tension across the surface of the healing wound.

Significant alterations in plasma copper, zinc, and the acute phase reactant ceruloplasmin have been documented following severe thermal injury.[44] Depressions in serum copper levels appear to be directly related to the extent of injury and parallel serum levels of the copper transport protein ceruloplasmin.[45] Similar depressions in serum zinc levels have also been documented in burn patients but are not as clearly related to burn size.[46] Copper is an essential nutrient, and an integral component of numerous enzymes, including lysyl oxidase, which is required for collagen crosslinking.[47] Without this enzymatic reaction, optimal wound healing is inhibited due to reduced connective tissue strength. Copper deficiency can manifest as neutropenia, leukopenia, bone demineralization, or impaired immune function.[48] It is apparent that the maintenance of normal copper levels and lysyl oxidase activity in the burn patient is critical for proper wound healing and immune function.

Zinc plays an important role in cell division.[49] It is necessary for RNA and DNA synthesis and acts as an unspecific mitogen in lymphocytes. Excess zinc can also produce the opposite effect on lymphocyte activity. Zinc has been demonstrated in mast cells, platelets, and macrophages, and 20 percent of the body stores reside in skin.[49, 50] While the relationship of serum zinc levels to wound healing is not fully documented, investigators studying burn patients exhibiting depressed zinc levels suggest that this deficiency is correlated with poor skin graft take and delayed wound healing.[51, 52] The micronutrient deficiencies seen in burn patients result from decreased intake, increased losses from the wound and in urine, and increased requirements due to use as cofactors in enzymatic reactions that have increased activity. As a result, there is now a consensus that vitamin and trace metal supplementation should be provided acutely to all patients hospitalized for serious burn injuries. Ideally, micronutrient determinations should be obtained in burn patients (especially those with injuries greater than 60 percent TBSA) soon after admission and routinely throughout their hospital course. Specific supplements should be administered when indicated.[25]

Cardiovascular Response

Barring the presence of significant inhalation injuries, patients with extensive burn injuries (those involving more than 30 percent TBSA) exhibit substantial depressions in cardiovascular performance that appear to be directly related to the extent of injury. Experimental studies investigating the basis for this early suppression have suggested the following mechanisms: (1) increased capillary permeability in the area of the burn wound[53]; (2) a generalized cell-membrane defect causing intracellular fluid shifts[54]; (3) increased interstitial osmotic pressure of burned tissues[53]; and (4) depressed myocardial contractility and decreased left ventricular function.[55]

Although direct thermal injury is responsible for many irreversible changes noted in the burn wound circulation, remote permeability alterations in uninjured cutaneous beds are also observed.[13] Histamine, serotonin, kinins, prostaglandins, thromboxane, oxygen radicals, and lipid peroxides have been cited by several investigators as the substances responsible for these local and remote alterations in vascular permeability,[9-12, 35] and these vasoactive mediators are noted to be substantially increased soon after injury. Burn-mediated intravascular volume losses attributed to these mediators are usually limited to the first 24 hours after injury, are directly related to the surface area of thermal injury,[56] and can lead to significant hypovolemia and burn shock in severe burns not treated with fluid resuscitation.

Several fluid resuscitation "formulas" have been used to maintain cardiovascular performance in burn patients, but all inevitably result in burn wound edema because of the marked increase in permeability of the microcirculation in burned tissues.[56] While hypertonic saline (250 mmol sodium per liter) and early colloid infusion appear to reduce burn edema, such measures cannot completely eliminate this response.[57, 58] The use of specific inflammatory antagonists in reversing the sequelae of burn shock has been largely unsuccessful. In one series, administration of cimetidine one half hour after a severe experimental burn injury reduced the fluid requirements for optimal cardiac output by 70 percent.[59] Further studies of this treatment suggest that cimetidine-mediated inhibition of the cytochrome P-450 oxidase enzyme systems may be responsible for improved cardiovascular performance after thermal injury.[60] Cytochrome P-450 is a significant mediator of lipid peroxidation following thermal injury[60] and an important pathway for arachidonic acid metabolism.[61] The effects of cytochrome P-450 metabolites on vascular permeability, myocardial contractility, and cardiovascular performance after thermal injury have not been fully documented.

A complex interrelationship exists among fluid retention, cardiovascular performance, and patient survival following severe burn injuries requiring massive fluid resuscitation,[62, 63] and for this reason the search for pertinent biochemical and physiological parameters for cardiovascular performance in this setting continues. It is obvious that multiple processes contribute to the onset of hypovolemia and burn shock. Pharmacological therapies for burn shock treatment will continue to be an active area of investigation.

Immune Response

Alterations of the cellular and humoral components of the immune system in the patient with severe thermal injury have been a major area of investigation. Burn wound sepsis and associated organ system failure continue to be the leading cause of death due to burns.[64] Lungs and the burn wound are the most frequent sites of infection, and opportunistic gram-negative organisms are the most common cause of fatal infections.[65] The incidence of fungal infections after severe burns may be decreasing as the result of a decreased use of prophylactic systemic antibiotics. However, of particular concern are the isolated outbreaks of wound infections caused by methicillin-resistant *Staphylococcus aureus*. Epidemics involving this organism have prompted closings of burn treatment facilities in an effort to break the cycle of cross-contamination that initiates widespread colonization.

Systemic antibiotics should be used only in conjunction with microbiological identification of sensitive organisms associated with a documented infection. Quantitative (full-thickness) burn wound biopsies documenting more than 10^5 organisms per gram of tissue warrant appropriate systemic antibiotic coverage.[66] Topical antimicrobial treatment of the burn wound continues to be the most generally accepted and utilized method of burn wound infection control. Newer formulations of high-concentration, slow-release topical agents impregnated in porous, nonadherent dressings are improving the ease of wound care (and decreasing the frequency of burn dressing changes) while providing adequate antimicrobial control.[67, 68] New topical agents such as chlorhexidine gluconate and norfloxacin[69] will hopefully minimize the problems of bacterial resistance that have been encountered with other established agents.

Investigations of the mediation of the altered immune response in burn patients have generally involved four areas: (1) the products of the injury itself, which are released into the circulation from the wound, (2) endogenous immunoregulatory molecules (e.g., prostaglandins), (3) immunologically active substances from exogenous sources (e.g., bacterial endotoxins), and (4) immune depression resulting as a side effect of burn treatment (e.g., the use of topical agents with suppressive activity).[70] While it is certain that the release of endogenous molecules with immunological activity is triggered after burn injury, it appears that the products of arachidonic acid metabolism are probably among the most important. Prostaglandins, which are found in large amounts in burned tissues, are potent cytokines, which, along with the leukotrienes, have immunoregulatory properties.[59]

Besides the endogenous mediation of the immune response by the burn wound, several other alterations or deficiencies of the humoral and cellular defense mechanisms following severe thermal injury have been documented. Among these are impaired phagocytic (macrophage) function,[71] decreased neutrophil chemotaxis,[72] impaired neutrophil phagocytosis and bacterial killing,[60, 73] impaired lymphocyte response to mitogen stimulation,[72] increased populations of suppressor T-cell lymphocytes,[73-76] decreased interleukin-2,[74] and decreased fibronectin and gamma globulin.[75, 77]

While the interrelationship of these altered immune mechanisms has not been fully documented, it is certain that the unhealed burn wound promotes the maintenance of this imbalanced state. Only temporary resistance to sepsis can be afforded by antibiotic therapy, intravenous immunoglobulins, and topical agents. Notwithstanding infection control measures and contributing external factors, the resistance to infection in the burn patient is ultimately related to techniques of wound management and the timely closure of the burn wound. The speed of closure has been shown to influence the survival of the severely burned, septic patient,[78] with mortality rates displaying institutional variance. These facts clearly emphasize that while the burn injury may have significant impact on the resistance to infection, timely excision and closure must remain the highest priority. This is not surprising since the injury is the skin wound. *Closure of the wound cures the patient.* One cannot wait and rely on the natural processes of epithelialization and contraction to accomplish closure.

MECHANISMS OF REPAIR

Burns cause a variable degree of destruction of the two skin layers, the surface epithelium (epidermis) and the deeper cells and matrix of the dermis and subdermal structures. Depending on the regenerative potential of the various cellular layers and the dimensions of the wound, various methods of repair are initiated to facilitate primary healing of the wound. In general, burns heal by three mechanisms: epithelialization, granulation tissue formation, and contraction. While the resurfaced epithelium is the sine qua non of a healed burn wound, it is the fibroblast and its product, collagen, that are crucial to the repair of the burn wound connective tissue matrix (dermis) that will support the epithelial cells or grafted skin. Therefore, it is important to investigate the factors that alter the burn wound connective tissue matrix. To facilitate understanding of the complex mechanisms that control this process (i.e., epithelialization, granulation tissue formation, and contraction), we will consider them as phases of a process rather than undertaking an exhaustive examination of each one.

Epithelialization

Epithelialization is initiated by the mitotic activity of basal cells located in the stratum spinosum of undamaged normal epithelium.[79] This activity is observed at the margin of the wound and from the viable remaining skin appendages (i.e., hair follicles and sweat glands). Increased epidermal mitotic activity is apparent within 42 hours after trauma with the hair follicle appearing to be the most important source of epidermal cells.[80] The production of proteolytic enzymes allows these new cells to migrate over the base of the burn eschar or blister.[81] While some controversy exists as to the benefit of the intact blister with regard to the concentrations of thromboxane,[81] prostaglandins, and leukotrienes[82] that may affect local burn wound edema and perfusion, the rate of epithelialization within the blister appears to be twice that seen in similar desiccated areas.[83] Epithelial cell migration does not require the presence of a complete basement membrane, which is later re-formed by the epidermis, although fibronectin is present as an adhesion molecule. Granulation tissue formation appears to complement epithelial cell migration by providing a proper substratum for cell nourishment, as new epidermal cells can migrate only an estimated 1 cm from the site of cell proliferation.[83] Ultimately, surface epithelialization is completed following the differentiation of the migrated epithelial cells that have covered the burn scar.[81, 82]

Epidermal growth factor (EGF), a single-chain polypeptide hormone isolated from human urine and from the submaxillary glands of the mouse,[84] is reported to stimulate epithelial cell proliferation and keratinization both in vivo and in vitro.[84] Studies of the effectiveness of EGF in enhancing wound healing after partial-thickness burns have only recently demonstrated potential efficacy for the application of peptide growth factors to the partial-thickness burn wound. Schultz and colleagues,[85] studying EGF, transforming growth factor-α (TGF-α), and vaccinia virus growth factor (VGF), demonstrated that topical application of TGF-α or VGF in antibiotic cream (1% silver sulfadiazine) to partial-thickness burns accelerated epidermal regeneration in comparison with untreated or vehicle-treated burns. TGF-α and VGF possess sequential homology to EGF and activate a common tyrosine kinase–linked receptor. Low levels of both TGF-α and VGF were more effective than EGF in stimulating epidermal regeneration. Clinical studies document accel-

erated healing of split-thickness skin graft donor sites (10.75 days for controls vs. 8.1 days for EGF treatment) following application of recombinant human epidermal growth factor (hEGF) in silver sulfadiazine cream.[86] Similar findings have also been observed with trials using hEGF in a saline vehicle.[86] In this regard, the use of polypeptide growth factors such as hEGF appears to hold promise for accelerated repair of partial-thickness cutaneous injuries.

Granulation Tissue Formation

In deeper partial-thickness or full-thickness burn injuries, a period of collagen formation and contraction is observed prior to wound closure. Granulation tissue gets its name from the granulated appearance that results from the reforming capillary buds and loops. Within this tissue fibroblasts invade the base of the wound, deposit collagen, and provide a structural matrix for the contraction of the wound edges. This timely modification of the injured dermis and subdermal tissues is crucial to the development of neovascularization and continued fibroblast infiltration, which are required for contraction and wound epithelialization.

Hunt and associates[87] have identified the wound macrophage as the cell that directly influences healing of the injured dermis through the release of various factors that promote neovascularization and granulation tissue formation and that also promote enhanced epithelial migration from the skin appendages. (These factors are discussed in detail in Chapter 16.) Angiogenic factor, secreted by the hypoxic macrophage at the wound edge or surface,[88] initiates neovascularization and appears to be a chemoattractant for mesenchymal cells and vascular endothelial cells that migrate to the wound edge to form new blood vessels. The release of angiogenesis factor is suppressed by a high tissue partial pressure of oxygen and stimulated by low oxygen partial pressure.[89] The presence of the overlying burn eschar suppresses angiogenesis and granulation tissue formation even in the presence of low oxygen partial pressure. At the burn wound surface where the partial pressure of oxygen is increased, the burn wound macrophage releases macrophage-derived growth factor (MDGF), which stimulates fibroblast mitosis and the deposition of collagen, fibronectin, and glycosaminoglycan.[90] Because these activities are enhanced by increased oxygen availability, angiogenesis, neovascularization, and established local blood flow must precede this phase of granulation tissue formation.[90] Additional enhancement of this response is observed in the presence of a platelet-derived growth factor (PDGF), which appears to have properties of both angiogenesis factor and MDGF.[91]

The optimal environment for wound healing is therefore one in which (1) burn eschar is removed (to minimize inhibition of angiogenesis and granulation tissue formation); (2) subsurface wound oxygen partial pressure is high (to stimulate secretion of MDGF and fibroblast deposition of collagen and glycosaminoglycans); and (3) surface bacterial contamination is minimized (to enhance graft take and minimize protein degradation by proteases released by activated neutrophils phagocytosing bacteria).[92] As previously noted, the synergistic increase in lactate concentrations and oxygen delivery is also important in supporting increased collagen deposition for dermal repair.

Contraction

The process of wound contraction involves interaction of fibroblasts, myofibroblasts, and collagen deposition. Burn wound contraction develops as a result of progressive collagen deposition beneath the granulation tissue of the burn wound. Myofibroblasts observed in the granulating wound appear to contain contractile elements that may contribute to burn wound contracture formation and burn scar hypertrophy (elevation).[93] Recent observations, however, suggest that wound contraction and the reorganization of the connective tissue matrix may result predominantly from the action of fibroblasts acting as individual units.[94] Burn scar contraction progresses through a combination of the shortened contracted state of fibroblasts and myofibroblasts and the increased deposition of mucopolysaccharides, chondroitin sulfate, and ground substance, which ultimately results in a fused, raised, firm collagen mass that limits tissue motion.[95] Mast cells are found in increased numbers in unhealed burn wounds and contribute to the deposition of mucopolysaccharides, chondroitin 4-sulfate, and histamine.[96] Histamine has also been demonstrated to stimulate the growth of cultured human fibroblasts.[97]

Burn scar hypertrophy is a common complication of the healed, deep partial-thickness burn wound. It is usually observed at about 3 weeks after final wound closure and is stable at 8 to 12 weeks. Hypertrophic scar maturity or regression may slightly improve over the next 1 to 2 years.

Studies of scar hypertrophy have established the existence of an inverse relationship between the myofibroblast population and the amount of dermis grafted in a partial-thickness wound.[98] For this reason, many have advocated the employment of burn wound excision and grafting in wounds that may potentially become hypertrophic scars (e.g., greater than 3 weeks healing time, early hypertrophic response, full-thickness burn wounds). Nonsurgical measures that have been used to treat the hypertrophic scar include pressure[99] and intralesional injection of triamcinolone.[100]

While wound contraction is usually an obligate force of the healing process, the burn scar contracture, in most instances, has very little functional or aesthetic value. Overall, treatment modalities aimed at improving the appearance of hypertrophic, contracted burn scars have had little success and are not without complications. For these reasons the treatment plan should exclude the promotion of chronic areas of granulation tissue formation and burn scar hypertrophy. If feasible, such areas, especially in regions of aesthetic importance, should receive early excision and appropriate split graft or flap coverage. If properly performed, these techniques will give results superior to those achieved by the unchecked development of the hypertrophic, contracted burn scar. Alternatively, a delayed approach to such reconstruction is also reasonable as long as the healing process does not adversely affect function. The key is that the reconstructive plan be initiated at a time when the surgical insult will be minimized for the best functional and cosmetic result.

CLOSING THE BURN WOUND

Perhaps more than in any other area of medicine, survival of the burn patient is dependent upon expeditious wound healing. *Closure of the burn wound is the treatment of the disease process, in contrast to management of a wound that is only a complication of another primary disease process.* Thus, it is not surprising that much of the emphasis on burn care centers on wound closure. In addition, modern advancements in early resuscitation allow for survival of patients with larger TBSA burns, creating a need for wound closure in patients who previously would have died before closure became an issue. This, as well as simultaneous advancements in the fields of biomaterials and cell culture techniques, has contributed to the present interest in skin substitutes.

The development of skin substitutes is really the history of skin grafting. This has been the subject of detailed reviews[101–104] and will be only briefly summarized here. Table 32–1 presents the terminology of skin grafting.[101]

The first recorded solution to the problem of skin replacement was the use of pedicle flaps.[101, 102] While the initial use of pedicle flaps has often been attributed to the ancient Egyptians and Greeks, the first clear description was recorded by the Indian surgeon Susruta in the 2nd century B.C. It appears that Susruta may have also utilized free skin grafts, but unfortunately his methods fell into disuse. In 1804, Baronio of Milan published his report of successful free grafting of full-thickness sheep skin. In 1823, Bunger reportedly completed the first successful human skin graft but it was not until Reverdin's "epidermic grafting" of a thumb tip in 1869 that the method was widely accepted. The subsequent detailed histological study of the "postage stamp" grafts of Thiersch in 1886 contributed additional scientific understanding of the method.[101–103]

Many of the early efforts at skin grafting involved autografts, which were not adequate for the large areas needing coverage in the burn patient. Appropriately, the first recorded successful cadaver donor allograft was performed on a burn patient in 1881 by Girdner.[101, 102] The skin was obtained from a fresh corpse and applied to a 10-year-old boy who suffered lightning burns. Noting that the grafts degraded, he repeated the procedure until the wounds healed. In 1942, J.B. Brown reported the application of allografts as a life-saving measure for massive burns,[105] and the technique became a part of modern medical care of the burn patient. However, it was not until the studies of Gibson and Medawar[106] in 1943 that it was understood that the donor skin was rejected and the wound healed by host epithelium.

While progress proceeded in allograft techniques, others were employing the use of xe-nografts. In 1682, Canaday attempted to use water lizard skin as a skin substitute.[101, 102] In the intervening 300 years, a variety of other species were used and by the 1960s porcine xenograft was competing with allografts.[107, 108] However, initial enthusiasm has been tempered by the knowledge that it serves as a biological dressing rather than a true skin substitute and its value may lie more in its collagen than in its living cells.[101, 109] While presently not used to treat full-thickness burns, it continues to be utilized for management of superficial burns[101, 110] and in toxic epidermal necrolysis[111] and in combination with autograft.[112]

Application of allografts or xenografts was aided by improvements in storage techniques. Early efforts at refrigerated storage in saline allowed viability for up to 2 weeks.[101] Subsequent investigations utilized lyophilization and standard freezing.[113] By 1970 storage in a glycerol solution in liquid nitrogen was reported to maintain large quantities of allograft for as long as 6 months.[114]

With the widespread use of autografts, allografts, and xenografts for management of the burn patient, survival and cosmetic and functional results were dramatically improved. However, certain problems remain. Allograft and xenograft ultimately do not substitute for the victim's skin but rather provide functional coverage until autografts can be placed. In large burns this is typically accomplished using the Tanner mesh procedure,[115] which gives a less than ideal cosmetic result. In burns approaching 100 percent of body surface area, this process requires months to accomplish since a small portion of the body surface must provide coverage for the rest of the body, requiring consecutive harvests at intervals that allow the donor site to regenerate. Despite the tremendous success of allograft and xenograft coverage, the concern for disease transmission with such biological materials will always be present. Burn surgeons await the development of a product that can decrease the present high cost of burn care while improving the morbidity, mortality, and cosmetic results (see Table 32–2).

Table 32–1. TERMINOLOGY OF SKIN GRAFTING*

Greek	Latin	Definition
Xenograft	Heterograft	A graft transferred from one species to another
Allograft	Homograft	A graft transferred between different members of the same species
Autograft	Isograft	A graft transferred from one place to another on the same individual

*The literature of skin grafting is sometimes confusing due to the mixing of Greek and Latin prefixes that refer to the association of graft donor and recipient.[101]

Skin Substitutes

The literature on "skin substitutes" or "artificial skin" is confusing since the terms have no unanimously accepted definition that distinguishes such products from wound dressings, especially biological dressings. Clearly, dressings have some of the properties of artificial skin (Table 32–2). For example, modified polyvinyl chloride dressings (e.g., OPsite) have good moisture-vapor characteristics, fine-mesh gauze has adequate adherence, and silver nitrate–soaked gauze is antibacterial, yet none of these is an "artificial skin." To be an artificial skin, the product must have some or all of the characteristics listed in Table 32–2, and some or all of it must ultimately be accepted biologically by the host as "self" and remain with the host for an extended period of time as a part of or modifying the normal metabolic processes of turnover. Even this definition does not adequately deal with some intermediate products such as Biobrane. Biobrane* consists of a silicone membrane, knitted nylon fabric covalently bonded to porcine dermal collagen peptides.[116–118] It appears that this product becomes involved in the biological processes of the healing skin wound since it inhibits wound

*Woodruff Laboratories, Inc., Santa Ana, CA.

Table 32–2. CHARACTERISTICS OF A SKIN SUBSTITUTE

Essential Characteristics
Physical
    Proper water flux
    Bacterial barrier
    Proper suturing characteristics
    Adherence to graft bed
    Appropriate bending rigidity
    Adequate tear strength
    Appropriate modulus of elasticity, surface energy

Biological
    Sterile
    Controlled biodegradation
    Nontoxic
    Nonantigenic
    Minimal inflammatory or foreign body response

Desirable Characteristics
    Improve cosmetic result (minimize scarring and contraction)
    Minimize pain
    Allow growth of skin appendages
    Inexpensive
    Available
    Facilitate angiogenesis

Modified from Burke JF, Yannas IV, Quinby WC Jr, et al: Successful use of a physiologically acceptable artificial skin in the treatment of extensive burn injury. Ann Surg 194:413–428, 1981.

contraction.[119] Nonetheless, as it is short-term and similar to allografts, it should be considered a dressing.

An artificial skin should take into account that skin is not a homogeneous organ. Much as the adrenal gland has a medulla and a cortex with different functions, the skin has an epidermis and dermis, each with its own physical and biological properties. The epidermis is four cell layers thick with the outer stratum corneum providing the primary barrier to water, chemical toxins, and bacteria. The characteristics of the epidermis vary with anatomical location. For example, the stratum corneum is thick and inflexible on the palms and soles and thin and flexible on the dorsa of the hands and feet. The epidermis is a metabolically active cell layer, particularly in regard to carbohydrate metabolism, and is the primary glycogen storage organ in the fetus before induction of liver enzymes at birth.[120] The dermis consists of an organized layer of primarily collagen and glycosaminoglycans and forms a structural framework for the epidermis, blood vessels, and skin appendages, provides a mechanical barrier to trauma, and is metabolically active in terms of protein and vitamin D metabolism.[121]

Table 32–2 lists both the essential and the desirable (but nonessential) characteristics of an artificial skin.[104, 109, 110, 121] The essential characteristics can be further subdivided into physical and biological characteristics. Some of the physical properties such as providing proper transfer of water (water flux) and an adequate bacterial barrier are the properties of the normal skin that the artificial skin must replace. Other properties are those necessary for "healing" of the artificial skin. It is essential that the new skin adequately adhere and have an appropriate peel strength, tear strength, surface energy, and modulus of elasticity to maintain contact with the wound bed and remain intact until it is firmly incorporated by the host. Bending rigidity is also an integral part of adherence, since it is this property that allows appropriate draping of the artificial skin over concave and convex surfaces. The biological properties include sterility, nontoxicity, and nonantigenicity. It is essential that the skin incite minimal inflammatory or foreign body response, since this might additionally stress an already compromised host. While it is not necessary (and perhaps not even desirable) that a skin substitute remain intact indefinitely, its biodegradation must proceed at a rate that allows it to perform its necessary functions before replacement or removal. In this case the rate of biodegradation not only involves the host's ability to degrade the artificial skin but also the rate of degradation by bacterial enzymes. Indeed, it is crucial that the skin substitute be resistant to bacterial degradation to avoid providing additional substrate for bacterial growth.

One may also delineate a separate group of desirable but nonessential characteristics. While ideally a skin substitute minimizes pain, scarring, and wound contraction, allows growth of skin appendages, facilitates angiogenesis, and improves the cosmetic result, these are not essential in a life-threatening situation. A skin substitute should be less expensive than current methods of excision and grafting. Nonetheless, if the ultimate result were superior in terms of morbidity, mortality, and aesthetics, one might choose to use it despite its expense. Finally, the issue of availability has at least two facets. First, the skin substitute should be universally available to all burn physicians and not require unusual means of preservation or preparation or have such a short shelf-life that its widespread use would be inhibited. To optimize its potential as a life-saving device in burn care it should be ready for use in the first 3 days after patient admission since this is when the first round of excision and grafting is done.[101, 122]

The skin equivalents may be categorized as primarily epidermal, dermal, or both and as having autogenous, xenogenous, or allogenic sources. This is not surprising, since these represent the two layers of skin and the historical sources of skin grafts for the burn patient. Table 32–3 describes selected skin equivalents that are discussed below.

Several improvements in epidermal culture techniques during the early 1970s allowed the development of the epidermal grafts (Table 32–3) in use in the 1980s. First, it was discovered that growing epidermal cells with lethally irradiated 3T3 cells allowed for serial subcultures of human cells, that the 3T3 cells inhibited the growth of other fibroblasts, and that the epidermal cells cultured in this fashion differentiate in a manner similar to that in normal epidermis.[123] Finally, the addition of epidermal growth factor and agents that increase cAMP to the culture media allowed a rate of amplification (1000- to 10,000-fold in 3 to 4 weeks) that made cultured epithelial grafts practical for burn wound care.[104, 123, 124]

While early grafting methods were evaluated mainly in animal models,[125] O'Connor and coworkers[126] reported the first application in burn patients. In this study, two patients with 80 and 40 percent body surface area burns each received eight grafts of approximately 2.0 to 2.5 cm diameter prepared in collaboration with Howard Green. It was found that the grafts behaved like thin split-thickness skin grafts. A subsequent study in two pediatric burn patients with 97 and 98 percent TBSA burns (83 and 89 percent full-thickness) confirmed these results and reported a 60 to 80 percent graft take.[127] This group has recently reported follow-up of 21 pediatric patients from 6 days to 5 years covered in part with cultured epidermal autografts (CEAs).[128] Full-thickness wounds excised to fascia and treated with CEA were histologically compared to meshed split-thickness autograft (MSTA) areas. They reported that differentiation into a fully stratified epidermis occurred by 6 days postgrafting with CEA. Rete ridges appeared from 5 to 18 months posttransplantation, depending on the site of origin of the cells but were reportedly not observed in the majority of MSTA interstice controls. De novo formation of the dermal-epidermal junction was accomplished in 3 to 4 weeks and anchoring fibrils were present at 1 week. These authors described the observed anchoring fibrils as thinner and more sparse than those in normal skin even at 1 year but similar to those of age-matched MSTA interstices. Langerhans cells

Table 32–3. COMPARISON OF SKIN EQUIVALENTS

	Epidermis	Dermis	Source	Advantages	Disadvantages
Burke/Yannas[122, 142, 143]	Silastic-auto-graft	Collagen; chondroitin-6-PO$_4$	Processed xeno-graft	Immediate availability; improved cosmesis	Requires autografting
Gallico/Green/Compton[127–129]	Cell culture	—	Autogenous	Improved cosmesis	Delayed availability; durability
Ehrlich/Bell[134]	Cell culture	Collagen	Autogenous	—	Rapid biodegradation; delayed availability
Cuono[140, 141]	Cell culture	Human dermis	Autogenous epidermis; allogenic dermis	—	Delayed availability
Hefton[137]	Cell culture	Human dermis	Allogenic	Immediate availability	Requires ultimate host epithelial replacement

reappeared in 1 week and pigmentation occurred 2 weeks to 7 months after grafting. Pathological changes observed were primarily parakeratosis and dyskeratosis with no evidence of transformed or premalignant cells. They also reported that by 3 years the underlying connective tissue had developed a bilayered structure of organized collagen. By 5 years this "dermis" had elastin comparable to normal skin and a complex vascular structure. No hair follicles or glandular structures were identified. The effect on burn wound contraction was not described, but in a separate application of cultured epithelial autografts to children with giant congenital nevi, contraction was inhibited less than with split-thickness skin grafts.[129] Figure 32–3 shows the histological aspects of burn wound grafting with this material.

Other investigators preparing epidermal autografts have had mixed results. Graft takes ranged from 0 to 100 percent and there were problems with strength and durability that may have been the result of abnormal anchoring fibrils.[130-133] These varying degrees of clinical success require further evaluation. Nonetheless, these initial suggestions of the induction of a neodermis hold exciting potential.

An alternative approach using autogenous cells to provide both an epidermal and dermal equivalent was developed by Bell and associates.[134] Host fibroblasts obtained by biopsy are first cultured in a collagen lattice to form a dermal equivalent to which epidermal cells obtained by biopsy are added. In 2 to 4 days this skin equivalent is ready for grafting. Initial animal studies suggested the formation of a dermis with some organization and the ability to block wound contraction. Adnexal structures and pigment cells were absent. Subsequent modification and application to human burn patients have had disappointing results, as 70 to 90 percent of the graft lysed by the second day.[135] In addition, it took 3 to 4 weeks to prepare a 100 cm^2 graft.[134] Improvement in the dermal equivalent stability and rate of production is necessary before this skin equivalent can be used clinically.

As previously mentioned, allogenic skin grafts are ultimately rejected, making it seem unlikely that allogenic cultured epidermal grafts would fare any better. However, it was discovered that in vitro epidermal cultures lose their Langerhans and endothelial cells and their associated class II antigens, which are implicated targets in the rejection of allogenic skin grafts.[136] Hefton and colleagues published their results with three burn patients receiving 9 × 6 cm^2 allogenic cultured grafts.[137] They reported good graft take and cosmetic result. Subsequent application to skin ulcers by other investigators revealed healing patterns suggesting that the epithelial cells of the wound came from the

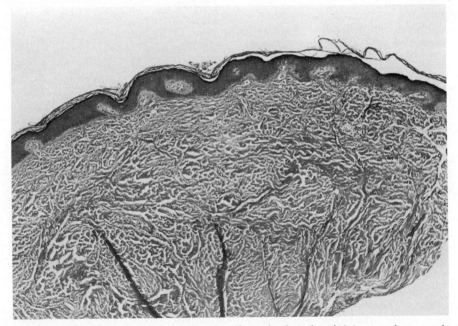

Figure 32–3. Hematoxylin and eosin stain of a groin skin–derived cultured graft 3½ years after transplantation. The tissue sample shows normal epidermal morphology with all normal strata and rete ridges. The underlying wound bed shows significant remodeling with bilayered distribution of collagen and a three-dimensional, basket-weave organization of the deep "dermal" layer. The vasculature is also remodeled with a regular array of hairpin-loop capillaries extending up between epidermal rete ridges.

host rather than from the allogenic cultured graft.[136, 138] More recently, using in situ hybridization techniques for the Y chromosome, Brain and colleagues demonstrated that in the bed of patients grafted with cultured allogenic cells of the opposite sex, only cells of the same sex could be found,[139] which suggests that the benefit of cultivated allogenic cells comes from the influence on wound healing rather than successful graft take.

An alternative approach is the use of a composite autologous-allogeneic skin substitute. Unlike the autologous or allogeneic skin substitutes previously discussed, this type acts as both a dermal and an epidermal substitute. In the first report, an adult patient with a 55 percent TBSA burn underwent total burn excision and placement of cryopreserved allograft skin from four donors on the third postinjury day.[140] Epidermis was harvested and cultured. On days 32 and 42, allografted skin was stripped of epidermis and subsequently resurfaced with cultured autologous cells. Follow-up in this and one other patient showed no evidence of rejection, inflammatory reaction, or adverse consequence to the patient.[141] By 120 days, anchoring fibrils were found. The presence of dermal appendages, rete pegs, and melanocytes and the effects on wound contraction were not reported. The theoretical advantages of providing a substitute dermis compared to cultured autologous cells alone include the potential for reduced wound contraction, increased skin durability, and possible improved cosmetic result. Further experience will determine whether these theoretical advantages are a practical reality.

An entirely different approach was taken by Burke and Yannas. They faced the reality that no skin substitute could be truly permanent since all human tissues are undergoing constant turnover. Instead, the authors' hypothesis stated that "the anatomic construction and chemical composition of the grafted artificial dermis would act as a model for the synthesis of a dermis-like structure whose physical properties would resemble dermis more than they resembled scar."[122] After carefully evaluating the physical and biological properties of skin and the properties required of a skin substitute (see Table 32–2), they chose to create a product having the bilaminar properties of skin.[122, 142, 143] The artificial dermis would act as the interface with the host tissue while the "epidermis" would be responsible for controlling water loss and bacterial invasion. Based on optimal physical and biological characteristics, a dermis was created from a well-defined mixture of native

bovine collagen and chondroitin-6-phosphate, a mixture that provided the proper modulus of elasticity and optimized biodegradation. To allow invasion of fibroblasts and achieve the proper rate of biodegradation, it was essential to control pore size and crosslinking, respectively. The epidermal equivalent was created from a 0.1 mm thick layer of liquid silicone applied to the artificial dermis making a firm bond with curing.[142, 143]

In the first clinical report, 10 burn patients underwent placement of this artificial skin on 15 to 60 percent of the body surface area with other areas treated with conventional autografts.[122] At approximately 2 to 3 weeks the silastic layer was peeled off and thin, meshed autograft (0.004 inch) placed. No inflammatory or foreign body response occurred and the final result was a durable skin with decreased hypertrophic scarring and wound contraction. Histologically (Fig. 32–4), the "neodermis" has a more open, loosely woven structure than typical scars. As early as 3 weeks after grafting, there is an epidermal appearance similar to rete pegs. Hair follicles and glandular structures do not regenerate.

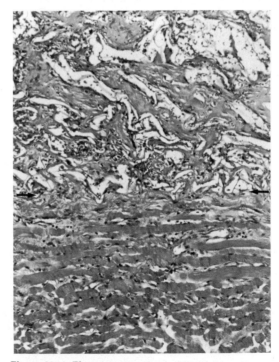

Figure 32–4. Photomicrograph of artificial skin of Burke and Yannas approximately 30 days postgrafting. The arrow marks the junction of the artificial dermis and muscle. The neodermis has the appearance of organized dermis rather than scar. (From Burke JF, Yannas IV, Quinby WC Jr, et al: Successful use of a physiologically acceptable artificial skin in the treatment of extensive burn injury. Ann Surg 194:413–428, 1981.)

In a subsequent study of 21 adult patients treated with this artificial skin, the likelihood of survival was approximately twice that of 22 patients managed without it.[144] While the number of patients was not statistically significant, this is the first indication that a skin substitute can have an impact on survival. An ongoing, prospective multicenter trial is needed to further evaluate its therapeutic efficacy.

While this bilaminar product appears to fulfill the goal of creating a scaffold for the formation of a neodermis, it has the disadvantage of ultimately requiring autografting, unlike the epidermal cultures. However, since only very thin split-thickness autografts are required, the donor site may be harvested more frequently, allowing faster definitive resurfacing. Until epithelial grafting is complete, the silicone artificial epidermis may provide a protective barrier for as long as 180 days.[144] Unlike cultured epithelial autografts, this product is available immediately, obviating the need to wait 3 to 4 weeks for cells to expand in culture. Thus, it may provide early, effective wound closure with the potential to minimize the physiological stress and complications of the open wound.

Initial investigation is under way on a stage 2 product in which a suspension of autogenous epithelial cells will be used to "seed" the dermal equivalent. Should this prove feasible in human patients, it would eliminate the need for eventual autografting.

CONCLUSION

The goals of the burn wound treatment are (1) obtaining epithelial coverage of the burn wound; (2) preventing burn scar contracture; and (3) preventing burn scar hypertrophy. A comprehensive approach to burn care will involve many of the modalities discussed in other sections of this text. Nonetheless, as a basis for the utilization of these modes one must insure that the burn wound environment has been optimally structured to promote the survival of epithelial appendages, excise and graft areas of delayed healing or early scar hypertrophy, and design functional splinting and range-of-motion protocols to prevent contractures.

Future treatment modalities for the burn patient will likely involve drugs that pharmacologically antagonize the altered vascular permeability and myocardial performance that accompany burn shock; such therapy should reduce burn edema, improve burn wound healing, and reduce early morbidity and mortality. Drugs will also be used to modify the hyper-

metabolic response of the early postresuscitation period, allowing more efficient utilization of caloric expenditure and reduced protein catabolism. Finally, the employment of a new class of burn wound dressings impregnated with polypeptide growth factors, antimicrobials, and a new category of anti-inflammatory/immune-enhancing agents will, respectively, provide for faster wound healing, reduce burn wound colonization, and modify the wound-mediated stimuli that initiate cellular and humoral immune depression. The development of skin substitutes along with advances in the preparation of rejection-free allograft will also substantially improve wound care, not only in the area of burn wound closure but also for other traumatic or disease states requiring significant surface coverage. The ultimate goal is to somehow prevent serious burn injuries from happening at all. Until that time, however, we must continue our efforts to promote the speedy return of the victims of burn tragedy to an acceptable, functional, and meaningful existence.

References

1. Mortiz AR: Studies of thermal injury. III. The pathology and pathogenesis of cutaneous burns. An experimental study. Am J Pathol 23:915, 1947.
2. Meryman HT: Mechanics of freezing in living cells. Science 124:515, 1956.
3. Washburn B: Frostbite. What it is. How to prevent it. Emergency treatment. N Engl J Med 266:974, 1962.
4. Weatherly-White RCA, Knize DM, Geisterfer DJ, et al: Experimental studies in cold injury. V. Circulatory hemodynamics. Surgery 66:208, 1969.
5. Ehrlich HP, Trelstad RL, Fallon JT: Dermal vascular patterns in response to burn or freeze injury in rats. Exp Mol Pathol 34:281, 1981.
6. Jackson D MacG: The diagnosis of the depth of burning. Br J Surg 40:588, 1953.
7. Zawacki BE: The natural history of reversible burn injury. Surg Gynecol Obstet 139:867, 1974.
8. Boykin JV, Eriksson E, Pittman RN: In vivo microcirculation of a scald burn and the progression of postburn dermal ischemia. Plast Reconstr Surg 66:191, 1980.
9. Robson MC, DelBecarro EJ, Heggers JP: The effects of prostaglandins on the dermal microcirculation after burning and the inhibition of the effects by specific pharmacologic agents. Plast Reconstr Surg 63:781, 1979.
10. Moncada S, Needleman P, Bunting S, et al: Prostaglandin endoperoxide and thromboxane generating systems and their selective inhibition. Prostaglandins 12:323, 1976.
11. Harms BA, Bodai BI, Smith M, et al: Prostaglandin release and altered microvascular integrity after burn injury. J Surg Res 31:274, 1981.
12. Wilhelm DL: Mechanisms responsible for increased vascular permeability in acute inflammation. Agents Actions 3:297, 1973.

13. Saez JC, Ward PH, Gunther B, et al: Superoxide radical involvement in the pathogenesis of burn shock. Circ Shock 12:229, 1984.
14. Sasaki J, Cottam G, Baxter C: Lipid peroxidation following thermal injury. J Burn Care Rehab 4:251, 1983.
15. Boykin JV, Eriksson E, Sholley MM, et al: Histamine-mediated delayed permeability response after scald burn inhibited by cimetidine or cold-water treatment. Science 209:815, 1980.
16. Boykin JV, Eriksson E, Sholley MM, et al: Cold-water treatment of scald injury and inhibition of histamine-mediated burn edema. J Surg Res 31:111, 1981.
17. Boykin JV, Crute SL: Mechanisms of burn shock protection after severe scald injury by cold-water treatment. J Trauma 22:859, 1982.
18. Tyler G: Treatment of special burns. In Hummel RP (ed): Clinical Burn Therapy. A Management and Prevention Guide. Boston, John Wright, 1982, pp 193–238.
19. Thomas S, Walker S, Coleman R, et al: Assessment of burn wound depth: Comparison of assessment methods. Presented at the Twentieth Annual Meeting of the American Burn Association, Seattle, WA, March 25, 1988.
20. Heimbach DM, Afromavitz MA, Engrav LH: Burn depth estimation—man or machine? J Trauma 24:373, 1984.
21. Goans RE, Cantrell JH, Meyers FB: Ultrasonic pulse-echo determination of thermal injury in deep dermal burns. Med Phys 4:259, 1977.
22. Deitch EA, Wheelahan TM, Rose MP, et al: Hypertrophic burn scars: Analysis and variables. J Trauma 23:895, 1983.
23. Novick M, Gard DA, Hardy SB, et al: Burn scar carcinoma: A review and analysis of 46 cases. J Trauma 17:809, 1977.
24. Wilmore DW, Aulick LII: Metabolic changes in burned patients. Surg Clin North Am 58:1173, 1978.
25. Molnar JA, Wolfe RR, Burke JF: Burns: Metabolism and Nutritional Therapy in Thermal Injury. In Schneider HA, Anderson CE, Coursin DB (eds): Nutritional Support in Medical Practice, 2nd ed. New York, Harper & Row, 1983.
26. Gump FE, Kinney JM: Caloric and fluid losses through the burn wound. Surg Clin North Am 50:1235, 1970.
27. Zawacki BF, Spitzer KW, Mason AD, et al: Does increased evaporative water loss cause hypermetabolism in burn patients? Ann Surg 171:236, 1970.
28. Wolfe RR, Durkot MJ, Allsop JR, et al: Glucose metabolism in severely burned patients. Metabolism 28:1031, 1979.
29. Burke JF, Wolfe RR, Mullany CJ, et al: Glucose requirements following burn injury. Ann Surg 190:274, 1979.
30. Wolfe RR, Herndon DN, Jahoor F, et al: Effect of severe burn injury on substrate cycling by glucose and fatty acids. N Engl J Med 317:403, 1987.
31. Wilmore DW, Long JM, Mason AD, et al: Catecholamines: Mediator of the hypermetabolic response to thermal injury. Ann Surg 180:653, 1974.
32. Jahoor F, Herndon DN, Wolfe RR: The role of insulin and glucagon in the response of glucose and alanine kinetics in burn-injured patients. J Clin Invest 78:807, 1986.
33. Herndon D: Mediators of metabolism. J Trauma 21:701, 1981.
34. Caldwell FT, Bowser BH, Crabtree JH: The effect of occlusive dressings on the energy metabolism of severely burned children. Ann Surg 1983:579, 1981.
35. Hunt TK, Niinikoski J, Zederfeldt B: Role of oxygen in repair processes. Acta Chir Scand 138:109, 1972.
36. Korn HN, Wheeler ES, Miller TA: Effect of hyperbaric oxygen on second-degree burn wound healing. Arch Surg 112:732, 1977.
37. Perrins DJD: A failed attempt to limit tissue destruction in scalds of pig skin with hyperbaric oxygen. In Wada J, Iwa T (eds): Proceedings of the Fourth International Congress on Hyperbaric Medicine. Baltimore, Williams & Wilkins, 1970, pp 381–387.
38. Im MJ, Hoopes JE: Energy metabolism in healing skin wounds. J Surg Res 10:459, 1970.
39. Hunt TK: The wound environment: Control of collagen synthesis and angiogenesis. American College of Surgeons Postgraduate Course, Wound Healing: Current Concepts and Applications, San Francisco, October 13–14, 1987.
40. Levene CI, Bates CJ: The effect of hypoxia on collagen synthesis in cultured 3T6 fibroblasts and its relationship to the mode of action of ascorbate. Biochem Biophys Acta 444:4456, 1976.
41. Jensen JA, Hunt TK, Scheuenstuhl H, et al: Effect of lactate, pyruvate and pH on secretion of angiogenesis and mitogenesis factors by macrophages. Lab Invest 54:574, 1986.
42. Levenson SM, Upjohn HL, Preston JA, et al: Effect of thermal burns on wound healing. Ann Surg 146:357, 1957.
43. Cohen IK, Diegelmann RF: Wound healing in cosmetic surgery: An overview. In Rudolph R (ed): Problems in Aesthetic Surgery. St. Louis, CV Mosby, 1986, pp 1–13.
44. Shewmake KB, Talbert GE, Bowser-Wallace BH, et al: Alterations in plasma copper, zinc, and ceruloplasmin levels in patients with thermal injury. J Burn Care Rehab 9:13, 1988.
45. Boosalis MG, McCall JT, Solem LD, et al: Serum copper and ceruloplasmin levels and urinary copper excretion in thermal injury. Am J Clin Nutr 44:899, 1986.
46. Sanchez-Agreda M, Cimorra GA, Mariona M, et al: Trace elements in burned patients: Studies of zinc, copper and iron contents in serum. Burns 4:28, 1977.
47. Harris ED, Gonnerman WA, Savage JE, et al: Connective tissue amine oxidase: II. Purification and partial characterization of lysyl oxidase from chick aorta. Biochem Biophys Acta 341:322, 1974.
48. Committee on Dietary Allowances, Food, and Nutrition Board, Commission on Life Science, National Research Council: Recommended Dietary Allowances, 9th ed. Washington, DC, National Academy Press, 1980.
49. Riordan JF: Biochemistry of zinc. Symposium on trace elements. Med Clin North Am 60:661, 1976.
50. Chvapil M: Effects of zinc on cells and biomembranes. Symposium on trace elements. Med Clin North Am 60:799, 1976.
51. Shakespeare PG: Studies on the serum levels of iron, copper, and zinc, and the urinary excretion of zinc after burn injury. Burns 8:358, 1981.
52. Pories WJ, Mansour EG, Plecka FR, et al: Metabolic factors affecting zinc metabolism in the surgical patient. In Prasad AS, Oberleas D (eds): Trace Elements in Human Health and Disease. Zinc and Copper, vol 1. New York, Academic Press, 1976, pp 123–136.
53. Arturson G: Microvascular permeability to macromolecules in thermal injury. Acta Physiol Scand (Suppl) 463:111, 1979.
54. Baxter CR: Fluid volume and electrolyte changes in the early postburn period. Clin Plast Surg 1:693, 1974.
55. Horton JW, Baxter CR, White J: The effect of aging

on the cardiac contractile response to unresuscitated thermal injury. J Burn Care Rehab 9:41, 1988.

56. Carvajal HF, Linares HA, Brouhard BH: Relationships of burn size to vascular permeability changes in rats. Surg Gynecol Obstet 149:193, 1979.

57. Monafo WW, Chunktrasakul C, Ayvazian VH: Hypertonic sodium solutions in the treatment of burn shock. Am J Surg 126:778, 1973.

58. Demling RH: Fluid resuscitation after major burns. JAMA 250:1438, 1983.

59. Boykin JV, Crute SL, Haynes BW: Cimetidine therapy for burn shock: A quantitative assessment. J Trauma 25:864, 1985.

60. Boykin JV, Manson NH: Mechanisms of cimetidine protection following thermal injury. Am J Med 83:76, 1987.

61. Davis KL, Schwartzman ML, Solangi K, et al: Competitive inhibition of arachidonic acid with cimetidine on purifeid cytochrome P-450. Fed Proc 46:866, 1987 (abstr).

62. Carlson RG, Miller SF, Finley RK, et al: Fluid retention and burn survival. J Trauma 27:127, 1987.

63. Carlson RG, Finley RK, Miller SF, et al: Fluid retention during the first 48 hours as an indicator of burn survival. J Trauma 26:840, 1986.

64. Marshall WG Jr, Dimick AR: The natural history of major burns with multiple subsystem failure. J Trauma 23:102, 1983.

65. Demling RH: Infections following burns. In Hoeprich P (ed): Infectious Diseases. New York, Harper & Row, 1984, pp 1348–1351.

66. Marvin JA, Heck EL, Loebl EC, et al: Usefulness of blood cultures in confirming septic complications in burn patients: Evaluation of a new culture method. J Trauma 15:657, 1975.

67. Modak S, Fox P, Stanford J, et al: Silver sulfadiazine-impregnated biologic membranes as burn wound covers. J Burn Care Rehab 7:422, 1986.

68. Deitch E, Sittig K, Heimbach D, et al: Results of a multicenter study on the safety and efficacy of DI-MAC, a new delivery system for silver sulfadiazine. Presented at the Twentieth Meeting of the American Burn Association, Seattle, WA, March, 1988.

69. Holder IA, Knoll CA, Wesselman J: Norfloxacin and silver-norfloxacin as topical and antimicrobial agents: results of in vitro susceptibility testing against bacteria and Candida sp isolated from burn patients. J Burn Care Rehab 7:479, 1986.

70. Ninnemann JL: Trauma, sepsis, and the immune response. J Burn Care Rehab 8:462, 1987.

71. Alexander JW, Ogle CK, Stinnet JD, et al: A sequential, prospective analysis of immunologic abnormalities and infection following severe thermal injury. Ann Surg 188:809, 1978.

72. Davis JM, Dineen P, Gallin JI: Neutrophil degranulation and abnormal chemotaxis after thermal injury. J Immunol 124:1467, 1980.

73. Carpenter AB, Boykin JV, Crute SL, et al: The acridine orange fluorochrome microassay: A new technique for quantitation of neutrophil function in burned patients. J Trauma 26:389, 1986.

74. Miller CL, Baker CC: Changes in lymphocyte activity after thermal injury: The role of suppressor cells. J Clin Invest 63:202, 1979.

75. Baker CC, Miller CL, Trunkey DD: Predicting fatal sepsis in burn patients. J Trauma 19:641, 1979.

76. Ninnemann JL, Stock AE, Condie JT: Induction of prostaglandin synthesis-dependent suppressor cells with endotoxin: Occurrence in patients with thermal injuries. J Clin Immunol 3:142, 1983.

77. Lanser ME, Saba TM, Scovill WA: Opsonic glycoprotein (plasma fibronectin) levels after burn injury: Relationship to extent of burn and development of sepsis. Ann Surg 192:776, 1980.

78. Wolfe RA, Roi LD, Flora JD, et al: Mortality differences and speed of wound closure among specialized burn care facilities. JAMA 250:763, 1983.

79. VanWinkle W: The epithelium in wound healing. Surg Gynecol Obstet 125:131, 1967.

80. McMinn RMH: Wound healing. In Beck F, Lloyd JB (eds): The Cell in Medical Science, vol 4. New York, Academic Press, 1976, pp 321–356.

81. Heggers JP, Ko F, Robson MC, et al: Evaluation of burn blister fluid. Plast Reconstr Surg 65:798, 1980.

82. Dobke MK, Hayes EC, Baxter CR: Leukotrienes LTB$_4$ and LTC$_4$ in thermally injured patients' plasma and burn blister fluid. J Burn Care Rehabil 8:189, 1987.

83. Odland G, Ross R: Human wound repair. I. Epidermal regeneration. J Cell Biol 32:231, 1967.

84. Starkey RM, Cohen S, Orth DN: Epidermal growth factor: Identification of a new hormone in human urine. Science 189:800, 1979.

85. Schultz GS, White M, Mitchell R, et al: Epithelial wound healing enhanced by transforming growth factor-alpha and vaccinia growth factor. Science 235:350, 1987.

86. Schultz G: Personal communication.

87. Hunt TK, Andrews WS, Halliday B, et al: Coagulation and macrophage stimulation of angiogenesis and wound healing. In Dineen P, Hildick-Smith P (eds): The Surgical Wound. Philadelphia, Lea & Febiger, 1981.

88. Banda MJ, Knighton DR, Hunt TK, et al: Isolation of a nonmitogenic angiogenesis factor from wound fluid. Proc Natl Acad Sci USA 79:7773, 1982.

89. Martin BM, Gimbrone MA, Unanue ER, et al: Macrophage derived growth factor: Production by cultured human mononuclear blood cells. Fed Proc 40:335, 1981.

90. Hunt TK, Pai MP: Effect of varying ambient oxygen tensions on wound metabolism and collagen synthesis. Surg Gynecol Obstet 135:561, 1972.

91. Knighton DR, Hunt TK, Thakral KK, et al: Role of platelets and fibrin in the healing sequence: An in vivo study of angiogenesis and collagen synthesis. Ann Surg 196:379, 1982.

92. Alvarez OM, Mertz PM, Eaglstein WH: The effect of occlusive dressings on collagen synthesis and re-epithelialization in superficial wounds. J Surg Res 35:142, 1983.

93. Bauer PS, Larson DL, Stacy TR: The observation of myofibroblasts in hypertrophic scars. Surg Gynecol Obstet 141:22, 1975.

94. Ehrlich HP: Do myofibroblasts produce the contractile forces which organize connective tissue matrices? Presented at the Twentieth Meeting of the American Burn Association, Seattle, WA, March, 1988.

95. Rudolph R: Location of the force of wound contraction. Surg Gynecol Obstet 148:547, 1979.

96. Kischer CW, Bunce H, Shetlar MR: Mast cell analysis in hypertrophic scars, hypertrophic scars treated with pressure and mature scars. J Invest Dermatol 70:355, 1978.

97. Russell JD, Russell SB, Trupin KM: The effect of histamine on the growth of cultured fibroblasts isolated from normal and keloid tissue. J Cell Physiol 93:389, 1977.

98. Rudolph R: Inhibition of myofibroblasts by skin grafts. Plast Reconstr Surg 63:473, 1979.

99. Larson DL: Techniques for decreasing scar formation and contractures in the burned patient. J Trauma 11:807, 1971.

100. Ketchum LD, Cohen IK, Masters FW: Hypertrophic scars and keloids. Plast Reconstr Surg 53:140, 1974.
101. Atnip RG, Burke JF: Skin coverage. Curr Prob Surg 20:624, 1983.
102. Saunders JBdeCM: A conceptual history of transplantation. In Najarian JS, Simmons RL (eds): Transplantation. Philadelphia, Lea & Febiger, 1972, pp 3–25.
103. Maltz M: Evolution of Plastic Surgery. New York, Froben Press, 1946.
104. Gallico GG, O'Connor NE: Cultured epithelium as a skin substitute. Clin Plast Surg 12:149, 1985.
105. Brown JB: Massive repairs of burns with thick split skin grafts: Emergency "dressings" with homografts. Ann Surg 115:658, 1942.
106. Gibson T, Medawar PB: The fate of skin homografts in man. J Anat 77:299, 1943.
107. Ersek RA, Lorio J: The most indolent ulcers of the skin treated with porcine xenografts and silver ions. Surg Gynecol Obstet 158:431, 1984.
108. Bromberg BE, Song IC, Mohn MP: The use of pigskin as a temporary biologic dressing. Plast Reconstr Surg 36:80, 1965.
109. Tavis MJ, Thornton J, Danet R, et al: Current status of skin substitutes. Surg Clin North Am 58:1233, 1978.
110. Pruitt BA, Levine NS: Characteristics and uses of biologic dressings and skin substitutes. Arch Surg 119:312, 1984.
111. Griswold JA, Molnar JA: Toxic Epidermal Necrolysis. In Martyn JA (ed): Acute Management of the Burned Patient. WB Saunders, Philadelphia, 1990, pp 128–137.
112. Yue-Liang D, Shu-Sung P, De-Zhen W, et al: Clinical and histological observations on the application of intermingled auto- and porcine-skin heterografts in third degree burns. Burns 9:381, 1981.
113. Mider GB, Morton JJ: The effect of freezing in vitro on some transplantable mammalian tumors and on normal rat skin. Am J Cancer 35:902, 1939.
114. Bondoc CC, Burke JF: Clinical experience with viable frozen human skin and frozen skin bank. Ann Surg 174:371, 1971.
115. Tanner JC, Vandput J, Ollery JF: The meshed skin graft. Plast Reconstr Surg 34:287, 1964.
116. Tavis MJ, Thornton JW, Bartlett RH, et al: A new composite skin prosthesis. Burns 7:123, 1979.
117. McHugh TP, Robson MC, Heggers JP, et al: Therapeutic efficacy of Biobrane in partial- and full-thickness thermal injury. Surgery 100:661, 1986.
118. Purdue GF, Hunt JL, Gillespie RW, et al: Biosynthetic skin substitute versus frozen human cadaver allograft for temporary coverage of excised burn wounds. J Trauma 27:155, 1987.
119. Foresman PA, Tedeschi KR, Rodeheaver GT: Influence of membrane dressings on wound contraction. J Burn Care Rel Res 7:398, 1986.
120. Montagna W, Parakkaol PF: The Structure and Function of Skin, 3rd ed. New York, Academic Press, 1974.
121. Eil C, Liberman UA, Rosen JF, et al: A cellular defect in hereditary vitamin-D-dependent rickets type II: Defective nuclear uptake of 1,25-dihydroxyvitamin D in cultured skin fibroblasts. N Engl J Med 304:1588, 1981.
122. Burke JF, Yannas IV, Quinby WC Jr, et al: Successful use of a physiologically acceptable artificial skin in the treatment of extensive burn injury. Ann Surg 194:413, 1981.
123. Green H, Hehinde O, Thomas J: Growth of cultured human epidermal cells into multiple epithelia suitable for grafting. Proc Natl Acad Sci USA 76:5665, 1979.
124. Rheinwald JG, Green H: Epidermal growth factor and the multiplication of cultured human epidermal keratinocytes. Nature 265:421, 1977.
125. Igel HJ, Freeman AE, Boeckman CR, et al: A new method for covering large surface area wounds with autografts. Arch Surg 108:724, 1974.
126. O'Connor NE, Mulliken JB, Banks-Schlegel S, et al: Grafting of burns with cultured epithelium prepared from autologous epidermal cells. Lancet 1:75, 1981.
127. Gallico GG III, O'Connor NE, Compton CC, et al: Permanent coverage of large burn wounds with autologous cultured human epithelium. N Engl J Med 311:448, 1984.
128. Compton CC, Gill JM, Bradford DA, et al: Skin regenerated from cultured epithelial autografts on full-thickness burn wounds from 6 days to 5 years after grafting: A light, electron microscopic and immunohistochemical study. Lab Invest 60:600, 1989.
129. Gallico GG III, O'Connor NE, Compton CC, et al: Cultured epithelial autografts for giant congenital nevi. Plast Reconstr Surg 84:1, 1989.
130. Herzog SR, Meyer A, Woodley D, et al: Wound coverage with cultured autologous keratinocytes: Use after burn wound excision, including biopsy followup. J Trauma 28:195, 1988.
131. Woodley DT, Peterson HD, Herzog SR, et al: Burn wounds resurfaced by cultured epidermal autografts show abnormal reconstitution of anchoring fibrils. JAMA 259:2566, 1988.
132. Kumagai N, Nihina H, Tanabe H, et al: Clinical application of autologous cultured epithelia for the treatment of burn wounds and burn scars. Plast Reconstr Surg 82:99, 1988.
133. Hunyadi J, Farkas B, Bertenyi C, et al: Keratinocyte grafting: A new means of transplantation for full-thickness wounds. J Dermatol Surg Oncol 14:75, 1988.
134. Bell E, Ehrlich HP, Sher S, et al: Development and use of a living skin equivalent. Plast Reconstr Surg 67:386, 1981.
135. Wassermann D, Schlotterer M, Toulon A, et al: Preliminary clinical studies of a biological skin equivalent in burned patients. Burns 14:326, 1988.
136. Phillips TJ, Kehinde O, Green H, et al: Treatment of skin ulcers with cultured epidermal allografts. J Am Acad Dermatol 21:191, 1989.
137. Hefton JM, Madden MR, Finkelstein JL, et al: Grafting of burn patients with allografts of cultured epidermal cells. Lancet 2:428, 1983.
138. Leigh IM, Purkis PE, Navsaria HA, et al: Treatment of chronic venous ulcers with sheets of cultured allogenic keratinocytes. Br J Dermatol 117:591, 1987.
139. Brain A, Purkis P, Coates P, et al: Survival of cultured allogeneic keratinocytes transplanted to deep dermal bed assessed with probe specific for Y chromosome. BMJ 298:917, 1989.
140. Cuono C, Langdon R, McGuire J: Use of cultured epidermal autografts and dermal allograft as skin replacement after burn injury. Lancet 1:1123, 1986.
141. Cuono CB, Langdon R, Birchall N, et al: Composite autologous-allogeneic skin replacement: Development and clinical application. Plast Reconstr Surg 80:626, 1987.
142. Yannas IV, Burke JF, Warpehoski M, et al: Design principles and preliminary clinical performance of an artificial skin. Biomaterials: Interfacial phenomena and applications. Adv Chem 199:475, 1982.
143. Yannas IV, Burke JF, Gordon PL, et al: Design of an artificial skin: II. Control of chemical composition. J Biomed Mater Res 14:107, 1980.
144. Tompkins RG, Hilton JF, Burke JF, et al: Increased survival after massive thermal injuries in adults: Preliminary report using artificial skin. Crit Care Med 17:734, 1989.

33

CLINICAL MANAGEMENT OF NONHEALING WOUNDS

W. Thomas Lawrence, M.D.

As discussed in previous chapters, a healed wound is the product of several separate but related processes. In order for a wound to heal, hemostatic and inflammatory mechanisms must be intact, mesenchymal cells must migrate to and proliferate in the wounded area, angiogenesis and epithelialization must occur, and collagen must be synthesized, crosslinked, and aligned properly to provide strength to the healed wound. In open wounds, contraction must take place as well. All of these processes must occur in proper sequence for optimal wound healing.

The nonhealing wound is a result of an impairment in one or more of these processes. It is important to consider which aspect of wound healing biology has been altered when analyzing a chronic nonhealing wound. Some factors leading to nonhealing wounds may affect more than one aspect of the wound healing process. In other cases, one aspect of healing may be influenced directly while subsequent wound healing processes are impeded as a result of the primary impairment. An impairment of one of the earlier aspects of healing such as inflammation will interfere with all subsequent wound healing processes. Therefore, impaired inflammation may manifest itself as inadequate angiogenesis, mesenchymal cell chemotaxis and proliferation, epithelialization, wound contraction, and collagen synthesis and remodeling.

In different types of wounds, different biological phenomena of the wound healing process are more or less important. For example, in a partial-thickness dermal injury, epithelialization alone is most critical. In an excisional or open wound, wound contraction and epithelialization are of primary importance. In an incisional wound, collagen synthesis and remodeling are vital for providing wound strength. Analysis of which aspect of healing is most important in a particular wound will help to identify the defect in healing.

Wound healing is a preferred biological process. Although it can be inhibited by a variety of factors, it is difficult to completely halt healing. Therefore when faced with a wound that won't heal, a limited correction of a healing problem may be enough. An ideal wound healing milieu may not be necessary, and this is fortuitous because not all factors that impair healing are reversible.

The factors that lead to impaired healing can be classified as intrinsic and extrinsic (Table 33–1). Intrinsic, or local, factors are characteristics

Table 33–1. FACTORS THAT IMPAIR HEALING

Intrinsic Factors	Extrinsic Factors
Infection	Hereditary healing disorders
Foreign bodies	Nutritional deficiencies
Ischemia	Distant malignancies
Cigarette smoking	Old age
Venous insufficiency	Diabetes
Radiation	Jaundice
Mechanical trauma	Alcoholism
Local toxins	Uremia
Cancer	Glucocorticoid steroids
	Chemotherapeutic agents
	Other medications

of the wound itself and include infection, foreign bodies, ischemia, smoking, venous insufficiency, radiation, mechanical irritation, local toxins, and cancer. Some of these factors are related; for example, the effects of radiation are at least partially a result of tissue ischemia. Extrinsic, or constitutional factors, are characteristics of the patient that have local effects on wound healing. Extrinsic factors include several congenital syndromes, nutritional factors, distant malignancies, old age, diabetes, jaundice or renal disease, and some medications such as glucocorticoid steroids and chemotherapeutic agents. Each of these factors is individually considered here, although some are discussed more thoroughly in other chapters.

INTRINSIC FACTORS

Infection

In wound infection the inflammatory response is prolonged and the healing process is retarded. Later wound healing processes such as epithelialization, contraction, and collagen deposition do not occur or occur in a very limited fashion. Wounds will not heal until infection is controlled.

Infection represents an imbalance between the host's defense system and the quantity of bacteria in the wound. Humans normally live in symbiosis with a large number of bacteria. Normal dry skin contains 10 to 1000 bacteria per gram of tissue while skin in exposed and moist areas contains up to 100,000 bacteria per gram of tissue.[1, 2] Human saliva contains up to 100 million bacteria per milliliter,[3] and stool also has a heavy bacterial load.

The human body has several protective mechanisms that limit bacterial invasion and proliferation in normal tissues. The stratum corneum of the skin is a compact physical barrier to bacterial invasion.[2] Dryness limits staphylococcal proliferation, but when the skin becomes excessively dry, it can crack and allow bacterial invasion.[4] Staphylococci proliferate readily in a moist environment such as macerated skin. Sebaceous secretions contain bactericidal and fungicidal fatty acids that limit infection.[5] The dilution of these cutaneous fatty acids that occurs with edema renders the patient or extremity more susceptible to infection. Skin is also rich in lysozymes, which hydrolyze bacterial cell membranes and further limit the possibility of infection.[6] The skin and its appendages produce other products that inhibit bacterial growth, including lactic and uric acid.[7]

The cilia of the tracheobronchial tree tend to expel bacteria, and the IgA and enzymes in the tracheobronchial secretions limit bacterial growth in that anatomical location.[6] The acidic pH of the stomach and vagina hinders bacterial growth and invasion through these portals.[4, 6]

The immune system normally acts as a significant barrier to bacterial invasion.[6] Both neutrophils and macrophages phagocytize bacteria and B lymphocytes generate antibodies that neutralize toxin and that, with complement, can lead to bacterial destruction. T lymphocytes are cytotoxic without complement. The combination of the natural barriers to infection and the immune system provides ample protection against bacterial invasion in most cases.

Infection can develop when body defenses are weakened, thus allowing a normal bacterial load to become overwhelming. Such a weakness may be a result of breakdown of one or more of the normal barriers to infection or an immune deficiency. Alternatively, the bacterial challenge may be greater than that which the body can effectively handle. In normal patients, the critical number is 100,000 bacteria per gram of tissue, above which the body loses control over proliferation and invasion. This number has been indirectly defined by several studies at the United States Army Institute of Surgical Research and elsewhere.[8–11] Therefore, a bacterial load of greater than 100,000 per gram of tissue is indicative of infection. This threshold number of bacteria holds true for all bacterial species other than group B streptococcus, which can cause infection in lesser quantities.[12] Although the invading bacteria can come from endogenous or exogenous sources, the bacteria that cause wound infections after burns and bowel surgery are usually endogenous.[13–15]

Diagnosis of infection can be accomplished by quantitative wound biopsy cultures,[16] which require 24 to 48 hours for results. However, a simpler rapid slide technique can tell within 1 hour whether or not more than 100,000 bacterial per gram of tissue are present in a wound.[17]

The value of the quantitation of the bacterial count has been repeatedly demonstrated. When bacterial counts are below 100,000 per gram of tissue, acute wounds will almost universally heal without infection.[18] If counts are greater, one can delay closure[19] or cover the wound with a skin graft until the bacterial count has been reduced.[20] Infections with wound breakdown almost always develops when bacterial counts are greater than 100,000 per gram of tissue.

Nonbacterial infections occasionally cause nonhealing. Syphilis, tuberculosis, and fungal diseases have all been associated with nonhealing wounds.

Infection is one of the primary reasons why wounds do not heal. Almost all of the other factors that can cause a nonhealing wound do so either entirely or partially by predisposing the wound to infection. Infection is therefore one of the primary final common pathways of nonhealing.

Foreign Bodies

While the presence of a foreign body can contribute to nonhealing, it is not by itself sufficient to prevent healing. Clearly most patients with synthetic heart valves, prosthetic vascular grafts, pacemakers, and breast implants do not have chronic, nonhealing wounds. Foreign bodies provide a nidus for bacterial growth. A small amount of bacteria, such as that found in normal skin, can cause infection when a foreign body is present. This fact was experimentally demonstrated by Elek,[21, 22] who produced purulence when approximately 100 staphylococci were dried onto a stitch that was placed in the skin. In contrast, greater than 1,000,000 staphylococci were required to generate pus when bacteria alone were injected subcutaneously. Edlich and associates demonstrated that some sutures are more potent adjuvants of bacterial proliferation than others.[23] Roettinger and colleagues showed that some foreign bodies such as liquid silicone have little ability to potentiate infection.[24] Therefore, one can conclude that all foreign bodies are not equivalent in their ability to function as bacterial adjuvants.

Even biological materials can at times function as foreign bodies. Hematomas can potentiate infection with relatively low quantities of bacteria.[25] Similarly, in a comminuted, compound fracture of the tibia, a bone fragment devascularized by the injury may die and act as a foreign body, thereby becoming an adjuvant for bacterial growth, subsequent infection, and inhibition of healing.

Once an infection has developed in the presence of a foreign body, eradication is difficult if not impossible without removal of the foreign body.

Inadequate Blood Supply

An adequate supply of oxygen and nutrients is required for normal wound healing and is delivered to the wound via the vascular system. The supply of these substances can vary at the wound site for three reasons. First, the supply of the material may be limited. This is generally not a problem with oxygen, though at extremely low hemoglobin concentrations, oxygen-carrying capacity may be limited. Supply can be a problem for nutrients, and this will be discussed subsequently. Second, the perfusion pressure provided by the heart may be inadequate as a result of either cardiac failure or inadequate intravascular volume. Hunt and co-workers demonstrated that tissue oxygenation dropped dramatically in dogs with experimentally induced hypovolemia, and that restoration of normal circulating volume led to improved tissue oxygenation after a slight delay.[26] Anemia alone is not an important determinant of tissue oxygenation or healing capacity.[26, 27] Third, the local vascular system may be impaired as a result of either local damage due to trauma or, more commonly, to a generalized process such as atherosclerosis. Problems with either the pump or the peripheral circulation manifest locally in the wound as relative tissue hypoxia.

Like infection, tissue hypoxia is another final common pathway through which other factors limit healing. Oxygen is required for aerobic metabolism and energy production. Although anaerobic metabolism is possible in a hypoxic wound environment, the quantity of energy that can be generated by this mechanism is inadequate for normal healing. The rate of fibroblast proliferation is likewise influenced by the oxygen concentration.[28, 29] Oxygen is also required for hydroxylation of lysine and proline during collagen synthesis.[30] Without adequate hydroxylation, collagen thermal stability is significantly impaired, leading to diminished wound strength. The overall rate of collagen synthesis has also been demonstrated to be inhibited in vitro by hypoxia.[31] The only aspect of healing facilitated by hypoxia is angiogenesis.[32]

Hypoxia has impaired healing in several wound models. Niinikoski first demonstrated that collagen accumulated in cellulose sponges in rats at a rate correlated with inspired oxygen tension,[28] and Hunt and Pai obtained similar results using a wound cylinder model.[33] Stephens and Hunt showed that the tensile strength of incisional wounds varied with inspired oxygen tension.[34]

In addition to its direct effect on wound healing biology, hypoxia also impairs the body's defense mechanisms against bacterial invasion. Oxygen is required by neutrophils for the creation of free oxygen radicals that kill bacteria.[35] The susceptibility of wounds to infection was found to directly correlate with oxygen concentration in two experimental models.[36, 37]

Clinically, Wagner and associates demonstrated that the healing of below knee amputations was significantly correlated with a higher midcalf transcutaneous oxygen measurement.[38] In another study, oxygen electrodes were implanted into a group of nonhealing wounds, and the Po_2 of the wound areas was found to range from 5 to 20 mmHg as compared to control tissue values of 30 to 50 mmHg.[39] An adequate tissue oxygen level is clearly required for wound healing to occur.

Ulcers resulting from arterial insufficiency and hypoxia characteristically occur on the distal lower extremity. They are painful and often covered with eschar. The wound base of ulcers induced by arterial insufficiency is generally pale and covered with fibrinous material and there is usually no granulation tissue. Surrounding skin is generally atrophic and hairless. These ulcers are frequently associated with claudication and, in extreme cases, rest pain.

Smoking

Smoking limits functional tissue perfusion through several mechanisms. It induces cutaneous vasoconstriction as demonstrated by skin temperature measurements,[40] plethysmography,[41] and direct observation of the capillary bed.[42] This vasoconstriction may be due to the direct effect of one or more constituents of cigarette smoke, the indirect effect of the increased catecholamine levels elicited by smoking,[43] or possibly both mechanisms. In addition, cigarette smoke contains 3 to 6 percent carbon monoxide, which binds to hemoglobin in the pulmonary capillaries, producing carboxyhemoglobin. Carboxyhemoglobin levels in smokers range from 1 to 20 percent.[44] In addition to limiting blood oxygen-carrying capacity, elevated carboxyhemoglobin levels have been associated with endothelial changes[44, 45] and increased platelet adhesiveness[46] that can lead to additional limitation of local blood flow. Chronic cigarette use is associated with increased rates of atherosclerosis, further contributing to decreased tissue oxygenation.[47]

In the rabbit ear model, nicotine has been demonstrated to slow wound contraction when injected intraperitoneally twice a day.[48] It has not been determined whether nicotine impairs healing by limiting perfusion or by some other mechanism.

Venous Insufficiency

Many chronic leg wounds are a result of venous insufficiency. The venous system of the lower extremity consists of a superficial system and a deep system with perforators that connect them. The superficial system includes the long and short saphenous veins and runs in the subcutaneous tissues, while the deep system includes the anterior and posterior tibial and peroneal veins and runs within the muscular compartments of the leg. Valves within the venous system direct blood from the superficial to the deep veins and back to the heart. The flow of blood within the deep system is facilitated by the pumping action of the calf muscles during physical activity. An episode of deep venous thrombosis can lead to destruction of the valves within the veins, which allows blood to flow in a retrograde fashion from the deep to the superficial system through the perforators. Valvular incompetence also limits the ability of calf muscles to direct blood back to the heart. Blood instead pools in the lower extremity, and back pressure in the capillary bed leads to edema. Fibrin is deposited around the capillaries, which may limit the transmission of oxygen and nutrients to tissue.[49] Pressure produced by back flow in the perforators causes ischemia and at times ulceration of the overlying skin. Venous ulcers are most commonly seen directly over the larger perforators cephalad to the medial malleolar region. These ulcers often fail to heal because of persistent venous hypertension and its effects. They are characteristically covered with red to purple granulation tissue and are surrounded by thickened, edematous, hemosiderin-stained tissue.

Radiation

The reaction of the skin to radiation is dose dependent, and the nature of the reaction changes with time.[50] Most therapeutic radiation is given in 20 to 30 fractions of 200 to 300 rads to a total dose of 6000 rads or less over a 5 to 6 week period. The early response to radiation is an inflammatory reaction with erythema, swelling, warmth, and tenderness. At doses greater than 4000 rads, moist desquamation with bullae and ulceration is sometimes seen. After conclusion of the treatment, these ulcers generally heal.

As the acute radiation reaction subsides, chronic changes develop.[50, 51] Pigmentation of the area may change, and epithelial appendages including sebaceous glands and hair follicles are generally destroyed by radiation, resulting in dryness and alopecia. The epidermis is thinned, rete pegs are absent, and dysplastic keratinocytes may be seen. The blood vessels in the upper dermis are irregularly dilated, causing telangiectasias. There is an overall decrease in the quantity of blood vessels. Various degrees of myointimal proliferation are seen in the arterioles of the subdermal plexus, and this proliferation causes partial obstruction and sometimes thrombosis of the blood vessels. Increasing fibrosis is noted in the dermis, and the dermal collagen is very dense and irregular. Many fibroblasts are present that on electron microscopy appear damaged with degenerating mitochondria, multiple cytoplasmic vacuoles, crystalline inclusions, and a dilated endoplasmic reticulum. Many elastotic fibers are found in the dermal stroma. Grossly the tissue is firm and fixed with a thin, fragile epidermis.

Radiation-damaged skin is easily damaged, producing nonhealing wounds. The base of these often painful ulcers is generally covered with fibrinopurulent material with little granulation tissue. Histologically, there is little inflammatory reaction or evidence of angiogenesis. The mechanism of ulcer formation is unclear, although many observers feel that ulcers are the result of ischemia due to the obliterative endarteritis of the microvasculature.[52] Damaged fibroblasts and collagen may also contribute to ulceration.[53]

One can speculate that radiation ulcerations fail to heal for several reasons. First, the fibroblasts and other cells in the treated area are damaged and may not be able to respond normally to the stimulus of a wound. Second, the deranged stroma may prevent normal migration of inflammatory and mesenchymal cells to and from the wound. In addition, transmission of signal peptides from the circulation to cells and from one cell to another may be altered by the stromal abnormalities. Third, the area is relatively ischemic, limiting the healing process through mechanisms previously described. As a secondary effect of ischemia, the irradiated tissue is predisposed to infection, which further impairs healing.

Mechanical Trauma

Chronic trauma, both intentional and unintentional, is another cause of impaired healing. Factitious ulcers are nonhealing wounds that result from chronic intentional trauma from an instrument or from scratching or biting. Factitious ulcers are seen in conjunction with psychiatric disorders of varying severity and are discussed in Chapter 29.

Unintentional trauma that results in a chronic wound is often due to anesthesia in the affected area. The classic example of this type of lesion is the pressure sores seen in spinal cord–injured patients that develop over weightbearing bony prominences. The anatomical area at risk depends on the positioning of the patient; for example, the ischial region is primarily at risk during sitting, while the sacrum, heels, scapulae, and occiput are primarily at risk during recumbency. The majority of these lesions develop in the ischial, trochanteric, and sacral regions.[54, 55] It has been suggested that spinal cord–injured patients have impaired healing capacity in their insensate areas, but this concept was questioned by Diegelmann and coworkers,[56] who demonstrated normal healing in the lower extremities of paraplegics.

The primary cause of pressure sores is pressure-induced ischemia in the affected area, with friction[57] and shearing[58] contributing secondarily. Whenever pressure over tissue exceeds capillary filling pressure (32 mmHg), tissue blood flow is impaired due to collapse of the capillaries.[59] Although tolerance to ischemia varies in different types of tissue,[60] all tissues can tolerate ischemia for limited periods of time.[61] When capillary pressure is only slightly exceeded, the pressure can be tolerated for a longer period than when the pressure applied to the tissue is much higher. Low pressures maintained for long periods induce more damage than high pressures for short periods, however. During recumbency or sitting, pressures large enough to induce pressure sores are produced over bony prominences.[62] Sensate individuals unconsciously or consciously move intermittently and thereby limit prolonged pressure to any one anatomical area. Patients with spinal cord injuries lose the ability to unconsciously relieve pressure, and unless they consciously relieve pressure, ischemic tolerance is exceeded in tissue overlying bony prominences and tissue death ensues. Kosiak demonstrated that relief of pressure to an area for 5 to 10 minutes every 2 hours can prevent pressure sores.[63] Less severe pressure-induced tissue injuries can sometimes heal, although more extensive injuries result in ulceration. These ulcers frequently do not heal because of persistent exposure to excess pressure. Moreover, the relative ischemia induced by pressure makes these areas susceptible to infection, which can compound the problem.

Diabetics characteristically develop neurotrophic ulcers over the metatarsal heads.[64] Diabetic neuropathy diminishes the ability to sense excess pressure on the weightbearing portions of the foot so movement to relieve pressure is not stimulated and pressure ulcerations develop. Improperly fitting shoes can exacerbate such problems.

Iatrogenic Nonhealing Wounds

Many agents that health care providers place on wounds actually impede healing. Rodeheaver and co-workers[65] and Custer and associates[66] demonstrated that washing a wound with Betadine soap or pHisoHex soap increased the likelihood of infection and nonhealing. Chlorhexidine digluconate, a component of Hibiclens, has been demonstrated to impede healing in incisional and abrasion wound models in pigs[67] and in incisional wounds in rats.[68] Hypochlorite solutions, of which Dakin's solution is an example, have been demonstrated to impair neutrophil migration,[69] to kill fibroblasts in culture,[70] and to impair healing in a rabbit ear chamber model.[71] Branemark examined several wound models histologically after irrigation with various agents and found that alcohol-containing solutions were extremely toxic to tissues. Hydrogen peroxide, ammonia compounds, hand soap, iodine solutions, and hexachlorophene were not benign but were less toxic in his systems.[72, 73]

Other agents can produce nonhealing wounds when injected subcutaneously into local tissues. Doxorubicin (Adriamycin) is a potent and oft used chemotherapeutic agent that occasionally inadvertently extravasates during intravenous administration. This drug persists in tissues for protracted periods, producing ischemic-appearing ulcers with shaggy, necrotic bases that heal very slowly if at all.[74, 75] The mechanism of injury is unclear: doxorubicin may bind to DNA and limit cell replication, and it may also limit wound contraction.[76] Pentazocine injections produce a severe necrotizing vasculitis and nonhealing wounds.[77] The bite of the brown recluse spider produces another wound that demonstrates limited healing due to a local toxin.[78] Excision of the toxin-affected area is frequently required in order to achieve healing after all of these injuries.

Cancer

Always considered in the differential diagnosis of a nonhealing wound, malignancy can be a primary skin cancer such as a basal cell cancer, a squamous cell cancer, a carcinoma of one of the epithelial appendages, or a malignant melanoma. Basal and squamous cell carcinomas can sometimes arise in chronic wounds resulting from other etiologies. These scar carcinomas, termed Marjolin's ulcers, arise after an average of 30 or more years and are more aggressive than usual skin cancers.[79] Noncutaneous tumors such as sarcomas can also present as nonhealing skin wounds. In addition, hematological malignancies including leukemias occasionally have cutaneous manifestations.

Cancer can also function as an extrinsic factor, and this is discussed in the following section.

EXTRINSIC FACTORS

Hereditary Healing Disorders

Several genetic disorders have an impact on wound healing. *Ehlers-Danlos syndrome* (cutis hyperelastica) is characterized by an inability to form normal collagen. There are at least ten variants of the syndrome with various severities and pathophysiologies.[80] The enzyme or biochemical deficiency producing many of the types is still unknown, with the mode of inheritance varying from type to type. The classic signs and symptoms are thin, lax, friable skin with prominent veins, hyperextensible joints, and "onion skin" scars covered by thin, silvery, atrophic epithelium most commonly seen over the knees and shins. Patients with less severe variants of the syndrome demonstrate only thin skin that is somewhat soft, while in the more extreme variants the skin tears apart under minimal stress. Gastrointestinal problems, including bleeding, hiatal hernia, intestinal diverticulae, and rectal prolapse, are common in some variants of the syndrome. Patients with the more severe types can develop aneurysms, cardiac valve incompetence, and corneal and joint dislocations. Ehlers-Danlos syndrome must be considered in patients with soft skin that tears easily and in younger patients with recurrent hernias and a coagulopathy, which is often coexistent.

Epidermolysis bullosa is characterized by blistering and ulcerations.[81, 82] There are both autosomal dominant and autosomal recessive variants of the disorder with several subtypes of each. The basic pathophysiology is a defect in tissue adhesion within the epidermis, basement membrane, or dermis resulting in tissue separation and blistering with minimal trauma. The different subtypes are characterized by different anatomical areas within the skin where tissue adhesion breaks down, and these differences contribute to variations in the extent and severity of tissue involvement. The majority of these ulcers will heal spontaneously through contraction, but hand deformities may result from secondary healing in some of the subtypes.

Several inherited disorders result in "soft" connective tissue that may make surgery and healing more difficult but are not universally associated with complications. *Marfan's syndrome*, in which there is an undefined defect in collagen crosslinking, is an example of this type of disorder. Marfan's syndrome is associated with tall stature, arachnodactyly, lax ligaments, myopia, scoliosis, pectus excavatum, and often dissecting aneurysms, which can be fatal and should be repaired. Patients with *osteogenesis imperfecta* also have soft connective tissue, most likely as a result of a defect in collagen maturation. These patients present with blue sclerae, hernias, thin skin, easy bruising, and osseous problems. Surgery can be successfully carried out on these patients.

Progeria, Werner's syndrome, and *homocystinuria* are inherited syndromes with dermatological manifestations that are associated with accelerated atherosclerosis, which can limit healing and potentially cause ulcers. Homocystinuric patients also have a poorly defined collagen crosslinking defect that can further contribute to poor healing. Not all inherited syndromes with cutaneous manifestations produce impaired healing, however. Patients with pseudoxanthoma elasticum and cutis laxa have abnormal, lax skin, but healing is generally uncomplicated.

Nutrition

It has been known for some time that malnutrition is associated with impaired healing.[83] Because specific nutrients are required for different aspects of the wound healing process, different nutrient deficiencies will have an impact on different parts of the healing process. In addition, inadequate nutrition is associated with an increased likelihood of infection.

Since collagen, the primary component of scar, is a protein, adequate protein intake is needed to provide the amino acids required for collagen synthesis. A deficiency in protein intake results in a wound healing impairment.[84, 85] Protein malnutrition may also affect healing indirectly by altering the function of inflammatory cells.[86] Williamson and coworkers[87] have suggested that sulfur-containing amino acids such as methionine and cystine are the most critical, and they believe that replenishment of cystine alone may be adequate to correct a healing impairment resulting from protein deficiency. This finding has been questioned by Irvin,[88] and others have promoted arginine as a pivotal amino acid.[89]

If inadequate quantities of fat and carbohydrate are provided, all normal metabolic functions including wound healing are slowed, and protein is broken down for energy.[90] Essential fatty acids are also required for normal healing, and the healing of skin incisions and burns has been demonstrated to be deficient in animals fed a diet deficient in these nutrients.[91]

Wound healing and collagen synthesis are significantly impaired in vitamin C deficiency.[92] Hydroxylation of the lysine and proline moieties within the collagen triple helix requires vitamin C as well as iron, oxygen, and α-ketoglutarate. If vitamin C is deficient, hydroxylation is impaired. In addition, if lysine is underhydroxylated, crosslinking is impaired, resulting in decreased wound strength. Resistance to infection is also diminished in scorbutic individuals.[93] Although incisional wounds in scorbutic animals are weak, wound contraction may proceed normally,[94] thereby demonstrating that collagen synthesis and wound contraction are distinct phenomena.

Vitamin A is also necessary for normal healing, although the pathophysiology of vitamin A deficiency is unknown. In wounds in vitamin A–deficient experimental animals, epithelialization is slowed, collagen synthesis is deficient, and collagen crosslink formation is impaired.[95] Vitamin A also seems to be important in glycosaminoglycan metabolism[96] and modulation of the immune system.[97]

Other vitamins are less important in wound healing. The role of B vitamins in wound healing is not clear, although a deficiency of thiamine has been associated with impaired healing in experimental animals.[98] Administration of vitamin E impairs wound healing in rats,[99] although its specific role in normal wound healing is poorly defined. Vitamin K is required for normal blood coagulation, and while deficiency is not associated with a specific defect in healing, the formation of a hematoma is a severe deterrent to the healing process. Vitamin D is required for normal calcium metabolism and is therefore necessary for normal bone healing.

Minerals are required for normal healing as well. Magnesium, copper, calcium, selenium, and manganese are among those known to be involved as cofactors to enzymes that are involved in various aspects of healing. The effect of deficiencies of these minerals on healing has not been extensively examined. While iron-deficient animals have been demonstrated in some studies to show impaired healing,[100] this finding has been questioned.[101] A zinc deficiency is associated with impaired granulation tissue formation[102] and healing.[103] Since zinc is a necessary cofactor of DNA polymerase and reverse transcriptase, the healing impairment associated with zinc deficiency may be due to an inhibition of cellular proliferation.

Distant Malignancy

The tumor-bearing state has been associated with impaired healing for a number of reasons.[85] Cancer, especially in advanced states, is associated with cachexia, which is characterized by weight loss, anorexia, asthenia, and malnutrition.[104] Although the mechanisms by which cancer produces anorexia are unknown, it is reversible by tumor removal.[105] In addition, intra-abdominal solid tumors can mechanically impair gastrointestinal function and further limit nutrient utilization.

The metabolism of cancer-bearing patients may be altered as well. Glucose turnover is increased in many cases, and this is often associated with glucose intolerance resulting in inefficient energy utilization.[106] Protein metabolism is frequently affected, causing increased muscular protein breakdown, hepatic gluconeogenesis, and intrahepatic protein synthesis.[107] Solid tumors require protein for growth, and the protein requirements of cancer patients are often increased. The quantity of amino acids in the venous effluent from sarcoma-bearing extremities is diminished as compared to that from nontumor-bearing extremities, suggesting active uptake of amino acids by the tumor.[108] Fat is not utilized efficiently as an energy source in many cancer patients; tumor-bearing animals accumulate fat at the expense of other tissues.[109] All of these metabolic changes combine to effectively limit the availability of nutrients for wound healing.

Inflammatory cell function is also altered by the tumor-bearing state. Such changes can affect the wound healing process by limiting the availability of inflammatory cell-derived growth factors, which normally stimulate healing.

Age

Carrell and DuNuoy studied wounded soldiers in World War I and demonstrated that wounds in 20-year-old patients contracted more quickly than those in 30 year olds, and those in 30-year-old patients contracted more quickly than in 40 year olds.[110] It was subsequently demonstrated that the incidence of wound dehiscence after duodenal ulcer surgery increased nearly linearly with age.[111] These clinical observations support the concept that older individuals heal more slowly than younger people.

The rate of epithelialization in induced blisters was found to be much faster in younger subjects.[112] Howes and Harvey evaluated bursting strength in abdominal wounds of old and young rats and determined that the wounds of young rats gained strength more quickly than those in older rats.[113] This finding was confirmed in a more recent study.[114] Wound disruption force was compared in small groups of patients older than or younger than 70 years and found to be reduced in the older patients.[115] Similarly, less granulation tissue was noted to accumulate within implanted cellulose sponges in old as compared to younger patients.[116] Granulation tissue from younger rats demonstrates a higher rate of metabolic activity as measured by oxygen consumption.[117] These experimental findings confirm the clinical observation that older patients heal more slowly than younger ones.

Diabetes

The diabetic patient has many problems that predispose to wound healing complications, including neuropathy, atherosclerosis, and an increased incidence of infection. In a review of 23,649 patients, diabetics were found to have five times the risk of infection in clean incisions than nondiabetics.[118] Uncontrolled diabetes has been demonstrated to impair wound healing in several models. Collagen accumulates at a slower rate in wound cylinders in diabetic animals,[119] and breaking strength is diminished in incisional wounds.[120] Both collagen synthesis and vascular ingrowth are decreased in an ear puncture wound model in diabetic rabbits.[121] Epithelialization may not be impaired, however. Some speculate that the primary defect in healing in uncontrolled diabetics results not from direct interference with collagen synthesis[122] but indirectly through impairment of the phagocytic function of granulocytes[123–125] and decreased granulocyte chemotaxis.[126] These defects in granulocyte function may also predispose to infection. The reduction in mechanical strength and collagen formation in wounds can be improved by correcting the hyperglycemia with insulin.[127–129]

As mentioned, hyperglycemia is not the only

aspect of diabetes that contributes to impaired healing. Neuropathy can lead to ulcerations over the metatarsal heads as a result of unsensed pressure. Atherosclerosis, which has a more peripheral distribution in diabetics than in non-diabetics,[130] contributes to tissue hypoxia, a problem previously discussed. Diabetics develop increased thickening and permeability of the capillary basement membranes and a decrease in the absolute number of capillaries in tissue. Such capillary changes may further limit blood flow[131, 132] and compound hypoxia.

Jaundice, Alcoholism, and Uremia

Ellis and Heddle noted an increased incidence of wound dehiscence and hernias in patients operated upon to relieve obstructive jaundice,[133] although others have disagreed.[134] Irvin and colleagues demonstrated a higher incidence of wound dehiscence in patients with obstructive jaundice due to cancer but not in jaundiced patients with stone disease.[135] The effect of obstructive jaundice on wound healing has been experimentally examined by several investigators. Bayer and Ellis[136] demonstrated decreased wound breaking strength in abdominal wounds in rats with obstructive jaundice. In gastric wounds, angiogenesis was subjectively diminished in the jaundiced animals, although wound breaking strength was normal. Arnaud and co-workers[137] also demonstrated a healing impairment with obstructive jaundice, although Greaney and associates[138] could not substantiate these results in a similar model. Greaney did show diminished collagen accumulation in the wounds of jaundiced animals, however.

In a separate study, healing was examined in a sponge model in mice chronically fed alcohol.[139] Chronic alcohol use was associated with slower cellular ingrowth and collagen accumulation in this model.

Wound healing has also been examined in both uremic rats[140] and humans.[141] In rats, the breaking strength of incisional wounds and the bursting strength of intestinal anastamoses were impaired. In humans, healing as reflected by hydroxyproline content of implantable Gore-Tex wound healing tubes showed significant diminution in the uremic patients at days 5 and 7 postimplantation.

It therefore appears that jaundice, alcoholism, and uremia can all slow the wound healing process, although the mechanisms of the impairments are unclear.

Glucocorticoid Steroids

Glucocorticoid steroids are used to treat a wide variety of connective tissue disorders, dermatological disorders, transplant rejection, and cancer. Patients taking hydrocortisone, prednisone, and prednisolone characteristically have thin, fragile skin and impaired healing.[142, 143] Sandberg demonstrated that cortisone must be given within 3 days prewounding and 2 days postwounding to have a significant effect on wound breaking strength in incisional wounds.[144] These steroids affect virtually all aspects of the healing process and have been shown to decrease strength in incisional wounds,[142, 145] to inhibit wound contraction,[146, 147] and to impede epithelialization.[146] Open wounds in patients taking glucocorticoid steroids are covered with pale granulation tissue.

Chemotherapeutic Agents

Impaired wound healing would be expected with the use of chemotherapeutic agents since they impede cellular proliferation. In addition to reducing the proliferation of mesenchymal cells directly involved in wound healing, chemotherapeutic agents most likely indirectly affect healing by producing thrombocytopenia and leukopenia. Diminished availability of platelets and inflammatory cells would be expected to limit the quantities of growth factors available to participate in wound healing. In addition, leukopenia renders the patient more susceptible to infection, which can further inhibit wound healing. Chemotherapeutic agents can also impair healing by contributing to malnutrition through their side effects of nausea, vomiting, and diarrhea and by damaging the gastrointestinal lining.[148]

The effects of many of the specific chemotherapeutic agents on the healing process have been examined in experimental models.[149] The data suggest that nitrogen mustard, cyclophosphamide, methotrexate, BCNU, and doxorubicin are the most potent healing inhibitors. There is a limited amount of data evaluating combinations of agents, although these would be expected to be more toxic than individual agents. Clinical studies have less clearly defined the degree of impairment induced by chemotherapeutic agents. Clinical trials evaluating nitrogen mustard, cyclophosphamide, thiotEPA, 5-fluorouracil, vincristine, doxorubicin, actinomycin-D, cytosine arabinoside, mercaptopurine, and cis-platinum for the treatment of a variety of tumors have provided little evidence that these agents significantly impair wound healing. Less pronounced clinical effects may be a result of the timing of the administration of chemotherapeutic agents in relation to surgery. For example, doxorubicin is a more potent wound healing inhibitor when delivered preoperatively rather than postoperatively.[150]

Other Drugs

The effect of a few additional drugs on the wound healing process has been examined. Cyclosporine impaired healing in an incisional model and in a PVA sponge model,[151] although another study did not confirm the findings in a cellulose sponge model.[152] Perioperative cephalosporins have also been demonstrated to impair healing in an abdominal wound model.[153] *Corynebacterium parvum* has been associated with impaired healing in incisional wounds.[154] It is conceivable that many as-yet untested drugs also impair the wound healing process.

Miscellaneous Causes

There are a variety of additional pathological states that can lead to chronic ulcers. In sickle cell anemia, sickling in the peripheral circulation can cause local vascular occlusion, ischemia, and tissue breakdown. These ulcers characteristically occur on the lower leg and commonly heal and recur. Other hematological disorders such as thalassemia and cryoglobulinemia can cause local vascular occlusion and chronic ulceration. Ulcerations are sometimes seen as a local manifestation of vasculitides secondary to rheumatoid arthritis, collagen vascular disease, and rarely hypertension. Pyoderma gangrenosum, which occurs with ulcerative colitis and occasionally other conditions, presents initially as pustulelike lesions and subsequently ulcerates. The lesions generally heal as the bowel condition improves. Diabetic necrobiosis lipoidica can lead to painful, well-demarcated chronic ulcerations in the pretibial region. Painful ulcers of the thighs, fingers, and legs are sometimes seen in association with hyperparathyroidism. Chronic ulcerations can be seen with a variety of primary dermatological conditions.

EVALUATION OF THE NONHEALING WOUND

In order to effectively treat the nonhealing wound, an accurate diagnosis of the factors limiting healing is required. As in the evaluation of any patient, the primary diagnostic tools are the history and physical examination. From the history, one can determine if this is the first nonhealing wound the patient has had or whether this is a recurrent problem. One can also determine how long the wound has existed, whether it is painful, whether it is improving, worsening, or staying the same, and what treatment modalities have been utilized in the past and with what effect. One can find out whether the area has been irradiated or if it is subject to pressure. One can inquire as to the patient's age as well as any coexistent problems such as diabetes, liver disease, renal dysfunction, cardiac or peripheral vascular disease, hypertension, neuropathies, rheumatoid arthritis, or connective tissue diseases.

If the initial history is negative, one can look for symptoms that may suggest one of these problems. For example, polyuria and polydipsia suggest diabetes, a history of jaundice indicates liver disease, and chest pain, shortness of breath, nocturnal dyspnea, or the need for pillows suggests cardiac disease. In addition, one can inquire about claudication or pain in an extremity that might point to peripheral vascular disease, persistent edema that suggests venous disease, or generalized skin or joint problems that may indicate a rheumatic or dermatological disorder. A drug history can provide information about whether the patient is taking glucocorticoid steroids, chemotherapeutic agents, or other medications that may inhibit healing. An employment history can indicate the amount of sun exposure to the involved area. Most skin cancers occur in areas with significant sun damage, such as the head, neck, and hands, and are seen more frequently in patients who spend a great deal of time outdoors, such as farmers. A travel history should be obtained because some wounds can result from unusual fungal infections that are common in tropical areas. A positive family history may suggest a hereditary disorder. A social history can provide information regarding cigarette and alcohol usage.

Next, the wound is examined. The location and size are noted along with the nature of the tissue. Wounds resulting from arterial disease are characteristically found on the distal lower extremity and have pale or grey nongranulating tissue at the base. Wounds resulting from radiation may look similar but are located in the treated area. Wounds due to vasculitides appear well demarcated with pale bases and are often painful. Ulcerations resulting from venous insufficiency are most commonly found on the ankle and are generally covered with red to purple granulation tissue. Pressure ulcers are found over weightbearing areas and generally extend deep to the underlying bony prominence. Foreign bodies should be sought, which may be traumatically embedded in the area, placed surgically, or the product of an injury such as dead bone or other tissue.

One must examine the tissue surrounding the wound. Lower extremities with arterial insufficiency will have thin, hairless skin without edema. The peripheral pulses are a good index of peripheral arterial patency. Venous insufficiency and lymphedema, which is less commonly associated with ulcers, are characterized by swelling. Venous insufficiency can also produce bluish pigmentation of the soft tissues surrounding the wound as a result of hemosiderin deposits. Jaundice will result in generalized yellow pigmentation. Irradiated tissue appears thin, dry, and hairless with telangiectasias. The tissues should be examined for evidence of trauma and for signs of infection, such as erythema, tenderness, heat, and swelling.

Vital signs are taken since fever, hypertension, and an irregular pulse may all be clues to wound etiology. The remaining skin is evaluated for other nonhealing wounds, which would suggest a generalized rather than a purely local problem. If the skin is loose and distensible or blisters easily, the patient may have a hereditary healing disorder. Malnutrition is suggested by thin skin, brittle hair that is falling out, pale conjunctivae, and a cachectic body habitus. Connective tissue or dermatological diseases may present as generalized skin or joint problems. The heart and lungs need to be examined to make sure heart sounds are normal and that there is no evidence of pulmonary edema or hypoxia from cardiac dysfunction. Glucocorticoid steroids can produce a characteristic body habitus with centralized obesity, a buffalo hump, moon facies, acne, and hirsutism.

After the history and physical examination, one can proceed with testing. If arterial insufficiency is suspected, Doppler examination of the extremities is indicated. Radiography may be indicated to look for foreign bodies or underlying bony pathology. A complete blood count will reveal an elevated white count, suggesting infection, white cell abnormalities indicative of a hematological problem such as

leukemia, or a hemoglobin level so low (<21) that oxygen-carrying capacity may be diminished. Serum chemistries can diagnose hyperglycemia (diabetes), an elevated creatinine and BUN (renal problems), and elevated liver function tests (hepatic dysfunction). Serum albumin, protein, and transferrin will give an idea of the nutritional status of the patient. Arterial blood gases are occasionally useful to indicate how well the blood is oxygenated. A wound biopsy is often indicated both for quantitative culture to consider the possibility of infection and for histological evaluation for malignancy.

One positive finding in the history, physical examination, or testing process should not cause the examining physician to abort the remainder of the evaluation process. Healing difficulties are often multifactorial.

MANAGEMENT OF NONHEALING WOUNDS

An accurate diagnosis of the factors impairing healing is a prerequisite for the successful treatment of a nonhealing wound. Not all factors limiting healing in a given patient can be corrected. For example, there is no specific therapy for the healing deficiency present in patients with Ehlers-Danlos syndrome, and there is no way to make older patients younger. Some agents limiting healing may be required for the treatment of coexistent problems and therefore cannot be discontinued; chemotherapeutic agents for cancer and glucocorticoids for rheumatic disorders are examples. Moreover, the patient may simply refuse to give up cigarettes or alcohol.

Once the contributory factors have been identified, treatment can be instituted. Benefit may be derived from improved management of contributing factors even though the primary disease cannot be cured. For example, patients with diabetes and renal and liver disease will benefit from careful dietary management, and some problems such as infection can be attacked directly. Once local conditions have been optimized, smaller wounds will generally heal by secondary intention. Larger wounds can then be closed by direct approximation, skin grafts, or flaps, depending on the clinical situation and the nature of the wound.

Management of Intrinsic Factors

Optimal local wound management depends on the nature of the wound. Surgical debridement is indicated for wounds containing nonviable tissue, toxins such as doxorubicin, or foreign material. If the material in question cannot be surgically debrided, wet to dry dressings are often effective. Wide mesh gauze is applied to a wound while wet and allowed to dry. The saline in the dressing combines with the wound exudate, and as the dressing dries, the dressing becomes enmeshed in the upper wound layers, and any nonviable material will be removed along with the dry dressing. This process should be repeated at least every 6 to 8 hours until debridement is complete.

For partial-thickness skin injuries such as those resulting from abrasions or harvesting of skin grafts, epithelialization is the primary means of closure. The purpose of a dressing placed on such a wound is to optimize the epithelialization process. If left untreated, a scab will form and barring infection, the wound will epithelialize under the scab. However, epithelialization under a scab does not occur as quickly as it does under a moist dressing.[155] Both impregnated and unimpregnated gauze dressings are used for partial-thickness injuries. Salomon and co-workers[156] evaluated a number of these dressings in a rat model and concluded that epithelialization proceeded more quickly under Xeroform and Scarlet Red than other gauze dressings. In humans, Gemberling and associates found no difference among Xeroform, Scarlet Red, plain gauze, and petroleum gauze, although all dressings were superior to no dressing.[157] Winter and associates reported that epidermal cells migrate sooner and complete resurfacing of a wound occurs more quickly in the moist environment under a polyethylene film than in the dry environment under a scab.[155, 158] Healing of partial-thickness wounds under polyurethane films (OPsite), hydrocolloid dressings (Duoderm), wet to dry dressings, and no dressing was compared by Alvarez and colleagues in a pig model.[159] Significantly accelerated epithelialization was noted under the polyurethane film and hydrocolloid dressing as compared to no dressing. Wet to dry dressings showed no significant advantage over no dressing. Varghese and co-workers[160] have demonstrated that although oxygen can penetrate the polyurethane film dressings, the P_{O_2} is low under both film and hydrocolloid dressings under normal conditions, suggesting that oxygen permeability is not an important dressing characteristic. Barnett and colleagues[161] reported accelerated epithelialization of skin graft donor sites in humans under Tegaderm and OPsite occlusive dressings as compared to fine mesh gauze dressings. Their patients also reported

that the occlusive dressings were much more comfortable. Brady and associates[162] compared OPsite, Scarlet Red, Jelonet (a coarse mesh paraffin gauze), and Vaseline petroleum gauze with an exposure technique on donor sites. Epithelialization was accelerated under Jelonet, Vaseline petroleum gauze, and OPsite as compared to wounds treated with Scarlet Red or left open. Hydrocolloid dressings have also been used with success on full-thickness leg ulcers where wound contraction as well as epithelialization was involved.[163] (Chapter 34 discusses the functions and characteristics of different types of dressings in greater detail.)

It can be concluded that partial-thickness injuries heal most readily and with least pain under an occlusive dressing. However, bacteria also proliferate under occlusive dressings, and one must be wary of infection with their use.[164, 165] With many nonhealing wounds, additional contributing factors have to be treated before one can rely on an occlusive dressing alone to yield a healed wound.

For infected wounds, the goal of treatment is to decrease the bacterial count of the wound tissue. Robson and colleagues[166] have demonstrated in a rat model that bacterial counts in wounds are not effectively lowered by systemic antibiotics. However, systemic antibiotics are useful for the treatment of cellulitis surrounding a wound, and they may be indicated in the immunocompromised host to prevent cellulitis and sepsis. For the wound itself, topical treatment is much more effective at lowering the bacterial count. Simply leaving the wound dressed for more than 4 days will often result in a decreased bacterial count, a fact that was discovered empirically during the Vietnam War when delayed primary closure was popularized and experimentally validated by Edlich and associates.[167]

Dressing changes of almost any type will decrease the bacterial count of a wound. Saline-soaked gauze, Betadine, biological dressings, dextranomer, and antibacterial agents have all been demonstrated to lower the bacterial count in wounds.[168–171]

A number of agents with specific antibacterial activity have been utilized in the management of burns and other infected tissue. One of the earlier antibacterial agents was 0.5% silver nitrate, which is active against a broad spectrum of bacteria.[172] Its primary disadvantages are that the silver stains tissues, dressings, and everything else it touches and that it is hypotonic and leaches electrolytes from normal tissues, producing hyponatremia and hypochloremia. Sulfamylon is another agent effective against a broad spectrum of bacteria. It penetrates wounds better than most other antibacterial agents,[173] but it has the disadvantages of producing local pain and generating a metabolic acidosis (it is a carbonic hydrase inhibitor). Both silver nitrate and Sulfamylon have the additional disadvantage of impeding epithelialization.[174] Silver sulfadiazine was developed to combine the benefits of silver nitrate and Sulfamylon.[175, 176] It is effective against a wide spectrum of bacteria and does not cause pain, produce electrolyte or acid-base abnormalities, or stain surrounding tissues and bed clothes. Silver sulfadiazine has the added advantage of accelerating epithelialization.[177]

Other less commonly used antibacterial agents are nitrofurazone, which has a high incidence of allergic reactions, and gentamicin cream, which is effective against *Pseudomonas aeruginosa* but leads to the development of resistant strains with protracted use.[169] Povidone-iodine has also been used as an antibacterial in wound management.[168] Kucan and colleagues[168] compared the speed with which dressing changes with silver sulfadiazine, povidone-iodine, and physiological saline could reduce bacterial counts to less than 100,000 per gram of tissue. They determined that the bacterial count could be reduced most universally and expeditiously with dressing changes with silver sulfadiazine, but all dressing change modalities were effective.

In most common wound situations, closure can be successfully carried out after the bacterial count has decreased to less than 100,000 per gram of tissue in the wound. As mentioned, Robson demonstrated that when infected wounds are treated until the bacterial count is less than 100,000 per gram, delayed closure can be successfully carried out more than 90 percent of the time.[19, 178] He also demonstrated that graft take can be obtained in wounds with bacterial counts below 100,000 per gram of tissue.[20, 179] In an infected small or superficial wound, secondary healing will occur under an occlusive dressing after infection has been eliminated, and formal wound closure is not needed.

Some local conditions that limit healing are not amenable to correction via dressing changes. One example is the irradiated wound. While local infection can be controlled, healing is still limited due to the radiation-induced tissue damage. The patient with an exposed joint or vascular prosthesis poses another difficult problem in that significant morbidity is associated with removal of such vital prostheses. Wounds involving osteomyelitis due to either a poststernotomy sternal infection or a severe tibial fracture are also difficult to close. All of these wounds have one thing in common—hypoxia. Muscle and musculocutaneous flaps can bring tissue with a vigorous new blood supply to such wounds and can contribute to wound healing in these difficult situations. Mathes and associates[180] were able to successfully close 50 of 54 problem wounds resulting from osteomyelitis, pressure sores, soft tissue defects, and osteoradionecrosis using muscle and myocutaneous flaps. Jurkiewicz and colleagues[181] dramatically improved morbidity and mortality and successfully closed sternal wounds after infection using muscle flaps. Greenberg and co-workers[182] and Lesavoy and associates[183] have both described the salvage of patients with exposed joint prosthesis using muscle and myocutaneous flaps. Arnold and Pairolero[184] obtained successful closure of irradiated chest wounds, and Hodgkinson and Shephard[185] closed wounds with exposed Goretex grafts using local muscle flaps.

Chang and Mathes[186] found that musculocutaneous flaps as compared to random flaps demonstrated an increased ability to withstand a bacterial challenge in dogs. The musculocutaneous flaps decreased the bacterial count in infected wound cylinders placed beneath them to a greater degree and in addition generated a higher oxygen concentration in the cylinders.

Vitamin A has also been demonstrated to reverse the healing impairment induced by radiation.[187, 188] Pretreatment with vitamin E has likewise been shown to limit the healing deficit produced by radiation.[189] Topical aloe vera, which is derived from the aloe vera cactus, has been suggested to improve healing of radiation ulcers as well.[190] Other substances such as ginseng,[191] d-penicillamine,[192] proline analogues,[193] and anti-inflammatory compounds such as chloroquine[194] may favorably influence the reaction to radiation, although the effects of these agents on wound healing have not been examined.

The patient with peripheral vascular disease also requires more than dressing changes. The history and physical examination as well as the Doppler examination should indicate whether the patient might benefit from surgical intervention to correct the tissue hypoxia. Rest pain, disabling claudication, and nonhealing wounds are indications for surgery in these patients. Wounds that will not form granulation tissue and remain covered with fibrinous material in spite of good local management generally require a better blood supply. The blood pressure at the ankle and the index between blood pressures at the ankle and the arm can help to indicate when healing will occur.[195, 196] Ulcers associated with an ankle to arm index of less than 0.45 usually do not heal without revascularization. The calcified vessels of diabetics can give falsely high ankle pressures in spite of low blood flow due to their incompressibility. An arteriogram will provide necessary information regarding the location of vascular occlusive lesions in surgical candidates, and the vascular surgeon can then design a reconstructive surgical plan to bring more blood to the involved extremity. A better blood supply combined with appropriate local wound management generally leads to a healed wound.

Patients will often refuse or fail to stop smoking, and even if they do stop, the chronic pulmonary damage and atherosclerosis that have already developed may not be reversible. Cessation of smoking will improve blood flow to some extent, however, and has been associated with the healing of previously nonhealing wounds in some cases.[197]

There is no way to reconstruct the venous system for the patient with venous insufficiency as can be done for the patient with arterial insufficiency. The surgeon must rely on controlling infection and creating an environment conducive to wound contraction and epithelialization. Edema control has been helpful in obtaining healing in the setting of venous insufficiency.[198] Control of edema may increase transcutaneous PO_2 and improve tissue perfusion. Unna boots, which control edema, create a warm moist enviornment, and contain bacteriostatic zinc oxide, have been successfully used in the management of smaller, uninfected venous ulcers. Wound excision and grafting are frequently required to close larger ulcers due to venous insufficiency, and bacterial control is a necessary prerequisite to such surgery. The excision should generally be at the fascial level and should include the excess scar that frequently surrounds chronic venous stasis ulcers. Ligation of underlying perforators during the excision may help decrease the likelihood of recurrence. Great care must be taken postoperatively to limit edema in order to avoid graft loss.

Many chronic wounds induced by pressure respond well to limiting pressure to the affected area, infection control, and management of secondary contributing problems such as spasticity, skin maceration, and malnutrition. Pressure distributing beds have accelerated healing of these wounds.[199] Constant effort is required to reduce pressure on insensate areas in spinal cord–injured and diabetic patients to limit recurrence of the lesions. Pressure-distributing seat cushions, mattresses, and shoes should be utilized prophylactically by susceptible patients.

The most difficult aspect of the management of the patient with factitious ulcers is establishing the diagnosis (see Chapter 29). Once this has been done, protection of the wound generally leads to healing.

Obtaining a diagnosis is also critical for the patient with cancer. Most skin cancers are effectively treated by surgical excision, although the margin of excision varies with the size of the lesion and the histological diagnosis.

Management of Extrinsic Factors

The extrinsic factors contributing to nonhealing are generally more difficult to control than the intrinsic ones. The patient with advanced cancer may benefit from surgical palliation, chemotherapy, or radiation, although the latter two also impair healing. There is no specific treatment for any of the inherited healing disorders such as Ehlers-Danlos syndrome or epidermolysis bullosa. The patient with epidermolysis bullosa does benefit from meticulous skin care directed at limiting blistering, however. One must be alert to the possibility of skin cancers, which develop fairly frequently in patients with more severe variants of epidermolysis bullosa.

In contrast, nutritional deficiencies, once diagnosed, can be specifically addressed. The patient with generalized malnutrition characterized by low serum albumin, protein, and transferrin must be fed high-calorie meals to reverse the healing impairment. Ideally the meals are taken orally, though intravenous total parenteral nutrition can be useful when oral intake is impossible.[200] A high-calorie meal with 50 to 60 percent carbohydrate and 1.5 to 2.0 grams of protein will provide adequate protein and sufficient carbohydrate so that protein is not used as an energy source. Improvement in nutrition has been demonstrated to reverse malnutrition-induced healing defects.[201–203] Specific vitamin, mineral, or nutrient deficiencies can also be corrected by supplementation (see Chapter 15).

Alcoholics should be encouraged to discontinue excessive alcohol intake to at least stabilize their liver damage. These patients frequently have nutritional deficiencies as well. Limiting protein intake may benefit some patients with severe hepatic cirrhosis due to alcohol or other causes. There is experimental evidence that oral bile salts may help reverse the healing deficit induced by obstructive jaundice.[204]

As mentioned, the healing impairment in diabetes is improved by better control of blood sugar through diet, oral hypoglycemic agents, and insulin,[129, 205, 206] but this will not necessarily reverse a diabetic neuropathy or improve peripheral circulation. Better blood sugar control, though helpful, does not obviate the need for careful foot care, including pressure modification devices when needed and peripheral vascular revascularization when indicated. Vitamin A supplements have also been suggested to reverse the healing impairment induced by diabetes, though the mechanism is not clear.[207]

Vitamin A has also been demonstrated to effectively reverse the healing impairment induced by corticosteroids.[208, 209] As discussed, steroids impair virtually all phases of the wound healing process, and vitamin A can reverse all aspects of the impairment other than wound contraction. The recommended systemic dose is 25,000 IU per day. Topical application of vitamin A may also reverse the inhibitory effects of steroids on the healing of open wounds.[210] Anabolic steroids reverse the corticosteroid-induced healing impairment in a similar manner.[211] Unlike vitamin A and anabolic steroids, the tetrachlorodecaoxygen-anion complex can reverse the inhibitory effects of steroids on wound contraction as well as the other aspects of wound healing.[212]

Few agents have been found to ameliorate the healing deficiencies associated with chemotherapeutic agents. Vitamin A has been shown to reverse the inhibitory effects of cyclophosphamide,[213] and leucovorin specifically antagonizes the negative effects of methotrexate on healing.[214] The healing impairment induced by doxorubicin can be modified by delivering it postoperatively instead of preoperatively.[150]

WOUND HEALING ACCELERATORS

For some time, investigators have been searching for a way to accelerate the healing process in normal as well as healing-impaired individuals. Many therapies have been tried, but with little success.[215] Promising results have been obtained in some studies with vitamin C, however.[216, 217]

There is currently a great deal of interest in growth factors as potential wound-healing stimulants. A number of these factors have been identified and purified. Transforming growth factor-β (TGF-β) was one of the first to be considered. It accelerated the accumulation of collagen and DNA in wound chambers in rats[218] and appeared to be the most potent single factor in reversing doxorubicin-induced healing impairment in a wound chamber model, with combinations of TGF-β, platelet-derived growth factor (PDGF), epidermal growth factor (EGF), and insulin being more effective than any individual factor.[219] Curtsinger and associates demonstrated that TGF-β in a collagen vehicle could reverse a doxorubicin-induced healing deficit in incisional wounds as well.[220] Mustoe and co-workers found that TGF-β accelerates the healing process in incisional wounds in normal rats,[221] and this was corroborated by Brown and colleagues.[222]

There is also a great deal of interest in PDGF, which has been shown to accelerate the healing in diabetic ulcers[223] and more recently in incisional wounds.[224] Wound breaking strengths of incisional wounds remained higher than controls for a more protracted period with PDGF than with TGF-β.[225] Knighton has shown that a platelet product can cause nonhealing ulcers to heal in humans.[226]

EGF accelerated closure of full-thickness skin injuries to rabbit ears in 1979.[227] EGF was examined in a polyvinyl sponge model[228, 229] and a hollow sponge model,[230] and it accelerated the rate of cell and collagen accumulation in both. It also increased the rate of epithelialization in partial-thickness wounds in pigs.[231] Recently, it has been shown to increase the rate of epithelialization in human skin graft donor sites.[232]

Other factors that have been evaluated include basic fibroblast growth factor (bFGF), transforming growth factor-α (TGF-α), and fibronectin. Intra-incisional administration of bFGF on postwounding day 3 accelerated healing in a linear wound model.[233] TGF-α increased the rate of healing of a partial-thickness wound in pigs,[234] and fibronectin accelerated closure of excisional wounds in rats.[235]

Several unanswered questions remain regarding optimal dosage and vehicles for the various growth factors. It may be that one factor may be optimal for one type of wound and another for a different type; one may be useful at one time and another at a different point after wounding. Current research is addressing these questions. Thus far, although these factors show great promise, there is insufficient evidence to justify their routine clinical use.

CONCLUSION

Many factors, both local and systemic, can contribute to a nonhealing wound. The key to successful treatment is accurate diagnosis of the factors contributing to the healing deficiency. Once these have been identified, healing conditions can be optimized through local wound management and control of systemic disorders. Although not all inhibiting factors can be effectively eliminated, most wounds will heal eventually with proper management because wound healing is a preferred biological process. In the future, growth factors may improve the management of nonhealing wounds.

References

1. Kligman AM: The bacteriology of normal skin. In Wolcott BW, Rund DA (eds): Skin Bacteria and Their Role in Infection. New York, McGraw-Hill 1965, pp 13–21.
2. Edlich RF, Rodeheaver GT, Morgan RF, et al: Principles of emergency wound management. Ann Emer Med 17:1284–1302, 1988.
3. Peebles K, Boswick JA Jr, Scott FA: Wounds of the hand contaminated by human or animal saliva. J Trauma 20:383–389, 1980.
4. Robson MC, Krizek TJ, Heggers JP: Biology of surgical infection. Curr Probl Surg 10:1–62, 1973.
5. Ricketts CR, Squire JR, Topley E: Human skin lipids with particular reference to the self sterilising power of the skin. Clin Sci 10:89–110, 1951.
6. Heggers JP: Natural host defense mechanisms. Clin Plast Surg 6:505–513, 1979.
7. Robson MC: Burn sepsis. Crit Care Clin 4:281–298, 1988.
8. Lindberg RB, Moncrief JA, Switzer WE, et al: The successful control of burn wound sepsis. J Trauma 5:601–616, 1965.
9. Teplitz C, Davis D, Mason AD, et al: Pseudomonas burn wound sepsis. I. Pathogenesis of experimental Pseudomonas burn wound sepsis. J Surg Res 4:200–216, 1964.
10. Kass EH: Asymptomatic infections of the urinary tract. Trans Ass Am Physicians 69:56–64, 1956.
11. Bendy RH, Nuccio PA, Wolfe E, et al: Relationship of quantitative bacterial counts to healing of decubiti. Effect of gentamicin. Antimicrob Agents Chemother 4:147–153, 1964.
12. Robson MC, Heggers JP: Surgical infection. II. The β-hemolytic Streptococcus. J Surg Res 9:289–292, 1969.
13. Heggers JP, Robson MC: Infection control in burn patients. Clin Plast Surg 13:39–47, 1986.
14. Phillips LG, Heggers JP, Robson MC: The effect of endogenous skin bacteria on burn wound infection. Ann Plast Surg 23:35–38, 1989.
15. Robson MC, Funderburk MS, Heggers JP, et al: Bacterial quantification of peritoneal exudates. Surg Gynecol Obstet 130:267–271, 1970.
16. Robson MC, Heggers JP: Bacterial quantification of open wounds. Milit Med 134:19–24, 1969.
17. Heggers JP, Robson MC, Ristroph JD: A rapid method of performing quantitative wound cultures. Milit Med 134:666–667, 1969.
18. Robson MC, Duke WF, Krizek TJ: Rapid bacterial screening in the treatment of civilian wounds. J Surg Res 14:426–430, 1973.
19. Robson MC, Heggers JP: Delayed wound closure based on bacterial counts. J Surg Oncol 2:379–383, 1970.
20. Krizek TJ, Robson MC, Kho E: Bacterial growth and skin graft survival. Surg Forum 18:518–519, 1967.
21. Elek SD: Experimental staphylococcal infections in the skin of man. Ann NY Acad Sci 65:85–90, 1956.
22. Elek SD, Conen PE: The virulence of Staphylococcus pyogens for man. A study of the problems of wound infection. Br J Exper Pathol 38:573–586, 1957.
23. Edlich RF, Panek PH, Rodeheaver GT, et al: Physical and chemical configuration of sutures in the development of surgical infections. Ann Surg 177:679–688, 1973.
24. Roettinger W, Edgerton MT, Kurtz LD, et al: Role of inoculation site as a determinant of infection of soft tissue wounds. Am J Surg 126:354–358, 1973.
25. Krizek TH, Davis JH: The role of the red cell in subcutaneous infection. J Trauma 5:85–95, 1965.
26. Hunt TK, Zederfeldt BH, Goldstick TK, et al: Tissue oxygen tensions during controlled hemorrhage. Surg Forum 18:3–4, 1967.
27. Heughan C, Grislis G, Hunt TK: The effect of anemia on wound healing. Ann Surg 179:163–167, 1974.
28. Niinikoski H: Effect of oxygen supply on wound healing and formation of granulation tissue. Acta Physiol Scand (Suppl) 334:1–72, 1969.
29. Kenny GE, Fink BR: The growth response of cells in culture to oxygen. Fed Proc 25:297, 1966 (abstract).
30. Udenfried S: Formation of hydroxyproline in collagen. Science 152:1335–1340, 1966.
31. Kao K-Y, Hitt WE, Dawson RL, et al: Connective tissue. VIII. Factors affecting collagen synthesis by sponge biopsy connective tissue. Proc Soc Exper Biol (NY) 113:762–766, 1963.
32. Knighton DR, Silver IA, Hunt TK: Regulation of wound-healing angiogenesis: Effect of oxygen gradients and inspired oxygen concentration. Surgery 90:262–270, 1981.
33. Hunt TK, Pai MP: The effect of varying ambient oxygen tensions on wound metabolism and collagen synthesis. Surg Gynecol Obstet 135:561–566, 1972.
34. Stephens FO, Hunt TK: Effect of changes in inspired oxygen and carbon dioxide tensions on wound tensile strength: An experimental study. Ann Surg 173:515–519, 1971.
35. Hohn DC, Hunt TK: Oxidative metabolism and microbicidal activity of rabbit phagocytes: Cells from wounds and from peripheral blood. Surg Forum 26:85–87, 1975.
36. Hunt TK, Linsey M, Grislis G, et al: The effect of ambient oxygen tension on wound infection. Ann Surg 181:35–39, 1975.
37. Knighton DR, Halliday B, Hunt TK: Oxygen as an antibiotic. The effect of inspired oxygen on infection. Arch Surg 119:199–204, 1984.
38. Wagner WH, Keagy BA, Kotb MM, et al: Noninvasive determination of healing of major lower extremity amputation: The continued role of clinical judgement. J Vasc Surg 8:703–710, 1988.
39. Sheffield PJ: Tissue oxygen measurements with respect to soft tissue wound healing with normobaric and hyperbaric oxygen. Hyperbaric Oxygen Rev 6:18–46, 1985.
40. Roth GJ, McDonald JB, Sheard C: The effect of cigarettes and of intravenous injections of nicotine on the electrocardiogram, basal metabolic rate, cutaneous temperature, blood pressure, and pulse rate of normal persons. JAMA 125:761–767, 1944.
41. Bruce JW, Miller JR, Hooker DR: The effect of smoking upon the blood pressures and upon the volume of the hand. Am J Physiol 24:104–116, 1909.

42. Wright IS, Moffat D: The effects of tobacco on the peripheral vascular system. JAMA 103:315–323, 1934.
43. Cryer PE, Haymond MW, Santiago JV, et al: Norepinephrine and epinephrine release and adrenergic mediation of smoking-associated hemodynamic and metabolic events. N Engl J Med 295:573–577, 1976.
44. Astrup P, Kjeldsen K: Carbon monoxide, smoking and atherosclerosis. Med Clin North Am 58:323–350, 1973.
45. Kjeldsen K, Astrup P, Wanstrup J: Ultra-structural intimal changes in the rabbit aorta after a moderate carbon monoxide exposure. Atherosclerosis 16:67–82, 1972.
46. Birnstingl MA, Brinson K, Chakrabarti R: The effect of short-term exposure to carbon monoxide on platelet stickiness. Br J Surg 58:837–839, 1971.
47. Sackett DL, Gibson RW, Bross IDJ, et al: Relation between aortic atherosclerosis and the use of cigarettes and alcohol: An autopsy study. N Engl J Med 279:1413–1420, 1968.
48. Mosely LH, Finseth F, Goody M: Nicotine and its effect on wound healing. Plast Reconstr Surg 61:570–574, 1978.
49. Moosa HH, Falanga V, Steed DL, et al: Oxygen diffusion in chronic venous ulceration. J Cardiovasc Surg 28:464–467, 1987.
50. Fajardo LF, Berthrong M: Radiation injury in surgical pathology. III. Salivary glands, pancreas, and skin. Am J Surg Pathol 5:279–296, 1981.
51. Rudolph R, Arganese T, Woodward M: The ultrastructure and etiology of chronic radiotherapy damage in human skin. Ann Plast Surg 9:282–292, 1982.
52. Teloh HA, Mason ML, Wheelock MD: Histopathologic study of radiation injuries to the skin. Surg Gynecol Obstet 90:335–348, 1950.
53. Grant RA, Cox RW, Kent CM: The effects of gamma irradiation on the structure and reactivity of native and crosslinked collagen fibers. J Anat 115:29–43, 1973.
54. Conway H, Griffith BH: Plastic surgery for closure of decubitus ulcers in patients with paraplegia. Am J Surg 91:946–975, 1956.
55. Danseareau JG, Conway H: Closure of decubiti in paraplegics. Plast Reconstr Surg 33:474–480, 1964.
56. Diegelmann RF, Lindblad WJ, Hussey RW, et al: Analysis of fibrogenic processes in denervated tissues of spinal cord injury patients. Plast Reconstr Surg 83:309–313, 1989.
57. Dinsdale SM: Decubitus ulcers: Role of pressure and friction in causation. Arch Phys Med Rehab 55:147–152, 1974.
58. Reichel S: Shearing force as a factor in decubitus ulcers in paraplegics. JAMA 166:762–763, 1958.
59. Landis E: Studies of capillary blood pressure in human skin. Heart 15:209–228, 1930.
60. Nola GT, Vistnes LM: Differential response of skin and muscle in the experimental production of pressure sores. Plast Reconstr Surg 66:728–733, 1980.
61. Husain T: An experimental study of some pressure effects on tissues with reference to the bed-sore problem. J Pathol Bacteriol 66:347–358, 1978.
62. Lindan O, Greenway RM, Piazza JM: Pressure distribution on the surface of the human body: I. Evaluation in lying and sitting positions using a "bed of springs and nails." Arch Phys Med Rehab 46:378–385, 1965.
63. Kosiak M: Etiology and pathology of ischemic ulcers. Arch Phys Med Rehab 40:62–69, 1959.
64. Barrett JP, Mooney V: Neuropathy and diabetic pressure lesions. Orthop Clin North Am 4:43–47, 1973.
65. Rodeheaver G, Bellamy W, Kody M, et al: Bactericidal activity and toxicity of iodine-containing solutions in wound. Arch Surg 117:181–186, 1982.
66. Custer J, Edlich RF, Prusak M, et al: Studies in the management of the contaminated wound. V. An assessment of the effectiveness of pHisoHex and Betadine surgical scrub solutions. Am J Surg 121:572–575, 1971.
67. Saatman RA, Carlton WW, Hubben K, et al: A wound healing study of chlorhexidine digluconate in pigs. J Surg Res 6:1–6, 1986.
68. Mobacken H, Wegstrom C: Interference with healing of rat skin incisions treated with chlorhexidine. Acta Derm Venereol (Stockh) 54:29–34, 1974.
69. Kozol RA, Gillies C, Elgebaly SA: Effects of sodium hypochlorite (Dakin's solution) on cells of the wound module. Arch Surg 123:420–423, 1988.
70. Lineaweaver W, Howard R, Soucy D, et al: Topical antimicrobial toxicity. Arch Surg 120:267–270, 1985.
71. Brennan SS, Leaper DJ: The effect of antiseptics on the healing wound: A study using the rabbit ear chamber. Br J Surg 72:780–782, 1985.
72. Branemark P-J, Albrektsson B, Lindstrom J, et al: Local tissue effects of wound disinfectants. Acta Chir Scand (Suppl) 357:166–176, 1976.
73. Branemark P-J, Ekholm R, Albrektsson B, et al: Tissue injury caused by wound disinfectants. J Bone Joint Surg 49A:48–62, 1967.
74. Luedke DW, Kennedy PS, Rietschel RL: Histopathogenesis of skin and subcutaneous injury induced by Adriamycin. Plast Reconstr Surg 63:463–465, 1979.
75. Rudolph R, Stein RS, Pattillo RA: Skin ulcers due to Adriamycin. Cancer 38:1087–1094, 1976.
76. Rudolph R, Suzuki M, Luce JK: Experimental skin necrosis produced by Adriamycin. Cancer Treat Rep 63:529–537, 1979.
77. Cosman B, Feliciano WC, Wolff M: Pentazocine ulcers. Plast Reconstr Surg 59:255–259, 1977.
78. Wasserman GS, Anderson PC: Loxoscelism and necrotic arachnicism. J Toxicol Clin Toxicol 21:451–472, 1984.
79. Arons MS, Lynch JB, Lewis SR, et al: Scar tissue carcinoma. I. A clinical study with special reference to burn scar carcinoma. Ann Surg 161:170–188, 1966.
80. Uitto J, Murray LW, Blumberg B, et al: Biochemistry of collagen diseases. Ann Intern Med 105:740–756, 1986.
81. Moynahan EJ: The treatment and management of epidermolysis bullosa. Clin Exper Dermatol 7:665–672, 1982.
82. Cuono C, Finseth F: Epidermolysis bullosa: Current concepts and management of the advanced hand deformity. Plast Reconstr Surg 62:280–285, 1978.
83. Howes EL, Briggs H, Shea R, et al: Effect of complete and partial starvation on the rate of fibroplasia in the healing wound. Arch Surg 27:846–858, 1933.
84. Thompson WD, Ravdin IS, Frank IL: Effect of hypoproteinemia on wound disruption. Arch Surg 36:500–518, 1938.
85. Devereaux DF, Thistlewaite PA, Thibault LF, et al: Effect of tumor bearing and protein depletion on wound breaking strength in the rat. J Surg Res 27:233–238, 1979.
86. Smythe PM, Brereton-Stiles GG, Grace HJ, et al: Thymolymphatic deficiency and depression of cell-mediated immunity in protein-calorie malnutrition. Lancet 2:939–943, 1971.
87. Williamson MB, McCarthy TH, Fromm HJ: Relation of protein nutrition to the healing of experimental wounds. Proc Soc Exper Biol Med 77:302–305, 1951.
88. Irvin TT: The effect of methionine on colonic healing in malnourished rats. Br J Surg 63:237–240, 1976.
89. Seifter E, Rettura G, Barbul A, et al: Arginine: An essential amino acid for injured rats. Surgery 84:224–230, 1978.

90. Levenson SM, Seifter E: Dysnutrition, wound healing, and resistance to infection. Clin Plast Surg 4:375–388, 1977.

91. Hulsey TK, O'Neill JA, Neblett WR, et al: Experimental wound healing in essential fatty acid deficiency. J Pediatr Surg 15:505–508, 1980.

92. Lanman TH, Ingalls TH: Vitamin C deficiency and wound healing. Experimental and clinical study. Ann Surg 105:616–625, 1937.

93. Meyer E, Meyer MB: The pathology of Staphylococcus abscess in vitamin C–deficient guinea pigs. Bull Johns Hopkins Hosp 74:98–118, 1944.

94. Grillo HC, Gross J: Studies in wound healing. III. Contraction in vitamin C deficiency. Proc Soc Exper Biol Med 101:268–270, 1959.

95. Freiman M, Seifter E, Connerton C, et al: Vitamin A deficiency and surgical stress. Surg Forum 21:81–82, 1970.

96. Shapiro SS, Mott DJ: Modulation of glycosaminoglycan synthesis by retinoids. Ann NY Acad Sci 359:306–321, 1981.

97. Cohen BE, Till G, Cullen PR, et al: Reversal of postoperative immunosuppression in man by vitamin A. Surg Gynecol Obstet 149:658–662, 1979.

98. Alvarez OM, Gilbreath RL: Effect of dietary thiamine on intermolecular collagen crosslinking during wound repair: A mechanical and biochemical assessment. J Trauma 22:20–24, 1982.

99. Ehrlich HP, Tarver H, Hunt TK: Inhibitory effects of Vitamin E on collagen synthesis and wound repair. Ann Surg 175:235–240, 1972.

100. Bains JW, Crawford DT, Ketcham AS: Effect of chronic anemia on wound tensile strength. Correlation with blood volume, total red blood cell volume and proteins. Ann Surg 164:243–246, 1966.

101. Macon WL, Pories WJ: The effect of iron deficiency on wound healing. Surgery 69:792–796, 1971.

102. Fernandez-Madrid F, Prasad AS, Oberleas D: Effect of zinc deficiency on nucleic acids, collagen, and noncollagenous protein of the connective tissue. J Lab Clin Med 82:951–961, 1973.

103. Chvapil M: Zinc and wound healing. In Zedeffeldt B (ed): Symposium on Zinc. Lund, Sweden, AB Tika, 1974.

104. Holroyde CP, Reichard GA Jr: General metabolic abnormalities in cancer patients: Anorexia and cachexia. Surg Clin North Am 66:947–956, 1986.

105. Norton JA, Moley JF, Green MV, et al: Parabiotic transfer of cancer anorexia/cachexia in male rats. Cancer Res 45:5547–5552, 1985.

106. Chlebowski RT, Heber D: Metabolic abnormalities in cancer patients: carbohydrate metabolism. Surg Clin North Am 66:957–968, 1986.

107. Kurzer M, Meguid MM: Cancer and protein metabolism. Surg Clinics North Am 66:969–1001, 1986.

108. Norton JA, Burt ME, Brenna MF: In vivo utilization of substrate by human sarcoma-bearing limbs. Cancer 45:2934–2939, 1980.

109. McAndrew PF: Fat metabolism and cancer. Surg Clin North Am 66:1003–1012, 1986.

110. DuNuoy P, Carrell A: Cicatrization of wounds. J Exper Med 34:339–348, 1921.

111. Ostenreich N, Selmanowitz VJ: Levels of biological function with aging. Trans NY Acad Sci 31:992–1012, 1969.

112. Grove GL: Age-related differences in healing of superficial skin wounds in humans. Arch Dermatol Res 272:381–385, 1982.

113. Howes EL, Harvey SC: The age factor in the velocity of the growing of fibroblasts in the healing wound. J Exper Med 55:577–590, 1932.

114. Holm-Pedersen P, Viidik A: Tensile properties and morphology of healing wounds in young and old rats. Scand J Plast Reconstr Surg 6:24–35, 1972.

115. Sandblom P, Peterson P, Muren A: Determination of the tensile strength of the healing wound as a clinical test. Acta Chir Scand 105:252–257, 1953.

116. Vijanto J: A sponge implantation method for testing connective tissue in surgical patients. Acta Chir Scand 135:297–300, 1969.

117. Eaglstein WH: Wound healing and aging. Clin Geriatr Med 5:183–188, 1989.

118. Cruse PJE, Foord RA: A prospective study of 23,649 surgical wounds. Arch Surg 107:206–210, 1973.

119. Goodson WH, Hunt TK: Studies of wound healing in experimental diabetes mellitus. J Surg Res 22:221–227, 1977.

120. Prakash A, Pandit PN, Sharma LK: Studies in wound healing in experimental diabetes. Int Surg 59:25–28, 1974.

121. Arquilla ER, Weringer EJ, Nakajo M: Wound healing: A model for the study of diabetic microangiopathy. Diabetes (Suppl) 25:811–819, 1976.

122. Goodson WH, Hunt TK: Wound healing and the diabetic patient. Surgery Gynecol Obstet 149:600–608, 1979.

123. Bybee JD, Rogers DE: The phagocytic activity of polymorphonuclear leukocytes obtained from patients with diabetes mellitus. J Lab Clin Med 64:1–13, 1964.

124. Nolan CM, Beaty HN, Bagdade JD: Further characterization of the impaired bactericidal function of granulocytes in patients with poorly controlled diabetes. Diabetes 27:889–894, 1978.

125. Bagdade JD, Root RK, Bugler RJ: Impaired leukocyte function in patients with poorly controlled diabetes. Diabetes 23:9–15, 1974.

126. Mowat AG, Baum J: Chemotaxis of polymorphonuclear leukocytes from patients with diabetes mellitus. N Engl J Med 284:621–627, 1971.

127. Gottrup F, Andreassen TT: Healing of incisional wounds in stomach and duodenum: The influence of experimental diabetes. J Surg Res 31:61–68, 1981.

128. Weringer EJ, Kelso JM, Tamai IY, et al: Effects of insulin on wound healing in diabetic mice. Acta Endocrinol 99:101–108, 1982.

129. Yue DK, McLennan S, Marsh M, et al: Effects of experimental diabetes, uremia, and malnutrition on wound healing. Diabetes 36:295–299, 1987.

130. Strandness DE, Priest RE, Gibbons GE: Combined clinical and pathologic study of diabetic and non-diabetic peripheral arterial disease. Diabetes 13:366–372, 1964.

131. Siperstein MD: Studies of muscle capillary basement membrane in normal subjects, diabetic and prediabetic patients. J Clin Invest 47:1973–1999, 1973.

132. Trap-Jensen J: Increased capillary permeability to 131-Iodine and (51-Cr) EDTA in the exercising forearm of long term diabetics. Clin Sci 39:39–49, 1970.

133. Ellis H, Heddle R: Does the peritoneum need to be closed at laparotomy? Br J Surg 64:733–736, 1977.

134. Keill RH, Keitzer F, Nichols WK, et al: Abdominal wound dehiscence. Arch Surg 106:573–577, 1973.

135. Irvin TT, Vassilakis JS, Chattopadhyay DK, et al: Abdominal wound healing in jaundiced patients. Br J Surg 65:521–522, 1978.

136. Bayer I, Ellis HL: Jaundice and wound healing: An experimental study. Br J Surg 63:392–396, 1976.

137. Arnaud J-P, Humbert W, Eloy M-R, et al: Effect of obstructive jaundice on wound healing. Am J Surg 141:593–596, 1981.

138. Greaney MG, Van Noort R, Smythe A, et al: Does obstructive jaundice adversely affect wound healing? Br J Surg 66:478–481, 1979.

139. Benveniste K, Thut P: The effect of chronic alcoholism on wound healing. Proc Soc Exper Biol Med 166:568–575, 1981.
140. Colin JF, Elliot P, Ellis H: The effect of uraemia upon wound healing: An experimental study. Br J Surg 66:793–797, 1979.
141. Goodson WH III, Lindenfeld SM, Omachi RS, et al: Chronic uremia causes poor healing. Surg Forum 33:54–56, 1982.
142. Howes EL, Plotz CM, Blunt JW, et al: Retardation of wound healing by cortisone. Surgery 28:177–181, 1950.
143. Taubenhaus M, Ambromin GD: The effects of the hypophysis, thyroid, sex steroids, and the adrenal cortex upon granulation tissue. J Lab Clin Med 36:7–18, 1950.
144. Sandberg N: Time relationship between administration of cortisone and wound healing in rats. Acta Chir Scand 127:446–455, 1964.
145. McNamara JJ, Lamborn PJ, Mills D, et al: Effect of short term pharmacologic doses of adrenocortical therapy on wound healing: Ann Surgery 170:199–202, 1969.
146. Hunt TK, Ehrlich HP, Garcia JA, et al: The effect of vitamin A on reversing the inhibitory effect of cortisone on the healing of open wounds in animals. Ann Surg 170:633–641, 1969.
147. Stephens FO, Dunphy JE, Hunt TK: Effect of delayed administration of corticosteroids on wound contraction. Ann Surg 173:214–218, 1971.
148. McAnena OJ, Daly JM: Impact of antitumor therapy on nutrition. Surg Clin North Am 66:1213–1228, 1986.
149. Shamberger RC, Devereaux DF, Brennan MF: The effect of chemotherapeutic agents on wound healing. Int Adv Surg Oncol 4:15–58, 1981.
150. Lawrence WT, Talbot TL, Norton JA: Preoperative or postoperative doxorubicin hydrochloride (Adriamycin): Which is better for wound healing? Surgery 100:9–12, 1986.
151. Fishel R, Barbul A, Wasserkrug HL, et al: Cyclosporine A impairs wound healing. J Surg Res 34:572–575, 1983.
152. Nemlander A, Ahonen J, Wiktorowicz K, et al: Effect of cyclosporine on wound healing. Transplantation 36:1–5, 1983.
153. Sher KS, Scott-Conner CE, Montany PF: Effect of cephalosporins on fascial healing after celiotomy. Arch Surg 155:361–365, 1988.
154. Greenhalgh D, Gamelli RL, Foster RS Jr, et al: Inhibition of wound healing by Corynebacterium parvum. J Surg Res 41:209–214, 1986.
155. Winter GD: Formation of scab and rate of epithelialization of superficial wounds in the skin of the domestic pig. Nature 193:293–294, 1962.
156. Salomon JC, Diegelmann RF, Cohen IK: Effect of dressings on donor site epithelialization. Surg Forum 25:516–517, 1974.
157. Gemberling RM, Miller TA, Caffee H, et al: Dressing comparison in the healing of donor site. J Trauma 16:812–814, 1976.
158. Hinman CC, Maibach HI, Winter GD: Effect of air exposure and occlusion on experimental skin wounds. Nature 200:377–378, 1963.
159. Alvarez OM, Mertz PM, Eaglstein WH: The effect of occlusive dressings on collagen synthesis and reepithelialization in superficial wounds. J Surg Res 35:142–148, 1983.
160. Varghese MC, Balin AK, Carter M, et al: Local environment of chronic wounds under synthetic dressings. Arch Dermatol 122:52–57, 1986.
161. Barnett A, Berkowitz RL, Mills R, et al: Comparison of synthetic adhesive moisture vapor permeable and fine mesh gauze dressings for split-thickness donor sites. Am J Surg 145:379–381, 1983.
162. Brady SC, Snelling CFT, Chow G: Comparison of donor site dressings. Ann Plast Surg 5:238–243, 1979.
163. Friedman SJ, Su WPD: Management of leg ulcers with hydrocolloid occlusive dressings. Arch Dermatol 120:1329–1336, 1984.
164. Katz S, McGinley K, Leyden JJ: Semipermeable occlusive dressing. Arch Dermatol 122:58–62, 1986.
165. Mertz PM, Eaglstein WH: The effect of a semiocclusive dressing on the microbial population in superficial wounds. Arch Surg 119:287–289, 1984.
166. Robson MC, Edstrom LE, Krizek TJ, et al: The efficacy of systemic antibiotics in the treatment of granulating wounds. J Surg Res 16:299–306, 1974.
167. Edlich RF, Rogers W, Kasper G, et al: Studies in the management of the contaminated wound. I. Optimal time for closure of contaminated open wounds. II. Comparison of resistance to infection of open and closed wounds during healing. Am J Surg 117:323–329, 1969.
168. Kucan JO, Robson MC, Heggers JP, et al: Comparison of silver sulfadiazine, povidone-iodine and physiologic saline in the treatment of chronic pressure sores. J Am Ger Soc 29:232–235, 1981.
169. Moncrief JA: Topical therapy for control of bacteria in the burn wound. World J Surg 2:151–165, 1978.
170. Freeman BG, Carwell GR, McGraw JB: The quantitative study of the use of dextranomer in the management of infected wounds. Surg Gynecol Obstet 153:81–86, 1981.
171. Robson MC, Samburg JL, Krizek TJ: Quantitative comparison of biologic dressings. J Surg Res 14:431–434, 1973.
172. Moyer CA, Brentano L, Gravens DL, et al: Treatment of large burns with 0.5 per cent silver nitrate solution. Arch Surg 90:812–867, 1965.
173. Moncrief JA: Use of topical antibacterial therapy in the treatment of the burn wound. Arch Surg 92:558–565, 1966.
174. Bellinger CG, Conway H: Effects of silver nitrate and Sulfamylon on epithelial regeneration. Plast Reconstr Surg 45:582–585, 1973.
175. Fox CL: Silver sulfadiazine: A new topical therapy for Pseudomonas in burns. Arch Surg 96:184–188, 1968.
176. Fox CL: Topical therapy and the development of silver sulfadiazine. Surg Gynecol Obstet 157:82–88, 1983.
177. Geronemus RG, Mertz PM, Eaglstein WH: Wound healing: The effects of topical antimicrobial agents. Arch Dermatol 115:1311–1314, 1979.
178. Robson MC, Shaw RC, Heggers JP: The reclosure of postoperative incisional abscesses based on bacterial quantification of the wound. Ann Surg 171:279–282, 1970.
179. Robson MC, Krizek TJ: Predicting skin graft survival. J Trauma 13:213–217, 1973.
180. Mathes SJ, Feng L-J, Hunt TK: Coverage of the infected wound. Ann Surg 198:420–429, 1983.
181. Jurkiewicz MJ, Bostwick J III, Hester TR, et al: Infected median sternotomy wound: Successful treatment with muscle flaps. Ann Surg 191:738–744, 1980.
182. Greenberg B, LaRossa D, Lotke PA, et al: Salvage of jeopardized total-knee prosthesis: The role of gastrocnemius muscle flap. Plast Reconstr Surg 83:85–89, 1989.
183. Lesavoy MA, Dubrow TJ, Wackym PA, et al: Muscle-flap coverage of exposed endoprostheses. Plast Reconstr Surg 83:90–96, 1989.
184. Arnold PG, Pairolero PC: Surgical management of the

radiated chest wall. Plast Reconstr Surg 77:605–612, 1986.

185. Hodgkinson DJ, Shephard GH: Coverage of exposed Gore-Tex dialysis access graft with local sublimis myocutaneous flap. Plast Reconstr Surgery 69:1010–1012, 1982.

186. Chang N, Mathes SJ: Comparison of the effect of bacterial inoculation in musculocutaneous and random-pattern flaps. Plast Reconstr Surg 70:1–9, 1982.

187. Levenson SM, Gruber CA, Rettura G, et al: Supplemental vitamin A prevents the acute radiation-induced defect in wound healing. Ann Surg 200:494–512, 1984.

188. Winsey K, Simon RJ, Levenson SM, et al: Effect of supplemental vitamin A on colon anastamotic healing in rats given preoperative irradiation. Am J Surg 153:153–156, 1987.

189. Taren DL, Chvapil M, Weber CW: Increasing the breaking strength of wounds exposed to preoperative irradiation using vitamin E supplementation. Int J Nutr Res 57:133–137, 1987.

190. Ashley FL, O'Loughlin BJ, Peterson R, et al: The use of aloe vera in the treatment of thermal and irradiation burns in laboratory animals and humans. Plast Reconstr Surg 20:383–396, 1957.

191. Takeda A, Katoh N, Yonezawa M: Restoration of radiation injury by ginseng. III. Radioprotective effect of thermostable fraction of ginseng extract on mice, rats, and guinea pigs. J Rad Res 23:150–167, 1982.

192. Ward WF, Shih-Hoellwarth A, Tuttle RD: Collagen accumulation in irradiated rat lung: Modification by D-penicillamine. Radiology 146:553–537, 1983.

193. Ohuchi K, Chang LF, Tabachnick J: Radiation fibrosis of guinea pig skin after β irradiation and an attempt at its suppression with proline analogs. Rad Res 79:273–288, 1979.

194. Chung J, Song CW, Yamaguchi T, et al: Effect of anti-inflammatory compounds on β-irradiation induced radiodermatitis. Dermatologica 144:97–107, 1972.

195. Faris I, Duncan H: Skin perfusion pressure in the prediction of healing in diabetic patients with ulcers or gangrene of the feet. J Vasc Surg 4:536–540, 1985.

196. Sage R, Doyle D: Surgical treatment of diabetic foot ulcers. A review of forty-eight cases. J Foot Surg 23:102–111, 1984.

197. Mosely LH, Finseth F: Cigarette smoking: Impairment of digital blood flow and wound healing in the hand. Hand 9:97–101, 1977.

198. Myers MB, Rightor M, Cherry G: Relationship between edema and healing rate of stasis ulcers of the leg. Am J Surg 124:666–668, 1972.

199. Allman RA, Walker JM, Hart MK, et al: Fluidized beds or conventional therapy for pressure sores? Ann Int Med 107:641–648, 1987.

200. Alverdy J, Sang H, Sheldon GF: The effect of parenteral nutrition on gastrointestinal immunity. The importance of enteral stimulation. Ann Surg 202:681–684, 1985.

201. Haydock DA, Hill GL: Impaired wound healing response in surgical patients receiving intravenous nutrition. Br J Surg 4:320–323, 1987.

202. Mullen JL, Buzby GP, Matthews DC, et al: Reduction of operative morbidity and mortality by combined preoperative and postoperative nutritional support. Ann Surg 192:604–613, 1980.

203. Steiger E, Daly JM, Allen TR, et al: Postoperative intravenous nutrition: Effects on body weight, protein regeneration, wound healing, and liver morphology. Surgery 73:686–691, 1973.

204. Askew AR, Bates GJ, Balderson G: Jaundice and the effect of sodium taurocholate taken orally upon abdominal wound healing. Surg Gynecol Obstet 159:207–209, 1984.

205. Prakash A, Pandit PN, Sharma LK: Studies in wound healing in experimental diabetes. Int Surgery 59:25–28, 1974.

206. Andreassen TT, Oxlund H: The influence of experimental diabetes and insulin treatments on the biochemical properties of rat skin healing wounds. Acta Chir Scand 153:405–409, 1987.

207. Seifter E, Rettura G, Padawer J, et al: Impaired wound healing in streptozotocin diabetes: Prevention by supplemental vitamin A. Ann Surg 194:42–49, 1981.

208. Ehrlich HP, Tarver H, Hunt TK: Effects of vitamin A and glucocorticoids upon inflammation and collagen synthesis. Ann Surg 177:222–227, 1973.

209. Ehrlich HP, Hunt TK: Effects of cortisone and vitamin A on wound healing. Ann Surg 167:324–328, 1968.

210. Hunt TK, Ehrlich HP, Garcia JA, et al: Effects of vitamin A on reversing the inhibitory effect on cortisone on healing of open wounds in animals and man. Ann Surg 121:569–571, 1971.

211. Ehrlich HP, Hunt TK: The effects of cortisone and anabolic steroids on the tensile strength of healing wounds. Ann Surg 170:203–206, 1969.

212. Hatz RA, Kelley SF, Ehrlich HP: The tetrachlordecaoxygen complex reverses the effect of cortisone on wound healing. Plast Reconstr Surg 84:953–959, 1989.

213. Stratford F, Seifter E, Rettura G, et al: Impaired wound healing due to cyclophosphamide alleviated by supplemental vitamin A. Surg Forum 31:224–225, 1980.

214. Calnan J, Davies A: The effect of methotrexate (Amethopterin) on wound healing: An experimental study. Br J Cancer 19:505–512, 1965.

215. Morgan JE: Topical therapy of pressure sores. Surgery Gynecol Obstet 141:945–947, 1975.

216. Taylor TV, Rimmer S, Day B, et al: Ascorbic acid supplementation in the treatment of pressure-sores. Lancet 2:544–546, 1974.

217. Ringsdorf WM, Cheraskin E: Vitamin C and wound healing. Oral Surg 53:231–236, 1982.

218. Sporn MB, Roberts AB, Shull JH, et al: Polypeptide transforming growth factors isolated from bovine sources and used for wound healing in vivo. Science 219:1329–1331, 1983.

219. Lawrence WT, Sporn MB, Gorschboth C, et al: The reversal of an Adriamycin induced healing impairment with chemoattractants and growth factors. Ann Surg 203:142–147, 1986.

220. Curtsinger LJ, Pietsch JD, Brown GL, et al: Reversal of Adriamycin-impaired wound healing by transforming growth factor-beta. Surgery Gynecol Obstet 168:517–522, 1989.

221. Mustoe TA, Pierce GF, Thomason A, et al: Accelerated healing of incisional wounds in rats induced by transforming growth factor-beta. Science 237:1333–1336, 1987.

222. Brown GL, Curtsinger LJ, White M, et al: Acceleration of tensile strength of incisions treated with EGF and TGF-β. Ann Surg 208:788–794, 1988.

223. Grotendorst GR, Martin GR, Pencev D, et al: Stimulation of granulation tissue formation by platelet-derived growth factor in normal and diabetic rats. J Clin Invest 76:2323–2329, 1985.

224. Pierce GF, Mustoe TA, Senior RM, et al: In vivo incision wound healing augmented by platelet-derived growth factor and recombinant c-sis gene homodimeric proteins. J Exp Med 167:974–987, 1988.

225. Pierce GF, Mustoe TA, Lingelbach J, et al: Platelet-

derived growth factor and transforming growth factor-β enhance tissue repair activities by unique mechanisms. J Cell Biol 109:429–440, 1987.

226. Knighton DR, Ciresi KF, Fiegel VD, et al: Classification and treatment of chronic nonhealing wounds: Successful treatment with autologous platelet-derived wound healing factors (PDWHF). Ann Surg 204:322–330, 1986.

227. Franklin JD, Lynch JB: Effects of topical applications of epidermal growth factor on wound healing: Experimental study in rabbit ears. Plast Reconstr Surg 64:766–770, 1979.

228. Buckley A, Davidson JM, Kamerath CD, et al: Sustained release of epidermal growth factor accelerates wound repair. Proc Natl Acad Sci USA 82:7340–7344, 1985.

229. Buckley A, Davidson JM, Kamerath CD, et al: Epidermal growth factor increases granulation tissue formation dose dependently. J Surg Res 43:322–328, 1987.

230. Laato M, Niinikoski J, Gerdin B, et al: Stimulation of wound healing by epidermal growth factor: A dose dependent effect. Ann Surg 203:379–381, 1986.

231. Brown GL, Curtsinger L, Brightwell JR, et al: Enhancement of epidermal regeneration by biosynthetic epidermal growth factor. J Exp Med 163:1319–1324, 1986.

232. Brown GL, Nanney LB, Griffen J, et al: Enhancement of wound healing by topical treatment with epidermal growth factor. N Engl J Med 321:76–79, 1989.

233. McGee G, Davidson JM, Buckley A, et al: Recombinant fibroblast growth factor accelerates wound healing. J Surg Res 45:145–153, 1988.

234. Schultz GS, White M, Mitchell R, et al: Epidermal wound healing enhanced by transforming growth factor-alpha and vaccinia growth factor. Science 235:350–352, 1987.

235. Cheng CY, Martin DE, Leggett CG, et al: Fibronectin enhances healing of excised wounds in rats. Arch Dermatol 124:221–225, 1988.

34

WOUND DRESSINGS: DESIGN AND USE

David M. Wiseman, Ph.D., M.R. Pharm. S.,
David T. Rovee, Ph.D., and Oscar M. Alvarez, Ph.D.

The history of wound care began with man's first injury. The desire to heal is perhaps reflected in the instinctive licking response, which may cleanse a wound by irrigation and the application of lysozyme and IgA or even accelerate healing by the application of epidermal or nerve growth factors (EGF, NGF).[1, 2]

Possibly the earliest examples of wound management are recorded in the Edwin Smith (c. 1500 B.C.) and Ebers (c. 1550 B.C.) papyri,[3] which describe the use of fresh flesh, fat, honey, and castor oil as dressings or adhesive plaster to appose wound edges. The primary objective in wound care, however, has always been the promotion of rapid wound healing with the best functional and cosmetic result.

FUNCTIONS OF A WOUND DRESSING

The principal function of a wound dressing is to provide an optimum healing milieu. Major changes occur in the wound environment at different stages during healing. To optimize the healing processes that take place in each of these stages may require different dressings. The dramatic changes in wound healing may be represented narratively by the following triptych:

In the first act of repair, the acute inflammatory events limit damage and clear the stage for subsequent repair to take place. Wounds must be protected from further damage, infec-

tion must be controlled, and debris must be cleared. In the second act, or proliferative phase, formation of fibrovascular granulation tissue and epithelialization occur. An optimal wound environment must be provided to allow rapid repair and regeneration. The triptych is completed by remodeling and maturation of scar tissue.

How does a dressing fit the specifications of this scenario? A wound must be isolated from the harmful external environment before healing can begin. The act of covering a wound mimics the barrier function of the epithelium. Hemostasis limits blood loss and the dissemination of microbes and toxins. A simple compression dressing promotes hemostasis and limits edema, reducing pain and improving gas and solute exchange between blood and tissue.

The nonspecific nature of inflammation results in tissue damage. Vascular leakage, the release and activation of lytic enzymes, free radical generation, oxygen consumption, and the sensitization of nerve endings are all disruptive to tissue.[4] Thus any measure that limits inflammation should promote wound healing, provided that it compromises neither the ability to resist infection nor essential macrophage function.

Infected wounds do not heal as quickly or as simply as noninfected wounds.[5] Significant numbers (10^3 to 10^4) of commensal microflora are found in a healing wound,[6] apparently without adverse effect. In occluded wounds these numbers increase (10^6 to 10^8) with a shift to gram-negative flora. There have been suggestions[7] that *Staphylococcus aureus* (but not other staphylococci) actually enhances wound healing (breaking strength) by inciting an "optimal" inflammatory response.

The distinction between "contamination" and "infection" will determine whether or not healing takes a complicated course. Infection is defined as contamination by pathogens that cannot be controlled by body defenses. Practically, wound sepsis occurs when more than 10^5 pathogens are present per gram of wound tissue,[8] impairing healing.[9] Thus a dressing cannot sterilize a wound but rather creates the conditions for reducing the pathogenic load by preventing overgrowth and colonization or by delivering antimicrobial agents to the wound.

In general, infection impedes wound healing by damaging tissue and by promoting inappropriate and excessive inflammation. The ability to resist infection is compromised by bacterial toxins (Table 34–1). Subsequent wound repair is delayed by the extension of inflammation: bacterial cell wall products and enzymes fix complement, destroy tissue, and activate or recruit neutrophils and macrophages.[4] Further discussion of wound sepsis can be found in specific texts.[10, 11]

Wound debris may be removed by debridement, irrigation, and absorption of exudate into a dressing. This reduces the requirement for phagocytic and autolytic debridement and removes a potential substrate for microbial growth.

CONTROL OF THE WOUND ENVIRONMENT

Occlusion

Dressing design for the second and third phases of wound healing is based principally on the manipulation of hydration and oxygen tension within the wound. Occlusion is a concept central to the evolution of wound dressings. It refers to the relative ability of a wound dressing to transmit gases and water vapor from a wound surface to the atmosphere. Numerous comparisons have been made between occluded and exposed wounds.[12–17]

Occlusion affects both epidermis and dermis. Exposed wounds are more inflamed and necrotic than occluded wounds in early stages of repair. Later, the dermis of exposed wounds is more fibroplastic, fibrotic, and scarred. Dermal collagen synthesis is enhanced in occluded wounds although not necessarily associated with

an increase in tensile strength.[18] Epithelial cell migration is enhanced by occlusion, although the magnitude and duration of the epithelial mitotic response are decreased.[15]

An occlusive dressing appears to function by limiting tissue desiccation and secondary damage (Fig. 34–1).[19] By maintaining a moist environment, epidermal barrier function is rapidly restored.[20] Interestingly, this effect may be noted by the faster rate of epithelialization in humid climates compared with that in arid ones.[21]

A scab forms when serous exudate dries, incorporating inflammatory cells, wound debris, and a layer of desiccated dermal tissue. The scab bonds wound and dressing surfaces, making dressing removal painful and traumatic.[20] Epithelialization is delayed in open wounds because epithelial cells are forced to migrate below the eschar, through the difficult terrain of dehydrated dermis, instead of taking the easy route of a moist occluded wound bed.[20] This moist environment is also conducive to the migration of defensive and reparative cells such as macrophages. It has been suggested that the scar left by an occlusively dressed wound is more cosmetically acceptable than that left by an exposed wound.[17]

Occlusion, however, must be carefully controlled. The same environment that enhances healing may enhance pathogenic growth. Thus, occlusion is contraindicated in infected and highly exudative wounds[22] and should be used with care in immunocompromised patients (e.g., in burns). Even clean wounds should be monitored for infection. Thus, some degree of moisture vapor permeability must be provided to prevent the possibility of exceeding the absorbency limits of the dressing, with resultant overheating, maceration, and microbial growth.[23]

Large numbers of microbes may be found in occluded wounds.[23–25] Even on normal skin, bacterial growth occurs beneath occlusion.[23, 26] In deliberately inoculated human skin wounds, occlusion supports bacterial growth, although without apparent detriment to healing.[22] In an uncomplicated wound such as a donor site, occlusion may decrease the incidence of infection slightly.[27] Control of wound pH may be a key to controlling pathogens under occlusion: a low pH (5.8 to 6.6) may be desirable[28] and may have a positive influence on epithelialization.[29]

Oxygen

The studies of Silver, Hunt, and their associates have illuminated the role of oxygen in

Table 34–1. BACTERIA INVOLVED IN WOUND SEPSIS AND THEIR PRINCIPAL MECHANISMS OF TOXICITY

Organism	Source	Wound Site	Toxicity
GRAM-POSITIVE			
Staphylococcus aureus (pyogenes) (aer, f anaer)*	Skin, nasopharynx, nosocomial	Burns, pustules, boils, wounds	Necrotizing hemolysins, exfoliatin, hyaluronidase, coagulase, catalase, lipase, plasminogen activator, protein A (activates complement)
Staphylococcus epidermidis (f) *(albus)* (aer, f anaer)	Skin, nose UGT	Cannulations, small skin wounds	Catalase
Peptococcus sp. (anaer)	GIT	GIT, peritonitis	
Streptococcus pyogenes (aer, f anaer)	BPT	Septicaemia, cellulitis	Pyogenic, hemolysins, hyaluronidase, leukocidin, plasminogen activator, erythrogenic toxins, DNAase
Streptococcus faecalis (enterococci) (aer, f anaer)	GIT		Nonhemolytic
Peptostreptococcus sp. (anaer)	BPT, UGT, GIT		Non- or slightly hemolytic
Clostridia welchii (perfringens) (s, b, anaer)	Soil, clothing, GIT, faeces, soil	Deep necrotic, hypoxic, acidotic wounds	Hemolysins, collagenases, hyaluronidase, lecithinase C, exotoxin, H_2 and CO_2 production (fermentation), gas gangrene, collagenase, hyaluronidase Co-exist with aerobes.
Cl. tetani (s, b, anaer) *Cl. oedematiens (novyi); Cl. septicum*	Soil, GIT		Tetanus exotoxin
GRAM-NEGATIVE			
Pseudomonas aeruginosa (b, f aer)	Water, soil, air, GIT, skin, UGT, nosocomial	Burns, UGT, wound sepsis	Leukocidin, exotoxin, endotoxin,‡ hemolysin, macrophage toxin, phospholipase C, elastase
Escherichia coli (b, aer, f anaer)	GIT, nosocomial	UGT, peritonitis, GIT	Endotoxin
Klebsiella pneumoniae (b, aer, f anaer)	Upper BPT, nosocomial		Endotoxin
Enterobacter sp. (b, f anaer)	UGT, GIT		Endotoxin
Proteus vulgaris (b, aer, f anaer)	GIT, UGT	UGT/wounds	Endotoxin
Proteus mirabilis (b aer, f anaer)	GIT, UGT, nosocomial	UGT/wounds	Endotoxin
Bacteroides fragilis (b, anaer)	GIT	Abcesses, peritonitis, UGT	Fibrinolysins, hyaluronidase, neuraminidase
Bacteroides melaninogenicus (anaer)	Mucous membranes		
Fusobacterium sp. (b, anaer)	Mouth	Oral, GIT	

*aer = aerobe; anaer = anaerobe; b = bacilli (rods); BPT = bronchopulmonary tract; f = facultative; GIT = gastrointestinal tract; s = spore forming; UGT = urogenital tract.

†Exotoxins are rapidly secreted proteins of some gram-positive organisms that have a specific pathophysiological effect.

‡Endotoxins are slowly diffusing toxins, mainly structural components (lipopolysaccharides) of gram-negative organisms that induce fever and activate a variety of immune and clotting cascades.

Data from references 4, 153, 154.

wound healing (see also Chapter 16).[30, 31] Perfusion and oxygenation of wounded tissue are vital to repair. Oxygen inhibits anaerobic growth and is required by phagocytes for the generation of microbicidal free radicals,[32] although it also inhibits macrophage angiogenic function.[30]

The requirement for oxygen seems to conflict with that for hypoxia. Since it is only practical to raise tissue P_{O_2} at the wound edges, the enhanced delivery of oxygen has the following effects: (1) neither central wound hypoxia nor central wound macrophage angiogenic activity are altered; (2) microbial clearance from the

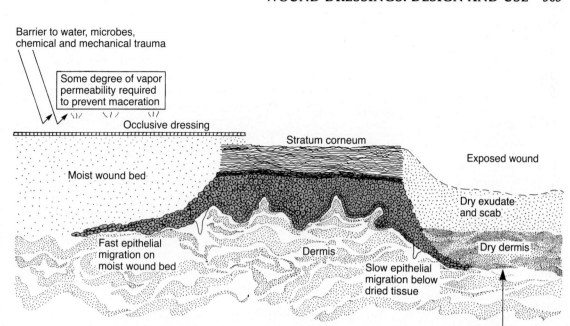

Figure 34–1. Wound healing under an occlusive dressing. (Adapted from Winter GD, Scales JT: Effect of air drying and dressings on the surface of a wound. Nature 197:91–92, 1963.)

wound is facilitated; and (3) fibroblast metabolism is promoted. Such enhancement of tissue Po_2 by adequate perfusion, hydration, and the inspiration of hyperbaric oxygen has been advocated for wound treatment and has been suggested to be as effective as antibiotics in reducing infection.[32, 33]

Although the beneficial effects of local oxygen administration have been discussed,[34–36] this treatment is controversial and raises further questions about the requirement for oxygen permeability in a dressing. Oxygen diffusion into normal adult human dermis from the atmosphere is insufficient to raise Po_2, although it may be sufficient in small mammals. Furthermore, wound exudate and active leukocytes present a formidable barrier for oxygen diffusion.[35] Studies in vitro have shown that optimal epidermal cell growth occurs at atmospheric oxygen concentrations of 10 to 50 percent[37–39] suggesting that increased epithelial oxygenation might enhance epithelialization. In full-thickness wounds the Po_2 under oxygen-permeable polyurethane films was only slightly raised compared with that under totally occlusive hydrocolloid dressings (4.5 mmHg vs. 0 mmHg).[28] However in abrasion wounds, epithelial oxygenation could be manipulated during the first few days after wounding, before the reconstitution of the oxygen-impervious stratum corneum and a dermal vasculature.[35]

What difference does this make to the rate of epithelialization? Rates of epithelialization under dressings correlate not with their known oxygen permeabilities but (inversely) with their moisture vapor transmission rates (Table 34–2). Thus it appears that oxygen permeability is not an essential attribute of a dressing.

The ability of an oxygen-permeable dressing to prevent anaerobic infection is controversial, since the oxygen permeability of plastic films (especially those coated with adhesive) is dramatically reduced in vivo, compared with in vitro.

It must be emphasized that occlusion should be used only on clean wounds in patients whose underlying pathology has been addressed.

Patient Comfort

The documented reduction of pain by dressings[27, 40–42] is a benefit that should not be undervalued (Table 34–3). The mechanism of analgesia by dressings is unclear, although reduction of inflammation and the protection of nerve endings may be important factors.

Heat losses are limited by the insulating effect of a dressing. Low temperature may have a specific effect on healing per se, due to a decrease in metabolic activity and to vasoconstriction. Healing in human partial-thickness

Table 34–2. THE EFFECT OF DRESSING OXYGEN AND MOISTURE VAPOR TRANSMISSION RATES ON EPITHELIALIZATION

Dressing	Oxygen Permeability (cm³/m²/24 hrs)	MVTR* (g/m²/24 hrs)	Increased Healing Rate (%)†
Hydrocolloid dressing (Duoderm, Squibb)‡	~0	~0	36%
Polyvinylidene (Saran 101 or 18, Dow Chemical)‡	15	3.1	31%
Polythylene (Clysar EH, Glad, Dupont)§	5037	13.9	24%
Polyurethane‖	2736	1095	25%
Human skin		300	—

All measurements at room temperature and pressure.
*Moisture vapor transmission rate.
†Increase in epithelial healing rates in partial-thickness wounds, compared to untreated wounds.[62]
‡See Alvarez et al.[18]
§Data from Films, sheets and laminates. Cordura, San Diego, 1979. Data are quoted per 0.001 inch thickness. Typical experimental films are 0.002–0.003 inches thick. This difference does not materially affect the relationships shown here.
‖Alvarez OM, unpublished observations.

wounds occurs optimally at 37 to 39°C. Below 26°C there is little epithelialization and above 42°C there is cell death.[43] A raised ambient temperature also has the effect of increasing skin surface Po_2.[35] Thus, although heat lamp treatment of wounds has been advocated, the dangers of desiccation and burning outweigh the benefits.

Toxicity, allergenicity, and overall safety are also important considerations in dressing design. Lint granulomata have been associated with the use of surgical swabs.[44, 45] However, refinements in woven and nonwoven technology, as well as the trend away from the use of cottons as primary dressings, has reduced this problem.

Table 34–3. THE EFFECT OF DRESSINGS ON WOUND PAIN*

Dressing Type	Study A†	Study B‡
Gauze	ND§	4.7
Exposed wounds	4.0	ND
Duoderm	1.3	ND
Tegaderm	ND	1.6
Bioclusive		
Transparent Dressing	1.5	ND
OPsite	1.6	1.6

*Pain scores scale (0 = no pain, 10 = extreme pain)
†Alvarez OM, Delannoy OA: The value of moist wound healing: A comparative assessment of new synthetic dressings. Am Acad Dermatol, Dec 1988 (abstract), suction blister wounds
‡Barnett et al,[40] donor site wounds
§ND, not determined

A transparent dressing should permit wound inspection without traumatic and time-consuming redressing, although pus and wound fluid accumulation may obscure inspection. Nonadherent dressings applied with tape may be removed painlessly and atraumatically.

Both ergonomic and economic aspects of wound care profoundly affect the compliance and confidence of nurses and patients. A dressing should be simple to apply, conform to body contours, and allow the patient to move[41] and to bathe. The high unit cost of certain dressings may be far outweighed by the cost of frequent dressing changes and nursing time necessitated by the use of seemingly cheaper materials.[46, 47] Cosmetically, the well-dressed and odorless wound provides comfort and confidence to a patient and the health care team.

EXPERIMENTAL EVALUATION OF WOUND HEALING

Various parameters are used to evaluate wound repair. Although nonspecific, wound DNA content and granulation tissue weight have been used to reflect granulation tissue formation.[48, 49] Tensile strength, collagen content, and synthesis are used to measure fibrogenesis. Epithelialization has been determined by the examination of serial sections,[12] by timing scab displacement or resurfacing,[50] and by measuring water vapor loss.[13] Sodium bromide or trypsin solutions have been used to separate dermis and epidermis, allowing an examination of epithelialization[50] and measurement of epidermal tensile strength.[14] Epidermal proliferation is assessed by the enumeration of mitotic figures following metaphase arrest[15, 20] or by the determination of DNA content or synthesis.[51, 52]

Its similarity to human skin in regard to morphology and repair has made the guinea pig plantar surface a useful model for incision wounds.[13, 14] Pigskin is also similar to human skin, and the large surface area lends itself to multiple trials on one animal.[50, 53] In the extrapolation of data from animal models it is noteworthy that human wounds do not generally heal by contraction. However in small laboratory mammals, the panniculus carnosus and the loose attachments between dermis and fascia permit free cuticular movement.[54, 55]

TYPES OF WOUND DRESSINGS

The lexicon of terms used to describe the many wound dressings available can be confusing. These terms are based on composition, physical properties, or usage and are not necessarily mutually exclusive. Figure 34–2 illustrates the design of several types of dressings. Table 34–4 classifies commercially available dressings using the terms described below. Tables 34–6 and 7 use this classification to summarize the appropriate uses of each dressing (see also the section "Which Dressing for Which Wound").

Primary and Secondary Dressings

All dressings can be classed as either primary or secondary types. A primary dressing is placed in direct contact with the wound and may provide absorptive capacity and prevent desiccation, infection, and adhesion of the secondary dressing to the wound. A secondary dressing is placed over a primary dressing to provide further protection, absorptive capacity, compression, and occlusion. The selection of materials for primary or secondary dressings is governed by the particular application. Cotton or rayon are most commonly used. They are inexpensive and can be manufactured in many configurations such as bandages, sponges, gauzes, tubular bandages, and stockings.

Absorbent Dressings

The accumulation of wound fluid to the point of flooding has severe consequences, including maceration and bacterial overgrowth.[23] Thus an absorbent dressing should imbibe exudate but without inebriation. If this "strikethrough" occurs, a channel is formed for microorganisms to enter the wound from the outside.

Cotton, wool, sponge, and moss have all been used as absorbent dressings. Even sawdust has been used to absorb pus and to pack abscesses; soft wood sawdust was recommended, possibly because it contains antimicrobial resins. Other absorbent materials that have been used include chitin and chitosan (from the exoskeletons of crustaceans),[56] alginates, pectin, gelatin, gels of the Pluronics series (triblock polymers of poly[oxypropylene] and poly[ethylene oxide]),

carboxymethylcellulose, karaya gum, and starch acrylonitriles.[57–59]

An absorbent dressing should be designed to match the exudation characteristics of the wound it is meant to cover: acute wounds exude maximally at about 24 hours following injury, while chronic wounds (e.g., leg ulcers) exude slowly at first (after debridement/dressing change) and then at a maximal plateau starting at 48 to 72 hours (Fig. 34–3). Thus, hydrocolloid dressings, which do not absorb rapidly at first, are of little use in an acute exudative wound (Fig. 34–4).

Nonadherent Dressings

Nonadherent dressings are designed to not stick to the wound. Gauze is often impregnated with paraffin, petroleum jelly, or KY Jelly for use as a nonadherent dressing. However, the impregnant may wear off, necessitating a dressing change.[60] A secondary dressing should be used with a nonadherent dressing to seal the wound edge to prevent desiccation and the entrance of pathogens.

In addition to the impregnated gauze type, often nonadherent dressings consist of an absorbent pad faced by a perforated nonadherent film layer. There have been some anecdotal reports of these dressings sticking to the wound, possibly because of epithelial ingrowth through the holes in the film layer or via a dried exudate. Even when slits have been used instead of holes, epithelial ingrowth may occur. Such adherence may be reduced by keeping the dressing moist at all times, even at the expense of some absorbency. Alternatively, the use of an ointment underneath the dressing may prevent adherence.

A distinction should be made between adherence to dry and to wet surfaces. Some "adhesive" backed film dressings do not stick to the wet wound surface, but adherence to the dry regenerated epithelium may cause disruption upon removal. Thus film dressings should be allowed to separate spontaneously from the healed wound.[41, 61] Plain gauze dressings will adhere to exudative wounds and this property has been used traditionally as a means of debridement, by removing the debris-encrusted dressing. This practice is counterproductive, however, since granulation tissue and regenerated epithelium are also removed.

Occlusive/Semiocclusive Dressings

The terms "occlusive" and "semiocclusive" (or "semipermeable") are used synonymously.

A NONADHERENT, NONABSORBENT DRESSING

Paraffin/petrolatum-coated gauze

B NONADHERENT, ABSORBENT DRESSING

Porous polyethylene film (nonadherent)

Absorbent cotton and/or rayon pad

C NONADHERENT, ABSORBENT, OCCLUSIVE DRESSING (HYDROCOLLOID)

Polyurethane film

Semiopen cell foam

Hydrocolloid/adhesive layer

D NONADHERENT ABSORBENT, OCCLUSIVE DRESSING (HYDROGEL)

Polyethylene film

Nylon support mesh

Hydrogel

E NONADHERENT, ABSORBENT, SEMIOCCLUSIVE DRESSING (COMPOSITE)

Polyurethane film

Exudative reservoir

Perforated polyurethane film

Acrylic adhesive

Polyurethane film

Absorbent pad

Acrylic adhesive

Nonadherent perforated membrane

F SEMIOCCLUSIVE, NONABSORBENT TRANSPARENT FILM DRESSING

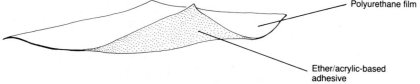

Polyurethane film

Ether/acrylic-based adhesive

Figure 34–2. Dressing construction and design.

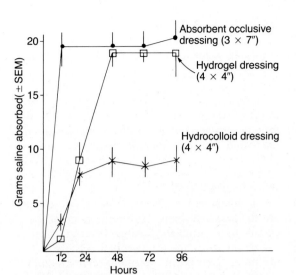

Figure 34–3. Absorptive capacity of some occlusive dressings. A dressing of the indicated size was weighed and placed over the top of a beaker (4.5 cm diameter) containing 40 ml of isotonic saline solution. The beaker was inverted and dressings were removed at various times after inversion. The dressings were weighed and the amount of liquid absorbed calculated. Each point indicates the mean of triplicate determinations.

Some water vapor permeability is desirable to prevent exudate puddling, although this may be aspirated from underneath the dressing. Occlusive/semiocclusive dressings provide an excellent environment for a clean, minimally exudative wound and can be used to protect uninvolved tissue from an exudative wound.

Experimentally polyvinylidene (Saran) and polyethylene (Glad) films increase epidermal healing by 31 and 24 percent, respectively, in certain wounds compared to untreated control (see Table 34–2).[62, 63] Adhesive polyurethane film dressings are probably the most common type in this category.[64] They increase epidermal healing by 18 to 20 percent compared with untreated control in porcine partial-thickness wounds,[62] although the re-injury caused by daily redressing necessitated by the experimen-

tal protocol reflects a true enhancement of about 25 percent. Clinically, faster healing rates are also observed in a variety of skin wounds[27, 65–67] using polyurethane dressings compared with traditional dressings.

Film dressings are waterproof and impervious to microbes but permeable to water vapor (and oxygen). They are prone to wrinkling, and the formation of channels allows microbes to enter the wound from its margins.[25] Thus it is important to obtain an "edge seal" around the wound, by degreasing and drying the skin surrounding the wound and framing the wound with at least 2 inches of dressing.[68, 69]

The tissue beneath a film dressing may have a yellow gelatinous appearance reminiscent of pus. Unless the wound is infected (in which case it is likely to be inflamed), this appearance reflects healthy autolytic debridement of the moist wound bed. Difficulty in handling film dressings has also been overcome by specially designed application systems.[70] Adhesive films have also been used to protect areas vulnerable to pressure, friction, or shear ulceration and for infusion or cannulation sites.[70] Hydrocolloid dressings are also occlusive (usually totally occlusive), as are a number of tapes used to fix gauze into place.

Hydrophilic/Hydrophobic Dressings

"Hydrophilic" and "hydrophobic" are terms often used to describe components of composite dressings. A primary hydrophilic layer is designed to absorb exudate, either directly or by capillary transposition to an absorbent layer. A hydrophobic backing renders the dressing waterproof and averts strike-through. In trilayered dressings, a hydrophilic layer is sandwiched between two hydrophobic layers, the lower of which is moisture (or moisture vapor) permeable and nonadherent.

Hydrocolloid and Hydrogel Dressings

Hydrocolloid and hydrogel dressings are attempts to combine the benefits of occlusion and absorbency. One approach has been the use of absorbent, hydrophilic hydrocolloids or hydrogels ("gels") formulated as sheets or pastes.

Hydrocolloids and hydrogels form complex structures with the dispersion medium (water). Hydrocolloids are dispersions of discrete parti-

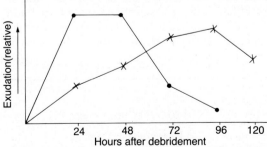

Figure 34–4. Exudative characteristics of acute and chronic wounds. Crosses indicate chronic wounds; circles denote acute wounds.

cles around which water molecules and solvated ions form a shell-like structure. Fluid absorption occurs principally by particle swelling and enlargement of this structure. The hydrocolloid mass of these dressings consists of gumlike materials such as guar or karaya, sodium carboxymethylcellulose, and pectin bound by an adhesive such as polyisobutylene.

Hydrocolloid dressings display wet tack (adhesion to a wet surface) because of particle swelling. This property facilitates atraumatic removal. The dry tack of hydrocolloid dressings is due to an adhesive such as polyisobutylene that is inactivated by moisture. The dry tack retained by the dressing around the wound preserves the edge seal. Exudate absorption by most hydrocolloid dressings results in the formation of a yellow/brown gelatinous mass that remains on the wound after dressing removal. This may be irrigated from the wound and should not be confused with pus.

Hydrogels are complex lattices in which the dispersion medium is trapped rather like water in a "molecular" sponge.[71] The hydrogel is typically a crosslinked polymer such as polyvinylpyrrollidone. Hydrogel dressings are nonadherent and have a high water content. Backed by a semipermeable film, hydrogels allow a high rate of evaporation without compromising wound hydration, which makes them useful in burn treatment.

Hydrogels and hydrocolloids have been reported to increase epidermal healing by 30–36 percent compared with untreated partial thickness wounds[62] and in full-thickness wounds.[72] Hydrocolloids and hydrogels can be supported by a foam or film layer and can be truly occlusive.[73] In liquefying, hydrogels and hydrocolloids conform to the wound and their removal is atraumatic. There has however been one report of epithelial damage on removal of hydrocolloid dressings,[61] and it is probably inadvisable to use hydrocolloid dressings (but not hydrogels) on wounds located on hairy surfaces.

Absorbable Materials

Absorbable materials are degraded in vivo. Particularly useful internally as hemostats, these materials include collagen, gelatin, oxidized cellulose, and oxidized regenerated cellulose.[74, 75] Collagen sponges have been used as wound dressings[72, 76, 77] and gelatin is a component of some hydrocolloid dressings. However, oxidized (regenerated) cellulose does not appear to be useful as an external wound dressing.

Medicated Dressings

Dressings have long been used as drug delivery devices. A plethora of exotic wound medications can be found in the materia medica of orthodox medicine as well as in popular folklore.[78-84] Agents that enhance epidermal resurfacing (with percentage increase compared with untreated control) include benzoyl peroxide (20% w/v) cream (33%), cod liver oil (33%), allantoin (37%), zinc oxide ointment (20%), and shark liver oil (16%).[62]

The most commonly applied medicaments are the antimicrobials. However, some of these agents may influence healing in a way that is unrelated to their antimicrobial activity.[85] For example, Neosporin ointment contains polymyxin B, bacitracin-zinc, and neomycin. While this ointment has been reported to increase epithelialization by 28 percent, such enhancement seems to be attributable to bacitracin-zinc. Zinc oxide ointment is also able to enhance epithelialization by up to 20 percent.[62] For other agents (e.g., silver sulfadiazine cream), the effect of the vehicle may be an important contributory factor.[24, 85]

The efficacy of topical antibiotics and disinfectants[86, 87] has been shown in several studies. However, some are of the opinion that wound infection should be treated systemically, inter alia, because of the problems of skin sensitization and microbial resistance.[60]

WHICH DRESSING FOR WHICH WOUND?

The use of classical materials in wound management may be described as "passive" since an environment is being created for a wound to heal itself. Correct selection from the wide choice of dressings is essential for optimal healing. Dressing selection is based upon an overall wound care strategy (Table 34–4) and consideration of the likelihood of drainage and/or infection. The classification by Cruse and Foord[88] is particularly helpful in the case of infection. Dressing changes should be made as

Table 34–4. WOUND CARE STRATEGY

Deal with underlying pathology (including infection)
Cleanse and debride wound
Determine wound type, depth and degree of exudation
Absorb exudation by appropirate dressing
Occlude the wound as soon as possible
Appose the wound edges as soon as possible (in healing by primary intention)

frequently as demanded by the accumulation of fluid and debris, overload of absorbent materials, degree of infection, and exhaustion or inactivation of medicaments.

A list and classification of commercially available dressings is presented in Table 34–5. We have compiled a chart showing the current clinical uses of various dressing types (Table 34–6). This is not necessarily based on the product license defined by the United States Food and Drug Administration. In all cases each manufacturer should be consulted as to the precise composition and usage of their particular products.

FUTURE DEVELOPMENTS

Growth Factors and Cytokines

Fundamental studies of wound healing have illuminated the interactions among cells, cytokines, and structural components of tissue. Purified wound factors are now available. There is the pharmacological vision of cytokine application to a wound, pre-empting cytokine endogenous synthesis and coordination. In problematic wounds this may be defective.

These ideas may not be so novel, merely their manner of execution. Eristratus (c. 300 B.C.) was unwittingly the first to advocate the use of growth factors in wound healing by the application of bird brain extracts to snake bites.[3] Brain tissue contains, among others, the acidic and basic fibroblast growth factors.[89, 90]

In the integration of biotechnology and wound management, we have the opportunity to coapt the frontiers of realism with those of idealism. A conventional dressing provides an optimal environment for repair and limited regeneration and establishes realistic standards of wound care. Using growth and differentiation factors, it is now possible to aim for the idealistic goal of true functional regeneration. At the very least we can strive to improve the quality of repair in such a way as to achieve *functionally regenerative repair*.

The biology of growth and differentiation factors with putative roles in healing—transforming growth factors, insulin-like growth factors, fibroblast growth factors, platelet-derived growth factor, tumor necrosis factor, angiogenesis factors, epidermal growth factor, interleukin-1, epibolin, and the interferons—has been reviewed extensively[90–97] (see also Chapters 4, 5, and 14).

The use of connective tissue elements in dressings or tissue substitutes may provide a scaffold for *functionally regenerative repair*. Many structural elements affect cells involved in healing (macrophages, fibroblasts, endothelial and epithelial cells), including the collagens entactin, vinculin, laminin, fibrin, fibronectin, hyaluronic acid, heparan sulfate, and heparin.[98–104]

Conceptual as well as practical problems have retarded the introduction of therapeutic products based on cytokines and growth factors. Practically there are the pharmaceutical problems of stability, formulation, and delivery of proteinaceous materials to an enzymatically hostile environment. More importantly, however, are conceptual problems associated with misconstruing the objectives and expectations underlying the use of the new products. To attain the goal of *functionally regenerative repair* requires the solution of two main problems.

First, in the delivery of agents to a wound, the temporal and spatial nature of regeneration and repair must be respected, requiring perhaps a cocktail of growth factors and their delivery by a suitably primed organ graft. The second problem concerns the assessment of healing and our expectations. In chronic indolent wounds it is reasonable to hope that by using growth factors we can reverse certain underlying pathologies to the point where "normal" repair can proceed. In such a system, assessment of wound repair by conventional means (epithelialization, wound closure, and granulation tissue formation) is acceptable. However in otherwise healthy individuals, we may be disappointed if we expect a faster rate of repair than can be obtained by sound wound care and use of dressings (implicit in this statement is the assumption that conventional dressings and wound treatments are used to their fullest potential). The paradigm of *functionally regenerative repair* requires a new agenda of assessment, the central question being "What does a regenerating tissue look like?" rather than "What does a good repair look like?"

Some recent reports have described the effects of growth factors in wound models. Epidermal growth factor (EGF) has been effective (usually by frequent or slow-release delivery) in the acceleration of healing in split-thickness excision or burn wounds in pigs,[105] in subcutaneously implanted sponges,[48] and in rat tendons.[106] In rabbit ear wounds Franklin and Lynch[107] reported faster and more extensive epithelialization, as well as a diminished con-

Table 34–5. COMMERCIALLY AVAILABLE DRESSINGS*

Dressing Type	Name and Manufacturer	Description
Adherent, Absorbent, Nonocclusive		Many absorbent woven and nonwoven gauze products are available. Gauzes are based on cotton and/or rayon (regenerated cellulose)
Nonadherent, Nonabsorbent, Nonocclusive	Adaptic (Johnson & Johnson Medical, Inc.)	Knitted cellulose acetate impregnated with petrolatum emulsion
	Aquaphor (Beiersdorf)	Impregnated gauze
	Jelonet (Smith and Nephew)	Paraffin tulle gras gauze
	N-Terface (Winfield)	Polyethylene-based mesh
	Transite (Smith and Nephew)	Fenestrated film
	Vaseline (Chesebrough-Pond's)	Petrolatum gauze
Nonadherent, Absorbent, Nonocclusive	Melolin (Smith and Nephew)	Nonadherent perforated poly(ethylene terephtalate) film backed by absorbent cellulosic/acrylic layer
	NA Dressing (Johnson & Johnson Patient Care, Ltd., United Kingdom)	Knitted cellulose acetate fabric
	Release (Johnson & Johnson Medical, Inc.)	Lightly absorbent rayon pad sandwiched between porous polyethylene film
	Scherisorb (Schering)	Pourable nonadherent hydrogel, removable by irrigation; mild to moderate exudation only
	Silicone NA Dressing (Johnson & Johnson Patient Care, Ltd., United Kingdom)	Knitted cellulose acetate fabric with silicone coating
	Sorbsan (Steriseal)	Calcium alginate material; soluble gel forms on absorption of exudate; mild to moderate exudation
	Telfa (Kendall)	Cotton sandwiched between perforated nonadherent poly(ethylene terephthalate) sheets
	Other products in this category include Coraderm (Armour), Lyofoam (Ultra), Primaderm (Calgon), and Synthaderm (Derma-lock)	
Nonadherent, Absorbent, Occlusive/ Semiocclusive		
Hydrocolloid Dressings	Comfeel Ulcus (Coloplast)	Absorbent carboxymethylcellulose/ adhesive layer backed by a polyurethane film; requires fixture with tape; also available as powder and paste containing guar, xanthan, and carboxymethylcellulose
	Duoderm (Granuflex in United Kingdom, Squibb)	Hydrocolloid layer composed of gelatin, pectin, sodium carboxymethylcellulose, and adhesive polyisobutylene; truly occlusive to gases and bacteria; backed by hydrophobic foam
	Johnson & Johnson Ulcer Dressing (Johnson & Johnson Medical, Inc.)	Hydrocolloid layer containing carboxymethylcellulose, karaya gum, silica, and polyisobutylene, backed by PVC foam sheet
	Other hydrocolloid dressings include Biofilm (Biotrol), Intact (Bard), Intrasite (Smith and Nephew), Restore (Hollister), and Ultec (Sherwood)	
Composite Dressings	Tegaderm Pouch Dressing (3M)	Inner fenestrated film; exudate accumulates in pouch formed by outer film layer, which transmits water vapor only at high levels; not strictly an "absorbent" dressing, although it has the same effect, i.e., displaces wound exudate away from wound
	Viasorb (Sherwood)	Cotton polyester pad contained within a polyurethane sleeve; wound surface is slit fenestrated
	Other composite dressings include Lyofoam (Ultra) and Transigen (Smith and Nephew)	

Table 34–5. COMMERCIALLY AVAILABLE DRESSINGS* *Continued*

Dressing Type	Name and Manufacturer	Description
Hydrogel Dressings	Geliperm (Geistlich-Pharma/Fougera)	Hydrogel of polyacrylamide and agar (96% water); moist sheet, dry material, and gel; tape required for fixation
	Vigilon (Bard)	Crosslinked polyethylene oxide hydrogel (95% water) between two polyethylene films; nonadherent, gas-permeable; both film layers can be removed to enhance evaporation but may not exclude bacteria; tape required for fixation
	Other hydrogel dressings include Bard Absorption Dressing (Bard), Cutinova Gelfilm (Beiersdorf), and Elastogel (Southwest Technologies)	
Semiocclusive/Occlusive, Nonabsorbent	Bioclusive (Johnson & Johnson Medical, Inc.)	Transparent polyurethane film with acrylic adhesive
	Blisterfilm (Chesebrough Pond's)	Polyurethane film with perimeter adhesive for atraumatic removal
	Opsite (Smith and Nephew)	Polyurethane film with polyether adhesive
	Tegaderm (3M)	Polyurethane film, acrylic adhesive
	Other products in this category include Acuderm (Acme United), Co Film (Chesebrough-Pond's) Ensure-It (Deseret) Opraflex (Professional Medical Products), Pharmaseal Transparent Dressing (Pharmaseal), Polyskin (Kendall), Uniflex (Howmedica/Pfizer), and Visulin (Beghin Say)	
Biological Dressings	Biobrane (Woodroof Laboratories)	Silicone-nylon/collagen bilayer composite; depending on chosen porosity can be used on heavily or lightly exudative wounds
	E. Z. Derm (Genetic Labs)	Porcine xenograft, crosslinked collagen, stable at room temperature; contains silver as antimicrobial; recommended for use as a short-term dressing (i.e., daily changes) until adherence, when it may be allowed to slough off spontaneously
Medicated Dressings	Bactigras (Smith and Nephew)	Chlorhexidine tulle gras
	Inadine (Johnson & Johnson Patient Care, Ltd., United Kingdon)	Rayon dressing impregnated with 10% povidone iodine ointment
	Actisorb (Johnson & Johnson Patient Care, Ltd., United Kingdon)	Nylon faced odor, and exudate activated charcoal cloth absorbent dressing
	Actisorb Plus (Johnson & Johnson Patient Care, Ltd., United Kingdon)	Activated charcoal cloth containing an antibacterial silver salt
	Odor Absorbent Dressing (Hollister)	Tea-bag–like structure containing activated charcoal deodorant
	Scarlet Red Dressing (Chesebrough-Pond's)	Lanolin/olive oil/petrolatum impregnated gauze, containing scarlet red
	Tegaderm Plus (3M)	Contains idophor
	Xeroform (Chesebrough-Pond's)	Absorbent gauze impregnated with bismuth tribromophenate in petrolatum base
Hemostats, Absorbable	Collagen hemostats include Avitene (Alcon), Helistat (Helitrex) Hemopad (Astra), Instat (Johnson & Johnson Medical, Inc.) Oxycell (Parke-Davis) (Oxidised cellulose), Surgicel, and Nu-Knit (Johnson & Johnson Medical, Inc.) (Oxidised regenerated cellulose).	
Powders and pastes	A number of absorbent powders or pastes are available that are poured into the wound, absorb exudate, are somewhat occlusive, and may later be irrigated from the wound. These include Bard Absorption Dressing (Bard), Comfeel Granules (Coloplast), Debrisan Wound Cleaning Beads and Debrisan Wound Cleaning Paste (Johnson & Johnson Medical, Inc.), Duoderm Granules (Squibb), and Intact (Bard).	

*The authors have attempted to give accurate descriptions of composition and use of commercially available wound dressings. We do, however, advise that the manufacturer should be consulted as to the precise composition and licensed usage of their products. The products described may be trademarks or registered trademarks of their respective companies.

Table 34–6. DRAINAGE AND DRESSINGS IN CLEAN WOUNDS

Drainage	Dressing
None	Semiocclusive dressing
Mild (1–2 ml/day)	Semiocclusive or absorbent nonadherent dressing
Moderate (3–5 ml/day)	Non-adherent primary layer* plus absorbent secondary layer plus an occlusive dressing to protect normal tissue
Heavy (>5 ml/day)	Non-adherent primary layer plus highly absorbent secondary layer plus an occlusive dressing to protect normal tissue

*The term "layer" connotes the use of either a commercially available composite dressing or an extemporaneously prepared dressing.

traction in EGF-treated wounds. This is perhaps a simple example of *functionally regenerative repair*. In other reports, EGF has failed to enhance wound healing significantly.[108–111]

Fibroblast growth factor (FGF) in various forms has been reported to stimulate wound healing or its components in sponge implant[49, 112] or blister healing[109] models. The same effect was seen with platelet-derived growth factor (PDGF)[113, 114] and a crude extract of platelet-derived wound healing factors (PDWHF),[115, 116] both alone[117] and in combination with other factors such as insulin-like growth factor-1 (IGF-1).[113] Another factor derived from platelets is transforming growth factor-β (TGF-β). When applied in a collagen gel TGF-β increased the rate of healing in a rat incision model.[118] Additionally, factors isolated from placenta and uterus have been shown to have potential as healing-promoting agents.[119–121]

Nonproteinaceous, low molecular weight (<1000 daltons) substances should be easier to formulate and deliver to a wound, and these include several angiogenic factors.[122–124] One of these factors may influence healing when injected at a remote site.[125]

Skin Grafts and Biosynthetic Membranes

The skin graft shares many of the problems of other types of organ graft: the use of an autograft is traumatic to an already compromised patient; donor or cadaver homografts are frequently rejected and pigskin grafts are usually removed after several days. Several types of artificial skin are under investigation: composites of connective tissue elements and synthetic materials,[126, 127] grafts of epidermal cells,[128–131] dermal cells,[132] or biosynthetic tissue

substitutes.[133] (For a complete discussion of artificial skin in burn patients, see Chapter 32.)

Sponges of type I collagen have been used experimentally[72] and clinically[77] as wound dressings/artificial skins in full-thickness but not partial-thickness wounds. These sponges reduced wound contraction and scarring and increased the rate of epithelialization. The mechanism of healing enhancement seems to be related to the physical rather than the chemical form of the sponge since milled collagen powder is ineffective.[76] Human amnion has been used as a treatment for burns and chronic leg ulcers.[134–137] Amnion possesses many ideal features of a dressing: it is somewhat occlusive, highly conforming, and releases a number of growth and angiogenic factors.[124]

THE INTERNAL WOUND DRESSING

The wound dressing to this point has been considered only in terms of treatment of the skin wound. The possibility for improvement in the rate and quality of internal repair lends itself to the concept of the internal wound dressing (IWD). Some examples of IWD use are described here, and additional information may be found in Chapter 35.

- To supplement the use of sutures or staples, tissue adhesive or fibrin glue[138, 139] may strengthen a suture line or reduce the requirement for sutures and the trauma caused by their use. In tissue that is difficult to suture, such as the spleen, kidney, or liver, tissue glue provides an alternative to partial resection.
- To improve the strength of supporting structures. Steel or polypropylene meshes are used to strengthen the abdominal wall following excision.[140, 141] Biodegradable materials such as collagen, polyglactin, or polydioxanone are used to replace the hepatic, splenic,[142] and renal capsules.[143] Vascular prostheses may be fabricated from bio-erodible materials; an interesting example is the incorporation of an endothelial cell growth factor (ECGF) to promote intimal regeneration.[144, 145]
- To promote hemostasis. Absorbable hemostatic sponges are made from gelatin, collagen, and oxidized regenerated cellulose.[74, 75] These materials promote hemostasis by providing a thrombogenic surface on which platelets may aggregate and fibrin may polymerize.

Table 34–7. WHICH DRESSING FOR WHICH WOUND?

Types of Dressings*

Wound Drainage	Types of Wounds	Adherent, Absorbent	Nonadherent, Nonabsorbent†	Nonadherent Absorbent	Hydrocolloids	Occlusive Absorbent Composites	Hydrogels§	Occlusive Nonabsorbant
Heavy (>5 ml/day)	Penetrating abdominal trauma Draining incisions Large excisions Stage 3–4 leg ulcer	Use with nonadherent primary dressing	Use with absorbent secondary dressing					
Moderate (3–5 ml/day)	Stage 3–4 ulcer‡ (above knee—pressure sore) Stage 2 ulcer (leg) Excisions—deep PT‖ Dermabrasion (large) Drainage incisions	Use with nonadherent primary dressing	Use with absorbent secondary dressing					
Light (1–2 ml/day)	Excisions—(curettage/shallow PT) Dermabrasion (small) Stage 2 ulcer‡ (above knee—pressure sore) Burns (outpatient) Dry incisions							
None	Partial thickness Stage 1 ulcer Minor burns Minor excisions Minor abrasions Minor incisions							
Protection	Areas liable to develop pressure sores Cannulation sites							

*Shading indicates that the particular dressing is recommended for the corresponding wound.
†Maintain moisture to prevent adherence
‡Ulcers on lower extremities tend to exude more heavily than similar wounds in sacral or trochanter areas.
§Tape is required to fix hydrogel dressings in place.
‖PT = partial thickness.

- To prevent adhesion formation. Fibrovascular adhesions complicate gynecological, intestinal,[146, 147] tendon,[148] and cardiac surgery.[149] Several factors have been implicated in adhesion formation: foreign body reactions to lint and starch, serosal damage due to handling, ischemia and tension imposed by suturing and handling, and impaired fibrinolysis.[146] Adhesion prevention has been approached in several ways:[146, 150] (1) reduction of fibrin deposition using heparin and fibrinolytic agents; (2) inhibition of fibroblast proliferation and collagen deposition using antihistamines or steroids; (3) use of careful surgical technique including meticulous hemostasis; and (4) separation of organs using omentum, amnion, oiled silk, or viscous intraperitoneal instillates. Curiously, fibrin glue has been suggested as a means to prevent adhesion formation,[139] possibly by sealing any exudative sources of fibrinogen. That these methods have met with limited success is indicative of the multiple and poorly understood etiology of adhesion formation. Recently however, a resorbable fabric of oxidized regenerated cellulose was shown to reduce the incidence, extent, and severity of adhesions in animals and clinical models.[151,152] The efficacy of the material was enhanced in the presence of heparin.

CONCLUSION

The subject of dressings and wound management has been complicated by the bewildering number of wound dressings available to the physician, surgeon, and nurse. The purpose of this chapter has been to explain why certain dressings are used (or should be used) on certain kinds of wounds and to provide insights into future forms of wound care involving growth factors. For this technology to realize its full potential one must think of healing not as "wound repair," but as *functionally regenerative repair*. Finally, with the evolution of bioresorbable and biocompatible materials, there are many opportunities for the development of "internal wound dressings," introducing the possibility of internal *functionally regenerative repair*.

For those individuals interested in keeping abreast of developments in the area of wound dressings, a quarterly newsletter is currently being published called "The Dressing Times." It is produced by The Welsh Centre for the Quality Control of Surgical Dressings, East Glamorgan Hospital, Church Village, Pontypridad, Mid Glamorgan, Wales.

References

1. Niall M, Ryan GB, O'Brien BM: The effect of epidermal growth factor on wound healing in mice. J Surg Res 33:164–169, 1982.
2. Li AK, Koroly MJ, Schattenkerk ME, et al: Nerve growth factor. Acceleration of the rate of wound healing in mice. Proc Natl Acad Sci USA 77:4379–4381, 1980.
3. Elliott IMZ: A Short History of Surgical Dressings. London, Pharmaceutical Press, 1964.
4. Taussig M: Processes in Pathology and Microbiology, 2nd ed. Oxford, Blackwell, 1984.
5. Bucknall TE, Cox PJ, Ellis H: Burst abdomen and incisional hernia—prospective study of 1129 major laparotomies. Br Med J 284:931–933, 1982.
6. Mertz PM, Eaglstein WH: The effect of a semiocclusive dressing on the microbial population in superficial wounds. Arch Surg 119:287–289, 1984.
7. Levenson SM, Kan-Gruber D, Gruber C, et al: Wound healing accelerated by Staphylococcus aureus. Arch Surg 118:310–320, 1983.
8. Robson MC, Heggars JP: Quantitative bacteriology and inflammatory mediators in soft tissue. In Hunt TK, Heppenstall RB, Pines E, et al (eds.): Soft and Hard Tissue Repair: Biological and Clinical Aspects. New York, Praeger, 1984, pp 483–507.
9. Krizek TJ, Robson MC, Kho E: Bacterial growth and skin graft survival. Surg Forum 18:518–519, 1967.
10. Altemeier WA, Burke JF, Pruitt BA, et al: Manual on control of infection in surgical patients. Philadelphia, JB Lippincott, 1976.
11. Kerstein MD: Management of surgical infection. Mount Kisco, NY, Futura, 1980.
12. Winter GD: Formation of the scab and the rate of epithelisation of superficial wounds in the skin of the young domestic pig. Nature 193:293–294, 1962.
13. Bothwell JW, Rovee DT: The effect of dressings on the repair of cutaneous wounds in humans. In Harkiss KJ (ed): Surgical Dressings and Wound Healing. London, Crosby Lockwood, 1971, pp 78–97.
14. Rovee DT, Miller CA: Epidermal role in the breaking strength of wounds. Arch Surg 96:43–52, 1968.
15. Rovee DT, Kurowsky CA, Labun J: Local wound environment and epidermal healing. Arch Dermatol 106:330–334, 1972.
16. Hinman CD, Maibach HI: Effect of air exposure and occlusion on experimental human skin wounds. Nature 200:377–378, 1963.
17. Linsky CB, Rovee DT, Dow T: Effect of dressings on wound inflammation and scar tissue. In Dineen P, Hildick-Smith G (eds): The Surgical Wound. Philadelphia, Lea & Febiger, 1981, pp 191–205.
18. Alvarez OM, Mertz PM, Eaglstein WH: The effect of occlusive dressings on collagen synthesis and epithelisation in superficial wounds. J Surg Res 35:142–148, 1983.
19. Winter GD, Scales JT: Effect of air drying and dressings on the surface of a wound. Nature 197:91–92, 1963.
20. Winter GD: Healing of skin wounds and the influence of dressings on the repair process. In Harkiss KJ (ed): Surgical Dressings and Wound Healing. London, Crosby Lockwood, 1971, pp 46–60.
21. Bothwell JW, Rovee DT, Downes AM, et al: The

effects of climate on the repair of cutaneous wounds in humans. In Maibach HI, Rovee DT (eds): Epidermal Wound Healing. Chicago, Year Book Medical Publishers, 1972, pp 255–266.

22. Katz S, McGinley K, Leyden JJ: Semipermeable occlusive dressings: Effects on growth of pathogenic bacteria and reepithelization of superficial wounds. Arch Dermatol 122:58–62, 1986.

23. Scales JT, Towers AG, Goodman N: Development and evaluation of a porous surgical dressing. Br Med J 2:962–968, 1956.

24. Eaglstein WH, Mertz PM, Alvarez OM: Effect of topically applied agents on healing wounds. Clin Dermatol 2:112–115, 1984.

25. Mertz PM, Marshall DA, Eaglstein WH: Occlusive wound dressings to prevent bacterial invasion and wound infection. J Am Acad Dermatol 12:662–668, 1985.

26. Aly R, Shirley C, Cunico B, et al: Effect of prolonged occlusion on the microbial flora, pH, carbon dioxide and transepidermal water loss on human skin. J Invest Dermatol 71:378–381, 1978.

27. May SR: Physiology, immunology and clinical efficacy of an adherent polyurethane wound dressing OP-site. In Wise DL (ed): Burn Wound Coverings, vol II. Boca Raton, FL, CRC Press, 1984, pp 53–78.

28. Varghese MC, Balin AK, Carter M, et al: Local environment of chronic wounds under synthetic dressings. Arch Dermatol 122:52–57, 1986.

29. Eisinger M, Soo Lee J, Hefton JM, et al: Human epidermal cell culture. Growth and differentiation in the absence of dermal components or medium supplements. Proc Natl Acad Sci USA 76:5340–5344, 1979.

30. Knighton DR, Oredsson S, Banda M, et al: Regulation of repair. Hypoxic control of macrophage mediated angiogenesis. In Hunt TK, Heppenstall RB, Pines E, et al: Soft and Hard Tissue Repair: Biological and Clinical Aspects. New York, Praeger, 1984, pp 41–49.

31. Silver IA: Cellular microenvironment in healing and non-healing wounds. In Hunt TK, Heppenstall RB, Pines E, et al: Soft and Hard Tissue Repair: Biological and Clinical Aspects. New York, Praeger, 1984, pp 50–66.

32. Hunt TK, Halliday B, Knighton DR, et al: Impairment of microbicidal function in wounds: Correction with oxygenation. In Heppenstall RB, Hunt TK, Pines E, et al: Soft and Hard Tissue Repair: Biological and Clinical Aspects. New York, Praeger, 1984, pp 455–468.

33. Bass BH: The treatment of varicose leg ulcers by hyperbaric oxygen. Postgrad Med J 46:407–408, 1970.

34. Fischer BH: Topical hyperbaric oxygen treatment of pressure sores and skin ulcers. Lancet 2:405–408, 1969.

35. Silver IA: Oxygen tension and re-epithelization. In Maibach HI, Rovee DT (eds): Epidermal Wound Healing. Chicago, Year Book Medical Publishers, 1972, pp 291–305.

36. Kaufman T, Alexander W, Nathan P, et al: Microclimate wound chamber. Topical treatment of experimental deep burns with humidified oxygen. Surg Forum 33:607–609, 1982.

37. Bullough WS, Johnson M: Epidermal mitotic activity and oxygen tension. Nature 167:488, 1951.

38. Karasek MA: In vitro culture of human skin epithelial cells. J Invest Dermatol 47:533–540, 1966.

39. Horikoshi T, Balin AK, Carter DM: Effect of oxygen on the growth of human epidermal keratinocytes. J Invest Dermatol 86:424–427, 1986.

40. Barnett A, Berkowitz RL, Vistnes LM: Comparison of synthetic adhesive moisture vapor permeable and fine mesh gauze dressings for split thickness skin graft donor sites. Am J Surg 145:379–381, 1983.

41. James JH, Watson AC: The use of Opsite, a vapor permeable dressing, on skin graft donor sites. Br J Plast Surg 28:107–110, 1975.

42. Friedman SJ, Su WPD: Management of leg ulcers with hydrocolloid occlusive dressing. Arch Dermatol 120:1329–1336, 1984.

43. Gimbal NS, Farris W: Skin grafting. Arch Surg 92:554–557, 1966.

44. Tinker MA, Teicher I, Burdman D: Cellulose granulomas and their relationship to intestinal obstruction. Am J Surg 133:134–139, 1977.

45. Brittan RF, Studley JGN, Parkin JV, et al: Cellulose granulomatous peritonitis. Br J Surg 71:452–453, 1984.

46. Conkle W: Op-site dressing. New approach to burn care. J Emerg Nurs 7:148–152, 1981.

47. Trelease C: A cost effective approach for promoting skin healing. Nursing Economics 4:265–266, 1986.

48. Buckley A, Davidson JM, Kamerath CM, et al: Sustained release of epidermal growth factor accelerates wound repair. Proc Natl Acad Sci USA 82:7340–7344, 1985.

49. Davidson JM, Klagsbrun M, Hill K, et al: Accelerated wound repair, cell proliferation and collagen accumulation are produced by a cartilage-derived growth factor. J Cell Biol 100:1219–1227, 1985.

50. Eaglstein WH, Mertz PM: New method for assessing epidermal wound healing. The effect of triamcinolone acetonide and polyethylene film occlusion. J Invest Dermatol 71:382–384, 1978.

51. Diegelmann RF, Cohen IK, Salomon JC: Measurement of epithelial DNA synthesis during reepithelization. J Surg Res 24:45–51, 1978.

52. Im MJC, Hoopes JE: Measurement of epithelial production in human skin wounds. J Surg Res 24:52–56, 1978.

53. Winter GD, Clarke DW: The pig as a laboratory animal for the study of wound healing and surgical dressings. In Harkiss KJ (ed): Surgical Dressings and Wound Healing. London, Crosby Lockwood, 1971, pp 61–69.

54. Peacock EE, van Winkle W: Contraction. In Peacock EE, van Winkle W (eds): Surgery and Biology of Wound Repair. Philadelphia, WB Saunders, 1970, pp 49–74.

55. Brody GS, Peng STJ, Landel RF: The etiology of hypertrophic scar contracture. Another view. Plast Reconstr Surg 67:673–679, 1981.

56. Balassa LL, Prudden JF: Applications of chitin and chitosan in wound healing acceleration. In Muzzarelli RAA, Parne ER (eds): Proc 1st Int Conf on Chitin and Chitosan. Cambridge, MIT Press, 1978.

57. Schmolka I: Artificial skin. I. Preparation and properties of Pluronic F-127 gels for treatment of burns. J Biomed Mater Res 6:571–582, 1972.

58. Nalbandian RM, Henry RL, Balko KW, et al: Pluronic F-127 gel preparation as an artificial skin in the treatment of third degree burns. J Biomed Mater Res 21:1135–1148, 1987.

59. De Riel S: Assessment of burn wound therapy systems. In Wise DL (ed): Burn Wound Coverings, vol I. Boca Raton, FL, CRC Press, 1984, pp 1–38.

60. Harkiss KJ: Cost analysis of dressing materials used in venous leg ulcers. Pharm J 235:268–269, 1985.

61. Zitelli JA: Delayed wound healing with adhesive wound dressings. J Derm Surg Oncol 10:709–710, 1984.

62. Alvarez OM: Pharmacological and environmental modulation of wound healing. In Uitto J, Perejda AJ (eds): Connective Tissue Disease. Molecular Pathology of the Extracellular Matrix. New York, Marcel Dekker, 1987, pp 367–384.

63. Sirvio LM, Grussing DM: The effect of gas permeability of film dressings on wound healing. J Invest Dermatol 93:528–531, 1989.

64. Thomas S, Loveless P, Hay NP: Comparative review of the properties of six semipermeable film dressings. Pharm J 240:785–787, 1988.

65. Falanga V: Occlusive wound dressings. Arch Dermatol 124:872–877, 1988.

66. Lobe TE, Anderson GF, King DR: An improved method of wound management for pediatric patients. J Pediatr Surg 15:886–889, 1980.

67. Hien NT, Prawer SE, Katz HI: Facilitated wound healing using transparent film dressing following Mohs micrographic surgery. Arch Dermatol 124:903–906, 1988.

68. Alling P, North AF: Polyurethane film for coverage of skin graft donor sites. J Oral Surg 39:970–971, 1981.

69. Weymuller EA: Dressings for split thickness skin graft donor sites. Plast Laryngoscope 91:652–653, 1981.

70. Eaglstein WH, Mertz PM, Falanga V: Occlusive dressings. Am Fam Phys 35:211–216, 1987.

71. Rawlins EA: Bentley's Textbook of Pharmaceutics, 8th ed. London, Balliere-Tindall, 1977.

72. Leipziger LS, Glushko V, DiBernardo B, et al: Dermal wound repair. Role of collagen matrix implants and synthetic polymer dressings. J Am Acad Dermatol 12:409–419, 1985.

73. Thomas S, Loveless P: Moisture vapour permeability of hydrocolloid dressings. Pharm J 241:806, 1988.

74. Arand AG, Sawaya R: Intraoperative chemical hemostasis in neurosurgery. Neurosurgery 18:223–233, 1986.

75. Browder IW, Litwin MS: Use of absorbable collagen for hemostasis in general surgical patients. Am Surg 52:492–494, 1986.

76. Leipziger LS, Glushko V, Shafaie F, et al: Inhibition of wound contraction by an acellular collagen matrix derived from bovine tendon. J Invest Dermatol 82:435, 1984 (abstract).

77. Zitelli JA: Wound healing for the clinician. Adv Dermatol 2:243–268, 1987.

78. Majno G: The Healing Hand. Cambridge, Harvard University Press, 1975.

79. Mikulic MA: Treatment of pressure ulcers. Am J Nurs 80:1125–1128, 1980.

80. Rudolph R: Wound treatments, nostrums and hokums. In Rudolph R, Noe JM (eds): Chronic Problem Wounds. Boston, Little, Brown, 1983, pp 47–51.

81. Efem SEE: Clinical observations on the wound healing properties of honey. Br J Surg 75:679–681, 1988.

82. Keswani MH, Vartak AM, Patil A, et al: Histological and bacteriological studies of burn wounds treated with boiled potato peel dressings. Burns 16:137–143, 1990.

83. Middleton KR, Seal D: Sugar as an aid to wound healing. Pharm J 235:757–758, 1985.

84. Topman JD: Sugar paste in treatment of pressure sores, burns, and wounds. Pharm J 241:118–120, 1988.

85. Geronemus RG, Mertz PM, Eaglstein WH: Wound healing—the effects of topical antimicrobial agents. Arch Dermatol 115:1311–1314, 1979.

86. Leyden J, Kligman A: Rationale for topical antibiotics. Cutis 28:515–528, 1978.

87. Leyden JJ, Stewart R, Kligman AM: Updated in vivo methods for evaluating topical antimicrobial agents on human skin. J Invest Dermatol 72:165–170, 1979.

88. Cruse PJ, Foord R: The epidemiology of wound infection. A ten year prospective study of 62,939 wounds. Surg Clin North Am 60:27–40, 1980.

89. Gospodarowicz D, Bialecki A, Greenburg G: Purification of the fibroblast growth factor activity from bovine brain. J Biol Chem 253:3736–3743, 1978.

90. Gospodarowicz D, Neufeld G, Schweigerer L: Molecular and biological characterization of fibroblast growth factor, an angiogenic factor which also controls the proliferation and differentiation of mesoderm and neuroectoderm cells. Cell Diff 19:1–7, 1986.

91. Cohen S: The epidermal growth factor. Cancer 51:1787–1791, 1983.

92. Folkman J, Klagsbrun M: Angiogenic factors. Science 235:442–447, 1987.

93. Goustin AS, Leof EB, Shipley GI, et al: Growth factors and cancer. Canc Res 46:1015–1029, 1986.

94. Le J, Vilcek J; Tumor necrosis factor and interleukin 1. Cytokines with multiple overlapping biological activities. Lab Invest 56:234–248, 1987.

95. Schor AM, Schor SL: Tumor angiogenesis. J Pathol 141:385–413, 1983.

96. Sporn M, Roberts A: Peptide growth factors and inflammation, tissue repair and cancer. J Clin Invest 78:329–332, 1986.

97. Stenn KS: Epibolin: A protein of human plasma that supports epithelial cell movement. Proc Natl Acad Sci USA 78:6907–6911, 1981.

98. Ford HR, Hoffman RA, Wing EJ, et al: Characterization of wound cytokines in the sponge matrix model. Arch Surg 124:1422–1428, 1989.

99. Alstadt SP, Hebda PA, Chung AE, et al: Effect of basement membrane entactin on epidermal attachment and growth. J Invest Dermatol 88:55–59, 1987.

100. Clark RAF, Lanigan JM, DellaPelle P, et al: Fibronectin and fibrin provide a provisional matrix for epidermal cell migration during wound reepithelialization. J Invest Dermatol 79:264–269, 1982.

101. Clark RAF, DellaPelle P, Manseau E, et al: Blood vessel fibronectin increases in conjunction with endothelial cell proliferation and capillary ingrowth during wound healing. J Invest Dermatol 79:269–276, 1982.

102. Dvorak HF, Harvey SV, Estrella P, et al: Fibrin containing gels induce angiogenesis. Lab Invest 57:673–686, 1987.

103. Grinnell F: Fibronectin and wound healing. J Cell Biochem 26:107–116, 1984.

104. Woodley DT, O'Keefe EJ, Prunieras M: Cutaneous wound healing: A model for cell matrix interactions. J Am Acad Dermatol 12:420–433, 1985.

105. Brown GL, Curtsinger L, Brightwell JR, et al: Enhancement of epidermal regeneration by biosynthetic epidermal growth factor. J Exp Med 163:1319–1324, 1986.

106. Franklin TJ, Gregory H, Morris WP: Acceleration of wound healing by recombinant human urogastrone (epidermal growth factor). J Lab Clin Med 108:103–108, 1986.

107. Franklin JD, Lynch JB: Effects of topical application of epidermal growth factor on wound healing. Plast Reconstr Surg 64:766–770, 1979.

108. Arturson G: Epidermal growth factor in the healing of corneal wounds, epidermal wounds and partial thickness scalds. Scand J Plast Surg 18:33–37, 1984.

109. Fourtanier AY, Courty J, Muller E, et al: Eye-derived growth factor isolated from bovine retina and used for epidermal wound healing in vivo. J Invest Dermatol 87:76–80, 1986.

110. Leitzel K, Cano C, Marks JG, et al: Growth factors and wound healing in the hamster. J Dermatol Surg Oncol 11:617–622, 1985.
111. Thornton JW, Hess CA, Cassingham V, et al: Epidermal growth factor in the healing of second degree burns: A controlled animal study. Burns 8:156–160, 1982.
112. Buntrock P, Buntrock M, Marx I, et al: Stimulation of wound healing, using brain extract with fibroblast growth factor (FGF) activity. Exp Pathol 26:247–254, 1984.
113. Lynch SE, Nixon JC, Colvin RB, et al: Role of platelet-derived growth factor in wound healing. Synergistic effects with other growth factors. Proc Natl Acad Sci USA 84:7696–7700, 1987.
114. Pierce GF, Mustoe TA, Senior RM, et al: In vivo incisional wound healing augmented by platelet-derived growth factor and recombinant c-*sis* gene homodimeric proteins. J Exp Med 167:974–987, 1988.
115. Knighton DR, Fiegel VD, Austin LL, et al: Classification and treatment of chronic nonhealing wounds. Ann Surg 204:322–330, 1986.
116. Knighton DR, Gersi K, Fiegel VD, et al: Stimulation of repair in chronic nonhealing cutaneous ulcers: A prospectively randomized blinded trial using platelet-derived wound healing formula. Surg Gynecol Obstet 170:56–60, 1990.
117. Grotendorst G, Martin GR, Pencev D, et al: Stimulation of granulation tissue formation by platelet derived growth factor in normal and diabetic rats. J Clin Invest 76:2323–2329, 1985.
118. Mustoe TA, Pierce GF, Thomason A, et al: Accelerated healing of incisional wounds in rats induced by transforming growth factor β. Science 237:1333–1336, 1987.
119. Burgos H, Herd A, Bennett JP: Placental angiogenic and growth factors in the treatment of chronic varicose ulcers: Preliminary communication. J Soc Med 82:598–599, 1989.
120. Burgos H, Lindenbaum ES, Beach D et al: Effect of decidua angiogenic factors on experimental dermis allografts. Burns 15:310–314, 1989.
121. Lindenbaum ES, Kaufman T, Beach D, et al: Uterine angiogenic factor induces vascularization of collagen sponges in guinea-pigs. Burns 15:225–229, 1989.
122. Weiss JB, Elstow SF, Hill CR, et al: Low molecular weight angiogenesis factor. A growth factor not unique to tumors which activates procollagenase. Prog Appl Microcirc 4:76–87, 1984.
123. Goldsmith HS, Griffith AL, Kupferman A, et al: Lipid angiogenic factor from omentum. JAMA 252:2034–2036, 1984.
124. Burgos H: Angiogenic factor from human term placenta. Purification and partial characterisation. Eur J Clin Invest 16:486–493, 1986.
125. Goldsmith HS, Griffith AL, Catsimpoolas N: Increased vascular perfusion after administration of an omental lipid fraction. Surg Gynecol Obstet 162:579–583, 1986.
126. Yannas IV, Burke JF, Warpehoski M, et al: Prompt long term functional replacement of skin. In Wise DL (ed): Burn Wound Coverings, vol II. Boca Raton, FL, CRC Press, 1984, pp 28–33.
127. Woodroof EA: Biobrane—a biosynthetic skin prosthesis. In Wise DL (ed): Burn Wound Coverings, vol II. Boca Raton, FL, CRC Press, 1984, pp 1–26.
128. O'Conner NE, Gallico G, Compton C, et al: Grafting of burns with cultured epithelium prepared from autologous epidermal cells. In Hunt TK, Heppenstall RB, Pines E, et al (eds): Soft and Hard Tissue Repair:
129. Eisinger M, Kraft ER, Fortner JG: Wound coverage by epidermal cells grown in vitro. In Hunt TK, Heppenstall RB, Pines E, et al (eds): Soft and Hard Tissue Repair: Biological and Clinical Aspects. New York, Praeger, 1984, pp 293–310.
130. Hunyadi J, Farkas B, Bertenyi C, et al: Keratinocyte grafting. Covering of skin defects by separated autologous keratinocytes in a fibrin net. J Invest Dermatol 89:119–120, 1987.
131. Green H, O'Conner NE: Cultured cells for the regeneration of epidermis by grafting. In Wise DL (ed): Burn Wound Coverings, vol I. Boca Raton, FL, CRC Press, 1984, pp 39–45.
132. Krueger WWO, Goepfert H, Romsdahl M, et al: Fibroblast implantation enhances wound healing as indicated by breaking strength determinations. Otolaryngology 86:804–811, 1978.
133. Bell E, Sher S, Hull B, et al: The reconstitution of living skin. J Invest Dermatol 81:2s-10s, 1983.
134. Bennett JP, Matthews R, Faulk WP: Treatment of chronic ulceration of the legs with human amnion. Lancet 1:1153–1156, 1980.
135. Faulk WP, Stevens PJ, Burgos H, et al: Human amnion as an adjunct in wound healing. Lancet 1:1156–1157, 1980.
136. Walker BB: Use of amniotic membranes for burn wound coverage. In Wise DL (ed): Burn Wound Coverings, vol I. Boca Raton, FL, CRC Press, 1984, pp 56–83.
137. Sawhney P: Amniotic membrane as a biological dressing in the management of burns. Burns 15:339–342, 1989.
138. Spotnitz WD, Mintz PD, Avery N, et al: Fibrin glue from stored human plasma. Am Surg 53:460–462, 1987.
139. Lindenberg S, Steenhoft P, Sorensen SS, et al: Studies on the prevention of intra-abdominal adhesion formation by fibrin sealant. Acta Chir Scand 151:525–527, 1985.
140. Ellis H: The abdominal wall. In Bucknall TE, Ellis H (eds): Wound Healing for Surgeons. London, Balliere Tindall, 1984, pp 124–142.
141. Jenkins SD, Klamer TW, Parteka JJ, et al: A comparison of prosthetic materials used to repair abdominal wall defects. Surgery 94:392–398, 1983.
142. Davies GC, Dixon JM: The liver, bile ducts, pancreas and spleen. In Bucknall TE, Ellis H (eds): Wound Healing for Surgeons. London, Balliere Tindall, 1984, pp 180–205.
143. Buchsbaum HJ, Christopherson W, Lifshitz S, et al: Vicryl mesh in pelvic floor reconstruction. Arch Surg 120:1389–1391, 1985.
144. Greisler HP, Kim DU, Dennis JW, et al: Compound polyglactin 910/polypropylene small vessel prostheses. J Vasc Surg 5:572–583, 1987.
145. Greisler HP, Klosak JJ, Dennis JW, et al: Biomaterial pretreatment with ECGF to augment endothelial cell proliferation. J Vasc Surg 5:393–402, 1987.
146. Ellis H: The causes and prevention of intestinal adhesions. Br J Surg 69:241–243, 1982.
147. Raftery AT: Serosae. In Bucknall TE, Ellis H (eds): Wound Healing for Surgeons. London, Balliere Tindall, 1984, pp 143–160.
148. Hutton P, Ferris B: Tendons. In Bucknall TE, Ellis H (eds): Wound Healing for Surgeons. London, Balliere Tindall, 1984, pp 286–296.
149. Vander Salm TJ, Okike ON, Marsicano TH, et al: Prevention of postoperative pericardial adhesions. Arch Surg 121:462–467, 1986.

150. Montz FJ, diZerega GS: Postsurgical mesothelial repair. In DeCherney A, Hazeltine F (eds): Physiology and Pathophysiology in Reproductive Surgery. New York, CK Hall Press, 1985.
151. Linsky CB, Diamond MP, Cunningham T, et al: Adhesion reduction in the rabbit uterine horn model using an absorbable barrier, TC7. J Reprod Med 32:17–20, 1987.
152. INTERCEED (TC7) Adhesion Barrier Study Group: Prevention of postsurgical adhesions by INTERCEED (TC7), an absorbable adhesion barrier: A prospective randomized multicenter clinical study. Fertil Steril 51:933–938, 1989.
153. Documenta Geigy Scientific Tables. 6th ed. Manchester, Geigy Pharmaceutical, 1962.
154. Raahave D, Friss-Moller A, Bjerre-Jepsen K, et al: The infective dose of aerobic and anaerobic bacteria in postoperative wound sepsis. Arch Surg 121:924–929, 1986.

35

SURGICAL DEVICES IN WOUND HEALING MANAGEMENT

Richard F. Edlich, M.D., George T. Rodeheaver, Ph.D., and John G. Thacker, Ph.D.

The surgeon's ultimate goal is to restore the physical integrity and function of the injured or diseased tissue. While this would best be achieved by regeneration, wound restoration usually results from the deposition of scar tissue. The surgeon should attempt to control the fibrous tissue synthesis stage of healing for optimal production of scar. By having a detailed knowledge of the biology of wound repair, the surgeon may improve wound closure, reducing deformity and dysfunction.

In the quest to reconstitute the damaged tissue, one must appreciate the consequences of its devastation. Whether the tissue injury will be limited to the initial wounding depends on the outcome of the interaction between the contaminants and the surgical wound. In the event that the contaminants are very reactive, a relatively insignificant wound may become a catastrophe. This outcome can be averted by the implementation of well-devised surgical care based on the biology of wound repair and infection.

The major focus of this chapter is on the technical considerations involved in wound repair and infection. This chapter has been specifically written for students of surgery who view themselves as artisans, cultivating and practicing the "science of surgery" and for the interested basic health scientist who wishes an

overview of the mechanical aspects of wound repair. As with any master craftsperson, the surgeon must understand the tools of the profession. The link between a surgeon and surgical equipment is a closed kinematic chain in which the surgeon's power is converted into finely coordinated motion. The ultimate goal of this interlinking is perfection of the surgical discipline.

Students of surgery must not read this chapter looking for support of prejudices, but rather in search for ways in which they can affect changes that might improve their results. We have tried to identify surgical principles that are fundamental truths that guide surgical practice. These truths must always stand the test of time or be replaced by new and improved concepts of wound care.

During surgery, the surgeon must make judgments that frequently tip the balance in favor of either infection or healing per primum. A large number of clinical and experimental studies have provided evidence of the influence of various technical considerations on the ultimate fate of the wound. We make specific recommendations, based on the biology of wound repair and infection, on the management of the surgical wound.

SURGICAL INCISION

Surgeons unconsciously separate the concept of injury from that of surgery. This division of

These clinical and experimental research investigations have been supported by generous gifts from the Texaco Philanthropic Foundation, White Plains, NY.

thought may provide the surgeon with a false sense of confidence that the consequences of injury are indeed distinct from those of surgery, when, in fact, they are identical in most aspects.

The outcome of both injury and surgery can be predicted by applying concepts of power, work, and force that were first appreciated in the 17th century. Surgeons simply employ various principles of energy transfer and mechanical, thermal, and radiant energy in a planned procedure to achieve an anticipated result. If the surgeon does not appreciate and control the sources of energy employed, an operation becomes an assault similar in nature to a traumatic injury. The "complete" surgeon must harness and control the sources of energy and force and appreciate their potentially destructive effects. Clinically, one of the most important consequences of any wounding process is that the divided edges of the wound are more susceptible to infection than unwounded tissue.[1] The magnitude of this enfeebled resistance will vary with the mechanism of wounding.

Mechanical Energy

Of all energy sources employed, the surgeon is most familiar with mechanical energy, which is that required to move an object. When performing surgery, the surgeon applies a carefully controlled force of a planned magnitude to divide tissue. This shearing force is delivered to the tissue by scissors or scalpel. To divide tissue with scissors, the surgeon applies a shearing force of equal magnitude in opposite directions, in two adjacent parallel planes separated by a small distance. A scalpel cuts tissue by applying a shearing force in only one direction. Because the volume of tissue contacted by these instruments is extremely small, very little energy is required to produce tissue failure.

The configuration of the cutting edge of a scalpel is designed to accomplish a specified surgical task using a prescribed technique. Despite all the technical advances in scalpel design, the ultimate performance of the scalpel depends on the surgeon's technical skill. The experienced surgeon who is cognizant of the scalpel's performance and the anatomy of tissue can cut to the desired depth with one sweep of the blade, making a wound that is very resistant to the development of infection, with 10^6 or more bacteria being necessary to cause infection.[1] The surgeon who does not appreciate the potential of his instrument and is unfamiliar with the structural configuration of the tissue will generally cut with multiple strokes of the knife. Such repeated passages of the scalpel through tissue damage local defenses and invite infection.[1]

While the decision to discontinue the use of a scalpel blade during an operation is usually related to blade dulling, some surgeons discard a blade after it contacts what they believe to be a source of contamination. A ritual practice in surgery has been to discard the sharp blade following its use on skin due to fear that it introduces skin contaminants into the depths of the wound. Jacobs[2] reported that scalpels are almost always sterile after cutting skin and need not be discarded. The influence of the use of only one knife, instead of two, on the postoperative wound infection rate was not evaluated in that study. Hasselgren and colleagues initiated the first controlled clinical trial in which the incidence of wound infection was recorded following the use of one or two knives for the skin incision.[3] When the skin incision was made by only one knife, the incidence of infection in 277 patients was 3.6%. A comparable rate of infection (5.5%) was encountered in 309 patients whose skin incisions were made by two separate knives. This difference was not significantly different.

Electrical Energy

Electricity is another source of energy that the surgeon has learned to use constructively in surgery. Electricity is the flow of electrons from one atom to another. The electrons set in motion by the electric force (voltage) may collide with each other and generate heat, transforming electrical energy into thermal energy. The amount of heat developed by a conductor varies directly with its resistance. The magnitude of resistance to electron flow varies widely in different tissues, with the high resistance of bone and low resistance of muscle to electron flow cases in point. The control and localization of the heating effect of electrical current is the fundamental basis for electrosurgery.

Involuntary spasmodic contractions of muscle in response to a low-frequency electrical stimulus subside as the frequency of the applied current is increased above 60 Hz. At frequencies between 0.5 and 1.0 megacycle, no muscle response is noted. In addition, high-frequency current can flow along paths that virtually block the 60-cycle current. The frequency of the current generated in electrosurgery is 250,000 to 2,000,000 Hz. Research in electrosurgery has focused predominantly on electronic technology with only theoretical clinical application. In the future, comprehensive research investigations must be undertaken to relate these modern technological advances to clinical performance.

The ability of the high-frequency current to damage tissue depends on its concentration or density. As the current density increases, its heating effect becomes more pronounced. The size of the active monopolar electrode is deliberately kept small so that concentrated heating will occur at its point of contact with tissue. Following contact, the current is dispersed to the return (ground) electrode, which encounters low current density and no tissue heating. The distribution of the current can be even more precisely controlled by making the active electrode bipolar rather than monopolar. The use of bipolar electrodes, usually in the form of forceps, delineates the tissue through which the current will pass. Bipolar electrodes contain two electrodes and contact the tissue at two points; current flows into the tissue through one arm of the forceps and back out through the other. The entire current is confined to the small area between the two ends of the forceps and no return electrode is needed.

When undamped high-frequency current is passed through tissue, the active electrode acts as a bloodless knife. The cells at the edge of the resultant wound literally disintegrate. Away from the plane of cutting, one can see elongated tissue cells as well as histological evidence of a mild thermal injury. Blood vessels at the wound edge are usually thrombosed, accounting for the hemostatic effect of the high-frequency current. This histological evidence of tissue damage is also associated with an increased susceptibility of the wound to infection. The wound made by electrosurgery in experimental studies was approximately three times more susceptible to infection than wounds made with the stainless steel scalpel.[4] In a prospective clinical study by Cruse and Foord, the use of electrosurgery almost doubled the infection rates of surgical wounds.[5] Although there is no prospective study comparing electrosurgery to the scalpel for cutting the fascia, Greenberg and associates believe that cutting the fascia with electrosurgery may have caused fascial necrosis in six of eight reported dehiscences.[6]

In massive excisional surgery (e.g., large soft-tissue tumors, debridement of third-degree burns), the threat of blood loss frequently outweighs the risk of subsequent infection. In burn wound excisions, Levine and his associates[7] reported that the operative blood loss during electrosurgical excision was approximately 50 per cent less than that encountered during scalpel excision. The operative time was de-creased by half by eliminating the additional time required to obtain hemostasis after the scalpel was used.

When the oscillations are damped, the current accomplishes hemostasis without cutting. This type of current causes a rapid dehydration of living cells, and the affected tissue is fused into a structureless homogeneous mass with a hyalinized appearance. The bleeding vessels within the tissue become thrombosed, resulting in hemostasis.

The technique of electrocoagulation has considerable influence on the magnitude of injury. The use of bipolar coagulation is a more precise method of hemostasis that limits the tissue injury encountered with the more traditional monopolar coagulation. Ferguson has noted that an equivalent current passed through a monopolar electrode caused approximately three times as much necrosis of the surrounding tissue as the use of bipolar coagulation.[8]

From surgery's beginning and well into the 19th century, cautery heated over a bed of hot coals was regularly used to control hemorrhage as well as to serve as an antiputrefactive agent. Surgeons can now cut tissue with new heated scalpels whose temperature can be controlled within narrow limits. Levenson and colleagues reported that the heated scalpel allowed excision of third degree burns in pigs and human subjects with much smaller blood loss compared with the usual cold scalpel.[9] Skin grafts applied immediately after excision had excellent rates of success similar to those of grafts applied immediately after excision with the unheated scalpel. These investigators reported that the heated knife did not interfere with the wounds' ability to resist infection.[9] In wounds in experimental animals made by either a heated or unheated scalpel and then contaminated with 100 million *Pseudomonas aeruginosa* or *Staphylococcus aureus*, no infection developed in either group. The absence of infection in wounds made either by the heated or unheated scalpel is difficult to explain because the inoculum used was 100 times greater than the infective dose for these pathogens in soft tissues. Consequently, inoculation of 100 million organisms should have resulted in gross evidence of infection in all wounds. Moreover, Levenson and colleagues reported that the heated scalpel had limited adverse effects on wound repair.[9] Using a temperature of 180°C, the breaking strengths of wounds made by the hot scalpel did not differ significantly from those in wounds made by the cold scalpel 7, 14, 25, 28, and 42 days after wounding. The only statistically significant difference ($p < 0.05$) between the breaking strengths of incisions made by the unheated scalpel was noted at 21 days and modestly favored the conventional scalpel. The innocuous effects of the heated scalpel could not be confirmed by our laboratory.[10] Using scalpels heated to a considerably lower temperature than that employed in Levenson's study,[9] we found that the heated knife impaired the wounds' resistance to infection and interfered with healing.

Radiant Energy

As a result of recent scientific advances, surgeons can now employ energy from light as a scalpel, making use of one of the many forms of radiant or electromagnetic energy. Such energy consists of photons that are both waves and particles. Once it is absorbed by tissue, radiant energy is converted into heat that rapidly increases the temperature of a small volume of tissue. This precise thermal injury results in a relatively bloodless division of tissue. The concept of light as a source of energy is realized in lasers. Light waves emitted from lasers are coherent and so nearly parallel that they can travel for miles in a straight line without spreading apart or converging. This coherent light provides tremendous pulses of power that do not diminish over great distances.

This energy source is now being used by some surgeons to cut tissue. Lasers used in surgery get their energy from rotation and vibration of electrons in the CO_2 molecule with a resultant emission of light having a wavelength of 10.6 μ. These infrared waves are then directed along an articulated arm and into a handpiece by means of mirrors located in precision rotary joints. A lens in the handpiece focuses the energy to a point less than 1 mm in diameter, which allows the beam to cut through skin and soft tissue. Despite this technological advance, laser surgery is limited by the cumbersome design of the surgical arm as well as an insufficient level of power. When maneuverability is required, laser surgery is difficult and time consuming.

The hemostatic effect of the laser scalpel makes it especially suited for massive surgical excisions. In a clinical series of 26 patients subjected to burn wound excision, Levine and co-workers reported that the blood loss encountered with scalpel excisions was nearly 3.3 times greater than that with laser surgery,[7] and electrosurgical excision had 1.67 times the blood loss of laser excision. The superior hemostatic effect of the laser over that of electrosurgery is

associated with increased damage to the tissue defenses, however. Experimental wounds made by a laser were approximately ten times more susceptible to infection than those made by electrosurgery.[4] This infection-potentiating effect of the laser scalpel mitigates against its use for incisional surgery. Fortunately, the tissue damage resulting from either electrosurgery or the laser does not interfere with the "take" of autografts or homografts on wound beds with low bacterial counts ($<10^6$ bacteria per gram of tissue).

MECHANICAL CLEANSING

The surgeon commonly employs mechanical forces to rid the wound of bacteria and other particulate matter retained on the wound surface by adhesive forces. For such forces to be successful they must exceed the adhesive forces of the contaminants. The two basic modes employed by the surgeon to cleanse wounds are hydraulic forces and direct contact.

In irrigation, the hydraulic forces of the irrigating stream act on particulate matter in the wound. The magnitude of the hydraulic forces is a function of the relative velocities and the configuration of the particle. When subjected to the same irrigating stream, particles with a smaller frontal surface area will encounter less force than particles with a similar configuration but a greater surface area. Consequently, it takes significantly less hydraulic pressure to rid the wound of large foreign bodies than it does to remove bacteria.

The level of hydraulic forces applied to the particle will also increase considerably as the velocity of the irrigating stream is raised. The simplest and most practical methods of raising the velocity are to increase the pressure within the irrigating syringe and to enlarge the internal diameter of the needle. Small syringes (5, 12 ml) are clinically impractical because delivery of large volumes of fluid would require an extended irrigation time. Therefore, the preferred method of increasing the velocity of an irrigating stream is to use a larger bore needle. Irrigation fluid delivered through a large bore needle generates a significantly greater irrigation force at a surface than fluid delivered through a small bore needle.

The pressure exerted by fluid delivered through a 19 gauge needle by a 35 ml syringe is 8 psi.[11] Irrigation pressures of this magnitude or higher are classified "high pressure," while irrigation pressures below this level, as obtained with a bulb syringe, are designated as "low pressure." These definitions have important clinical implications. High-pressure irrigation successfully cleanses the wound of small particulate matter, bacteria, and soil infection potentiating fractions, and as a result, the infection rate of experimentally contaminated wounds is reduced. In contrast, low-pressure syringe irrigation, even with large volumes of fluid, has negligible capacity to remove small particles (bacteria), but has measurable therapeutic effect in removing large particulate matter, such as detached devitalized tissue.

Despite the advantages of high-pressure irrigation, several theoretical objections have been raised against its routine use. One commonly expressed concern is that foreign bodies on the surface of the wound may be disseminated more deeply into the wound as a result of high-pressure irrigation. On the basis of recent experimental studies, this fear appears to be unfounded.[12] Consequent to high-pressure irrigation, the bacteria remain at the surface of the wound even though the irrigant solution may disseminate deeply into the tissues. The tissue penetration of a high-pressure irrigating stream is predominantly in a lateral direction similar to that encountered with a jet parenteral injection.

However, concern that high-pressure irrigation can damage tissue defenses appears to be justified. Pulsatile or syringe irrigation results in trauma to the tissues, which makes the wound more susceptible to experimental infection. This finding serves to remind the surgeon that high-pressure irrigation should not be performed indiscriminately, but should be reserved for heavily contaminated wounds. In such wounds, the benefits of this cleansing technique outweigh the increased risk of infection, resulting in a marked decrease in the number of bacteria and uncomplicated healing of the wound without clinical infection.

In the clinical setting, high-pressure irrigation is accomplished with an inexpensive disposable irrigation assembly consisting of a 19 gauge plastic needle attached to a 35 ml syringe. Sterile electrolyte solution (usually 250 ml of 0.9% sodium chloride) is delivered through a one-way valve attached to the syringe barrel via standard intravenous plastic tubing. The tip of the needle, fastened to the syringe filled with saline, is placed perpendicular and as close as possible to the surface of the wound; then the surgeon exerts maximal force to the syringe plunger to deliver the irrigant to the wound.

Another force often employed by surgeons to cleanse a wound is direct mechanical contact in which force is exerted by applying a solid object to the particle to effect its removal. An example is scrubbing a dirty wound with a sponge. This technique has proven to be an effective means of removing bacteria from wounds. Unfortunately, despite this benefit, scrubbing the wound with a saline-soaked sponge does not decrease the incidence of infection.

Tissue trauma inflicted by the sponge impairs the wound's ability to resist infection and allows the residual bacteria to elicit an inflammatory response. The magnitude of the damage to the local tissue resistance is correlated with the porosity of the sponge. Sponges with a low porosity are more abrasive and exert more damage to the wound than do those with a higher porosity. The addition of a nontoxic surfactant, such as poloxamer 188, to a sponge minimizes tissue damage while maintaining the bacterial removal efficiency of mechanical cleansing. Consequently, the use of a surfactant-soaked sponge reduces the incidence of infection in contaminated wounds in experimental animals.[13]

In a recent clinical trial involving more than 3000 patients, wound treatment with poloxamer 188 was accomplished without discernible toxic effects or allergic reactions. This considerable clinical experience is consistent with the investigations demonstrating that this surfactant does not result in any significant damage to either the wound's resistance to infection and healing or to the cellular components of blood.[14] A potential shortcoming of poloxamer 188 is that it exhibits no antibacterial activity. Consequently, skin cleansing with poloxamer 188 should be supplemented by immediate antibiotic treatment in wounds that are prone to infection.

The potential toxicity of several commercially available surgical scrub solutions has been recognized by other investigators.[13] The irritant effect of these solutions can be easily appreciated by any surgeon by adding the surgical scrub solutions to blood and then observing the cellular integrity of the components of blood.[14] Exposure of blood to either Hibiclens or Betadine surgical scrub solution damaged its cellular components. Following contact with the Iodophor surgical scrub solution, no cellular components were identified. The significant damage to red blood cells resulted in considerable hemolysis (8 gm% hemoglobin). In contrast, Hibiclens' deleterious effects on blood was most pronounced with white blood cells, which were completely destroyed. Lesser but significant effects on red blood cells were detected. After exposure to Hibiclens, an approximate 2 logarithmic decrease in red blood cell count was encountered with a rise in plasma hemoglobin to 1.2 g per cent. Toxicity to the cellular components of blood was not noted with poloxamer 188. This incriminating evidence, however, has not dampened the enthusiasm of some surgeons for these toxic scrub solutions in wounds. With the advent of a safe and effective surfactant, it is inconceivable that some surgeons continue to use these toxic agents. Those who continue to pursue this dangerous course should be reminded again of the surgical dictum that has stood the test of times, "The only solution that should be placed in a wound is one that can be safely poured in the surgeon's eye."[15]

HEMOSTATIC AGENTS

Topical hemostatic agents have found wide applications in a variety of surgical procedures. They can effectively control bleeding from large areas of cancellous bone[16] and are often used to stop bleeding from vascular anastomoses before additional sutures are placed.[17] Bleeding from splenic, hepatic, and renal injuries can also be arrested by application of these agents.[18–20]

A wide variety of topical hemostatic agents have been used clinically to reduce bleeding and include the following: Beeswax,* stabilized fibrin and collagen paste,† oxidized cellulose (OC),‡ oxidized regenerated cellulose (ORC),§ absorbable gelatin foam (AGF) or powder (AGP),‖ microfibrillary collagen (MC),¶ bovine thrombin (BT),** and fibrin glue. OC is an absorbable oxidized cellulose that is available in either cotton type pledgets or gauzelike pads or strips. ORC is an absorbable knitted fabric prepared by the controlled oxidation of regenerated cellulose. AGF is a pliable, nonantigenic foam from specifically treated, purified gelatin solution and is capable of absorbing and holding within its meshes many times its weight of whole blood. This latter product is also available as a powder (AGP). MC is an absorbable agent prepared as a dry, fibrous, water-insoluble, partial hydrochloric acid salt of purified bovine corium collagen. In its manufacture, swelling of the native collagen fibrils is controlled by ethyl

*Ethicon, Inc., Somerville, NJ.
†Ethnor, Ethicon, Ltd., Edinburgh, Scotland.
‡Oxycel, Deseret Medical, Inc., Sandy, UT.
§Surgicel, Johnson and Johnson Products, Inc., New Brunswick, NJ.
‖Gelfoam, The Upjohn Co., Kalamazoo, MI.
¶Avitene, American Critical Care, McGaw Park, IL.
**Thrombostat, Parke, Davis & Co., Detroit, MI.

alcohol to permit noncovalent attachment of hydrochloric acid to amine groups on the collagen molecule and preservation of its essential morphology. BT is produced through a conversion reaction in which prothrombin is activated by tissue thromboplastin in the presence of calcium chloride. After standardization of potency by dilution, thrombin solution is sterilized by filtration, poured into vials, dried from the frozen state, and sealed under aseptic conditions. BT can be combined with an equal volume of fibrinogen concentrate to produce fibrin glue by the reaction:

$$\text{Fibrinogen} \xrightarrow{\text{Thrombin}} \text{Fibrin monomer} \xrightarrow[\substack{\text{Factor XIII} \\ \downarrow Ca^{++}}]{} \text{Fibrin polymer}$$

The reaction can be enhanced by reconstitution of BT in 40 mM calcium chloride.

Beeswax has been used almost exclusively to arrest bleeding from the cut edges of cancellous bone. Its use was first described by Horsley in 1882.[21] The most commonly used bone wax currently available has a formula of refined beeswax 88% (w/w) and isopropyl palmitate 12% (w/w). The hemostatic action of bone wax is physical, as the wax tamponades the bleeding edges of the cut bone. Unwanted accompaniments to its hemostatic benefit are a foreign body giant cell response, persistence of wax at the bony site for years, and a physical barrier to bony union.[22] Acting as a foreign body, bone wax significantly impairs the ability of cancellous bone to kill bacteria.[23]

In 1977, Lawrie reported a new absorbable bone hemostatic sealant containing stabilized fibrin, soluble collagen, glycerol, and dextran that had the consistency of putty.[24] Its hemostatic effect appears to be by tamponade, but both the fibrin and collagen may contribute to local hemostasis. It was a more efficient hemostatic agent than bone wax and it did not interfere with bone healing.[25] Absorption was complete within 3 weeks. The effect of this stabilized fibrin and collagen paste on bacterial clearance has not been examined.

In experimental studies, Cobden and colleagues evaluated the efficacy of MC, BT-soaked AGF, and BT powder as topical hemostatic agents for bleeding cancellous bone.[16] All three agents significantly reduced bleeding compared with the controls, with MC being the most effective. At 3 months, there was no evidence that MC and BT-soaked AGF interfered with bone healing. Their influence on infection in this clinical setting was not investigated.

Most experimental studies have demonstrated that the absorbable hemostatic agents damaged tissue defenses and invited the development of infection. Jenkins and his colleagues pointed out that in the presence of contamination or infection, AGF may act as a culture medium and may influence the development and propagation of infection.[26, 27] The experiments of Cipolla and Narat demonstrated that AGF and OC intensified infection due to *Staphylococcus aureus* in the subcutaneous tissue of dogs.[28] Moistening these absorbable agents with penicillin did not prevent infection. However, intramuscular administration of penicillin in oil inhibited the potentiation of infection caused by the absorbable hemostatic agents. Hinman and Babcock reported that OC and AGF enhanced the incidence of infection of contaminated nephrotomy incisions as compared to control wounds without the hemostatic agent subjected to a comparable amount of the suspension of feces.[29]

It was possible to produce a dose response curve for ORC by varying the quantity employed and by maintaining a constant bacterial inoculum which emphasizes the importance of using the minimal amount of ORC consistent with satisfactory hemostasis. No such dose response curve could be obtained for MC because significant infection occurred at even the smallest doses studied. Because ORC and MC were equally effective in controlling bleeding from raw surfaces, the advantage of ORC as compared to MC from the standpoint of infection makes it the superior hemostatic agent.[30]

Laufman and Method showed the deleterious effects of placing AGF and OC in contact with anastomoses of the large intestine in dogs.[31] They believed that the increased incidence of perforation and peritonitis with topical hemostatic agents was due to their ability to act as a culture medium for bacteria. In another experimental study, Uhrich demonstrated that OC did not prevent leakage from the large intestinal anastomotic line when a single through-and-through suture end-to-end anastomosis was performed in dogs.[32] In addition, OC appeared to promote the growth of bacteria in the infected peritoneal cavity. Chamberlain and co-workers demonstrated that absorbable gelatin sponge in apposition to an intestinal anastomosis increased the risk of peritonitis and fatal perforation in dogs.[33] Impregnation of this sponge with crystalline penicillin was effective in preventing perforation of the anastomosis and local abscess formation.

In contrast to the other investigations that document an infection-potentiating effect for topical hemostatic agents, Dineen[34–36] and Dineen and Kuchta[37] reported that ORC reduced the bacterial population in vitro and in vivo. Its mode of antibacterial action was explained, in part, by its low pH. In vitro, most of its activity was blocked by the addition of sodium hydroxide. These researchers also showed that ORC prevented infection in several different experimental models.[34–37] In contaminated subcutaneous wounds in guinea pigs, Dineen found that ORC prevented the development of infection.[34] AGF had no demonstrable antibacterial activity in wounds subjected to comparable bacteria inocula. Dineen reported that ORC prevented sepsis following an intravenous bacterial challenge.[35] In dogs with Teflon aortic patches, wrapping the area of the Teflon patch with ORC before the bacterial challenge reduced the bacterial contamination of the patches as compared to animals without ORC. Similarly, ORC decreased the level of contamination in splenotomy sites as compared to AGF following an intravenous injection of a bacterial inoculum.[36] In another experimental model that simulated the clinical situation of infected subdiaphragmatic blood clots, animals treated with ORC showed longer survival times and no development of abscesses and/or peritonitis following an intravenous bacterial challenge as compared to control animals or those treated with either AGF or MC who died within 5 days of frank peritonitis and/or abdominal abscess.[37]

European surgeons have had broad experience with a variety of surgical applications of fibrin glue, a biological adhesive prepared from commercially pooled human plasma.[38, 39] Hemostatic use of the glue can be facilitated by combination with an AGF. The Food and Drug Administration has not approved this product for use because of a high associated risk of hepatitis and acquired immunodeficiency syndrome from the pooled human plasma used in the production of fibrinogen, an essential component of the glue. However, it is possible to produce a fibrin glue from the patient's own blood, thereby circumventing this problem.

DRAINS

Use of surgical drainage in a clinical setting requires a delicate weighing of potential benefits and harmful effects. The obvious beneficial effect of drainage is its ability to evacuate potentially harmful collections of certain fluids like pus, blood, bile, and gastric and pancreatic juices from wounds or body cavities. Pus is detrimental to the healing wounds. Hippocrates noted poor healing in wounds with collections of purulent exudate. Carrel and Hartmann found that when a surgical wound became infected, repair was arrested or regressed.[40] Carrel also noted that an abscess far removed from the site of a healing clean wound delayed its healing.[41] A similar effect was obtained when sterile pus was injected under the skin of an animal while the healing of a wound was observed. In an experimental study, Smith and Enquist reported that subacute staphylococcal wound infection in animals initiated profound gross, histological, and biochemical changes in wound healing, as well as in other tissues distant from the site of infection.[42] The infected wounds were weaker than the control wounds in the early postoperative period. Consequently, pus within a wound or body cavity exerts many deleterious effects on the host and should be removed whenever a localized collection can be drained.

Sterile collections of blood per se are not major irritants to tissues, but hemoglobin enhances bacterial virulence. Animal studies with dogs and rats performed by Davis and Yull have demonstrated that an intraperitoneal injection of Escherichia coli (10^8 to 10^{11} organisms) was not lethal.[43] However, if hemoglobin at a concentration of 4 g per cent or greater was added to the inoculum, approximately 70 per cent of the animals died within 24 hours. The precise mechanisms by which hemoglobin enhances infection had defied definition until the recent studies of Pruett and his colleagues.[44] They demonstrated that leukotoxins resulted from E. coli growth in solutions of pure hemoglobin. These leukotoxins severely damaged neutrophils and accounted for the infection-potentiating effect of hemoglobin in experimental peritonitis. There was no experimental support for the hypothesis that hemoglobin provided a nutritional boost to the growth of E. coli. Red blood cells also enhance subcutaneous infection in experimental animals. Krizek and Davis found that when red blood cells were injected into the same subcutaneous tissue site as E. coli, a serious and often fatal infection occurred, whereas the infection with bacteria alone proved relatively innocuous.[45] In addition, the heme moiety of hemoglobin may contribute to the production of oxygen free radicals that can produce direct cell damage.[46]

There is also no doubt that collections of bile and gastric juice are harmful. In a recent report, Cohn and colleagues reviewed the pathophysiology of bile peritonitis.[47] Leakage of sterile bile into the peritoneal cavity caused a generalized exudation of protein-rich fluid. Gallbladder bile was considerably more irritating than hepatic bile, presumably because it was more concentrated. Rewbridge and Hrdina demonstrated that the inflamed and injured intestinal wall permitted transmigration of enteric and clostridial organisms which grew rapidly in the bile-laden fluid.[48] The presence of bacteria severely potentiated the damaging effects of the bile, leading to a virulent peritonitis. Therefore, extravasated bile should always be removed from the peritoneal cavity.

The spillage of gastric contents into the peritoneal cavity inflicts a severe injury. Initially, the process is a sterile one, the inflammatory reaction of the peritoneum being attributable to the corrosive properties of acid and pepsin. The damaging effects of pancreatic juices on tissues are also well documented by Thal and his associates,[49] as well as others.[50] Enzymes liberated during the early stages of hemorrhagic pancreatitis or traumatic injury to the pancreas can digest fats, carbohydrates, and proteins. The major proteolytic enzymes are secreted in inactive forms, trypsinogen and chymotrypsinogen. They are then activated by either trypsin or intestinal kinases. Peritoneal inflammation and widespread fat necrosis result from enzymatic digestion by spilled potent proteolytic enzymes.

The obvious beneficial effect of drainage is its ability to evacuate collections of these harmful fluids from either wounds or body cavities. When the fluids must be removed against gravity, active drainage resulting from an applied vacuum is required. When the vacuum is applied directly to the wound or body cavity without an external vent, closed wound drainage results. The efficiency of this drainage system can be improved by adding a second lumen to the tube that serves as an external vent.[51] This double lumen tube, known as a sump tube, prevents occlusion of the tube fenestrations by collapsed tissue.

Despite the advantages of vented drainage, we have been hesitant to use sump tubes for drainage of either cavities or wounds because of the dangers of retrograde contamination of particulate matter and bacteria passing through the air vent into the wound or cavity that contains a culture-rich medium. This hazard has been eliminated by attaching a filter to the air vent lumen of the sump tube.[51]

The performance of the vented drainage tube has also been enhanced by coating its surfaces with a new hydrogel coating[52] formed by a reaction of polyvinylpyrrolidone and an isocyanate prepolymer.* Being a hydrogel, it absorbs

_____

*Axiom Medical, Inc., Paramount, CA.

water and has a low coefficient of friction. This surface coating limits the adherence of blood clots to the drain and facilitates its removal from the wound.

Recent advances in interventional radiology have demonstrated the value of percutaneous aspiration (PCA) and drainage (PCD) in patients with abscesses. Catheter drainage is performed by a modified Seldinger technique, with the passage of the catheter being monitored by either ultrasound or computed tomography.[53] The indications for the technique can be diagnostic, palliative, or therapeutic. Cytological and microbiological examination of the aspirate can detect the presence of malignancy as well as the responsible pathogen. Palliation is defined as temporary control of the infection in which the clinical infection is relived, but the infectious process is not cured until an elective operative procedure is performed. PCD is therapeutic in a well-localized, unilocular bacterial abscess with a success rate of 96 per cent.[54] While PCD appears to be the preferred method of management of the latter abscess, it is uniformly unsuccessful in treating collections that contain semisolid or solid particulate matter (e.g., organized hematoma, parapancreatic phlegmon, fungal infections, necrotic infected tumor metastases).

In instances in which no definite localized collection of fluid exists, drainage must be considered prophylactic, and its potential harmful effects become more important. Drains act as retrograde conduits through which skin contaminants gain entrance into the wound. Cerise and associates performed a splenectomy in rabbits and inoculated the skin around the drain tract with type 6 streptococcus, taking care not to inoculate the drain.[55] Twenty per cent of the animals had positive intraperitoneal cultures at 24 hours, and 56 per cent at 72 hours, compared to a positive culture rate of only 5 per cent in undrained animals.

The air vent in a sump tube provides another potential conduit for organisms. Baker and Borchardt[56] demonstrated that the degree of contamination was proportional to the degree of suction applied. When continuous suction was employed at 10 psi, airborne contamination occurred, but lowering the vacuum pressure attached to suction eliminated this airborne contamination. Plugging the vents with cotton or gauze or use of a synthetic air filter provided the same benefit.[57]

The presence of drains impairs tissue resistance to infection. In an experimental study by Magee and associates, placement of drains within experimental wounds exposed to subinfective inoculations of bacteria greatly enhanced the rate of wound infection compared to that in undrained controls.[57] Both Silastic and Penrose drains dramatically enhanced the infection rate of soft-tissue wounds in guinea pigs. The rate of infection when the drain was brought out through the wound was similar to the rate when the drain lay entirely within the wound, suggesting a deleterious effect of the drain per se.

Studies of the impairment of wound healing in the presence of drains have been performed with intestinal anastomoses. Berliner and his associates performed proximal and distal intestinal anastomoses in dogs, draining one anastomosis in each dog.[58] Three of the 20 nondrained anastomoses leaked compared to 11 to 20 drained anastomoses and, of these, anastomotic disruption proved fatal in four cases. Manz and his colleagues confirmed the damaging effects of drains on colonic anastomoses in dogs.[59] Of 20 dogs with Penrose drainage at their anastomoses, 9 died of anastomotic disruption and peritonitis, and the remainder had extensive adhesions as well as varying degrees of stricture formation. All dogs with drainage had evidence of bacterial contamination at the site of the anastomosis at the necropsy, while the control dogs had only filmy adhesions and no stricture formation.

SKIN CLOSURE

The technique of skin closure selected depends on the type of wound. There are essentially two types of skin wounds. One type is characterized by a loss of tissue, while the other has no evidence of tissue loss. In the latter, primary closure can be accomplished simply by reapproximating the divided skin edges by a variety of methods. For wounds with associated tissue loss, grafts or flaps are often required to close the defect. This chapter discusses only the use of devices for attaining the reapproximation of divided skin.

Timing of Closure

The timing of the closure is critical. Immediate closure should be reserved for (1) wounds resulting from elective procedures classified as either clean, refined-clean, or clean-contaminated, and (2) traumatic wounds that have not been contaminated by feces, saliva, purulent exudate, or soil. Immediate approximation of the skin edges of this group of wounds should be accompanied by an extremely low infection rate (less than 5 per cent, regardless of the closure technique employed).

Open wound management with delayed primary closure is recommended for wounds that have a high risk of infection following primary closure. The principles of delayed primary closure arose from the experience of military surgeons, who learned repeatedly over the centuries that immediate closure of battle wounds frequently resulted in infection and that such wounds were best left open until delayed primary closure could be undertaken. All emergency war wounds, regardless of their appearance, are candidates for delayed primary closure. In these cases, the wound should be explored to remove foreign bodies, to rule out the presence of damage to specialized structures (e.g., vessels, nerves, bone), and to relieve increased compartmental pressure that may follow edema or slow bleeding into a fascia-enclosed muscle compartment. The removal of devitalized tissue is advisable, but in practice is difficult as its definition is unclear. Wounds contacted by feces, saliva, purulent exudates, or soil infection potentiating fractions are also candidates for open wound management. When wound care is delayed for more than 6 hours, open management is recommended due to the increased risk of infection.

The rationale for delayed primary closure is that the healing open wound will gain resistance to infection and permit an uncomplicated closure. The reparative process associated with this developing resistance to infection in the open wound undergoing primary closure is associated with accelerated skin healing. In addition, Johnson and associates showed that secondary closure of the subcutaneous tissue and skin results in stronger fascial strength than that obtained by primary closure.[60]

Methods and Materials

Adhesives, staples, tapes, and sutures can all provide an accurate and secure approximation of the skin edges. Ideally, the choice should be based on the biological interaction of the materials employed, the tissue configuration, and the biomechanical properties of the wound. The tissue should be held in apposition until the tensile strength of the wound is sufficient to withstand stress. A common theme of the few reportable investigations is that all biomaterials placed within the tissue damage the host defenses and invite infection.

Adhesives

Cyanoacrylate tissue adhesives have been advocated for repair of organs or as hemostatic agents in emergency or mass combat casualty situations.[61-63] Mathes and Terry demonstrated that methyl-2-cyanoacrylate adhesive caused successful hemostasis in 14 of 16 longitudinal nephrotomies in dogs.[62] The adhesive failed to achieve adequate hemostasis in two nephrotomies and capsule sutures were required to stop bleeding. Microscopic examination of the nephrotomies treated with the adhesive revealed extensive scar formation. One kidney contained several calculi, measuring 2 to 4 mm in diameter, which probably resulted from the adhesive entering the renal calyx. Fein and co-workers compared the efficacy of suture repair of a kidney in experimental animals to that repaired with n-butyl cyanoacrylate.[64] The principal advantage of cyanoacrylate closure was the speed with which hemostasis and repair were achieved. The disadvantage included failure of hemostasis caused by excessive bleeding, increased adhesions at the surgical site and increased incidence of calculi. It was concluded that the tissue adhesive will be a useful adjunct in the management of renal injuries once a more suitable monomer is found.

Furka and colleagues described an experimental procedure for closing longitudinal nephrotomy incisions that employed a tissue adhesive and eliminated the need for sutures in the renal parenchyma.[65] The tissue adhesive, histoacryl-N-blau, permitted approximation of the two halves of the organ without sutures. The incision was then covered by regenerated cellulose impregnated with a minimal amount of tissue adhesive. During the incision and closure, the hilum was temporarily constricted with noncrushing clamps. This technique produced rapid and reliable hemostasis followed by complete absorption of the hemostatic agents. The use of currently available tissue adhesives should be approached with caution because the polymer acts as a barrier between the growing edges of the wound, which delays healing and increases susceptibility to infection.[66]

Fibrin glue has also been used as an adhesive for wound repair. Ihara and co-workers demonstrated the effects of fibrin sealant as a hemostatic and fixational agent in incisional skin wounds and transplants in burn patients.[67] Jørgensen and associates examined the mechanical strength of rat skin incisions treated with fibrin glue.[68] Their results demonstrated that the fibrin sealant provided mechanical strength in the initial period (0 to 4 days) of healing, while the control wounds possessed little independent strength. They also showed that the fibrin sealant delayed the development of mechanical strength at 20 days after wounding, but did not interfere with wound repair after 42 days of healing.

Clips and Staples

The surgeon's burgeoning interest in clips and staples for wound closure has provided the impetus for an increasing number of scientific studies on their influence on the biology of wound repair and infection. In 1971, Stephens and colleagues compared the breaking strength of wounds approximated by continuous sutures of 4-0 monofilament stainless steel wire to those closed by Michel clips using rats as the experimental animal.[69] Seven days after closure, the breaking strength of the wounds closed by Michel clips (602 ± 29.8 g) was significantly greater than that of wounds approximated by wire (488.8 ± 27.7 g) (p < 0.01). Early removal of wire sutures on the third postoperative day was associated with a greater breaking strength (674.0 ± 27.0 gm) than that encountered in wounds in which the sutures were left in the wound for 7 days (506.7 ± 23.0 g) (p < 0.001). In similar studies, Myers and colleagues reported that early removal of sutures was associated with an increase in breaking strength of the skin wounds.[70]

The results from the investigation by Stephens and co-workers[69] contrast dramatically with those reported by Harrison and associates[71] who found skin clips to have a deleterious effect on wound healing in piglet wounds examined at the fifth, seventh, and fourteenth postoperative days. Wounds approximated by clips had a significantly lower tensile strength at all stages than those approximated by interrupted 2-0 monofilament nylon sutures. Comparison of the strength of 14 day wounds in which clips had been removed after only 7 days showed them to be significantly stronger than similar wounds in which the clips had been retained for the entire 14 day period. Retention of the nylon sutures during the second week of healing produced no significant change in strength as compared to similar wounds in which the sutures were removed early. Harrison and co-workers noted progressive ulceration at the site of contact of clip teeth to the skin that may account for the deleterious effects on wound healing.[71]

More recently, Jewell and associates compared the healing of sutured wounds to that of stapled wounds in the rat.[72] The skin incisions

in one experimental group were closed with regular size Proximate* staples implanted at 5 mm intervals, while skin incisions in the remaining group were approximated by interrupted 4-0 monofilament nylon sutures placed at 5 mm intervals. Staples and sutures were removed from the wounds on the seventh postoperative day. They reported no significant difference between the mean breaking strength of wounds with either staples or sutures at 10, 42, and 180 days after closure. However, there was a significant difference in the breaking strength at 21 days, with the sutured wounds being slightly stronger than the stapled wounds.

Chvapil examined the influence of staple configuration on the magnitude of tissue injury and the biology of wound repair.[73] He tested the hypothesis that arcuate staples elicited different tissue reactions than rectangular staples. His analysis indicated a more uniform distribution of stresses in the nonlinear elastic environment around the arcuate staple and accumulation of stresses (crowding of the tissue elements) at the rectangular corner of a staple.

It was surprising that Chvapil and colleagues reported that the magnitude of tissue injury inflicted by the staples did not correlate with the magnitude of the breaking strength of skin incisions in the neck, abdomen, and groin in pigs closed separately by the three different staples.[73] Wounds closed by the rectangular staple (Premium†) exhibited a significantly greater breaking strength than that of wounds closed by either the arcuate staple or a different brand of rectangular staple (Proximate), irrespective of the anatomical location of the incision.

The limited tissue damage inflicted by the arcuate staple as compared to the rectangular staple did not appear to minimize the pain of staple penetration or removal. In a clinical study by Silloway and co-workers, rectangular and arcuate staples were implanted into the medial aspect of the forearm of eight healthy volunteers.[74] After staple implantation and extraction, the patients were asked to grade the severity of the pain using a numerical scale. The pain associated with staple implantation was significantly greater than that caused by staple removal. However, the configuration of the staple did not influence the magnitude of pain associated with either staple implantation or removal. While the subjects tolerated implantation of four staples, they were reluctant to have implantation of additional staples without infiltration anesthesia.

---

*Ethicon, Inc., Somerville, NJ.
†US Surgical Corp, Norwalk, CT.

There is uniform agreement that wounds closed by staples exhibit a superior resistance to infection than wounds contaminated by the least reactive suture. In an experimental study, Johnson and colleagues compared the resistance to infection of contaminated wounds approximated by either tapes, rectangular (Premium) staples, or sutures.[75] Wounds closed by tape exhibited the greatest resistance to infection, followed by the stapled wounds, and then the sutured wounds. The superiority of tape closure was evident at all levels of contamination except 5×10^7, at which all wounds were destined to develop infection regardless of the closure technique. In the presence of lower bacterial inocula, wounds approximated by staples exhibited a lower rate of infection than with the least reactive nonabsorbable suture, monofilament nylon. The infection rate in these wounds correlated with the wound bacterial counts. Sutured wounds exhibited the highest bacterial counts, followed by stapled wounds and then taped wounds. When the infection rate of wounds reached 100 per cent, the bacterial counts did not differ significantly.

The superior resistance of stapled wounds to infection as compared to sutured wounds was confirmed by the experimental study of Stillman and colleagues.[76] In contaminated wounds in mice, stapled wounds displayed a lower incidence of infection than wounds approximated by either percutaneous sutures (4-0 silk, 4-0 monofilament nylon, 4-0 polyglycolic acid) or subcuticular sutures (4-0 polyglycolic acid).

In a recent study, we examined the influence of the staple configuration as well as its depth of implantation on the resistance of the wound to infection in experimental animals.[107] The results demonstrated that neither factor significantly altered the tissue's resistance to infection. Even though we were not able to demonstrate any deleterious effects of deeply implanted staples on the tissue defenses, it is important to remember that staple cross members that are flush with the skin can result in permanent transverse scars ("cross-hatching").

A variety of disposable skin stapling devices are now commercially available for use in surgery. The selection of a skin stapler by a surgeon will be determined primarily by its mechanical performance. Ideally, the device should be designed so that it does not obstruct the surgeon's view of the wound edge. Moreover, the stapler should have a prepositioning mechanism that permits the surgeon to hold the staple securely during its formation. The configuration of the stapler should also allow the position of its cartridge to be adjusted manually to facilitate placement of the staple, and there should be an ejector spring that automatically releases the staple. Finally, the handling characteristics of the stapler should be such that the surgeon can easily implant a large number of staples without becoming fatigued.

Sutures

Sutures remain the most common method of approximating the divided edges of the tissue. Selection of a suture material is based on its biological interaction with the wound as well as its mechanical performance in vivo and in vitro. Measurements of the in vivo degradation of sutures separate them into two general classes.[77] Sutures that undergo rapid degradation in tissues, losing their tensile strength within 60 days, are considered absorbable; those that maintain their tensile strength for longer than 60 days are nonabsorbable sutures. This terminology is somewhat misleading, because even some nonabsorbable sutures (e.g., silk, cotton, nylon) lose their tensile strength during this 60 day time interval. Postlethwait measured the tensile strength of implanted nonabsorbable sutures during a period of 2 years.[78] Silk lost approximately one half of its tensile strength in 1 year and had no strength at the end of 2 years; cotton lost 50 per cent of its strength in 6 months, but still had 30 to 40 per cent of its strength at the end of the 2 years; and nylon lost approximately 25 per cent of its original strength throughout the 2 year observation period.

Some nonabsorbable sutures are made from natural fibers include silk, cotton and linen, while modern chemistry has developed a variety of synthetic fibers, including polyamides (nylon), polyesters (Dacron), polyolefins (polyethylene, polypropylene), and polybutester. The latter suture is a block copolymer that contains poly(butylene) terephthalate (84%) and poly(tetramethylene ether) glycol terephthalate (16%). The nonabsorbable sutures may also be characterized by their physical configuration. Sutures constructed from one filament are called monofilament sutures (nylon, polyethylene, polypropylene, polybutester, and stainless steel); those containing multiple fibers are called multifilament sutures (nylon, polyester, stainless steel, silk, and cotton).

The absorbable sutures are made from either the submucosa of sheep or bovine small intestine (gut) or from reconstituted collagen manufactured from tendon collagen of beef (collagen). This collagenous tissue is treated in an aldehyde solution, which crosslinks and strengthens the suture, making it more resistant to enzymatic degradation. Suture materials treated in this way are called plain gut or collagen. If the suture is additionally treated in chromium trioxide, it becomes chromic gut or collagen, which is more highly crosslinked than plain gut or collagen and more resistant to absorption. The plain gut and collagen and chromic gut and collagen sutures are composed of several plies that have been twisted slightly, machine ground, and polished to yield a relatively smooth surface and monofilament-like diameter. Despite the development of modern manufacturing processes, these collagen sutures still have the shortcomings of variable strength and unpredictable absorption.[79] The eventual reduction in tensile strength of these sutures is caused by enzymatic degradation by acid hydrolytic and collagenolytic enzymes. Salthouse and colleagues have demonstrated that gut and collagen resorb due to sequential attacks by lysosomal enzymes.[80] In most locations, this degradation is started by acid phosphatases, with leucine amniopeptidase playing a more important role later in the absorption period. Collagenase was also thought to contribute to the enzymatic degradation of these gut or collagen sutures.

A search for a synthetic substitute for collagen or gut sutures began in the 1960s,[81] and procedures were soon perfected for the synthesis of high molecular weight polyglycolic acid and the next homologue in this series of alpha polyesters, polylactic acid, which led to the development of the polyglycolic acid and polyglactin 910 sutures.[82] The copolymers of polyglactin 910 are prepared by polymerizing nine parts of glycolide with one part of lactide, while the polyglycolic acid sutures are produced from the homopolymer. Because of the inherent rigidity of these copolymers, monofilament sutures produced from polyglactin 910 or polyglycolic acid sutures are too stiff for surgical use and can be used as a monofilament suture only in the very finest size. Consequently, these high molecular weight polymers are extruded into thin filaments and braided. The polyglycolic acid and polyglactin 910 sutures lose their strength in tissues during a 4 week after implantation.

The surfaces of these synthetic sutures are coated to decrease their high coefficient of friction.[83] The coating on the polyglycolic acid suture is the absorbable surface lubricant, poloxamer 188. The polyglactin 910 suture is coated with an absorbable mixture of calcium stearate and a copolymer of lactic acid (65%) and glycolic acid (35%).

A monofilament absorbable suture, polydioxanone, has been developed by polymerizing the monomer in the presence of a suitable catalyst.[84] This polymer is processed into small granules and melt-extruded through appropriate dies into monofilaments of the desired size. Another synthetic absorbable monofilament suture is glycolide trimethylene carbonate (GTMC) suture.[85] GTMC is a linear copolymer made by reacting trimethylene carbonate (TMC) and glycolide with diethylene glycol as an initiator and stannous chloride dihydrate as the catalyst. The strength of these monofilament sutures is maintained in vivo much longer than that of the braided synthetic absorbable suture. These monofilament sutures retain approximately 70% of their breaking strength following implantation for 28 days and 13 per cent of their original strength at 56 days. In contrast, braided absorbable sutures retain only 1 to 5 per cent of their strength at 28 days.

The direct correlation of molecular weight and breaking strength of the synthetic absorbable sutures with both in vivo and in vitro incubation implies a similar mechanism of degradation. Because in vitro incubation gives only a buffered aqueous environment, the chemical degradation of these sutures appears to be by nonenzymatic hydrolysis of the ester bonds. In contrast, gut or collagen sutures, being proteinaceous substances, are degraded primarily by the action of proteolytic enzymes.

All sutures damage the local tissue defenses to infection, and several mechanisms have been implicated.

1. The trauma of inserting a needle is sufficient to cause an inflammatory response.

2. The physician's suturing technique is crucially important. Sutures tied too tightly impair blood supply and cause tissue necrosis.[82]

3. Sutures that penetrate the intact skin provide an avenue for wound contamination via the perisutural cuff.

4. The presence of the suture material itself increases the tissue's susceptibility to infection. The effect of this local injury on tissue defenses is related to the type of suture within the wound (e.g., diameter, length) and to its chemical reaction.

The infection-potentiating effects of suture materials are listed in Table 35–1. Synthetic absorbable sutures elicit the least inflammatory response of the absorbable sutures, followed by plain gut, and then chromic gut. Of the nonabsorbable sutures, nylon and polypropylene are the least reactive. The infection-potentiating effect of the polybutester suture has not been reported.

Table 35–1. INFECTION POTENTIATING EFFECT OF SURGICAL SUTURES

Absorbable	Nonabsorbable
Synthetic*	Nylon (polypropylene)
Plain gut	Dacron (coated or noncoated)
Chromic gut	Metal
	Silk

*Listed in order of reactivity.

The relatively high infection rates encountered with either monofilament or multifilament stainless steel sutures may be the result of either their chemical or their physical configuration. Stainless steel is not generally as inert as pure polymers and undergoes degradation in vivo. In addition, metallic sutures are so stiff that movement induces tissue damage and impairs the wound's ability to resist infection.

Sutures made of natural fibers potentiate infection more than any other nonabsorbable sutures, which correlates with the tissue's reaction to these sutures in clean wounds. It would appear from these experimental studies that the use of silk and cotton should be avoided in wounds having known gross bacterial contamination.

Surprisingly, our studies indicated that the physical configuration of the suture had a relatively unimportant role in the development of infection.[77] Although the incidence of infection in contaminated tissue containing monofilament sutures was lower than in those containing multifilament sutures, these differences were not statistically significant. Using a model similar to that reported by our laboratory, Sharp and associates reported that synthetic sutures potentiated infection less than the nonsynthetic sutures.[86] The synthetic monofilament sutures were associated with lower rates of infection than encountered with the multifilament synthetic sutures exposed to the same bacterial inocula. The superiority of the synthetic absorbable sutures over the naturally occurring gut sutures was also evident using this model.

Proper selection and placement of sutures is critical, because failure of the suture itself, or the tissue through which it passes, will permit the wound to reopen. A series of recent investigations have re-evaluated suture-tying techniques and should be consulted.[87–89]

The selection of the technique for sutural closure is influenced by the wound's configuration and biomechanical properties as well as other special circumstances. In general, the techniques of sutural closure of skin can be divided into two types. In one technique, sutures (percutaneous) are passed through the epidermis and dermis. In the other, the suture (dermal or subcuticular) reapproximates the divided edges of the dermis without penetrating the epidermis. Occasionally, dermal and percutaneous sutures are used together. Dermal or percutaneous sutures can be employed either as continuous ("running") or interrupted sutures. In a running suture, the loops are connected and are tied or otherwise fixed only at the ends of the incision. In interrupted suturing, each stitch is a separate knotted loop that has no connection with adjacent loops.

Percutaneous sutures of either monofilament nylon or polypropylene are excellent for skin closure of skin wounds because they exert the least damage to the wound defenses.[77] The polybutester type of suture has unique mechanical performance characteristics that may be advantageous for skin closure.[90] This new monifilament suture exhibits distinct differences in elongation as compared to other sutures, with low forces yielding significantly greater elongation than in other monofilament sutures. In addition, its elasticity is superior, allowing the suture to return to its original length once the load is removed.

Percutaneous sutures are recommended for closure of stellate lacerations resulting from crush injuries. In these wounds, meticulous percutaneous suture closure of the skin edges approximates the wound more exactly than does tape. Closing these wounds often is like putting together a jigsaw puzzle, and tapes have little practical value. Undoubtedly, the more accurate approximation of skin edges by skillfully applied sutures leads to a more pleasing cosmetic result.

Because the magnitude of the suture's damage of the local tissue defenses is related to the quantity of the suture within the wound (e.g., diameter, length), we employ the most narrow diameter suture (5-0 or 6-0) whose strength is sufficient to resist disruption of the skin wound. By approximating the midportion and the bisected portions of the unclosed wound with percutaneous sutures, the least length of suture can be employed in the skin closure. An interrupted dermal suture placed in each quadrant of the wound subjected to strong static and dynamic skin tensions provides sufficient strength to permit early suture removal. Sutural closure of the adipose tissue beneath the skin should be avoided.[91] Obliteration of this potential dead space between the cut edges of adipose tissue by even the least reactive suture increases the incidence of infection.

In closing wound edges of different thickness, the needle should be passed through one edge of the wound and drawn out before re-entering through the other side. This will ensure that the needle will be inserted at comparable levels on each side of the wound. Unless appropriate adjustment of the bite is made on the thinner side, uneven coaptation of the skin will occur, resulting in a step-off scar.

Dermal (subcuticular) sutures, either interrupted or continuous, can be used alone or as adjuncts to percutaneous sutures in wounds subjected to strong skin tensions as an added precaution against disruption of the wound. Some surgeons prefer a synthetic absorbable suture for dermal closure, while others favor a synthetic nonabsorbable suture. When continuous nonabsorbable sutures are employed, they should be removed before the eighth day after wound closure to prevent the development of needle puncture scars.

Percutaneous sutures should be avoided in favor of dermal sutures (1) in infants or children frightened at the prospects of suture removal, (2) when follow-up appointments are difficult to keep, and (3) when wounds are covered by casts. When dermal closure alone is used, it is advisable to immediately tape skin closures to the wound edges to produce a more accurate approximation of the epidermis.

The influence of dermal suture closure on the wound infection rate is the subject of debate. Certainly, dermal suture closure reduces or totally prevents the normal serosanguinous discharge noted on surgical dressings that can serve as a culture medium for bacteria. In a prospective clinical trial by Foster and co-workers in 127 patients after appendectomy, wound infection were significantly more common with dermal polyglycolic acid sutures than with percutaneous interrupted nylon sutures.[92] In another clinical study by Hopkinson and Bullen involving 184 patients after appendectomy, the infection rate in wounds closed with interrupted polypropylene sutures did not differ from that of wounds approximated by continuous dermal polypropylene sutures.[93] However, there is general agreement that wounds subjected to continuous dermal (subcuticular) closure are more resistant to exogenous bacterial contamination than wounds closed by percutaneous sutures.[94] The percutaneous suture serves as an avenue for the migration of bacteria from the skin surface into the wound. After infection develops beneath the dermal skin closure, the collecting purulent exudate spreads preferentially between the divided edges of fat rather than penetrating the sutural closure, and by the time infection becomes clinically apparent, it has involved the entire extent of the wound.

This situation is distinct from the localized collections of purulent discharge encountered in infected taped closed wounds. In the latter circumstance, the purulent discharge first exits between its wound edges before spreading between the divided layers of adipose tissue.

Another concern about continuous dermal nonabsorbable suture is that suture pull-out may require considerable force that may break the suture and cause discomfort. Several technical considerations may facilitate suture removal.[95] First, polypropylene suture is advocated over other monofilament sutures because its surface displays the lowest coefficient of friction facilitating removal. In addition, the continuous dermal polypropylene sutures should be surfaced as a percutaneous suture every 5 to 6 cm to allow shorter segments of the suture to be removed. Suture pull-out by elastic traction applied over minutes to hours is considerably easier than manual traction. Despite the immediate aesthetically pleasing appearance of dermal skin closure, it does not improve the cosmetic appearance of the scar.[96]

However, the type of sutures used to approximate fascia (galea aponeurotica) has considerable influence on the width and depth of skin scars. In a study by Nordström and Nordström of a group of patients undergoing scalp excision for correction of androgenic alopecia, polypropylene sutures reduced the postoperative stretching and depth of skin scars more than did comparable size polyglycolic acid sutures.[97]

Another approach to reducing the static skin tensions on the wound is to undermine its edges prior to closure. Despite common clinical usage of this technique, there has been only one experimental study that objectively evaluated its effects on wound closure. In this in vivo study, McGuire identified the directional orientation of the static skin tensions by observing the oval distortion of 6 mm circular skin biopsy sites in pigs.[98] At each location, the immediate change in the shape of the resulting defect indicated the magnitude and directional properties of the static skin tensions. The direction of the static skin tension lines corresponded to the long axis of the defects. Wounds made parallel to these static skin tension lines required less force and work to close initially, retracted less with initial excision, and benefited more from undermining than similar wounds oriented perpendicular to the static skin tension lines. Because undermining the wound margin decreases the forces required for wound closure, it should limit the width of the ultimate scar. However, this benefit must be weighed against the potential damage to the skin blood supply that may limit the host's defenses and invite infection. Consequently, we reserve undermining for wounds that are subjected to strong static and dynamic tensions with low levels of bacterial contamination during elective surgical procedures.

The selection of needles for suture closure is another important consideration. We recommend precision point cutting edge needles manufactured from stainless steel alloy American Society of Testing Materials (ASTM) 45500.[99] The strong yield and tensile strengths of this alloy permit the production of needles that are sharper and stronger (e.g., resistant to bending or breakage) than comparable size needles manufactured from other stainless steel alloys (ASTM 42000, ASTM 42200).

Tape

The superior resistance to infection of taped wounds as compared to sutured wounds makes tape closure a significant clinical tool.[100] The incidence of infection of contaminated wounds whose edges are approximated even with the least reactive suture is significantly higher than the infection rate of taped wounds subjected to a comparable level of contamination. The ease with which wounds can be closed by tape varies according to the anatomical and biomechanical properties of the wound site. Linear wounds in skin subjected to minimal static and dynamic tensions are easily approximated by tape. The relatively lax skin of the face and abdomen are amenable to wound closure by tapes. Contrary to the usual expectation, tape closure without sutures is more easily accomplished in obese patients. The thick cut edges of adipose tissue tend to evert the skin, facilitating tape skin closure. The taut skin of the extremities, subjected to frequent dynamic joint movements, requires that tape skin closures be supplemented with dermal sutures. The copious secretions from the skin of the axilla, palms, and soles also discourage tape adherence.

The difficulties encountered in performing sutureless tape closure of wounds subjected to strong tensions can be explained by the deformation of skin at the periphery of the wound. When the skin is cut, its inherent tensions retract its edges. As with any elastic membrane, the shrinkage in surface area of the skin is greatest at the wound margin and becomes progressively less as the distance from the wound increases. The extent of these changes is directly related to the magnitude of the static and dynamic forces within the skin. The use of dermal sutures prior to taping stretches the skin

to its uninjured dimensions and makes application of tape skin closures considerably easier. In wounds subjected to weak skin tensions, tape skin closure can be accomplished without the use of reinforcing dermal sutures. In such cases, the tape is first attached to the skin at one wound edge, and the other wound edge is pulled toward the taped edge before the remaining portion of the tape is applied to the skin.

When tape skin closures are employed to close linear lacerations subjected to weak tensions, the cosmetic results are excellent and many patients will require no further surgery. This method avoids the discomfort of suture removal and the development of suture puncture scars. An additional bonus is that the patient need not be subjected to the painful injection of the local anesthetic agent required for suturing. Scar revision, if needed later, can be done after some weeks or months under much more ideal conditions than in the Emergency Department. In elective surgery, the sedation will be better, the chance of contamination is reduced, and the blood supply of the damaged tissue can be more accurately determined. All of these factors lead to a superior aesthetic result with less emotional trauma to the patient and only a single visit to the operating theater. This closure technique is presently being used on approximately 10 per cent of the patients with lacerations seen in our medical center.

In the child or woman with glabrous skin, tape skin closures are good for closing transverse lacerations over the brow, under the chin, or across the malar prominence. After definitive taping, most of these wounds will heal with an imperceptible scar. In an editorial, McDowell advocates the use of tape skin closures for such wounds[101] and points out that "there is little reason to put these crying and upset children through a long and complicated surgical procedure, and their family through an exhausting financial and emotional wringer."

An ideal surgical wound closure tape would have the following performance characteristics.[102] It should be strong enough, even when wet, to withstand the forces disrupting the wound. Its adhesive should be sufficiently aggressive to adhere securely to the wound and maintain approximation of the wound edges. While a secure bond to skin is necessary for wound security, it also appears to be beneficial for the tape to stretch slightly under constant stress; this elongation under moderate loads reduces the shear forces on the underlying edematous skin, thereby preventing blister formation. Finally, the tape construction should provide an environment on the skin surface that is antithetical to bacterial growth. Bacterial proliferation under a tape may be a source of infection during the time in which epidermization of the wound is incomplete.

Wound closure tapes will not adhere to excessively wet skin. Drying with a gauze sponge sometimes does not completely remove wet exudate, and the residual fluid continues to impair tape adhesion. If not excessive, this can be overcome by applying an adhesive adjunct, such as compound benzoin tincture, to the skin prior to tape application, which enhances the immediate adhesion of the tape closures to the skin and reduces the chance for tape dislodgement. Inadvertent spillage of this adjunct should be avoided because it impairs the wound's ability to resist infection. To minimize the chance of contamination, the adhesive adjunct is applied in a thin film to the skin at the wound edge utilizing applicator sticks.

POSTOPERATIVE WOUND CARE

Postoperative wound care should optimize healing and should be tailored to the type of wound. In primarily closed wounds, the surgical dressing acts as a barrier against exogenous bacteria. Soaking with serum permits passage of bacteria through the dressing. Saturation of a dressing with fluid that wets both inner and outer surfaces, is called fluid strike-through. As long as its outer surface remains dry, however, a dressing will remain an effective barrier to bacterial contamination.

The length of time that dry dressing should cover the closed wound is based on knowledge of the period during which the wound is susceptible to bacterial penetration. Sutured wounds, as they heal, become increasingly resistant to the development of infection following surface contamination.[103] Swabbing the surface of the wound with either *Staphylococcus aureus* or *Escherichia coli* during the first 48 hours after closure caused localized gross infections. Contamination after the third postoperative day did not produce gross infection in the sutured wound. Thus barrier dressings are useful to protect the fresh incision from surface contamination in the first few days. Thereafter, removal of the dressing permits daily inspection and palpation of the wound.

Wounds closed with tape have a greater capacity to resist infection than do sutured

wounds.[104] Even immediate contamination seldom causes infection in any taped wounds. This resistance to infection after surface contamination reduces the need for protective dressings during the postoperative period in wounds free of sutures. In a real sense, the skin suture has the objectionable features of a small drain.

Another important purpose of some dressings is to exert pressure on the underlying tissues to minimize accumulation of intercellular fluid and limit the dead space. The application of pressure dressings is easiest on convex surfaces (e.g., skull, extremity). Maximal pressure should be applied to the wound site, as well as distal to it. Proximal to the wound, pressure is decreased to minimize any chance of compromising the venous or lymphatic return.

Due to its bulk, a pressure dressing will immobilize what it covers. This has the benefit of reducing lymphatic flow, thereby minimizing the spread of the wound microflora. Furthermore, immobilized tissue demonstrates the best resistance to the growth of bacteria. Whenever possible, the site of injury should be elevated above the patient's heart, to limit the accumulation of fluid in the wound interstitial spaces. The injured wound with little edema proceeds more rapidly to complete rehabilitation than does the markedly edematous wound.

Most importantly, dressings must provide a physiological environment that is conducive to epithelial migration from the wound edges across the surface of the fresh wound. When an area of epidermis is lost, water begins at once to evaporate from the exposed dermal tissue. The exudate on the surface dries and becomes the outer layer of the scab, which does not prevent water from evaporating from the dermis underneath. The surface of the dermis itself progressively dries (within 18 hours). This dry scab and dermis resist migration of epidermal cells, which must seek the underlying fibrous tissue of the upper reticular layer of dermis where enough moisture remains to support cellular viability.[105]

When the wound is covered by a dressing that prevents or delays evaporation of water from the wound surface, the scab and underlying dermis remain moist. Epidermal cells can easily migrate through the moist scab over the surface of the dermis. Under such dressings, epithelialization is more rapid, and no dry dermis is sacrificed.

The water vapor–permeable dressing would seem to be ideal for coverage of primarily closed wounds and has been usefully employed in the treatment of donor sites, mesh grafts, and dermabraded skin.[106] Unfortunately, excessive exudate may make it difficult to keep the dressing in place, and the moist exudate, while providing an ideal medium for epidermal repair, is also a suitable culture medium for the multiplication of microorganisms.

A complete discussion of the use of dressings is provided in Chapter 34.

CONCLUSION

The ultimate goal of wound care is to restore the physical integrity and function of the injured tissue. Whether the tissue injury will be limited to the initial wound depends on the outcome of the interaction between the viable and nonviable contaminants and the wound. A catastrophic outcome can be averted by a well-devised treatment plan based on the biology of wound repair and infection.

References

1. Edlich RF, Rodeheaver GT, Thacker JG: Technical factors in the prevention of infections. In Simmons RL, Howard RJ (eds): Surgical Infectious Diseases. New York, Appleton-Century-Crofts, 1982, p 449.
2. Jacobs HB: Skin knife—deep knife: The ritual and practice of skin incisions. Ann Surg 179:102, 1974.
3. Hasselgren PO, Hagberg E, Malmer H, et al: One instead of two knives for surgical incision. Does it increase the risk of postoperative wound infection? Arch Surg 119:917, 1984.
4. Madden JE, Edlich RF, Custer JR, et al: Studies in the management of the contaminated wound. IV. Resistance to infection of surgical wounds made by knife, electrosurgery, and laser. Am J Surg 119:222, 1970.
5. Cruse PJE, Foord R: A five-year prospective study of 23,649 surgical wounds. Arch Surg 107:206, 1973.
6. Greenburg AG, Saik RP, Peskin GW: Wound dehiscence. Pathophysiology and prevention. Arch Surg 114:143, 1979.
7. Levine NS, Peterson HD, Hugh D, et al: Laser, scalpel, electrosurgical and tangential excisions of third degree burns. A preliminary report. Plast Reconstr Surg 56:286, 1975.
8. Ferguson DJ: Advances in the management of surgical wounds. Surg Clin North Am 51:49, 1971.
9. Levenson SM, Gruber DK, Gruber C, et al: A hemostatic scalpel for burn debridement. Arch Surg 117:213, 1982.
10. Keenan KM, Rodeheaver GT, Kenney JG, et al: Surgical cautery revisited. Am J Surg 147:818, 1984.
11. Stevenson TR, Thacker JG, Rodeheaver GT, et al: Cleansing the traumatic wound by high pressure syringe irrigation. J Am Coll Emerg Phys 5:17, 1976.
12. Wheeler CB, Rodeheaver GT, Thacker JG, et al: Side-effects of high pressure irrigation. Surg Gynecol Obstet 243:775, 1976.
13. Faddis D, Daniel D, Boyer J: Tissue toxicity of antiseptic solutions. A study of rabbit articular and periarticular tissues. J Trauma 17:895, 1977.
14. Bryant CA, Rodeheaver GT, Reem EM, et al: Search for a non-toxic surgical scrub solution for periorbital laceration. Ann Emerg Med 13:317, 1984.
15. Bränemark PI, Albrektsson B, Lindstrom J, et al: Local tissue effects of wound disinfectants. Acta Chir Scand (Suppl) 357:166, 1966.
16. Cobden RH, Thrasher EL, Harris WH: Topical hemostatic agents to reduce bleeding from cancellous bone. A comparison of microcrystalline collagen, thrombin, and thrombin-soaked gelatic foam. J Bone Joint Surg 58A:70, 1976.
17. Abbott WM, Austen WG: Microcrystalline collagen as a topical agent for vascular surgery. Surgery 75:925, 1974.
18. Hanisch MG, Guerriero WG: The use of microfibrillar collagen hemostat for control of renal bleeding. J Urol 119:312, 1978.
19. Morgenstern L: Microcrystalline collagen used in experimental splenic injury. Arch Surg 109:44, 1974.
20. Morgenstern L, Michel SL, Austin E: Control of hepatic bleeding with microfibrillar collagen. Arch Surg 112:941, 1977.
21. Horsley V: Historical note: Horsley and bone wax. Surg Neurol 9:366, 1978.
22. Brightmore TGJ, Haves P, Humble J, et al: Hemostasis and healing following median sternotomy. Br J Surg 62:152, 1975.
23. Johnson P, Fromm D: Effects of bone wax on bacterial clearance. Surgery 89:206, 1981.
24. Lawrie P: Unpublished work. Ethicon, Ltd., Research Unit, Edinburgh.
25. Harris P, Cappernauld I: Clinical experience in neurosurgery with Absele: A new absorbable hemostatic bone sealant. Surg Neurol 13:231, 1980.
26. Jenkins HP, Janda R, Clarke J: Clinical and experimental observations on the use of gelatin sponge or foam. Surgery 20:124, 1946.
27. Jenkins HP, Senz EH, Owen HW, et al: Present status of gelatin sponge for the control of hemorrhage. With experimental data on its use for wounds of the great vessels and the heart. JAMA 132:614, 1946.
28. Cipolla AF, Narat JK: Effect of absorbable sponges on infection. An experimental study. Surgery 24:828, 1948.
29. Hinman F, Babcock KO: Local reaction to oxidized cellulose and gelatin hemostatic agents in experimentally contaminated renal wounds. Surgery 26:633, 1949.
30. Hait MR, Robb CA, Baxter CR, et al: Comparative evaluation of Avitene microcrystalline collagen. Am J Surg 125:284, 1973.
31. Laufman H, Method H: Effect of absorbable foreign substance on bowel anastomosis. Surg Gynecol Obstet 86:669, 1948.
32. Uhrich GL: Effect of oxidized cellulose in the protection of the suture line in intestinal anastomoses in dogs. Arch Surg 59:326, 1949.
33. Chamberlain BE, Delmonico JE, Gregg RO: Effect of Gelfoam on the integrity of intestinal anastomosis. Am J Surg 82:462, 1951.
34. Dineen P: Antibacterial action of oxidized regenerated cellulose. Surg Gynecol Obstet 142:481, 1976.
35. Dineen P: The effect of oxidized regenerated cellulose on experimental intravascular infection. Surgery 82:576, 1977.
36. Dineen P: The effect of oxidized regenerated cellulose on experimental infected splenotomies. J Surg Res 23:114, 1977.
37. Kuchta N, Dineen P: Effect of absorbable hemostats on intraabdominal sepsis. Infect Surg 2:441, 1983.
38. Spotnitz WD, Mintz PD, Avery N, et al: Fibrin glue from stored human stored plasma. An inexpensive

and efficient method for local blood bank preparation. Am Surg 53:460, 1987.

39. Spotnitz WD, Dalton MS, Baker JW, et al: Reduction of perioperative haemorrhage by anterior mediastinal spray application of fibrin glue during cardiac operations. Ann Thor Surg 44:529, 1987.

40. Carrel A, Hartmann A: Cicatrization of wounds. I. The relation between the size of a wound and the rate of its cicatrization. J Exper Med 24:429, 1916.

41. Carrel A: Cicatrization of wounds. XII. Factors initiating regeneration. J Exper Med 34:425, 1921.

42. Smith M, Enquist IF: A quantitative study of impaired healing resulting from infection. Surg Gynecol Obstet 125:965, 1967.

43. Davis JH, Yull AB: A toxic factor in abdominal injury. II. The role of the red cell component. J Trauma 4:84, 1964.

44. Pruett TL, Rotstein OD, Fiegel VD, et al: Mechanism of the adjuvant effect of hemoglobin in experimental peritonitis. VIII. A leukotoxin is produced by *Escherichia coli* metabolism in hemoglobin. Surgery 96:375, 1984.

45. Krizek TJ, Davis JH: The role of the red cell in subcutaneous infection. J Trauma 5:85, 1965.

46. Angel MF, Narayanan K, Swartz WM, et al: The etiologic role of free radicals in hematoma-induced flap necrosis. Plast Reconstr Surg 77:795, 1986.

47. Cohn I Jr, Cotlar M, Atik M, et al: Bile peritonitis. Ann Surg 152:827, 1960.

48. Rewbridge AG, Hrdina LS: The etiological role of bacteria in bile peritonitis. An experimental study in dogs. Proc Soc Exper Biol Med 27:528, 1929–1930.

49. Thal A, Perry JF Jr, Egner W: A clinical and morphologic study of forty-two cases of fatal acute pancreatitis. Surg Gynecol Obstet 105:191, 1957.

50. Howard JM, Singh LM: Peritoneal fluid pH after perforation of peptic ulcers: The myth of "acid-peritonitis." Arch Surg 87:483, 1983.

51. Golden GT, Roberts TL, Rodeheaver GT, et al: A new filtered sump tube for wound drainage. Am J Surg 128:716, 1975.

52. Pearce RSC, Rodeheaver GT, Edlich RF: Evaluation of a new hydrogel coating for drainage tubes. Am J Surg 148:301, 1984.

53. Ferrucci JT Jr, Mueller PR, Harbin WP: Percutaneous transhepatic biliary drainage. Technique, results, and applications. Radiology 135:1–13, 1980.

54. Pruett TL, Rotstein OD, Crass J, et al: Percutaneous aspiration and drainage for suspected abdominal infection. Surgery 96:731, 1984.

55. Cerise EJ, Pierce WA, Diamond DL: Abdominal drains: Their role as a source of infection following splenectomy. Ann Surg 171:764, 1970.

56. Baker BH, Borchardt KA: Sump drains and airborne bacteria as a cause of wound infections. J Surg Res 17:407, 1974.

57. Magee C, Rodeheaver GT, Golden GT, et al: Potentiation of wound infection by surgical drains. Am J Surg 131:547, 1976.

58. Berliner SD, Burson LC, Lear PE: Use and abuse of intraperitoneal drains in colon surgery. Arch Surg 89:686, 1964.

59. Manz CW, LaTendresse C, Sako Y: The detrimental effects of drains on colonic anastomoses: An experimental study. Dis Colon Rectum 13:17, 1970.

60. Johnson BW, Scott PG, Brunton JL, et al: Primary and secondary healing in infected wounds. An experimental study. Arch Surg 117:1189, 1982.

61. Marable SA, Wagner DE: The use of rapidly polymerizing adhesives in massive liver resection. Surg Forum 13:264, 1962.

62. Mathes GL, Terry JW Jr: Non-suture closure of nephrotomy. J Urol 89:122, 1963.

63. Morgenstern L, Kahn FH, Weinstein IM: Subtotal splenectomy in myelofibrosis. Surgery 60:336, 1966.

64. Fein RL, Matsumoto T, Soloway HB: Renal injury: Suture versus n-butyl-cyanoacrylate tissue adhesive spray repair. Invest Urol 8:12, 1970.

65. Furka I, Bornemissza GY, Miko I: Use of absorbable material for closure of experimental longitudinal nephrotomy. Intern Urol Nephrol 8:107, 1976.

66. Edlich RF, Thul J, Prusak M, et al: Studies in the management of the contaminated wound. VIII. Assessment of tissue adhesives for repair of contaminated tissue. Am J Surg 122:394, 1971.

67. Ihara N, Sozaki K, Tanaka H, et al: Application of fibrin glue to burns. Its haemostatic and skin transplant fixation affects in the excised wound. Burns 10:396, 1984.

68. Jørgensen PH, Jensen KH, Andreassen TT: Mechanical strength in rat skin incisional wounds treated with a fibrin sealant. J Surg Res 42:237, 1987.

69. Stephens FO, Hunt TK, Dunphy JE: Studies of traditional methods of care on the tensile strength of skin wounds in rats. Am J Surg 122:78, 1971.

70. Myers MB, Cherry G, Heinburger S: Augmentation of wound tensile strength by early removal of sutures. Am J Surg 117:338, 1969.

71. Harrison I, Williams DF, Cuschieri A: The effect of metal clips on the tensile properties of healing skin wounds. Br J Surg 62:945, 1975.

72. Jewell ML, Sato R, Rahija R: A comparison of wound healing in wounds closed with staples versus skin sutures. Contemp Surg 22:29, 1983.

73. Chvapil M: Personal communication.

74. Silloway KA, Morgan RF, Kenney JG, et al: Arcuate staple: Its influence on pain of staple penetration and removal. Am J Surg 150:612, 1985.

75. Johnson A, Rodeheaver GT, Durand LS, et al: Automatic disposable stapling devices for wound closure. Ann Emerg Med 10:631, 1981.

76. Stillman RM, Marino CA, Seligman SJ: Skin staples in potentially contaminated wounds. Arch Surg 119:821, 1984.

77. Edlich RF, Panek PH, Rodeheaver GT, et al: Physical and chemical configuration of sutures in the development of surgical infection. Ann Surg 177:679, 1973.

78. Postlethwait RW: Long-term comparative study of nonabsorbable sutures. Ann Surg 171:892, 1970.

79. Laufman H, Rubel T: Synthetic absorbable sutures. Surg Gynecol Obstet 145:597, 1977.

80. Salthouse TN, Williams JA, Willigan DA: Relationship of cellular enzyme activity to catgut and collagen suture absorption. Surg Gynecol Obstet 129:691, 1969.

81. Frazza EJ, Schmitt EE: A new absorbable suture. J Biomed Mater Res 1:43, 1971.

82. Rodeheaver GT, Thacker JG, Edlich RF: Mechanical performance of polyglycolic acid and polyglactin 910 synthetic absorbable sutures. Surg Gynecol Obstet 153:835, 1981.

83. Rodeheaver GT, Thacker JG, Owen J, et al: Knotting and handling characteristics of coated synthetic absorbable sutures. J Surg Res 35:525, 1983.

84. Ray JA, Doddi N, Regula D, et al: Polydioxanone (PDS), a novel monofilament synthetic absorbable suture. Surg Gynecol Obstet 153:497, 1981.

85. Katz AR, Mukherjee DP, Kaganov AL, et al: A new synthetic monofilament absorbable suture made from polytrimethylene carbonate. Surg Gynecol Obstet 161:213, 1985.

86. Sharp WV, Belden TA, King PH, et al: Suture resistance to infection. Surgery 91:61, 1982.

87. Thacker JG, Rodeheaver GT, Kurtz L, et al: Mechanical performance of sutures in surgery. Am J Surg 133:713, 1977.
88. Tera H, Åberg C: Tensile strength of twelve types of knot employed in surgery, using different suture materials. Acta Chir Scand 142:1, 1976.
89. Holmlund DEW: Knot properties of surgical suture materials. A model study. Acta Chir Scand 140:355, 1974.
90. Rodeheaver GT, Nesbit WS, Edlich RF: Novafil.™ A dynamic suture for wound closure. Ann Surg 204:193, 1986.
91. deHoll D, Rodeheaver G, Edgerton MT, et al: Potentiation of infection by suture closure of dead space. Am J Surg 127:716, 1974.
92. Foster GE, Hardy EG, Hardcastle JD: Subcuticular suturing after appendicectomy. Lancet 1:1128, 1977.
93. Hopkinson GB, Bullen BR: Removable subcuticular skin suture in acute appendicitic: A prospective comparable suture. Br Med J 284:869, 1982.
94. Polglase A, Nayman J: A comparison of incidence of infection following the use of percutaneous and subcuticular sutures: An experimental study. Aust NZ J Surg 47:423, 1977.
95. Pham S, Rodeheaver GT, Dang M-C, et al: Ease of continuous dermal suture removal. J Emerg Med 8:539, 1990.
96. Winn HR, Jane JA, Rodeheaver G, et al: Influence of subcuticular sutures on scar formation. Am J Surg 133:257, 1977.
97. Nordström REA, Nordström RM: Absorbable versus nonabsorbable sutures to prevent postoperative stretching of wound area. Plast Reconstr Surg 78:186, 1986.
98. McGuire MF: Studies of the excisional wound: I. Biomechanical effects of undermining and wound orientation on closing tension and work. Plast Reconstr Surg 66:419, 1980.
99. Abidin MR, Towler MA, Nochimson GD, et al: A new quantitative measurement for surgical needle ductility. Ann Emerg Med 18:64, 1989.
100. Edlich RF, Tsung MS, Rogers W, et al: Studies in the management of the contaminated wound. I. Technique of closure of such wounds together with a note on a reproducible experimental model. J Surg Res 8:585, 1968.
101. McDowell AJ: Extravagent treatment of garden variety lacerations. Plast Reconstr Surg 63:111, 1979.
102. Rodeheaver GT, Halverson JM, Edlich RF: Mechanical performance of wound closure tapes. Ann Emerg Med 12:203, 1983.
103. Panek PH, Prusak MP, Bolt D, et al: Potentiation of wound infection by adhesive adjuncts. Am Surg 38:343, 1972.
104. Schauerhamer RA, Edlich RF, Panek P, et al: Studies in the management of the contaminated wound. VII. Susceptibility of surgical wounds to postoperative bacterial contamination. Am J Surg 122:74, 1971.
105. Winter GD: Formation of the scab and the rate of epithelization of superficial wounds in the skin of the young domestic pig. Nature 193:293, 1962.
106. James JH, Watson ACH: The use of OPsite®, a vapor permeable dressing, on skin graft donor sites. Br J Plast Surg 28:107, 1975.
107. Edlich RF, Becker DG, Thacker JG, et al: Scientific basis for selecting staple and tape skin closures. Clin Plast Surg 17:571, 1990.

INDEX

Page numbers in *italics* refer to illustrations; page numbers followed by t refer to tables.

Allografts *(Continued)*
　plus cultured autologous dermis, for burn
　　　wounds, 536
　skin, cadaver donor, 532
　　storage of, 532
Allyl alcohol, hepatocyte injury and, 417
Allysines, in collagen crosslink formation, 158–
　159, *159*
Aloe vera, topical, for infected radiation wounds,
　553
Alveolitis, fibrosing, 519
Alveolus(i), after acute lung injury, 399, *401*
　anatomy of, 398, *399*
　inflammation of, in chronic pulmonary fibrosis,
　　403–404
　macrophage-derived growth factor of, mesen-
　　chymal cell replication and, 404
　repair of, 400, 402t, 402–407
　　therapies promoting, 410
Amino acids, early research in, 16
　in diseased liver, 423
　in wound environment, 275–276
　wound healing and, 250–251
Aminoguanidine, in diabetes, 253
Aminopeptidase cleavage site, abnormalities of,
　in Ehlers-Danlos syndrome type VII, 168,
　168–169
4-Aminophenyl mercuric acetate (APMA),
　collagenase activation by, 186
　inducing conformational change in procollagen,
　185
β-Aminopropionitrile (BAPN), collagen
　crosslinking inhibited by, 225, 306, 311–313
　for keloids, 506
　metabolism of, 312
　topical, experimental studies of, 312–313
Amnion, human, as wound dressing, 574
Amniotic fluid, structure and function of, fetal
　health and, *329*, 330–331
　wound contraction and, 335–336
Amputation, of vertebrate appendage,
　epimorphic regeneration after, 24–28, *25*
Anabolic steroids, for reversal of healing
　impairment due to corticosteroids, 555
Anastomoses, esophageal, complications with,
　441–442
　gastrointestinal, healing of, 441–445
　　local factors influencing, 444–445
　　systemic factors influencing, 443–444
　topical hemostatic agents and, 587
Anatomists, surgical, early, 13–14
Anesthesia, first use of, 14–15
Angiogenesis, 77–95. See also
　Neovascularization.
　abnormal morphology in, 82–83
　after acute lung injury, 409
　angiogenic factor(s) in, 83–86
　　angiogenin as, 86
　　heparin-binding, 83–85, 89
　　in burn wounds, 530
　　lipids as, 86
　　macrophage-derived, 409
　　prostaglandins as, 86
　　transforming growth factor-α as, 85
　　transforming growth factor-β as, 85–86, 284
　　tumor necrosis factor-α as, 85
　　types of, 83
　ascorbic acid and, 254, 256
　assays of, 79–80
　at fracture site, 359

Angiogenesis *(Continued)*
　cell types inducing, 86–87, *87*
　cellular components of, 80–83
　clinical applications of research into, 89–90
　direct and indirect, 83, *84*
　endothelial cell chemotaxis and, 242, 409
　extracellular matrix molecules modulating, 87–
　　89
　fetal, 333
　hyaluronic acid and, 338
　macrophages and, 276–277, 409
　models for study of, 79–80
　monokines and, 283
　oxygen and, 89
　sequential steps in, 80–81, *82*
　tumor, 82–83
Angiotensin-converting enzymes, scleroderma
　and, 519
Antebrachial cutaneous nerve, lateral and medial,
　for nerve autografting, 464–466
Antibiotics, first uses of, 15
　in burn patients, 552–553
　　systemic, 529
　　topical, 529
　in medicated dressings, 570
Antibodies, against endothelial cells, in
　scleroderma, 516
Antigens, bullous pemphigoid, 117, 121, 147
　MHC, in immune response, 282
　proteoglycans and, 203
Antihistamines, for keloids, 503
Antineoplastic drugs, wound healing and, 351
α₁–Antiprotease, inhibition of serine elastases by,
　228
Antlers, deer, regeneration of, 30, 34–38
Appendage, amputated, epimorphic regeneration
　of, 24–28, *25*
Arabic learning, in Middle Ages, 11
Arachidonic acid, epidermal maturation and, 297
　metabolism of, 45–46, 292–293. See also *Eico-
　　sanoids.*
　　in burn injury, 528–529
　platelet-derived growth factor and, 68
　production and metabolism of, 293
　　lipoxygenase pathway of, 298–300
Arginine, in wound microenvironment, 275–276,
　279
　wound healing and, 250–251, 263, 352, 547
Arm, reattachment of, reinnervation with, 475,
　476–477
Arteries, elastin production by, 232–233
Arteriolar reactions, in burn injury, 524–525
Arteriovenous malformations, angiogenesis with,
　82
Arthrochalasia multiplex, 167–168
Arthro-ophthalmopathy, hereditary, defective
　collagen synthesis and, 170
Ascorbic acid, collagen biosynthesis and, 155, 160
　elastin synthesis and, 225, 229
　gastrointestinal anastomotic complications and,
　443
　glucocorticoid effect on procollagen synthesis
　　and, 309
　hyperglycemia and, 252–253
　in burn patients, 527
　in Crohn's disease, 439
　wound healing and, 254, *254–255*, 256–260,
　　257–259, 350, 547
Aspartate, substituted for glycine, in type III
　collagen gene, 165

Collagen *(Continued)*
  telopeptide regions of, 135–136, *142*, 142–143, 158–159, *159*
  fibrils of, anchoring, *170*
    as substrate for collagenase assay, 180–181
    defective, 170, *170*
    exclusion of water from, 186
    formation of, 158, *159*, 177, *178*
      in Ehlers-Danlos syndrome, 164
    in tendon and ligament, 384
    of epineurium, 451
    properties of, 177
  folding of, definition of, 130
  general considerations in, 131–133
  molecular, 138–141
    conformational forms in, 141, *141*
    C-terminal globular domains in, 141
    triple helix formation in, 130, 139–140, *139–140*, 155–156
    features of, *140*, 140–141
    in osteogenesis imperfecta, 161–162, *162*
  wound healing and, 146–147
  X-Pro bonds in, helix formation and, 139–140
  thermal stability of, 165, 167, 177–178, 543
    tests for, 162
  type I, defective, 162–163, 169
    failure of cleavage by aminopeptidase in, 168, *168–169*
    fiber formation in, 143
    in epidermal wound closure, 122, 122t
    in hepatic fibrosis, 425, 428
    in interstitium after acute lung injury, 406
    in liver, 419–420
    in osteogenesis imperfecta, *161–162*, 161–163
    in scleroderma, 518
    in tendon and ligament, 384
    procollagen, glycosylation of molecules of, 156, *157*
    propeptide cleavage of, 158, *158*
    sponges of, as artificial skin, 574
    steroid treatment and, 308–309
  type II, defective, 169–170
    in wound healing, 147
    mutations in, 169–170
  type III, in Ehlers-Danlos syndrome, 164–165
    in hepatic fibrosis, 428
    in interstitium after acute lung injury, 406
    in liver, 419–420
    in scleroderma, 518
    in wound healing, 147
    propeptide cleavage of, 158, *158*
    steroid treatment and, 308–309
  type IV, additional chains of, 131, 132t
    aggregates of, 144–145, *145*
    chain structure in, 136–137
    collagenase cleavage site on, 137
    crosslinking in, 136–137
    C-terminal nontriplet segment in, 137
    in epidermal wound closure, 122, 122t
    in hepatic fibrosis, 427
    in lamina densa, 118
    in liver, 419–420
    in migrating epithelium, 121
    molecular structure of, 141, *141*
    of basement membrane, 433–434
    repetitive triplet domain in, 137
  type V, in bowel wall, 434
    in Crohn's disease, 438

Collagen *(Continued)*
  in epidermal wound closure, 122, 122t
  in migrating epithelium, 121
  in wound healing, 147
  type VI, aggregate formation of, 145, *145*
    features of, 137
  type VII, aggregate formation of, *145*, 145–146
    chain structure in, 138
    defective, disorders due to, 170–171
    in fibrils under hemidesmosomes, 118
    mutations in, 170–171
  type VIII, chains in, 131, 132t
  type IX, features of, 138
    fiber size regulation in, 144
    interaction of with type II, 138
    molecular structure of, 141, *141*
  type XII, fiber size regulation in, 144
  type XIII, chains in, 131, 132t
  types of, 131, 132t
  wound contraction and, 98
Collagen gels, fibroblast reorganization of, 214, 215
  for in vivo studies of growth factor effects, 244
Collagen genes, chromosomal localization of, 131, 132t
  collagen biosynthesis regulation by, 160
  expression of, agents altering, 160
    steroid treatment and, 308, *309*
  fibrillar, organization of, 152, *154*
  mutations in, connective tissue disorders due to, 160–161
    Ehlers-Danlos syndrome due to, 163–169
    in type II collagen, 169–170
    in type VII collagen, 170–171
    osteogenesis imperfecta due to, 161–163
  nomenclature of, 152
  nonfibrillar, 152–153
  sizes of, 152
  structure of, 152–154
  transcription of, 153–154, *154*
    lactate effect and, 277
  translation of, 154
  type I, COL1A1, 160, 168, *168*
    COL1A2, 160
  type II, COL2A1, 170
    defective, 169–170
  type III, COL3A1, 165, *167*
Collagenases, activation of, 184–186
  angiogenic factors and, 88
  assay of, 180–183, *181*
    methods of, 180–182, *181*
      immunologic, 182–183
    requirements for, 180
    substrate for, 180, 182, 183
    zymography for, 182
  biologic inhibition of, 186–188
  biologic reagents for, 184
  degradation of sutures by, 593
  fibroblast, in epidermolysis bullosa, 441
    vs. granulocyte collagenase, 184
  function of, 177–178, *179*
  granulocyte, vs. fibroblast collagenase, 184
  in collagen degradation, 137, 159
    rate-limiting step in, 178–179
  in hepatic fibrosis and cirrhosis, 425–426
  in human skin, 179–180, 190, 190t
  in keloids, 503
  in inflammation, 44, 46
  in tissue repair, 53
  nature of, 183–184

Endoplasmic reticulum, molecular collagen
structure and, 139
rough. See *Rough endoplasmic reticulum.*
Endothelial cell growth factor, in internal wound
dressing, 574
Endothelial cells, capillary, after acute lung
injury, 408–409
endoneurial, 454
in angiogenesis, 80–81, *82*
pericyte inhibition of, 87
chemotactic factors for, 242
cold injury and, 524
collagen synthesis and degradation and, 88
fibrotic liver collagen produced by, 423
growth factors and, 84, 405
Ia expression of, interferon-γ and, 51
in hemostasis, interleukin-1 and, 46–47
in inflammatory response, 42
in scleroderma, 515–517
in wound healing, 240
vascular, 77
lymphokine effects on, 284, 286t
Endothelial relaxing factor, 279
Endothelium, capillary, structure of, 398, *399*
Energy expenditure, in burn patients, 526
oxygen and, 543
Entactin, in hepatic extracellular matrix, 419
Enzyme-linked immunosorbent assay (ELISA),
for collagenase, 182–183
Enzymes, in proline and lysine hydroxylation in
collagen biosynthesis, 155
of neutrophilic granules, bactericidal activity
of, 44
extracellular degradative activity of, 44
proteolytic, damaging effects of, 588
degradation of sutures by, 593
Epidermal cells. See also *Epithelial cells.*
collagenolytic activity and, 190
cytoskeletal machinery for movement of, 124
gap junctions in, 121
migration of, with moist dressings, 597
Epidermal growth factor, as chemotactic factor,
239, *239*, 242, 244
as wound healing stimulant, 555
collagenase inhibition by, 189
diabetes and, 253
epidermal wound closure and, 123t
fibroblast chemotaxis and, 70–71, 239, *239*
in epithelialization in burn wound repair, 530
in lung repair, 407
in wound healing, 571, 574
receptor for, 70
scleroderma fibroblast sensitivity to, 514–515
transforming growth factor-α and, 49, 85
Epidermis. See also *Skin.*
artificial skin characteristics and, 533
autografts of, for burn wounds, 534–535
cell movement in, initiation of, 123–124
morphology of, 118–119
sheet migration as, biochemical and biophysical parameters of, 121–123
models of, 119, *120*
development of, 117
in deer antler development, 37
in occluded vs. open wounds, 563
in rabbit ear regenerative model, 32–33, *33*
in tissue repair vs. epimorphic regeneration, 27
maturation of, eicosanoid activity and, 297
stratification in, 115, *116*
structure and properties of, 115, *116*, 117, 344

Epidermis *(Continued)*
with hydrocolloid and hydrogel dressings, 570
Epidermolysis bullosa, cancer and, 554
dystrophic, defective collagen fibrils in, 170,
170
healing response to, 441
impaired wound healing with, 546–547
phenytoin for, 189
Epimorphic regeneration, as growth mechanism,
24–28
nerve supply and, 26
prerequisites for, 24–26
vs. tissue repair, 27–28
Epineurium, lymphatics of, 454
of peripheral nerves, 451, *452*
direct suture repair of, 463–464, *464*
Epithelial cells. See also *Basal epidermal cells;
Epidermal cells.*
gastrointestinal, 433
movement of, in burn wound repair, 530
in wound closure, 118–119
initiation of, 123–124
morphology of, 118–119
sheet migration of, 119, *120*, 121–123
biochemical and biophysical factors affecting, 121–123
Epithelial growth factor, in wound healing, 90
Epithelialization, 115–127. See also
Reepithelialization.
aging and, 353
eicosanoid activity and, 297
experimental evaluation of, 566
in burn wound repair, 530
in open wounds, 563
in wound healing, 348
in fetus, 333
wound dressings and, 552
medicated, 570
oxygen permeability and, 565, 566t
Epithelium, alveolar, after acute lung injury,
399–400, *401*, 407–408
structure of, 398, *400*
characteristics of, 115
gastric, repair of, 435
in burn wound repair, 530
wound dressing mimicking, 562, 563, 565
Eriksson, E., 17
Eristratus, wound dressings of, 571
Erosions, intestinal, 435–436, *436*
Erythroblastosis fetalis, 328
Erythrocytes, infection enhanced by, 588
Erythropoiesis, atrophy and functional demand
and, 23
Estrogens, in fetal lung maturation, 330
placental synthesis of, 330
Ethnor, 586
Excoriators, neurotic, 492
Exercises, range of motion, for inhibition of scar
contractures, 110
Exoglycosidases, 201
Extracellular matrix. See also *Collagen.*
angiogenesis and, 87–89
cell behavior and, 209
collagen and, BAPN and, 312
fetal, 333–334
fibroblast reorganization of, 103–104
heparan sulfate proteoglycans and, 203
hepatic, 418–420
in hepatic fibrosis, 426–427
in burn wounds, 529

H

Metabolism (Continued)
  in cancer patients, impaired wound healing
    and, 548
  in mammals, regenerative ability and, 29–30
  in trauma, 318–321
  in wound repair, 248–274, 324
    of carbohydrates, 251–253
    of fats, 253–254
    of fat-soluble vitamins, 261–265
    of proteins, 249–251
    of trace minerals, 265–266
    of water-soluble vitamins, 254–261
  ¹⁵N glycine, 249
  of keloids, 502
  resistance to infection and, 268, 268
  with burn injury, 526–528
Metalloenzymes, elastases type of, 228
Metalloproteinases, 183
  tissue inhibitors of. See TIMP (tissue inhibitor
    of metalloproteinases).
Metchnikoff, Elie, 15
Methionine, wound healing and, 250
7-Methylguanosine, in transcription of collagen
    genes, 153–154
Methylprednisolone (Depo-Medrol), wound
    healing and, 308
MHC antigens, in immune response, 282
Michel clips, for skin closure of wounds, 591
Micronutrients, metabolism of, in burn patients,
    527
Microvasculature, in burn injury, 524–525
  of hepatic lobule, 416, 416
Middle Ages, medical knowledge during, 11–12
Minerals, wound healing and, 265–266, 547–548
Mitoattractants, epidermal growth factor as, 242
  platelet-derived growth factor as, 242
Mondeville, Henry de, 12
Monocyte-derived neutrophil chemotactic factor,
    52
Monocytes. See also Macrophages.
  chemotaxis ofs, 44–45, 49
  in inflammatory response, 44–48, 347
  in scleroderma, 517
  in wounds, 275
  interferon-γ effects on, 50, 50–51
  product(s) of, in acute inflammation, cachectin
    as, 47–48
      collagenase as, 46
      colony-stimulating factor as, 48
      interleukin-1 as, 46–47, 47
      transforming growth factor as, 49, 85
      tumor necrosis factor as, 47–48
    in chronic inflammation, 52
    stimulated by interferon-γ, 50
Monokines. See also Cytokines; Lymphokines.
  released by macrophages at wound site, 283–
    284, 285t
Mononuclear cell factor, in cartilage repair, 376
  in connective tissue metabolism, interleukin-1
    and, 47
Montpelier, medical school of, 11
Morton, William T. G., use of ether by, 14–15
Mouse, Algire chamber in, as model for
    angiogenesis, 79
  tight skin, as model for role of fibroblasts in
    wound contraction, 100–101
Moxibustion, 5
mRNA. See Ribonucleic acid (RNA), messenger.
Mucopolysaccharides, in burn wound contracture
    formation, 531

Mucopolysaccharides (Continued)
  in skin in scleroderma, abnormalities of, 513
Mucopolysaccharidoses, proteoglycan degradation
    in, 201
Mucosa, gastrointestinal, inflammation of, 435–
    436, 436
  postoperative healing of, 443
  structure and function of, 433–434
Multilineage-CSF. See also Interleukin-3.
  functions of, 48, 51
Multiple organ failure syndrome, acute lung
    injury with, 397
Munchausen's syndrome, 490–491
Muscle, action potentials of, compound, after
    entubulation nerve repair, 470, 470–474,
    472–473
  in nerve conduction studies, 455
  denervated, fibrillation potentials in, 455
    on electromyography, 454–455
  electromyographic activation of, 454–455
  glycogen breakdown in, in trauma, 319–321
  granuloma in, metabolism of, 319–320
  skeletal, atrophy and functional demand and,
    23–24
Muscle cells, smooth. See Smooth muscle cells.
Muscle flaps, for infected problem wounds, 553
  fracture repair and, 371, 371
Muscularis mucosa, in Crohn's disease, 438
  of gastrointestinal tract, 434, 435
Muscularis propria, of gastrointestinal tract, 434
Myeloperoxidase, in microbicidal activity of
    neutrophils, 43
Myofibroblast anchoring substance, 99
Myofibroblasts, absence in fetal wounds, 335–
    336
  characteristics of, 99
  hepatic, 418
  in burn wound contracture formation, 531
  in keloids, 502
  in tissue culture, cell lines derived from, 107–
    108
  in wound closure, 104
  in wound contraction, 99–112, 105–110, 332,
    349
    animal models of, 105, 105
    location in experimental animals and hu-
      mans, 106–107
    vs. fibroblasts, 99–104
  skin grafts and, 111
  wound tension and, 110
Myosin, in epidermis, 121
  light chain of, in chemotactic response of fibro-
    blasts, 239, 239

N
NADPH oxidase system, in neutrophils, 43,
    43
Navicular bone, fracture repair of, 371
N-cadherin, 462
NCAM (neural cell adhesion molecule), 462
Necrobiosis lipoidica, diabetic, impaired wound
    healing with, 550
Necrosis, hepatic, 422–423
Needles, used for suture closure, 596
Neodymium-yttrium-aluminum-garnet (Nd:YAG)
    laser surgery, for keloids, 505
Neosporin, in medicated dressing, 570
Neovascularization. See also Angiogenesis.